BMA

VASCULAR SURGERY
Principles and Practice
FOURTH EDITION

VASCULAR SURGERY

PRINCIPLES AND PRACTICE

FOURTH EDITION

EDITED BY

SAMUEL ERIC WILSON
Department of Surgery
University of California, Irvine
Irvine, California, USA

JUAN CARLOS JIMENEZ
Division of Vascular Surgery
University of California, Los Angeles
Los Angeles, California, USA

FRANK J. VEITH
Department of Surgery
New York University Medical Center
New York, New York, USA
and
Department of Surgery
Cleveland Clinic
Cleveland, Ohio, USA

A. ROSS NAYLOR
Department of Vascular Surgery
Leicester Royal Infirmary
Leicester, UK

JOHN A.C. BUCKELS
Department of Surgery
University of Birmingham
and
Queen Elizabeth Hospital
Birmingham, UK

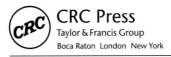

CRC Press
Taylor & Francis Group
Boca Raton London New York

CRC Press is an imprint of the
Taylor & Francis Group, an **informa** business

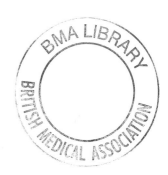

CRC Press
Taylor & Francis Group
6000 Broken Sound Parkway NW, Suite 300
Boca Raton, FL 33487-2742

© 2017 by Taylor & Francis Group, LLC
CRC Press is an imprint of Taylor & Francis Group, an Informa business

No claim to original U.S. Government works

Printed and bound in India by Replika Press Pvt. Ltd.

Printed on acid-free paper
Version Date: 20160824

International Standard Book Number-13: 978-1-4822-3945-4 (Pack - Book and Ebook)

Visit the Taylor & Francis Web site at
http://www.taylorandfrancis.com

and the CRC Press Web site at
http://www.crcpress.com

This one is for Ellie, Sam and Camille.

Samuel Eric Wilson

For Dr. Carlos and Ana Jimenez, my parents and inspirations for my medical career.

Juan Carlos Jimenez

I have four people who have supported my career throughout and who deserve an acknowledgement: my wife Carol and my associates Jackie Simpson, Julie Harris and Jamie McKay.

Frank J. Veith

To my three mentors, Jetmund Engeset, Vaughan Ruckley and Peter Bell.

A. Ross Naylor

Contents

SECTION IV: ANEURYSMS

SECTION V: CEREBROVASCULAR DISEASE

SECTION VI: VISCERAL ARTERIAL DISEASE

Preface

When the first edition of *Vascular Surgery: Principles and Practice* was planned three decades ago, we could not have anticipated the revolution that was about to occur in vascular surgery. On reflection, the changes brought by endovascular methods evolved progressively from 'Jeffersonian research' – the application of innovation to solve practical problems. Beginning with Dotter's recanalization experiments in dilation of obstructed arteries and his human application, leading to Gruentzig's critical balloon catheter modifications, the stage was set for rapid advancement. Peripheral arterial stents were made from stainless steel and nitinol, and percutaneous angioplasty began to replace bypass operations for arterial occlusive disease. Endovascular repair of aortic aneurysms was the most dramatic advance reducing operative mortality to one quarter of open repair and reducing hospitalization to 1 or 2 days.

Throughout all of this change, vascular surgeons, more than any other surgical specialty, have supported their practice with rigorous clinical trials. For example, in occlusive disease percutaneous angioplasty was compared to bypass operation and carotid endarterectomy to medical management. In aneurysmal disease, repair was randomized to observation for small aortic aneurysms and endovascular to open repair. Some specialties having major changes to less invasive technology have seen numbers of procedures multiply, whereas having well-defined indications for intervention, as in aneurysm repair and carotid endarterectomy, has not led to proliferation in these procedures. More than anything, this signifies the need for vascular surgeons to remain involved in research – both basic and clinical – ultimately ensuring the public health.

Vascular surgery continues to evolve. No doubt questions such as the role of carotid stenting, repair of type II endoleaks, prevention of myointimal hyperplasia or designing a better arterial replacement will be answered in the next decade.

The goal of this text is to set out current standards in practice. We recognize these may change in the years ahead, but the methods we describe have been selected to last for the remainder of this decade. Proven patient management is emphasized, relying heavily on clinical trial research. Procedures are described and an atlas of open procedures included, but it is not a text of personal operative descriptions. Rather the discussions are directed at diagnosis, indications, methods of intervention and expected outcomes. We hope this work will be useful for the practicing vascular surgeon, resident in training or anyone inquiring into our field.

Indeed, the reader will find vascular surgery has evolved dramatically since the first edition of this text was published in 1987. Vascular surgery has seen a remarkable transformation from a specialty which dealt with the natural history of vascular disease and its treatment primarily by open procedures to a specialty which has kept the focus it had while mastering the major components of improved imaging and endovascular treatments. This fourth edition of *Vascular Surgery: Principles and Practice* has incorporated these advances while maintaining the specialty's past assets. Since natural history and open surgery will always be a component of optimal care for patients with vascular diseases, this mix of the old and the new will make this edition a valuable resource for all vascular surgeons and others interested in the optimal care of vascular patients.

Lastly, we thank the authors who have given so generously of their time, knowledge and experience, which made this book possible.

Samuel Eric Wilson
Juan Carlos Jimenez
Frank J. Veith
A. Ross Naylor
John A.C. Buckels

Contributors

Stefan Acosta
Department of Vascular Surgery
Lund University
Lund, Sweden

Mostafa Albayati
Cardiovascular Division
King's College London
London, United Kingdom

Mark M. Archie
Division of Vascular and Endovascular Surgery
University of California, Los Angeles
Los Angeles, California

Enrico Ascher
Department of Surgery
Lutheran Medical Center
New York, New York

Ojan Assadian
Department of Surgery
University of Huddersfield
Huddersfield, United Kingdom

Ali Azizzadeh
Department of Cardiothoracic & Vascular Surgery
and
Memorial Hermann Heart & Vascular Institute
McGovern Medical School
The University of Texas Health Sciences Center at Houston
Houston, Texas

Richard Azzaoui
Department of Vascular Surgery
Centre Hospitalier Régional Universitaire de Lille
Lille, France

Hisham S. Bassiouny
Chicago, Illinois

Robert Bennion
Department of Surgery
University of California, Los Angeles
Los Angeles, California

Jos C. van den Berg
Service of Interventional Radiology
Ospedale Regionale di Lugano, sede Civico
Lugano, Switzerland

and

Department of Radiology
University of Bern
Bern, Switzerland

Bertram M. Bernheim
Department of Surgery
Johns Hopkins University School of Medicine
Baltimore, Maryland

Martin Björck
Department of Surgical Sciences
Uppsala University
Uppsala, Sweden

James H. Black III
Division of Vascular Surgery and Endovascular Therapy
and
Johns Hopkins Hospital and Johns Hopkins Medical
Institutions
Baltimore, Maryland

Paul H. Blair
Belfast Vascular Centre
Belfast Health & Social Care Trust
Belfast, Northern Ireland

Laura T. Boitano
Department of Surgery
Harvard Medical School
Boston, Massachusetts

Gert J. de Borst
Department of Vascular Surgery
University Medical Center Utrecht
Utrecht, the Netherlands

John A.C. Buckels
Department of Surgery
University of Birmingham
and
Queen Elizabeth Hospital
Birmingham, United Kingdom

John G. Carson
Division of Vascular Surgery
University of California, Davis
and
Department of Veteran Affairs Health System
Mather, California

Neal S. Cayne
Department of Surgery
New York University Medical Center
New York, New York

Ankur Chandra
Division of Vascular and Endovascular Surgery
Scripps Clinic/Scripps Green Hospital
La Jolla, California

Benjamin B. Chang
Department of Surgery
Albany Medical College
and
Albany Medical Center Hospital
Albany, New York

David C. Chang
Department of Surgery
Harvard Medical School
Boston, Massachusetts

Roberto Chiesa
Department of Vascular Surgery
Vita-Salute San Raffaele University
Milan, Italy

Elizabeth L. Chou
School of Medicine
University of California, Irvine
Orange, California
and
Massachusetts General Hospital
Boston, Massachusetts

Sophia Chun
Veterans Healthcare Administration (VHA) Spinal Cord Injury
and Disorders System of Care
Veterans Affairs Central Office
Washington, DC

Efrem Civilini
Department of Vascular Surgery
Vita-Salute San Raffaele University
Milan, Italy

W. Darrin Clouse
Division of Vascular and Endovascular Surgery
Harvard Medical School
Boston, Massachusetts
and
Uniformed Services University of the Heath Sciences
Bethesda, Maryland

Anthony J. Comerota
Jobst Vascular Institute
ProMedica Toledo Hospital
Toledo, Ohio
and
University of Michigan
Ann Arbor, Michigan

Alexander J. Continenza
The Yakes Vascular Malformation Center
Englewood, Colorado

Michol A. Cooper
Johns Hopkins University School of Medicine
Baltimore, Maryland

Jeffrey D. Crawford
Department of Surgery
Oregon Health & Science University
Portland, Oregon

R. Clement Darling III
Department of Surgery
Albany Medical College
and
Division of Vascular Surgery
Albany Medical Center Hospital
and
The Institute for Vascular Health and Disease
Albany Medical Center Hospital
Albany, New York

Alun Huw Davies
Academic Section of Vascular Surgery
Imperial College London
London, United Kingdom

Robert S.M. Davies
Department of Vascular Surgery
Leicester Royal Infirmary
Leicester, United Kingdom

Ralph G. DePalma
Office of Research and Development
US Department of Veterans Affairs
Washington, DC
and
Department of Surgery
Uniformed Services University of the Health Sciences
Bethesda, Maryland

Brian G. DeRubertis
Department of Surgery
University of California, Los Angeles
Los Angeles, California

J.R. De Siqueira
University of Leeds
Leeds, United Kingdom

Adam Doyle
Division of Vascular Surgery
University of Rochester
Rochester, New York

Joseph DuBose
Division of Vascular & Trauma Surgery
University of California, Davis
Davis, California

Julie A. Freischlag
Human Health Sciences
and
School of Medicine
University of California Davis Health System
Sacramento, California

J. Timothy Fulenwider
Gainesville, Georgia

Karan Garg
Department of Surgery
Montefiore Medical Center
Bronx, New York

Nicholas J. Gargiulo III
Department of Surgery
Montefiore Medical Center
New York, New York

Dmitri V. Gelfand
Department of Vascular Surgery
Sutter Medical Group
Roseville, California

Bruce L. Gewertz
Department of Surgery
Cedars-Sinai Health System
Los Angeles, California

David L. Gillespie
Department of Vascular and Endovascular Surgery
Southcoast Health
Fall River, Massachusetts

and

Department of Surgery
Uniformed Services University
Bethesda, Maryland

James A. Gillespie
Department of Surgery
St George's Hospital
University of London
London, United Kingdom

Ian Gordon
Department of Surgery
University of California, Irvine
Irvine, California

Michael J. Gough
Department of Vascular Surgery
University of Leeds
Leeds, United Kingdom

Jean de Ville de Goyet
Bambino Gesù Childrens Hospital
Tor Vergata Roma University
Roma, Italy

Adam M. Gwozdz
Cardiovascular Division
King's College London
London, United Kingdom

George Hamilton
Royal Free London NHS Foundation Trust
Great Ormond Street Hospital for Children NHS
Foundation Trust
and
University College London Medical School
London, United Kingdom

Denis W. Harkin
Belfast Vascular Centre
Belfast Health & Social Care Trust
Belfast, Northern Ireland

Stéphan Haulon
Department of Vascular Surgery
Centre Hospitalier Régional Universitaire de Lille
Lille, France

Adrien Hertault
Department of Vascular Surgery
Centre Hospitalier Régional Universitaire de Lille
Lille, France

Jonathan R. Hiatt
Department of Surgery
University of California, Los Angeles
Los Angeles, California

Michael S. Hong
Division of Vascular Surgery
University of California, Davis
Davis, California

Julius H. Jacobson II
Division of Vascular Surgery & Endovascular Therapy
Johns Hopkins University School of Medicine
Baltimore, Maryland

Ieuan Harri Jenkins
Imperial College Healthcare NHS Trust London
London, United Kingdom

Juan Carlos Jimenez
Division of Vascular Surgery
University of California, Los Angeles
Los Angeles, California

Nii-Kabu Kabutey
Division of Vascular and Endovascular Surgery
University of California, Irvine
Irvine, California

Khushboo Kaushal
Department of Internal Medicine
University of California, San Diego
San Diego, California

Jerry J. Kim
Department of Surgery
Harbor-University of California Los Angeles Medical Center
Torrance, California

Paul B. Kreienberg
Albany Medical Center Hospital
Albany, New York

David A. Kulber
Division of Plastic Surgery
Cedars-Sinai Medical Center
and
Division of Plastic and Reconstructive Surgery
University of Southern California
Los Angeles, California

Gregg S. Landis
Long Island Jewish Medical Center
New Hyde Park, New York

Gregory J. Landry
Department of Surgery
Oregon Health & Science University
Portland, Oregon

Sujin Lee
Veterans Affairs Long Beach Spinal Cord Injury/Disorders
Center
and
Memorial Care Rehabilitation Institute
Long Beach Memorial Hospital
Long Beach, California

Timothy K. Liem
Department of Surgery
Oregon Health & Science University
Portland, Oregon

Evan C. Lipsitz
Department of Surgery
Montefiore Medical Center
New York, New York

Dennis Malkasian
Department of Neurosurgery
University of California
Los Angeles and Irvine, California

James M. Malone
College of Medicine
The University of Arizona
Tucson, Arizona

and

Scottsdale Healthcare-Shea
Scottsdale, Arizona

Jorges Mascaro
Department of Surgery
Queen Elizabeth Hospital
Birmingham, United Kingdom

Blandine Maurel
Department of Vascular Surgery
Centre Hospitalier Régional Universitaire de Lille
Lille, France

Germano Melissano
Department of Vascular Surgery
Vita-Salute San Raffaele University
Milan, Italy

Hynek Mergental
Liver Unit
Queen Elizabeth Hospital
Birmingham, United Kingdom

Doran Mix
Division of Vascular Surgery
University of Rochester
and
Kate Gleason College of Engineering
Rochester Institute of Technology
Rochester, New York

Bijan Modarai
Cardiovascular Division
King's College London
London, United Kingdom

Samuel R. Money
Department of Surgery
Mayo Clinic College of Medicine
Phoenix, Arizona

Nariman Nassiri
Department of Surgery
Harbor-University of California Los Angeles Medical Center
Torrance, California

A. Ross Naylor
Department of Vascular Surgery
Leicester Royal Infirmary
Leicester, United Kingdom

Andrea T. Obi
Department of Surgery
University of Michigan
Ann Arbor, Michigan

Mark E. O'Donnell
Department of Surgery
Mayo Clinic College of Medicine
Phoenix, Arizona

Adam Z. Oskowitz
Department of Surgery
University of California, Los Angeles
Los Angeles, California

Madhukar S. Patel
Harvard Medical School
Massachusetts General Hospital
Boston, Massachusetts

Benjamin O. Patterson
St Georges Vascular Institute
St Georges Hospital
London, United Kingdom

Bruce A. Perler
Department of Surgery
Johns Hopkins Hospital
Baltimore, Maryland

Seshadri Raju
The Rane Center at St. Dominic
Jackson, Mississippi

Enrico Rinaldi
Department of Vascular Surgery
Vita-Salute San Raffaele University
Milan, Italy

Darin J. Saltzman
Department of Surgery
University of California, Los Angeles
Los Angeles, California

Naveed Saqib
Department of Cardiothoracic and Vascular Surgery
University of Texas
and
Memorial Hermann Heart & Vascular Institute
Houston, Texas

Michael D. Sgroi
Department of Surgery
University of California, Irvine
Irvine, California

Aamir S. Shah
Division of Thoracic and Cardiac Surgery
Cedars-Sinai Medical Center
Los Angeles, CA

Dhiraj M. Shah
Department of Surgery (Vascular)
Albany Medical College
Albany, New York

Maxim E. Shaydakov
Jobst Vascular Institute
ProMedica Toledo Hospital
Toledo, Ohio

Meryl A. Simon
University of California, Davis
Davis, California

Robert B. Smith III
School of Medicine
Emory University
Atlanta, Georgia

Jonathan Sobocinski
Department of Vascular Surgery
Centre Hospitalier Régional Universitaire de Lille
Lille, France

Rafaëlle Spear
Department of Vascular Surgery
Centre Hospitalier Régional Universitaire de Lille
Lille, France

James C. Stanley
Section of Vascular Surgery
University of Michigan
Ann Arbor, Michigan

Ankur Thapar
Academic Section of Vascular Surgery
Imperial College London
London, United Kingdom

Matt M. Thompson
Department of Vascular Surgery
St Georges Hospital
London, United Kingdom

Giovanni Tinelli
Department of Vascular Surgery
Centre Hospitalier Régional Universitaire de Lille
Lille, France

Geoffrey S. Tompkins
Redwood Orthopaedic Surgery Associates
Santa Rosa, California

Frank J. Veith
Department of Surgery
New York University Medical Center
New York, New York

and

Department of Surgery
Cleveland Clinic
Cleveland, Ohio

Cristine S. Velazco
Division of Vascular and Endovascular Surgery
Mayo Clinic College of Medicine
Phoenix, Arizona

Christian de Virgilio
Department of Surgery
Harbor-University of California Los Angeles Medical Center
Torrance, California

Thomas W. Wakefield
Department of Surgery
University of Michigan
Ann Arbor, Michigan

Michael L. Wall
Department of Vascular Surgery
Flinders Medical Centre
Bedford Park, South Australia, Australia

Bruce A. Warden
Department of Pharmacy
Oregon Health & Science University
Portland, Oregon

Russell A. Williams
Department of Surgery
University of California, Irvine
Irvine, California

Samuel Eric Wilson
Department of Surgery
University of California, Irvine
Irvine, California

Chengpei Xu
Department of Surgery
School of Medicine
Stanford University
Stanford, California

Alexis M. Yakes
The Yakes Vascular Malformation Center
Englewood, Colorado

Wayne F. Yakes
The Yakes Vascular Malformation Center
Englewood, Colorado

Jane K. Yang
Division of Vascular and Endovascular Surgery
University of California, Los Angeles
Los Angeles, California

Caroline A. Yao
Division of Plastic and Reconstructive Surgery
University of Southern California
Los Angeles, California

Christopher K. Zarins
Department of Surgery
Stanford University
Stanford, California

Max Zegelman
Department of Vascular and Thoracic Surgery
Krankenhaus Nordwest
and
J. W. Goethe University Frankfurt
Frankfurt am Main, Germany

SECTION I

Assessment of Vascular Disease

The evolution of vascular surgery

JAMES C. STANLEY

CONTENTS

Contemporary vascular surgery evolved slowly over many years with notable exceptions that catapulted new paradigms into clinical practice. Most landmark contributions occurred during the last half of the twentieth century, resulting from a better understanding of the physiologic consequences of vascular disease, the availability of heparin anticoagulation, the introduction of synthetic grafts, the development of non-invasive testing, an improved anatomic imaging and the maturation of technical skills in complex open surgical and endovascular procedures. Although vascular surgery had its beginning in many other disciplines, it has evolved into a finite specialty with a defined body of knowledge and established standards of practice. The history of vascular surgery is best addressed by reviewing three specific time periods: antiquity to the end of the nineteenth century, the early twentieth century and the last half of the twentieth and the early twenty-first century.

A select group of listings of landmark contributions have been created as a reference to the historical events affecting certain aspects of vascular surgery, including aortic occlusive disease (Table 1.1); nonanatomic revascularization of the lower extremities (Table 1.2); femoral, popliteal and tibial arterial occlusive disease (Table 1.3); aortic aneurysms (Table 1.4); femoral and popliteal artery aneurysms (Table 1.5); splanchnic and renal arterial disease (Table 1.6); cerebrovascular disease recognition and basis for treatment (Table 1.7); cerebrovascular disease–surgical treatment (Table 1.8); and venous disease (Table 1.9).

Many of the aforenoted events represent first-time accomplishments in the specialty; others were simply benchmark contributions to the care of patients with vascular diseases. Many clinicians and clinical scientists have added both depth and breadth to our knowledge of vascular surgery but are not included in the aforenoted listings because of this review's brief nature. Four earlier historical works have been published that offer additional insight into the evolution vascular surgery.[1–4]

ANTIQUITY TO THE END OF THE NINETEENTH CENTURY

Arterial disruptions due to trauma and ruptured aneurysms were confronted by the ancients, whose earliest vascular surgical procedures related to controlling bleeding from these vessels.[3] Perhaps, the first recorded reports on this topic were from India, where Sushruta used hemp fibres for blood vessel ligations around 700 BC.[5] Celsus made an important contribution in the first century, when he ligated vessels both above and below the site of injury and then transected the involved vessel so that it might retract from the wound, thus lessening the risk of hemorrhage which often accompanied wound infections. A century later, Galen had ligated many vessels and Antyllus ligated both entering and exiting vessels of an aneurysm, but infection continued to compromise such efforts.

Venous disease was also well recognized by the ancients, including Hippocrates, who recommended treating venous varicosities with compressive dressings and avoidance of standing.[3] Celsus used bandages and plasters to treat venous ulcerations in the first century and Galen suggested multiple ligations as a therapeutic intervention in the second century. Little change occurred in the management of venous disease over the next 1500 years.

The dark ages of European history witnessed few advances in vascular surgery. It wasn't until the sixteenth century that Ambroise Pare successfully ligated vessels in the battlefields at Danvilliers and used stringent agents to lessen wound infections.[6] This was a major contribution in the treatment of controlling hemorrhage from arteries and veins.

During the eighteenth century, considerable efforts were extended to the treatment of aneurysms, led by John Hunter, who made many extraordinary contributions to the scientific classification and treatment of vascular diseases.[7-10] One of his more noteworthy accomplishments involved ligation of the femoral artery for the treatment of a popliteal artery aneurysm. This procedure provided the impetus for his interest in the relevance of the collateral circulation in the extremities.

During the ensuing nineteenth century, many other physicians described arterial ligature in the management of aneurysms. One of the most inventive of those practitioners was Ashley Cooper,[11,12] a student of Hunter, who ligated the carotid artery for an aneurysm in 1805.[13] The patient subsequently died, but he undertook a second successful ligation for the same disease 3 years later in 1808.[14] Cooper also ligated the aorta for an iliac artery aneurysm and treated a femoral artery aneurysm by ligation during this same era. Shortly thereafter, in 1817, Valentine Mott ligated the innominate artery for a subclavian aneurysm.[15] Mott also ligated the common iliac artery for an external iliac artery aneurysm in 1820. His work, performed in New York City, was some of the earliest vascular surgery undertaken in the United States.

Rudolph Matas was a widely recognized contributor to vascular surgery towards the end of the nineteenth century.[16] In 1888, he successfully performed a brachial artery aneurysm endoaneurysmorrhaphy.[17] His technique of ligating the entering and exiting vessels from within the aneurysm proved essential in preserving collateral vessels and maintaining the viability of distal tissues. Matas applied this procedure to the treatment of aortic aneurysms in the next century.

Chronic occlusive disease came to the forefront during the nineteenth century, when Barth described claudication for the first time in 1835, affecting a patient with an aortic thrombosis.[18] His report went unrecognized for many decades, but clearly established the concept that arterial obstructions could cause chronic symptoms amenable to later reconstructive procedures.

In 1896, a critical contribution to the understanding of vascular diseases came about with Wilhelm Roentgen's initial discovery of x-rays,[19] followed 3 months later by an actual arteriogram performed in an amputated upper extremity.[20] It would be decades before the usefulness of arteriography would become apparent in clinical practice.

Jaboulay and Briau successfully performed an end-to-end reanastomosis of the carotid artery in 1896.[21] This was remarkable, given the previously held belief that sutures placed in a vessel would result in its early thrombosis. John Murphy, a year later in 1897, described a successful end-to end arterial anastomosis of a femoral artery that had been injured with a gunshot wound with development of a pseudoaneurysm.[22] His case followed considerable experimental work with vascular anastomoses in both canine and bovine subjects and set the stage for subsequent advances in the succeeding century.

EARLY TWENTIETH CENTURY

Alexis Carrel, a student of Jaboulay, had an early interest in vascular anastomoses.[23,24] Carrel came to the United States shortly after the turn of the century and joined Charles C. Guthrie in the Department of Physiology at the University of Chicago.[25,26] These two individuals took the concept of inserting a vein into the arterial circulation and demonstrated that such was feasible in animal experiments.[27-29] Together they co-authored 28 papers. This work was the basis of Carrel's receiving the Nobel Prize in Medicine and Physiology in 1912.

Given an awareness of the novelty of successful vascular anastomoses performed in the laboratory, Jose Goyanes resected a patient's popliteal artery aneurysm and replaced it with a popliteal vein graft in 1906.[30] This was considered the first clinically successful arterial reconstruction using a vein graft.

The treatment of aortic aneurysms at the beginning of the twentieth century continued to involve non-reconstructive procedures. Instillation of large amounts of wire into an aneurysm as a means of inducing thrombosis and external wrapping to limit aneurysmal expansion proved inadequate and was soon discarded as acceptable therapy. Rudolph Matas, who successfully ligated the infrarenal aorta for the treatment of an aortic aneurysm in 1923,[31] reported his life's experience in 1940 with 62 similar operations for aneurysms with a commendable mortality of only 15%.[32] Although the natural history of untreated aortic and peripheral aneurysms became better defined during the early twentieth century, adequate treatment would not become commonplace until the second half of the century.

The management of lower extremity ischemia advanced quickly towards the end of the first half of the twentieth century. In 1946, Juan Cid dos Santos undertook a number of extensive endarterectomies for arteriosclerotic arterial occlusions.[33,34] He is often credited as the founder of arterial endarterectomy, although similar procedures had been performed earlier by Bazy and colleagues for aortic occlusive disease.[35] Endarterectomy was a landmark contribution to the evolution of vascular surgery.

In 1948, Jean Kunlin performed a successful femoropopliteal bypass with reversed autogenous saphenous vein and established a therapeutic approach that continues to present times.[36] William Holden, 6 months following Kunlin's achievement, was first in the United States to perform a lower extremity bypass with vein,[37] and his success was followed by that of many others.

Although not directly related to treating lower extremity ischemia, the surgical therapy of thoracic isthmic coarctations during the early mid-twentieth century established the feasibility of clamping the aorta and undertaking its operative reconstruction. Clarence Crafoord, in 1944, first resected the coarcted segment and reconstructed the aorta with an end-to-end anastomosis.[38] Robert Gross did the same in 1945,[39] and in 1948 he replaced the coarcted aortic segment with a homograft.[40,41] These achievements allowed others to treat aortoiliac occlusive disease later with much greater confidence.

Attention to diseases of the distal aorta followed Rene Leriche's 1923 report on the clinical manifestations of thrombotic occlusion of the arteriosclerotic aortic bifurcation.[42] His experience with the treatment of this disease was later described in a widely heralded report of 1948.[43] The treatment of aortoiliac occlusive disease by operative means progressed rapidly thereafter during the last half of the century.

Recognition of diseases affecting the renal artery during the first half of the twentieth century would wait many years before they were successfully treated surgically. Harry Goldblatt, in elegant studies performed in the 1920s and 1930s, documented that renal artery constrictions in experimental animals caused hypertension.[44] In 1938, the clinical relevance of his observations became apparent when Leadbetter and Burkland removed a small ischemic kidney in a child with renal artery occlusive disease and cured his severe hypertension.[45] Unfortunately, the next few decades saw many kidneys removed without benefit, namely, because the careful selection of patients having a renin-mediated form of hypertension was undeveloped and vascular procedures for reconstructing the renal arteries were non-existent.

The classic description of occlusive disease of the splanchnic arteries causing intestinal angina was proposed in J. Englebert Dunphy's classic paper of 1936.[46] He recognized the importance of postprandial abdominal pain as a manifestation of arteriosclerotic narrowings of the major arteries to the gut and noted its potential to eventuate in intestinal infarction. As was the case with renal artery disease, many years would pass before the successful vascular surgical treatment of intestinal angina occurred.

During the first half of the twentieth century, the role of the extracranial internal carotid artery as a cause of stroke received little attention. There were a number of reasons for this. First, cerebral angiography, initially performed by Egas Moniz in 1927,[47] was not to be used as a diagnostic test for many decades to come. Second, neck vessels were rarely examined during routine autopsy studies, and the existence of extracranial carotid artery arteriosclerosis was usually overlooked. In fact, the most commonly perceived cause of a cerebrovascular accident during the mid-century was thrombosis of the middle cerebral artery, with no understanding that thromboembolism from the region of the carotid bulb often played a role in the occlusive process.

The treatment of venous diseases was one of the mainstays of practice among physicians during the first half of the twentieth century. Varicose veins were known to have plagued man since antiquity, and external compression continued to be the basis of most therapies at the close of the century. A noteworthy contribution in that regard was the plaster dressing introduced by Unna, which became the forerunner of the dressing carrying his name a century later.[48] In 1905, Keller undertook stripping of extremity veins[4] and Babcock in the same time period developed an intraluminal stripper for vein removal.[49]

John Homans subsequently made many observations that advanced our understanding of venous disease. During the century's second decade, he emphasized the importance of saphenofemoral vein ligation in the prevention of varicosities.[50,51] A little more than 20 years later, in 1938, Robert Linton described the importance of incompetent communicating veins and subsequently developed a technique for subfascial ligation of these perforating veins.[52] More direct surgical interventions on the veins themselves to prevent venous hypertension would await another 3 decades.

The lethal nature of pulmonary emboli was well known in the early twentieth century, and prevention of this complication of venous thrombosis became important. In 1934, Homans advocated femoral vein ligation to prevent pulmonary embolism.[53] By 1945, ligation of the inferior vena cava (IVC) was reported by Northway, Buxton and O'Neill as a means of preventing fatal pulmonary embolism.[54,55] Ligation of the cava for prevention of septic emboli had been reported a few years earlier.[56]

A major advance in the evolution of vascular surgery during the early twentieth century was the introduction of translumbar aortography in 1929 by Reynaldo dos Santos.[57] Imaging of blood vessels was to prove essential to the continued advancement of vascular surgery. A second major advance was the use of heparin anticoagulation to prevent perioperative thromboses that affected the vast majority of vascular interventions during the very early twentieth century. Although heparin had been discovered in 1918 by Jay McLean in W. H. Howell's laboratory,[58] it was not purified and readily available for use until the 1930s and 1940s. It was only then that its value in treating arterial thromboses became widely recognized.[59,60]

Thus, the first half of the twentieth century witnessed the ability to approximate injured vessels, removal of arteriosclerotic plaque by the technique of endarterectomy and replacement of chronically diseased arteries with bypass grafts, all under the influence of anticoagulation. These achievements laid the foundation for the many advances of the last half of the twentieth century in vascular surgery.

THE LAST HALF OF THE TWENTIETH CENTURY AND THE EARLY TWENTY-FIRST CENTURY

More recent times have been born witness to profound changes in the practice of vascular surgery. These events are best discussed by addressing the individual contributions unique to specific disease entities.

Aortoiliac arteriosclerotic occlusive disease

Treatment of arteriosclerotic aortic disease was first successfully undertaken by Jacques Oudot in 1950 with a homograft replacement of a thrombosed aortic bifurcation.[61,62] With the recognition of homograft degeneration and the initial use of synthetic grafts, this form of aortic reconstruction fell into disuse.

Although the earliest aortoiliac endarterectomy may have been performed by Bazy and colleagues,[35] this technique was first undertaken in 1951 in the United States by Norman Freeman[63] and shortly thereafter popularized by his former colleague in practice, Edwin Wylie.[64,65]

The introduction of synthetic bypass grafts for the management of aortic diseases changed treatment dramatically, and for the next 40 years, these grafts, serving as aortofemoral bypasses, were the most common means of treating aortoiliac occlusive diseases.[66–73]

Nonanatomic revascularization procedures also evolved during the 1950s and 1960s for the treatment of aortoiliac occlusive lesions in high-risk situations. These unconventional interventions were used most often in reoperations for an infected or failed earlier bypass, avoidance of a hostile abdomen or concerns about the operative hazards of a more extensive procedure. Many types of nonanatomic procedures were developed over a short period of time.

The first of these nonanatomic reconstructions was by Jacques Oudot in 1951, who performed a crossover ilioiliac arterial bypass.[74] Subsequently, Norman Freeman used an endarterectomized superficial femoral artery in 1952 to perform a femorofemoral arterial crossover bypass.[75] An iliac artery to contralateral popliteal artery bypass was constructed by McCaughan and Kahn in 1958.[76] However, little attention was paid to these operations by most practitioners in the earlier days of contemporary vascular surgery.

It was in the 1960s that nonanatomic procedures became popular, after reports by Veto of a femorofemoral arterial crossover bypass in 1960,[77] as well as by Blaisdell and Hall of an axillofemoral bypass using a synthetic graft in 1962.[78] An important contribution to the latter procedure came from Lester Savage, who in 1966 added a crossover femorofemoral arterial bypass to a unilateral axillofemoral bypass as a means of revascularizing both lower extremities.[79] Although unrelated to the primary treatment of aortoiliac occlusive disease, the performance of an obturator bypass, first reported by Guida and Moore in 1969,[80] allowed lower extremity revascularizations with avoidance of an otherwise hostile groin area.

Endovascular interventions provided the most important major advance in the treatment of aortoiliac occlusive disease during the last quarter of the twentieth century, becoming widely used in the 1990s. This technology evolved from the pioneering work of Charles Dotter who reported on percutaneous coaxial dilation of peripheral arteries in 1964[81] and Andreas Gruentzig, who introduced percutaneous twin-lumen balloon angioplasty in 1974.[82] Treatment of iliac artery stenoses by balloon dilation markedly reduced the frequency with which open aortobifemoral bypass procedures were undertaken, and the use of balloon-assisted intraluminal stents developed by Palmaz in 1988[83] lessened the risk of complications associated with dissections. The rapid application of stent technology to angioplasty of iliac artery lesions followed during the next decade.[84]

Infrainguinal arteriosclerotic occlusive disease

Jean Kunlin reported 17 patients who had undergone autogenous vein lower extremity revascularizations in 1951.[85] Just 3 years after, he performed the first such operation. This was followed by similar bypass procedures in the United States by many surgeons including Julian, Lord, Dale, DeWeese, Linton, Darling and Szilagyi that confirmed the utility of reversed saphenous vein femoropopliteal reconstructions. Extension of vein graft procedures to the more distal infrageniculate arteries was first reported by Palma, who undertook a femorotibial bypass in 1956.[86] This too was followed with similar revascularizations by many others.

The use of the saphenous vein in situ after rendering its valves incompetent was first reported by Karl Hall in 1962.[87] This technology saw limited use until 1979, when Robert Leather and his colleagues introduced a new valve cutter for in situ revascularizations.[88] Subsequently, the procedure became widely used during the next decade.

Table 1.1 Aortic and aortoiliac occlusive disease.

Reynaldo dos Santos	1929	Translumbar aortography
Clarence Crafoord	1944	Thoracic coarctation resection, aortic reanastomosis
Rene Leriche	1948	Treatment of thrombotic occlusion of atherosclerotic aortic bifurcation, first described in 1923
Robert Gross	1949	Homograft replacement of thoracic aortic coarctation
Jacques Oudot	1950	Homograft replacement of thrombosed aortic bifurcation
Norman Freeman	1951	Aortoiliac endarterectomy; followed shortly thereafter in 1951 by Wylie, who popularized the open technique first described by Bazy and colleagues in 1949
Julio Palmaz	1988	Balloon-assisted stenting of arterial stenoses

Table 1.2 Nonanatomic revascularization of the lower extremities.

Jacques Oudot	1951	Ilioiliac bypass
Norman Freeman	1952	Femorofemoral bypass with endarterectomized superficial femoral artery
J.J. Mccaughan Jr., S. F. Kahn	1958	Iliopopliteal bypass
R. Mark Veto	1960	Femorofemoral bypass
F. William Blaisdell, A.D. Hall	1962	Axillofemoral bypass
Lester Sauvage	1966	Axillobifemoral bypass
P.M. Guida, S.W. Moore	1969	Obturator bypass

Table 1.3 Femoral, popliteal and tibial arterial occlusive disease.

Joao Cid dos Santos	1946	Femoral endarterectomy
Jean Kunlin	1948	Reversed autogenous saphenous vein femoral popliteal bypass
Eduardo Palma	1956	Femoral–tibial bypass with vein
Karl Hall	1962	In situ saphenous vein bypass
Thomas Fogarty	1963	Balloon-catheter embolectomy
Charles Dotter	1964	Percutaneous angioplasty (coaxial)
	1969	Percutaneous arterial endograft (experimental)
Peter Martin	1971	Extended profundoplasty
Herbert Dardik	1976	Use of human umbilical vein grafts in lower extremity revascularizations
Robert Leather	1979	In situ saphenous vein bypass popularized with introduction of new valve cutter
Dierk Maass	1982	Percutaneous expandable endoprosthesis
John Simpson	1985	Percutaneous transluminal atherectomy
Adair Bolia	1989	Percutaneous subintimal arterial recanalization

Although some have questioned the advantage to these reconstructions, their use in many distal revascularization procedures appeared valid.

An alternative biologic graft for use instead of autogenous vein was the tanned human umbilical vein, reported initially by Herbert Dardik in 1976.[89] Late aneurysmal changes in these grafts led to their eventual disuse. Although utilization of Dacron grafts for lower extremity reconstructions waned with the success of vein revascularizations, the introduction of extruded polytetrafluoroethylene (PTFE) grafts caused a resurgence in synthetic graft use for the treatment of lower extremity ischemia. In two hallmark papers, John Bergan, Frank Veith, Victor Bernhard and their colleagues demonstrated the utility of PTFE grafts for femoropopliteal reconstructions, with lesser benefits when used for distal infrageniculate procedures.[90,91]

The importance of the profunda femoris artery was initially reported in 1971 by Peter Martin, who described an extended profundoplasty as a means of improving blood flow to the ischemic extremity.[92]Although unrelated to his report, the importance of the profunda femoris artery in completing the distal anastomosis of an aortofemoral bypass was well recognized during the same time period, and an extension of the graft limb onto this vessel became standard practice.

The endovascular approach in managing lower extremity peripheral arterial occlusive became popular around the turn of the century. The spectrum of these less-invasive interventions ranged from simple balloon angioplasty of a focal superficial femoral artery stenosis to more complex subintimal recanalizations that were proposed by Adair Bolia in 1989.[93] Subsequently, catheter-directed mechanical atherectomy for more severe occlusive disease was introduced by John Simpson in 1985.[94] A variety of such devices are now used in contemporary practice to remove obstructing arteriosclerotic plaque. Percutaneous placement of a prosthetic graft, initially proposed by Dotter in 1969,[95] became clinically relevant in 1982 with the publication by Maass on the use of catheter-implanted expandable endografts.[96] Later, stenting both diseased vessels and endografts with self-expanding devices was advanced by Rabkin's 1989 report on the use of nitinol stents in humans.[97]

Embolic arterial occlusions of the lower extremity

One of the major advances in vascular surgery was introduced in Thomas Fogarty's 1963 report on balloon-catheter extractions of thromboembolic material from distant vessels.[98] Given the risks of open procedures for saddle aortic emboli that often followed a myocardial infarction and the difficulties in removing emboli originating from atrial fibrillation in the smaller arteries of the leg, the ability to remove occlusive material through a femoral artery under local anaesthesia must be considered a sentinel contribution to the discipline of vascular surgery.

Aortic aneurysms

The lethal nature of aortic aneurysms led to many direct therapeutic advances, once clamping of the aorta was recognized to be tolerable and the postoperative management of these patients became better. Charles Dubost was the first to successfully treat an abdominal aortic aneurysm in 1951.[99] He replaced the aneurysm with a thoracic aortic homograft in a relatively complex procedure. Shortly thereafter, in 1953, Michael DeBakey and Denton Cooley replaced a thoracic aortic aneurysm with a similar homograft.[100] These reconstructions occurred during a time of considerable interest in the use of homografts for a variety of vascular procedures. The inevitable degenerative changes affecting these conduits led to their later abandonment in the clinical practice of aortic surgery, although in contemporary times they have been used in cases of infection when replacing the aorta.

Aortic aneurysm treatment changed dramatically shortly after Arthur Voorhees, Arthur Blakemore and Alfred Jaretzki reported the successful implantation of Vinyon-N cloth grafts in animals in 1951.[72] Two years later, in 1953, they used this type of graft in a patient with a ruptured aortic aneurysm

who subsequently died of a myocardial infarction. However, their case was made, and in 1954 they described the use of this type of synthetic graft in 17 patients.[101] Unfortunately, this nylon material proved too brittle. Conduits constructed of Teflon and Dacron were subsequently developed, with the latter being popularized by DeBakey in the mid-1950s. Operative refinements involved lessening the risk of graft-enteric erosions by covering the implanted graft with the aneurysm shell, which in earlier times was usually excised in toto, and using synthetic sutures rather than silk, which with its deterioration led to late anastomotic separations of the graft from the vessel and eventual development of pseudoaneurysms. An important innovation in the therapy of aortic aneurysmal disease was the 1974 reported success of E. Stanley Crawford in using intraluminal grafts rather than bypass grafts to treat thoracoabdominal aneurysms that involved the renal and splanchnic arteries.[102]

The most important advance in aortic surgery during recent decades followed the publication by Volodos in 1988 on the use of an endograft to treat a traumatic aneurysm of the aorta.[103] This work and its implication to clinical practice went relatively unnoticed until 1991 when Juan Parodi reported using an endograft to treat an abdominal aortic aneurysm.[104] These former contributions, especially Parodi's, revolutionized the management of aortic aneurysms, and the subsequent decade witnessed many contributions to this new paradigm of vascular surgery. In 1994, this technology expanded the use of endografts in the treatment of ruptured abdominal aortic aneurysms.[105] A major and necessary improvement in the endovascular treatment of abdominal aortic aneurysms was modular prostheses, introduced by Chuter in 1994.[106,107] One of the most

Table 1.4 Aortic aneurysms.

Rudolph Matas	1923	First successful ligation for treatment of abdominal aortic aneurysm; unsuccessful attempt by Ashley Cooper in 1817
Charles Dubost	1951	Homograft replacement of abdominal aortic aneurysm
Arthur Voorhees, Arthur Blakemore, Alfred Jaretzki	1952	Development of synthetic graft (Vinyon-N) in experimental subjects; first clinical results with these grafts reported in 1953
Michael DeBakey, Denton Cooley	1953	Homograft replacement of thoracic aortic aneurysm
Michael DeBakey	1955	Repair of abdominal aortic aneurysm with prosthetic grafts
E. Stanley Crawford	1974	Intraluminal graft repair of thoracoabdominal aneurysms
Nicholas Volodes	1988	Endograft treatment of traumatic thoracic aortic aneurysm
Juan Parodi	1990	Endograft treatment of abdominal aortic aneurysm
Timothy Chuter	1994	Modular endograft treatment of aortic aneurysm
Syed Yusuf	1994	Endograft treatment of ruptured aortic aneurysm

Table 1.5 Femoral and popliteal artery aneurysms.

Ashley Cooper	1808	Femoral aneurysm ligation (patient lived 18 years)
Jose Goyanes	1906	Popliteal aneurysm excision, replaced with vein (first vein bypass graft used in clinical practice)
Michael Marin	1994	Endovascular stent–graft exclusion of popliteal artery aneurysm

valuable applications of this technology was the placement of endovascular stent grafts in the treatment of degenerative thoracic aortic aneurysms, as initially reported by Michael Dake in 1994.[108] It is an understatement to note that endovascular interventions have had a major impact on patient care and indeed the very definition of vascular surgery.

The common association of femoral and popliteal artery aneurysms with aortic aneurysms, especially in male patients, was clearly established in the last half of the twentieth century.[109–111] Their clinical management during recent decades was advanced by lytic therapy for thrombosed popliteal artery aneurysms before the operative bypass and aneurysm exclusion was performed. Endovascular placement of an endoluminal graft to exclude a popliteal aneurysm was first reported by Marin and his colleagues in 1994,[112] although the exact circumstances have not been defined when this technology is best pursued.

Renal artery occlusive disease

The first renal artery endarterectomy was performed by Norman Freeman in 1953,[113] a procedure popularized later by Edwin Wylie and his colleagues.[114] Nevertheless, aortorenal bypass using autogenous saphenous vein, first performed by Marion S. DeWeese in 1958, was subsequently more widely used than endarterectomy.[115] Stoney and his colleagues favoured using autologous iliac artery for reconstructing the renal arteries,[116] and DeCamp's first successful nonanatomic renal revascularization by a splenorenal bypass in 1957 offered yet another alternative means of renal revascularization.[117]

Despite these early contributions, the surgical treatment of renal artery occlusive disease was uncommon until after a series of publications from the Cooperative Study of Renovascular Hypertension in the mid-1970s.[118–122] Shortly thereafter, large surgical series appeared which firmly established the appropriateness of operation for renovascular hypertension.[123,124] During the same time period, a definitive classification of renal artery occlusive disease followed two publications, one in 1971[125] and the other in 1975.[126]

Andreas Gruntzig and his colleagues reported the first successful percutaneous balloon dilation of an arteriosclerotic renal artery occlusive lesion in 1978.[127] This technology had caused major changes in the management of renovascular hypertension by the close of the twentieth century. Continued clinical experience confirmed that endovascular-performed angioplasty is preferred for the treatment of most adult fibrodysplastic renal artery disease. Although the use of stents is technically efficacious in treating many arteriosclerotic ostial stenoses, this technology has received little support from a number of prospective trials including a recent study by Cooper and his colleagues in 2014 comparing percutaneous transluminal angioplasty to drug therapy alone.[128] However, considerable controversy surrounds a potential bias in many of the former studies regarding patient selection entering the trials.

Splanchnic artery occlusive disease

Acute intestinal ischemia, usually a consequence of embolism to the superior mesenteric artery, continued to be a lethal illness throughout latter half of the twentieth century. Klass in 1951 was the first to successfully treat acute intestinal ischemia by performance of a superior mesenteric artery embolectomy.[129] The operative treatment of both acute and chronic intestinal ischemia leading to today's endarterectomy and bypass procedures was subsequently advanced by Shaw and Mikkelsen with their colleagues in the late 1950s.[130,131] Additional experience during the last few decades of the twentieth century

Table 1.6 Splanchnic and renal arterial disease.

Renal artery disease		
Harry Goldblatt	1929	Established importance of renal artery occlusion and secondary hypertension
W.F. Leadbetter, G.E. Burkland	1938	Nephrectomy for renovascular hypertension (first treated case of renovascular hypertension)
Norman Freeman	1953	Renal artery endarterectomy
Marion DeWeese	1959	Aortorenal bypass with autogenous vein
Andreas Gruntzig	1978	Percutaneous renal artery balloon dilation
Splanchnic artery disease		
J. Englebert Dunphy	1936	Description of chronic intestinal ischemia
J. Klass	1951	Superior mesenteric artery embolectomy
R.S. Shaw, E.P. Maynard	1958	Operative treatment of acute and chronic intestinal ischemia
W.P. Mikkelsen	1959	Operative treatment of chronic intestinal ischemia
J. Furrer	1980	Percutaneous balloon angioplasty of the superior mesenteric artery

affirmed the generally accepted tenets that aortomesenteric bypasses with synthetic grafts were preferable to vein graft reconstructions and that multiple vessel revascularizations were more likely to provide greater long-term benefits than single-vessel reconstructions.

As has been evident in other vascular territories, endovascular therapy has become part of the therapeutic armamentarium in treating splanchnic arterial occlusive disease. The first percutaneous angioplasty in the treatment of chronic intestinal ischemia was reported by Furrer and Gruntzig and their colleagues in 1980.[132] The surgical management of intestinal ischemia due to splanchnic arteriosclerosis must be considered somewhat anecdotal compared to treatment of other vascular diseases. In fact, no large clinical studies exist that properly compare the differing therapeutic options. The same conclusion applies to the therapy of many splanchnic artery aneurysms, with few definitive experiences reported since two widely quoted reviews were published in the 1970s.[133,134]

Cerebrovascular disease

Miller Fisher reported autopsy findings in 1951 that for the first time presented irrefutable evidence that extracranial carotid artery bifurcation arteriosclerosis was likely to be a common cause of a stroke.[135] This led to a series of remarkable advances in the surgical treatment and prevention of stroke. The first reported operation for carotid artery stenotic disease was in 1951 by Raul Carrea, Mahelz Molins and Guillermo Murphy, who resected the affected carotid artery and reanastomosed the internal carotid artery to the external carotid artery.[136] Three years later, in 1954, Felix Eastcott, George Pickering and Charles Rob reported a similar procedure with resection of the diseased carotid bifurcation and a reanastomosis of the internal carotid artery to the common carotid artery.[137] In 1953, the first conventional carotid endarterectomy was performed by Michael DeBakey.[138] One year later, in 1954, Davis, Grove and Julian reported having performed the first innominate artery endarterectomy,[139] and in 1958,

Table 1.7 Cerebrovascular disease: recognition and basis for treatment.

Egas Moniz	1927	Cerebral angiography.
Miller Fisher	1951	Post-mortem exam of 373 patients suggested arteriosclerosis of the extracranial carotid artery bifurcation might be a common cause of cerebrovascular accident.
Henry Barnett	1991, 1998	NASCET documented benefit of surgical therapy for symptomatic stenotic lesions greater than 50%.
Robert Hobson	1993	Surgical benefit documented for select treatment of asymptomatic carotid artery stenosis.
James O'Toole	1993	Asymptomatic carotid artery study documented surgical benefit for asymptomatic lesions greater than 70%.
J.S. Yadav	2004	Randomized trial comparing carotid artery stenting and endarterectomy in high-risk patients.

Table 1.8 Cerebrovascular disease: surgical treatment.

Raul Carrea, Mahelz Molins, Guillermo Murphy	1951	Resected arteriosclerotic carotid, with external to internal carotid reanastomosis (first operation for carotid stenotic disease)
Michael DeBakey	1953	Carotid artery endarterectomy
H.H.G. (Felix) Eastcott, George Pickering, Charles Robb	1954	Resected carotid bifurcation, with common carotid to internal carotid reanastomosis
C. Lyons, G. Galbraith	1956	Subclavian–carotid artery bypass
J.B. Davis, W.J. Grove, O.C. Julian	1954	Innominate artery endarterectomy
Michael DeBakey, George Morris, G.L. Jordan, Denton Cooley	1957	Innominate–subclavian–carotid arterial bypass
Stanley Crawford, Michael DeBakey, William Fields	1958	Vertebral artery endarterectomy and bypass
M. Gazi Yasargil, Hugh A. Krayenbuhl, Julius H. Jacobson II	1970	Extracranial–intracranial arterial bypass
Klaus D. Mathias	1977	Percutaneous angioplasty of carotid artery stenosis
Donald Bachman, Robert Kim, Klaus D. Mathias	1980	Percutaneous angioplasty of subclavian artery stenosis

E. Stanley Crawford, Michael DeBakey and William Fields reported endarterectomy as a means of treating vertebral artery occlusive disease.[140]

The benefits of treating cerebral ischemic syndromes with a bypass were also first recognized during the mid-1950s. Lyons and Galbraith in 1956 performed a subclavian-to-carotid artery bypass,[141] and in 1958, Michael DeBakey and his associates reported an innominate artery to subclavian and carotid arterial bypass.[142] A vertebral artery bypass was also reported by Crawford, DeBakey and Fields that same year. A more dramatic approach to these diseases was by an extracranial–intracranial arterial bypass, championed by Yasargil and his colleagues in the early 1970s.[143] This has been used infrequently following a still-controversial clinical study of the technique published by Henry Barnett and his colleagues in 1989.[144]

One of the most important effects on the surgical treatment of carotid artery arteriosclerosis resulted from a series of well-designed and well-conducted prospective clinical studies initially published in the 1990s that better defined the indication for endarterectomy procedures. The first, the North American Symptomatic Carotid Endarterectomy Trial (NASCET), led by Henry Barnett, was published initially in 1991 and updated in 1998.[145,146] These studies documented the benefit of carotid endarterectomy in lessening the risk of subsequent stroke in patients with symptomatic stenotic lesions greater than 50%. Two other studies, one from Europer[147] and the other from veterans' hospitals in the United States,[148] supported the NASCET conclusions.

The beneficial effects of carotid endarterectomy in preventing stroke in patients with asymptomatic carotid stenoses greater than 70% was subsequently reported by James O'Toole and Robert Hobson.[149,150] Although some may dispute the details of any of these studies, the benefits of a carefully performed carotid endarterectomy in a properly selected patient were definitively established.

Carotid endarterectomy at the conclusion of the twentieth century was the most common vascular operation performed in the United States, but it was soon to be challenged by percutaneous endovascular interventions. The first angioplasty for carotid artery disease was reported in 1977 by Mathias,[151] but it wasn't acclaimed to be an appropriate alternative to endarterectomy until decades later when a number of clinical trials were reported; perhaps, the most influential being published in 2004 and 2008 by Yadav and colleagues.[152,153] At the close of the last century, the introduction of percutaneous carotid artery dilation and stenting was touted as a reasonable alternative to carotid endarterectomy. However, its exact role in the clinical arena has yet to be clearly established.

Less controversy exists regarding endovascular dilation and stenting of the proximal subclavian artery for the treatment of vertebrobasilar symptoms evident in the subclavian steal syndrome. Percutaneous angioplasty of subclavian stenoses was first reported in 1980 by Bachman and Kim[154] and Mathias.[155] Although these initial procedures involved balloon dilation alone, the use of stenting in succeeding years became part of most interventions.

Venous disease

Prevention of embolization and venous hypertension arising from deep venous thromboses led to a number of important surgical interventions during the last half of the twentieth century. Although ligation of the IVC had been performed earlier for prevention of pulmonary embolism and often was used as the treatment of choice for septic emboli, the morbidity of this therapy was considerable.

In 1958, Marion S. DeWeese was the first to partially interrupt the vena cava for the prevention of pulmonary emboli, using a suture plication technique.[156,157] In 1967, Kazi Mobin-Uddin introduced an umbrella device to trap emboli in transit.[158,159] His remarkable innovation was followed by Lazar Greenfield's conical vena cava filter,[160] which was initially placed through the jugular vein with an open procedure but was later inserted percutaneously through a femoral vein route. Subsequently, other caval devices have been developed to trap emboli from the lower body veins. The reduction in fatal pulmonary embolism using vena cava filters represents a major accomplishment of vascular surgeons.

Treatment of venous hypertension in the last half of the twentieth century focused on both direct venous reconstructive surgery and less-invasive procedures for interrupting incompetent perforating veins. In 1952, Jean Kunlin performed a saphenous vein bypass of an obstructed external iliac artery vein,[161] and 6 years later, Eduardo Palma performed a saphenofemoral vein crossover bypass.[162] A more distal decompressive procedure, a saphenopopliteal vein bypass, was accomplished by Husni in 1970.[163]

Endovascular disobliteration of thrombosed extremity veins with subsequent catheter-based dilation, usually with stenting, is a direct means of reducing venous hypertension but has had limited applicability in clinical practice. However, endovascular interventions for obstructions affecting the more major veins have been pursued in cases of severe venous hypotension. The first stenting of the vena cava in such a setting was reported in 1986 by Gianturco and his colleagues.[164]

Reducing elevated venous pressures in the lower extremity by reconstructing the vein's valves was introduced by Robert Kistner, who successfully performed venous valvuloplasty procedures,[165,166] and Taheri who was the first to undertake transplantation of a venous valve.[167] Hauer in 1985 reported on the endoscopic interruption of incompetent perforating veins that contributed to elevated venous pressures at the ankle.[168] Durable treatment of venous hypertension and its complications, including cutaneous ulcerations, continues to challenge the current clinical skills of physicians.

Surgical elimination of lower extremity varicose veins by means other than stripping was advanced after a 1944 report on foam sclerotherapy,[169] with the later development of various sclerosing agents. Subsequently, an early form of radiofrequency ablation was introduced

Table 1.9 Venous disease.

Prophylactic prevention of pulmonary embolism		
John Holmans	1934	Femoral vein ligation
O. Northway, Robert Buxton, E. O'Neill	1944	IVC ligation
Marion S. DeWeese	1958	Suture plication of the IVC
Kazi Mobin-Uddin	1967	Transvenous IVC umbrella filter
Lazar J. Greenfield	1974	Percutaneous IVC conical–strut filter
Correction of venous hypertension		
Robert Linton	1938	Subfascial division of incompetent perforating veins
Jean Kunlin	1952	Saphenous vein bypass of obstructed external iliac vein
Eduardo Plama	1958	Saphenofemoral vein crossover bypass
E.A. Husni	1970	Saphenopopliteal vein bypass
Robert Kistner	1975	Valvuloplasty
S.A. Taheri	1982	Vein–valve transplant
G. Hauer	1985	Endoscopic interruptions of incompetent perforating veins
C. Charnsangavej	1986	Endovascular stenting of the vena cava
Removal of varicose veins		
W.W. Babcock	1905	Intraluminal stripper for vein removal
John Homans	1916	Saphenofemoral vein ligation
E.J. Orbach	1944	Foam sclerotherapy
M. Politowski	1966	Radiofrequency venous ablation
C. Bone	1999	Laser venous ablation

in 1966[170] followed by laser venous ablation in 1999.[171] Both interventions have been part of the endovascular approach to the contemporary management of venous disease.

THE FUTURE

The diagnosis of vascular disease in the early decades of the current millennium is likely to evolve dramatically with genetic testing that will identify patients at risk for various arteriosclerotic occlusive disorders, matrix problems leading to aneurysms and other vascular diseases. This will revolutionize the selection of patients for early interventions, both medical and surgical, and will affect vascular surgery more than any other advance since the introduction of contemporary imaging techniques, vascular grafts and heparin anticoagulation.

The practice of vascular surgery, especially in industrial nations during the early decades of the twenty-first century, will be impacted by increasing costs of health care, a greater number of patients needing treatment as the population ages and the involvement of third parties in controlling affordable medical practice. Given society's greater medical literacy and availability of the internet, there will also be an increasing patient demand for better care in relation to outcomes. Vascular surgery, because of its easily documented clinical end points, should be the beneficiary of evidence-based care.

Finally, there will be complementary and competing practices in the new millennium. This will likely result in the establishment of true multidisciplinary care and the elimination of those disciplines unable to adapt to new paradigms of practice. Vascular surgery can ill afford to not adapt to change. This relates to training and certification in a bureaucratic era, where benefits of treatment, and surgical intervention in particular, must outweigh the risk of alternative therapies. Durable benefits must be afforded patients. The evolution of vascular surgery has been one of enormous success. The challenge now is how to best enhance and advance the knowledge base and practice patterns enacted by our discipline's forebears.

REFERENCES

1. Barker WF. A history of vascular surgery. In: Moore WF, ed. *Vascular Surgery: A Comprehensive Review*, 5th ed. Philadelphia, PA: Saunders, 1998, pp. 1–19.
2. Dale WA, Johnson G Jr., DeWeese JA. *Band of Brothers: Creators of Modern Vascular Surgery*. Chelsea, MI: BookCrafters, 1996.
3. Friedman SG. *A History of Vascular Surgery*. New York: Futura, 1989.
4. Thompson JE. History of vascular surgery. In: Norton JA, Bollinger RR, Chang AE, Lowry SF, Mulvihill SJ, Pass HI, Thompson RW, eds. *Surgery: Basic Science and Clinical Evidence*. New York: Springer-Verlag, 2001, pp. 969–985.
5. Prakash UBS. Sushruta of ancient India. *Surg Gynecol Obstet*. 1978;146:263–272.

6. Hamby W. *The Case Reports and Autopsy Records of Ambrose Pare*. Springfield, IL: Charles C. Thomas, 1960.

7. Chitwood WR Jr. John and William Hunter on aneurysms. *Arch Surg*. 1977;112:829–836.

8. Lambert. Extract of a letter from Mr. Lambert, surgeon at Newcastle Upon Tyne, to Dr. Hunter; giving an Account of a new Method of treating an Aneurysm. Read June 15, 1761. *Med Obs Inq*. 1762;2:360.

9. Perry MO. John Hunter-triumph and tragedy. *J Vasc Surg*. 1993;17:7–14.

10. Schlechter DC, Bergan JJ. Popliteal aneurysm: A celebration of the bicentennial of John Hunter's operation. *Ann Vasc Surg*. 1986;1:118–126.

11. Brock RC. The life and work of Sir Astley Cooper. *Ann R Coll Surg Engl*. 1969;44:1.

12. Rawling EG. Sir Astley Paston Cooper, 1768–1841: The prince of surgery. *Can Med Assoc J*. 1968;99:221–225.

13. Cooper A. A second case of carotid aneurysm. *Med Chir Trans*. 1809;1:222–233.

14. Cooper A. Account of the first successful operation performed on the common carotid artery for aneurysm in the year 1808 with the postmortem examination in the year 1821. *Guy's Hosp Rep*. 1836;I:53–59.

15. Rutkow JM. Valentine Mott (1785–1865) the father of American vascular surgery: A historical perspective. *Surgery*. 1979;85:441–450.

16. Cordell AR. A lasting legacy: The life and work of Rudolph Matas. *J Vasc Surg*. 1985;2:613–619.

17. Matas R. Traumatic aneurysm of the left brachial artery. *Med News Phil*. 1888;53:462.

18. Barth. Observation d'une Obliteration Complete de l·aorte Abdominale Recuillie Dans le Service de M Louis, Suivie de Reflections. *Arch Gen Med*. 1835;8:26–53.

19. Roentgen WK. Ueber eine neue Art von Strahlen. *Nature*. 1896;53:274.

20. Haschek E, Lindenthal OT. Ein Beitrag zur praktischen Verwerthung der Photographie nach Roentgen. *Wien Klin Wochenschr*. 1896;9:63.

21. Jaboulay M, Briau E. Recherches Experimentales Sur la Suture ct al Greffe Arterielle. *Lyon Med*. 1896;81:97–99.

22. Murphy JB. Resection of arteries and veins injured in continuity-end-to-end suture-experimental and clinical research. *Med Res*. 1897;51:73.

23. Carrel A. La Technique Operatoire des Anastomoses Vasculaires et de la Transplantation des Visceres. *Lyon Med*. 1902;98:850.

24. Carrel A, Moullard J. Anastomose Bout a Bout de la Jugulaire et de la Caroticle Primitive. *Lyon Med*. 1902;99:114.

25. Edwards WS, Edwards PD. *Alexis Carrel, Visionary Surgeon*. Springfield, IL: Charles C. Thomas, 1974.

26. Harbison SP. The origins of vascular surgery: The Carrel-Guthrie letters. *Surgery*. 1962;52:406–418.

27. Carrel A, Guthrie CC. Uniterminal and Biterminal Venous Transplantations. *Surg Gynecol Obstet*. 1906;2:266–286.

28. Carrel A, Guthrie CC. Resultats du 'Patching' des Arteres. *C R Soc Biol*. 1906;60:1009.

29. Guthrie CC. *Blood Vessel Surgery and Its Applications*. London, UK: Longmans Green, 1912.

30. Goyanes J. Nuevos Trabajos de Cirugia Vascular. Substitution Plastica de las Arterias por las Venas, 0 Arterioplastia Venosa, Applicada, como Nuevo Metodo, al Tratamiento de los Aneurismas. *El Siglo Med*. 1906 September;346:561.

31. Matas R. Aneurysm of the abdominal aorta at its bifurcation into the common iliac arteries. A pictorial supplement illustrating the history of corinne D, previously reported as the first recorded instance of cure of an aneurysm of the abdominal aorta by ligation. *Ann Surg*. 1940;112:909–922.

32. Matas R. Personal experiences in vascular surgery: A statistical synopsis. *Ann Surg*. 1940;112:802–839.

33. dos Santos JC. Sur la Desobstruction des Thromboses Arterielles Anciennes. *Mem Acad Surg*. 1947;73:409–411.

34. dos Santos JC. From embolectomy to endarterectomy or the fall of a myth. *J Cardiovasc Surg*. 1976;17:113–128.

35. Bazy L, Hugier J, Reboul H et al. Techniques des 'Endarterectomies' or Arterities Obliterantes Chroniques des Membres Inforieures, des Iliaques, et de L' aorte Abdominale Inferieur. *J Chir*. 1949;65:196–210.

36. Kunlin J. Le Traitement de L'arterite Obliterante par la Greffe Veineuse. *Arch Mal Coeur*. 1949;42:371.

37. Holden WD. Reconstruction of the femoral artery for arteriosclerotic thrombosis. *Surgery*. 1950;27:417–422.

38. Crafoord C, Nylin G. Congenital coarctation of the aorta and its surgical treatment. *J Thorac Surg*. 1945;14:347–361.

39. Gross RE. Surgical correction for coarctation of the aorta. *Surgery*. 1945;18:673–678.

40. Gross RE, Hurwitt ES, Bill AH Jr., Pierce EC II. Preliminary observations on the use of human arterial grafts in the treatment of certain cardiovascular defects. *N Engl J Med*. 1948;239:578–579.

41. Gross RE. Treatment of certain aortic coarctations by homologous grafts: A report of 19 cases. *Ann Surg*. 1951;134:753–758.

42. Leriche R. Des Obliterations Arterielles Hautes (Obliteration de la Terminaison de l'aorte) Comme Cause des Insuffisancces Circulatoires des Membres lnferieurs. *Bull Mem Soc Chir*. 1923;49:1404–1406.

43. Leriche R, Morel A. The syndrome of thrombotic obliteration of the aortic bifurcation. *Ann Surg*. 1948;127:193–206.

44. Goldblatt H, Lynch J, Hanzal RF, Summerville WW. Studies on experimental hypertension. I. The production of persistent elevation of systolic blood pressure by means of renal ischemia. *J Exp Med*. 1934;59:347–379.

45. Leadbetter WF, Burkland GE. Hypertension in unilateral renal disease. *J Urol*. 1037;39:661–726.

46. Dunphy JE. Abdominal pain of vascular origin. *Am J Med Sci.* 1935;192:109–113.

47. Moniz E. L'encephalographic Arterielle son Importance dans la Loalisation des Tumeurs Cerebrales. *Rev Neurol.* 1927;2:72–90.

48. Unna PG. Ueber Paraplaste: Eine neue Form medikamentoser Pilaster. *Wien Med Wschr.* 1895;46:1854.

49. Babcock WW. A new operation for the extirpation of varicose veins. *N Y Med J.* 1907;86:153–156.

50. Homans J. The operative treatment of varicose veins and ulcers, based upon a classification of these lesions. *Surg Gynecol Obstet.* 1916;22:143–158.

51. Homans J. The etiology and treatment of varicose ulcer of the leg. *Surg Gynecol Obstet.* 1917;24:300–311.

52. Linton RR. The communicating veins of the lower leg and the operative treatment for their ligation. *Ann Surg.* 1938;107:582–593.

53. Homans J. Thrombosis of the deep veins of the lower leg causing pulmonary embolism. *N Engl J Med.* 1934;211:933–997.

54. Northway O, Buxton RW. Ligation of the inferior vena cava. *Surgery.* 1945;18:85–94.

55. O'Neill EE. Ligation of the inferior vena cava in the prevention and treatment of pulmonary embolism. *N Engl J Med.* 1945;232:641–646.

56. Collins CG, Jones JR, Nelson WE. Surgical treatment of pelvic thrombophlebitis. *New Orleans Med Surg J.* 1943;95:324–329.

57. dos Santos R, Lamas A, Pereirgi CJ. L'arteriographie des Membres de L'aorte et ses Branches Abdominales. *Bull Soc Nat Hir.* 1929;55:587.

58. Howell WH. Two new factors in blood coagulation-heparin and proantithrombin. *Am J Physiol.* 1918;47:328–341.

59. Murray G. Heparin in surgical treatment of blood vessels. *Arch Surg.* 1940;40:307–325.

60. Murray GWG, Best CH. The use of heparin in thrombosis. *Ann Surg.* 1938;108:163–177.

61. Oudot J. La Greffe Vasculaire dans les Thromboses du Crrefour Aortique. *Presse Med.* 1951;59:234–236.

62. Oudot J, Beaconsfield P. Thrombosis of the aortic bifurcation treated by resection and homograft replacement: Report of five cases. *Arch Surg.* 1953;66:365–374.

63. Freeman NE, Leeds FH. Vein inlay graft in treatment of aneurysm and thrombosis of abdominal aorta: Preliminary communication with report of 3 cases. *Angiology.* 1951;2:579–587.

64. Wylie EJ Jr., Kerr E, Davies O. Experimental and clinical experiences with the use of fascia lata applied as a graft about major arteries after thromboendarterectomy and aneurysmorrhaphy. *Surg Gynecol Obstet.* 1951;93:257–272.

65. Wylie EJ. Thromboendarterectomy for arteriosclerotic thrombosis of major arteries. *Surgery.* 1952;32:275–292.

66. DeBakey ME, Cooley DA, Crawford ES, Morris CG Jr. Clinical application of a new flexible knitted dacron arterial substitute. *Arch Surg.* 1957;74:713–724.

67. Edwards WS, Tapp S. Chemically treated nylon tubes as arterial grafts. *Surgery.* 1955;38:61–70.

68. Julian OC, Deterling RA, Dye WS, Bhonslay S, Grove WJ, Belio ML, Javid H. Dacron tube and bifurcation prosthesis produced to specification: II. Continued clinical use and the addition of microcrimping. *Arch Surg.* 1957;78:260–270.

69. Sauvage LR, Berger K, Wood SJ, Nakagawa Y, Mansfield PB. An external velour surface for porous arterial prostheses. *Surgery.* 1971;70:940–953.

70. Szilagyi DE, France LC, Smith RF, Whitcomb JG. Clinical use of an elastic dacron prosthesis. *Arch Surg.* 1958;77:538–551.

71. Voorhees AB Jr. The development of arterial prostheses: A personal view. *Arch Surg.* 1985;120:289–295.

72. Voorhees AB Jr., Jaretzki A, Blakemore AH. The use of tubes constructed from vinyon "N" cloth in bridging arterial defects: A preliminary report. *Ann Surg.* 1952;135:332–336.

73. Wesolowski SA, Dennis CA, eds. *Fundamentals of Vascular Grafting.* New York: McGraw-Hill, 1963.

74. Oudot J. Un Deuxiemecas de Greffe de la Bifurcation Aortque Pour Thrombose da la Fourche Aortique. Mem. *Acad Chir.* 1951;77:644–645.

75. Freeman NE, Leeds FH. Operations on large arteries: Application of recent advances. *Calif Med.* 1952;77:229–233.

76. Mccaughan JJ Jr., Kahn SF. Cross-over graft for unilateral occlusive disease of the iliofemoral arteries. *Ann Surg.* 1960;151:26–28.

77. Yetto RM. The treatment of unilateral iliac artery obstruction with a trans-abdominal subcutaneous femorofemoral graft. *Surgery.* 1962;52:342–345.

78. Blaisdell FW, Hall AD. Axillary-femoral artery bypass for lower extremity ischemia. *Surgery.* 1963;54:563–568.

79. Sauvage LR, Wood SJ. Unilateral axillary bilateral femoral bifurcation graft: A procedure for the poor risk patient with aortoiliac disease. *Surgery.* 1966;60:573–577.

80. Guida PM, Moore SW. Obturator bypass technique. *Surg Gynecol Obstet.* 1969;128:1307–1316.

81. Dotter CT, Judkins MP. Transluminal treatment of arteriosclerotic obstruction: Description of a new technique and a preliminary report of its application. *Circulation.* 1964;30:654–670.

82. Gruentzig AR, Hopff H. Perkutaner Rekanalisation Chronischer Arterieller Verschluss mit Einem Neuen Dilatations Katheter. *Dtsch Med Wschr.* 1974;99:2502.

83. Palmaz JC, Tio FC, Schatz RA, Alvarado R, Res C, Garcia O. Early endothelialization of balloon-expandable stents: Experimental observations. *J Intervent Radiol.* 1998;3:119–124.

84. Palmaz JC, Richter G, Noeldge G et al. Intraluminal stenting of atherosclerotic iliac artery stenosis: Preliminary report of a multicenter study. *Radiology*. 1998;168:727–731.

85. Kunlin J. Le Traitement de L'ischemie Arteritique par la Greffe Veineuse Longue. *Rev Chir*. 1951;70:206.

86. Palma EC. The treatment of arteritis of the lower limbs by autogenous vein grafts. *Minerva Cardioangiol Eur*. 1960;8:36–49.

87. Hall KV. The great saphenous vein used in situ as an in arterial shunt after extirpation of the vein valves. *Surgery*. 1962;51:492–495.

88. Leather RP, Powers SR Jr., Karmody AM. The reappraisal of the in situ saphenous vein arterial bypass: Its use in limb salvage. *Surgery*. 1979;86:453–461.

89. Dardik H, Miller N, Dardik A, Ibrahim IM, Sussman B, Silvia M, Berry M, Wolodiger F, Kahn M, Dardik I. A decade of experience with the glutaraldehyde-tanned human umbilical cord vein graft for revascularization of the lower limb. *J Vasc Surg*. 1988;7:336–346.

90. Bergan JJ, Veith FJ, Bernhard VM, Yao JST, Flinn WR, Gupta SK, Scher LA, Samson RH, Towne JB. Randomization of autogenous vein and polytetrafluoroethylene grafts in femoral distal reconstruction. *Surgery*. 1982;92:921–930.

91. Veith FJ, Gupta SK, Ascer E, White-Flores S, Samson RH, Scher LA, Towne JB, Bernhard JJ. Six-year prospective multicenter randomized comparison of autologous saphenous vein and expanded polytetrafluoroethylene grafts in infrainguinal arterial reconstructions. *J Vasc Surg*. 1986;3:104–114.

92. Martin P, Renwick S, Stephenson C. On the surgery of the profunda femoris artery. *Br J Surg*. 1971;55:539–542.

93. Bolia A, Brennan J, Bell PR. Recanalization of femoro-popliteal occlusions: Improving success rate by subintimal recanalization. *Clin Radiol*. 1989;40:325.

94. Simpson JB, Johnson DE, Thapliyal HV, Marks DS, Braden LJ. Transluminal atherectomy: A new approach to the treatment of atherosclerotic vascular disease. *Circulation*. 1985;72(Suppl. 2):111–146.

95. Dotter CT. Transluminally-placed coilspring endarterial tube grafts: Long-term patency in canine popliteal artery. *Invest Radiol*. 1969;4:327–332.

96. Maass D, Kropf L, Egloff L, Demierre D, Turina M, Senning A. Transluminal implantation of intravascular "double helix" spiral prostheses: Technical and biological considerations. *ESAO Proc*. 1982;9:252–256.

97. Rabkin JK. New types of technology in roentgenosurgery. IX. All-Unions Konress-Uber Frotschritte in der Roentgen-Chirurgie. Moskau, Russia, 1989.

98. Fogarty TJ, Cranley JJ, Krause RJ, Strasser ES, Hafner CD. A method for extraction of arterial emboli and thrombi. *Surg Gynecol Obstet*. 1963;116:241–244.

99. Dubost C, Allary M, Oeconomos N. Resection of an aneurysm of the abdominal aorta: Reestablishment of the continuity by preserved human arterial graft, with results after six months. *Arch Surg*. 1952;64:405–408.

100. DeBakey ME, Cooley DA. Successful resection of aneurysm of thoracic aorta and replacement by graft. *J Am MedAssoc*. 1953;152:673–676.

101. Blakemore AH, Voorhees AB Jr. The use of tubes constructed from vinyon "N" cloth in bridging arterial defects experimental and clinical. *Ann Surg*. 1954;140:324–334.

102. Crawford ES. Thoracoabdominal aortic aneurysms involving renal, superior mesenteric and celiac arteries. *Ann Surg*. 1974;179:763–772.

103. Volodos NL, Karpovich IP, Shekhanin VE, Troian VI, Iakovenko LF. A case of distant transfemoral endoprosthesis of the thoracic artery using a self-fixing synthetic prosthesis in traumatic aneurysm. *Grudn Khir*. 1988;6:84–86.

104. Parodi J, Palrnaz JC, Barone HD. Transfemoral intraluminal graft implantation for abdominal aortic aneurysms. *Ann Vasc Surg*. 1991;5:491–499.

105. Yusuf SW, Whitaker SC, Chuter TAM, Wenham PW, Hopkinson BR. Emergency endovascular repair of leaking aortic aneurysm (letter). *Lancet*. 1994;344:1645.

106. Chuter TAM. Transfemoral aneurysm repair (DM Thesis). Nottingham, UK: University of Nottingham, 1994.

107. Scott RAP, Chuter TAM. Clinical endovascular placement of bifurcated graft in abdominal aortic aneurysm without laparotomy. *Lancet* 1994;343:413.

108. Dake MD, Miller DC, Semba CP, Mitchell RS, Walker PJ, Liddell RP. Transluminal placement of endovascular stent-grafts for the treatment of descending thoracic aortic aneurysms. *N Engl J Med*. 1994;331:1729–1734.

109. Diwan A, Sarkar R, Stanley JC, Zelenock GB, Zelenock GB, Wakefield TW. Incidence of femoral and popliteal artery aneurysms in patients with abdominal aortic aneurysms. *J Vasc Surg*. 2000;31:863–869.

110. Graham LM, Zelenock GB, Whitehouse WM Jr., Erlandson EE, Dent TL, Lindenauer SM, Stanley JC. Clinical significance of arteriosclerotic femoral artery aneurysms. *Arch Surg*. 1980;115:502–507.

111. Whitehouse WM Jr., Wakefield TW, Graham LM, Kazmers A, Zelenock GB, Cronenwett JL. Limb threatening potential of arteriosclerotic popliteal artery aneurysms. *Surgery*. 1983;93:694–699.

112. Marin ML, Veith FJ, Panetta TF, Cynamon J, Bakal CW, Suggs WD, Wengerter KR, Barone HD, Schonholz C, Parodi JC. Transfemoral endoluminal stented graft repair of a popliteal artery aneurysm. *J Vasc Surg*. 1994;19:754–757.

113. Freeman NE, Leeds FH, Elliot WG, Roland SI. Thromboendarterectomy for hypertension due to renal artery occlusion. *J Am Med Assoc.* 1954;156:1077–1079.

114. Wylie WJ, Perloff DL, Stoney RJ. Autogenous tissue revascularization techniques in surgery for renovascular hypertension. *Ann Surg.* 1969;170:416–428.

115. Stanley JC. Surgical treatment of renovascular hypertension. *Am J Surg.* 1997;174:102–110.

116. Stoney RJ, DeLuccia N, Ehrenfeld WK, Wylie WK. Aortorenal arterial autografts: Long-term assessment. *Arch Surg.* 1981;116:416–422.

117. DeCamp PT, Snyder GH, Bost RB. Severe hypertension due to congenital stenosis of artery to solitary kidney: Correction by splenorenal arterial anastomosis. *Arch Surg.* 1957;75:1023–1026.

118. Bookstein JJ, Abrams HD, Buenger RE, Reiss MD, Lecky JW, Franklin SS, Bleifer KH, Varady PD, Maxwell MH. Radiologic aspects of renovascular hypertension. Part 2. The role of urography in unilateral renovascular disease. *J Am Med Assoc.* 1972;220:1225–1230.

119. Bookstein JJ, Abrams HL, Buenger RE, Reiss MD, Lecky JW, Franklin SS, Bleifer KH, Varady PD, Maxwell MH. Radiologic aspects of renovascular hypertension. Part 3. Appraisal of arteriography. *J Am Med Assoc.* 1972;221:368–374.

120. Bookstein JJ, Maxwell MH, Abrahams HL, Buenger RE, Lecky J, Franklin SS. Cooperative study of radiologic aspects of renovascular hypertension: Bilateral renovascular disease. *J Am Med Assoc.* 1977;237:1706–1709.

121. Foster JH, Maxwell SS, Bleifer KH, Trippel OH, Julian OC, DeCamp PT, Varady PD. Renovascular occlusive disease: Results of operative treatment. *J Am Med Assoc.* 1975;231:1043–1048.

122. Franklin SS, Young JD, Maxwell MH, Foster JH, Palmer JM, Cerny J, Varady PD. Operative morbidity and mortality in renovascular disease. *J Am Med Assoc.* 1975;231:1148–1153.

123. Foster JH, Dean RH, Pinkerton JA, Rhamy RL. Ten years experience with surgical management of renovascular hypertension. *Ann Surg.* 1973;177:755–766.

124. Ernst CB, Stanley JC, Marshall FF, Fry WJ. Autogenous saphenous vein aortorenal grafts: A ten-year experience. *Arch Surg.* 1972;105:855–864.

125. Harrison EG Jr., McCormack LJ. Pathology classification of renal arterial disease in renovascular hypertension. *Mayo Clin Proc.* 1971;46:161–167.

126. Stanley JC, Gewertz BL, Bove EL, Sottiurai V, Fry WJ. Arterial fibrodysplasia: Histopathologic character and current etiologic concepts. *Arch Surg.* 1975;110:551–556.

127. Gruntzig A, Kuhlmann U, Vetter W, Lutolf U, Meier B, Siegenthaler W. Treatment of renovascular hypertension with percutaneous transluminal dilatation of a renal-artery stenosis. *Lancet.* 1978;1:801–802.

128. Cooper CJ, Murphy TP, Cutlip DE, Jamerson K, Henrich W, Reid DM, Cohen DJ, for the CORAL Investigators. Stenting and medical therapy for atherosclerotic renal-artery stenosis. *N Engl J Med.* 2014;370:13–22.

129. Klass J. Embolectomy in acute mesenteric occlusion. *Ann Surg.* 1951;134:913–917.

130. Shaw RS, Maynard EP. Acute and chronic thrombosis of the mesenteric arteries associated with malabsorption: Report of two successful cases treated by thromboendarterectomy. *N Engl J Med.* 1958;258:874–878.

131. Mikkelsen WP, Zaro JA. Intestinal angina: Report of a case with preoperative diagnosis and surgical relief. *N Engl J Med.* 1959;260:912–914.

132. Furrer J, Gruntzig A, Kugelmeier J, Goebel N. Treatment of abdominal angina with percutaneous dilatation of an arteria mesenterica superior stenosis. *Cardiovasc Intervent Radiol.* 1980;3:43–44.

133. Deterling RA. Aneurysm of the visceral arteries. *J Cardiovasc Surg.* 1971;12:309–322.

134. Stanley JC, Thompson NW, Fry WJ. Splanchnic artery aneurysms. *Arch Surg.* 1970;101:689–697.

135. Fisher M. Occlusion of the internal carotid artery. *Arch Neurol Psychiatry.* 1951;65:346–377.

136. Carrea R, Molins M, Murphy G. Surgical treatment of spontaneous thrombosis of the internal carotid artery in the neck: Carotid-carotideal anastomosis: Report of a case. *Acta Neurol Latinoamer.* 1955;I:71–78.

137. Eastcott HHG, Pickering GW, Rob CG. Reconstruction of internal carotid artery in a patient with intermittent attacks of hemiplegia. *Lancet.* 1954;2:994–996.

138. DeBakey ME. Successful carotid endarterectomy for cerebrovascular insufficiency: nineteen year follow-up. *J Am Med Assoc.* 1975;233:1083–1085.

139. Davis JB, Grove WJ, Julian OC. Thrombotic occlusion of the branches of the aortic arch, Martorell's syndrome: Report of a case treated surgically. *Ann Surg.* 1956;144:124–126.

140. Crawford ES, DeBakey ME, Fields WS. Roentgenographic diagnosis and surgical treatment of basilar artery insufficiency. *J Am Med Assoc.* 1958;168:514.

141. Lyons C, Galbraith G. Surgical treatment of atherosclerotic occlusion of the internal carotid artery. *Ann Surg.* 1957;146:487–498.

142. DeBakey ME, Morris GC, Jordan GL, Cooley DA. Segmental thrombo-obliterative disease on branches of aortic arch. *J Am Med Assoc.* 1958;166:998–1003.

143. Yasargil MC, Krayenbuhl HA, Jacobson JH II. Microneurosurgical arterial reconstruction. *Surgery.* 1970;67:221–233.

144. Extracranial intracranial Bypass Study Group. Failure of extracranial-intracranial anterior bypass to reduce the risk of ischemic stroke. *N Engl J Med.* 1985;313:1191–1200.

145. North American Symptomatic Carotid Endarterectomy Trial Collaborators. Beneficial effect of carotid endarterectomy in symptomatic patients with high-grade carotid stenosis. *N Engl J Med.* 1991;325:325–453.

146. Barnett HJ, Taylor DW, Eliasziw M et al. Benefit of carotid endarterectomy in patients with symptomatic moderate or severe stenosis. *N Engl J Med.* 1998;339:1415–1425.

147. European Carotid Surgery Trialists' Collaborative Group. MRC European carotid surgery trial: Interim results for symptomatic patients with severe (70–99%) or with mild (0–29%) carotid stenosis. *Lancet.* 1991;337:1235–1243.

148. The Veterans Affairs Cooperative Studies Program 309 Trialist Group, Mayberg MR, Wilson SF, Yatsu F, Weiss DG, Messina L, Hershey LA. Carotid endarterectomy and prevention of cerebral ischemia in symptomatic carotid stenosis. *J Am Med Assoc.* 1991;266:3259–3295.

149. Executive Committee for the Asymptomatic Carotid Atherosclerosis Study. Endarterectomy for asymptomatic carotid artery stenosis. *J Am Med Assoc.* 1995;273:1421–1428.

150. The Veterans Affairs Cooperative Study Group, Hobson RW II, Weiss DG, Fields WS, Goldstone J, Moore WS, Towne JB, Wright CB. Efficacy of carotid endarterectomy for asymptomatic carotid stenosis. *N Engl J Med.* 1993;328:221–227.

151. Mathias K. A new catheter system for percutaneous transluminal angioplasty (PTA) of carotid artery stenoses. *Fortschr Med.* 1977;95:1007–1011.

152. Yadav JS, Wholey MH, Kuntz RE et al. Protected carotid-artery stenting versus endarterectomy in high-risk patients. *N Engl J Med.* 2004;351:1493–1501.

153. Gurm HS, Yadav JS, Fayad P et al. Long-term results of carotid stenting versus endarterectomy in high-risk patients. *N Engl J Med.* 2008;358:1572–1579.

154. Bachman DM, Kim RM. Transluminal dilatation for subclavian steal syndrome. *Am J Roentgenol.* 1980;135:995–996.

155. Mathias K, Staiger J, Thron A, Spillner G, Heiss HW, Konrad-Graf S. Percutaneous transluminal dilation of the subclavian artery. *Dtsch Med Wochenschr.* 1980;105:16–18.

156. DeWeese MS, Hunter DC Jr. A vena cava filter for the prevention of pulmonary emboli. *Bull Soc Int Chir.* 1958;1:1–19.

157. DeWeese MS, Kraft RO, Nichols KW. Fifteen-year clinical experience with vena cava filter. *Ann Surg.* 1973;173:247–257.

158. Mobin-Uddin K, Smith PE, Martinez LD, Lombardo CR, Jude JR. A vena cava filter for the prevention of pulmonary embolus. *Surg Forum.* 1967;18:209–211.

159. Mobin-Uddi K, McLean R, Bolooki H et al. Caval interruption for prevention of pulmonary embolism: Long-term results of a new method. *Arch Surg.* 1969;99:711–715.

160. Greenfield LJ, Peyton MD, Brown PP, Elkins RC. Transvenous management of pulmonary embolic disease. *Ann Surg.* 1974;180:461–468.

161. Kunlin J. The reestablishment of venous circulation with grafts in cases of obliteration from trauma or thrombophlebitis. *Mem Acad Clin.* 1953;79:109.

162. Palma EC, Esperon R. Vein transplants and grafts in the surgical treatment of the post phlebitis syndrome. *J Cardiovasc Surg.* 1960;1:94–107.

163. Husni EA. In situ saphenopopliteal bypass graft for incompetence of the femoral and popliteal veins. *Surg Gynecol. Obstet.* 1970;2:279–284.

164. Charnsangavej C, Carrasco CH, Wallace S, Wright KC, Oyawa K, Richli W, Gianturco C. Stenosis of the vena cava: preliminary assessment of treatment with expandable metallic stents. *Radiology.* 1986;161:295–298.

165. Kistner R. Surgical repair of a venous valve. *Straub Clin Proc.* 1968;34:41–43.

166. Kistner R. Surgical repair of the incompetent femoral vein valve. *Arch Surg.* 1975;110:1336–1342.

167. Taheri SA, Lazar L, Elias S, Marchand P, Heffner R. Surgical treatment of postphlebitic syndrome with vein valve transplant. *Am J Surg.* 1982;144:221–224.

168. Hauer G. The endoscopic subfascial division of the perforating veins-preliminary report. *Vasa.* 1985;14:59–61.

169. Orbach EJ. Sclerotherapy of varicose veins-utilization of an intravenous air block. *Am J Surg.* 1944;66:362–366.

170. Politowski M, Zelazny T. Complications and difficulties associated with electrocoagulation treatment of varices of lower extremities. *Pol Przegl Chir.* 1966;38:519–522.

171. Bone C. Tratamiento Endoluminal de las Varices con Laser de Diodo: Studio preliminary. *Rev Patol Vasc.* 1999;5:35–46.

2

Pathophysiology of human atherosclerosis

CHRISTOPHER K. ZARINS and CHENGPEI XU

CONTENTS

Atherosclerosis is a degenerative process of the major human elastic and muscular arteries. It is characterized by the formation of intimal plaques consisting of lipid accumulations, smooth-muscle and inflammatory cells, connective tissue fibres and calcium deposits. Morbidity associated with atherosclerosis arises from plaque enlargement or degeneration. Plaque enlargement may obstruct the lumen, resulting in stenosis and impairment of blood flow. Sudden obstruction of the lumen may result from the dissection of blood from the lumen into or under the plaque or hemorrhage within the plaque from vasa vasorum. Plaque ulceration may result in embolization of plaque elements or thrombus formation on the disrupted intima. Thrombosis may also occlude atherosclerotic vessels without obvious plaque disruption due to local modifications of flow. Finally, atrophy of the media, often associated with atherosclerotic disease, may result in weakening of the artery wall with aneurysmal dilatation, mural thrombosis and rupture.

Atherosclerosis is a generalized disorder of the arterial tree associated with a number of recognized predisposing risk factors, including altered serum lipid and lipoprotein profiles, hypertension, cigarette smoking, diabetes mellitus and lifestyle. However, the clinical expression of atherosclerosis tends to be focal, with clinical symptoms caused by localized interference with circulation occurring in several critical sites. In addition, the morphologic features underlying morbidity and mortality vary somewhat depending on location. In the coronary arteries, for example, stenosis and thrombosis tend to reduce flow or cause sudden catastrophic occlusion, principally at the site of lesion formation, while at the carotid bifurcation, plaque ulceration and thrombosis often cause characteristic symptoms by embolization to distal cerebral vessels. Extensive disease, often with multiple focal occlusive stenoses, is characteristic of peripheral vascular disease of the lower extremities, while aneurysm formation is a major feature of abdominal aortic disease. While there is a large body of descriptive clinical and experimental knowledge with regard to the general appearance of atherosclerotic lesions, the precise initiating and perpetuating pathogenic mechanisms in human beings remain obscure, and the factors which determine human lesion composition, rate of lesion enlargement, lesion organization and lesion disruption remain to be elucidated.

In this chapter, we discuss both the structural features of the artery wall and the hemodynamic factors which may relate to the pathogenesis, localization and disruption of plaques, and we review the principal features of human lesion composition and configuration. These considerations should help to provide insight into the clinical consequences of differences in plaque localization and composition and serve as a basis for the critical evaluation of currently available methods for the quantitative assessment of human lesions.

STRUCTURE OF THE ARTERY WALL

The artery wall consists of three concentric layers or zones. From the lumen outward, these are the intima, the media and the adventitia (Figure 2.1).

Intima

The intima extends from the luminal endothelial lining to the internal elastic lamina. The endothelium is formed by a continuous monolayer of flat, usually elongated polygonal cells, which tend to be aligned in the direction of blood flow. In areas of slow, reversing or nonlaminar flow, endothelial cells tend to assume a less clearly oriented configuration.[1] Edges of adjacent endothelial cells overlap, with the downstream edges of most endothelial cells overriding

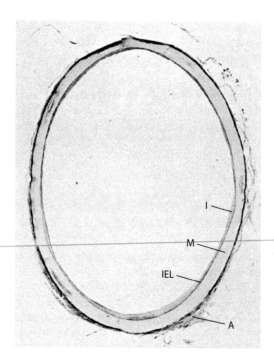

Figure 2.1 Transverse section of a normal human superficial femoral artery. Note intima (I), media (M) and adventitia (A). The intima and media are separated by the internal elastic lamella (IEL).

their immediate downstream neighbours much like the shingles on a roof. Cytoplasmic bridges, surface ridges and microvillus projections as well as interendothelial gaps, stomata or open junctions between endothelial cells have been described. These features are, however, largely absent from vessels which have been fixed while distended and which have not been manipulated prior to fixation.[2] A protein coating, the glycocalyx, overlies the luminal surface. Immediately beneath the endothelium is a closely associated fibrillar layer, the basal lamina. This structure is thought to form a continuous bond between the endothelial cells and the subendothelial connective tissue matrix. Numerous focal attachments are also present between endothelial cells and the underlying internal elastic lamina,[3] while less prominent focal attachments are also formed with other fibres in the intima. The extensive basal lamina provides a supple, pliable junction well adapted to permit bending and changes in diameter or configuration associated with pulse pressure without disruption or detachment of the endothelium. The focal, tight, relatively rigid junctions may prevent downstream slippage or telescoping, which could result from the shear stresses imposed by blood flow. Between the basal lamina and the internal elastic lamina, the intima in most locations normally contains a few scattered macrophages, smooth-muscle cells and connective tissue fibres.

Since the endothelial cell layer is the immediate interface between the bloodstream and the underlying artery wall, it is subjected to normal forces exerted by blood pressure and to shearing or drag forces resulting from blood flow. Experimentally, imposed shearing stresses in excess of 400 dyn/cm^2 in canine aortas have resulted in morphologic evidence of endothelial injury or disruption and in increased endothelial permeability.[4] Other observations have failed to reveal evidence of endothelial injury in areas normally subjected to comparable or higher levels of shear stress,[5] suggesting that endothelial cells may withstand relatively high shearing stresses without ill effect in some locations (Figure 2.2).

Endothelial cells exposed to continuous high-flow conditions, such as in arteries supplying an arteriovenous fistula, are activated, whereas the endothelial cells in arteries with decreased flow are inactivated. Endothelial activation is characterized by lumen protrusions, increase of cytoplasmic organelles, abluminal protrusions, basement membrane degradation, internal elastic lamina degradation and sproutings in the capillaries. These are ultrastructurally comparable to angiogenesis. Endothelial inactivation is characterized by the decrease of endothelial cell number with apoptosis, which is ultrastructurally comparable to angioregression.[6,11]

The endothelial layer has been considered to function as a thrombosis-resistant surface as well as a selective interface for diffusion, convection and active transport of circulating substances into the underlying artery wall. Endothelial cells play a critical role in the physiology and pathophysiology of vascular disorders.[7] They respond

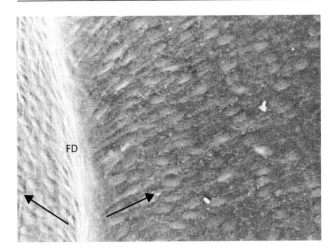

Figure 2.2 Scanning electron micrograph of a monkey aortic ostial flow divider (FD). The FD is an area subjected to high shear stress. The endothelial cells are intact and elongated in the direction of flow with no disruption. Arrows indicate direction of blood flow.

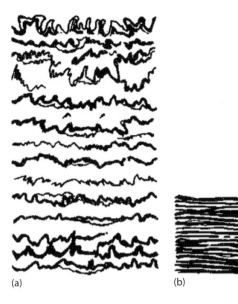

(a) (b)

Figure 2.3 Tracing of elastic fibres in transverse sections of rabbit aortic media. (a) A transverse section of a collapsed aorta demonstrating wavy elastic lamellae and increased thickness of each lamellar unit and increased total thickness of the media. (b) A rabbit aorta fixed while distended. Note the straight elastic fibres and thickness of the media.

to hemodynamic stresses and may transduce an atheroprotective force[8] by regulating the ingress, egress and metabolism of lipoproteins and other agents that may participate in intimal plaque initiation and progression.[9,10] Endothelial cells have been shown to participate in an array of metabolic and biosynthetic functions related to thrombosis, prostaglandin formation and smooth-muscle contraction.[11] Detachment of endothelial cells with persistence of the basal lamina does not necessarily result in occlusive thrombus formation. Although a layer of thrombocytes appears to deposit on the denuded basal lamina, large aggregates and fibrin deposits may require the exposure of collagen fibres and other deeper mural components.[12]

Media

The media extends from the internal elastic lamina to the adventitia. Although an external elastic lamina demarcates the boundary between media and adventitia in many vessels, a distinct external elastic lamina may not be present, particularly in vessels with a thick and fibrous adventitial layer. The outer limit of the media can nevertheless be distinguished in nearly all intact arteries, for in contrast to the adventitia, the media consists of closely packed layers of smooth-muscle cells in close association with elastin and collagen fibres. Elastic fibres of the media are predominantly wavy or undulating on cross sections of collapsed arteries but appear as relatively straight bands or lamellae in fully distended vessels (Figure 2.3). The smooth-muscle cell layers are composed of groups of similarly oriented cells, each surrounded by a common basal lamina and a closely associated interlacing basketwork of

collagen fibrils, which tighten about the cell groups as the media is brought under tension.[13] This configuration tends to hold the groups of cells together and prevents excessive stretching or slippage. In addition, each cellular subgroup or fascicle is encompassed by a system of similarly oriented elastic fibres. Focal tight attachment sites between smooth-muscle cells and elastic fibres are normally abundant. In the aorta, the juxtaposition of similarly oriented musculoelastic fascicles results in the appearance on transverse sections of layers of continuous elastic lamellae and intervening smooth-muscle layers. In addition to the pericellular network of fine collagen fibrils, thicker, crimped collagen bundles weave between adjacent lamellae. The elastic fibres are relatively extensible and allow for some degree of compliance; they recoil during the cardiac cycle and tend to distribute mural tensile stresses uniformly. The thick collagen fibre bundles provide much of the tensile strength of the media and, because of their high elastic modules, limit distension and prevent disruption (Figure 2.4).

The aortic elastin lamella and its corresponding smooth-muscle layer has been termed a lamellar unit. With increasing mammalian species size, the adult aortic radius increases, with a corresponding increase in medial thickness and in the number of transmural lamellar units (Figure 2.5).[14] The total tangential tension exerted on the wall is closely approximated by the product of the distending pressure and the radius (law of Laplace). Since aortic pressure is similar for most adult mammals and individual medial layers tend to be of similar thickness regardless of

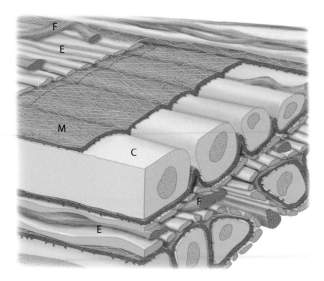

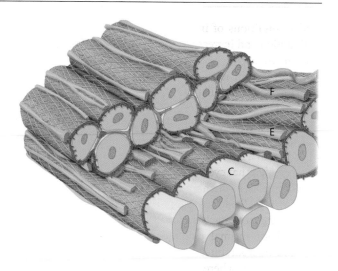

Figure 2.4 Diagrammatic representation of the microarchitecture of the media of the aortic wall. The long axes of the smooth-muscle cells (C) are oriented circumferentially or perpendicular to the long axis of the artery. Each cell is surrounded by a matrix (M) consisting of basal lamina and a fine meshwork of collagen fibrils. Groups or layers of smooth-muscle cells are surrounded by circumferentially oriented elastic fibres (E), which appear as almost continuous sheets on transverse section of the artery. Wavy collagen bundles (F) course between the successive facing elastic fibre layers. (Adapted from Clark JM and Glagov S, *Arteriosclerosis*, 5, 19, 1985. With permission.)

Figure 2.6 Diagrammatic representation of microarchitecture of the wall of a muscular artery. The long axes of the smooth-muscle cells (C) of the media are oriented circumferentially or perpendicular to the long axis of the artery. Cells are surrounded by a matrix of basal lamina and collagen fibrils. Elastin fibre systems (E) are less prominent. Collagen bundles (F) are interspersed. Compared to elastic arteries (see Figure 2.4), muscular arteries have a greater number of smooth-muscle cells and relatively fewer collagen and elastin fibres. (Adapted from Clark JM and Glagov S, *Arteriosclerosis*, 5, 19, 1985. With permission.)

species, there is a very nearly linear relationship between adult aortic radius and the number of medial fibrocellular lamellar units. On the average, the tangential tension per aortic lamellar unit is close to 2000 dyn/cm.

Smaller *muscular arteries* contain relatively less collagen and elastin and more smooth-muscle cells than the aorta and the proximal, larger elastic arteries. The musculoelastic fascicles, which are very prominent in elastic arteries, are also present in muscular arteries and are generally aligned in the direction of the tensile forces (Figure 2.6). However, because of the preponderance of smooth-muscle cells, they are less clearly demarcated and the layering of the media is less distinct.[15] Medial thickness and the number of layers is nevertheless closely related to the radius, and the average tension per layer tends to be constant for homologous vessels in mammals.[16] In addition, the relative proportion of collagen and elastin varies between muscular and elastic arteries. The media of the proximal aorta and that of the major brachiocephalic elastic arteries contain a larger proportion of elastin and a lower proportion of collagen than the abdominal aorta or the distal peripheral vessels.[17] The proximal major vessels are therefore more compliant than the abdominal aorta but also are more friable and prone to tear with suturing.

Medial smooth-muscle cells, in addition to synthesizing the collagen and elastin fibres, which determine the mechanical properties of the aortic wall, are actively engaged in metabolic processes that contribute to wall tone and may be related to susceptibility to plaque formation.[18]

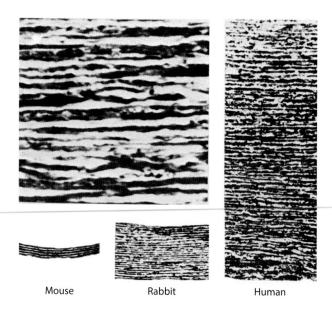

Mouse   Rabbit   Human

Figure 2.5 Aortic lamellar architecture in three mammals. With increasing species size, the aortic radius increases. There is a corresponding increase in medial thickness due to an increase in the number of medial lamellar units. (A) Higher-power view of transverse section of media demonstrating lamellar architecture.

Under conditions of increased pulse pressure, increased wall motion and increased wall tension, which exist proximal to an aortic coarctation, medical smooth-muscle cell metabolism is increased, as is plaque formation.[19] Conversely, when wall motion, pulse pressure and smooth-muscle cell metabolism are decreased, as in areas distal to a severe arterial stenosis, intimal plaque formation is inhibited, despite the continued presence of strong atherogenic stimuli such as marked hyperlipidemia.[20] In vitro studies have revealed that cyclic stretching of smooth-muscle cells grown on elastin membranes results in increased biosynthetic activity,[21] and acute arterial injury experiments have revealed that an intact, metabolically active media may be required for intimal plaque formation.[22] The composition and microarchitecture of the media are designed to ensure stability, whereas the metabolic state of the media appears to be an important factor in the pathogenesis of atherosclerotic lesions.

Adventitia

Although the boundary between media and adventitia is usually distinct, even in the absence of a well-defined external elastic lamina, the outer limit of the adventitia may be difficult to identify, for it is often continuous with the surrounding perivascular connective tissues. Although the aorta and pulmonary trunk are normally invested by relatively little adventitial fibrous connective tissue and are closely associated with mediastinal or retroperitoneal adipose tissue and lymph nodes, the adventitia of some of the major arteries, such as the renal and mesenteric branches, are composed of prominent layers of elastic and collagen fibres and may be thicker than the associated media. Compared to the media, cells in the adventitia are relatively sparse and most are fibroblasts. For the normal aorta, removal of the adventitia has little effect on static pressure–volume relationships. In muscular arteries, however, where connective tissue fibres are relatively sparse in the media and smooth-muscle contraction may regulate vessel diameter and play a role in maintaining circumferential tensile support, a thick, structured adventitia may serve to provide significant tethering and axial tensile support, prevent excessive dilatation and dampen the cyclic changes in tangential tension associated with the pulse pressure wave. In instances where a large, intimal atherosclerotic plaque overlies an atrophic media, a thickened adventitia may be the principal mural structural component of the artery wall (see Figure 2.7). During carotid or femoral endarterectomy, the entire intima and extensive portions of remaining media may be removed, leaving only the adventitia to provide support.

The adventitia is also the primary source of vasa vasorum and may play a prominent role in arteritis and periaortitis[23] as well as in the inflammatory component of atherosclerosis.[24] Adventitial responses may also be important in the artery wall response to balloon injury and angioplasty.[25,26]

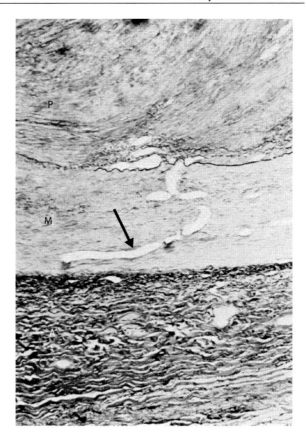

Figure 2.7 Transverse section of superficial femoral artery. Note the prominent adventitial (A) thickening and vasa vasorum (arrow) penetrating through media (M) into plaque (P).

ARTERY WALL NUTRITION

The adventitia of all of the major elastic and muscular arteries contains vasa vasorum – i.e., small arteries, arterioles, capillaries and venous channels – which are presumed to participate in the nutrition of the artery wall. Except for the aorta, however, precise relationships among vasa supply, vessel location, diameter, wall thickness and architecture have not been established. The aortic media is nourished directly from the lumen and may also be perfused by means of vasa vasorum from the adventitial side. Passage through the lining endothelium is apparently sufficient to nourish the inner 0.5 mm of the adult mammalian aortic media, which corresponds to approximately 30 medial fibrocellular layers.[27] Thus, the aortic media of a small mammal such as the rat or rabbit, which is less than 0.5 mm thick and has fewer than 30 medial lamellar layers, contains no medial vasa vasorum and is nourished largely from the intimal side. Large mammals such as pigs, sheep and horses have an aortic media with more than 30 medial lamellar layers. The inner 30 aortic layers in such species are avascular, but the remaining outer medial lamellar units contain vasa vasorum (Figure 2.8). Aortic vasa vasorum arise from major arterial branches close to their origins and usually enter the media at right angles. Within the media, the vasa tend to be oriented axially in

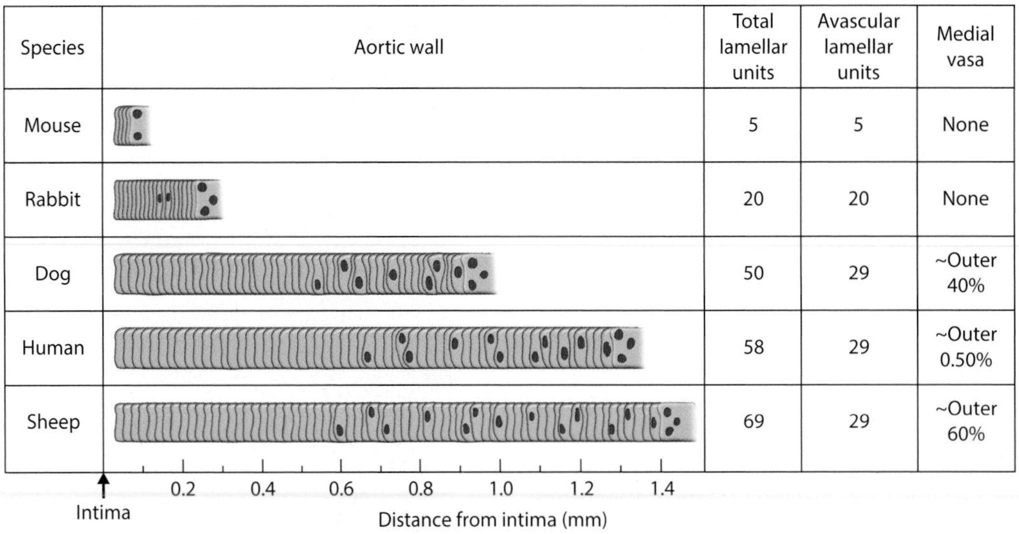

Species	Aortic wall	Total lamellar units	Avascular lamellar units	Medial vasa
Mouse		5	5	None
Rabbit		20	20	None
Dog		50	29	~Outer 40%
Human		58	29	~Outer 0.50%
Sheep		69	29	~Outer 60%

Intima   0.2   0.4   0.6   0.8   1.0   1.2   1.4

Distance from intima (mm)

Figure 2.8 Relationship between aortic medial lamellar architecture and vasa vasorum blood supply to outer portion of the media in different species. (Reproduced from Glagov S, Hemodynamic risk factors: Mechanical stress, mural architecture, medial nutrition and the vulnerability of arteries to atherosclerosis, in: Wissler RW and Geer JC, eds., *The Pathogenesis of Atherosclerosis*, Williams & Wilkins, Baltimore, MD, 1972, pp. 166–199. With permission.)

several branching levels. The average tension per medial lamellar unit for aortas that contain medial vasa tends to be somewhat higher than for aortas without vasa, suggesting that the presence of nutritive vessels within the media permits each lamellar unit to function at a somewhat higher level of tensile stress. The human abdominal aorta appears to be exceptional when compared to aortas of other mammals, since it is more than 0.5 mm thick but contains fewer than 30 layers.[28] It is not furnished with

medial vasa vasorum, although the estimated tensile stress per layer is in the range of those aortas with medial vasa (Figure 2.9). The implication of this situation with respect to atherosclerosis and aneurysm formation is discussed in the following text. Although mural stresses and deformations associated with hypertension may impair medial vasal flow,[29] the details of aortic media microarchitecture, which permit intramural vasa vasorum to remain open under normal conditions despite the cyclic

Comparison of human thoracic and abdominal aorta

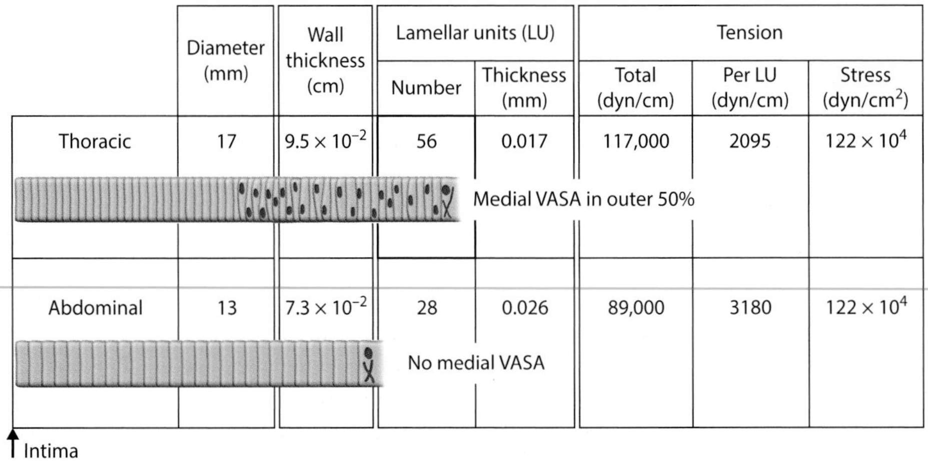

	Diameter (mm)	Wall thickness (cm)	Lamellar units (LU)		Tension		
			Number	Thickness (mm)	Total (dyn/cm)	Per LU (dyn/cm)	Stress (dyn/cm^2)
Thoracic	17	9.5×10^{-2}	56	0.017	117,000	2095	122×10^4
				Medial VASA in outer 50%			
Abdominal	13	7.3×10^{-2}	28	0.026	89,000	3180	122×10^4
				No medial VASA			

Intima

Figure 2.9 The human thoracic aorta has medial vasa vasorum in the outer lamellae, and each lamellar unit supports approximately 2095 dyn/cm. The human abdominal aorta, however, has 28 lamellar units and has no medial vasa, and each lamellar unit supports about 3180 dyn/cm. This architectural difference may be important in the vulnerability of the abdominal aorta to atherosclerosis and aneurysm formation. (Reproduced from Glagov S, Hemodynamic risk factors: Mechanical stress, mural architecture, medial nutrition and the vulnerability of arteries to atherosclerosis, in: Wissler RW and Geer JC, eds., *The Pathogenesis of Atherosclerosis*, Williams & Wilkins, Baltimore, MD, 1972, pp. 166–199. With permission.)

compressive and shearing stresses within the artery wall, have not been clarified. Vasa vasorum have been identified in atherosclerotic arteries and, in particular, within atherosclerotic plaques. Although vasa vasorum in atherosclerotic plaques have been supposed to underlie disruptive lesion hemorrhages,[30] relationships among lesion size, composition and complications and the presence of vasa vasorum are not clear.

AGE-RELATED CHANGES IN THE ARTERY WALL

Focal intimal thickenings, including cushions or pads at or near branch points, have been observed in infants and fetuses. Many of these tend to be modified and incorporated into the media during growth, and most are therefore likely to represent local changes in vessel wall organization related to redistributions of tensile stress associated with developmental changes in diameter, length and geometric configuration.[31]

Progressive fibrocellular diffuse intimal thickening, on the other hand, proceeds from infancy to old age, differing considerably in both extent and degree in different locations in the arterial tree.[32,33] This process tends to be more or less uniform about the vessel circumference and is not limited to areas about branch ostia, bifurcations or the inner aspects of curves. Although the component cells tend to be oriented axially in straight portions of arteries, the organization and composition of thickened intima resemble to some extent that of the underlying media (Figure 2.10). The lumen may not, however, be significantly narrowed by this process, for, while the condition may produce an artery wall with an intima thicker than the media, the process tends to be concentric, accumulation of lipid is not a prominent feature, there is no focal stenosis and the vessel lumen may actually be larger than normal. Diffuse intimal thickening is, nevertheless, especially evident in those vessels that tend to be susceptible to clinically significant atherosclerotic disease.[34] There is, however, little evidence to indicate that diffuse intimal thickening is necessarily a precursor of the formation of atherosclerotic lesions. With advancing age, the internal elastic lamina of the aorta and of the large arteries may show gaps, splits and fragmentation as well as calcium salt deposits. In addition, neoformation of elastin within the thickened intima or in plaques may result in the accumulation of many layers of elastic fibres in the intima.

In general, arteries tend to increase in diameter, elongate and become tortuous with age. Age-related changes include intimal and medial thickening, arterial calcification and increased deposition of matrix substances, thus leading to increased wall stiffness that significantly contributes to an increase in systolic blood pressure.[35]

Diffuse, apparently irreversible enlargement, when marked, is called ectasia. The common form of diffuse and extensive ectasia of the aorta and large arteries parallels a relative overall increase in matrix fibre accumulation,[36]

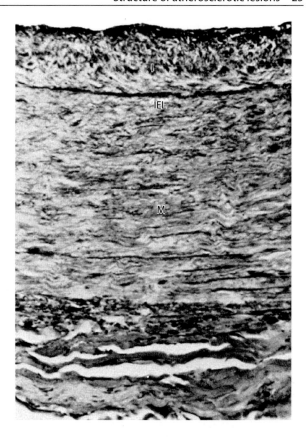

Figure 2.10 Transverse section of coronary artery of an 18-year-old accident victim demonstrating diffuse intimal thickening (I). Note that the organization and composition of the thickened intima resembles the underlying media (M). IEL represents the internal elastic lamina.

including an increase in collagen content, a decrease in elastin content, a calcification of the elastic fibres and a decrease in compliance of the wall. While elongation and tortuosity of the vessel may be quite marked, the diffuse and extensive form of moderate ectasia is not necessarily associated with serious consequences. When complications occur, they are generally attributable to associated atherosclerosis and/or the formation of aneurysms.[37]

STRUCTURE OF ATHEROSCLEROTIC LESIONS

Atherosclerotic lesions may begin in childhood or adolescence and enlarge progressively over years or decades without associated symptoms. Although intimal plaques are evident in arteries of nearly all adults coming to autopsy in much of the world, little is known concerning the factors which determine individual differences in plaque morphology or govern the gradual or sudden transition from asymptomatic plaques to those which enlarge sufficiently to cause obstruction to flow, ulcerate or induce occlusive thrombosis or aneurysm formation. On the basis of morphologic appearance and composition, human lesions are usually classified as *fatty streaks* or fibrous 'raised' *plaques*. Transitional forms have also been identified. While fatty streaks are not associated with symptoms, raised plaques are more complex and are associated with the alterations which underlie circulatory compromise.

Fatty streaks

Fatty streaks are relatively flat, fairly well-demarcated patches or minute yellow foci which may appear soon after birth and are seen on the luminal surface of most aortas of individuals over the age of 3 years (Figure 2.11).[38] Fatty streaks are found with increasing frequency between the ages of 8 and 18, becoming most numerous around puberty. These formations are not, however, limited to young persons and may be seen at any age adjacent to or even superimposed upon fibrous plaques. Fatty streaks consist largely of intimal lipid-laden cells (foam cells) and variable quantities of matrix materials beneath an intact endothelium. The extent to which fatty streaks are precursors of subsequent complex, fibrous, progressive atherosclerotic lesions remains unresolved.[39] There is evidence that many human fatty streaks may be evanescent, for the distribution of fatty streaks seen in young individuals does not coincide entirely with the distribution of fibrous plaques seen later in life. It has also been found that cells in human fatty streaks are not monotypic with respect to isoenzyme content[40] but that advanced lesions are composed of cells which contain extensive regions of cellular monotypia.[41] These findings have suggested that focal events occurring in some fatty streaks may result in cellular proliferation with the persistence of lesions and the subsequent formation of the more complex fibrous plaques, while other fatty streaks resolve.

Intimal thickening can reflect an adaptive response to diminish lumen calibre under conditions of reduced flow or can be a response designed to augment wall thickness when tensile stress increases.[42,43] Focal intimal thickenings have been observed in infants and fetuses at or near branch points and probably represent local remodelling of vessel wall organization related to growth and the associated redistribution of tensile stress.[44] Diffuse fibrocellular intimal thickening can occur as a more generalized phenomenon without a clear relationship to branches or curves and may result in a diffusely thickened intima that is considerably thicker than the media. Lipid accumulation is not a prominent feature in such intimal thickening, and the lumen remains regular and normal or slightly larger than normal in diameter.[33] Although there is little direct evidence that diffuse intimal thickening is a precursor of lipid-containing atherosclerotic plaques, both intimal thickening and plaques tend to occur in similar locations, and intimal thickening is most evident in vessels that are especially susceptible to atherosclerosis.[34,45] Evidence has also been presented that diffuse forms of intimal thickening do not develop uniformly and that foci of relatively rapid thickening undergo dystrophic changes, which give rise to necrosis and other features characteristic of plaques.[46] The relationship of these findings to usual atherosclerosis remains to be defined.

Fibrous plaques

Fibrous plaques do not usually appear until the second decade of life and may not become the predominant lesion type until the fourth decade. The endothelial lining appears to be intact over most uncomplicated lesions, i.e., lesions without evidence of disruption, ulceration, hemorrhage or thrombus formation. Although plaque composition varies considerably with respect to the relative proportions of the usual lesion components, a predominant mode of composition and organization can be discerned. There is frequently a relatively compact zone of connective tissue fibres and smooth-muscle cells immediately beneath the endothelium known as the fibrous cap (Figure 2.12). Deeper in the central portion of the plaque and beneath the fibrous cap is a zone of variable composition and consistency known as the *necrotic core* or *centre*. It contains amorphous debris, lipid-containing cells with morphologic and functional characteristics of either smooth-muscle cells or macrophages,[47] extracellular lipids including droplets and cholesterol crystals,

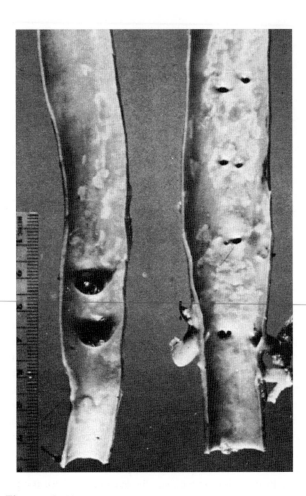

Figure 2.11 Fatty streaks in aorta of 45-year-old patient.

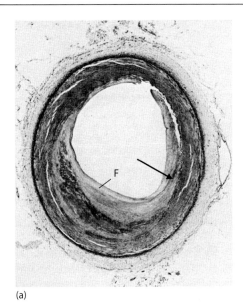

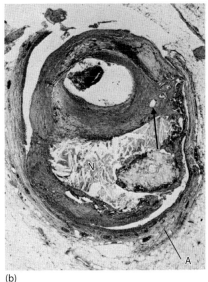

(a)   (b)

Figure 2.12 (a) Transverse section of superficial femoral arteries demonstrating fibrous plaque with prominent fibrous cap (F). Note the thinning of media below the thickest portion of the plaque. Note the formation of a new elastic lamina (arrow) near the lumen. (b) Plaque with prominent necrotic centre (N) medial thinning and thickened adventitia (A). Note the vasa vasorum (arrow) penetrating into plaque and fibrous cap.

calcium salts and myxoid deposits. In addition, matrix fibres, including elastin, collagen, finer fibrillar material and structures resembling basal lamina as well as amorphous ground substance, are evident. The fibrous cap may become quite thick and form a well-organized fibrocellular, layered structure, which may even include a subendothelial elastic lamina. Thrombi formed on lesions as well as fibrin deposits are also incorporated into lesions. Vasa vasorum penetrate from the adventitia or from the lumen to supply the plaque[30] and fibrous cap (Figure 2.7) and to organize thrombotic deposits. There may be thinning and attenuation of the media below the intimal lesion such that the atheromatous deposit and the media bulge outwards towards the adventitia. Some advanced lesions, particularly those associated with aneurysms, may appear to be atrophic and relatively acellular, consisting of dense fibrous tissue, prominent calcific deposits and only minimal evidence of a necrotic centre. Calcification is a prominent feature of advanced plaques and may be quite extensive, involving both the superficial and deeper reaches of the plaques. Although there is no consistent relationship between plaque size or complexity and the degree of calcification, calcific deposits are most prominent in plaques of older individuals and in areas, such as the abdominal aortic segment and coronary arteries, where plaques form earliest.[48] Advanced lesions are called fibrocalcific, lipid rich, fibrocellular, necrotic, myxomatous, etc., depending on their morphologic features. The presence of large quantities of lipid, necrotic material and cells would tend to make a lesion soft and friable, in contrast to the hard or brittle consistency of a mainly fibrocalcific lesion with an intact and prominent fibrous cap.

Lesion complications

Although it tends to isolate the advanced lesion from the lumen, the fibrous cap may be very thin or virtually absent. It may also be interrupted or disrupted focally, exposing underlying lesion contents to the bloodstream and favouring the formation of thrombi or the penetration of blood from the lumen into the lesion. Since advanced atherosclerotic lesions often contain vasa vasorum, these vessels may rupture and result in hemorrhage into the lesion and degeneration of plaque contents. Degeneration and ulceration of plaques are most common at the sites at greatest risk of advanced lesion formation. Thus, the consequences to the circulation of lesions in those areas derive not only from the tendency to progressive stenosis but also from the effects of lesion complications, leading to rapid or sudden local occlusion or to distal embolization of thrombi or atheromatous fragments. Direct relationships among lesion composition, age of the lesion, lesion complication and the presence of particular risk factors remain to be demonstrated. Excision of lesions obtained during surgical procedures and at autopsy has revealed complications which may be related spatially and temporally to documented clinical manifestations.[49] It should also be noted, however, that lesions studied at autopsy and not associated with known clinical manifestations may show evidence of earlier complications, including hemosiderin deposits from hemorrhages, partially organized thrombi and inflammatory cells such as macrophages, lymphocytes, plasma cells and giant cells.[50,51] These findings indicate that lesions may progress through stages potentially severe enough to induce clinical morbidity but that local tissue reactions may be adequate, at least temporarily, to contain the injury.

CONFIGURATION OF LESIONS

The perception that advanced atherosclerotic lesions protrude or bulge into the arterial lumen is suggested by angiographic or ultrasonic views of arteries in longitudinal projections which reveal narrowing of the lumen. *En face* observations of the luminal surface of arteries opened at operation or autopsy also reveal plaques as projecting elevations, and transverse sections of unopened but undistended atherosclerotic arteries may show narrow, crescentic or slitlike arterial lumens. These perceptions may be somewhat misleading, for the absence of distending pressure results in partial collapse of the arterial lumen and corresponding deformation of both the artery wall and the plaque. Progressive distension of the normal aorta from zero to diastolic pressure results in a nearly twofold increase in aortic radius, a fourfold increase in lumen cross-sectional area and a 50% reduction in wall thickness (see Figure 2.3).[52] Similar findings are evident for other arteries. Beyond diastolic pressure, there is little change in artery wall configuration or lumen diameter in keeping with the mechanical properties related to the connective tissue fibre content and organization of the media as outlined earlier. Examination of atherosclerotic arteries fixed while distended reveals that the lumen on transverse section is almost always round or oval and only rarely irregular, triangular or slitlike.[53] Sequential transverse sections through distended vessels with narrowings on axial projections reveal that the lumen is round even in areas of marked stenosis. In addition, plaques are most often eccentric with respect to the cross section of the artery wall and, under the conditions of normal distension, do not usually protrude into the lumen as mound-like projections but tend instead to bulge outwards from the lumen. The luminal surface of the fibrous cap is therefore usually concave on transverse section, corresponding to the curvature of the adjacent uninvolved artery wall. As a consequence, the external or outer contour of the artery tends to become oval while the corresponding lumen remains circular (Figure 2.13). As long as the fibrous cap is intact, the necrotic centre is effectively sequestered from the lumen and the circular configuration of the lumen is preserved. Thus, while plaques may appear as focal projections into the lumen on angiographic images, cross-sectional views reveal rounded lumen contours and a concave luminal profile of the plaque.[54] Circular lumen profiles may also be evident in excised undistended and unopened rigid atherosclerotic arteries when plaques are completely encircling and largely fibrocalcific. Irregular transverse lumen contours on sonograms or distended arteries examined in cross section generally correspond to recent or resolving plaque disruptions ulcerations or thrombus deposition.

The structural changes with atherosclerosis are currently considered degenerative phenomena, which primarily involve a sequence of reactions within the intima and include monocyte recruitment and macrophage formation, lipid deposition, smooth-muscle cell migration, proliferation and extracellular matrix synthesis. The molecular and

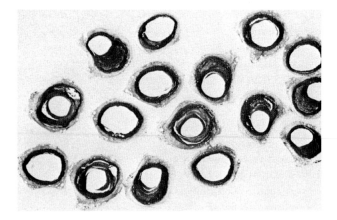

Figure 2.13 Multiple transverse sections at 0.5 cm intervals through a 10 cm segment of superficial femoral artery. Despite the presence of large intimal plaques, the lumen remains rounded. The external vessel contour becomes oval as the artery locally dilates to accommodate the enlarging lesion.

cellular mechanisms underlying the disease cascade have been thoroughly investigated in experimental animals and cell culture. These molecular and cellular mechanisms are closely related with the structure of healthy human arteries and the pathological events occurring during the atherosclerotic process which has been examined by both transmission and scanning electron microscopy.[55]

ENLARGEMENT OF ATHEROSCLEROTIC ARTERIES

The formation of intimal plaque does not necessarily lead to stenosis and obstruction of the arterial lumen. Atherosclerotic arteries may compensate for increasing plaque deposits by enlarging, and such enlargement can maintain a normal or near-normal lumen calibre when the cross-sectional area of the intimal plaque does not exceed approximately 40% of the area encompassed by the internal elastic lumina.[56] Larger plaques tend to be completely encircling and result in lumen stenosis. Compensatory arterial enlargement has been demonstrated in human coronary arteries,[56–60] carotid arteries,[61,62] superficial femoral arteries[63,64] and abdominal aortas.[65–67] Enlargement has also been demonstrated in experimental atherosclerosis in the coronary,[68,69] carotid[70] and superficial femoral arteries of primates and in the coronary artery of pigs.[71,72] However, different segments of the arterial tree respond differently to increasing intimal plaque.[73] In the distal left anterior descending coronary artery, arterial enlargement occurs more rapidly than intimal plaque deposition. This may result in a net increase in lumen area rather than lumen stenosis in the most severely diseased arteries.[57] Individual variation has also been demonstrated in the superficial femoral artery.[74] Thus, it appears that the development of lumen stenosis, the maintenance of a normal lumen cross-sectional area or the development of an increase in lumen diameter is determined by the relative rates of plaque growth and artery enlargement.[75] Reduction in artery size can also result in the development of lumen stenosis, and this phenomenon has been demonstrated in vivo with intravascular ultrasound.[76] Further study of this phenomenon of artery enlargement or reduction in size, particularly in regions associated with great morbidity related to plaque deposition, is needed in order to fully understand the processes involved in the development of atherosclerotic stenoses and aneurysms. Although plaques may occur in straight vessels away from branch points, they are usually located at bifurcations or bends, where variations in hemodynamic conditions are especially likely to occur.[77] The mechanism by which this enlargement occurs is not clear. Possible explanations include the effects of altered blood flow on the segment of artery wall which is free of plaque formation or direct effects of the plaque on the subjacent artery wall. Flow-mediated arterial enlargement is limited by competitive matrix metalloproteinase inhibition in a dose-dependent fashion.[78–80]

Normal arteries respond to changes in wall shear stress[81,82] with increase[83] or decrease[84,85] in lumen diameter. This response appears to be dependent on the presence of an intact endothelial surface[86] and may be mediated through endothelial-derived vasoactive agents.[87] Whether enlargement of atherosclerotic arteries in response to increasing intimal plaque occurs by a similar mechanism is unknown. Focal narrowing of the lumen caused by intimal plaque may result in a local increase in wall shear stress, which may stimulate endothelial-dependent arterial dilation.[88] Since most atherosclerotic plaques are eccentric, the relatively uninvolved sections of artery wall may respond normally to shear stress stimuli despite an extensive lesion on the opposite wall. Under these circumstances, enlargement of the free wall would act to promote the further development of eccentricity. Adaptive enlargement may fail if the plaque becomes concentric and rigid with no responsive free wall.

Alternatively, atherosclerotic artery enlargement may develop as a result of plaque-induced involutional changes in the underlying media. Thinning of the media is commonly seen beneath atherosclerotic plaques, and dissolution of the support structure of the artery wall may result in outward bulging of the plaque.[89] Under these circumstances, direct effects of the plaque on the underlying wall promote enlargement. The observation of apparent overcompensation with excess enlargement in the distal left anterior descending coronary artery in humans is consistent with a direct effect of the plaque on the artery wall, as are morphologic evidences of outward plaque bulging. The balance between plaque deposition and artery enlargement is likely to be an important determinant whether lumen calibre remains normal or whether lumen stenosis or ectasia develops.

In experimentally produced arteriovenous fistulae, the afferent artery has been shown to enlarge just enough to restore shear stress to baseline levels.[83] Wall shear stress thus appears to act as a regulating signal to determine artery size, and this response is dependent on the presence of an intact endothelial surface.[86,90–92] The response is mediated by the release of endothelial-derived relaxing factor or nitric oxide.[87,93] Thus, the endothelium functions as a mechanically sensitive signal-transduction interface between the blood and the artery wall.[94,95] Nitric oxide (NO) plays an important role in both the acute and chronic increase in vessel calibre in response to the increased flow.[96,97] Inhibition of NO synthesis by means of a long-term oral administration of L-NAME can inhibit flow-induced arterial enlargement.[98,99]

Atherosclerotic arteries are also capable of enlarging in response to increases in blood flow and increase in wall shear stress, but this process may be limited.[56] Atherosclerotic artery enlargement is further discussed later in this chapter. The nature and mechanisms of the artery wall–adaptive processes which allow arteries to adjust lumen diameter are currently being actively investigated. Understanding the mechanism and limits of the adaptive process and identification of the consequences for the vessel wall of shear stress that is persistently higher or lower than normal will be of value in clinical efforts to maintain normal lumen calibre.

LOCALIZATION OF ATHEROSCLEROTIC LESIONS

Several major arterial sites are particularly prone to the development of advanced atherosclerotic lesions, while others are relatively resistant. The coronary arteries, carotid bifurcation, infrarenal abdominal aorta and iliofemoral vessels are particularly susceptible, while the mesenteric, renal, intercostals and mammary arteries tend to be spared.[100]

The apparently selective localization of plaques which evolve to cause clinical symptoms has been attributed to local differences in vessel wall metabolism, structure and permeability and to differences in local hemodynamic patterns.

Since many plaques tend to form in relation to branch points and bends where flow profiles have been shown to undergo deviations from unidirectional laminar flow, various flow features related to these changes have been implicated in plaque localization. These include elevated shear stress,[4] turbulence,[101,102] flow separation[103] and low shear stress.[104,105] Elevated shear stress has been thought to contribute to plaque initiation by causing endothelial injury. The resulting exposure of intimal connective tissue to the bloodstream would favour platelet deposition and release of platelet growth factor, thereby including focal intimal thickening by stimulating smooth-muscle cell proliferation.[106] Variations in shear stress direction associated with pulsatile flow may favour increased endothelial permeability by direct mechanical effects on cell junctions, whereas relatively high unidirectional shear stresses may not be injurious[107] and may even favour endothelial mechanical integrity.[108] Endothelial cells are normally aligned in the direction of flow[109] in an overlapping arrangement.[110]

Cyclic shifts in the relationship between shear stress direction and the orientation of intercellular overlapping borders may disturb the relationships between ingress and egress of particles through junctions. This hypothesis agrees well with reports of increased permeability of cultured, confluent endothelial cells subjected to changes in shear stress[111] as well as increased permeability to Evans blue dye in relation to differences in endothelial cell orientation,[112] which may be associated with different flow patterns. Oscillatory shear stress has also been shown to influence endothelium and nitric oxide synthase expression[113] and stimulate adhesion molecule expression in cultured human endothelial cells.[114]

Heart rate has been implicated as an independent risk factor in coronary atherosclerosis and is discussed further in the section dealing with the coronary arteries. Reduction in heart rate in experimental atherosclerosis has been shown to retard carotid plaque progression.[115,116]

Turbulence may, however, develop in association with stenoses and irregularities of the flow surface caused by atherosclerotic plaques, but turbulence is located distal to the lesion, not at the lesion. Experimentally produced stenoses reveal that turbulence is greatest two to four vessel diameters distal to the stenosis in an area that frequently develops poststenotic dilatation but does not readily develop diet-induced plaques.[117–119] Thus, turbulence per se has not been shown to be an initiating factor in atherogenesis. Nevertheless, turbulence may play a role in plaque disruption or thrombogenesis. Further investigation is needed to establish these relationships. Evidence that these are major initiating or sustaining mechanisms in human or experimental plaque formation has not been forthcoming. Experimental observations reveal no evidence of endothelial damage or disruption over early developing experimental foam cell lesions,[10] suggesting that endothelial denudation is not an important initiating factor in plaque pathogenesis.

Clinical observations suggest that plaques localize first in areas of low shear stress, such as on the upstream rather than the downstream rim of aortic ostia (Figure 2.14). Quantitative correlative studies of flow profiles and early plaque formation in the human carotid bifurcation suggest that flow separation, reduced flow rate, reduced shear stress and departures from unidirectional laminar flow may be the important hemodynamic factors in plaque pathogenesis.[120] At the carotid bifurcation, for example, plaques do not begin in the vicinity of the flow divider where flow velocity is high, laminar and unidirectional throughout the cardiac cycle. Plaques are formed earliest and are most advanced opposite the flow divider, where flow velocity and shear stress are low (Figure 2.15). Under conditions of pulsatile flow, flow reversal occurs in the same area, particularly during the downstroke of systole with oscillation in wall shear stress direction.[121] These flow-field disturbances may be associated with prolonged residence time of atherogenic particles such as lipids or mitogens at sites which are prone to plaque formation. Although reduced velocity and shear stress, departures from unidirectional laminar flow and flow reversal appear to favour plaque formation, turbulence as such does not appear to be a factor. Areas of high

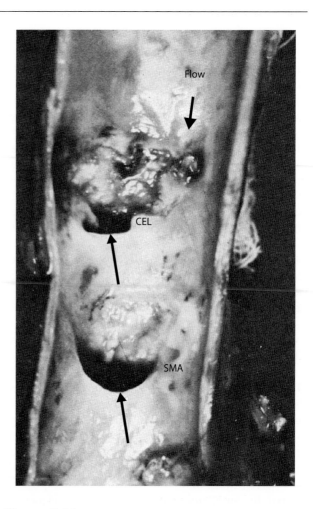

Figure 2.14 Ostia of celiac artery and superior mesenteric artery of human aorta. Note the prominent plaque formation at upstream rim of the ostia with no plaque formation on the flow divider (arrows), which is exposed to high shear stress.

turbulence which occurs immediately distal to experimental stenoses are not sites of preferential lesion formation.[122] Such findings also suggest that an increase in flow velocity and shear in a developing atherosclerotic stenosis could tend to retard further plaque formation.

Since the development of complex flow patterns and shear stress reversal occurs during systole, an elevated heart rate may be expected to be associated with the acceleration of plaque formation at sites of predilection, for increased heart rate would prolong the relative time spent in systole. This effect would be expected to be particularly important in the coronary arteries, where systolic flow is biphasic. Experimental studies reveal that lowered heart rate has a profound effect on retarding the development of diet-induced coronary artery[123] and carotid artery[70,124] plaques. Clinical epidemiologic studies have revealed heart rate to be a primary independent risk factor for coronary and cardiovascular mortality on both men and women.[125] The combined protective effects of increased flow velocity and reduced heart rate are consistent with the known protective effects of regular exercise against coronary artery disease in humans.

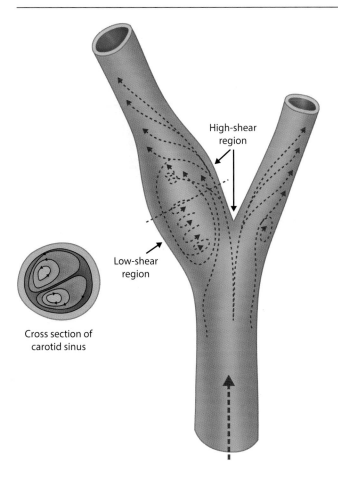

in combination with the branching angle results in a flow profile in which a large area of flow separation is formed along the outer wall of the sinus (Figure 2.15).

Secondary and tertiary flow patterns, vortex formation and oscillations in the angle of the flow vector occur at the side walls of the sinus.[121] Intimal plaques are deposited early in life in this region. As plaques enlarge at the outer wall, the geometric configuration of the lumen is modified so that other flow patterns may develop which favour plaque formation on the side and inner walls. In its most advanced and stenotic form, the disease may involve the entire circumference of the sinus, including the region of the flow divider, but plaques are commonly largest and most complicated at the outer and side walls of the carotid bifurcation (Figure 2.16). The hemodynamic conditions which exist at the carotid bifurcation may also influence the surface characteristics of existing carotid plaques and contribute to their tendency to ulcerate and embolize.

Carotid plaques producing high-grade stenosis exhibit features of intraplaque hemorrhage, ulceration, thrombosis, lumen surface irregularity and calcification.[128] These micro-anatomic features are present in plaques removed from

Figure 2.15 Blood flow patterns in the human carotid bifurcation. There is a large area of slow flow, flow separation, low shear stress and disordered flow patterns in the internal carotid sinus opposite the bifurcation flow divider. Plaques localize in this area. The area of high shear stress at the flow divider is relatively spared of plaque formation. (Reproduced from Zarins CK et al., Atherosclerotic plaque distribution and flow velocity profiles in the carotid bifurcation, in: Bergan JJ and Yao JST, eds., *Cerebrovascular Insufficiency*, Grune & Stratton, New York, 1983, pp. 19–30. With permission.)

CAROTID BIFURCATION PLAQUES

Intimal thickening is found in the carotid sinus or carotid bulb early in life, and atherosclerotic lesions are common at this site in adults. Although extensive, complex and complicated plaques may be present in the carotid bifurcation, particularly within the sinus, there is little plaque formation in the immediately proximal common carotid artery or the internal carotid artery immediately distal to the sinus. Within the bony canal in the base of the skull, lesions are unusual, but the basilar artery and the proximal segments of the cerebral arteries about the circle of Willis are commonly involved. The distribution of lesions about the bifurcation is probably associated with hemodynamic conditions which derive from the special geometry at this site.[120,126,127] The internal carotid sinus is a localized region which has a cross-sectional area twice that of the immediately distal internal carotid segment. This configuration

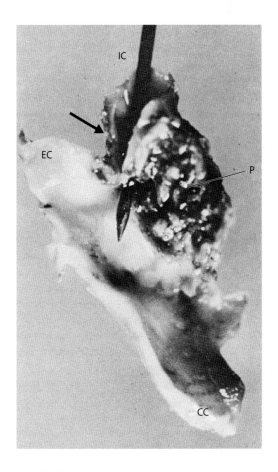

Figure 2.16 Longitudinal section of carotid endarterectomy specimen. Note the marked plaque formation (P) on the outer wall of internal carotid (IC) sinus. This corresponds to the area which is exposed to low flow velocity and low shear stress. The inner wall (arrow) has minimal intimal thickening. External carotid (EC), common carotid (CC).

symptomatic and asymptomatic patients and appear to be related to plaque size. Ulceration and surface thrombi that may lead to cerebral embolization are prominent features in markedly stenotic plaques even when symptoms are absent. These observations indicate that the disruptive processes that underlie plaque instability appear to be closely associated with plaque size rather than plaque composition.[129]

Quantitative morphologic studies of human carotid bifurcations have demonstrated increased intimal thickness in association with lumen enlargement with resultant preservation of normal tangential mural tension.[130,131] The factors that differentiate a normal adaptive intimal thickening from an inappropriate intimal hyperplastic response resulting in lumen stenosis at a vascular anastomosis are not well understood. Techniques to precisely measure stresses in the artery wall are now available and will help define the role of mechanical forces in artery wall response.[132,133]

AORTIC ATHEROSCLEROSIS

Plaques are regularly found in the adult human thoracic aorta, but they are often less abundant, more discrete, less complicated and less calcific than in the abdominal aortic segment of the same individual. Although plaques tend to deposit about intercostal branch ostia, significant occlusive lesions of the thoracic aorta do not develop and thoracic aorta aneurysms are unusual. The infrarenal abdominal aortic segment, on the other hand, is particularly prone to the early occurrence of plaques and occlusive disease as well as to the development of marked medial atrophy, calcification and aneurysmal dilation with mural thrombus formation.

The differing susceptibilities of the thoracic and abdominal aorta to atherosclerosis and to aneurysmal dilation may be due to differences in architecture, composition and nutrition of the artery wall as well as to differences in the distribution of mechanical stresses. As noted previously, the thoracic aorta is thicker and has a greater number of medial lamellar units than the abdominal aorta, in keeping with its greater diameter and tangential wall tension.[15] The thoracic aorta contains a greater relative proportion of elastin and a lower proportion of collagen than the abdominal aorta.[13] The increased stiffness of the abdominal aorta is associated with an elevated pulse pressure that could result in altered medial smooth-muscle metabolism and increased susceptibility to plaque deposition.[134,135] In addition, differences exist with respect to wall nutrition that could result in different propensities to atherogenesis and to different responses of the media to mechanical stress.[136]

The outer two-thirds of the thoracic aortic media is well perfused by intramural vasa vasorum, whereas the inner 30 lamellar units are nourished by diffusion from the lumen. The abdominal aorta, however, is nourished only from the lumen and lacks medial vasa vasorum; moreover, the tension per layer is much larger than for the thoracic segment.[2] These factors may place the medial smooth-muscle cells of the abdominal aorta at a relatively higher risk for ischemic injury. Intimal plaque formation may

increase the diffusion distance from the lumen and induce reparative and healing processes, which may promote lipid uptake and further plaque formation. Penetration of vasa vasorum into atherosclerotic plaque has been demonstrated and may further promote a proliferative response in the artery. Thus, the composition and microarchitecture of the media and the metabolic state of the media smooth-muscle cells may be important factors in determining differential susceptibilities of the aorta to atherosclerosis.[134]

Flow conditions in the aorta may also predispose it to plaque formation. The thoracic aorta is exposed to relatively high rates of flow, with obligatory flow to the cerebral, upper extremity and visceral arterial beds, including the renal arteries, which deliver one quarter of the cardiac output at rest. By contrast, blood flow in the infrarenal aorta may be highly variable, with volume flow largely dependent on muscular activity of the lower extremities. Under modern conditions of motorized transport and an increasingly sedentary lifestyle, the abdominal aortic segment is likely to be subjected to relatively reduced blood flow velocities over the long term. The abdominal aorta would therefore be exposed to the adverse hemodynamic forces of low flow velocity, low wall shear stress and prolonged particle residence time and oscillation of wall shear.[137,138] Each of these factors would act to favour plaque formation.[139] Experimental flow studies in models of the human abdominal aorta reveal that these adverse hemodynamic conditions can be eliminated or minimized by hemodynamic conditions that prevail during exercise.[140]

ANEURYSM FORMATION

The association between atherosclerosis and abdominal aortic aneurysm formation has long been recognized in humans. However, the mechanisms by which the atherosclerotic process may be associated with aneurysmal dilation are not well defined. A number of other etiologic factors have been proposed, including increased proteolytic enzyme activity[141–143] and genetic abnormalities leading to deficiencies in connective tissue structure and function.[144,145] Although some investigators have questioned a role for atherosclerosis in aneurysm formation, evidence for its importance is increasing.

Most aneurysms are localized to the infrarenal abdominal aortic segment, where aortic atherosclerosis is usually most advanced. Plaque formation in this region may further impair diffusion of nutrients to the aortic wall, resulting in atrophy of the underlying aortic wall. Plaque deposition is accompanied by compensatory enlargement of the aorta, as described earlier in this chapter. Under these circumstances, the plaque may provide structural support to the aortic wall. Subsequent plaque atrophy may leave an enlarged aorta with a thinned wall unable to support wall tension as aneurysmal enlargement progresses. Ingrowth of vasa vasorum into the media and plaque occurs commonly in occlusive aortic atherosclerosis (Figures 2.17 and 2.18). However, under conditions where

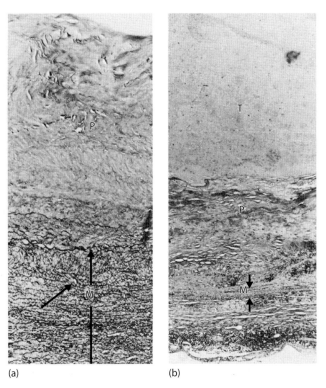

(a)   (b)

Figure 2.17 (a) Transverse section of abdominal aorta demonstrating intimal plaque (P) with preservation of underlying media (M) with its lamellar architecture. Vasa vasorum (arrow) are present in the media. (b) Aneurysm with marked medial atrophy (M), delineated by arrows, fibrous plaque (P) and large mural thrombus (T).

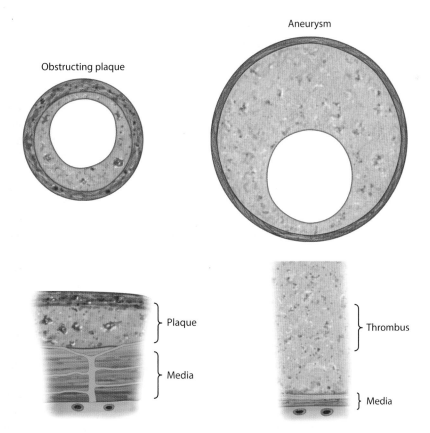

Figure 2.18 Obstructing plaques in the abdominal aorta are characterized by ingrowth of vasa vasorum to nourish the media and plaque. Aneurysms are relatively devoid of vasa with atrophy of the aortic wall. A deficiency of medial nutrition may be a factor in aneurysm pathogenesis. (Reproduced from Zarins CK and Glagov S, Aneurysms and obstructive plaques: Differing local responses to atherosclerosis, in: Bergan JJ and Yao JST, eds., *Aneurysms: Diagnosis and Treatment*, Grune & Stratton, New York, 1982, pp. 61–82. With permission.)

vasa vasorum are absent, impaired nutrition of plaque and media may result in atrophy of both the plaque and the artery wall with aneurysmal enlargement.[146]

Experimental studies confirm the importance of the medial lamellar architecture in the pathogenesis of aneurysms[147] and reveal that diet-induced atherosclerosis may result in the destruction of the media and in aneurysm formation.[148,149]

A controlled trial of cholesterol-lowering therapy in monkeys revealed plaque regression, thinning of the media and aneurysmal dilation of the abdominal aorta.[150] These observations suggest that the formation of abdominal aortic aneurysms may complicate the atherosclerotic process under special experimental and human clinical conditions. Aneurysms appear at a relatively late phase of plaque evolution, when plaque regression and medial atrophy predominate, rather than at earlier phases when cell proliferation, fibrogenesis and lipid accumulation characterize plaque progression. Macrophages and proteolytic enzymes during this phase of atherosclerotic artery wall degeneration may provide the mechanisms whereby dissolution of the aortic wall occurs. Individual differences in plaque evolution reflecting differences in both the rate and duration of plaque formation and plaque regression and in tissue and cell responses to the atherogenic process are likely to be major determinants of individual susceptibility to aneurysm formation. Microarchitectural differences in artery wall structure as well as local mechanical conditions related to geometry, blood flow and blood pressure are likely to be major determinants of aneurysm localization.[151] These factors may be modulated by genetic predisposition and by local injurious,[22] hemodynamic,[152,153] metabolic and tensile stresses.

SUPERFICIAL FEMORAL ARTERY STENOSIS

The arteries of the lower extremities are frequently affected by atherosclerotic plaques, while vessels of similar size in the upper extremities are spared. In addition to differences in hydrostatic pressure, the arteries of the lower extremities are subjected to more marked variations in flow rate, depending on the level of physical activity. Similar to the situation that prevails in the abdominal aorta, sedentary lifestyles would tend to favour low flow rates and lead to increased plaque deposition in vessels of the lower extremities. Cigarette smoking and diabetes mellitus are the risk factors most closely associated with atherosclerotic disease of the lower extremities.[154] The manner in which these factors and the special hemodynamic conditions are mutually enhancing in the vessels of the lower extremities remains to be elucidated. Of the arteries of the lower extremity, the superficial femoral artery is most commonly the site of multiple stenotic lesions, while the profunda femoris tends to be spared. The superficial femoral artery is a major conduit with relatively few proximal branches,

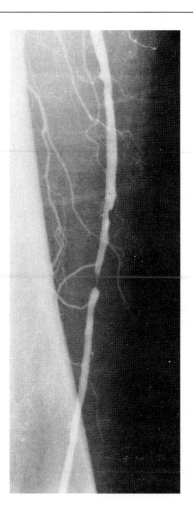

Figure 2.19 Focal stenosis of superficial femoral artery at adductor hiatus.

and flow velocity is likely to be relatively slow on the average, varying in relation to activity of the calf muscles during walking or running. The profunda femoris is a smaller, muscular vessel with many branches to lower extremity muscles; flow velocity is likely to be relatively high under normal conditions. Plaques in the superficial femoral artery have not been shown to occur preferentially at branching sites, but stenotic lesions tend to appear earliest at the adductor hiatus, where the vessel is straight and branches are few (Figure 2.19). Repeated mechanical trauma, limitations on vessel compliance or alterations in the adaptive enlargement process associated with the closely applied adductor magnus tendon[63] may contribute to the selective localization of occlusive disease in this position.

CORONARY ARTERY ATHEROSCLEROSIS

The coronary arteries are particularly prone to develop atherosclerosis.[155] The special hemodynamic features of the coronary circulation, including the marked excursions in flow rate during the cardiac cycle, the geometric configuration of the vessels and their branches, the mechanical torsion and flexions of the vessels associated with cardiac motion and the special reactivity of coronary artery smooth muscle to vasoactive substances and nervous impulses, have been suggested as predisposing factors that could underlie individual differences in lesion distribution. The selective involvement of the left coronary artery opposite the flow divider at the bifurcation of the left circumflex indicates that hemodynamic relationships similar to those that prevail at the carotid bifurcation also occur in the coronary arteries. In addition, compared to other vessels, there are two pulses of flow during systole. Since the oscillatory changes in fluid shear are related to the downstroke phase of the systolic pulse,[121] an increase in heart rate may exert a greater effect on atherogenesis in the coronary arteries than elsewhere in the arterial tree. Recent studies suggest that reduced heart rate retards the development of experimental, diet-induced plaques.[70,123,124,156] These observations are consistent with clinical observations of a reduced risk of cardiovascular mortality in men and women with a lower heart rate.[125]

QUANTITATIVE EVALUATION OF ATHEROSCLEROSIS

Quantitative clinical assessment of atherosclerosis by modern diagnostic methods may include evaluation of several distinct but related aspects of involvement.[157] These include the extent of the disease process, i.e., the degree to which a given artery segment or arterial bed is involved by the disease and/or the number of distinguishable lesions present in a vessel or group of vessels (Figure 2.20). Irregularities and strictures of lumen contour on angiograms as well as on ultrasonic and axial tomographic images, and the presence of calcifications have been considered to be major indicators of extent of disease. A second quantifiable feature that bears directly on the consequences to the circulation is the severity of the disease, as reflected in the degree of luminal stenosis. Usual estimates are expressed as percent stenosis, based on comparisons between lumen diameter at a definite

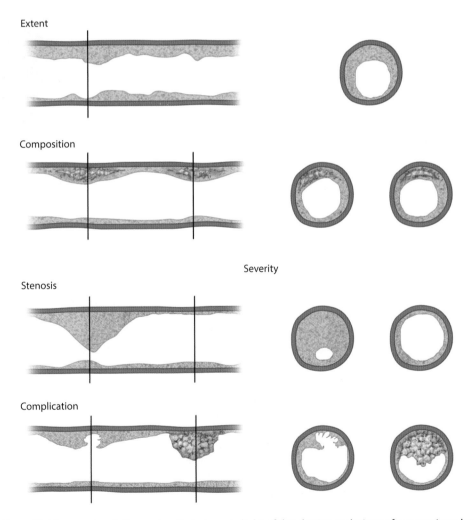

Figure 2.20 Quantifiable aspects of atherosclerotic lesions. In light of developing techniques for assessing plaque size, configuration and composition in vivo, the use of more precise terms for the description of lesions could improve validation and clinical pathologic correlative studies. The extent implies a degree of involvement of a particular vessel or arterial bed, while severity implies interference with flow and reduction of perfusion. Both stenosis (narrowing of the lumen) and complication (plaque disruption, hemorrhage or thrombosis) determine severity regardless of the extent of disease. Lesion composition may be important in predisposing to complication.

narrowing and an immediately adjacent segment which appears to be uninvolved. Another discernible index of the atherosclerotic process, independent of both extent of involvement and severity of stenosis, is lesion complication. This includes ulceration, necrosis, thrombosis and plaque hemorrhage. Finally, quantitative information concerning lesion composition may be obtained. This includes calcification, frequently revealed by clinical visualization methods and estimates of lipid, cell and matrix fibre content, usually estimated from histologic sections.

Most often, quantitative descriptions of atherosclerosis deal with the severity of disease, or *percent stenosis*, of a lesion imaged by angiography. Since angiography can only demonstrate the opacified artery lumen, the degree of stenosis is calculated by comparing lumen diameter at the narrowest point to an apparently 'disease-free' area in the same vessel. In addition to errors in projection, resolution and magnification, errors may arise if the apparently normal zone is involved by advanced intimal plaques. In comparing sequential angiograms, further errors may result if arteries dilate as atherosclerosis progresses. Such a response to progressing disease has been demonstrated in experimental[68] and human atherosclerosis.[54]

Ultrasonic imaging of arteries has the capability of visualizing not only the lumen of the vessel but also the artery wall.[158] Other imaging techniques such as computed tomography and nuclear magnetic resonance have similar potential to visualize the plaque. It is important, however, to recognize the difference in definition of percent stenosis by these imaging techniques compared to angiography (Figure 2.21) when assessing validation studies.

Gross morphologic and histologic examinations of atherosclerotic arteries have the advantage of direct visualization and inspection of the lumen, plaque and artery wall. However, redistension of the collapsed artery wall during fixation is necessary in order to restore in vivo configuration.[54] Failure to do so has led to a misperception that angiography 'underestimates' the degree of stenosis when compared to postmortem examination.[159] Calculation of percent stenosis from histologic cross sections of arteries is usually performed by comparing the lumen cross-sectional area to the area encompassed by the internal elastic lamina, the presumed lumen size before the plaque developed (Figure 2.21). This difference in definition of percent stenosis may make comparison to other methods difficult. In addition, if vessel enlargement occurred during plaque enlargement, the internal elastic lamina landmark may not accurately represent the 'true lumen'. Furthermore, accurate quantitative correlation of plaque cross-sectional area as measured on histologic sections with in vivo clinical measurements requires corrections to account for tissue shrinkage during fixation and processing.[54]

Although plaques may vary a good deal in composition, methods for assessing the distribution of plaque components in vivo are not yet sufficiently sensitive or specific to permit the establishment of criteria for predicting which lesions are likely to enlarge or ulcerate and which lesions will remain relatively stable. Methods that

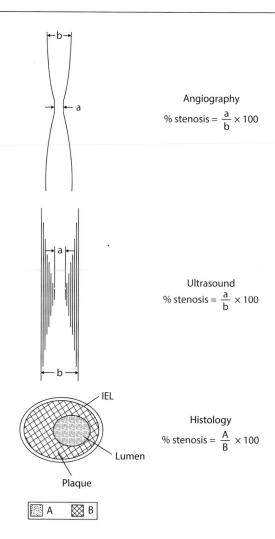

Figure 2.21 Different methods of measuring and defining percent stenosis. Including more quantitative in vivo measurements of lumen diameter, plaque and artery wall thickness, plaque composition, plaque disruption and thrombosis. For the present, attempts to quantitate atherosclerotic disease in the living patient or from histologic sections in order to evaluate treatment programmes dealing with prevention, regression or early detection must take appropriate account of the features of plaque and vessel morphology outlined earlier. In particular, the outward sequestration effect, the persistence of a circular lumen which may approximate normal dimensions despite the presence of a large plaque, the association of plaque formation with enlargement of the vessel and the need for fixation under pressure must be considered.

provide direct information about actual plaque size and composition are developing rapidly and are likely to gain increased application. These include real-time ultrasound imaging, reconstructions from computerized tomography and nuclear magnetic resonance and positron imaging. Thus, more accurate assessments of the extent of disease may be available in the future, including more quantitative in vivo measurements of lumen diameter, plaque and artery wall thickness, plaque composition, plaque disruption and thrombosis. For the present, attempts to quantitate atherosclerotic disease in the living patient or from histologic sections in order to evaluate treatment programmes dealing with prevention, regression or early detection must take appropriate account of the features of plaque and vessel morphology outlined earlier. In particular, the outward sequestration effect, the persistence of a circular lumen which may approximate normal dimensions despite the presence of a large plaque, the association of plaque formation with enlargement of the vessel and the need for fixation under pressure must be considered.

REFERENCES

1. Flaherty JT, Pierce JE, Ferrans VJ, Patel DJ, Tucker WK, Fry DL. Endothelial nuclear patterns in the canine arterial tree with particular reference to hemodynamic events. *Circ Res.* 1972;30:23–33.

2. Clark JM, Glagov S. Evaluation and publication of scanning electron micrographs. *Science.* 1976;192:1360–1361.

3. Ts'ao CH, Glagov S. Basal endothelial attachment. Tenacity at cytoplasmic dense zones in the rabbit aorta. *Lab Invest.* 1970;23:510–516.

4. Fry D. Acute vascular endothelial changes associated with increased blood velocity gradients. *Cir Res.* 1968;22:165–197.

5. Zarins CK, Taylor KE, Bomberger RA, Glagov S. Endothelial integrity at aortic ostial flow dividers. *Scan Electron Microsc.* 1980:249–254.

6. Sho E, Nanjo H, Sho M, Kobayashi M, Komatsu M, Kawamura K, Xu C, Zarins CK, Masuda H. Arterial enlargement, tortuosity, and intimal thickening in response to sequential exposure to high and low wall shear stress. *J Vasc Surg.* 2004;39:601–612.

7. Cines DB, Pollak ES, Buck CA et al. Endothelial cells in physiology and in the pathophysiology of vascular disorders. *Blood.* 1998;91:3527–3561.

8. Traub O, Berk BC. Laminar shear stress: Mechanisms by which endothelial cells transduce an atheroprotective force. *Arterioscler Thromb Vasc Biol.* 1998;18:677–685.

9. Schwartz CJ, Valente AJ, Sprague EA, Kelley JL, Nerem RM. The pathogenesis of atherosclerosis: An overview. *Clin Cardiol.* 1991;14:11–16.

10. Taylor KE, Glagov S, Zarins CK. Preservation and structural adaptation of endothelium over experimental foam cell lesions: Quantitative ultrastructural study. *Arteriosclerosis.* 1989;9:881–894.

11. Jaffe EA. *Biology of Endothelial Cells.* Boston, MA: Martinus Nijhoff; 1984.

12. Masuda H, Kawamura K, Nanjo H et al. Ultrastructure of endothelial cells under flow alteration. *Microsc Res Tech.* 2003;60:2–12.

13. Clark JM, Glagov S. Structural integration of the arterial wall. I. Relationships and attachments of medial smooth muscle cells in normally distended and hyperdistended aortas. *Lab Investig.* 1979;40:587–602.

14. Wolinsky H, Glagov S. A lamellar unit of aortic medial structure and function in mammals. *Circ Res.* 1967;20:99–111.

15. Clark JM, Glagov S. Transmural organization of the arterial media: The lamellar unit revisited. *Arteriosclerosis.* 1985;5:19–34.

16. Glagov S. Hemodynamic risk factors: Mechanical stress, mural architecture, medial nutrition and the vulnerability of arteries to atherosclerosis. In: Wissler RW, Geer JC, eds. *The Pathogenesis of Atherosclerosis.* Baltimore, MD: Williams & Wilkins; 1972, pp. 164–199.

17. Fischer GM, Llaurado JG. Collagen and elastin content in canine arteries selected from functionally different vascular beds. *Circ Res.* 1966;19:394–399.

18. Pomerantz KB, Hajjar DP. Eicosanoids in regulation of arterial smooth muscle cell phenotype, proliferative capacity, and cholesterol metabolism. *Arteriosclerosis.* 1989;9:413–429.

19. Davis HR, Runyon-Hass A, Zarins CK. Interactive arterial effects of hypertension and hyperlipidemia. *Fed Proc.* 1984;43:711.

20. Lyon RT, Zarins CK, Glagov S. Artery wall motion proximal and distal to stenoses. *Fed Proc.* 1985;44:1136.

21. Leung DY, Glagov S, Mathews MB. Cyclic stretching stimulates synthesis of matrix components by arterial smooth muscle cells in vitro. *Science.* 1976;191:475–477.

22. Bomberger RA, Zarins CK, Glagov S. Medial injury and hyperlipidemia in development of aneurysms or atherosclerotic plaques. *Surg Forum.* 1980;31.

23. Parums DV, Chadwick DR, Mitchinson MJ. The localisation of immunoglobulin in chronic periaortitis. *Atherosclerosis.* 1986;61:117–123.

24. Wilcox JN, Scott NA. Potential role of the adventitia in arteritis and atherosclerosis. *Int J Cardiol.* 1996;54(Suppl.):S21–S35.

25. Barker SG, Tilling LC, Miller GC, Beesley JE, Fleetwood G, Stavri GT, Baskerville PA, Martin JF. The adventitia and atherogenesis: Removal initiates intimal proliferation in the rabbit which regresses on generation of a 'neoadventitia'. *Atherosclerosis.* 1994;105:131–144.

26. Shi Y, O'Brien JE Jr., Ala-Kokko L, Chung W, Mannion JD, Zalewski A. Origin of extracellular matrix synthesis during coronary repair. *Circulation.* 1997;95:997–1006.

27. Wolinsky H, Glagov S. Nature of species differences in the medial distribution of aortic vasa vasorum in mammals. *Circ Res.* 1967;20:409–421.

28. Wolinsky H, Glagov S. Comparison of abdominal and thoracic aortic medial structure in mammals: Deviation of man from the usual pattern. *Circ Res.* 1969;25:677–686.

29. Heistad DD, Marcus ML, Law EG, Armstrong ML, Ehrhardt JC, Abboud FM. Regulation of blood flow to the aortic media in dogs. *J Clin Invest.* 1978;62:133–140.

30. Paterson JC. Vascularization and hemorrhage of the intima of arteriosclerotic coronary arteries. *Arch Pathol.* 1936;22:313.

31. Fleischmann D, Hastie TJ, Dannegger FC, Paik DS, Tillich M, Zarins CK, Rubin GD. Quantitative determination of age-related geometric changes in the normal abdominal aorta. *J Vasc Surg.* 2001;33:97–105.

32. Wilens SL. The nature of diffuse intimal thickening of arteries. *Am J Pathol.* 1951;27:825.

33. Movat HZ, More TH, Haust MD. The diffuse intimal thickening of the human aorta with aging. *Am J Pathol.* 1958;34:1023.

34. Tejada C, Strong JP, Montenegro MR et al. Distribution of coronary and aortic atherosclerosis by geographic location, race and sex. *Lab Investig.* 1968;15:5009.

35. Nicita-Mauro V, Maltese G, Nicita-Mauro C, Basile G. Vascular aging and geriatric patient. *Minerva Cardioangiol.* 2007;55:497–502.

36. Mendez J, Tejada C. Chemical composition of aortas from guatemalans and north americans. *Am J Clin Pathologe.* 1969;51:598–602.

37. Bilato C, Crow MT. Atherosclerosis and the vascular biology of aging. *Aging.* 1996;8:221–234.

38. Mitchell JRA, Schwartz CJ. Study of cardiovascular disease at necropsy. In: Mitchell JRA, Schwartz CJ, eds. *Arterial Disease.* Oxford, UK: Blackwell Scientific; 1965, pp. 377–396.

39. McGill HC Jr. Atherosclerosis: Problems in pathogenesis. In: Paoletti R, Gotto AM, eds. *Atherosclerosis Reviews.* New York: Raven Press; 1977, pp. 27–65.

40. Pearson TA, Dillman JM, Solex K, Heptinstall RH. Clonal markers in the study of the origin and growth of human atherosclerotic lesions. *Circ Res.* 1978;43:10–18.

41. Benditt EP, Benditt JM. Evidence for a monoclonal origin of human atherosclerotic plaques. *Proc Natl Acad Sci USA.* 1973;70:1753–1756.

42. Glagov SB, Bassiouny HS, Giddens DP, Zarins CK. Intimal thickening: Morphogenesis, functional significance and detection. *J Vasc Invest.* 1995;1:2.

43. Glagov S, Zarins CK, Masawa N, Xu CP, Bassiouny H, Giddens DP. Mechanical functional role of non-atherosclerotic intimal thickening. *Front Med Biol Eng.* 1993;5:37–43.

44. Wilens SL. The nature of diffuse intimal thickening of arteries. *Am J Pathol.* 1951;27:825–839.

45. Glagov S, Bassiounyz N, Masawa N, Giddens DP, Zarins CK. Induction and composition of intimal thickening and atherosclerosis. *Vasc Med.* 1993;293–296.

46. Tracy RE, Kissling GE. Age and fibroplasia as preconditions for atheronecrosis in human coronary arteries. *Arch Pathol Lab Med.* 1987;111:957–963.

47. Stary HC. The intimal macrophage in atherosclerosis. *Artery.* 1980;8:205–207.

48. Rifkin RD, Parisi AF, Folland E. Coronary calcification in the diagnosis of coronary artery disease. *Am J Cardiol.* 1979;44:141–147.

49. Imparato AM, Riles TS, Mintzer R, Baumann FG. The importance of hemorrhage in the relationship between gross morphologic characteristics and cerebral symptoms in 376 carotid artery plaques. *Ann Surg.* 1983;197:195–203.

50. Glagov S, Bassiouny HS, Giddens DP, Zarins CK. Pathobiology of plaque modeling and complication. *Surg Clin North Am.* 1995;75:545–556.

51. Glagov S. Intimal hyperplasia, vascular modeling, and the restenosis problem. *Circulation.* 1994;89:2888–2891.

52. Wolinsky H, Glagov S. Structural basis for the static mechanical properties of the aortic media. *Circ Res.* 1964;14:400–413.

53. Glagov S, Zarins CK. Quantitating atherosclerosis: Problems of definition. In: Gene Bond M, ed. *Clinical Diagnosis of Atherosclerosis.* New York: Springer-Verlag; 1983, pp. 11–35.

54. Zarins CK, Zatina MA, Glagov S. Correlation of postmortem angiography with pathologic anatomy: Quantitation of atherosclerotic lesions. In: Bond MG, Insull W Jr., Glagov S, eds. *Clinical Diagnosis of Atherosclerosis.* New York: Springer-Verlag; 1983, pp. 283–303.

55. Perrotta I. Ultrastructural features of human atherosclerosis. *Ultrastruct Pathol.* 2013;37:43–51.

56. Glagov S, Weisenberg E, Zarins CK, Stankunavicius R, Kolettis GJ. Compensatory enlargement of human atherosclerotic coronary arteries. *N Engl J Med.* 1987;316:1371–1375.

57. Zarins CK, Weisenberg E, Kolettis G, Stankunavicius R, Glagov S. Differential enlargement of artery segments in response to enlarging atherosclerotic plaques. *J Vasc Surg.* 1988;7:386–394.

58. Losordo DW, Rosenfield K, Kaufman J, Pieczek A, Isner JM. Focal compensatory enlargement of human arteries in response to progressive atherosclerosis. In vivo documentation using intravascular ultrasound. *Circulation.* 1994;89:2570–2577.

59. Vavuranakis M, Stefanadis C, Toutouzas K, Pitsavos C, Spanos V, Toutouzas P. Impaired compensatory coronary artery enlargement in atherosclerosis contributes to the development of coronary artery stenosis in diabetic patients: An in vivo intravascular ultrasound study. *Eur Heart J.* 1997;18:1090–1094.

60. Nakamura Y, Takemori H, Shiraishi K, Inoki I, Sakagami M, Shimakura A, Usuda K, Kubota K, Takata S, Kobayashi K. Compensatory enlargement of angiographically normal coronary segments in patients with coronary artery disease: In vivo documentation using intravascular ultrasound. *Angiology.* 1996;47:775–781.

61. Bonithon-Kopp C, Touboul PJ, Berr C, Magne C, Ducimetiere P. Factors of carotid arterial enlargement in a population aged 59 to 71 years: The eva study. *Stroke.* 1996;27:654–660.

62. Crouse JR, Goldbourt U, Evans G, Pinsky J, Sharrett AR, Sorlie P, Riley W, Heiss G. Risk factors and segment-specific carotid arterial enlargement in the atherosclerosis risk in communities (aric) cohort. *Stroke*. 1996;27:69–75.

63. Blair JM, Glagov S, Zarins CK. Mechanism of superficial femoral artery adductor canal stenosis. *Surg Forum*. 1990;41:359–360.

64. Pasterkamp G, Borst C, Post MJ, Mali WP, Wensing PJ, Gussenhoven EJ, Hillen B. Atherosclerotic arterial remodeling in the superficial femoral artery. Individual variation in local compensatory enlargement response. *Circulation*. 1996;93:1818–1825.

65. Zarins CK, Xu C, Glagov S. Clinical correlations of atherosclerosis: Aortic disease. In: Fuster V, ed. *Syndromes of Atherosclerosis: Correlations of Clinical Imaging and Pathology*. Armonk, NY: Futura Publishing; 1996, pp. 33–42.

66. Zarins C, Xu C, Glagov S. Aneurysmal and occlusive atherosclerosis of the human abdominal aorta. *J Vasc Surg*. 2001;33(1):91–96.

67. Zarins CK, Xu C, Glagov S. Atherosclerotic enlargement of the human abdominal aorta. *Atherosclerosis*. 2001;155:157–164.

68. Bond MG, Adams MR, Bullock BC. Complicating factors in evaluating coronary artery atherosclerosis. *Artery*. 1981;9:21–29.

69. Clarkson TB, Prichard RW, Morgan TM, Petrick GS, Klein KP. Remodeling of coronary arteries in human and nonhuman primates. *J Am Med Assoc*. 1994;271:289–294.

70. Beere PA, Glagov S, Zarins CK. Experimental atherosclerosis at the carotid bifurcation of the cynomolgus monkey: Localization, compensatory enlargement, and the sparing effect of lowered heart rate. *Arterioscler Thromb*. 1992;12:1245–1253.

71. Armstrong ML, Heistad DD, Marcus ML, Megan MB, Piegors DJ. Structural and hemodynamic response of peripheral arteries of macaque monkeys to atherogenic diet. *Arteriosclerosis*. 1985;5:336–346.

72. Holvoet P, Theilmeier G, Shivalkar B, Flameng W, Collen D. LDL hypercholesterolemia is associated with accumulation of oxidized LDL, atherosclerotic plaque growth, and compensatory vessel enlargement in coronary arteries of miniature pigs. *Arterioscler Thromb Vasc Biol*. 1998;18:415–422.

73. Birnbaum Y, Fishbein MC, Luo H, Nishioka T, Siegel RJ. Regional remodeling of atherosclerotic arteries: A major determinant of clinical manifestations of disease. *J Am Coll Cardiol*. 1997;30:1149–1164.

74. Wong CB. Atherosclerotic arterial remodeling in the superficial femoral artery: Individual variation in local compensatory enlargement response. *Circulation*. 1997;95:279–280.

75. Keren G. Compensatory enlargement, remodeling, and restenosis. *Adv Exp Med Biol*. 1997;430:187–196.

76. Smits PC, Bos L, Quarles van Ufford MA, Eefting FD, Pasterkamp G, Borst C. Shrinkage of human coronary arteries is an important determinant of de novo atherosclerotic luminal stenosis: An in vivo intravascular ultrasound study. *Heart*. 1998;79:143–147.

77. Ravensbergen J, Ravensbergen JW, Krijger JK, Hillen B, Hoogstraten HW. Localizing role of hemodynamics in atherosclerosis in several human vertebrobasilar junction geometries. *Arterioscler Thromb Vasc Biol*. 1998;18:708–716.

78. Karwowski JK, Markezich A, Whitson J, Abbruzzese TA, Zarins CK, Dalman RL. Dose-dependent limitation of arterial enlargement by the matrix metalloproteinase inhibitor RS-113,456. *J Surg Res*. 1999;87:122–129.

79. Masuda H, Zhuang YJ, Singh TM, Kawamura K, Murakami M, Zarins CK, Glagov S. Adaptive remodeling of internal elastic lamina and endothelial lining during flow-induced arterial enlargement. *Arterioscler Thromb Vasc Biol*. 1999;19:2298–2307.

80. Sho E, Sho M, Singh TM, Nanjo H, Komatsu M, Xu C, Masuda H, Zarins CK. Arterial enlargement in response to high flow requires early expression of matrix metalloproteinases to degrade extracellular matrix. *Exp Mol Pathol*. 2002;73:142–153.

81. Zarins CK, Zatina MA, Giddens DP, Ku DN, Glagov S. Shear stress regulation of artery lumen diameter in experimental atherogenesis. *J Vasc Surg*. 1987;5:413–420.

82. Kamiya A, Togawa T. Adaptive regulation of wall shear stress to flow change in the canine carotid artery. *Am J Physiol*. 1980;239:H14–21.

83. Masuda H, Bassiouny H, Glagov S, Zarins C. Artery wall restructuring in response to increased flow. *Surg Forum*. 1989;XL:285–286.

84. Guyton JR, Hartley CJ. Flow restriction of one carotid artery in juvenile rats inhibits growth of arterial diameter. *Am J Physiol*. 1985;248:H540–H546.

85. Singh TM, Zhuang Y-J, Masuda H, Zarins CK. Intimal hyperplasia in response to reduction of wall shear stress. *Surg Forum*. 1997;48:445–446.

86. Langille BL, O'Donnell F. Reductions in arterial diameter produced by chronic decreases in blood flow are endothelium-dependent. *Science*. 1986;231:405–407.

87. Furchgott RF. Role of endothelium in responses of vascular smooth muscle. *Circ Res*. 1983;53:557–573.

88. Zarins CK. Adaptive responses of arteries. *J Vasc Surg*. 1989;9:382.

89. Glagov S, Zarins C, Giddens DP, Ku DN. Hemodynamics and atherosclerosis. Insights and perspectives gained from studies of human arteries. *Arch Pathol Lab Med*. 1988;112:1018–1031.

90. Pohl U, Holtz J, Busse R, Bassenge E. Crucial role of endothelium in the vasodilator response to increased flow in vivo. *Hypertension*. 1986;8:37–44.

91. Hull SS Jr., Kaiser L, Jaffe MD, Sparks HV Jr. Endothelium-dependent flow-induced dilation of canine femoral and saphenous arteries. *Blood Vessels.* 1986;23:183–198.

92. Rubanyi GM, Romero JC, Vanhoutte PM. Flow-induced release of endothelium-derived relaxing factor. *Am J Physiol.* 1986;250:H1145–H1149.

93. Koller A, Sun D, Huang A, Kaley G. Corelease of nitric oxide and prostaglandins mediates flow-dependent dilation of rat gracilis muscle arterioles. *Am J Physiol.* 1994;267:H326–H332.

94. Davies PF. Flow-mediated endothelial mechano-transduction. *Physiol Rev.* 1995;75:519–560.

95. Cooke JP, Rossitch E Jr., Andon NA, Loscalzo J, Dzau VJ. Flow activates an endothelial potassium channel to release an endogenous nitrovasodilator. *J Clin Invest.* 1991;88:1663–1671.

96. Holtz J, Forstermann U, Pohl U, Giesler M, Bassenge E. Flow-dependent, endothelium-mediated dilation of epicardial coronary arteries in conscious dogs: Effects of cyclooxygenase inhibition. *J Cardiovasc Pharmacol.* 1984;6:1161–1169.

97. Miller VM, Burnett JC Jr. Modulation of no and endothelin by chronic increases in blood flow in canine femoral arteries. *Am J Physiol.* 1992;263:H103–H108.

98. Tronc F, Wassef M, Esposito B, Henrion D, Glagov S, Tedgui A. Role of no in flow-induced remodeling of the rabbit common carotid artery. *Arterioscler Thromb Vasc Biol.* 1996;16:1256–1262.

99. Guzman RJ, Abe K, Zarins CK. Flow-induced arterial enlargement is inhibited by suppression of nitric oxide synthase activity in vivo. *Surgery.* 1997;122:273–279; discussion 279–280.

100. Roberts JC, Moses C, Wilkins RH. Autopsy studies in atherosclerosis, I. Distribution and severity of atherosclerosis in patients dying without morphologic evidence of atherosclerotic catastrophe. *Circulation.* 1959;XX:511–519.

101. Stehbens WE. The role of hemodynamics in the pathogenesis of atherosclerosis. *Prog Cardiovasc Dis.* 1975;18:89–103.

102. Bharadvaj BK, Mabon RF, Giddens DP. Steady flow in a model of the human carotid bifurcation. Part I – Flow visualization. *J Biomech.* 1982;15:349–362.

103. Scharfstein H, Gutstein WH, Lewis L. Changes of boundary layer flow in model systems: Implications for initiation of endothelial injury. *Circ Res.* 1963;13:580–584.

104. Caro CG, Fitz-Gerald JM, Schroter RC. Atheroma and arterial wall shear: Observation, correlation and proposal of a shear dependent mass transfer mechanism for atherogenesis. *Proc Roy Soc Lond B Biol Sci.* 1971;177:109–159.

105. Tsao R, Jones SA, Giddens DP, Zarins CK, Glagov S. Measurement of particle residence time and particle acceleration in an arterial model by an automatic particle tracking system. *Proceedings, International Congress on High Speed Photography and Photonics,* Victoria, British Columbia, Canada, 1992.

106. Ross R, Harker L. Hyperlipidemia and atherosclerosis. *Science.* 1976;193:1094–1100.

107. Fry DL. Hemodynamic forces in atherogenesis. In: Scheinberg P, ed. *Cerebrovascular Disease.* New York: Raven Press; 1976, pp. 77–75.

108. De Keulenaer GW, Chappell DC, Ishizaka N, Nerem RM, Alexander RW, Griendling KK. Oscillatory and steady laminar shear stress differentially affect human endothelial redox state: Role of a superoxide-producing nadh oxidase. *Circ Res.* 1998;82:1094–1101.

109. Nerem RM, Levesque MJ, Cornhill JF. Vascular endothelial morphology as an indicator of the pattern of blood flow. *J Biomech Eng.* 1981;103:172–176.

110. Clark JM, Glagov S. Luminal surface of distended arteries by scanning electron microscopy: Eliminating configurational and technical artefacts. *Br J Exp Pathol.* 1976;57:129–135.

111. Dewey CF Jr., Bussolari SR, Gimbrone MA Jr., Davies PF. The dynamic response of vascular endothelial cells to fluid shear stress. *J Biomech Eng.* 1981;103:177–185.

112. Fry DL. Responses of the arterial wall to certain physical factors. *Ciba Found Symp.* 1973;12:93.

113. Ziegler T, Bouzourene K, Harrison VJ, Brunner HR, Hayoz D. Influence of oscillatory and unidirectional flow environments on the expression of endothelin and nitric oxide synthase in cultured endothelial cells. *Arterioscler Thromb Vasc Biol.* 1998;18:686–692.

114. Chappell DC, Varner SE, Nerem RM, Medford RM, Alexander RW. Oscillatory shear stress stimulates adhesion molecule expression in cultured human endothelium. *Circ Res.* 1998;82:532–539.

115. Bassiouny HS, Lee DC, Zarins CK, Glagov S. Low diurnal heart rate variability inhibits experimental carotid stenosis. *Surg Forum.* 1995;46:334–336.

116. Davies PF, Remuzzi A, Gordon EJ, Dewey CF Jr., Gimbrone MA Jr. Turbulent fluid shear stress induces vascular endothelial cell turnover in vitro. *Proc Natl Acad Sci USA.* 1986;83:2114–2117.

117. Khalifa AM, Giddens DP. Characterization and evolution poststenotic flow disturbances. *J Biomech.* 1981;14:279–296.

118. Coutard M, Osborne-Pellegrin MJ. Decreased dietary lipid deposition in spontaneous lesions distal to a stenosis in the rat caudal artery. *Artery.* 1983;12:182–198.

119. Kannel WB, Schwartz MJ, McNamara PM. Blood pressure and risk of coronary heart disease: The framingham study. *Dis Chest.* 1969;56:43.

120. Zarins CK, Giddens DP, Bharadvaj BK, Sottiurai VS, Mabon RF, Glagov S. Carotid bifurcation atherosclerosis. Quantitative correlation of plaque localization with flow velocity profiles and wall shear stress. *Circ Res.* 1983;53:502–514.

121. Ku DN, Giddens DP. Pulsatile flow in a model carotid bifurcation. *Arteriosclerosis.* 1983;3:31–39.

122. Bomberger RA, Zarins CK, Taylor KE, Glagov S. Effect of hypotension on atherogenesis and aortic wall composition. *J Surg Res.* 1980;28:402–409.

123. Beere PA, Glagov S, Zarins CK. Retarding effect of lowered heart rate on coronary atherosclerosis. *Science*. 1984;226:180–182.

124. Bassiouny HS, Zarins CK, Hovanessian A, Glagov, S. Heart rate and experimental carotid atherosclerosis. *Surg Forum*. 1992;XLIII:373.

125. Kannel WB, Kannel C, Paffenbarger RS Jr., Cupples LA. Heart rate and cardiovascular mortality: The framingham study. *Am Heart J*. 1987;113:1489–1494.

126. Wakhloo AK, Lieber BB, Seong J, Sadasivan C, Gounis MJ, Miskolczi L, Sandhu JS. Hemodynamics of carotid artery atherosclerotic occlusive disease. *J Vasc Interv Radiol*. 2004;15:S111–S121.

127. Rollo M, Tartaglione T, Pedicelli A, Settecasi C. Atherosclerosis of carotid and intracranial arteries. *Rays*. 2001;26:247–268.

128. Glagov S, Zarins CK. What are the determinants of plaque instability and its consequences? *J Vasc Surg*. 1989;9:389.

129. Bassiouny HS, Davis H, Massawa N, Gewertz BL, Glagov S, Zarins CK. Critical carotid stenoses: Morphologic and chemical similarity between symptomatic and asymptomatic plaques. *J Vasc Surg*. 1989;9:202–212.

130. Masawa N, Glagov S, Zarins CK. Quantitative morphologic study of intimal thickening at the human carotid bifurcation: I. Axial and circumferential distribution of maximum intimal thickening in asymptomatic, uncomplicated plaques. *Atherosclerosis*. 1994;107:137–146.

131. Masawa N, Glagov S, Zarins CK. Quantitative morphologic study of intimal thickening at the human carotid bifurcation: II. The compensatory enlargement response and the role of the intima in tensile support. *Atherosclerosis*. 1994;107:147–155.

132. Vito RP. *Measurement of Strain in Soft Biological Tissue Developments*. 1990.

133. Vito RP. *Stress Analysis of the Diseased Arterial Cross-Section*. 1990.

134. Stehbens WE. *Hemodynamics and the Blood Vessel Wall*. Springfield, IL: Charles C. Thomas; 1979.

135. Cozzi PJ, Lyon RT, Davis HR, Sylora J, Glagov S, Zarins CK. Aortic wall metabolism in relation to susceptibility and resistance to experimental atherosclerosis. *J Vasc Surg*. 1988;7:706–714.

136. Lyon RT, Runyon-Hass A, Davis HR, Glagov S, Zarins CK. Protection from atherosclerotic lesion formation by reduction of artery wall motion. *J Vasc Surg*. 1987;5:59–67.

137. Klocke FJ, Mates RE, Canty JMJ, Ellis AK. Coronary pressure-flow relationships. Controversial issues and probable implications. *Circ Res*. 1985;56:310–323.

138. Granata L, Olsson RA, Huvos A, Gregg DE. Coronary inflow and oxygen usage following cardiac sympathetic nerve stimulation in unanesthetized dogs. *Cir Res*. 1965;16:114–120.

139. Zarins CK, Glagov S, Giddens DP, Ku DN. Hemodynamic factors and atherosclerotic change in the aorta. In: Bergan JJ, Yao JST, eds. *Aortic Surgery*. Philadelphia, PA: W.B. Saunders; 1988, pp. 17–25.

140. Ku DN, Glagov S, Moore JE Jr., Zarins CK. Flow patterns in the abdominal aorta under simulated postprandial and exercise conditions: An experimental study. *J Vasc Surg*. 1989;9:309–316.

141. Dobrin PB, Baker WH, Gley WC. Elastolytic and collagenolytic studies of arteries. Implications for the mechanical properties of aneurysms. *Arch Surg*. 1984;119:405–409.

142. Menashi S, Campa JS, Greenhalgh RM, Powell JT. Collagen in abdominal aortic aneurysm: Typing, content, and degradation. *J Vasc Surg*. 1987;6:578–582.

143. Cohen JR, Mandell C, Margolis I, Chang J, Wise L. Altered aortic protease and antiprotease activity in patients with ruptured abdominal aortic aneurysms. *Surg Gynecol Obstet*. 1987;164:355–358.

144. Tilson MD. A perspective on research in abdominal aortic aneurysm disease with unifying hypothesis. In: Bergan JJ, Yao JST, eds. *Aortic Surgery*. Philadelphia, PA: Saunders; 1989, pp. 355–358.

145. Xu C, Zarins CK, Glagov S. Aneurysmal and occlusive atherosclerosis of the human abdominal aorta. *J Vasc Surg*. 2001;33:91–96.

146. Zarins CK, Glagov S. Aneurysms and obstructive plaques: Differing local responses to atherosclerosis. In: Bergan JJ, Yao JST, eds. *Aneurysms, Diagnosis and Treatment*. New York: Grune and Stratton, Inc.; 1982, pp. 61–82.

147. Zatina MA, Zarins CK, Gewertz BL, Glagov S. Role of medial lamellar architecture in the pathogenesis of aortic aneurysms. *J Vasc Surg*. 1984;1:442–448.

148. Zarins CK, Glagov S, Vesselinovitch D et al. Aneurysm formation in experimental atherosclerosis: Relationship to plaque evolution. *J Vasc Surg*. 1990;12:246–256.

149. Strickland HL, Bond MG. Aneurysms in a large colony of squirrel monkeys (*Saimiri sciureus*). *Lab Anim Sci*. 1983;33:589–592.

150. Zarins CK, Xu CP, Glagov S. Aneurysmal enlargement of the aorta during regression of experimental atherosclerosis. *J Vasc Surg*. 1992;15:90–98; discussion 99–101.

151. Glagov SZ, Zarins CK. Pathophysiology of aneurysm of formation. In: Kerstein M, Moulder PV, Webb WR, eds. *Aneurysms*. Baltimore, MD: Williams & Wilkins; 1983, pp. 1–18.

152. Zarins CK, Runyon-Hass A, Zatina MA, Lu CT, Glagov S. Increased collagenase activity in early aneurysmal dilatation. *J Vasc Surg*. 1986;3:238–248.

153. Goergen CJ, Johnson BL, Greve JM, Taylor CA, Zarins CK. Increased anterior abdominal aortic wall motion: Possible role in aneurysm pathogenesis and design of endovascular devices. *J Endovasc Ther*. 2007;14:574–584.

154. Gordon T, Kannel WB. Predisposition to atherosclerosis in the head, heart, and legs: The framingham study. *J Am Med Assoc*. 1972;221:661–666.

155. Glagov S, Rowley DA, Kohut R. Atherosclerosis of human aorta and its coronary and renal arteries. *Arch Pathol*. 1961;72:82–95.

156. Xu C, Zarins CK, Pannaraj PS, Bassiouny HS, Glagov S. Hypercholesterolemia superimposed by experimental hypertension induces differential distribution of collagen and elastin. *Arterioscler Thromb Vasc Biol.* 2000;20:2566–2572.

157. Strandness DE. Workshop overview. In: Bond MG, Insull W Jr., Glagov S, eds. *Clinical Diagnosis of Atherosclerosis.* New York: Springer-Verlag; 1983, pp. 1–9.

158. Greene ER, Eldridg MW, Voyles WF. Quantitative evaluation of atherosclerosis using doppler ultrasound. In: Bond MG, Insull W Jr., Glagov S, eds. *Clinical Diagnosis of Atherosclerosis.* New York: Springer-Verlag; 1983, pp. 8–168.

159. Isner JM, Kishel J, Kent KM, Ronan JA Jr., Ross AM, Roberts WC. Accuracy of angiographic determination of left main coronary arterial narrowing: Angiographic—Histologic correlative analysis in 28 patients. *Circulation.* 1981;63:1056–1064.

160. Zarins CK, Giddens DP, Glagov S. Atherosclerotic plaque distribution and flow velocity profiles in the carotid bifurcation. In: Bergan JJ, Yao JST, eds. *Cerebrovascular Insufficiency.* New York: Grune & Stratton; 1983, pp. 19–30.

3

Hemodynamics and non-invasive testing

DORAN MIX and ANKUR CHANDRA

CONTENTS

HEMODYNAMICS

Introduction

As dictated by biologic principles, once an aerobic organism's total cell mass is large enough that simple diffusion from the environment cannot provide the necessary components for cellular metabolism, a circulatory system is required. If you were to take a moment and try to design a circulatory system of your own, you will begin to realize that certain components are required. As the majority of cells in an organism find themselves in an aqueous environment, the most efficient design of a circulatory system is to provide bulk transport through flow of an aqueous solution. Most importantly, this circulatory system must provide bulk transport of required components of cellular metabolism and a means for the cell to expel toxic by-products. This bulk transport of metabolites must occur at a rate greater than or equal to the rate of cellular metabolism. In animals, the perfusion solution blood uses the basic chemical properties of iron in the form of hemoglobin to increase the capacity at which oxygen can be transported. By increasing the efficiency of the metabolite-carrying capacity, the flow rate of the blood is decreased so that the cells circulating in the blood are not destroyed by the forces within the blood vessel.

As its name implies, hemodynamics examines the nature of both blood flow and vessel wall mechanics within the human body using basic, Newtonian principles. It is easy to become quickly overwhelmed with mathematical equations when approaching the topic of hemodynamics. Therefore, it is helpful to break the topic into its fundamental concepts before attempting to memorize endless combinations of Greek letters. At its core, hemodynamics is nothing more than a form of energy accounting that invokes the law of conservation of energy. This law of physics states that the total energy in an isolated system cannot be created or destroyed but must be conserved over time. Another way to conceptualize this is if, at any given time, you add all the expended energy in a system to the energy remaining, it must always equal the original energy in the system. Applied to the circulatory system, if you take the original blood pressure in the system (original potential energy) and subtract it from the current blood pressure (remaining potential energy) in the system, the difference is the total energy lost through this portion of the circulation. These losses include blood velocity (kinetic energy), heat-generated (friction/thermal) energy and sound waves (mechanical energy). These energy transfers are dynamic, and, just as changes in pressure energy can be the source of changes in blood velocity, changes in blood velocity can be the source for changes in pressure energy. The only energy in a system that must remain constant is the total energy of the system.

There are many complex hemodynamic equations that go to great lengths to account for the precise location and events for every joule of energy in the circulatory system. For this chapter, we will invoke the equations that make intuitive sense in the hope that these concepts might help in solving practical clinical problems. Following our discussion of hemodynamics, we will examine the ways in which these theoretical principles are currently applied in the non-invasive vascular lab.

Newtonian mechanics

When first considering the concept of fluid energy, it should start with an understanding of Newton's second law of motion. This states that an object's acceleration (*a*) is directly proportional to the net force (*F*) working on the object and inversely proportional to the object's mass (*m*). Frequently, Newton's second law of motion is mathematically summarized as the definition of force:

$$Accleration(a) = \frac{Net\ force(F)}{Object\ mass(m)} = \frac{F}{m} \qquad (3.1)$$

$$F = mass * accleration = m * a$$

Intuitively, Newton's original statement makes more sense that for a given mass, a larger force will result in a greater acceleration, and conversely, for a given net force, a larger mass will result in a smaller acceleration.

When depicting Newton's second law, a common example is of a bowling ball falling off a cliff, where the mass of the bowling ball can be measured and the acceleration is provided by the gravitational force of the earth (Figure 3.1). In order to determine the conservation of energy in this system, we must first define what energy is. Mechanical energy can be defined as a force multiplied by a distance:

$$Energy = Force * Change\ in\ distance = F * \Delta d \quad (3.2)$$

The energy in the bowling ball exists in two forms of mechanical energy, potential energy and kinetic energy. The first form of energy, potential energy, is energy stored in the system. Consider holding the bowling ball off of a cliff without dropping it for which the ball has a potential energy stored within it created by gravitational

acceleration (*g*). The potential energy of this bowling ball system

$$Potential\ energy = F * h = (m * a) * h = m * g * h \qquad (3.3)$$

is defined by substituting the definition of force (3.1) with the mass of the bowling ball and gravitational acceleration (*g*). The distance (Δd) is the height (*h*) or time for which gravitational acceleration can continue to influence the object unopposed by other forces. Importantly, once the mass of the ball and gravitational field are defined, the only variable that can change the energy in the system is the height (*h*) of the ball from the ground.

If the bowling ball is released, the potential energy stored in the bowling ball is converted to downward motion. This downward motion is known as kinetic energy or the energy which is being actively consumed in the system. During the fall, the location of the bowling ball can be determined by the length of time the ball has been falling or the period of time that gravitational acceleration has acted on the ball:

$$\Delta distance = \frac{1}{2} * a * \Delta t^2 \qquad (3.4)$$

The kinetic energy in the system can also intuitively be defined as the distance the ball has travelled (3.4) because that distance defines the energy that has been used up by the bowling ball at a given point in time. The distance can be substituted into the definition of energy (3.2) to precisely calculate the kinetic energy of the system. This definition of kinetic energy

$$Kinetic\ energy = F * \Delta d = (m * a) * \left(\frac{1}{2} * a * \Delta t^2 \right) \quad (3.5)$$

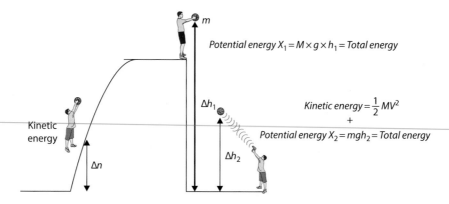

Figure 3.1 Newtonian mechanics as depicted by a bowling ball held off a cliff. Prior to release, the total energy of the bowling ball is all potential energy. Once released, the total energy of the ball is unchanged and equal to the sum of the kinetic energy as defined by its velocity and potential energy as defined by its height off the ground. In this example, the velocity of the bowling ball can be measured using a radar gun which utilizes the Doppler effect. The gun transmits a sound wave at a given frequency (depicted in red) and based on the velocity of the falling ball, the wave is reflected at a shifted frequency (depicted in green).

illustrates an important point about calculating energies in an experimental system. In our bowling ball experiment, mass is typically measured at the beginning of the experiment and assumed to be constant throughout the duration. Determining the change in time and the acceleration of a biologic system may be more complicated if not impossible without disrupting the system being studied. These potential errors in measurement propagate and lead to errors in system energy calculations. Certain variables, such as velocity, can be experimentally obtained with an instrument such as a speed gun, which derives velocity using the Doppler effect without largely changing the energy in the system. Algebraically, we could change our definition of kinetic energy (3.5) by rearranging the definition of acceleration

$$Acceleration(a) = \frac{v}{\Delta time} \quad or \quad \Delta time = \frac{v}{a} \quad (3.6)$$

to solve for change in time (Δt). This redefines kinetic energy based on the experimental measured value of velocity:

$$Kinetic\, energy = F * \Delta d = m * a * \left(\frac{1}{2} * \frac{v^2}{a} \right) = \frac{1}{2} * m * v^2 \quad (3.7)$$

The law of conservation of energy

$$Kinetic\, energy + Potential\, energy$$

$$= \frac{1}{2} * m * v^2 + m * g * h = Total\, energy \quad (3.8)$$

describes that the original total energy in the system, which was defined by the potential energy of the ball dangling off the cliff, must be equal to the summations of the potential and kinetic energies in the system at any point in time after the ball is dropped. If the total energy of the original system cannot be calculated, the summation of kinetic energy and potential energy at a given point in time (t_0) can be equated to the summation of kinetic energy and potential energy at any other time point (t_1) in the system

$$Kinetic\, energy_{t0} + Potential\, energy_{t0}$$

$$= Kinetic\, energy_{t1} + Potential\, energy_{t1} \quad (3.9)$$

The bowling ball example also implies that the potential energy found in the ball must itself be derived from some previously expanded source. In this case, the kinetic energy was spent carrying the bowling ball up the cliff. One of the finer points of hemodynamic study, which is commonly overlooked, is the fact that mass is the variable that determines the *maximum energy content* of a system.

This *mass–energy equivalence* is in part the relationship that Einstein was describing in his theory of *special relativity*

$$E = m * c^2 \quad (3.10)$$

and provides the link between biologic systems and celestial objects.

Fluid energy

POTENTIAL ENERGY

To transition the concept of the energies of a falling bowling ball to hemodynamic energies, it is imperative to remember is that a liquid, by its nature, is obligated to take the shape of its container. Therefore, it is easier to define a liquid by a volume and then calculate its mass. In order to calculate the mass of a given fluid, from a given fluid volume, we must know the density of the fluid in question:

$$\rho = \frac{Mass}{Volume} = \frac{m}{V} \quad (3.11)$$

The concept of blood density provides the first complicating factor in our attempt to understand human hemodynamics. Blood is a compressible, non-Newtonian fluid which means its density is a variable depending on the temperature, flow, disease state and patient. Blood is simplified to an incompressible, Newtonian fluid by the assumption that blood density in the macrovascular circulation is relatively constant. Therefore, when calculating a given patient's fluid-energy state, the density of blood is constant before and after transitions of energy states of interest.

When describing the potential energy of a human blood volume (3.2), both the force of a blood volume and the distance for which acceleration can work on that blood volume must be included. Clinically, the term force is not used, but rather the measured value of pressure

$$Pressure = \frac{Force}{Area} = \frac{F}{A} \quad (3.12)$$

which is force divided by area. It is critical to differentiate pressure and force since a force (F) can be used to produce a pressure when applied to an area (A), but the terms are not interchangeable. The next challenge is to define pressure as a potential energy. One might not think that pressure can be defined as energy but the act of obtaining an intravascular pressure measurement, with a *pressure transducer*, allows the conversion of one form of energy (pressure) to another (voltage). The very fact that pressure energy is *transduced* would imply that pressure is a form of energy. By multiplying the definition of pressure (3.12) by distance, pressure can be defined as a unit of energy divided by a volume. Thus, pressure can be conceptualized as *volumetric energy*:

$$Pressure = \frac{F}{A} = \frac{F*d}{A*d} = \frac{Potential\,energy}{Volume} \quad (3.13)$$

Because hemodynamics involves a fluid system, we can redefine pressure by substituting the definition of force and simplify the *mass per unit volume* term as the density of the fluid in the system:

$$Pressure = \frac{F*d}{A*d} = \frac{m*a*d}{V} = \rho*a*d \quad (3.14)$$

Applying Equation 3.14 to human anatomy allows for the definition of key hemodynamic terms. When a person stands up from a seated position, the static volume of blood filling their vessels will have a downward gravitational acceleration (g). The height difference of this blood column can be defined at any given point along the blood vessel and will produce a pressure that is proportional to the density of the blood itself. In the human circulatory system, the right atrium is defined at a height equal to zero; therefore, the reference pressure at the right atrium is also equal to zero. As the distance from the right atrium to the foot is defined opposite to the direction of gravitation acceleration, hydrostatic pressure is defined as negative or in a direction towards the ankle:

$$Hydrostatic\,pressure = -\rho*g*h \quad (3.15)$$

Hydrostatic pressure is analogous to a glass of water; if the glass's height is defined by the top of the glass, the pressure of water, and therefore the mass, is greatest at the bottom of the glass. Hydrostatic pressure can be the dominant pressure in a human leg based on the height of the person. Using known values of blood density and gravitational force, every centimetre below the right atrium creates ~0.8 mmHg of pressure. For an individual whose right atrium is 100 cm above the ankle, the hydrostatic pressure is approximately 80 mmHg. A clinical correlate is in critical limb ischemia and rest pain. When a patient places their leg in a dependent position, they create a height differential (Δh) and hydrostatic pressure, or volumetric energy, which results in increased peripheral flow through dermal capillary perfusion.

When a human stands, it would be an evolutionary disadvantage to have their lower extremity vessels expand and fill with their complete blood volume. In part, the vascular tree does not expand due primarily to the medial and adventitial layers of the vessel wall providing a balancing tensile force to this load. This force created by the blood vessel and applied over its area is called the static filling pressure and works opposite to the hydrostatic pressure; thus its sign is inverted:

$$Static\,filling\,pressure = \rho*g*h \quad (3.16)$$

In the artery, the static filling pressure is augmented by the biologic function of the arterial tissue. Whenever the smooth muscle cells of an arterial wall are stretched, special stretch-active ion channels, primarily in the arterioles, lead to contraction proportional to the stretch. This effect, known as the Bayliss effect or myogenic response, is not only important to augmenting the total peripheral resistance, but also in providing energy to maintain forward flow during the diastolic cycle.

It is important to note here that pressure, as derived earlier, is subtly different than clinical blood pressure. Hemodynamics describes events as idealized equations captured at a moment in time. Thus far, gravity has been the only acceleration applied to the blood volume. In the human arterial system, the primary source of energy in the human body is the *dynamic cardiac pressure* (P_{DC}) created by the contraction of the heart. Thus, the total potential energy in the circulatory system can be described by the sum of dynamic cardiac pressure (P_{DC}), hydrostatic pressure and static filling pressure. The clinically obtained blood pressure is a summation of all the pressures acting on the human circulatory system. Since pressure is the source of potential energy in the human circulatory system, velocity becomes the sink or consumer of this energy.

KINETIC ENERGY

Just as the potential energy of a bowling ball on a cliff can be translated into *volumetric energy* or pressure, the kinetic energy of the falling ball can be translated into *volumetric energy* as well. By substituting the definition of kinetic energy (3.7) based on velocity of a mass, and dividing by its volume, fluid kinetic energy is defined as the square of the fluid velocity multiplied by its density divided by two:

$$Fluid\,kinetic\,energy = \frac{Kinetic\,energy}{Volume} = \frac{\frac{1}{2}*m*v^2}{Volume} = \frac{1}{2}*\rho*v^2$$

$$(3.17)$$

Previously, we emphasized the importance of defining kinetic energy by a term that can be accurately measured without perturbing the system itself. In the bowling ball example, the Doppler effect with a radar gun is used to measure the velocity of the ball. Kinetic fluid energy is nearly negligible in a healthy subject but becomes the dominate energy sink in the disease state. Blood velocity is measured non-invasively in the vascular lab with the Doppler effect through duplex imaging. These measurements must be accurate to reduce the misidentification of disease when none exists.

TOTAL ENERGY

The law of conservation of energy can now be applied using the definitions of fluid potential energy and fluid kinetic energy to determine total fluid energy. This is known as Bernoulli's principle:

$$Total\,energy = Potential\,energy + Kinetic\,energy$$

$$Total\,fluid\,energy = \frac{Potential\,energy}{Volume} + \frac{Kinetic\,energy}{Volume}$$

$$Total\,fluid\,energy = Pressure + \frac{1}{2}*\rho*v^2$$

$$Pressure_{t0} + \frac{1}{2}*\rho*v_{t0}^2 = Pressure_{t1} + \frac{1}{2}*\rho*v_{t1}^2$$

$$Pressure_{t0} - Pressure_{t1} = \frac{1}{2}*\rho*v_{t1}^2 - \frac{1}{2}*\rho*v_{t0}^2$$

$$Pressure_{t0} - Pressure_{t1} = \frac{1}{2}*\rho*\left(v_{t1}^2 - v_{t0}^2\right)$$

(3.18)

A common clinical application of Bernoulli's principle is used to estimate a pressure drop across a stenosis in a blood vessel or cardiac valve through the change in velocity created by the stenosis (Figure 3.2). Bernoulli's continuity equation also illustrates an import difference between fluid flow and fluid kinetic energy. Fluid kinetic energy, and its velocity term, is commonly incorrectly considered synonymous with flow. Blood flow is often reported in litres per minute or, more simplistically, as a change in volume over a change in time:

$$Flow = \frac{\Delta Volume}{\Delta Time}$$

(3.19)

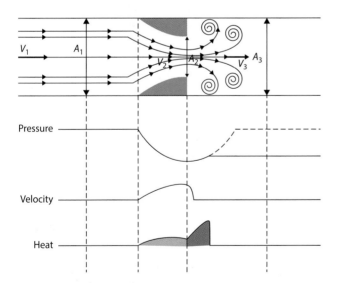

Figure 3.2 Depiction of a pressure drop created by a stenosis from the consumption of fluid potential energy or pressure with an increase in fluid kinetic energy or fluid velocity. Note that pressure does not return to its original energy state (as indicated by the red dotted line) secondary to the heat energy lost. Velocity must return to its original energy state as flow must be conserved, so $A_1 * V_1 = A_2 * V_2 = A_3 * V_3$. Heat loss occurs due to viscous energy loss (orange area under the heat curve) and expansion losses (green area under the heat curve).

In a cylindrical blood vessel, flow can also be defined by its geometric terms. That is, the volume of a cylinder is equal to the cross-sectional area of the cylinder multiplied by the cylinder's length over a given unit of time. The length-divided-by-time relationship is equivalent to velocity:

$$Flow = \frac{\Delta Volume}{\Delta Time} = \frac{Area * \Delta length}{\Delta Time} = Area * Velocity$$

(3.20)

The example of Bernoulli's Equation in Figure 3.2 depends on fluid flow being constant. If one compared the velocity of blood at an area ($Area_1$) before a stenosis to the velocity of the blood at the smallest area within the stenosis ($Area_2$), the velocity must increase in order for fluid flow to remain constant:

$$Flow = Area_1 * Velocity_1 = Area_2 * Velocity_2$$
$$= Area_3 * Velocity_3$$
$$And\,if$$
$$Area_1 = Area_3$$
$$Then$$
$$Velocity_1 = Velocity_3$$

(3.21)

Similarly, if the vessel area before ($Area_1$) and after ($Area_3$) the stenosis where equal, then the velocities before ($Velocity_1$) and after ($Velocity_3$) the stenosis would also be equal in order to maintain a uniform flow. Here, flow is constant, while velocity is dependent on changes in luminal area. Further distinguishing fluid flow from fluid kinetic energy is that fluid flow does not describe the physical properties of the fluid in transit. If, for example, a vessel with a radius of 1 cm had 1 L of water pushed through it versus 1 L of mercury over 1 minute, the flows (1 L/min) and velocity (318.3 cm/min) would be the same, but the kinetic energy of the mercury system would be greater due to the greater density of mercury. The key difference being that the definition of flow lacks the variable of mass which is needed to define energy. Therefore, the distinction between fluid flow and fluid kinetic energy should be clearly delineated.

Fluid energy loss

The application of Bernoulli's principle to a vessel stenosis would predict that the pressure before and after a vessel narrowing should be equivalent. Clinically, it is understood that pressure drops after a stenosis. This loss of energy is the effect of frictional energy loss in the form of heat. When blood is flowing within a vessel, friction occurs at two primary sites of interaction. The first interaction occurs at the blood-vessel wall interface and the second occurs as a result of red blood cells

(RBCs) rubbing against each other at varying velocities. Intuitively, the effect of blood-vessel wall interface is typically much greater than the effect of blood cell–blood cell interaction. In order to simplify fluid dynamic equations, the velocity of the blood at the vessel wall is assumed to approach zero. Within large blood vessels, only a few RBC, relative to the total number of cells in the cross-sectional area of the vessel, are on the periphery to interact with the vessel wall resulting in negligible frictional energy losses. In smaller vessels, a greater percentage of RBCs are interacting with the vessel wall, and thus, the frictional loss is greater. These frictional losses cause the RBC near the vessel wall to have less kinetic energy and, therefore, a lower velocity compared to the RBC in the centre of flow (Figure 3.3).

The RBC at the periphery also has a partial interaction with the next RBC towards the centreline of flow. These parallel *layers* of blood cell interactions exponentially decrease from the vessel wall to the centreline of flow, such that the kinetic energy and velocity of the blood in the centreline of flow is greatest. Viscosity (η) is the physical measurement of how strongly particles of flowing fluid interact with each other. When observing a flowing liquid, viscosity can roughly be determined by how much the fluid resists flow in that fluids with greater viscosity have greater resistance to flow. As the RBC at the periphery has less kinetic energy than the RBC at the centreline, the energy difference must have been translated into another form of energy. Due to the frictional interaction of the blood and vessel, the energy is lost as pressure energy and can be calculated using Poiseuille's equation:

$$Input\ force = \Delta P * A = \Delta P * \left(\pi * r^2\right)$$

$$Viscous\ force = \left(2 * \pi * r * L\right) * n * \frac{dv}{dr}$$

$$\Delta P * \left(\pi * r^2\right) - \left(2 * \pi * r * L\right) * n * \frac{dv}{dr} = 0 \qquad (3.22)$$

$$Q = \frac{\pi * \Delta P * R^4}{8 * n * L}$$

$$R = \frac{\Delta P}{Q} = \frac{8 * n * L}{\pi * R^4}$$

To derive Poiseuille's equation, the forces acting on the vessel are derived using a rearrangement of the definition of pressure (3.13).

The force produced by the pressure drop across the vessel is multiplied by the vessel cross-sectional area. The force produced by the viscous blood's interaction with the vessel wall is calculated by the area of the vessel lumen multiplied by the shear stress (τ) on the vessel wall:

$$Shear\ stress\ \tau\left(r\right) = \mu * \frac{dv}{dr} \qquad (3.23)$$

The velocity gradient term is then solved for flow through a cylinder.

It is shear stress that accounts for the viscous frictional loss of energy that occurs across a vessel with a given radius and length for a particular fluid flow. Complicating shear stress, as mentioned previously, is that blood is a heterogeneous, non-Newtonian fluid with a viscosity that varies with changes in velocity. In large vessels, however, blood behaves as a Newtonian fluid and shear stress is directly proportional to changes in velocities between adjacent flow layers. The endothelial layer also actively detects shear stress and modulates it via nitric oxide–mediated vasodilation. A clinical example of shear stress modulating vessel diameter is the arterial dilation that can occur proximal to a patent hemodialysis fistula. By increasing the vessel diameter, shear stress at the vessel wall is decreased. Shear stress has also been proposed to modulate angiogenesis via shear stress–regulated gene expression. At areas of changing vessel geometry, like the carotid bulb, where a component of the velocity profile must decrease secondary to the shape of the vessel, regions exist where the velocity profile and shear stress approach zero. These low-velocity eddy currents create an environment which is prone to the development of atherosclerotic plaques. Predicting the velocity profile across complex vessel geometries can be mathematically challenging but evolving computational fluid dynamic simulation tools allow for modelling of complex in vivo flow profiles (Figure 3.4).

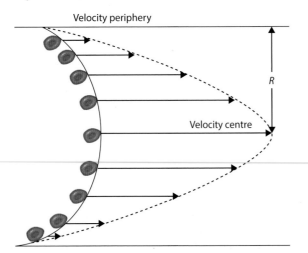

Figure 3.3 Laminar flow occurs in a parabolic shape as the interaction of the red blood cells with the vessel wall creates an energy loss that reduces the velocity of the blood at the periphery ($V_{periphery}$) where the velocity of blood in the centreline of flow ($V_{centreline}$) is relatively unopposed.

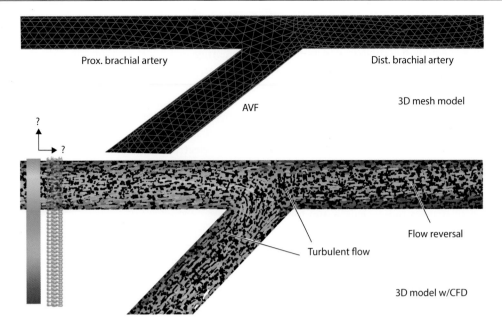

Figure 3.4 Example of computational fluid dynamic simulation tool used to simulate the complex flow patterns involved in steal syndrome. (From Chandra A et al., *Vascular*, 21(1), 54, February 2013.)

Because Poiseuille's equation is dependent on laminar or parabolic flow, it underestimates the pressure drop that occurs when flow becomes non-laminar. Once a flow pattern transitions from laminar to turbulent, the resulting pressure drop is the square of the flow rate. The Reynolds number (R_e) is an attempt to mathematically predict the fluid dynamic factors that regulate when fluid transitions from laminar parabolic flow to turbulent *plug flow*:

$$R_e = \frac{(2*R)*v*\rho}{\mu} \qquad (3.24)$$

Factors that directly affect the Reynolds number are vessel radius (R), mean flow velocity (v) and the ratio of fluid density to fluid viscosity (ρ/μ), also known as the kinematic viscosity. Typically, a Reynolds number of greater than 2000 will predict flow transition to turbulent flow. It is important to understand that the Reynolds number is simply a ratio which is dependent upon many additional factors. The most accurate method to determine when flow has transitioned is when a linear relationship stops between flow and pressure drop as predicted by Poiseuille's equation (Figure 3.5). Typically, turbulent flow does not occur within the human circulatory system, with the notable clinical exception of hemodialysis access. The classic thrill that is detected with the creation of hemodialysis access has been proposed to represent turbulence secondary to the high flow rate.

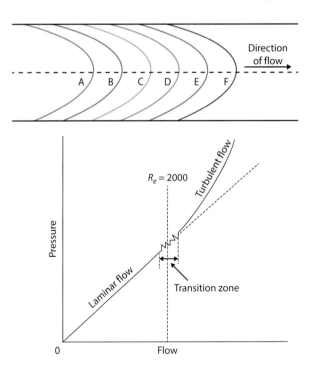

Figure 3.5 Graphical depiction of the Reynolds number when the pressure gradient across a vessel transitions from a linear pressure drop as related to fluid flow to an exponential pressure drop as related to fluid flow. Typically, a Reynolds number of 2000 is used to mark the transition, but the transition zone from laminar to turbulent flow can occur for a range of Reynolds numbers. The velocity profiles labelled (A) through (F) show the transition from laminar to turbulent flow. (From Nichols WW et al., *McDonald's Blood Flow in Arteries: Theoretic, Experimental, and Clinical Principles*, 5th ed., Hodder Arnold, London, UK, 2005.)

Vascular resistance

Frequently, Poiseuille's equation is compared to its electrical analogue, Ohm's law,

$$Voltage = Current * Resistance \quad or \quad V = I * R$$
$$Pressure = Flow * Resistance \quad or \quad \Delta P = Q * R, \tag{3.25}$$

in order to define vascular resistance. The concept of vascular resistance is also used to demonstrate the relationship between a pressure gradient that occurs across a stenosis in terms of stenosis radius, length and flow as demonstrated by Poiseuille's equation (3.22).

Resistance is directly proportional to length (L) and is inversely proportional to vessel radius to the 4th power. A practical application of this relationship dictates that a 50% stenosis reduces the pressure by a factor of 16, whereas a 75% lumen reduction would reduce the pressure by a factor of 256, showing the effect of radius change to an exponential power. For this same example, a stenosis whose length is doubled will only reduce the pressure by a factor of two. Additionally, there is a well-described relationship between increased flow across a fixed vascular stenosis and increased pressure gradient across that stenosis.

The human body can regulate vascular bed resistance to overcome certain disease states. The purpose of the circulatory system is to provide bulk transport for cellular metabolism and its by-products through regulation of blood flow. Flow can only be provided at the expense of kinetic energy, and kinetic energy can only be provided by a source of potential energy, in this case pressure. When an arterial stenosis is present, energy is lost due to viscous energy losses as well as heat losses that occur due to fluid inertia at both the entry and exit of the stenotic segment. The body has a large physiologic reserve and can autoregulate blood flow in many different terminal vascular beds. If a stenosis is *critical*, however, the pressure drop across the stenosis is too great for the distal vascular bed to compensate. This failure of autoregulation results in distal, vascular bed ischemia secondary to the loss of proximal potential energy or pressure.

Vascular resistance can be used to describe the effect of a stenosis within a vascular circuit. Stenoses that are found sequentially within the same vascular bed, or in series, have an additive effect on the pressure drop across a vessel. This effect occurs because the conservation of flow dictates that in a series, the flow across each stenosis must be equal, and so the energy lost at each stenosis is cumulative. This means that often multiple small stenoses, whose individual pressure drops would not cause distal ischemia, can result in tissue ischemia when located in series causing the same effect as one *critical stenosis*:

$$Series\ resistance = R_1 + R_2 + R_3 \tag{3.26}$$

The *in series* vascular resistance concept also offers insight into how procedures such as percutaneous angioplasty, stenting or endarterectomy provide therapeutic benefit. The *critical stenosis* is removed out of the series with the remaining vascular and replaced with a low-resistance-treated artery. Flow is restored without the loss of kinetic energy from the stenotic lesion.

Vascular resistances found in parallel also behave like their electrical analogues in that the parallel paths reciprocal resistances are additive:

$$\frac{1}{Total\ parallel\ resistance} = \frac{1}{R_1} + \frac{1}{R_2} + \frac{1}{R_3}$$

$$\frac{1}{Total\ parallel\ resistance} = \frac{1}{R_X} + \frac{N}{R_Y} \tag{3.27}$$

$$Total\ parallel\ resistance = \frac{R_Y * R_X}{R_Y + (R_X * N)}$$

Unlike a series circuit where the flow across each of the lesions must be uniform, a parallel circuit will allow flow to preferentially follow the path of the least resistance. The development of collateral circulation helps to illustrate how reciprocal resistances function. Imagine a hemodynamically significant vascular stenosis. The human body's physiologic response to a *critical stenosis* is to form high-resistance collateral pathways around the stenosis in order to re-establish distal flow. Collateral pathways are small channels with relatively high fixed resistance. In order for collaterals to compensate for their small size, a large number of collaterals form to decrease the net resistance of the obstructed path. As an example, consider a critically stenotic vessel with resistance (R_X) and (N) collateral arteries with a resistance (R_Y) that bypass the stenosis. Collateral arteries are small and their resistance is considered to be fixed. Even if R_Y is assumed to be 10 times that of R_X, one collateral pathway around the stenosis only reduces the resistance by 10%, but 5 collateral channels will reduce the overall resistance of the pathway by 45%. Remembering that vascular resistance is directly proportional to the pressure lost across a stenosis, these collateral pathways directly reduce the pressure lost across a lesion and increase the energy available for distal perfusion. Unlike in-line procedures, surgical bypasses work on the premise of providing a low-resistance, parallel pathway. By establishing a low-resistance bypass, the surgeon provides a high flow path thereby decreasing the overall pressure drop and energy lost across a critical lesion.

The human arterial tree is comprised of many vascular branches that contain multiple divisions and collateral pathways (Figure 3.6a). Physiologically, it is necessary to maintain a constant pressure at each of the bifurcations in the human arterial tree. Similar to a parallel circuit, the proximal inflow to a vascular branch must equal the summation of the flows in each of the bifurcations (Figure 3.6b). Branches, unlike parallel circuits, do not

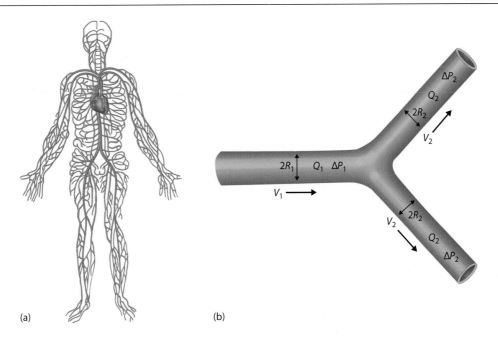

Figure 3.6 (a) The human arterial circulation is comprised of multiple branches with paths in both parallel and series circuits. (b) A theoretical model of each branch can be constructed based on Poiseuille's equation to determine what the ratio between the inflow vessel must be compared to the outflow vessels to maintain the same pressure at each division. (From Nichols WW et al., *McDonald's Blood Flow in Arteries: Theoretic, Experimental, and Clinical Principles*, 5th ed., Hodder Arnold, London, UK, 2005.)

share common distal nodes, so the pressure drop across each branch is variable. In order for pressure to remain constant at each division, Poiseuille's equation can be used to determine the ratio of the vessel's areas (A) that must be maintained to the number of branches (N) that allow for pressure at each division to be maintained. The inflow (Q_1) must equal the sum of all the flows (Q_2) within N branches. Solving for vessel radius, the ratio of the radius of the outflow vessel to the inflow vessel must equal the ratio of inflow velocity to outflow velocity divided by the number of branches:

$$Q_1 = N * Q_2 \quad \text{where } Q = V * A$$

$$V_1 * A_1 = N * V_2 * A_2 \quad \text{where } A = \pi * R^2$$

$$V_1 * \pi * R_1^2 = N * V_2 * \pi * R_2^2$$

$$\frac{V_1}{V_2} = N * \frac{R_2^2}{R_1^2} \tag{3.28}$$

$$\frac{R_2^2}{R_1^2} = \frac{\left(\dfrac{V_1}{V_2}\right)}{N}$$

This suggests that the velocity ratio between two branch points can be used to estimate the difference in radius between the inflow vessels and branches. Poiseuille's equation, applied to the principle that the inflow must equal the sum of the flows at the branch points, allows for the calculation of the expected change in pressure at a given branch point for a given change in radius:

$$Q_1 = N * Q_2$$

$$Q = \frac{\pi * \Delta P * R^4}{8 * n}$$

$$\frac{\pi * \Delta P_1 * R_1^4}{8 * n} = N * \frac{\pi * \Delta P_2 * R_2^4}{8 * n}$$

$$\frac{\Delta P_1}{\Delta P_2} = N * \frac{R_2^4}{R_1^4}$$

$$\frac{\Delta P_1}{\Delta P_2} = N * \left(\frac{R_2^2}{R_1^2}\right)^2 \tag{3.29}$$

$$\frac{\Delta P_1}{\Delta P_2} = N * \left(\frac{\left(\dfrac{V_1}{V_2}\right)}{N}\right)^2 = \frac{\left(\dfrac{V_1}{V_2}\right)^2}{N}$$

$$\frac{V_1}{V_2} = \sqrt{N} \text{ commonly } \sqrt{2}$$

If the ratio of radius is substituted for the previously calculated velocity ratio, we find that for pressure to remain constant ($P_1 = P_2$), the velocity ratios must equal the square root of the number of branches (N). Many times the branch point is a bifurcation and thus $N = 2$. For a bifurcation, if the inflow/outflow velocity ratio is less than 1.414 then pressure at the branch point will rise. Clinically, this ratio can be used to determine the estimated pressure at a branch point from an inflow vessel with a known pressure.

Pulsatile flow

Applying Ohm's law to hemodynamics is limited by many factors, most notably that the human circulatory system is not under steady flow but is a pulsatile system. Because blood has mass, it also has inertia, meaning that blood will resist acceleration and deceleration during the cardiac cycle. Additionally, blood occupies a 3D structure which is interacting with the vasculature and constantly changing direction due to vessel geometry. The continual forces that disrupt linear motion cause the vast majority of energy loss in the form of inertial energy losses. The blood vessels possess elastic properties resulting in expansion and contraction through the cardiac cycle. This elasticity is critical in maintaining blood pressure and perfusion during the prolonged period of normal diastole. This necessary quality was first illustrated by fire brigades in the eighteenth century. The problem was first described when firefighters placed hand-cranked pumps into local waterways attempting to pump water to burning buildings. Between cranks when water was not actively driven forward, flow at the end of the fire hose would stop. To remedy this, a *Windkessel* or capacitor full of air was placed between the pump and the hose. During forward pump flow (systole), the air would

be compressed and water would be actively driven forward by the pump. Between cranks when the pump is *refilling* (diastole), the compressed air would drive the water in the compliance chamber forward. In much the same manner, arteries store expansion energy proportional to the local blood volume during systole to contract and drive blood forward to maintain blood pressure during diastole. An equivalent circuit model which simulates this *capacitance* characteristic of elastic arteries can be constructed using an electrical capacitor. This capacitor is placed in a configuration known as the low-pass filter (Figure 3.7). When an electrical capacitor is added to a pulsatile (alternating current) circuit, charge can build up when the inflow is greater than the outflow and then discharge when the outflow falls. Using basic mechanical properties of the artery, a vessel electrical capacitance can be calculated:

$$\frac{2 * Radius * \left(\pi * Radius^2 * Length \right)}{Wall\,thickness * Elastic\,modulus} \tag{3.30}$$

Pulsatile flow also creates an interesting situation where the flow within a vascular segment is dependent on the time it takes the vessel to discharge the pressure stored

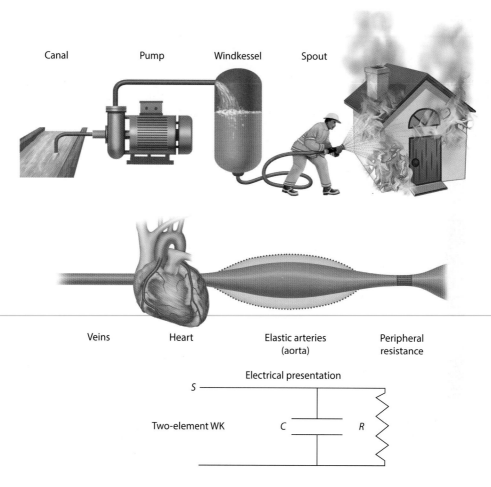

Figure 3.7 Windkessel hydraulic model and pulsatile electric circuit model. (Adapted from Westerhof N et al., *Med Biol Eng Comput*, 47(2), 131, February 2009.)

during systole (potential energy). In electronics, this time to discharge is known as tau (τ):

$$\tau = Resistance * Capacitance \qquad (3.31)$$

When a complex vascular circuit such as a hemodialysis fistula is simulated using vessel capacities, the time it takes for the proximal, distal and collateral vasculature to discharge during diastole can predict the pulsatile flow in the artery distal to the hemodialysis fistula. This is dependent on size and resistance of the arteriovenous anastomosis (Figure 3.8).[11]

Another interesting quality of pulsatile blood flow in elastic arteries is the relationship between the velocity of the blood and the energy reflected back at the next propagating pulsatile wave. To understand the concept of travelling waves of blood that produce reflected waves, consider a string tied to the wall. If the string is moved quickly up and down, it will create standing waves through the string. When the forward moving wave hits the wall, it will reflect back on the string as a wave moving in reverse. If the forward moving wave combines with the wave moving in reverse in phase, meaning both during an upward deflection of the string, then the amplitude of the combined wave created on the string will be additive causing the wave to double in size. If the waves combine so that the upward deflection of the forward moving wave combines with the downward deflection of the reverse moving wave, the waves will cancel each other making the string flat. As a result, the timing of the interaction of the two waves is critical in predicting the composite resulting waveform (Figure 3.9a).

Pressure waves are potential energy waves that move rapidly though the arterial circulation. If a blood vessel were an inelastic lead pipe, a pressure wave would move at the speed of sound both forward from the heart, as well as then reflecting back after striking a curved wall or vessel bifurcation. Because a vessel is distensible, some of the potential energy of the pressure wave is translated into outward wall movement, subsequently slowing the forward moving wave. The speed of this wave is known as the pulse wave velocity (PWV) and is a surrogate for disease-induced stiffness of the aorta. Elevated PWV has been studied to predict cardiovascular risk.

When analyzing the audible Doppler signal during an evaluation of the peripheral arteries, the velocity wave or kinetic energy is described as triphasic, biphasic or monophasic. The triphasic wave morphology represents arteries feeding high-resistance vascular beds and, by definition, has three distinct components. The first component represents antegrade velocity during systolic ejection. The second component of the waveform is a result of the previous cardiac cycle's pulse wave travelling backward after reflecting on high-resistance distal vascular beds causing a retrograde, or negative, velocity. The last component of the wave is the contraction of the elastic arteries during diastole resulting in antegrade velocity in end-diastole. The biphasic wave has antegrade velocity during the complete cardiac cycle from both systolic ejection and contraction of healthy vasculature without a velocity wave being reflected off distal high-resistance vascular beds. A biphasic wave can result from a proximal stenosis, vasodilation of an ischemic tissue bed or an end organ low-resistance distal vascular bed such as the brain or liver. Finally, a monophasic signal results from a proximal stenosis or occlusion causing the loss of the multiphasic wave associated with a normal cardiac cycle (Figure 3.9b).

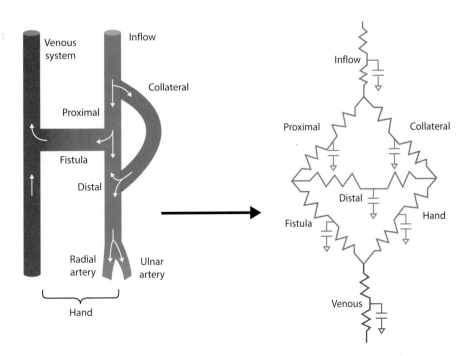

Figure 3.8 Complex electrical equivalent of a fistula model simulating both arterial resistance and capacitance. (From Chandra A et al., *Vascular*, 21(1), 54, February 2013.)

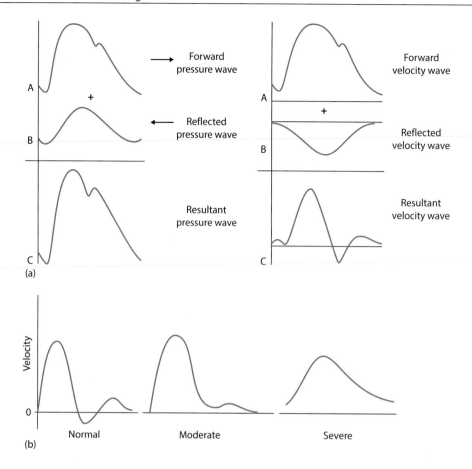

Figure 3.9 (a) Reflecting pressure and flow waves. (b) Doppler triphasic, biphasic and monophasic morphology.

Vessel wall dynamics

Not only can physics be used to describe the characteristics of blood flow, but it can also be used to describe the dynamic nature of the vessel wall. The complex hemodynamics of arterial dissection flap formation and propagation is under active study and provides two examples of the effect of hemodynamic energy on vessel wall dynamics. When a dissection begins, low-velocity blood separates the intimal and medial layers and enters a *false* lumen. This occurs simultaneously and parallel with high-velocity blood in the artery lumen. Just as an airplane wing relies on its curvature to create a high-velocity airstream resulting in a lower-relative pressure and lift, the dissection flap is pulled towards the higher velocity blood stream of the true lumen. This is encouraged by the relative higher pressure created by the slower velocity blood in the false lumen which subsequently propagates the dissection plane (Figure 3.10). It is therefore conceptually possible, in the clinical treatment of acute dissections, to inadvertently increase the velocity of the blood within the true lumen by agents that decrease peripheral vascular resistance, while attempting to decrease blood pressure. Within the false lumen, the law of conservation of energy underlies the further extension of the dissection flap. When kinetic energy in the form of velocity enters the false lumen, the blood velocity quickly approaches zero due to the lack of outflow. This incoming kinetic energy is suddenly and nearly entirely converted to potential energy in the form of pressure, a phenomena commonly described as 'water hammer'. This high pressure causes extension of the dissection flap into the true lumen causing the lumenal narrowing and increased velocity. This results in decreased true lumen pressure creating a cycle of further dissection propagation.

The risk of aneurysm rupture has been correlated to maximum aneurysm wall diameter. Laplace's law is often used to explain why wall tension increases with aneurysm diameter. Within a perfectly symmetric cylindrical aneurysm which was not ruptured (Figure 3.11), there are two forces in balance, the distention force and the retractile force:

$$Distending\ force = P_T * A \quad for\ which \quad A = 2 * r * l$$

$$Re\,tractile\ force = \sigma * 2 * (t * l)$$

$$Distending\ force = Retractile\ force$$

$$P_T * 2 * r * l = \sigma * 2 * (t * l)$$

$$P_T * r = \sigma * t$$

$$\sigma = \frac{P_T * r}{t}$$

(3.32)

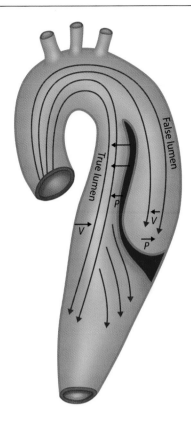

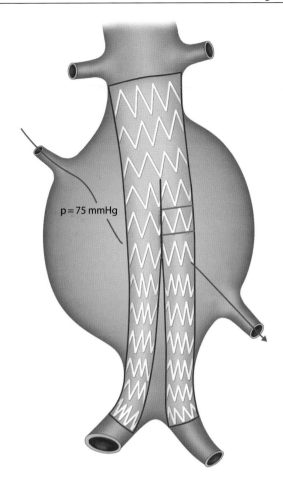

Figure 3.10 As predicted by the Bernoulli equation, dissection flap dynamics are much like an airplane wing where velocity of the blood in the true lumen is higher causing a decrease in pressure and lift on the flap. Additionally, the false lumen serves as an example of a *water hammer* when the velocity of the kinetic energy is converted completely into potential energy and increase pressure forcing the flap to continue to dissect.

Figure 3.12 Laplace's law applied to endoleak.

The distention force is the intraluminal pressure by blood applied to the area of the inner vessel wall. The retractile force is the transmural pressure applied across both the thickness of symmetrical blood-vessel walls, and the length of the blood vessel. By solving these two equations in equilibrium the transmural wall tension can be defined as directly proportional to the blood pressure and vessel diameter and inversely proportional to the wall thickness.

The practical application of Laplace's law can be used to define the risk of endoleaks in endovascular aneurysm repair. If an aneurysm is assumed to be a perfect 6 cm sphere, it's surface area can be calculated using the surface area of a sphere. If a type 2 endoleak were to transmit even a reduced systemic pressure (e.g. 75 mmHg) to the area of the aneurysm, the distention force of the aneurysm is equal to 113 N (Figure 3.12).

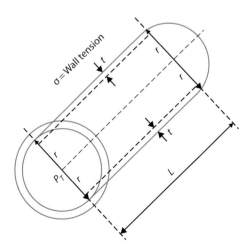

Figure 3.11 Depiction of Laplace's law. Distending force is the transluminal pressure or blood pressure (P_T) applied to a cross-sectional plane throughout the length (*l*) of a vessel (depicted in blue), in balance with the wall tension (σ) across the thickness of the vessel (*t*) in that same plane (depicted in green).

NON-INVASIVE TESTING

Introduction

The clinical study of hemodynamics in a non-invasive manner is made possible through the application of ultrasound principles and their resultant images. Prior to the 1960s, there was no method to non-invasively assess blood flow. The application of a continuous wave Doppler to assess blood flow was first applied in battlefield scenarios and then transitioned to routine clinical care. The use of piezoelectric crystals allowed for the transmission of ultrasonic waves into tissue which was then complemented by varying the pulse frequency of these waves with more sophisticated algorithms to generate visual images of the tissue being interrogated. Through the 1960s and 1970s, Dr. Eugene Strandness and his vascular surgery colleagues at the University of Washington further developed the application of Doppler principles to existing B-mode ultrasound to create Duplex imaging, thus revolutionizing vascular imaging to this day.[13] This section will cover the basic concepts of ultrasound physics and instrumentation, Doppler shift and duplex imaging. It is paramount to understand that the concepts of hemodynamics form the basis for the concepts of non-invasive testing discussed here.

Ultrasound instrumentation and physics

A clinical ultrasound machine involves three components, the probe (or transducer), a signal translation algorithm and a display. As such, the probe functions as the interface with the patient to send and receive sonographic information, the signal translation algorithm converts the received signal from the probe to functional clinical data, and the display is used to output these clinical data to the end user. An ultrasound probe is constructed using a small array of piezoelectric crystals. A piezoelectric crystal is a structure that reversibly changes its shape when kinetic energy in the form of an electric current is applied across it. The new shape of the crystal holds a small amount of stored mechanical energy and, if the applied current is rapidly varied, the transducer will produce sound waves at precise frequencies transmitted in the direction of probe orientation. Just as a piezoelectric device changes its shape under a current, if an external

mechanical force such as a sound wave is applied to the piezoelectric crystal, the crystal will create voltage which can be measured by the ultrasound machine. In this way, the piezoelectric crystals on an ultrasound transducer can both transmit a sound wave and then measure the sound wave that returns from any object the sound wave has come in contact with.

If the ultrasound probe continuously transmits and receives sound waves, it is a continuous wave Doppler. If the probe transmits sound waves in packets of varying lengths and frequencies and varies the window during which it receives (or 'listens' for) them, it is a pulse wave Doppler. The practical difference is that a continuous wave Doppler is not able to distinguish location or depth in tissue but requires far less computational effort in its signal translation algorithm and uses a speaker as its display to produce an audible Doppler signal. An example of a continuous wave Doppler is the bedside Doppler 'pencil' or probe. A pulse wave Doppler is able, through the decoding of the sound packets or pulses, to generate a visual result on a video display of both tissue structure (greyscale or brightness (*B*) mode of imaging) and blood velocity (Doppler effect). The standard clinical ultrasound machine which is able to generate images and blood velocity profiles is a pulse wave machine.

The generation of a velocity versus time waveform through pulse wave imaging is made possible through the application of a fast Fourier transform. This process allows the binning of discrete frequency data over time to generate a spectral waveform (Figure 3.13). This spectral waveform is converted to velocity through the Doppler equation, thus producing the velocity over time waveform which is interpreted clinically. Each major vessel that is typically interrogated in an attempt to define disease has unique spectral waveforms based on the target end organ of that vascular bed. Large clinical studies have derived various criteria to determine when a disease might exist in a given central (Table 3.1) or peripheral vascular structure (Table 3.2).

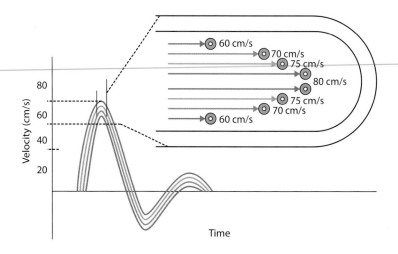

Figure 3.13 Frequency/velocity binning to generate a spectral Doppler waveform.

Table 3.1 Commonly used duplex velocity criteria for determining stenosis in various vascular beds.

Internal carotid artery occlusive disease
University of Washington criteria

Stenosis (%)	PSV	EDV	Spectral waveform
Normal	<125 cm/s	Not applicable	No broadening
1%–15%	<125 cm/s	Not applicable	Limited broadening in late systole
16%–49%	<125 cm/s	Not applicable	Broadening throughout systole
50%–79%	>125 cm/s	<140 cm/s	Broadening throughout systole
80%–99%	>125 cm/s	>140 cm/s	Broadening throughout systole
Occlusion	Undetectable	Undetectable	Undetectable

Consensus panel greyscale and Doppler criteria for carotid stenosis

Stenosis (%)	ICA PSV	Plaque estimate	ICA/CCA PSV	ICA EDV
Normal	<125 cm/s	None	<2.0	<40 cm/s
<50%	<125 cm/s	<50%	<2.0	<40 cm/s
50%–69%	125–230 cm/s	≥50%	2.0–4.0	40–100 cm/s
70%–99%	>230 cm/s	≥50%	>4.0	>100 cm/s
Total occlusion	Undetectable	No detectable lumen	Undetectable	Undetectable

Mesenteric occlusive disease
Celiac artery

Stenosis (%)	PSV	EDV	Spectral waveform
	Moneta criteria	Zwolak criteria	
Normal	90–110 cm/s	Not applicable	Low-resistance flow pattern
50%–70% (fasting)	<200 cm/s	≥55 cm/s	Low-resistance flow pattern
≥70% (fasting)	>200 cm/s	≥55 cm/s	Retrograde hepatic flow

Superior mesenteric artery

Stenosis (%)	PSV	EDV	Spectral waveform
	Moneta criteria	Zwolak criteria	
Normal	95–150 cm/s	>0	High-resistance flow pattern
50%–70% (fasting)	<275 cm/s	≥45 cm/s	Diastolic flow reversal
≥70% (fasting)	>275 cm/s	≥45 cm/s	Loss of diastolic flow reversal

Renal (Zierler and Strandness criteria)

Stenosis (%)	PSV	RAR PSV
Normal	<180 cm/s	<3.5
<60%	>180 cm/s	<3.5
≥60%	>180 cm/s	≥3.5
Total occlusion	Undetectable	Indeterminable

Sources: AbuRahma AF et al., *J Vasc Surg*, 55(2), 428, 2012; Cronenwett JL et al., *Rutherford's Vascular Surgery*, Philadelphia, PA, Saunders/Elsevier, 2010; Grant EG et al., *Radiology*, 229(2), 340, 2003; Pellerito J and Polak JF, *Introduction to Vascular Ultrasonography*, Philadelphia, PA, Elsevier, 2012; Spencer M, Full capability Doppler diagnosis, In: Spencer MP et al., eds. *Cerebrovascular Evaluation with Doppler Ultrasound*, Developments in Cardiovascular Medicine, Vol. 6, The Hague, the Netherlands, Springer, pp. 211–221, 1981; Spencer MP and Reid JM, *Stroke*, 10(3), 326, 1979; Zierler RE et al., *Am J Hypertens*, 9(11), 1055, 1996.

Abbreviations: ICA, Internal Carotid Artery; CCA, Common Carotid Artery; PSV, Peak Systolic Velocity; EDV, End Diastolic Velocity; RAR, Renal-Aortic Ratio of Peak Systolic Velocities.

Doppler shift and duplex imaging

Similar to a police officer indirectly measuring the speed of a car using a speed gun, the velocity of RBC can be non-invasively measured within a human blood vessel. The velocity of the RBC can ultimately be derived using the Doppler equation:

$$Velocity = \frac{c * (F_R - F_T)}{2 * F_T * \cos\theta} \quad (3.33)$$

The Doppler effect states that when an insonent sound wave reflects off of an object in motion, the frequency of the insonent sound wave will predictably change based on the velocity of the reflecting object. Solving the Doppler equation for velocity shows that the velocity of an RBC is directly proportional to the speed of sound in a given medium (c) and the difference in the transmitted frequency (F_T) and retuned frequency (F_R). This velocity is inversely proportional to two times transmitted frequency (F_T) multiplied by the cosine of the angle theta.

Table 3.2 Commonly used duplex velocity criteria for determination of peripheral vascular disease and monitoring of peripheral vascular interventions.

Peripheral arterial testing Ankle–brachial index			
ABI	**Symptoms**	**TBI**	**Symptoms**
>1.3	Non-compressible	≥0.8	No significant PAD
0.9–1.3	No significant PAD	0.2–0.5	Claudication
0.8–0.9	Mild PAD	<0.2	Rest pain
0.5–0.8	Claudication		
<0.5	Non-healing wounds		
<0.3	Rest pain		
Stenosis (%)	**PSV**	**Velocity ratio**	**Spectral waveforms**
<20%	<150	<1.5	Triphasic
20%–49%	150–200	1.5–2	Triphasic
50%–75%	200–300	2–4	Monophasic
>75%	>300 End-diastolic velocity >40	>4	Damped monophasic
Occlusion	Undetectable	Indeterminable	Undetectable

Peripheral bypass graft surveillance criteria				
Graft stenosis	**PSV**	**Velocity ratio**	**PSV distal to stenosis**	**Chang in ABI**
<50%	<80 cm/s	<2.0	>45 cm/s	<0.15
50%–70%	180–300 cm/s	>2.0	>45 cm/s	<0.15
>70%	>300 cm/s	>3.5	>45 cm/s	<0.15
>70% with low graft flow	>300 cm/s	>3.5	<45 cm/s	>0.15

Sources: Hiatt WR, *N Engl J Med*, 344(21), 1608, 2001; Hodgkiss-Harlow KD and Bandyk DF, *Semin Vasc Surg*, 26(2–3), 95, 2013.

Abbreviations: ABI, ankle–brachial index; TBI, toe–brachial index; PSV, peak systolic velocity.

Theta is the angle of insonation at which the sound wave hits the RBC.

As blood vessels run under the skin it is frequently impossible to interrogate RBC velocities perpendicular to

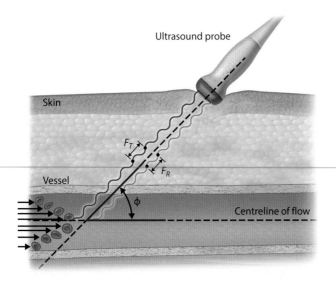

Figure 3.14 Geometry of transmitted frequency (F_T Green) and retuned frequency (F_R Orange) second to the Doppler shift created by the velocity of travelling red blood cells at an angle (θ) from the centreline of flow.

the direction of travel, as this would cause theta to equal 90° and the cosine of 90° is zero. In order to determine the true velocity of the RBC, the angle of insonation is kept as close to 60° as possible which yields a cosine value of 0.5 (Figure 3.14). Along similar lines, as theta approached 0°, the cosine would approach 1 resulting in artificially elevated results.

Intuitively, the Doppler equation makes sense as when a transmitted wave F_o collides into an RBC moving towards the transducer the transmitted wave will be compressed, making the returned frequency F_R larger, thus giving a positive sign to the difference between the returned and transmitted frequency ($F_R - F_T$). An RBC moving away from the transducer will result in a decrease in F_R which would yield a negative velocity. In duplex imaging, velocity direction is displayed as colour flow with a legend corresponding the colour and the direction (Figure 3.15).

FUTURE DIRECTIONS

1. Increased use of ultrasound imaging modalities that allow for the prediction of tissue mechanical properties.
2. Expanding use of ultrasound (microbubble) contrast to image microvascular structures, such as vasa vasorum or use of novel echo contrast agents linked to proteins that allow for in vitro tissue molecular imaging.
3. Improved use of new ultrasound imaging techniques, such as intravascular ultrasound and 3D ultrasound,

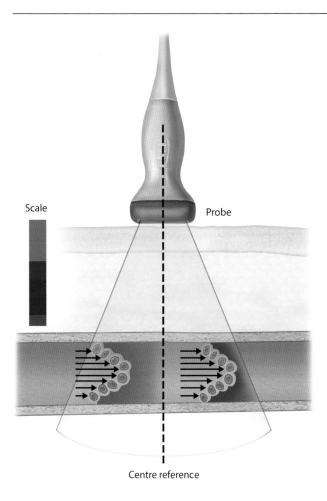

Scale

Probe

Centre reference

Figure 3.15 Colour flow Doppler encodes the velocity of the RBC's detected on the screen using a *colour scale*. In this example, positive velocities towards the probes centre reference are encoded in red and negative velocities away from the probes centre reference are encoded in blue.

and integration of ultrasound with other imaging modalities.
4. The use of ultrasound for not only diagnosis of vascular disease but also the use of ultrasound as a therapeutic modality or as the determinate when a therapeutic goal has been achieved.

KEY REFERENCES

1. Wixon CL. Vascular hemodynamics. In: Hallett JW, Mills JL, Earnshaw J, Reekers JA, Rooke T, eds. *Comprehensive Vascular and Endovascular Surgery*. Philadelphia, PA: Elsevier; 2009.

    Concise summary of vascular hemodynamics as well as physical principles that govern hemodynamic principles.
2. Nichols WW, O'Rourke MF, McDonald DA. *McDonald's Blood Flow in Arteries: Theoretic, Experimental, and Clinical Principles*, 5th ed. London, UK: Hodder Arnold; 2005.

    Definitive text of vascular hemodynamics and the experiments used to derive known hemodynamic phenomena. This text includes the derivation of theoretical principles as well as an extensive review of the experiments and interments used in those experiments.
3. Sumner DS. Essential hemodynamic principles. In: Rutherford RB, ed. *Vascular Surgery*, 4th ed. Philadelphia, PA: Saunders; 1995.

    A conscience summary of Dr. Strandness seminal work in the application of vascular hemodynamics to clinical practice.
4. Strandness DE Jr., Sumner DS. *Hemodynamics for Surgeons*. New York: Grune & Stratton, 1975.

    To date the most complete clinical text on the application of hemodynamic principles to vascular surgery.
5. Zierler RE. *Strandness's Duplex Scanning in Vascular Disorders*. Philadelphia, PA: Lippincott Williams & Wilkins; 2010.

    Complete review of using ultrasound to diagnose clinical pathology in vascular surgery.

REFERENCES

1. AbuRahma AF, Stone PA, Srivastava M et al. Mesenteric/celiac duplex ultrasound interpretation criteria revisited. *J Vasc Surg*. 2012 February;55(2):428–436.e6; discussion 35–36.
2. Chandra A, Mix D, Varble N. Hemodynamic study of arteriovenous fistulas for hemodialysis access. *Vascular*. 2013 February;21(1):54–62.
3. Cronenwett JL, Johnston W, Rutherford RB. *Rutherford's Vascular Surgery*. Philadelphia, PA: Saunders/Elsevier; 2010.
4. Grant EG, Benson CB, Moneta GL et al. Carotid artery stenosis: Gray-scale and Doppler US diagnosis – Society of Radiologists in Ultrasound Consensus Conference. *Radiology*. 2003 November; 229(2):340–346.
5. Hiatt WR. Medical treatment of peripheral arterial disease and claudication. *N Engl J Med* 2001 May 24;344(21):1608–1621.
6. Hodgkiss-Harlow KD, Bandyk DF. Interpretation of arterial duplex testing of lower-extremity arteries and interventions. *Semin Vasc Surg*. 2013 June–September;26(2–3):95–104.
7. Pellerito J, Polak JF. *Introduction to Vascular Ultrasonography*. Philadelphia, PA: Elsevier; 2012.
8. Spencer M. Full capability Doppler diagnosis. In: Spencer MP, Reid JM, Brockenbrough EC, eds. *Cerebrovascular Evaluation with Doppler Ultrasound*. Developments in Cardiovascular Medicine: Vol. 6. The Hague, the Netherlands: Springer; 1981, pp. 211–221.

9. Spencer MP, Reid JM. Quantitation of carotid stenosis with continuous-wave (C-W) Doppler ultrasound. *Stroke*. 1979 May–June;10(3):326–330.

10. Westerhof N, Lankhaar JW, Westerhof BE. The arterial Windkessel. *Med Biol Eng Comput*. 2009 February;47(2):131–141.

11. Wixon CL, Hughes JD, Mills JL. Understanding strategies for the treatment of ischemic steal syndrome after hemodialysis access. *J Am Coll Surg*. 2000 September;191(3):301–310.

12. Zierler RE, Bergelin RO, Davidson RC, Cantwell-Cab K, Polissar NL, Strandness D Jr. A prospective study of disease progression in patients with atherosclerotic renal artery stenosis. *Am J Hypertens*. 1996;9(11):1055–1061.

13. Blackshear WM, Phillips DJ, Thiele BL et al. Detection of carotid occlusive disease by ultrasonic imaging and pulsed Doppler spectrum analysis. *Surgery*. 1979;86:698–706.

4

Clinical examination of the vascular system

MICHAEL D. SGROI, ELIZABETH L. CHOU and SAMUEL ERIC WILSON

CONTENTS

INTRODUCTION

Vascular disease may involve the arterial, venous or lymphatic systems of the body. This chapter will review the physical examination of each of the circulatory systems, as well as typical exam findings in patients with common vascular diseases, such as peripheral arterial disease, chronic venous insufficiency and lymphedema. It should be noted, however, that vascular compromise is often multifactorial; thus a full physical exam is important on a patient with vascular disease because the aetiology may be secondary to another organ system. This chapter will only focus on the specific findings within the vascular system, but care should be taken to always start with a broad differential.

ARTERIAL PHYSICAL EXAMINATION

Pulse exam

The examination of the arterial vascular system begins with a pulse exam. To ensure consistency within one's practice, the pulse exam should be performed in a similar manner each time. No matter which location the examiner is evaluating, the patient should be positioned in a dependent, comfortable position to avoid tension, twitching or moving, which may cause inaccurate evaluation. The second and third fingers are used to evaluate the pulse. It is important to use the fingertips rather than the finger pad to prevent the examiner from feeling their own digital artery pulse. The same is true for avoiding the use of the thumb for pulse examination. In general, the larger the surface area used to detect a pulse, the greater the chance that the transmission of sensation may be misperceived and cause inaccurate diagnosis. Palpation should start light and increase gradually as needed. In a patient with vascular disease, a pulse examination should never exceed 5 seconds without releasing pressure and re-evaluating in a new location. This will reduce the likelihood of a falsely positive exam. Additionally, the examiner should always perform bilateral examination in the upper and lower extremities to evaluate for asymmetry.

The carotid pulse can be evaluated in the neck of the patient between the trachea and the sternocleidomastoid muscle. Pulsation can be appreciated from the base of the neck at the clavicle to the angle of the mandible. The patient should be instructed to turn their head towards the opposing side of the carotid being palpated. This allows for expansion of the examination area and assists in locating the carotid artery, particularly when evaluating obese patients with large necks. Palpation should be performed lightly at first, especially in the elderly, as increased pressure on the chemoreceptors of the carotid body may lead to bradycardia and hypotension. A careful examination may allow the examiner to appreciate the strength and pulse contour, thereby assisting with diagnosis of any abnormalities.

Upper extremity pulses typically examined include the brachial, radial and ulnar pulses. The brachial pulses are best palpated in the antecubital fossa of the elbow, medial to the biceps tendon. Below the elbow the brachial artery bifurcates into the radial ulnar arteries. The radial pulse can be palpated at the wrist near the base of the first digit. As the radial artery travels proximally, the pulse usually becomes more difficult to palpate as the radial artery runs deep within the proximal forearm below the flexor muscles. As a general rule, a systolic blood pressure of at least 70 mmHg is required for a palpable radial pulse.[1] The ulnar pulse is more difficult to palpate due to its deeper location at the wrist. Deep palpation is required for pulse evaluation. Both pulses are best appreciated by placing the arm in a comfortable position with the palm up and the wrist extended.

Pulses in lower extremity can be evaluated in three locations: the femoral, popliteal and pedal positions. The common femoral artery can be palpated just below the inguinal ligament. It is medial to the quadriceps muscles and between the femoral nerve and the femoral vein. In obese patients, anatomical landmarks may assist in finding the correct location. The anterior superior iliac spine and the pubic symphysis help locate the inguinal ligament. Halfway between these two points is the usual location of the femoral artery. Lateral rotation of the leg, retraction of the overhanging pannus and palpation with four fingers across can aid in detection. The popliteal artery is often more difficult to examine. It is most commonly located in the popliteal fossa between the medial and lateral epicondyles of the femur. It is often difficult to palpate because the overlying muscles may obscure the pulse. To better expose the artery, the examiner may hold the patients leg with both hands to reveal the entire fossa and palpate with underlying fingers. It is also important to help the patient relax the leg as much as possible, often in a mildly flex position to minimize the contraction of overlying muscles. The posterior tibial pulse can be appreciated posterior and inferior to the medial malleolus at Pimenta's point. This is an imaginary landmark at the midpoint between the medial malleolus and the insertion point of the Achilles tendon. Gentle pressure within this location should allow for adequate examination. The dorsalis pedis pulse is found on the dorsum of the foot usually just lateral to the extensor hallucis longus tendon. The absence of this pulse in young, healthy patients may not be pathological, as there is a 2%–3% incidence of congenitally absent foot pulses.[2]

Other arteries that can be palpated if necessary include the temporal artery, which is located superior and anterior to the ear, the occipital artery, which is 2 cm lateral from the midline at the base of the occiput, and the costal arteries in patients with coarctation of the aorta, which may be palpated at the base of the scapula and subcostally in the upper ribs.

Auscultation

Auscultation of normal vessels should reveal no sounds as there is no obstruction of blood flow. The presence of a bruit, which is secondary to turbulent blood flow within the vessel, represents an abnormality such as an arterial stenosis, extrinsic compression, aneurysmal dilatation or arteriovenous connection. The proximal location of a bruit defines the location of turbulent flow, but auscultation of the bruit may propagate for an additional 5 cm.

Larger vessels usually transmit lower-pitched bruits and small vessels transmit at a higher pitch. The severity of the stenosis correlates with the strength or volume of the transmitted bruit. Thus, severely stenotic vessels may convey a high-pitched, high-volume sound. Once an artery occludes, the bruit will likely disappear due to the absence of flow. The longevity of the bruit also carries significance. A bruit that extends into diastole implies an advanced stenosis.

Arteries examined by palpation may also be auscultated for evaluation of hemodynamic stability. There are additional vessels that may be examined by auscultation that may not be accessible by palpation including the subclavian and renal arteries. When there is a clinical suspicion for subclavian stenosis or renal artery stenosis, auscultation of bruit may help guide further diagnostic evaluation. Subclavian artery auscultation is performed with the patient sitting comfortably, looking forward, with the shoulders relaxed and hands resting on the lap. The bell of the stethoscope is lightly applied in each supraclavicular fossa. Exercising the ipsilateral arm with repetitive squeezing of rubber ball or other object for 30–60 seconds may aid in revealing a provoked bruit. Renal artery auscultation is evaluated by pressing the bell of the stethoscope deep into the abdomen above the umbilicus with the patient position supine. The patient may bend his/her legs at the knees to aid with relaxation. This exam may be difficult in large body habitus patients.

ADDITIONAL ARTERIAL EXAMINATIONS

Allen test

The radial and ulnar arteries are the main vessels supplying the hand. In most people, the two arteries are in continuity with each other through the deep and superficial palmar arches. Thus, in most people, adequate circulation can be obtained from just one of the two vessels; however, 5%–10% of the population has an incomplete arch. In those people, loss of one of the arteries can result in ischemia to the hand and fingers. The Allen test can help to demonstrate an incomplete arch. Occlusive pressure is applied to both the radial and ulnar arteries at the wrist. The patient is then instructed to open and close their hand to empty and venous system and create pallor at the hand. The examiner then releases one of the pulses. Skin colour should return to normal throughout the entire palmar surface within several seconds. The other branch of the arch is tested in a similar manner. If the palmar pallor does not resolve with release of one of the branches, the examiner can conclude that the patient has either an incomplete arch or an occlusion distal to where the artery is being released.

Examination of the skin

Variations in the skin presentation may suggest underlying vascular pathology. By examining both limbs, the examiner can evaluate the cause for asymmetry by comparing the affected limb with the unaffected one. Distinct skin changes can be seen in patients with ischemia, venous insufficiency and lymphedema. With regard to arterial skin changes manifested by acute and chronic limb ischemia, patients will have decreased capillary refill in the foot and toes. Refill time is more prominent in patients with acute limb ischemia due to inadequate time for development of collateral flow. Capillary refill greater than 3 seconds is indicative for decreased flow within the arterial system. Patients with chronic occlusive disease may demonstrate the absence of hair, thickened toenails, pallor and coolness to the skin. Chronic hypoperfusion may eventually lead to muscle and subcutaneous tissue atrophy. In patients with acute limb ischemia, pallor is often recognized at a point distal to the occlusion. There may also be a marked difference in skin temperature proximal and distal to occlusion. These findings may be able to assist the examiner in knowing the location of the occlusion prior to any imaging or entering of the operating room.

Arterial occlusive disease may lead to the formation of ischemic ulcers. The ulcers tend to be small, annular, pale and desiccated due to inadequate perfusion. The ulcers are typically located at the acral position of a limb, such as the toes, heel or fingertips. Unlike ulcerations secondary to neuropathy, ischemic ulcers are also painful. Diabetic ulcers also usually occur in locations of sustained pressure, bony prominences, callus formation or areas exposed to trauma. It is sometimes difficult to distinguish the aetiology of ulcers as most diabetics will also have peripheral vascular disease. Progression of ulceration leads to tissue necrosis and gangrene. Gangrene can be diagnosed by the observation of blackened, mummified tissue in a patient with vascular disease. Differentiation between dry and wet gangrene is important as the latter is a surgical emergency

due to infection, and debridement must be performed immediately to prevent systemic spread of infection and additional tissue compromise.

Changes in microcirculation from arterial compromise also manifest in skin presentation. Punctate lesions, splinter hemorrhages, and focal areas of cyanosis are indicative of microemboli. The lesions are usually 1 mm in diameter and painful. Microcirculatory infarcts may eventually lead to skin pitting. The cause of the microcirculatory disease may be from an array of different arterial sources including the heart, aorta and medium and small arterial vessels. Diagnosis of the underlying aetiology and source of emboli is most important. Common aetiologies include cardiac emboli, emboli from severe atherosclerosis of the aorta, microvascular disease such as diabetes or renal insufficiency and even vascular spasm as is the case for Raynaud's disease.

Positioning of the extremity

Dynamic positioning of the lower extremity may assist with diagnosing a vascular disease during the physical exam. On initial exam, the patient should be in a supine position with the examined limb in a comfortable location. Pallor of the lower extremity while in this horizontal position suggests critical limb ischemia. If a patient is placed in the seated position with the examined limb hanging off of the examination bed, one should see a difference in colour of the extremity due to restoration of dependent flow. Likewise, pallor that develops 15 seconds after elevating an extremity to 60° from supine suggests severe occlusive disease.

Upper extremity manoeuvres may undergo similar evaluation. For example, the thoracic outlet is a site of potential vascular interruption where vessels exit the chest to each arm. Care must be taken to differentiate arterial from neuropathic or venous thoracic outlet syndrome (TOS) in determining aetiology. Numbness and paresthesia in the absence of any loss of pulse or swelling to the arm suggest neuropathic origin. Loss of pulse within the extremity during hyperabduction of the arm suggests vascular origin. The Adson test, which consists of rotating the head and extending the neck towards the affected side, may elucidate symptoms in a patient with vascular compression. Further evaluation of TOS is discussed later in this chapter.

EXAMINATION FINDINGS IN PERIPHERAL ARTERIAL DISEASE

Peripheral arterial disease (PAD) is a term generally applied to atherosclerosis of limb vasculature. It is most commonly observed in the lower extremities. PAD is a broad term that can include asymptomatic patients, those with intermittent claudication (IC) or rest pain and critical limb ischemia. Patients with PAD should also be evaluated for coronary artery disease (CAD) due to the systemic nature of atherosclerotic disease. Likewise, CAD and PAD share similar risk factors, including male gender, age, smoking, diabetes, hypertension, renal insufficiency and hypercholesterolemia.[3] The prevalence of PAD increases with age, such that roughly 20% of patients over age 65 have PAD (including symptomatic and asymptomatic disease), which calculates to nearly 8 million Americans.[4,5] Due to the increasing average age of the population, the overall prevalence of PAD is also increasing.

Roughly 20%–50% of patients diagnosed with PAD are asymptomatic, though most have functional impairment to elicit vascular testing.[3] The first symptom that most patients experience is IC. The word claudication is derived from the Latin and French *claudication* and *claudico*, respectively, and was commonly used to describe a lame horse. Claudication is an exertion-induced pain that is relieved with rest. It is commonly described as a cramping, burning or aching pain. Often, patients will also talk about being fatigued for which they need to intermittently sit down and rest. Their limitation is not due to shortness of breath, but due to fatigue in the limb. The walking distance–limiting pain recurs in the same area with each provocation. Patients' description of their symptoms is important to determining aetiology. Given the frequent lifestyle limiting effect of IC, patients can often provide very detailed accounts of their symptoms.

The location of pain can be an important clue to the area of stenosis. Patients can often locate exactly when and where their pain starts. Symptoms often occur one level below the area of stenosis and generally occur in the most proximal muscle area with inadequate perfusion. For example, a patient with common iliac artery stenosis may experience buttock and thigh discomfort, while those with superficial femoral artery or popliteal stenosis will have calf and pedal discomfort.

Relief of the discomfort with rest is a hallmark finding in patients with IC. Patients are often very descriptive on how the pain is relieved. Frequent responses include relief while lying down, sitting or just standing still. They may also reveal the length of rest required until they can resume ambulation. Claudication symptoms gradually improve with rest. Most patients state that they will need to rest for 5–10 minutes before they are again pain free. Pain that is relieved immediately upon cessation of activity is likely not claudication and not related to poor perfusion. Pain that is relieved with positional changes or with activity is not likely the consequence of peripheral arterial disease, but rather of neuropathic or musculoskeletal origin.

Age of onset and disease progression can elucidate the potential course of their arterial occlusive disease. The presence of PAD in younger populations should prompt examination for aetiologies that can exacerbate the development and progression of atherosclerosis like hyperhomocysteinemia and familial hypercholesterolemia or other causes like vasculitides or arterial entrapment. Atherosclerosis is usually a disease of slow progression. The time course for disease evolution is over years. The initial symptoms generally occur during periods of extreme exertion and may remain undiagnosed. As the disease progresses, the process of plaque rupture and thrombosis may lead to periods of waxing and waning symptom progression. An acute onset of symptoms suggests a more critical problem that may require immediate intervention.

As time and disease progresses, patient symptoms may worsen. Rest pain occurs when the perfusion pressure during inactivity is inadequate to meet the basal requirements of the supplied tissue. The lack of blood flow can affect all tissue, including muscles, nerves, bone, subcutaneous tissue and skin. Pain is normally described in the most distal location of the limb, such as the toes or foot. In this group of patients, gravity appears to play a role in their symptoms. When the patient is in the supine position, such as during sleeping, the pain is worse because the legs are elevated. Pain is relieved when the legs are placed over the side of the bed and gravity assists with forward blood flow. Patients with this type of severe progression of disease may also have atrophy of limb musculature, hair loss, skin colour changes and possible non-healing open wounds due to chronic arterial insufficiency. The most painful areas are associated with tissue breakdown.

Along with the clinical examination for objective data when identifying a patient with PAD, subjective data is also helpful, especially in the context of determining the most appropriate method of treatment. There are multiple quality of life questionnaires that may be filled out by the patient to aid the examiner in understanding the severity of symptoms in the context of baseline level of physical activity. One such questionnaire is the Study Short Form 36 (SF-36),[6] which is a measure of physical and mental health functioning. Others are disease specific for PAD, such as the Vascular Quality of Life (VascuQOL),[7] the Walking Impairment Questionnaire (WIQ)[8] and the Peripheral Artery Questionnaire (PAQ).[9]

EXAMINATION FINDINGS FOR ACUTE LIMB ISCHEMIA

Sudden occlusion of a lower extremity artery often manifests with acute changes on physical exam. Acute limb ischemia may result from local thrombus formation or from an embolism originating at a more proximal site. A thorough history and physical examination is essential for the diagnosis of acute limb ischemia and particularly important for differentiating an embolic source from an arterial in situ thrombus. Patients with an arterial embolus often complain of sudden onset and significantly worsening pain. In many cases, patients will be able to describe the exact onset of pain. Most will not have prior PAD symptoms in the affected leg and are unlikely to have any symptoms in the contralateral limb. A thorough review of medical history looking for cardiac disease, atrial fibrillation or myocardial infarction is critical for determining a possible cardiac aetiology. Patients with in situ arterial thrombus, on the other hand, will often provide a history of claudication and acute worsening symptoms. These are often patients who have a history of atherosclerotic disease with eventual plaque rupture and thrombus formation. They may also have PAD symptoms in the contralateral limb, but likely not as severe. One should also always ask about a history of hypercoagulability to evaluate a genetic aetiology.

The usual time course for symptom development and progression in a patient with acute arterial occlusion is hours. Sudden and dramatic decreases in perfusion cause ischemic changes to the skin, musculature and nerves resulting in a classic description of acute limb ischemia as characterized by the 6 Ps: pain, pallor, paresthesia, pulselessness, paralysis and poikilothermia. Pain is often the first symptom. It can be intensified with both passive and active movement. As ischemic time ensues, the patient will start to manifest additional symptoms. Paresthesia in patients with acute ischemia presents as the inability to distinguish sensation between the first and second toes. Compared to the contralateral limb, the skin temperature of the affected limb will be significantly cooler. The severity of blood flow decrement will dictate the symptoms appreciated. The presence of nervous or musculature symptoms indicate a greater severity of disease. Based on these findings, the appropriate classification of acute limb ischemia may be assigned to guide further treatment (Table 4.1).[10]

Along with a thorough physical examination, further studies will be necessary in this group of patients. An ankle–brachial index should be performed on the bilateral lower extremities to first evaluate the severity of disease and obtain a pre-intervention objective baseline measurement. Afterwards, vascular imaging is useful to further evaluate the location of insult, as well as planning for potential intervention. In addition to these studies, an EKG and echocardiogram are helpful to determine possible embolic sources for occlusion.

EXAMINATION FINDINGS IN MESENTERIC ISCHEMIA

Mesenteric ischemia may present as an acute or chronic event and precipitate from compromised arterial or venous flow. Acute mesenteric ischemia, much like acute limb ischemia, is caused by sudden reduction in intestinal blood flow most commonly from arterial occlusion, vasospasm or hypoperfusion of the mesenteric vessels. Arterial obstruction due to acute embolic or thrombotic occlusion of the superior mesenteric artery is most often observed. Acute occlusive venous obstruction due to thrombosis of the superior mesenteric vein or segmental intestinal strangulation may also present in a similar manner. Patients with acute mesenteric ischemia have rapid onset of severe periumbilical abdominal pain that is out of proportion to findings on physical exam, characterized by sudden pain associated with minimal abdominal signs. Nausea and vomiting are common. In those with nonocclusive ischemia or insidious mesenteric vein thrombosis, symptoms may be present for days to weeks with nonspecific abdominal pain and nonspecific findings on abdominal exam. The vague physical exam findings will often correlate with the symptoms and risk factors associated with mesenteric ischemia in those of high suspicion. Risk factors such as atrial fibrillation, congestive heart failure, peripheral vascular disease and history of hypercoagulability or prior embolic event will strongly aid in further imaging studies to confirm clinical suspicion and appropriate intervention.

In contrast to acute mesenteric ischemia, patients with chronic mesenteric ischemia present with recurrent episodes of abdominal pain corresponding to intermittent episodes of increased circulatory intestinal demand. These episodes are frequently postprandial or during periods of exercise. Patients may have an extended history of weight loss due to development of food aversion from anticipated postprandial pain. Physical exam has a small role in the diagnosis of chronic mesenteric ischemia. Noninvasive duplex studies are more helpful in supporting the diagnosis if high

Table 4.1 Classification of acute limb ischemia.

Category	Description/prognosis	Findings		Doppler signals	
		Sensory loss	Muscle weakness	Arterial	Venous
I. Viable	Not immediately threatened	None	None	Audible	Audible
II. Threatened					
a. Marginally	Salvageable if promptly treated	Minimal (toes) or none	None	Inaudible	Audible
b. Immediately	Salvageable with immediate revascularization	More than toes, associated with rest pain	Mild, moderate	Inaudible	Audible
III. Irreversible	Major tissue loss or permanent nerve damage inevitable	Profound, anesthetic	Profound, paralysis (rigour)	Inaudible	Inaudible

Source: Rutherford RB et al., *J Vasc Surg*, 26, 517, 1997.

grade stenotic mesenteric vessels are observed. A full physical exam and history of these patients, however, will likely correspond with a long history of smoking and underlying peripheral vascular disease or coronary artery disease.

EXAM FINDINGS IN ABDOMINAL ANEURYSMS

The abnormal increase in the size of a blood vessel can augment its pulse. A vessel is aneurysmal when it increases in diameter by 150%. If the vessel has expanded less than this, it is defined as ectatic. Most aneurysms, particularly of the chest or abdomen, are found incidentally on radiographic imaging. Diagnosing an abdominal aneurysm through physical exam is possible, but difficult. The examiner should gradually increase pressure along the midline of a patient using all eight fingertips. Both sides of the aneurysm are usually pulsatile, allowing the examiner the ability to estimate the diameter of the mass. Detection is directly related to aneurysm size and inversely related to patient abdominal girth. Pulsatile expansion distal to the umbilicus indicates aneurysmal disease into the iliac artery system. Significant discomfort during the examination may represent recent expansion, inflammatory aneurysm or even rupture. Aneurysms in the extremities are most often present in the infra-popliteal region. These patients will more likely present with signs and symptoms of acute limb ischemia due to progressive thrombus accumulation in the aneurysm sac leading to acute occlusion or distal emboli, which most often necessitates immediate intervention.

MISCELLANEOUS DISEASES

Thoracic outlet syndrome

The patient that presents with positional claudication symptoms in the upper extremity may have TOS. TOS is a group of disorders that occurs due to compression of the neurovascular bundle at the superior thoracic outlet composed of the anterior and middle scalene muscle and first rib. Symptoms may be due to a primarily neurogenic, arterial or venous irritation at the thoracic outlet. In arterial TOS resulting in aneurysmal dilatation, the axillo-subclavian artery may undergo external compression from a cervical rib, abnormal insertion of the anterior scalene muscle or apposition of the clavicle and first rib during elevation of the arm above the shoulder. Common complaints include weakness, fatigue or heaviness of the arm with activities above the shoulder. Patients will often complain of the inability to comb or wash their hair, or clean in high places. Distal to the compression, the vessel may become aneurysmal. The aneurysm may then lead to further complications, such as distal embolization in the affected upper extremity.

Popliteal artery entrapment syndrome

IC is unusual among patients under the age of 50. In this group of patients, the examiner must consider popliteal entrapment syndrome. The popliteal artery is compressed by the medial belly of the gastrocnemius muscle in patients with this syndrome. They present with symptoms of claudication, particularly after long episodes of running or cycling. Due to the fact that these patients are normally healthy, the examiner is likely to have normal pulse exam when these patients are at rest. It is a diagnosis of exclusion.

Vasculitis

Inflammation of the blood vessel wall can cause the development of stenotic lesions, aneurysmal dilatation and constitutional symptoms. Important clinical entities that may lead to these abnormalities include Takayasu's arteritis, giant cell (temporal) arteritis and Buerger's disease (thromboangiitis obliterans).

Takayasu's arteritis is a rare inflammatory arteritis that affects predominately the aorta and its immediate branches.[11] This is a disease mostly found in young adults, with a predisposition towards Asian females. The vascular inflammation eventually leads to arterial thickening, stenosis and eventually fibrosis and thrombus formation. Pulses may be diminished. The clinical course of Takayasu's arteritis starts with non-constitutional symptoms, such as fever, lethargy, malaise and myalgias. The continued inflammatory changes to the vessels will then result in arterial insufficiency symptoms such as lower extremity claudication.

Giant cell (temporal) arteritis is an elastic artery vasculitis that tends to involve the branches of the thoracic aorta. This is a disease of the elderly, with the majority being diagnosed over the age of 70.[12] The patient may have a history of fever, fatigue, weight loss, headache and jaw claudication. These symptoms in conjunction with the following physical exam findings should raise a suspicion for temporal arteritis. Pulses may be diminished due to inflammation of large vessels. Temporal and other cranial arteries may be tender or thickened on palpation. An ophthalmologic exam may show a swollen pale disc and blurred margins consistent with ischemic optic neuropathy. These patients may also have decreased active range of motion in the shoulders, neck and hips due to limitation from pain. Bruit may also be auscultated in the carotid or supraclavicular areas due to inflammatory changes affecting hemodynamic flow. The gold standard for diagnosis is temporal artery biopsy, but biopsy should not delay treatment with steroids when there is high clinical suspicion. Delay may lead to potentially irreversible ocular ischemia.[13]

Buerger's disease, also known as thromboangiitis obliterans, is a nonatherosclerotic inflammatory disease affecting the small and medium arteries and veins of the extremities. It is most common among young smokers who present with distal extremity ischemia, digit ulcers or gangrene. Superficial thrombophlebitis often serves as a precursor to the disease. Digit ischemia is the most common manifestation accompanied by pain and discoloration of the digits, eventually progressing to ulceration and gangrene. Thus, a thorough history and physical exam usually reveals extensive smoking history and the presence of superficial venous nodules and cords at the early stage and ischemia of bilateral hands or feet in later stages. Physical exam alone, however, cannot distinguish occlusive disease due to Buerger's disease versus other aetiologies. Biopsy provides definitive diagnosis and clinical diagnosis is based on exclusion.[14]

VENOUS PHYSICAL EXAMINATION

In contrast to the arterial vascular system in which there are discrete signs and symptoms when disease is present, the venous physical examination is subtle and can be difficult to elucidate an underlying disease. Objective testing is commonly required for diagnosis.

All veins in the body drain into the central venous system and eventually back to the right atrium. The veins of the arm, head and neck and chest drain into the superior vena cava, while the veins of the abdomen and lower extremities drain into the inferior vena cava. The veins of the lower extremity are separated into the deep veins, the superficial veins and the perforators (or communicating veins). The deep veins of the lower extremity carry approximately 90% of the venous return.[15] The superficial veins carry little blood back to the central venous system and have little surrounding structural support. The two superficial veins of the lower extremity include the greater saphenous vein, which starts anterior to the medial malleolus and eventually drains into the deep system at the common femoral vein, and the lesser saphenous vein, which begins at the lateral foot distally and drains into the deep system at the popliteal fossa.

All veins have one-way valves to allow blood movement against gravity without backflow or pooling according to dependent positioning. If the valves of the venous system become incompetent, blood will move towards dependent areas causing pooling and stasis and sometimes compromising arterial perfusion. These changes manifest as venous disease, such as venous insufficiency, varicose veins and thrombosis.

The most common physical exam finding of an abnormal venous system is the presence of edema. Asymmetric swelling within the lower extremity will often be obvious when comparing to the opposite extremity. Symmetric swelling is often more difficult to appreciate but can be compared to relatively less dependent areas of the body. To evaluate pitting edema, the examiner should press firmly on the limb with their thumb for at least 5 seconds. Edema should be evaluated on the dorsum of the foot, behind each malleolus, and over the shins. A depression left by the pressure of the thumb is diagnostic of pitting edema. Pitting edema is graded on a 4-point scale from minimal to very marked.

Examination of the skin

Specific skin changes in the context of clinical history and patient risk factors can also suggest venous pathology and a narrowed aetiology. Specific changes in the colour of the skin can help to differentiate cellulitis or superficial thrombophlebitis from chronic venous insufficiency. In cellulitis, the affected area is usually warm, edematous and erythematous. It may or may not have purulent drainage or exudate. The edema may cause dimpling of the skin resembling an orange peel texture. Patients will frequently have a history of trauma or disruption of the skin barrier. Patients with superficial thrombophlebitis will also have tenderness, induration and erythema in an affected area, but there will also often be a palpable cord due to thrombus of the affected vein. Because chronic venous insufficiency is insidious in nature, the affected areas are less likely to be tender or have calor. There will also be the additional clues of telangiectasias, varicose veins, lipodermatosclerosis, venous ulcers and hyperpigmentation most often at the medial ankle. These specific changes are discussed further in the chronic venous insufficiency exam section later. Patients with chronic venous insufficiency, however, are also prone to develop stasis dermatitis characterized by a dry, scaly skin and inflammatory rash, which may be difficult to distinguish from cellulitis. Thus, chronicity of symptoms and thorough skin evaluation are important in determining the underlying aetiology.

Positioning of the extremity

Varying the dependent position of the affected extremity can help identify venous pathology. Rubor that significantly improves with extremity elevation is more consistent with venous stasis compared with erythema from infectious or inflammatory aetiology. Likewise, confirmation of edema is best appreciated after the patient has removed compression garments and has remained in a seated or standing position for 10–15 minutes. Improvement of lower extremity edema after elevation of the extremity affected above the level of the heart for the same amount of time is more consistent with venous insufficiency rather than lymphedema.

EXAMINATION FINDINGS IN ACUTE DEEP VENOUS THROMBOSIS

In addition to the prevalent chronic venous disorders that require a thorough physical exam, there are a few acute venous conditions that are important to recognize for timely intervention and prevention of irreversible tissue or vessel damage. Physical examination of lower extremity deep vein thrombosis may reveal a palpable cord consistent with a thrombosed vein, calf or thigh pain, unilateral swelling, superficial venous dilation or warmth, tenderness and erythema of the affected limb and area. Tenderness on deep palpation and a positive Homan's sign, characterized by calf pain on ankle dorsiflexion with knee extension, is suggestive, but not diagnostic. Thus, physical exam findings need to be used with validated algorithms such as the Wells score to minimize unnecessary additional testing, appropriate diagnosis and timely treatment if necessary.[16]

When thrombosis of the deep veins progresses to or includes complete occlusion of the proximal iliofemoral system, or completely compromises the deep venous system, the affected limb blanches, sometimes appearing white without cyanosis. The limb appears edematous and is tender to palpation. This set of conditions is known as phlegmasia alba dolens. Progression of the occlusion can lead to phlegmasia cerulean dolens, where both the deep and the major collateral veins are compromised and venous flow is shunted to the superficial system that is unable to compensate. This stage of occlusion is characterized by sudden severe pain, swelling, cyanosis and edema. Patients at this stage of occlusion are at high risk of massive pulmonary embolism even during anticoagulation. Occlusion of outflow can lead to arterial compromise and tissue ischemia, venous gangrene and compartment syndrome. Preventing and recognizing phlegmasia – through early DVT detection and treatment and physical exam – is imperative in avoiding delay in therapy and reducing mortality and limb loss associated with this condition.

EXAMINATION FINDINGS IN CHRONIC VENOUS INSUFFICIENCY

Patients with chronic venous insufficiency may have symptoms without significant physical exam findings or no symptoms with significant findings on physical exam. It is important to correlate these two areas to guide further studies and treatment planning. About 20% of patients with symptoms of chronic venous insufficiency such as feelings of limb heaviness, distention or pain have no visible clinical signs. Duplex exam in these patients may be helpful to identify functional disease. The remaining majority of patients will have signs or symptoms. Telangiectasias are most frequently seen in venous disease and consist of dilated intradermal venules less than one millimetre in diameter. Varicose veins can be seen and palpated due to their larger size (>3 mm in diameter), tortuosity and location in the subcutaneous fat. Edema is often present as well but is not a specific finding. Skin changes, specifically hyperpigmentation on the anterior lower leg due to hemosiderin deposition from extravasated red blood cells from damaged capillaries due to increased venous pressure, is a common sign in venous insufficiency. Lipodermatosclerosis may be present in those with severe venous insufficiency and consists of fibrotic changes to the subcutaneous tissue resulting in firm induration at the medial ankle that can circumferentially surround the ankle. These chronic inflammatory and fibrotic changes increase patient risk for developing dermatitis, cellulitis and ulceration due to

compromise of microvascular circulation. These complications are often seen in patients with chronic venous insufficiency and should not be treated in isolation, but instead with the underlying aetiology in mind.

LYMPHATIC PHYSICAL EXAM

The lymphatic system comprises of an extensive network of vessels that drain lymph fluid from bodily tissue and return it to the venous circulation. The lymph system starts peripherally as small capillaries that coalesce and drain centrally through an array of channels that are interposed by lymph nodes. The lymph fluid drains into the venous system through the right lymphatic duct and the thoracic duct at the origin of the subclavian vein. Like the venous system, lymph flow takes place in a low-pressure system that relies on local arterial pulsation, skeletal muscle contraction and unidirectional valves to prevent backward flow. The lymph system is evaluated in a similar fashion to the venous system with additional consideration of the lymph nodes and immune system. Disorders of the lymphatic system may be structural or immune related. Thus, correlating the physical exam with patient history is important to differentiate an underlying circulatory or immune pathology. The most common sign of circulatory lymphatic impairment is lymphedema, characterized by swelling. This condition can result from primary causes associated with congenital syndromes such as Turner syndrome, Klippel–Trenaunay–Weber syndrome or Noonan syndrome or secondary causes associated with trauma, scarring of lymphatic vessels or lymphatic blockage from tumour or infection.

EXAMINATION FINDINGS IN LYMPHEDEMA

Lymphatic impairment results in accumulation of interstitial fluids and swelling and distention of the affected limb. Edema due to lymphatic compromise is non-pitting and painless, compared to the pitting edema present in venous insufficiency. Temporary lymphedema may result from tight garments or shoes. Persistent distention may cause permanent connective tissue damage and chronic edema. Stagnant interstitial fluid, much like venous stasis, affects microcirculation and increases patient risk of infection and ulcer formation. A positive Stemmer sign, characterized by the examiner's inability to lift the skin of the affected limb or dorsum of the fingers or toes of the affected limb, is also indicative of lymphedema.[17] Measurement of the limb volume with water displacement or circumferential measurements may be helpful in monitoring response to therapy.

Key points

Always perform full physical exam due to the multifactorial aetiology of vascular disease.

The patient, limb or area of interest should be positioned for maximum exposure and comfort of the patient.

The underlying physiology and suspected condition under evaluation should always be considered. Use positioning to differentiate aetiologies with similar signs.

Abnormal pulse exam or auscultation of bruit should be correlated with clinical history and followed by additional directed questions or further diagnostic studies.

Acute ischemic conditions require recognition of key signs and symptoms for prompt treatment and further diagnostic studies.

- Acute limb ischemia: pain, pallor, paresthesia, pulselessness, paralysis and poikilothermia
- Acute mesenteric ischemia: pain out of proportion to exam
- Ruptured or leaking arterial aneurysm: tearing back pain, increased pain during exam and interval increase in pulsatile mass
- Phlegmasia: sudden blanching white limb and blue limb

In the case of acute limb ischemia, classification of the severity of limb ischemia may assist with the decision to intervene.

Most vasculitis will present as a diagnosis of exclusion, with further testing necessary to diagnose these inflammatory diseases.

Patients with severe venous insufficiency will oftentimes have a difficult exam to distinguish from arterial disease.

Arterial ulcers are more painful than venous ulcers.

Pitting edema is secondary to a vascular insufficiency, while non-pitting edema correlates with lymphatics.

REFERENCES

1. Deakin CD, Low JL. Accuracy of the advanced trauma life support guidelines for predicting systolic blood pressure using carotid, femoral, and radial pulses: Observational study. *Br Med J.* 2000; 321:673–674.

2. Robertson GS, Ristic CD, Bullen BR. The incidence of congenitally absent foot pulses. *Ann R Coll Surg Engl.* 1990;72:99–100.

3. Hirsch AT, Haskal ZJ, Hertzer NR et al. ACC/AHA 2005 Practice Guidelines for the management of patients with peripheral arterial disease (lower extremity, renal, mesenteric, and abdominal aortic): A collaborative report from the American Association for Vascular Surgery/Society for Vascular Surgery, Society for Cardiovascular Angiography and Interventions, Society for Vascular Medicine and Biology, Society of Interventional Radiology, and the ACC/AHA Task Force on Practice Guidelines (Writing Committee to Develop Guidelines for the Management of Patients With Peripheral Arterial Disease): Endorsed by the American Association of Cardiovascular and Pulmonary Rehabilitation; National Heart, Lung, and Blood Institute; Society for Vascular Nursing; TransAtlantic Inter-Society Consensus; and Vascular Disease Foundation. *Circulation.* 2006;113:e463–e654.

4. Hirsch AT, Criqui MH, Treat-Jacobson D et al. Peripheral arterial disease detection, awareness, and treatment in primary care. *J Am Med Assoc.* 2001;286:1317–1324.

5. Meijer WT, Hoes AW, Rutgers D, Bots ML, Hofman A, Grobbee DE. Peripheral arterial disease in the elderly: The Rotterdam Study. *Arterioscler Thromb Vasc Biol.* 1998;18:185–192.

6. Ware JE Jr., Sherbourne CD. The MOS 36-item short-form health survey (SF-36). I. Conceptual framework and item selection. *Med Care.* 1992;30:473–483.

7. Morgan MB, Crayford T, Murrin B, Fraser SC. Developing the vascular quality of life questionnaire: A new disease-specific quality of life measure for use in lower limb ischemia. *J Vasc Surg.* 2001;33:679–687.

8. McDermott MM, Liu K, Guralnik JM, Martin GJ, Criqui MH, Greenland P. Measurement of walking endurance and walking velocity with questionnaire: Validation of the walking impairment questionnaire in men and women with peripheral arterial disease. *J Vasc Surg.* 1998;28:1072–1081.

9. Spertus J, Jones P, Poler S, Rocha-Singh K. The peripheral artery questionnaire: A new disease-specific health status measure for patients with peripheral arterial disease. *Am Heart J.* 2004;147:301–308.

10. Rutherford RB, Baker JD, Ernst C et al. Recommended standards for reports dealing with lower extremity ischemia: Revised version. *J Vasc Surg.* 1997;26:517–538.

11. Maffei S, Di Renzo M, Bova G, Auteri A, Pasqui AL. Takayasu's arteritis: A review of the literature. *Intern Emerg Med.* 2006;1:105–112.

12. Huston KA, Hunder GG, Lie JT, Kennedy RH, Elveback LR. Temporal arteritis: A 25-year epidemiologic, clinical, and pathologic study. *Ann Intern Med.* 1978;88:162–167.

13. Delecoeuillerie G, Joly P, Cohen de Lara A, Paolaggi JB. Polymyalgia rheumatica and temporal arteritis: A retrospective analysis of prognostic features and different corticosteroid regimens (11 year survey of 210 patients). *Ann Rheum Dis.* 1988;47:733–739.

14. Mills JL, Porter JM. Buerger's disease: A review and update. *Semin Vasc Surg.* 1993;6:14–23.

15. Bickley LS, Szilagyi PG, Bates B. Chapter 11: The peripheral vascular system. In: Bickley LS, Szilagyi PG, eds. *Bates' Guide to Physical Examination and History Taking*, 9th ed. Philadelphia, PA: Lippincott Williams & Wilkins; 2007.

16. Wells PS, Anderson DR, Bormanis J et al. Value of assessment of pretest probability of deep-vein thrombosis in clinical management. *Lancet.* 1997;350:1795–1798.

17. Rockson SG. Diagnosis and management of lymphatic vascular disease. *J Am Coll Cardiol.* 2008;52:799–806.

5

A review for clinical outcomes research
Hypothesis generation, data strategy and hypothesis-driven statistical analysis

LAURA T. BOITANO and DAVID C. CHANG

CONTENTS

INTRODUCTION

Clinicians have an insatiable drive for definitive answers regarding clinical judgements they make every day. They also hold deep convictions and make clinical decisions based upon experience and training, which can only be shaken (modified) by convincing data. The days of relying upon the 'chart review' for guiding clinical practice have passed us by. How, then, can we answer important clinical questions using current tools from the rapidly developing world of outcomes research? This requires the conversion of an interesting clinical observation into an outcomes research question with a testable hypothesis, followed by an outcomes analysis with a research team.

The purpose of this book chapter is to first define outcomes research and to describe a 'protocol' or pathway, to facilitate this process. Akin to the formal method we teach, new physicians to conduct a history and physical (H&P) examination, a formal protocol such as described in this book chapter, will facilitate outcomes analyses. There are three main phases, study design, data preparation and data analysis, with multiple steps within each phase. The logic of the outcomes analysis process becomes clear if the steps proceed sequentially.

OUTCOMES RESEARCH

Before creating an outcomes research question and embarking on the pathway of outcomes analysis, it is essential to understand how outcomes research is different from other study types and which questions are best answered utilizing an outcomes analysis. The determinants of outcomes are threefold: the patient, provider and therapies. Traditional study techniques have focused on how the patient and therapies affect outcomes utilizing basic science and randomized controlled trials, respectively. Although outcomes research can be utilized for these traditional topics, its strengths lie in its ability to answer question about the provider variable in the equation, by looking at the higher-level issues at the national, regional, hospital and surgeon levels that would be difficult, if not impossible, to do with traditional study types.

To the extent that they examine these novel factors, outcomes research is more formally known as health services research; how the people of the system (patients, providers) at various levels (national, regional, individual) affect patient outcomes, expanding our understanding beyond patient factors and therapeutics choice and management.

STUDY DESIGN PHASE

The most important, and arguably the most difficult, phase of a study is its design phase. In fact, most problems with research studies arise in the very first step in this phase – asking the research question. An improperly framed research question will create difficult problems throughout the following steps of the project. Note that both the design phase and the data preparation phase will comprise the 'Methods' section of a manuscript.

Before framing the research question, one must determine whether the study will be a descriptive study or an analytical study.

A descriptive study is often employed when there is little established knowledge about the topic being studied in the research question, for instance, a rare or new occurrence, disease or procedure. A descriptive study is investigated using open-ended questions, typically beginning with 'what', 'where', 'when', 'who' or 'how'. For example, 'Who has the disease in question?' or 'What are the common co-morbidities of patients with the disease in question?' In this study, statistical testing is not applicable because there is no established expectation for any particular answer. Basic descriptive statistics are employed and a statistician will not be necessary.

In contrast, an analytical study is utilized when there are established data on the study topic. It requires 'closed-ended' questions, usually beginning with a verb: 'Is/ Was…' or 'Do/Does…' For example, 'Does race or gender affect the mortality of patients with the disease in question?' These studies call for a yes/no answer, and statistical testing is applicable.

The difference between open-ended questions for an inquiry in its earliest stage versus closed-ended questions in later stages can be compared to gathering H&P examination information from a patient. A patient interview begins with open-ended questions ('Tell me about your pain') but then moves on to closed-ended questions ('Was it dull?' 'Did you had a fever?' 'Was it in the left lower quadrant?') as the matrix of information narrows the differential diagnosis and creates a picture of the clinical situation.

Though the difference between the two study types may seem obvious, confusion arises when an attempt is made to make a comparison between two subsets within the same population. For example, if we want to know if there were more men or women who underwent open abdominal aortic aneurysm (AAA) repair last year, the percentage of women versus men would be a descriptive study, and p-values would not be relevant. This may appear to be a comparative study, but in fact, it is a descriptive study because both populations (men who undergo open AAA repair and women who undergo open AAA repair) are correlated and thus represent the same population. They are essentially flip sides of the same coin. Figure 5.1 may help to clarify. Note that in Figure 5.1a, there is really only one pie, even though we have divided that pie into multiple pieces (representing, for example, male patients vs. female patients). However, both slices of that pie are calculated with the same denominator,

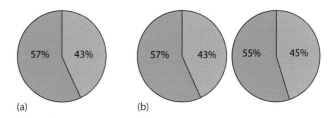

Figure 5.1 Conceptual illustration of the difference between a descriptive and an analytical analysis. (a) Depicts a descriptive study, where both ratios are calculated off of the same denominator, and thus, there is really only one study population. No formal statistical testing is applicable between 57 and 43%. (b) Depicts an analytical study, where there are two different study populations (i.e. the 55% is calculated off of a different denominator as the 57%). In that case, formal statistical testing is applicable to compare 55% versus 57%. (a) p-value is not applicable to compare different parts of the same populations. (b) p-value is applicable for comparing parts of two populations.

being patients who undergo open AAA repair. Any comparative statistics about them would be descriptive, and formal statistical testing would not be applicable.

To change the earlier question from a descriptive question to a 'testable' question, we could, for example, ask whether the male-to-female ratio has changed between last year and the year before. Then, one could calculate a p-value to compare the differences between the two ratios. The p-value in this instance would be interpreted as the probability that the observed finding is based on random chance alone and establishes whether the findings are significant; e.g. a p-value of 0.05 indicates that in that status quo, one would see the results that were found only 5% of the time, a p-value of 0.01 indicates that one would see the results that were found only 1% of the time and so on. Looking at Figure 5.1b, it shows that there are now two pies, so we can ask whether the proportion of one group is higher or lower in one pie than the proportion of that group in another pie and determine the significance of the observation using the p-value.

Step 1: Define the population using inclusion and exclusion criteria

Akin to determining eligibility criteria in a clinical trial, defining the inclusion criteria for a study population is usually fairly intuitive, but there are some nuances to consider. For example, in examining the risk factors for patient safety events in patients undergoing open AAA repair, it may be obvious that open AAA patients should be the study population. However, how should such patients be defined? Depending on the database (as described later), the definition of an open AAA patient may be as simple as all patients in the database if there is an open AAA registry. However, it may be more complicated if the database is a generic database such as an administrative database. In such a case, a set of diagnosis codes would be necessary to define these patients.

But not all open AAA patients culled from an administrative database would be pertinent to answering the study question. This is where it becomes important to craft appropriate exclusion criteria. These exclusion criteria are usually related to the outcome variable or the independent variable (outcome variable and independent variable will be defined in more detail later). For example, the risk factors for an event among patients who have the condition already cannot be studied. If the development of urinary tract infection (UTI) is to be studied, then patients who are admitted with UTIs would need to be excluded. Additionally, the risk factors cannot be studied in a population in which all possible variations in the independent variable that you want to test are not possible. For example, in the examination of the effect of insurance upon hospital admission status, patients over age 65 would have to be excluded, since they are all insured, and there are no uninsured patients in that population. Importantly, patients may be excluded for a combination of reasons. For example, ruptured AAA patients may be excluded from open AAA populations because the outcomes are known to be so poor and predictors of outcomes in ruptured patients are different from that of most open AAA patients.[1]

There is a difference, however, in simply not including certain patients in the inclusion criteria versus actually excluding the patients altogether. This is best explained with the use of Venn diagrams. For instance, the inclusion criteria could be aortic dissection (A) and AAA (B) (Figure 5.2a). Let's say instead, your inclusion criteria is only aortic dissections (Figure 5.2b); even though AAA was not part of the inclusion criteria, there are a group of patients who will be included with both a dissection and aneurysm. To actually isolate dissections without including aneurysms, AAA must be in the exclusion criteria (Figure 5.2c). This can easily be missed, so when thinking of inclusion criteria, one must consider associated conditions that may be grouped in by default.

The validity of a study depends, in large part, on how the study population is defined. Subtle differences in population definition can produce different results. For example, many administrative databases use the International Classification of Disease, Ninth Revision (ICD-9) coding system to classify both diagnoses and procedures. Most physicians in the United States are more familiar with the American Medical Association's Current Procedural Terminology (CPT) system for classifying procedures and think that the ICD-9 system only pertains to diagnosis codes, but in fact, there are ICD-9 diagnosis codes and procedure codes. There are, however, differences between the two systems; there are more CPT than ICD-9 procedure codes with multiple procedures often lumped into the same ICD-9 procedure code, thus making it difficult to identify certain procedures. This incongruity can lead to seemingly disparate study findings due to different ICD-9 procedure codes having been included in the inclusion criteria. To clarify such situations, the list of exact diagnosis and/or procedure codes used in the population definition should be included in the manuscript, either in the 'Methods' section or as a list in the 'Appendix'.

Step 2: Define subsets

In outcomes research, an answer is often generated based upon large heterogeneous populations. Subset analysis can ask and answer questions about more homogeneous groups (minorities, elderly, geographic area, etc.) within the larger set. Thus, outcomes research is actually less effective in showing that a treatment works in a large population (i.e. the efficacy issue), since it is difficult to control for all possible confounders retrospectively in a database.[2] Rather, the strength of outcomes research is in its generalizability (i.e. whether the treatment works in real-life situations or in every patient subpopulation). This has also been labelled the 'effectiveness' issue and makes outcomes research an important tool for comparative effectiveness research. For example, if 'A' works overall, does it also work in the elderly? Does it also work in minority populations? The latter is especially an important issue, given the absence of data regarding minority populations in the literature.[3,4]

Step 3: Define outcome variable(s)

Defining outcome variables is perhaps the most important step in designing a research question. Unfortunately, it is often inadequately addressed, or missed entirely. It is quite typical for people to ask, 'what are the outcomes for

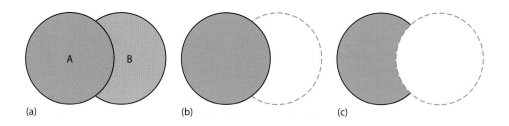

Figure 5.2 Conceptive illustration of the difference between inclusion and exclusion criteria. (a) Depicts inclusion criteria including both aortic dissection (A) and abdominal aortic aneurysm (AAA) (B). (b) Depicts inclusion criteria of only aortic dissection (A). There will be a population of individuals with both aortic dissection and AAA who are included. (c) Depicts inclusion criteria of only aortic dissection and exclusion criteria of AAA. This isolates aortic dissection for the study population.

xyz patients?' But such a question does not specify what the target outcome of interest actually is. An appropriate analytical research question requires the outcome to be specified up front: Is it mortality? Is it complications or a specific set of complications? Complications as an outcome is a perfect example of why the outcome variable needs to be specified up front: if you define 'complication' to include only two events, you will get a very different rate than if you included 10 events. Additionally, certain outcomes, particularly those with clinical subjectivity such as wound infection or sepsis, are notoriously difficult to define. It should be noted that outcome variables can include presentation status, treatment differences and discharge outcomes.

If the question was properly framed in the beginning, as a closed-ended question, then it usually becomes obvious what the outcome variable is. Once again, the importance of the initial framing of the question cannot be understated.

Outcomes research allows investigation of various outcome time points during a hospitalization. For instance, the research question can focus on an outcome that encompasses hospital presentation, hospital care, complications/associated procedural outcomes or discharge outcomes. For example, does gender, race, smoking, etc. affect the likelihood of having an amputation versus revascularization for critical limb ischemia? In this case, amputation and revascularization are the outcomes. An example of a research question focusing on presentation status is, 'Does gender, race, smoking, etc. affect presenting to the hospital as a rupture AAA?'

As will be described later, a study should have as few outcomes as possible, so they must be chosen very carefully. Each outcome of interest will require a fairly detailed analysis on its own. Having multiple outcomes may make the manuscript confusing. For example, the contributors leading to a deep vein thrombosis are likely to be different in the setting of sepsis versus wound dehiscence versus death. A study that attempts to examine all these different outcome variables is likely to be lengthy and difficult to digest.

Step 4: Define the primary comparison to be made

This is a critical feature for any analytical study. In a descriptive study, however, there is no comparison: the prevalence of x and y and the average of z in that population is simply described. An analytical study, on the other hand, requires that some comparison be made. For example, the question 'what is the mortality of xyz procedures in elderly patients?' would be in a descriptive study where statistical testing would not be applicable. The question 'are the elderly at elevated risk for mortality compared to younger patients following xyz procedure?' would be in a comparative study where a statistical comparison would be made between elderly patients and young patients. Specifying the comparison to be tested upfront also helps to avoid type I error; otherwise, the investigator runs the risk of trying additional analyses, which may lead to spurious findings.

Step 5: Define covariates/confounders

There are usually many factors that can influence an outcome variable of interest: these are termed covariates and confounders. For example, in comparing mortality rates of patients, the influence of age, gender, race, socio-economic status, location, etc. must be considered in addition to the primary comparison variable of interest. This highlights a fundamental difference between clinical trials methodology and outcomes research. Both are concerned with confounders, but each addresses them differently. Clinical trials methodology addresses the issue via randomization, creating an equal mix of all possible confounders in both comparison groups. Outcomes research, on the other hand, does not have this luxury, and so it needs to adjust for the influence of confounders statistically. This presents a problem, however, since you need to know that something is a confounder before you can add it to the analysis and adjust for it. For example, if hair colour were a determinant of mortality, but we did not know this and thus it was not collected and added to the database, then we would not be able to adjust for it in the analysis. This is a major difference between outcomes research compared to clinical trials, which is why this step is critical for outcomes researchers and relies on the knowledge from previous studies to identify all appropriate covariates. The strengths of an outcomes study depend on how many covariates can be identified and adjusted for.

DATA PREPARATION PHASE

Once the research question is defined, the next step is to prepare the data for analysis. It is often surprising how long and challenging this 'data preparation' or 'data cleaning' step can be. It is rare for an investigator to move straight from the research question to an analysis without needing to deeply analyze and qualify the relevant data. Additionally, it is important to take precaution at this phase to ensure patient confidentiality, by not including patient identifiers in the analytical file to be created. This issue may be less relevant when analyzing administrative databases or population databases but may be overlooked when accessing institutional clinical databases.

Note that both the design phase and the data preparation phase will comprise the 'Methods' section of a manuscript.

Step 1: Select the database(s)

The first step in the data preparation phase is to select the workhorse database. Depending upon the research question, an administrative database versus a clinical database needs to be chosen. Additionally, the Agency for Healthcare Research and Quality offers a user's guide to registries that can be used to evaluate patient outcomes.[5] An example of an administrative database would be the

Nationwide Inpatient Sample (NIS),[6] which is effective in answering questions regarding the cost of care. Examples of clinical databases would be the National Surgical Quality Improvement Program,[7] the Vascular Study Group of New England (VSGNE) database[8] or the Surveillance, Epidemiology, and End Results (SEER) database,[9] all of which contain more detailed clinical data. More than one databases may be suitable, or necessary, to address the question at hand.

Step 2: Link databases

The data that are needed to answer the research question may reside in different databases, in which case the linking of these databases will be necessary. This will require some identifiers that are common in both databases; for example when looking at hospital characteristics (teaching status, rural/urban location, volume, etc.) and their impact on patient outcomes, the patient database will need to be linked with the hospital database, probably via hospital identification numbers. For internal institutional databases, data are often scattered across multiple data sources (medical records, labs, radiology, etc.), and linking databases together with patient identifiers becomes necessary. In most cases, the need for identifiers to make this linkage will make it impossible for investigators to act without help, especially when dealing with population-level databases.[10–12] For example, since most population-level databases are de-identified, it is not possible to link the SEER database with NIS, which would be useful for answering questions about hospital care versus long-term outcomes. Fortunately, the federal government has recognized the need for such a linked database and has now released the SEER Medicare database for this purpose.

Step 3: Select data elements

The research question should guide the selection of data elements from those available within a particular database. Such selection involves looking up the reference manual or 'data dictionary', for each database, and matching the research question elements to their corresponding database definitions. This may be challenging, depending upon the clarity and rigor of the particular database. For example, the variable 'coronary artery disease' in the VSGNE database includes angina and myocardial infarction in its definition, but does not include patients who are asymptomatic but with intervention, i.e. coronary artery bypass.

Step 4: Generate new data elements

This is perhaps the most time-intensive phase of an outcomes study. It is common for the sought variables to not be defined in a way that immediately meets the need of the study at hand. As discussed earlier, for example the

definition of CAD in the VSGNE database may not fit the assumptions of the study at hand. It then becomes necessary to manually construct novel 'CAD' variable based upon information from a number of other variables, such as 'CABG', 'percutaneous coronary intervention' and 'stress' (which includes the results of stress test). This can become even more difficult if the variable of interest is somewhat amorphous. For example, for any outcomes study, it is important to adjust for patient 'co-morbidity'. However, there is no standard definition of co-morbidity that is universally accepted. To adjust for 'co-morbidity' would therefore involve literature research, identifying possible methods to measure 'co-morbidity' (preferably multiple methods) and then manually constructing that variable based on other information contained in the database about each patient. In this specific case of co-morbidity, the Charlson Index[13,14] or the Elixhauser Index,[15] among others, would be useful.

ANALYSIS PHASE

Following the process described later will produce the 'Results' section of the manuscript.

Step 1: Univariate descriptive analysis

The univariate descriptive analysis describes the entire study population. This analysis is employed in both descriptive and analytical studies. It is called 'univariate' analysis because the population is described one characteristic at a time: average age, proportion males, race, socio-economic status, insurance status, location, etc. This is important so that future readers can determine whether the study applies to their patients. Since this section is solely descriptive, no formal statistical testing is necessary or applicable. An example data table for a univariate analysis is presented in Table 5.1. A study which is only descriptive would likely end after this stage. Analytical studies will continue on through the next few steps.

Step 2: Bivariate analysis

The purpose of bivariate analysis is to report the differences between the comparison groups one characteristic at a time. For example, in comparing elderly versus younger patients, the data table will be a two-column table, with one column for elderly and another column for younger patients, and one row for every additional characteristic to be compared. An example is presented in Table 5.2. The term 'bivariate' analysis is used because for every statistical test performed, the relationship between two variables (i.e. between age and death rates, then between age and length of stay) is described statistically. It is at this phase of the analysis that statistical testing becomes critical. If the characteristic to be compared is a continuous variable (e.g. length of stay),

Table 5.1 Example of a univariate/demographics table.

Age	Median (interquartile range [IQR])
Gender	
Male	N, %
Female	N, %
Ethnicity	
White	N, %
Black	N, %
Hispanic	N, %
Asian	N, %
Intervention	
Intervention A	N, %
Intervention B	N, %
Median length of stay in days (IQR)	N (IQR)
Morbidity	N, %
Mortality	N, %

Table 5.2 Example of a bivariate analysis data table, presenting unadjusted comparison.

	Intervention A	Intervention B	
Age	Median (IQR)	Median (IQR)	p = 0.ttt
Gender			p = 0.ttt
Male	N, %	N, %	
Female	N, %	N, %	
Ethnicity			p = 0.ttt
White	N, %	N, %	
Black	N, %	N, %	
Hispanic	N, %	N, %	
Asian	N, %	N, %	
Length of stay in days	Median (IQR)	Median (IQR)	p = 0.ttt
Morbidity	N, %	N, %	p = 0.ttt
Mortality	N, %	N, %	p = 0.ttt

then tests (for mean) or Wilcoxon test (for median) can be applied.[16] If the characteristic to be compared is a categorical variable (e.g. live or die), then chi-square test can be applied. If the outcome of interest is survival over time, then a Kaplan–Meier analysis may be performed.

In the bivariate analysis, it is essential to avoid type I and II errors. A type I error occurs when there is incorrect rejection of the null hypothesis. For instance, if the null hypothesis is 'hair colour has no effect on aneurysm size', it asserts that there is a relationship between hair colour and aneurysm. If you look hard enough, you will find something. In clinical practice, this is the equivalent of incidentaloma on a CT scan. The converse of this is a type II error. In this case, there is an incorrect acceptance of the null hypothesis, reporting a p > 0.05. These errors occur

when there hasn't been a thorough enough investigation. In clinical practice, this would be an incomplete workup. An underpowered study can also lead to a type II error.

In outcomes analysis, the aforementioned tests are referred to as 'unadjusted' because the comparison is being made one variable at a time without accounting for confounders. In contrast, clinical trials often end their analyses here because comparison groups are matched in every way due to randomization. To further account for confounding variables, outcomes analyses proceed to the multivariable analysis. Thus, in outcomes analysis, further testing (as described later) must be employed. Unlike clinical trials where the comparison groups are equally matched secondary to randomization, further comparison groups are equally matched.

Step 3: Multivariable analysis

Multivariate analysis is the hallmark of outcomes research. In a nutshell, it allows investigators to compare disparate groups, by mathematically adjusting the differences (i.e. the confounders) between comparison groups so that they approach mathematical equivalence. Findings from multivariable analysis are also called 'adjusted' results. An example is presented in Table 5.3. Multivariate analysis is performed with multiple logistic regression steps for a categorical outcome variable (e.g. live or die) or multiple linear regressions for a linear outcome variable (e.g. length of stay). If the outcome of interest is survival over time, then Cox proportional hazards analysis will be used.

The validity of the results from an outcomes analysis rests on the strengths of this multivariable analysis – more specifically, on the number of confounders accounted for in this step. Therefore, it is important to list all the variables that are included in a multivariable analysis, discuss the rationale behind each of them and then discuss these

Table 5.3 Example of a multivariable analysis data table, showing adjusted risks of outcome.

	Odds or hazard ratio	95%CI	p-value
Age	X.xx	Y.yy – Z.zz	0.ttt
Gender			
Male	Reference		
Female	X.xx	Y.yy – Z.zz	0.ttt
Ethnicity			
White	Reference		
Black	X.xx	Y.yy – Z.zz	0.ttt
Hispanic	X.xx	Y.yy – Z.zz	0.ttt
Asian	X.xx	Y.yy – Z.zz	0.ttt
Intervention			
Intervention A	Reference		
Intervention B	X.xx	Y.yy – Z.zz	0.ttt

in the 'limitations' description in the 'Discussion' section regarding any variable that could not be accounted for in the study. The existence of unknown confounders should also be acknowledged (unlike clinical trials, which theoretically control for both known and unknown confounders via its randomization process, the possibility exists in outcomes analysis that there may be confounders that the world does not yet know about).

Many outcomes analyses end here at the multivariable analysis step. But to make a stronger case, subset analysis and sensitivity analysis should also be performed. It will demonstrate appropriate rigor.

Step 4: Subset analysis

The goal of subset analysis is to determine the generalizability of the findings. The idea is to repeat the analysis within every patient subgroup, to determine whether the findings are qualitatively the same in all patients. These subset analyses will eliminate the concern that the study may be a spurious finding.

This is especially important in outcomes research, where heterogeneous patients make up the study populations. For example, if A works overall, does it also work in the elderly? Does it also work in minority populations? This is analogous to the concept of 'clinical indications' in clinical medicine. In clinical statistics, the concept is called 'heterogeneity of treatment effects'.[17] The consistency of the findings across different patient subpopulations will not only make the case for generalizability of findings but also address one of the fundamental limitations of outcomes research: its inability to adjust for all confounders. If a finding is consistent across all patient populations, then the unknown confounders are probably not an issue. Since the prevalence of confounders is probably different in different patient subgroups, but the results are nevertheless qualitatively consistent across these groups, then these confounders will likely not alter the study findings. There will obviously be quantitative differences between different patient populations, so this effect will be stronger or weaker in different patient subgroups. The objective of subset analysis (and the next step, sensitivity analysis) is not to detect these minor differences, but rather, to detect whether there are qualitative differences – i.e. are the findings reversed in any patient subgroups? A few sentences regarding the presence or absence of qualitative differences should suffice.

Step 5: Sensitivity analysis

The objective of sensitivity analysis is to alter some key assumptions of the study, to determine if those changes will affect the conclusion. If the answer is no, it will strengthen the case that the study is not affected by methodological problems. Since there is often no consensus on what is the 'best' methodology, a study that goes ahead and uses multiple methodologies will eliminate any potential reviewer concern that one method is better than another. For example, if the data are adjusted for patient co-morbidities with the Charlson Index, the analysis could be repeated with the Elixhauser Index to determine if the results change qualitatively. Another approach would be to adjust for patient confounders with regular multiple regression analysis, and then with propensity score analysis, and see if the findings are equivalent.[18,19]

Again, as in subgroup analysis, there will likely be some quantitative differences (e.g. the difference between groups may be a little more or a little less), but hopefully, there will be no qualitative change in your conclusion. A few sentences regarding the presence or absence of qualitative differences in the 'Discussion' section should suffice.

LIMITATIONS

The major limitation with outcomes research is data accuracy, which is likely to be common. However, inaccuracies are likely to be randomly distributed so this is unlikely to bias the finding if the study was properly constructed with a hypothesis and a comparison group. Although somewhat counter-intuitive, data inaccuracies may actually strengthen the conclusion available from the study, because if a 'signal' can be detected in a 'noisy' dataset with many inaccuracies, one can conclude that the true signal would have been even larger, if the data were cleaner. Therefore, data inaccuracies are actually considered a form of conservative bias. In other words, data accuracy is less of a concern when it comes to large population analyses; it would be more important to consider sources of biases instead and how they would affect the study's conclusions.

CONCLUSION

A methodical protocol such as the one described here can facilitate converting an interesting clinical question into an outcomes research question with a testable hypothesis.

REFERENCES

1. Mani K, Bjorck M, Lundkvist J, Wanhainen A. Improved long-term survival after abdominal aortic aneurysm repair. *Circulation*. 2009;120:201–211.
2. Guller U. Surgical outcomes research based on administrative data: Inferior or complementary to prospective randomized clinical trials? *World J Surg*. 2006;30(3):255–266.
3. Ford JG, Howerton MW, Lai GY et al. Barriers to recruiting underrepresented populations to cancer clinical trials: A systematic review. *Cancer*. 2008 January 15;112(2):228–242.
4. Mosenifar Z. Population issues in clinical trials. *Proc Am Thorac Soc*. 2007 May;4(2):185–187; discussion 187–188.

5. Agency for Healthcare Research and Quality (AHRQ). *Registries for Evaluating Patient Outcomes: A User's Guide*. Rockville, MD: AHRQ; 2007.

6. HCUP Nationwide Inpatient Sample (NIS). Healthcare Cost and Utilization Project (HCUP). Agency for Healthcare Research and Quality, Rockville, MD, 2000–2001. Available at http://www.hcup-us.ahrq.gov/nisoverview.jsp.

7. National Surgical Quality Improvement Program (NSIP). American College of Surgeons, Chicago, IL. Available at https://acsnsqip.org/login/default.aspx.

8. Vascular Study Group of New England. Society of Vascular Surgery, Chicago, IL. Available at http://www.vascularweb.org/regionalgroups/vsgne/Pages/home.aspx.

9. Surveillance, Epidemiology, and End Results (SEER). National Cancer Institute, Rockville, MD. Available at http://seer.cancer.gov/.

10. Newcombe HB, Kennedy JM, Axford SJ, James AP. Automatic linkage of vital records. *Science*. 1959;130:954–959.

11. Cook LJ, Knight S, Olson LM, Nechodom PJ, Dean JM. Motor vehicle crash characteristics and medical outcomes among older drivers in Utah, 1992–1995. *Ann Emerg Med*. 2000;35:585–591.

12. Clark DE, Hahn DR. Hospital trauma registries linked with population-based data. *J Trauma*. 1999;47:448–454.

13. Charlson ME, Pompei P, Ales KL, MacKenzie CR. A new method of classifying prognostic comorbidity in longitudinal studies: Development and validation. *J Chronic Dis*. 1987;40:373–383.

14. Romano PS, Roos LL, Jollis JG. Adapting a clinical comorbidity index for use with ICD-9-CM administrative data: Differing perspectives. *J Clin Epidemiol*. 1993;46(10):1075–1079.

15. Elixhauser A, Steiner C, Harris DR, Coffey RM. Comorbidity measures for use with administrative data. *Med Care*. 1998;36:8–27.

16. Tassler PL, Dellon AL. A draught of historical significance. *Plast Reconstr Surg*. 1994 August;94(2):400–401.

17. Kravitz RL, Duan N, Braslow J. Evidence-based medicine, heterogeneity of treatment effects, and the trouble with averages. *Milbank Q*. 2004;82(4):661–687.

18. Rubin DB. *Multiple Imputation for Non-Response in Surveys*. New York: John Wiley & Sons, Inc; 1987.

19. Oyetunji TA, Crompton JG, Stevens KA, Efron DT, Haut ER, Chang DC, Cornwell EE, Crandall ML, Haider AH. Using multiple imputation to account for missing data in the National Trauma Data Bank (NTDB). *American Association for the Surgery of Trauma, Poster Presentation*, Maui, HI, September 2008.

SECTION II

Medical Treatment

6

Pathology and medical management of atherosclerotic vascular disease

RALPH G. DEPALMA

CONTENTS

Vascular surgeons mainly treat complications of atherosclerosis. That atherosclerosis is segmental in distribution effectively treated by bypass or removal of lesions is a uniquely surgical insight recognized over six decades ago.[1] However, atherosclerosis, also a systemic disease, remains dormant in arteries until a complication signals its presence. Not only does atherosclerosis progress in native arteries, it also affects newly placed grafts.[2] Surgical and endovascular arterial interventions do not prevent disease progression. Advances in medical management and understanding of atherogenesis offer prospects for primary prevention and effective secondary treatment based upon stabilization and regression of the atherosclerotic plaque. Peripheral arterial disease (PAD) is associated with increased cardiovascular disease (CVD) risk and mortality mainly due to stroke and myocardial infarction.[3] *PubMed* lists, at this time, over 104,000 citations for *atherosclerosis* and 4469 ongoing or completed *regression* studies in *Clinical Trials.gov*. Effective management of PAD requires understanding of the natural history of atherosclerotic lesions and principles of medical management. This chapter reviews the pathology of atherosclerosis and, in this context, outlines current medical management strategies for patients with atherosclerosis as a narrative review. Established as well as emerging scientific concepts of atherogenesis and its treatment will be considered.

ATHEROSCLEROTIC PLAQUE

Figure 6.1 shows a typical fibrous plaque containing a central lipid core with a fibrous or fibromuscular cap, macrophage accumulation and round-cell adventitial infiltration. The Greek word *atheroma* means porridge. *Sclerosis* means induration or hardening. These contrasting characteristics exist in varying degrees in distinct plaques, disease stages and individuals. Von Haller applied the term *atheroma* to the common type of plaque, which, on sectioning, exudes yellow pultaceous content.[4] Atherosclerotic plaques have been found in Egyptian mummies dating back to 1580 BCE.[5] These lesions consist of three main components: cholesterol, mainly in the form of cholesterol esters; cells, mainly smooth muscle, macrophages and other cell types; and fibrous proteins, mainly collagen, elastin and proteoglycans. Fibrin, blood components and calcification characterize advanced plaques. Lesions vary in composition, intensity and distribution; their variability can be appreciated even in a single site as in the carotid bifurcation.[6] Plaques sometimes exhibit mainly smooth-muscle cellular proliferation, collagen, and little lipid content, but more commonly, localized carotid plaques contain a necrotic core of lipid debris and blood elements. Heterogeneous compositional characteristics of carotid plaques relates to current controversy concerning efficacy of medical management as compared to surgical

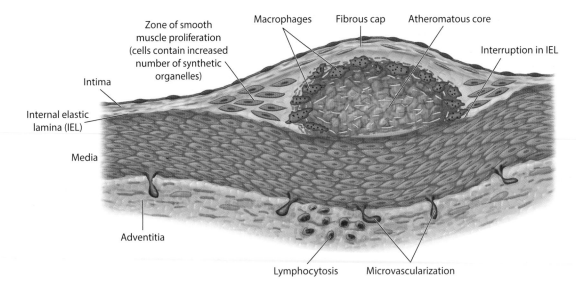

Figure 6.1 Schematic of a typical type IV atheroma. Note central lipid core, fibrous cap, accumulation of macrophages and zone of synthetically active smooth muscle at the *shoulders* of the core. Note tendency of the media to bulge outward, adventitial neovascularization and lymphocytic infiltration. (From DePalma RG, Pathology of atheromas, in: Bell PRF, Jamieson CW, Ruckley CV, eds., *Surgical Management of Vascular Disease*, W.B. Saunders, London, UK, 1992, pp. 21–34.)

or endovascular interventions for asymptomatic lesions.[7] Complicated plaques, which are calcified, ulcerated or necrotic, are intrinsically unstable. Plaques may expand due to intraplaque hemorrhage, or provoke thrombosis related to high-grade stenosis or sudden rupture of an overlying friable cap. Ulcerated plaques cause embolism of atherosclerotic debris. Embolism from presumably *asymptomatic* carotid plaques has been documented by intracranial ultrasound.[8] This finding predicts a high incidence of subsequent transient ischemic attacks, stroke and death. Resolution of issues concerning asymptomatic carotid lesions requires effective imaging which better delineate plaque pathology.[9]

ClinicalTrials.gov lists 40 ongoing studies for asymptomatic carotid disease. These also compare carotid artery stenting and carotid endarterectomy and concurrent medical management.[10] Understanding the nuances of atherosclerotic plaque progression, stabilization or regression relates to the unique dynamics of the plaque lipid atherosclerotic core and associated inflammatory responses.[11,12] These processes determine outcomes of medical interventions. A systematic review of 189 studies of plaque regression comprising 10,235 subjects studied with imaging techniques showed regression, when present, to relate directly to lipid core reduction, mainly induced by statin administration. Regressive changes were seen within an average of about 19.7 months.[13] Plaque regression and stabilization and clinical benefits relate to relatively small decreases in plaque volume and area. Decreased plaque lipid core volume mainly signals regression/stabilization related to improved clinical outcomes particularly in coronary artery disease. Regression/stabilization of plaques also associate with reduction of serum inflammatory biomarkers including C-reactive protein (CRP) and other biomarkers such as interleukin-6 (IL-6).[13,14]

PLAQUE EVOLUTION

Stary et al.[15] defined the initial pathology of fatty streaks, intermediate lesions of atherosclerosis and initial cellular alterations within the arterial wall. A second report further defined the pathology of advanced atherosclerosis, providing a taxonomy to describe disease severity.[16] Hypotheses relating to atherogenesis may be judged by their ability to predict measures to prevent or control this process. Measures to prevent initial plaque formation, important for primary prevention, are likely to be quite different from those needed later to treat advanced disease. Several evolutionary stages of lesions may coexist in single individuals and several pathways might lead to the characteristic fibrous plaque shown in Figure 14.1. For example, an early etiologic hypothesis suggested that viral infection[17] stimulated proliferation of smooth-muscle cells. Other hypotheses postulated initial immunologic or mechanical endothelial damage exposing subintimal smooth muscle to plasma and cellular components, with lipid accumulation and cellular infiltration occurring as subsequent events. However, early childhood and initial lesions in animal models are predominantly fatty. Plaques most often develop and progress beneath morphologically intact endothelium. Entry of low-density lipoprotein cholesterol (LDL-C) and macrophages into the subendothelium occur mainly in relation to increased blood cholesterol levels.

FATTY STREAKS

Fatty streaks, minimally raised, yellow lesions, occur in the aorta and coronary arteries of infants and children. They contain lipids deposited intracellularly within macrophages and smooth-muscle cells. Type I lesions are *microscopic*; they contain subintimal macrophages and a few foam cells. Type II lesions, in contrast, are *grossly* visible and slightly elevated. They stain for fat with Sudan III or IV. They exhibit an abundance of foam cells and lipid droplets, also within intimal smooth-muscle cells along with heterogeneous droplets of extracellular lipids. Type III intermediate lesions are bridges between the fatty streak and the prototypical atheromatous fibrous plaque. Sites and chronology of lesion appearance thus provide clues to early atherogenesis.

Type III lesions develop in characteristic expression–prone localities in the arterial tree,[18] in sites exposed to forces that cause increased LDL-C influx, particularly in areas of low shear stress.[19] It was important to recognize that fatty streak type II lipids are chemically similar to those of the plasma.[20] Plasma lipids enter the arterial wall in several ways: due to altered intimal permeability, increases in interstitial spaces within the intima, faulty metabolism of LDL-C by vascular cells, impeded transport of LDL-C from the intima to the media, increased plasma LDL-C concentrations or specific LDL-C binding to arterial wall connective tissue components, particularly intimal proteoglycans.[21] Experimental observations show LDL-C cholesterol intimal accumulation beneath intact endothelium well before lesions develop; observations identical to those early described in humans by Aschoff[22] and Virchow.[23]

Binding of monocytes to the endothelial lining and their diapedesis into the subintimal layer to become tissue macrophages are also important early atherogenic events.[24–26] Fatty streaks are populated by monocyte-derived macrophages. These lipid-engorged scavenger cells become foam cells, populating fatty streaks and more advanced plaques. The notion that LDL must be altered by oxidation or acetylation to be taken up by macrophages to become foam cells is a key concept.[27] Oxidized LDL-C (OxLDL) is a powerful chemoattractant for monocytes. Inflammatory responses have become central to thinking about pathogenesis and emerging treatment approaches. Another aspect of this concept suggests that endothelium itself might modify LDL-C to promote foam cell formation.

Interactions of plasma LDL within the arterial wall characterize the early stages of atherogenesis. Low-density lipoproteins traverse the endothelium mostly through receptor-independent transport, but also through cell breaks.[28] Endothelial cells,[29] smooth cells[30] and macrophages[31] are all capable of promoting LDL oxidation. OxLDL further attracts monocytes into the intima and promotes their transformation into macrophages. Macrophages produce cytokines including platelet-derived growth factor, transforming growth factor beta, interleukin-1 and other inflammatory cytokines such as TNFa, IL-6 and metalloproteases. OxLDL also induces gene products ordinarily unexpressed in normal vascular tissue including tissue factor, the cellular initiator of a coagulation cascade expressed by atheroma monocytes and foam cells.[32]

GELATINOUS PLAQUES

Intimal gelatinous lesions, also first described by Virchow,[23] are interesting variant lesions. Some believe that these are important progenitors of advanced atherosclerosis.[33,34] Investigation of these lesions showed that virtually all human plasma proteins, particularly hemostatic components, enter the arterial intima.[35] Gelatinous plaques are low in lipid content and translucent and neutral in colour, with central greyish or opaque areas. They occur most commonly in the aorta and separate easily from the underlying arterial wall without entering an endarterectomy plane. Cellularity is increased in transitional stages; these plaques sometimes contain smooth-muscle cells. They also contain substantial amounts of cross-linked fibrin, likely related to increased plasma fibrinogen levels along with other biomarkers such as CRP and Biglycan-mRNA found in smokers without additional risk factors for CVD.[36]

THE FIBROUS PLAQUE

The prototypical atherosclerotic lesion, the type IV fibrous plaque, contains large numbers of smooth-muscle cells and connective tissue forming a fibrous cap over its inner yellow atheromatous core (Figure 1 in Ref. 182). This soft core, composed of cholesterol esters, is thought to be derived from disrupted foam cells. A second type of particle contains both cholesterol and cholesterol esters. Early lesions contain lipids derived directly from LDL by enzymes which hydrolyze LDL cholesterol esters.[37] The composition and integrity of the fibrous cap is clinically relevant. It prevents intraluminal rupture of the soft core and its rupture was early observed as causing acute coronary thromboses.[38,39]

Type IV plaques appear after fatty streaks and Type III lesions, most often in the same anatomic locations. Fibrous plaques characterize clinically significant atherosclerosis. While other lesions might be their precursors, evolution from fatty streak to fibrous plaque is likely the common pathway of lesion development. Fibrous plaques might occasionally arise by conversion of a mural thrombosis into an atheroma.[40] While fibrous plaques protrude into the arterial lumen on fixed cut sections, abluminal or outward bulges occur when arteries are fixed at arterial pressure.[41] This process affects the entire arterial wall and characterizes early coronary and peripheral lesions in subhuman primates and humans.[42,43] The *prestenotic*, or minimally stenotic, phase of atherosclerosis makes quantifying plaque volume problematic using solely measures of luminal intrusion by arteriography. More precise measures involve the use of ultrasound or magnetic resonance imaging (MRI) which image the arterial wall itself. These methods are now increasingly used to assess plaque composition and morphology.[13]

Lipid arterial wall interactions are important in relationship to plaque inflammatory responses. Cholesterol esters in fatty streaks occur in the form of ordered arrays of *intracellular* lipid crystals. Lipids in more advanced plaques assume isotropic forms occurring *extracellularly*.[44] Extracellular cholesterol esters and oxysterols cause severe inflammatory tissue reactions. Plaque inflammation has been found to be involved with neutrophils as well as round cells, indicating more intense inflammation in advanced disease stages.[45] Arteries with fibrous plaques exhibit periarterial inflammation, fibrosis and infiltration of inflammatory cells which reflect disease severity.[46] Neovascularization from the adventitia, another potential source of plaque instability, characterizes advancing intermediate and fibrous plaque lesions. Atherosclerotic lesions contain immunoglobulin G (IgG) in large quantities along with other immunoglobulins and complement components. The contained IgG recognizes epitopes characteristic of oxidized LDL, indicating that inflammatory and immune processes relate to all stages of plaque development.[47] Inflammatory and immune process are associated with systemic effects; patients with carotid atherosclerosis have higher antibody levels of anti-OxLDL and IGM than comparable nonatherosclerotic controls.[48]

PROGRESSION TO COMPLICATED PLAQUES

Fibrous plaque progression causes complications of atherosclerosis: embolization, thrombosis and distal ischemia. The pathologic classification of advanced atherosclerotic lesions[16] considers extracellular lipid to be the precursor of the core of the type IV fibrous plaque. Type V lesions exhibit a thick layer of fibrous tissue and type VI lesions exhibit fissures, hematoma or thrombus representing far advanced disease. Aneurysms due to atherosclerosis have been included within the recent pathologic classification of advanced disease.[16] Aneurysm formation may represent unique small effect on genetic or immune responses to the atherosclerotic process.[49,50] A high prevalence of atherosclerotic risk factors along with coincident atherosclerotic involvement occurs in the usual patient with aneurysms.[51] Medical management is indicated as for patients with occlusive disease patterns, with the understanding that indications for intervention for aneurysmal disease are not delayed by medical management.

APPROACH TO TREATMENT

Epidemiologically defined risk factors may be viewed as etiologic factors but not in a strict sense. While it is useful to approach medical interventions that alter or minimize risk factors, it is also important to recognize that atherosclerosis comprises a spectrum of vascular pathology. Its etiology is not singular and univariate, but rather, it is complex and interactive. Atherosclerosis can be viewed as a family of closely related vascular disorders. Bodily patterns of involvement relate to specific risk factors associated with distinctly differing rates of progression.[52,53] Individual management will differ from one case to another. PAD usually afflicts older individuals; concurrent dyslipidemia may not be evident in these cases. However,

dyslipidemia will be found to have existed in the past. Risk factors are epidemiologically defined constructs. Their effects on vascular complications and disease prevalence are epidemiologically, rather than etiologically, defined.[54] Traditional risk factors include hyperlipidemia, primarily elevated levels of LDL-C, cigarette smoking, hypertension and diabetes mellitus along with male sex and age. Novel emerging risk factors include systemic inflammatory biomarkers. Younger patients present with more concurrent risk factors, including dyslipidemia, cigarette addiction and diabetes. Smoking is the most salient risk factor in presentation of PAD patients, particularly those requiring multiple vascular operations.[55] Complete cessation of this habit, a critical lifestyle alteration, must be insisted upon and effectively supported.

Lesion arrest, stabilization and regression

Regression of atherosclerosis in response to lowered serum cholesterol has been observed in autopsy studies of starved humans[22] and abundantly demonstrated in experimental animal studies.[56,57] Experiments confirming plaque regression related to aggressive lipid reduction had set the stage for the many plaque regression trials recently reviewed.[13] Imaging studies to measure regression include quantitative angiography, ultrasound and intravascular ultrasound, MRI and MRI/positron emission scanning. Experimental markers which detect and quantify plaque inflammatory responses are beginning to be exploited in clinical settings.[58,59] In experimental models, favourable plaque alterations can be documented by direct sequential observations using surgery and biopsy as well. Operational aspects confirming experimental plaque regression have used morphometric and biochemical measurements not possible to obtain in humans. Regressive plaque change occurs mainly by lipid egress from the lipid core. Plaque bulk and luminal intrusion can be reduced in dogs,[60,61] rhesus monkeys[62,63] and other species. Protein content may increase or decrease in involved vascular areas during regression.[63] Plaque fibrous protein increase during regression, while limiting plaque volume decrement, converts unstable plaques into more stable lesions. This process has been shown using pravastatin in an experimental model.[64] To produce consistent experimental arrest or regression, total serum cholesterol must be reduced below a threshold of ~200 mg/dL. Conversely, moderate serum cholesterol levels above which experimental lesions progress to ischemia, stroke and aneurysm formation occurred in canines observed over extended time periods.[65]

Serial observational imaging studies confirm human atherosclerotic plaque regression.[13] Decrements in luminal intrusion and plaque surface area, usually modest, range in single-digit values. More importantly, change in the proportion of the lipid core as related to total plaque volume decreases considerably. Human threshold lipid values for regression may approximate total serum cholesterol of 150–170 mg/dL with LDL-C levels of 100 mg/dL or less. Similar cholesterol levels prevail coincidentally in world populations in which atherosclerosis is virtually absent.[66,67] By contrast, based on long-term outcomes in the MRFIT trial,[68] cholesterol levels exhibited a continuous graded relationship (in contrast to threshold values) to long-term risk of coronary heart disease (CAD), CVD, all-cause mortality and a longer estimated life expectancy for young men with favourable serum cholesterol levels. These relationships will be further considered along with current controversy concerning medical management strategies targeting specific cholesterol levels.

Medical management

Lipid dynamics and inflammatory responses assume crucial roles in atherosclerosis and its complications which are reflected in blood biomarker levels. Statin treatment, in addition to reducing LDL-C, also reduces systemic inflammatory biomarkers. It promotes favourable changes in the atheroma and an increased survival documented in over 137 open or completed prospective trials listed in *ClinicalTrials.gov*.[69] The highly favourable results of the 2004 MRC/BHF heart protection study using simvastatin initiated the current era of widespread statin administration.[70] This trial included over 20,000 high-risk patients without elevated lipid levels. Recent American College of Cardiology/American Heart Association (ACC/AHA) cardiovascular guidelines in 2013 endorsed a novel paradigm of matching intensity of preventive methods with an individual's absolute risk (based in part upon ethnicity) using pooled cohort atherosclerotic cardiovascular risk equations[71] rather than using the National Cholesterol Educational Program (NCEPIII) lipid values for those at high risk including patients with PAD and diabetes.[72] NCEPIII targets values of LDL <100 mg/mL, with an optimal target goal of 70 mg/mL for high-risk individuals. The 2013 ACC/AHA guidelines instead propose implementation of cholesterol-lowering treatment using evidence-based therapy *without specific targets*, significantly increasing the number of patients recommended for cholesterol-lowering therapy.[73] ACC/AHA guidelines depend in the main upon randomized controlled trials, for example, showing prospective benefits of reduction of CRP and LDL-C as both affecting cardiovascular event rates with high-intensity statin intervention.[74] ATPIII, however, remains practical, in this authors opinion, to guide treatment of coexisting dyslipidemia. While the new recommendations appear on the surface conflicting, serial coronary studies of large numbers of individuals receiving high-intensity statin treatment studied with intravascular ultrasound showed regressive plaque effects and clinical outcomes, for example, as reported by Puri and Nissen in the coronary arteries[14,75] and favourable changes in carotid and femoral arteries summarized by Noyes and Thompson.[13]

Drug treatment

Statins, 3-hydroxy-3- methylglutaryl coenzyme H–reducing agents, lower LDL-C and exhibit pleiotropic actions which reduce inflammatory biomarkers. Statins are widely prescribed for high-risk patients with PAD or diabetes. Roberts[76] early editorialized that statin drugs are to atherosclerosis as what penicillin was to infectious disease. However, statin therapy requires caution concerning toxic effects. These include liver disorders, myopathy and other neuromuscular effects. A population study showed increased incidence of new onset diabetes particularly in women.[77] Another population-based study also showed that the risk of new onset diabetes rises with adherence to statin therapy but concluded that statin benefits outweigh risks.[78] These appear to be consensus opinions regarding statin risk and benefits. In support, an overview of 16 published trials including 29,000 subjects revealed no evidence for increased noncardiovascular deaths or cancer incidence.[79]

Currently available statins include atorvastatin (high-intensity dose 40–80 mg/dL q d; moderate-intensity dose 10–20 mg q d), rosuvastatin (high-intensity dose 20–40 mg; moderate-intensity dose 5–10 mg q d), fluvastatin 40 mg BID, lovastatin 40 mg, pitavastatin 2–4 mg, pravastatin 40–80 mg and simvastatin 20–40 mg q d.[80]

Comprehensive recommendations for dyslipidemia management recently summarized by the National Lipid Association[80] stress the need for primary interval screening for lipoprotein lipid levels. In the author's opinion, all patients presenting with atherosclerosis as well as individuals with risk factors should be screened to include inflammatory biomarkers as well. The presence of asymptomatic lesions detected by non-invasive screening indicates an urgent need for aggressive medical interventions. LDL-C comprises approximately 75% of the cholesterol carried by lipoprotein particles other than HDL. This percentage is lower in patients with elevated triglycerides. Desirable lipid levels as listed in these recommendations are as follows: Non-HDL-C <130 mg/dL (i.e. total cholesterol minus HDL-C), LDL-C < 100, HDL-C > 40 men and >50 women and triglycerides <150 mg/dL. Treatment of homozygous familial hypercholesterolemia requires additional measures. These patients present early in life mainly with coronary disease in contrast to the usual PAD patients who usually present much later in life. New agents for management of these disorders will be discussed later.

While statins comprise the cornerstone of medical intervention for atherosclerosis, statin intolerance or toxicity are serious challenges. Alternative therapies must be considered for such individuals. About 70% of long-term statin adherence has been described with about 30% of those discontinuing statins due to side effects.[13] In these cases, changing statin types and dosages can be considered. Beyond statins, alternative agents include fibrates, such as gemfibrozil and ezetimibe, bile acid sequestrants, n-3 fatty acids and niacin. The reader is referred to a recent expert review for the use of these agents.[81] Side effects of flushing with niacin, its potential to promote diabetes and its liver toxicity, remain problematic in this author's opinion. A recent randomized trial showed that niacin failed to reduce adverse vascular events.[82]

Cigarette smoking

This habit causes progression of PAD to amputation,[83] high mortality from ischemic heart disease,[84] failure of aortic[85] and femoral–popliteal grafts.[86] Smoking cessation, a most important intervention, must be insisted upon and facilitated in all patients. Cigarette smoking promotes atherosclerosis and graft thrombosis in multiple ways. Cigarette smoking causes increased platelet reactivity, promotes peripheral vasoconstriction and is associated with reduced HDL levels.[87] It is interesting to note that in populations in whom LDL-C levels remain exceedingly low, cigarette smoking may not be associated with a high incidence of atherosclerotic vascular disease. Smoking cessation clinical practice guidelines use motivational intervention strategies,[82] nicotine replacement and scheduled follow-up contacts. Nicotine-replacement therapy is most effective when used as part of a formal programme.[88] Following personal advice given by physicians to encourage smoking cessation at a single consultation, only an estimated 2% of all smokers successfully stopped smoking after 1 year.[89] Vascular specialists, recognizing the limitations of individual advice, should encourage and support institutional development of formal smoking cessation programmes. Nicotine replacement and bupropion administration provide improved results as compared to placebo therapy with counseling, which yielded only 19% compliance.[90] Bupropion exhibits a unique characteristic promoting prosexual effects[91] possibly facilitating smoking cessation by substituting one pleasure for another.

Hypertension

An evidenced-based management guide for hypertension to prevent myocardial infarction, stoke renal failure and death has been recently published.[92] Though not without controversy, evidence from controlled trials provide strong evidence to support treating hypertensives aged 60 years or older to a BP goal of <150/90 mmHg and hypertensives 30–59 years to a diastolic goal of <90 mmHg. Based on expert opinion the panel recommends a goal of <140/90 for the elderly.[92] Chronic hypertension accelerates experimental atherosclerosis,[93,94] and treatment of hypercholesterolemia and hypertension using combined drug therapy has been found to be effective in a primate model.[94] A recent Cochrane review summarized results of 8 RCTs of drugs in treatment of hypertensive PAD patients.[95] The rates of cardiovascular events, death, claudication symptoms and progression of PAD showed considerable variation of comparisons and outcomes.[95] The reviewers

concluded that evidence regarding choice of various antihypertensive drugs in people with PAD is poor, but that lack of data specificity should not detract from the overwhelming evidence on the benefits of blood pressure reduction.[92] Traditionally, sodium reduction and weight loss are feasible and safe in older people.[96] Interestingly, a meta-analysis addressing the controversy as to whether or not reduced sodium intake would decrease the blood pressure of a population did not support this recommendation as a population-based intiative.[97]

Control of hypertension prolongs life and reduces coronary mortality.[92] In affluent societies, hypertension relates to premature atherosclerotic disease risk independently of the risk factors of hyperlipidemia and cigarette smoking.[98] Hypertension is also linked to risk factor clustering: glucose intolerance, hyperinsulinemia, dyslipidemia and abdominal obesity. This cluster comprises the metabolic syndrome.[99] Treatment of this condition requires weight loss, exercise and possibly drug treatment for associated elevated triglycerides. Treatment of hypertension with thiazide diuretics require a caution in that this choice appeared to be disadvantageous in terms of coronary outcome in a subgroup of men with minor EKG abnormalities during the MRFIT trial.[100] Beta blockers require particular caution when initiated in the immediate preoperative period. While preoperative beta blockade started within 1 day of non-cardiac surgery prevents non-fatal MI, it also increases risks of post-operative stroke death, hypotension and bradycardia.[101] Recommended lifestyle alterations include weight reduction, reduced dietary sodium intake, reduced alcohol intake, increased physical activity and, possibly, increased calcium intake.[102] A meta-analysis of 147 trials showed that the use of beta blockers, angiotensin-converting enzyme (ACE) inhibitors, angiotensin receptor blockers, diuretics and calcium channel blockers in older people results in equivalent reductions of coronary and stroke events for given decreases in blood pressure.[103] Agent choice depends upon efficacy judged by blood pressure monitoring, tolerability and the presence of specific comorbidities, including kidney disease. The use of ACE inhibitor ramipril 10 mg daily, in a randomized placebo-controlled trial involving 212 PAD participants, was reported to increase walking times and quality of life after 24 weeks of treatment.[104]

Diabetes mellitus

Diabetes is one of the most important risk/pathogenetic factors promoting atherosclerosis. In its singular form, diabetes is associated with a pattern of infracural and coronary atherosclerosis.[52] An early diabetes control trial[105] showed favourable reduction in microvascular complications with *tight* control achieved by insulin use; unfortunately, this trial was not designed to study end points of macrovascular atherosclerotic complications. Tight control of diabetes with insulin and sulfonylureas, in a cross-sectional study of type 2 diabetics (T2DM), associates with increases in mortality and morbidity[106] suggesting targeting more liberal Hbg A1C values and avoiding overtreatment in persons at hypoglycemic risk, predominantly the elderly.[107]

With any given level of LDL, CHD risk has long been known to be tripled in diabetics relative to individuals without the disease,[108] a critical consideration in overall management, indicating a role for statins in this group.[68,108] Among patients with T2DM, traditional cardiovascular risk factors including age, sex, race and particularly smoking status are associated with the development of incident PAD.[110] Management of modifiable cardiovascular risk factors is a critical first step in approaching patients with PAD and T2DM. Treatment strategies include lifestyle and pharmacologic interventions targeting hyperglycemia, hypertension, dyslipidemia, obesity, cigarette smoking, prothrombotic factors and physical inactivity.[111]

Beyond primary interventions, several categories of drugs are the subject of many clinical trials. At this time (December 2014), 403 trials of these agents are listed on *Clinical Trials.gov* with over 54,553 subject listings in *PubMed*. Classes of drugs include biguanidines; metformin, which decreases the amount of glucose released from the liver; sulfonylureas meglitinides, which stimulate the pancreas to release more insulin; thiazolidinediones, which enhance insulin sensitivity; DPP 4 inhibitors, which lower glucose made by the body; and alpha-glucosidase inhibitors, which along with bile acid sequestrants lower intestinal glucose absorption. Combinations of these agents are used along with a new class of agents, sodium-glucose cotransport 2 inhibitors, which promote renal glucose excretion.[112] Selecting appropriate choices among this imposing array of agents is challenging; expert consultation is recommended. That being said, metformin is usually the first line agent used. This drug must be discontinued before angiographic studies using contrast media.[113]

Lifestyle factors: General considerations

Lack of exercise, obesity and psychological stress have been considered primary risk factors predisposing to atherosclerosis. A classic retrospective study reported that sedentary London bus drivers had a higher incidence of coronary disease than a matched cohort of their more physically active bus conductors.[114] The Framingham epidemiologic study[115] early showed the inverse relationship of overall mortality and cardiovascular mortality to be related to physical activity. This effect was small, however, as compared to that of the major risk factors of smoking, hypertension, diabetes and hyperlipidemia. Mortality in general obesity, associated with risk of sudden cardiac death in middle-aged, non-smoking individuals, appears to be mediated mainly by traditional cardiovascular risk factors. Central obesity measured by waist circumference and waist/hip ratio, as occurs with the metabolic syndrome (and T2DM), independently is associated with

sudden cardiac death as described in a recent multicenter prospective cohort study.[116] While non-intentional (observational) weight loss in patients with CAD is associated with an increase in clinical CVD events, intentional weight loss is associated with fewer clinical events in CAD.[116,117] Surprisingly, data concerning the efficacy of weight loss interventions specifically for PAD are lacking, though this advice is often given. Its effect may relate to reduction of accompanying risk factors.

Past psychological constructs associated coronary artery disease with type A behaviour – type A individuals exhibiting enhanced competitiveness, ambitiousness and a chronic sense of time urgency. The clinical picture comprises individuals that are 'dissatisfied with themselves and others, very ill-humoured, and easily angered or annoyed'. Clarkson[118] quoting Osler[119] who characterized the typical coronary patient as 'the robust, the vigorous in mind and body, the keen and ambitious man; whose engine is always at full-speed ahead'. Clarkson's primate experiments[118] showed that highly aggressive monkeys kept in chronically unstable social conditions developed more extensive coronary atherosclerosis than dominant monkeys living in unstressed social conditions. The type A psychological construct has been replaced by a newly coined type D personality type: a person who is anxious, irritable and insecure. Type D (Distressed) personality type in a case control study were reported to have a higher incidence in CHD[120] and plaque severity in a CT scanning study.[121] The relevance of these observations to PAD management relates to interactions of a negative personality type to the core role of traditional risk factors which coexist to a higher degree in these individuals. This personality type presents the clinician with compliance issues.

Exercise

The effects of exercise on treatment of atherosclerosis are considered from two viewpoints: preventative versus therapeutic use for claudication. Habitual physical activity has long been known to decrease the primary incidence of CHD.[122] Symptomatic improvement in claudication is due likely to improved muscular metabolism related to mitochondrial dysfunction associated with PAD.[123] Exercise training in PAD improves cardiorespiratory fitness, pain free and total flat walking distance.[124] Exercise should be recommended as an option for PAD patients in the absence of contraindications.[125] Exercise, however, has not been shown to cause atherosclerotic plaques stabilization or regression. Episodes of sudden death due to coronary atherosclerosis during strenuous exercise result from plaque disruption, a concern[126] for clinicians prescribing exercise for known CAD.

Exercise is a complex behaviour for which no standard measure exists similar to blood pressure measurement or lipid profile determination. Modern exercise research uses standard aerobic exercise programmes. For example, a quantitative exercise study compared the efficacy of dietary weight loss to exercise by measuring enhanced VO_2 max induced by exercise to a predetermined amount.[127] Quantitation of exercise described in multiple intervention studies is often difficult to assess, as is its contribution to observed favourable effects. Exercise is not sufficient to offset the deleterious effects of other risk factors such as elevated LDL-C, hypertension or smoking. Before prescribing or permitting strenuous exercise, stress testing and monitoring are recommended.

Exercise improves lipid profile and glucose metabolism, aids in weight reduction and, as mentioned, is effective in relief of claudication.[128–131] Computer models of flow dynamics of human aortas show that with increased flow, shear stress is normalized; early stages of atherosclerosis might be inhibited.[132] Favourable effects in clotting and platelet reactivity have been reported[133] along with improved fibrinolytic activity after strenuous exercise.[134]

Diet

The prior edition of this book in 2004[135] summarized results of four prospective dietary lipid lowering trials in CAD with end points of fatal and non-fatal coronary events in combination. Among those, only one, the Oslo trial, showed a statically significant reduction in these adverse outcomes.[136] Considerable interest continues in dietary interventions for primary prevention and treatment of established disease. To assess dietary intervention effects, patients with PAD should have baseline measures of lipids, inflammatory markers, fasting glucose and HbA1C. Blood samples should be obtained from stable ambulatory patients consuming their customary diet. Acute illnesses and procedures associated with hospitalization cause sudden, inexplicable decrements in total serum cholesterol levels. Early iterations of the Adult Treatment Panel for the National Cholesterol Guidelines recommended a stepwise treatment using a graded approach to a low-fat reduced-calorie diet before initiating drug treatment.[137] However, more frequently, statins are started as initial treatment. A vast literature on diet and atherosclerosis exists: 349 trials under this heading, predominantly related to supplement effects, appear on *ClinicalTrials.gov*. The heading diet and PAD lists 39 trials. While it is accepted that injudicious dietary habits cause premature death and chronic disease such as CVD, a myriad of distracting claims as to the benefits of one diet over another make the subject of dietary advice confusing.[138]

The author and associates[139] long ago advocated a diet low in sucrose, red or processed meat and dairy products, including eggs. These early recommendations were based upon a review of existing dietary literature and experiments clearly showing that plaque progression and regression related to elevation or reduction of lipid levels in animal models.[60–65] Experience with dietary-induced atherosclerosis in the rhesus monkey showed that addition of large quantities of cholesterol up to 20% by weight to Purina Monkey chow (5% crude fat, 15% protein, 5% fibre and 62% nitrogen-free extract and vitamins) caused only mild cholesterolemia and minor fatty streaks when fed over intervals of up to 2 years. In sharp contrast, a diet containing in grammes %, *egg yolk* 36.6%, *sucrose* 47.9%, soy protein 7.48%, along with nonnutritive fibre, salt and vitamin mix and crystalline cholesterol ~0.4% produced, within 24 months, elevation of cholesterol level from ~134 mg/dL at baseline to ~400 mg/dL and rapid development of intrusive atherosclerotic plaques.[62] The lipid pattern in the rhesus resembles that of human acquired non-familial type II hyperlipidemia. Triglycerides, in spite of weight gain, remained normal. Return to normal feeding caused visible regressive plaque changes within 6 months. Recognizing the limits of extrapolation from a subhuman primate model to free living humans, these findings prompted our recommendations to eliminate dietary sucrose by substituting whole fruit for desserts and to drastically reduce red meat consumption. We sought and found arteriographic evidence of human plaque regression when cholesterol reduction was combined with complete smoking cessation.[140] These experiments and case observations have influenced the author's clinical approach to dietary interventions for patients with vascular disease. But more systematic studies are needed.

An overwhelming number of proposed diets currently exist. These include low carbohydrate, low fat, low glycemic, mixed and balanced with animal and plant food, Palaeolithic, vegetarian and vegan.[138] The Mediterranean diet recently attracted considerable scientific attention based upon population survival studies[141] and its effect upon inflammatory biomarker reduction.[142] This diet is characterized by abundant olive oil consumption; high consumption of plant foods (fruits and vegetables); moderate wine intake with meals; moderate consumption of fish, seafood, yogurt, cheese, poultry and eggs; and very low red meat consumption. By contrast, a singular intervention for CVD consists of an austere diet, all plant based as well as complete abstinence from dairy products, oils and nuts of all types.[142] This diet was advised for 198 CVD patients followed for a mean of 3.7 years. A recent report from this group described angiographic lesion regression in some cases and clinical benefits with only one stroke among 177 strictly adherent subjects. By contrast, 13 of 21 non-adherent subjects had adverse CVD events.[142]

Antiplatelet and anticoagulant therapy

Atherothrombosis, clotting superimposed upon underlying plaque, causes ischemic cerebrovascular, coronary and PAD complications. Antiplatelet agents minimize or prevent these adverse events.[143] A voluminous literature concerning optimal aspirin dosages exists. The *Physicians' Health Study* initially showed that patients given with 325 mg of aspirin on alternate days had reduced CVD events and had the need for peripheral vascular surgery,[144] but were at risk of gastric effects and a slightly increased stroke risk. Aspirin dosages ranging from 74 to 159 mg daily are more effective than larger doses.[145] Aspirin in doses of 81 mg are convenient, readily available and preferred by the author. Concomitant use of clopidogrel combined with aspirin was based upon overall improved outcomes in the CAPRIE trial in a subset of participants with PAD which made the study positive.[146] A Cochrane review of 12 studies involving 12,168 patients reviewed evidence for efficacy of aspirin, clopidogrel and dipyridamole in PAD. This review suggested that first line evidence for aspirin in PAD is weak and that further research is needed to determine whether aspirin might be replaced with a different class of antiplatelet agent.[147] For symptomatic patients undergoing carotid endarterectomy, perioperative therapy should include aspirin with the addition of clopidogrel on a case-to-case basis. With carotid stenting and stenting in other vessels, aspirin and clopidogrel are recommended.[148,149]

Cilostazol, a phosphodiesterase 3 inhibitor, reportedly improved claudication without increased bleeding risk.[150] A case control study of 16 patients with carotid stenosis receiving 200 mg of cilostazol daily used MRI plaque imaging at 6 and 12 months. These investigators reported an increased fibrous component and decrease in the lipid necrotic core in carotid plaques with no change in plaque volume on ultrasonography.[151] This small study is unusual in that interventions that alter atherosclerotic plaques towards regression or stabilization usually use statins.

To test the hypothesis that long-term administration of high-dose antiplatelet agents would improve or prevent atherosclerotic plaque progression, our group used atherosclerotic rhesus monkeys on a diet high in sucrose and egg yolk receiving high dose (13.5 mg/kg aspirin and 15 mg/kg dipyridamole) for 12 months compared to controls on diet alone.[152] Serial platelet survival measurements between the two groups did not change during 58 months of progression of atherosclerosis, indicating a non-role for platelets in atherogenesis in this dietary model of atherosclerosis. Plaques in treated animals developed prominent necrotic lipid cores (Figure 6.2) and thromboses notably absent in control animals. These findings in a subhuman primate are alarming. Caution is clearly warranted in the use of high-dose antiplatelet interventions for human atherosclerosis. The effects of antiplatelet agents and Cox 2 inhibitors on human plaque morphology clearly require further study.

Aspirin, rather than anticoagulation, may be the best intervention for atheroembolism (blue toe syndrome), an uncommon condition related to ulcerated aortic plaques, the so-called shaggy aorta.[153] Anticoagulation makes matters worse and, in some cases, actually cause this condition. On the other hand, antiplatelet therapy with aspirin[154] and anticoagulants reportedly reduced the risk of graft occlusion and ischemic events after infrainguinal bypass surgery.[155] Major bleeding independently increases the risk of ischemic events indicating the need for caution when using antiplatelet agents.[156] In addition, certain pre-existing hypercoagulable states cause post-operative graft thrombosis. Patients with low levels of antithrombin III and proteins C and S and plasminogen abnormities require perioperative warfarin administration.[157]

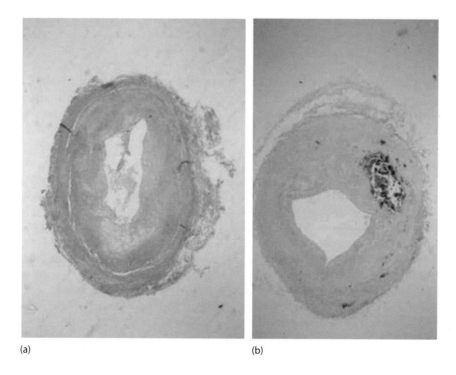

(a)   (b)

Figure 6.2 Effects of 12 months high dose aspirin/dipyridamol administration on atherosclerosis in rhesus monkey. Femoral arteries: (a) 58 months atherogenic diet; (b) diet plus 12 months aspirin/dipyridamol. (Adapted from DePalma RG et al., Failure of antiplatelet treatment in dietary atherosclerosis: A serial intervention study, In Gallo LL and Vahouny GV (eds.), *Cardiovascular Disease: Molecular and Cellular Mechanisms, Prevention, Treatment*, New York, Plenum Press, pp. 407–426, 1987.)

New horizons

REDUCTION OF LDL; NEW AGENTS

Extreme LDL-C reductions are now possible. The discovery of proprotein convertase subtilisin/kexin type 9 (PCSK9), a novel and unique advance, provides a new approach to LDL-C reduction. PCSK9 promotes LDL receptor degradation within hepatocytes to reduce the concentration of receptors on the surface of hepatocytes resulting in lower plasma LDL clearance.[158] Agents that inhibit PCSK9 cause reduction of LDL-C well below 70 mg/dL. PCSK9 inhibitors are monoclonal antibodies (evolocumab, alirocumab and bococizumab) that are given by injection. They are capable of reducing LDL-C in individuals with familial dyslipidemia otherwise resistant to statins.[159] At the time of this writing, these drugs await FDA approval prior to their widespread introduction.

REDUCTION OF INFLAMMATORY RESPONSES

Interleukin-6 is intimately involved in inflammation. Elevated blood levels of this cytokine along with CRP have been found to predict future myocardial infarction in a prospective observational study of over 14,000 apparently healthy men.[160] To test directly the inflammatory hypothesis, a low-dose methotrexate trial (CIRT) to reduce TNFa, IL-6 and CRP levels is recruiting participants.[161] The study will randomly allocate 7000 patients with myocardial infarction, type 2 diabetes or the metabolic syndrome to low-dose methotrexate (target 15–20 mg/week) or placebo for average follow-up of 3–5 years.[162]

IRON AND OXIDATIVE INJURY

Iron in its ferrous form, a powerful inflammatory and oxidizing agent, is postulated to promote progressive inflammatory diseases including CVD.[163] Its balance is regulated by hepcidin, a hormone promoting iron retention in macrophages, which in turn, may increase plaque iron content and inflammatory responses.[164] The Iron and Atherosclerosis Study, a prospective, randomized, controlled single-blinded clinical trial of iron reduction using phlebotomy in participants with PAD, tested the hypothesis that improved clinical outcomes might be achieved by ferritin reduction.[165] The primary outcome was all-cause mortality and secondary outcomes combined death plus non-fatal myocardial infarction and stroke. While overall results did not show a difference in outcomes related to phlebotomy, statistically significant improvement in primary and secondary outcomes with iron reduction occurred in younger participants, aged 43–61 years, and in smokers as compared to non-smokers.[165,166] The iron reduction effect and ferritin levels decreased with increasing age. Ferritin levels below 80 ng/mL, irrespective of phlebotomy intervention, correlated with favourable primary and secondary outcomes.[167] Elevated inflammatory cytokine signatures (IL-6, TNFa, CRP) were found in PAD participants as compared to levels in disease-free individuals.[168] Significant direct relationships between mortality, ferritin levels and inflammatory cytokines levels were found on completion of the 6-year study.[169] Statins for PAD, introduced during the trial, increased HDL/LDL ratios and reduced ferritin levels.[169,170] Improved clinical outcomes, however, were associated with lower ferritin levels rather than improved lipid status, an interesting observation that led to postulating a *statin–iron nexus*. Statins and ferritin reduction may both act similarly to reduce inflammatory processes.[170] Cross-sectional observations comparing outcomes in White and African American CSP 410 participants demonstrated significantly higher ferritin levels, lower red cell measures, serum iron and % transferrin saturations and differing responsiveness to iron reduction in African Americans as compared to White participants.[171] Higher rates of amputation are known to occur in African Americans despite controlling for co-morbidities, disease severity, surgeon and hospital performances.[172] Adverse CVD outcomes in African Americans may relate, in part, to racial differences in iron metabolism and greater sensitivity to diets high in iron content. These findings suggest that future studies be structured to include racial differences along with adaptive allocation using risk factors.[171]

HOMOCYSTEINEMIA

Homocysteine, a sulphur-containing amino acid, is formed during methionine metabolism. In excess, it has been considered an independent risk factor for several disorders including CVD.[173] While elevated homocysteine levels are reduced by folic acid intake, a meta-analysis of 8 randomized trials involving over 37,000 participants showed no effect on CVD outcomes, although homocysteine levels were reduced effectively.[174]

INFECTION

Cytomegalovirus (CMV) and *Chlamydophila pneumoniae* infections have been associated with atherosclerosis.[17] Comprehensive reviews have summarized interesting biologic evidence supporting relationships between infection and atherosclerosis including CMV, a ubiquitous virus.[175] Deleterious effects of infection might relate to inflammation and bacterial heat shock proteins which incite arterial inflammatory and autoimmune reactions.[176] While these molecular mechanisms remain of pathogenic interest, randomized prospective trials assessing the efficacy of antibiotics to prevent cardiovascular events have been negative.[177] Periodontal disease has also been suggested as a contributor to CVD. *ClinicalTrials.gov* lists current 11 studies concerning the results of periodontal treatment upon CVD outcomes. Substantive publications of any effect, positive or negative, have not been published.

MICROBIOME: GUT MICROBIOTA

Dietary nutrients with a trimethylamine (TMA) moiety such as choline, phosphatidylcholine and L-carnitine have been implicated experimentally in the development of atherosclerosis and CVD risks.[178] The mechanism relates to gut microbiota dependant formation of TMA and host transformation to TMA-O-Oxide (TMAO), a vascular irritant.

Studies in mice show critical roles for dietary choline interacting with gut flora to produce TMAO which then augments macrophage cholesterol accumulation and foam cell formation. Suppression of gut microflora in atherosclerosis-prone mice inhibited this sequence.[179] TMA-containing nutrients such as meat, egg yolk and high-fat dairy products interacting with the host microbiome enhance formation of the proatherogenic TMAO entity.[180,181] Alteration of the gut microbiome to address primary and secondary interventions for atherosclerosis will continue to attract attention, particularly as related to dietary interventions.

SUMMARY

This chapter considers medical management strategies from the standpoint atherosclerotic plaques characteristics and interventions promoting their stability or regression. I have highlighted comparative effectiveness issues and varying guideline recommendations and recommend screening and monitoring of associated lipid and inflammatory biomarkers as treatment goals. The last decade witnessed great progress in vascular imaging which, correlated with outcomes, provides objective means to observe direct effects of medical interventions on the disease process within arteries. The increasing use of non-invasive carotid imaging stimulated controversy and negative views about screening for asymptomatic individuals. This, in my opinion, is an unwarranted controversy. The ability to detect, define and measure plaque size, stability and content offers important clinical insights. Indeed, the presence of asymptomatic atherosclerosis calls for aggressive medical management. Vascular surgeons possess both visual and tactile understanding of the pathology of atherosclerosis with its wide spectrum of heterogeneous lesions and patterns. They are in a position to assess the effectiveness of medical treatments upon atherosclerotic plaques along with the need for prompt direct interventions for critical vascular lesions. While clinical assessments of comparative efficacy evolve, clinical choices for optimal care require case-by-case evaluation. Intelligent choice of medical management strategies combined with evidence-based interventions promise continued improvement in outcomes for patients with atherosclerosis.

DISCLAIMER

The opinions expressed are those of the author and not those of the Department of Veterans Affairs or the United States Government.

REFERENCES

1. DeBakey ME, Crawford ES, Cooley DA, Morris GC Jr. Surgical considerations of occlusive disease of the abdominal Aorta and iliac and femoral Arteries: Analysis of 803 cases. *Arch Surg.* 1958;148:306–324.

2. DePalma RG. Atherosclerosis in vascular grafts. In: Gotto AM, Paoletti R, eds. *Atherosclerosis Reviews.* New York: Raven Press; 1979; Vol. 6, pp. 147–177.

3. Criqui MH, Ninomiya JK, Wingard DL. Progression of peripheral arterial disease predicts cardiovascular disease morbidity and mortality. *J Am Coll Cardiol.* 2008;52:1736–1742.

4. Haimovici H, DePalma RG. Atherosclerosis: Biologic and surgical considerations. In: Haimovici H, Callow AD, Emst CB, Hollier LH, eds. *Vascular Surgery*, 3rd ed. Norwalk, CT: Appleton and Lange; 1989, pp. 161–167.

5. Ruffer MA. On arterial lesions found in Egyptian mummies (1580 BC–525 AD). *J Pathol Bacteriol.* 1911;15:453.

6. Imparato AM. The carotid bifurcation plaque: A model for the study of atherosclerosis. *J Vasc Surg.* 1986;3:249–255.

7. Parasekevas KI, Abbott AL, Veith FJ. Optimal management of patients with symptomatic and asymptomatic carotid artery stenosis: Work in progress. *Expert Rev Cardiovasc Ther.* 2014;12:437–441.

8. Lam TD, Lammers S, Munoz C et al. Diabetes, intracranial stenosis and microemboli in asymptomatic carotid stenosis. *Can J Neurol Sci.* 2103;40:177–181.

9. Abbott AL, Nicolaides AN. Improving outcomes in patients with carotid stenosis: Call for better research opportunities and standards. *Stroke.* 2015;46(1):7–8.

10. Clinical Trials.gov. Intervention for asymptomatic carotid disease. Accessed December 2014.

11. Guyton JR, Kemp KF. Development of the lipid-rich core in human atherosclerosis. *Arterioscler Thromb Vasc Biol.* 1996;16:4–11.

12. Ross R. Atherosclerosis is an inflammatory disease. *Am Heart J.* 1999;138:S419–S420.

13. Noyes AM, Thompson PD. Symptomatic review of the time course of atherosclerotic plaque regression. *Atherosclerosis.* 2014;234:75–84.

14. Puri R, Nissen SE, Libby P et al. C-reactive protein, but not low-density lipoprotein cholesterol levels, associate with coronary artery atheroma regression and cardiovascular events after maximally intensive statin therapy. *Circulation.* 2013;128:2395–2403.

15. Stary HC Chandler AB, Glagov S et al. A definition of initial fatty streak and intermediate lesions of atherosclerosis: A report from the committee on vascular lesions of the council on atherosclerosis. *Arterioscler Thromb.* 1994;14:840–856.

16. Stary HC, Chandler AB, Glagov S et al. A definition of advanced types of atherosclerotic lesions and a histological classification of atherosclerosis. *Arterioscler Thromb.* 1995;15:1512–1531.

17. Melnick JL, Adam E, DeBakey ME. Possible role of cytomegalovirus in atherogenesis. *J Am Med Assoc.* 1990;263:2204–2207.

18. Cornhill JF Hederick EE, Stary HC. Topography of human aortic sudanophilic lesions. *Monogr Atheroscler.* 1990;15:13–19.

19. Glagov S, Zarins C, Giddens DP et al. Hemodynamics and atherosclerosis: Insights and perspectives gained from studies of human arteries. *Arch Pathol Lab Med*. 1988;112:1018–1031.

20. Insull W Jr., Bartch GE. Cholesterol, triglyceride and phospholipid content of intima, media and atherosclerotic fatty streak in human thoracic aorta. *J Clin Invest*. 1966;45:513–523.

21. Chisolm GM, DiCarleto PE, Erhart, LA et al. Review of atherogenesis. In: Young JR, Graor RA, Olin JW, Bartholomew JR, eds. *Peripheral Vascular Diseases*. St. Louis, MO: Mosby-Year Book; 1991, pp. 137–160.

22. Aschoff, L. Atherosclerosis. In: Aschoff L, ed. *Lectures on Pathology*. New York: Hoeber Inc.; 1924, pp. 131–153.

23. Virchow, R. *Gesammelte Abhandlungen zur Wissenschaft-lichen Medizin*. Frankfurt am Main, Germany: Meidinger Sohn; 1856, pp. 496–497.

24. Fagiotto A, Ross R, Harker L. Studies of hypercholesterolemia in the nonhuman primate, I: Changes that lead to fatty streak formation. *Arteriosclerosis*. 1984;4:323–340.

25. Fagiotto A, Ross R. Studies of hypercholesterolemia in the nonhuman primate, II: Fatty streak conversion to fibrous plaque. *Arteriosclerosis*. 1984;4:341–356.

26. Gerrity RG. The role of monocyte in atherogenesis, I: Transition of blood borne monocytes into foam cells in fatty lesions. *Am J Pathol*. 1981;103:181–190.

27. Steinberg D, Parthasarathy S, Carew TE et al. Beyond cholesterol: Modifications of low density lipoprotein that increase its atherogenicity. *N Engl J Med*. 1989;320:915–924.

28. Wiklund O, Carew TF, Steinberg D. Role of the low density lipoprotein receptor in the penetration of low density lipoprotein into the rabbit aortic wall. *Arteriosclerosis*. 1985;5:135–141.

29. Steinbrecher UP. Role of Superoxide in endothelial-cell modification of low density lipoprotein. *Biochem Biophys Acta*. 1988;959:20–30.

30. Heinecke JW, Baker L, Rosen L, Chait A. Superoxide mediates modification of low density lipoprotein by arterial smooth muscle cells. *J Clin Invest*. 1986;77:757–761.

31. Parthasarathy S, Printz DJ, Boyd D et al. Macrophage oxidation of low density lipoproteins generates a form recognized by the scavenger receptor. *Arteriosclerosis*. 1986;6:505–510.

32. Brand K, Banka CL, Mackman N et al. Oxidized LDL enhances lipopolysaccharide induced tissue factor expression in human adherent monocytes. *Arterioscler Thromb*. 1994;14:790–797.

33. Haust DM. The morphogenesis and fate of potential and early atherosclerotic lesions in man. *Hum Pathol*. 1971;2:1–29.

34. Smith EB. Identification of the gelatinous lesion. In: Schettler G, Gotto HM, eds. *Atherosclerosis III*. New York: Springer-Verlag; 1983, pp. 170–173.

35. Smith EB. Fibrinogen, fibrin and fibrin degradation products in relation to atherosclerosis. In: Fidge NH, Vestel PJ, eds. *Atherosclerosis VII*. Amsterdam, the Netherlands: Elsevier Science; 1986, pp. 459–462.

36. Madraffino G, Imbalzano E, Mamone F et al. Biglycan expression in current cigarette smokers: A possible link between active smoking and atherogenesis. *Atherosclerosis*. 2014;237:471–479.

37. Baranowski A, Adams CW, High OB, Bowyer DB. Connective tissue responses to oxysterols. *Atherosclerosis*. 1982;41:255–266.

38. Davies MJ, Thomas A. Thrombosis and acute coronary artery lesions in sudden cardiac ischemic death. *N Engl J Med*. 1984;310:1137–1140.

39. Lee RT, Libby P. The unstable atheroma. *Arterioscler Thromb Vasc Biol*. 1997;17:1859–1867.

40. Duguid JB. Thrombosis as a factor in the pathogenesis of coronary atherosclerosis. *J Pathol*. 1946;58:207–212.

41. Glagov S, Zarins C. Quantitating atherosclerosis: Problems of definition. In: Bond MC, Insull W Jr., Glagov S, eds. *Clinical Diagnosis of Atherosclerosis: Quantitative Methods of Evaluation*. New York: Springer-Verlag; 1982, pp. 12–35.

42. Bond MG Adams MR, Bullock BC. Complicating factors in evaluating coronary artery atherosclerosis. *Artery*. 1981;9:21–29.

43. DePalma RG. Angiography in experimental atherosclerosis: Advantages and limitations. In: Bond MG, Insull W Jr., Glagov S, eds. *Clinical Diagnosis of Atherosclerosis: Quantitative Methods of Evaluation*. New York: Springer-Verlag; 1982, pp. 99–123.

44. Hata Y, Hower J, Insull, W Jr. Cholesterol ester-rich inclusions from human aortic fatty streak and fibrous plaque lesions of atherosclerosis. *Am J Pathol*. 1974;75:423–456.

45. Hartwig H, Silvestre-Roig C, Daemen M et al. Neutrophils in atherosclerosis: A brief overview. *Hamostaseology*. 2014;11:35.

46. Schwartz CJ, Mitchell JR. Cellular infiltration of human arterial adventitia associated with atheromatous plaques. *Circulation*. 1962;26:73–78.

47. Yla-Herttuala S, Palinski W, Butler S et al. Rabbit and human atherosclerotic lesions contain IgG that recognizes epitopes of oxidized LDL. *Atheroscler Thromb*. 1993;13:32–40.

48. Maggi E, Chiesa R, Milissano G et al. LDL oxidation in patients with severe carotid atherosclerosis: A study of In vitro and in vivo oxidation markers. *Atheroscler Thromb*. 1994;14:1892–1899.

49. Brown MJ. Genomic insights into abdominal aortic aneurysms. *Ann R Coll Surg Engl*. 2014;96:405–414.

50. McColgan P, Peck GE, Greenhalgh RM, Sharma P. The genetics of abdominal aortic aneurysms, a comprehensive meta analysis involving eight candidate genes in over 16,700 patients. *Int Surg*. 2009;94:350–358.

51. DePalma RG, Sidawy AN, Giordano JM. Associated etiological and atherosclerotic risk factors in abdominal aneurysms. In: Mannick JA, ed. *The Cause and Management of Aneurysm*. London, UK: W.B. Saunders; 1990, pp. 37–46.

52. DePalma RG. Patterns of peripheral atherosclerosis: Implications for treatment. In: Shepard J, ed. *Atherosclerosis: Developments, Complications and Treatment.* Amsterdam, the Netherlands: Elsevier Science; 1987, pp. 161–174.

53. DeBakey ME, Lawrie GM, Glaeser DH. Patterns of atherosclerosis and their surgical significance. *Ann Surg.* 1985;201:115–131.

54. Giordano JM. Vascular disease: Epidemiology and risk factors. In: Giordano JM, Trout HH III, DePalma RG, eds. *The Basic Science of Vascular Surgery.* New York: Futura; 1988, pp. 345–374.

55. DePalma RG, Sidawy AN, Giordano JM. Management of arterial risk factors in patients requiring multiple vascular operations. In: Veith FJ, ed. *Current Critical Problems in Vascular Surgery.* St. Louis, MO: Quality Medical Publishing; 1989, pp. 430–438.

56. DePalma RG, Insull W Jr., Bellon EM et al. Animal models for study of progression and regression of atherosclerosis. *Surgery.* 1972;72:268–278.

57. St. Clair RW. Atherosclerosis regression in animal models: current concepts of cellular and biochemical mechanisms. *Prog Cardiovasc Dis.* 1983;26:109–132.

58. Wenning C, Kloth C. Kuhlmann MT et al. Serial F-18-FDG PET/CT distinguished inflamed from stable plaque phenotypes in shear-stressed induced murine atherosclerosis. *Atherosclerosis.* 2014;234:276–282.

59. Gaemperli O, Shalhoub J, Owen DR. et al Imaging intraplaque inflammation in carotid atherosclerosis with 11C-PK11195 positron emission tomography/computed tomography. *Eur Heart.* 2012;33:1902–1910.

60. DePalma RG, Hubay CA, Insull W Jr., Robinson AV, Hartman PH. Progression and regression of experimental atherosclerosis. *Surg Gynecol Obstet.* 1970;131:633–647.

61. DePalma RG, Bellon EM, Klein L et al. Approaches to evaluating regression of experimental atherosclerosis. In: Manning GM, Haust MD, eds. *Atherosclerosis: Metabolic, Morphologic and Clinical Aspects.* New York: Plenum Publishing; 1977, pp. 459–470.

62. DePalma RG, Bellon EM, Koletsky S et al. Atherosclerotic plaque regression in a rhesus monkey induced by bile acid sequestrant. *Exp Mol Pathol.* 1979;31:423–439.

63. DePalma RG, Klein L, Bellon EM et al. Regression of atherosclerotic plaques in rhesus monkeys. *Arch Surg.* 1980;115:1268–1278.

64. Shiomi M, Ito T, Tsukada T et al. Reduction of serum cholesterol levels alters lesional composition of atherosclerotic plaques. *Arterioscler Thromb Vasc Biol.* 1995;15:1938–1944.

65. DePalma RG, Koletsky S, Bellon EM, Insull W Jr. Failure of regression of atherosclerosis in dogs with moderate cholesterolemia. *Atherosclerosis.* 1977; 27:297–310.

66. Schonfeld G. Inherited disorders of lipid transport. *Endocrinol Metab Clin North Am.* 1990;19:229–257.

67. LaRosa JC. Cholesterol lowering, low cholesterol and mortality. *Am J Cardiol.* 1993;72:776–786.

68. Stamler J, Daviglus ML, Garside DB et al. Relationship of baseline serum cholesterol levels in 3 large cohorts to long-term coronary, cardiovascular and all-cause mortality and to longevity. *J Am Med Assoc.* 2000;284:311–318.

69. ClincalTrials.gov. Statins and cardiovascular risk reduction. Accessed August 22, 2016.

70. Heart Protection Study Collaborative Group. MRC/BHF Heart Protection Study of cholesterol lowering with simvastatin in 20,536 high risk individuals: A randomized placebo-controlled trial. *Lancet.* 2002;360:7–22.

71. Stone NJ, Robinson J, Lichtenstein C et al. 2013 ACC/AHA guideline on the treatment of blood cholesterol to reduce atherosclerotic cardiovascular risk in adults: A report of the American College of Cardiology/American Heart Association Task Force on Practice Guidelines. *J Am Coll Cardiol.* 2014;63(25 Pt B):2889–2934.

72. Grundy SM. National Cholesterol Education Program (NCEP) – The National cholesterol Guidelines in 2001. Adult Treatment Panel (ATP) III. *Am J Cardiol.* 2002;90(8A):11i–21ii.

73. Smith JC Jr., Grundy SM. 2013 ACC/AHA guidelines recommends fixed dose strategies instead of targeted goals to lower blood cholesterol. *J Am Coll Cardiol.* 2014;64:601–612.

74. Ridker PM, Danielson E, Fonesca FA et al. Reduction in C-reactive protein and LDL cholesterol and cardiovascular event rates after initiation of rosuvastatin. *Lancet.* 2009;373:1172–1182.

75. Puri R, Nissen SE, Shao M et al. Impact of baseline lipoprotein and C reactive protein levels on coronary regression following high intensity statin therapy. *Am J Cardiol.* 2014 November 15;114(10):1465–1472.

76. Roberts WC. The underutilized miracle drugs: The statin drugs are to atherosclerosis what penicillin was to infectious disease. *Am J Cardiol.* 1996;78:377–378.

77. Carter AA, Gomes T, Camacho X et al. Risk of incident diabetes among patients treated with statins: Population based study. *Br Med J.* 2013;346:f2610.

78. Corrao G, Ibrahim B, Nicotra F et al. Statins and risk of diabetes: Evidence from a large population based study. *Diabetes Care.* 2014;37:2225–2232.

79. Herbert PR, Gazaino JM, Chan KS, Hennekens CH. Cholesterol lowering with statin drugs, risk of stroke, and total mortality: An overview of randomized trials. *J Am Med Assoc.* 1997;278:313–321.

80. Jacobson TA, Ito MK, Maki KC et al. National lipid association recommendations for patient centered management of dyslipidemia. *J Clin Lipidolog.* 2014;8:473–488.

81. Pang J, Chan DC, Watts GF. Critical review of non-statin treatments for dyslipidemia. *Expert Rev Cardiovasc Ther.* 2014;12:359–371.

82. McCarthy M. Niacin fails to reduce vascular events in a large randomized trial. *Br Med J.* 2014 July 22;349:g4774.

83. Juergens JL, Barker NW, Hines EA Jr. Arteriosclerosis obliterans: A review of 520 cases with special reference to pathogenic and prognostic factors. *Circulation*. 1960;21:188–195.

84. Gordon T, Castelli WP, Hjortand MC et al. Predicting coronary heart disease in middle-aged and older persons: The Framingham Study. *J Am Med Assoc*. 1977;238:497–499.

85. Wray R, DePalma RG, Hubay CA. Late occlusion of aortofemoral bypass grafts: Influence of cigarette smoking. *Surgery*. 1971;70:969–973.

86. Ameli FM, Stein M, Prosser RJ et al. Effects of cigarette smoking on outcome of femoropopliteal bypass for limb salvage. *J Cardiovasc Surg*. 1989;30:591–656.

87. Garrison RJ, Kannel WB, Feinleib M et al. Cigarette smoking and HDL cholesterol: The Framingham offspring study. *Atherosclerosis*. 1978;30:17–25.

88. The Agency for Health Care Policy and Research. Smoking cessation clinical practice guideline. *J Am Med Assoc*. 1996;275:1270–1289.

89. Law M, Tang JL. An analysis of the effectiveness of interventions to help people stop smoking. *Arch Intern Med*. 1995;155:1933–1941.

90. Hurt RD, Sachs DP, Glover ED et al. A comparison of sustained release bupropion and placebo for smoking cessation. *N Engl J Med*. 1997;337:1195–1202.

91. Modell JG, Katholi CR, Modell JD, DePalma RL. Comparative side effects of bupropion, fluoxetine, paroxetine and seratoline. *Clin Pharm Ther*. 1997;61:476–487.

92. James PA, Oparil S, Carter BL et al. 2014 evidenced-based guideline for the management of high blood pressure in adults: Report from the panel members appointed to the Eighth Joint National Committee (JNC8). *J Am Med Assoc*. 2014;311:507–520.

93. Koletsky S, Roland C, Rivera-Velez JM. Rapid acceleration of atherosclerosis in hypertensive rats on a high fat diet. *Exp Mol Pathol*. 1968;9:322–338.

94. Hollander W, Madoff I, Paddock J, Kirkpatrick B. Aggravation of atherosclerosis in a subhuman primate model with coarctation of the aorta. *Circ Res*. 1976;8(6 Suppl. 2):63–72.

95. Lane DA, Lip GY. *Cochrane Database Syst Rev*. 2013 December 4;12:CD003075.

96. Whilton PK, Appel LJ, Espeland MA et al. Sodium reduction and weight loss in the treatment of hypertension in older persons. *J Am Med Assoc*. 1998;279:839–845.

97. Gradual NA, Galloe AM, Garred P. Effects of sodium restriction on blood pressure, renin aldosterone, catecholamines, cholesterols and triglyceride: A meta-analysis. *J Am Med Assoc*. 1998;279:1383–1391.

98. Kannel WB. Hypertension and other risk factors in coronary heart disease. *Am Heart J*. 1987;114:918–925.

99. O'Neil S, O'Driscoll L. Metabolic syndrome: A closer look at the growing epidemic and its associated pathologies. *Obes Rev*. 2015 January;16(1):1–12.

100. Kezdi P, Kezdi PC, Khamis HJ. Diuretic induced long term hemodynamic changes in hypertension: A retrospective study in a MRFIT clinical center. *Clin Exp Hypertens*. 1992;14:347–365.

101. Wijeysundera DN, Duncan D, Nkonde-Price C et al. Perioperative beta blockade in noncardiac surgery: A systemic review for the 2014 ACC/AHA guideline. *J Am Coll Cardiol*. 2014;64:2406–2425.

102. Stone NJ. Lifestyle interventions in atherosclerosis. In: La Rosa JC, ed. *Medical Management of Atherosclerosis*. New York: Marcel Dekker; 1998, pp. 91–124.

103. Aronow WS. Treating hypertension and prehypertension in older people: When, whom and how. *Maturitas*. 2015 January;80(1):31–36.

104. Ahimastos AA, Walker PJ, Askew C et al. Effect of ramipril on walking times a quality of life among patients with peripheral arterial disease and intermittent claudication: A randomized controlled trial. *J Am Med Assoc*. 2013;309:453–460.

105. Diabetes Control and Complication Trial Research Group. The effect of intensive treatment of diabetes on the development and progression of long term complications in insulin dependent diabetes mellitus. *N Engl J Med*. 1993;329:977–986.

106. Aron D, Conlin PR, Hobbs C et al. *Ann Intern Med*. 2011;155:340–341.

107. Tseng CL, Soroka O, Maney M et al. Assessing potential glycemic overtreatment in persons at hypoglycemic risk. *J Am Med Assoc Intern Med*. 2014;174:259–268.

108. Bierman EI. Atherogenesis in diabetes. *Arterioscler Thromb*. 1992;12:647.

109. Katsiki N, Athyros VG, Daragiannis A, Mikhalidis DP. The role of statins in the treatment of type 2 diabetes mellitus: An update. *Curr Pharm Des*. 2014;20:3665–3674.

110. Althouse AD, Abbott JD, Forker AD et al. Risk factors for incident peripheral arterial disease in type 2 diabetes. *Diabetes Care*. 2014;37:1346–1352.

111. Lorber D. Importance of cardiovascular disease risk management in patients with type 2 diabetes mellitus. *Diabetes Metab Syndr Obes*. 2014;23:169–183.

112. Anderson SL. Dapagliflozin efficacy and safety: A perspective review. *Ther Adv Drug Saf*. 2014;5:242–254.

113. Cicero AF, Tartagni E, Ertek S. Metformin and its clinical use: New insights for an old drug in clinical practice. *Arch Med Sci*. 2012;8:907–917.

114. Morris JN, Heady JA, Raffle PAB et al. Coronary heart disease and physical activity of work. *Lancet*. 1953;2:1053–1057.

115. Dawber TR. *The Epidemiology of Atherosclerotic Disease: The Framingham Study*. Cambridge, MA: Harvard University Press; 1980.

116. Adabaq S, Huxley RR, Lopez FL et al. Obesity related risk of sudden cardiac death in the atherosclerosis risk in communities study. *Heart*. 2015 February;101(3):215–221.

117. Pack QR, Rodriguez-Escudero JP, Thomas RJ et al. The prognostic importance of weight loss in coronary artery disease: A systematic review and meta-analysis. *Mayo Clin Proc*. 2014;89:1368–1377.

118. Clarkson TB. George Lyman Duff memorial lecture: Personality, gender and coronary atherosclerosis of monkeys. *Arteriosclerosis.* 1987;7:1–8.

119. Osler W. The Lumeian lectures on angina pectoris. *Lancet.* 1910;1:839–844.

120. Christodoulo C, Douzenas A, Mommersteg PM. A case control validation of type D personality in Greek patients with stable coronary disease. *Ann Gen Psychiatry.* 2013;12(1):38.

121. Comapare A, Mommersteg PM, Faletra F et al Personality traits, cardiac risk factors, and their association with the presence and severity of coronary artery plaque in people with no history of cardiovascular disease. *J Cardiovasc Med.* 2014;15:423–430.

122. Powell KE, Thompson PD, Cabperson CJ, Kentrick JS. Physical activity and the incidence of coronary heart disease. *Ann Rev Public Health.* 1987;8:253.

123. Pepinos II, Judge AR, Selby JT et al. The myopathy of peripheral arterial occlusive disease. Functional and histomorphological changes and evidence of mitochondrial dysfunction. *Vasc Endovasc Surg.* 2007;41:481–489.

124. Parmenter BJ, Dieberg G, Smart NA. Exercise training for management of peripheral arterial disease: A systematic review and meta-analysis. *Sports Med.* 2015 February;45(2):231–244.

125. Has TL, Lloyd PG, Yang HT, Terjung RL. Exercise training and peripheral arterial disease. *Compr Physiol.* 2012;2:2933–3017.

126. Curfman GD. Is exercise beneficial – or hazardous – to your heart? *N Engl J Med.* 1993;32:1730–1731.

127. Katzel LI, Bleeker ER, Colman EG et al. Effects of weight loss vs aerobic exercise training on risk Factors for coronary disease in healthy, obese, middle aged and older men. *J Am Med Assoc.* 1995;274:1915–1921.

128. Jonason T, Jonzon B, Ringqvist I, Oman-Rydberg A. Effects of physical training on different categories of patients with intermittent claudication. *Acta Med Scand.* 1979;206:253–258.

129. Hiatt WR, Regensteiner JG, Hargarten ME et al. Benefit of exercise conditioning for patients with peripheral arterial disease. *Circulation.* 1990;81:602–609.

130. Gardner AW, Poehlman ET. Exercise rehabilitation programs for the treatment of claudication pain: A meta-analysis. *J Am Med Assoc.* 1995;274:975–980.

131. Williams LR, Ekers MA Collins PS, Lee JF. Vascular rehabilitation: Benefits of a structured exercise/risk modification program. *J Vasc Surg.* 1991;14:320–326.

132. Taylor CA, Hughes TJ, Zarins CK. Effect of exercise on hemodynamic conditions in the abdominal aorta. *J Vasc Surg.* 1999;29:1077–1089.

133. Wang J, Fen CJ, Chen, HI. Effects of exercise training and reconditioning on platelet function in men. *Arterioscler Thromb Vasc Biol.* 1995;15:1668–1674.

134. Eriksson M, Johnson O, Borman K. Improved fibrinolytic activity may be an effect of the adipocyte-derived hormones leptin and adiponectin. *Thromb Res.* 2008;122:701–708.

135. Depalma RG, Kowallek DL. Chapter 14: Medical management of atherosclerotic vascular disease. In: Hobson RW II, Wilson ES, Veith FJ, eds. *Vascular Surgery: Principles and Practice*, 3rd ed. New York: Marcel Dekker Inc.; 2004, pp. 249–272.

136. Rossouw JE, Rifkin BM. Does lowering serum cholesterol levels lower coronary heart disease risk? In: La Rosa JC, ed. *Endocrinology and Metabolism Clinics of North America.* Philadelphia, Pa: Saunders; 1990, Vol. 19(2), pp. 279–299.

137. Expert Panel on Detection, Evaluation, and Treatment of High Blood Cholesterol in Adults. Executive Summary of the Third National Cholesterol Education Program (NCEP). *J Am Med Assoc.* 2001;285:2486–2497.

138. Katz DL, Meller S. Can we say what diet is best for health? *Annu Rev Pub Health.* 2014;35:83–103.

139. DePalma RG, Hubay CA, Botti RE, Peterka JL. Treatment of surgical patients with atherosclerosis and hyperlipidemia. *Surg Gynecol Obstet.* 1970;131:313–322.

140. DePalma RG. Control and regression of atherosclerotic plaques (commentary). In: Dale WA, ed. *Management of Arterial Occlusive Disease.* Chicago, IL: Yearbook Medial Publishers; 1971, pp. 63–64.

141. Trichopoulou A, Costacou T, Barmis C, Trichopoulos D. Adherence to a Mediterranean diet and survival in a Greek population. *N Engl J Med.* 2003;348:2599–2608.

142. Essylstyn CB Jr., Gendy G, Doyle J et al. A way to reverse CAD? *J Fam Pract.* 2014;63:356–364.

143. Munger MA, Hawkins DW, Atherothrombosis: Epidemiology, pathophysiology, and prevention. *J Am Pharm Assoc.* 2003;44(2 Suppl.):S5–S12.

144. Goldhaber SZ, Manson JE, Stampfer MJ et al. Low dose aspirin and subsequent peripheral arterial surgery. *Lancet.* 1992;340:143–145.

145. Hennekens CH. Update on aspirin in the treatment of cardiovascular diseases. *Am J Manage Care.* 2002;8:S691–S700.

146. CAPRI Steering Committee. A randomized blinded trial of clopidogrel in patients at risk for ischemic events. *Lancet.* 1996;340:143–145.

147. Wong PF, Chong LY, Mikhalidis DP et al. Antiplatelet agents for intermittent claudication. *Cochrane Database Syst Rev.* 2011 November 9;11:CD001272.

148. Paciaroni M, Bogousslavsky J. Antithrombotic therapy in carotid stenosis: An update. *Eur Neurol.* 2014;73:51–56.

149. Comerota AJ, Thakur S. Antiplatelet therapy for vascular interventions. *Perspect Vasc Surg Endovasc Ther.* 2008;20:28–35.

150. Comerota AJ. Effect on platelet function of cilostazol, clopidogrel, and aspirin, each alone or in combination. *Atheroscler Suppl.* 2005;15:13–19.

151. Yamaguchi Oura M, Sasaki M, Ohba H et al. *J Stroke Cerebrovasc Dis.* 2014;23:2425–2430.

152. DePalma RG, Bellon EM, Manalo P, Bomberger RA. Failure of antiplatelet treatment in dietary atherosclerosis: A serial intervention study. In: Gallo LL, Vahouny GV, eds. *Cardiovascular Disease: Molecular and Cellular Mechanisms, Prevention, Treatment.* New York: Plenum Press; 1987, pp. 407–426.

153. DePalma RG. Atheroembolism. In: Stanley J, Veith FJ, Wakefield T, eds. *Current Therapy in Vascular and Endovascular Surgery.* St. Louis, MO: Elsevier; 2014, pp. 631–633.

154. Gassman AA, Degner BC, Al-Nouri O et al. Aspirin usage is associated with improved prosthetic infrainguinal graft patency. *Vascular.* 2014;22:105–111.

155. Geraghty AJ, Welch K. Antithrombotic agents for preventing thrombosis after infrainguinal bypass surgery. *Cochrane Database Syst Rev.* 2011 June 15;6:CD000536.

156. van Hattum ES, Algra A, Lawson JA et al. Bleeding increases the risk of ischemic events in patients with PAD. *Circulation.* 2009;120:1569–1576.

157. Donaldson MC, Weinberg DS, Belkin M et al. Screening for hypercoagulable states in vascular surgery practice. *J Vasc Surg.* 1990;11:825–831.

158. Horton JD, Cohen JC, Hobbs HH. PCSKp: A convertase that coordinates LDL catabolism. *J Lipid Res.* 2009; 50(Suppl.):S172–S177.

159. Mabichi H, Nohara A. Therapy: PCSK9 inhibitors for treating familial hypercholesterolemia. *Nat Rev Endocrinol.* 2015;11:8–9.

160. Ridker PM, Rifai N, Stampfer MJ, Hennekens CH. Plasma concentration of interleukin-6 and risk of future myocardial infarction among apparently healthy men. *Circulation.* 2000;101:1767–1772.

161. Ridker P. Testing the inflammatory hypothesis of atherothrombosis scientific rationale for the cardiovascular inflammation reduction trial (CIRT). *J Thromb Hemost.* 2009;7(Suppl. 1):332–339.

162. Everett BM, Pradhan AD, Solomon DH et al. Rationale and design of the cardiovascular inflammation reduction trial: A test of the inflammatory hypothesis of atherothrombosis. *Am Heart J.* 2013;166:199–207.

163. Kell DB. Iron behaving badly: Inappropriate iron chelation as a major contributor to the etiology of vascular and other progressive inflammatory and degenerative diseases. *BMC Med Genomics.* 2009;2:2.

164. Sullivan JL. Macrophage iron, hepcidin, and atherosclerotic plaque stability. *Exp Biol Med.* 2007;232:1014–1020.

165. Zacharski LR, Chow BK, Howes PS et al. Reduction of cardiovascular outcomes in patient with peripheral arterial disease, a randomized controlled trial. *J Am Med Assoc.* 2007;297:603–610.

166. DePalma RG, Zacharski LR, Chow BK, Shamayeva G, Hayes VW. Reduction of iron stores and clinical outcomes in peripheral arterial disease: Outcome comparisons in smokers and non-smokers. *Vascular.* 2013;21:233–241.

167. Zacharski LR, G. Shamayeva, Chow BK. Effect of controlled reduction of body iron stores on clinical outcomes in peripheral arterial disease. *Am Heart J.* 2011;162:949–957.

168. DePalma RG, Hayes VW, Cafferata HT et al. Cytokine signatures in atherosclerotic claudicants. *J Surg Res.* 2003;111:215–221.

169. DePalma RG, Hayes VW, Chow B, Shamayeva G, May PE, Zacharski L. Ferritin levels, inflammatory biomarkers and mortality in peripheral arterial disease: A substudy of the Iron (Fe) and Atherosclerosis Study (FeAST) Trial. *J Vasc Surg.* 2010;51:1498–1503.

170. Zacharski LR, DePalma RG, Shamayeva G, Chow BK. The statin-iron nexus: Anti-inflammatory intervention for arterial disease prevention. *Am J Public Health.* 2013 April;103(4):e105–e112.

171. Zacharski LR, Shamayeva G, Chow BK, DePalma RG. Racial differences in iron measures and outcomes observed during an iron reduction trial in peripheral arterial disease. *J Health Care Poor Underserved.* 2015 February;26(1):243–259.

172. Regenbogen SE, Gawande AA, Lipsitz SR et al. Do differences in hospital and surgeon quality explain racial disparities in lower-extremity vascular amputations? *Ann Surg.* 2009;250(3):424–431.

173. Mandaviya PR, Stolk L, Heil SG Homocysteine and DNA methylation: A review of animal and human literature. *Mol Genet Metab.* 2014;113:243–252.

174. Bazzano LA. No effect of folic acid supplementation on cardiovascular events, cancer or mortality after five years in people at increased cardio vascular risk. *Evid Based Med.* 2011;16:117–118.

175. High KP. Atherosclerosis and infection due to Chlamydia pneumoniae or cytomegalovirus: Weighing the evidence. *Clin Infect Dis.* 1999;28:746–749.

176. Lamb DJ, El-Sankary W, Ferns GA. Molecular mimicry in atherosclerosis, a role for heat shock protein. *Atherosclerosis.* 2003;167:177–185.

177. Stassen FR, Vainas T, Bruggeman CA. Infection and atherosclerosis: An alternative view on an outdated hypothesis. *Pharm Rep.* 2008;60:85–92.

178. Tang WH, Hazen SL. The contributory role of gut microbiota in cardiovascular disease. *J Clin Invest.* 2014;124:4204–4211.

179. Wang Z, Klipfell E, Bennett BJ et al. Gut flora of phosphatidylcholine promotes cardiovascular disease. *Nature.* 2011;472:57–63.

180. Brown JM, Hazen SL. Metaorganismal nutrient metabolism as a basis of cardiovascular disease. *Curr Opin Lipidol.* 2014;25:48–53.

181. Wilson Tang WH, Wang Z, Levinson BS et al. Intestinal microbial metabolism of phosphatidylcholine and cardio vascular risk. *New Engl J Med.* 2013;368:1575–1584.

182. DePalma RG. Pathology of atheromas. In: Bell PRF, Jamieson CW, Ruckley CV, eds. *Surgical Management of Vascular Disease.* London, UK: W.B. Saunders; 1992, pp. 21–34.

7

Thrombophilia as a cause of recurrent vascular access thrombosis in hemodialysis patients

KHUSHBOO KAUSHAL and SAMUEL ERIC WILSON

CONTENTS

According to the US Renal Data System 2014 Annual Data Report, the incidence of end-stage renal disease (ESRD) has now plateaued after steadily increasing over the past three decades.[1] Since 2000, there has been about a 57.4% increase in the size of the population undergoing hemodialysis and peritoneal dialysis. Among these patients on hemodialysis and peritoneal dialysis, hospitalization rates and average length of stay have been declining over recent years. Infection has become a more frequent cause of hospitalizations with an increase in 21.8% between 1993 and 2012. Other causes of hospitalizations, such as vascular access procedures, have been declining though continue to be prevalent. Vascular access–related complications account for 14%–17% of hospitalizations per year for dialysis patients with annual costs exceeding $1 billion in the United States.[2] Vascular access thrombosis is the most common and expensive hemodialysis complication.[3] In addition to vascular access thrombosis, patients maintained by chronic hemodialysis also are susceptible to other thrombotic complications such as ischemic heart disease and cerebral strokes.[4–6] Casserly and Dember, as well as Paulson, have suggested that thrombophilia may be a cause of dialysis access thrombosis in many ESRD patients.[7,8] Thrombophilia may be acquired, genetically determined or a combination of both and leads to a predisposition to thrombosis.[9] This chapter examines coagulation abnormalities in ESRD patients, focusing on thrombophilia and management of the hypercoagulable state in ESRD patients.

COAGULATION ABNORMALITIES IN ESRD

Hemodialysis patients are at increased risk for bleeding or thromboses.[10] The more common coagulation abnormality is a hemorrhagic tendency in uremia from a defect of primary hemostasis secondary to platelet dysfunction and altered platelet–vessel wall interactions.[10,11] Indeed, it is this coagulation abnormality that allows arteriovenous fistulas (AVFs) and grafts to function in ESRD patients, whereas in patients with normal clotting function, these would thrombose.

Insufficient knowledge about the association between renal insufficiency and inflammatory and procoagulant markers led Shlipak et al. in 2003 to evaluate eight inflammatory and procoagulant factors (C-reactive protein, fibrinogen, interleukin-6, intercellular adhesion molecule-1, factor VII, factor VIII, plasmin–antiplasmin and D-dimer).[12] They found that renal insufficiency had an independent correlation with increased levels of inflammatory and procoagulant biomarkers and may promote atherosclerosis and thrombosis in ESRD patients. These biochemical changes in hemodialysis patients lead to chronic activation of coagulation and result in a hypercoagulable state.[13] ESRD patients have higher levels of particular markers of coagulation activation, such as prothrombin fragment 1 + 2 and thrombin.[4] Furthermore, Hafner et al. suggest that the levels of the thrombin–antithrombin complex are associated with thrombosis of the extracorporeal hemodialysis circuit while the patient is undergoing hemodialysis.[14] In addition to high levels of coagulation activators, these patients also have lower levels of endogenous anticoagulants such as protein C, protein S and antithrombin III.[15,16]

Diabetic and nondiabetic ESRD patients have elevated procoagulatory activity, as indicated by increased platelet aggregation, increased D-dimer concentration, von Willebrand factor antigen and platelet factor 4.[17] Ambuhl et al. found elevated D-dimer levels, indicating that accelerated thrombin formation and unimpaired fibrinolytic activity, contributes to development of the hypercoagulable state.[18] They demonstrated that ESRD patients are in a procoaguable state and hemodialysis further stimulates coagulatory activity. Previous studies showed that human recombinant erythropoietin has an overall procoagulatory effect since it influences blood coagulation and fibrinolysis.[19,20] Ambuhl et al. confirmed these findings and also found that higher doses of erythropoietin were correlated with smaller amounts of prothrombin fragments.[18]

Vascular endothelium actively participates in hemostasis. Variations in the morphology of the blood flow and vessel wall in the AVF may disrupt hemostasis.[21,22] Erdem et al. investigated the molecular markers that activate and/or inhibit coagulation and fibrinolysis in patients with ESRD and assessed the effects AVF may have on endothelial surfaces and hemostasis.[4] For ESRD patients, the results showed activated coagulation markers and fibrinolysis in the systemic circulation. These findings suggest that turbulent flow of an AVF may be a factor that independently influences the coagulation and fibrinolytic cascades.

THROMBOPHILIA AS A CAUSE OF ACCESS FAILURE IN HEMODIALYSIS PATIENTS

Thrombophilia is suspected to be a potential cause of dialysis access thrombosis though the prevalence of thrombophilia in ESRD patients remains unclear.[5,23] A limited number of prior studies has looked at inherited or acquired thrombophilia and its relation to access thrombosis in ESRD patients though the results of these studies were contradictory.[23] Knoll et al. conducted a large and comprehensive case-control study that assessed the association between thrombophilic disorders and dialysis access thrombosis.[5] They measured concentrations of factor V Leiden, prothrombin gene mutation, factor XIII genotype, methylenetetrahydrofolate reductase genotype, lupus anticoagulant, anticardiolipin antibody, factor VIII, homocysteine and lipoprotein in hemodialysis patients. The most common genetic determinants were point mutations in the factor V and prothrombin genes.[24,25] This study demonstrated that the presence of thrombophilia increased risk for dialysis access thrombosis and further that each additional thrombophilic factor increased the likelihood of access thrombosis almost twofold.

Although a direct cause and effect in vascular access thrombosis has not been proven, it is clear that changes in hemostatic plasma protein enzymes may establish hypercoagulable states in patients on hemodialysis.[26–30] Nampoory et al. investigated changes in hemostatic risk factors that may contribute to hypercoagulability in patients on dialysis and hypothesizing that renal transplantation would be a highly effective treatment in patients with ESRD, examined the biologic effect renal transplantation had on hypercoagulability.[31] Those who had these access complications had significantly abnormal levels of lupus anticoagulant and activated protein C, protein S and protein C resistance in comparison with patients who did not experience vascular access thrombosis. It is noteworthy that renal transplantation appeared to correct these levels.

O'Shea et al. found antibodies associated with thrombosis and increased concentrations of factor VIII and fibrinogen, especially in patients with recurring vascular access thrombosis.[32] LeSar et al.'s study revealed a high correlation (81.8%) between thrombotic complications and hypercoagulability leading these authors to suggest that hypercoagulability is a major causative factor in graft thromboses that develop independent from anatomic causes.[33] Documentation of a hypercoagulable state in the ESRD patient with repeated access thrombosis, in the absence of anatomical abnormalities or extrinsic factors (e.g. compression), naturally leads one to consider therapeutic anticoagulation measures.

MANAGEMENT OF THE HYPERCOAGULABLE ESRD PATIENT

Better understanding of the pathogenesis of thrombosis will allow for more efficient treatment and the opportunity to prevent reoccurring complications.[33] Recognizing that fistula thrombosis may arise from both anatomic and nonanatomic causes, one should consider that hypercoagulable states may be a cause of vascular access thrombosis in selected patients in whom no anatomical abnormality can be found.[32] Diseases that cause hypercoagulability and their complications include antiphospholipid syndrome, antithrombin III deficiency, protein S deficiency, protein C deficiency, activated protein C resistance and erythropoietin deficiency.[33–39]

Aspirin, clopidogrel and warfarin are commonly used in patients with high prevalence of access thrombosis and cardiovascular disease.[40] Prior studies have conflicting findings regarding the benefits of anticoagulation in these patients. In their guide to management of thromboembolism in hemodialysis patients, Dorthy Lo et al. noted that trials of anticoagulants have not shown a benefit for prevention of access thrombosis.[13] Kaufman et al. reinforced this notion with a study of combinations of 75 mg of clopidogrel and 325 mg of aspirin that did not reduce prosthetic access thrombosis.[41] However, in patients with antiphospholipid syndromes, Rosove and Brewer and

Khamashta et al. found that the incidence of thrombotic events decreased with warfarin therapies of intermediate to high intensity.[42,43]

Anticoagulants may have the potential to increase vascular access graft patency[32] but at the cost of an increase in the likelihood of serious hemorrhagic complications in ESRD patients.[33,44,45] Chan et al. conducted a retrospective study that evaluated whether exposure to aspirin, clopidogrel and Coumadin affected survival in hemodialysis patients and found that patients who took these medications had significantly higher mortality.[40] In another study, Crowther et al. showed that warfarin increased major bleeding events in hemodialysis patients and 75 mg of clopidogrel did not confer benefits for autogenous access.[46]

After this selective review of literature which is often conflicting, we are unable to make a definite evidence-based recommendation on the use of anticoagulants to prevent access thrombosis. It seems prudent, however, to consider low-dose warfarin or antiplatelet agents in ESRD patients who suffer repetitive thrombosis of *lifeline* access sites. Precautions must be taken, monitoring of coagulation tests and avoidance of trauma, to minimize bleeding.

CONCLUSION

Thrombosis is one of the most common complications of vascular access, deserving further attention directed towards understanding of the multiple aetiologies and the contribution of thrombophilia to recurrent, otherwise unexplainable, access clotting. The ideal approach to decreasing the morbidity and costs of access thrombosis may be a combination of preventing endothelial and fibromuscular hyperplasia of outflow stenosis, along with the correction of hypercoaguability.[16,33]

REFERENCES

1. United States Renal Data System. USRDS 2014 annual data report: Atlas of end-stage renal disease in the United States. National Institutes of Health, National Institute of Diabetes and Digestive and Kidney Diseases, Bethesda, MD, 2014. http://www. usrds.org/adr.htm.
2. United States Renal Data System. The economic cost of ESRD, vascular access procedures, and Medicare spending for alternative modalities of treatment. *Am J Kidney Dis.* 1997;30:S160–S177.
3. Knoll GA, Wells PS, Young D. Thrombophilia and the risk for hemodialysis vascular access thrombosis. *J Am Soc Nephrol.* 2005;16:1108–1114.
4. Erdem Y, Haznedaroglu IC, Celik I et al. Coagulation, fibrinolysis and fibrinolysis inhibitors in haemodialysis patients: Contribution of arteriovenous fistula. *Nephrol Dial Transplant.* 1996;11:1299–1305.
5. Linder A, Charra B, Sherrad DJ et al. Accelerated atherosclerosis in prolonged maintenance hemodialysis. *N Engl J Med.* 1974;290:697–702.
6. Ansari A, Kaupke CJ, Vaziri ND et al. Cardiac pathology in patients with end stage renal disease maintained on haemodialysis. *Int J Artif Organs.* 1993;16:31–36.
7. Casserly LF, Dember LM. Thrombosis in end-stage renal disease. *Semin Dial.* 2003;16:245–256.
8. Paulson WD. Prediction of hemodialysis synthetic graft thrombosis: Can we identify factors that impair validity of the dysfunction hypothesis? *Am J Kidney Dis.* 2000;35:973–975.
9. Tripodi A, Mannucci PM. Laboratory investigation of thrombophilia. *Clin Chem.* 2001;47:1597–1606.
10. Holden RM, Harman GJ, Wang M et al. Major bleeding in hemodialysis patients. *Clin J Am Soc Nephrol.* 2008;3:105–110.
11. Ho SJ, Gemmel R, Brighton A. Platelet function testing in uraemic patients. *Hematology.* 2008;13:49–58.
12. Shlipak MG, Fried LF, Crump C et al. Elevations of inflammatory and procoagulant biomarkers in elderly persons with renal insufficiency. *Circulation.* 2003;107:87.
13. Lo DS, Rabbat CG, Clase CM. Thromboembolism and anticoagulant management in hemodialysis patients: A practical guide to clinical management. *Thromb Res.* 2006;118(3):385–395.
14. Hafner G, Klingel R, Wandel E et al. Laboratory control of minimal heparinization during hemodialysis in patients with a risk of hemorrhage. *Blood Coagul Fibrin.* 1994;5:221–226.
15. Lai KN, Yin JA, Yuen PM et al. Protein C, protein S, and antithrombin III levels in patients on continuous ambulatory peritoneal dialysis and hemodialysis. *Nephron.* 1990;56:271–276.
16. Nakamura Y, Chida Y, Tomura S. Enhanced coagulation – Fibrinolysis in patients on regular hemodialysis treatment. *Nephron.* 1991;58:201–204.
17. Gordge MP, Leaker BR, Rylance PB et al. Haemostatic activation and proteinuria as factors in the progression of chronic renal failure. *Nephrol Dial Transplant.* 1991;6:21–26.
18. Ambuhl P, Wuthrich R, Korte W et al. Plasma hypercoagulability in haemodialysis patient: Impact of dialysis and anticoagulation. *Nephrol Dial Transplant.* 1997;12:2355–2364.
19. Taylor JE, Belch JJF, McLaren M et al. Effect of erythropoietin therapy and withdrawal on blood coagulation and fibrinolysis in hemodialysis patients. *Kidney Int.* 1993;44:182–190.
20. Huraib S, Al-Momen AK, Gader AM et al. Effect of recombinant human erythropoietin (rhEPO) on the hemostatic system on chronic hemodialysis patients. *Clin Nephrol.* 1991;36:252–257.
21. Remuzzi G, Cavenaghi A, Mecca G, Donati M, DeGaetano G. Prostacyclin-like activity and bleeding in renal failure. *Lancet.* 1977;2:1195–1197.

22. Remuzzi G, Perico N, Zoja C, Coma D, Macconi D, Vigano D. Role of endothelium derived nitric oxide in the bleeding tendency of uremia. *J Clin Invest.* 1990;86:1768–1771.

23. Salmela B, Hartman J, Peltonen S. et al. Thrombophilia and arteriovenous fistula survival in ESRD. *Clin J Am Soc Nephrol.* 2013;8:962–968.

24. Bertina RM, Rosendaal FR. Venous thrombosis – The interaction of genes and environment. *N Engl J Med.* 1998;338:1840–1841.

25. Girndt M, Heine GH, Ulrich C et al. Gene polymorphism association studies in dialysis: Vascular access. *Semin Dial.* 2007;20:63–67.

26. Fodinger M, Mannhalter C, Pabinger I et al. Resistance to activated protein C (APC): Mutation at ARG 506 of coagulation factor V and vascular access thrombosis in haemodialysis patients. *Nephrol Dial Transplant.* 1996;11:668–672.

27. Prieto LN, Suki WN. Frequent hemodialysis graft thrombosis: Association with antiphospholipid antibodies. *Am J Kidney Dis.* 1994;23:587–590.

28. Brunet P, Ailland M, Marco MS et al. Antiphospholipids in hemodialysis patients: Relation between lupus anticoagulant and thrombosis. *Kidney Int.* 1995;48:794–800.

29. Sallam S, Wafa E, El-Gayar A, Sobh M, Salama O. Anticardiolipin antibodies in children on chronic haemodialysis. *Nephrol Dial Transplant.* 1994;9:1292–1294.

30. Prakash RM, Miller CC, Suki WN. Anticardiolipin antibody in patients on maintenance hemodialysis and its association with recurrent arteriovenous graft thrombosis. *Am J Kidney Dis.* 1995;26:347–352.

31. Nampoory MRN, Das KC, Johny KV et al. Hypercoagulability, a serious problem in patients with ESRD on maintenance hemodialysis, and its correction after kidney transplantation. *Am J Kidney Dis.* 2003;42:797–805.

32. O'Shea SI, Lawson JH, Reddan D et al. Hypercoagulable states and antithrombotic strategies in recurrent vascular access site thrombosis. *J Vasc Surg.* 2003;38:541–548.

33. LeSar CJ, Merrick HW, Smith MR. Thrombotic complications resulting from hypercoagulable states in chronic hemodialysis vascular access. *J Am Coll Surg.* 1999;189:73–79.

34. Bick RL, Baker WF. Antiphospholipid and thrombosis syndromes. *Semin Thromb Hemost.* 1994;20:3–15.

35. Bayston TA, Lane DA. Antithrombin: Molecular basis of deficiency. *Thromb Hemost.* 1997;78:339–343.

36. Schwarz HP, Fischer M, Hopmeier P et al. Plasma protein S deficiency in familial thrombotic disease. *Blood.* 1984;64:1297–1300.

37. Clouse LH, Comp PC. The regulation of hemostasis: The protein C system. *N Engl J Med.* 1986;314:1298–1304.

38. Svensson PJ, Dahlback B. Resistance to activated protein C as a basis for venous thrombosis. *N Engl J Med.* 1994;330:517–522.

39. Shen L, Dahlback B. Factor V and protein S as synergistic cofactors to activated protein C in degradation of factor VIIIa. *J Biol Chem.* 1994;269:18735–18738.

40. Chan KE, Lazarus M, Thadhani R et al. Anticoagulant and antiplatelet usage associates with mortality among hemodialysis patients. *J Am Soc Nephrol.* 2009;20:872–881.

41. Kaufman JS, O'Connor TZ, Zhang JH et al. Randomized controlled trial of clopidogrel plus aspirin to prevent hemodialysis access graft thrombosis. *J Am Soc Nephrol.* 2003;14:2313–2321.

42. Rosove MH, Brewer PM. Antiphospholipid thrombosis: Clinical course after the first thrombotic event in 70 patients. *Ann Intern Med.* 1992;117:303–308.

43. Khamashta MA, Cuadrado MJ, Mujic F et al. The management of thrombosis in the antiphospholipid-antibody syndrome. *N Engl J Med.* 1995;332:993–997.

44. Hirsh J, Warkentin TE, Shaughnessy SG et al. Heparin and low molecular-weight heparin: Mechanisms of action, pharmacokinetics, dosing, monitoring, efficacy, and safety. *Chest.* 2001;119:64S–94S.

45. Gerlach AT, Pickworth KK, Seth SK et al. Enoxaparin and bleeding complications: A review in patients with and without renal insufficiency. *Pharmacotherapy.* 2000;20:771–775.

46. Crowther MA, Clase CM, Margetts PJ et al. Low-intensity warfarin is ineffective for the prevention of PTFE graft failure in patients on hemodialysis: A randomized controlled trial. *J Am Soc Nephrol.* 2002;13:2331–2337.

8

Anticoagulants

JEFFREY D. CRAWFORD, BRUCE A. WARDEN and TIMOTHY K. LIEM

CONTENTS

INTRODUCTION

Care of the vascular surgical patient requires an updated, evidence-based approach to the management of anticoagulation. In addition to managing arterial and venous thrombi, vascular surgeons also must be adept at managing the frequently encountered co-morbid conditions of our patient population as well as careful perioperative and intraoperative decisions to balance the risk of bleeding and recurrent thrombosis. The homeostatic mechanisms governing this delicate and complex process are regulated by the endothelium, extracellular tissue and circulating blood proteins and cells. An in-depth review of the nuances and complex interactions of the coagulation cascade is beyond the scope of this chapter. This chapter reviews current FDA-approved anticoagulants, focusing on mechanisms of action and pharmacokinetics, indications and supporting data, important side effects, drug monitoring and reversal and perioperative management in an attempt to improve the care of the vascular patient. The recent introduction of several new anticoagulants and reversal agents makes this topic especially pertinent (Figure 8.1).

HEPARINS

Heparin is one of the oldest and most commonly used anticoagulants. Unfractionated heparin (UFH) continues to be broadly used despite the introduction of many new agents, largely due to its efficacy, safety, short half-life, reversibility, physician familiarity and low cost. UFH and the low-molecular-weight heparins (LMWH) are similar compounds with a common mechanism available only in parenteral formulations.[1] Heparins are heavily sulphated polysaccharides isolated from mammalian mucosal cells rich in mast cells (Table 8.1).[2]

Mechanism of action

Heparins prevent thrombosis by two primary mechanisms: increased activity of antithrombin and mobilization of tissue factor pathway inhibitor (TFPI).[1,3] Antithrombin is a potent inhibitor of clotting enzymes such as thrombin, factor Xa and other serine proteases of the coagulation cascade. The binding of heparin to AT induces a conformational change of the AT active site, rendering it more accessible to subsequent binding of other proteases of coagulation resulting in deactivation of clotting factors. *This binding of heparin to AT doubles the rate of factor Xa inactivation; however, it has no direct effect on thrombin levels (factor IIa).* Thrombin inhibition is achieved by formation of a ternary complex consisting of AT, heparin and thrombin.[4] A long polysaccharide tail, at least 18–20 saccharide units (present on nearly all UFH molecules and only ~50% of LMWH), is required to form this ternary structure holding AT and thrombin in close apposition to one another for complete thrombin inhibition (Figure 8.2).[5]

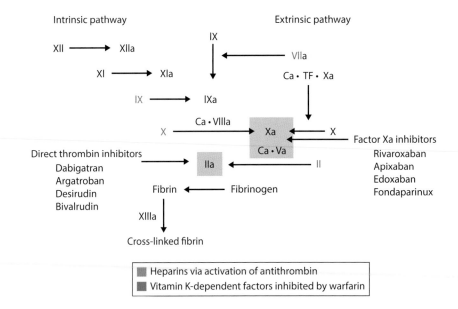

Figure 8.1 Coagulation cascade schematic.

The ability of heparin to bind AT is dependent upon a pentasaccharide moiety, common to all heparin-like agents including UFH, LMWH and fondaparinux. Therefore, each causes equal factor Xa inhibition. However, because LMWH consists of shorter heparin chains, its effect on thrombin inhibition is limited. Generally, UFH has 1:1 inhibition of Xa and IIa, whereas LMWH has 3–4:1 inhibition. Furthermore, fondaparinux entirely lacks this polysaccharide tail; thus, direct thrombin inhibition is not seen with this agent and fondaparinux is therefore classified as a factor Xa inhibitor (discussed in the succeeding text).

The second mechanism of action is a sixfold upregulation in the circulating concentration of TFPI.[6] TFPI is a serine protease inhibitor synthesized and secreted by endothelial cells. It forms a complex with factor Xa, VIIa and tissue thromboplastin, thereby preventing the conversion of factor X to Xa and factor IX to IXa. TFPI upregulation is most pronounced with longer heparin chains (UFH > LMWH > fondaparinux).[6,7]

FDA approval

UFH is approved for treatment of deep vein thrombosis (DVT)/pulmonary embolism (PE), disseminated intravascular coagulopathy (DIC), atrial fibrillation, DVT/PE prophylaxis and prophylaxis against catheter-related occlusion, thrombosis during cardiac surgery and extracorporeal and dialysis procedures. Despite widespread use, there is little level 1 evidence for UFH. Early trials demonstrated that an initial bolus, followed by a weight-based infusion of UFH at 18 U/kg/h, more effectively reduced the risk of recurrent venous or arterial thrombosis at 30 days.[8] Another trial demonstrated that

fixed-dose intravenous (IV) UFH was superior to weight-based subcutaneous (SC) UFH.[9] However, fixed-dose SC UFH proved to be non-inferior to twice-daily therapeutic LMWH injection for the treatment of DVT/PE suggesting that laboratory monitoring for therapeutic doses of SC UFH is not required.[10]

Nonetheless, UFH is utilized by vascular surgeons worldwide, most commonly administered intravenously prior to clamp placement for arterial reconstruction. The American College of Chest Physicians (ACCP) Clinical Practice Guidelines suggest immediate systemic anticoagulation with UFH in patients with acute limb ischemia prior to reperfusion therapy, despite a paucity of studies demonstrating improved outcomes in this setting (Level 2 Grade C).[11] UFH also has been studied in patients with claudication. There is no benefit in walking distance nor is there harm from bleeding complications, and its use is not recommended for claudication (Level 2 Grade C).[11,12]

LMWHs are approved for treatment and prophylaxis of DVT/PE, acute coronary syndrome. The LMWH tinzaparin also is approved for thrombosis prophylaxis with dialysis extracorporeal circuits and with indwelling IV lines.[13–16]

LMWH has been compared to UFH for treatment and prevention of non-ST elevation myocardial infarction (MI), and results are mixed. The American College of Cardiology/American Heart Association guidelines give equal recommendations for both, but most institutions still use UFH.[17,18] For VTE treatment, prospective randomized controlled trials have demonstrated superiority of LMWH over warfarin in cancer patients, reducing recurrence and propagation of DVT/PE.[19] Patients with malignancy requiring DVT/PE prophylaxis should receive

Table 8.1 Heparins.

| | UFH | LMWH | | |
		Enoxaparin (Lovenox®)	Dalteparin (Fragmin®)	Tinzaparin (Innohep®)
FDA-approved indications	1. DVT/PE prophylaxis 2. Prophylaxis in cardiac surgery, dialysis and extracorporeal procedures and against catheter-related clot 3. DIC treatment 4. DVT/PE treatment 5. AF	1. DVT prophylaxis following hip/knee arthroplasty, general surgery or medical patients 2. ACS 3. DVT treatment with/without PE	1. DVT prophylaxis following hip arthroplasty, general surgery or medical patients 2. ACS 3. DVT/PE treatment in cancer patients	1. DVT prophylaxis following hip/knee arthroplasty or general surgery 2. Prophylaxis against indwelling IV lines and HD circuit 3. DVT treatment wwo PE
Route of administration	SC; IV	SC; IV	SC	SC; IA or IV – for HD
Peak effect (hrs)	3	3–5	4	4–6
Half-life (hrs)	1–2	4.5–7	3–5	3–4
Renal clearance	Small amounts unchanged in the urine	Primary route: 40% of dose, 10% as active fragments	Primary route: >70% of dose in animal models	Primary route: 90% of dose in animal models
Dialyzable	No	No; not FDA approved, risk of accumulation, use not recommended	No; not FDA approved, risk of accumulation, use not recommended	No; not FDA approved, risk of accumulation, use not recommended
Hepatic/other clearance	Yes, but no CYP P450 involvement	Metabolized to small inactive fragments	None known	None
Dosing[a,b]	1. N/A 2. N/A 3. 10,000 U IV bolus, then 5,000–10,000 U (50–70 U/kg) IV q4–6 hrs or 5,000 U IV bolus, then 12.25–24.5 U/kg/hr IV 4. 80 U/kg IV bolus, then 18 U/kg/hr IV or 333 U/kg SC bolus, then 250 U/kg SC q12 hrs 5. IV as per #4[c]	1. N/A 2. 1 mg/kg SC q12 hrs or 1.5 mg/kg SC q24 hrs 3. 30 mg IV + 1 mg/kg SC q12 hrs	1. N/A 2. 120 U/kg SC q12 hrs 3. 200 U/kg SC q24 hrs for 1 month, then 150 U/kg every 24 hrs for months 2–6	1. N/A 2. N/A 3. 175 U/kg SC q24 hrs
Factors requiring dose adjustment	None	Renal	Renal[d]	Renal[d]

Sources: Dalteparin [Internet], Micromedex Healthcare Series, 2014 [cited September 20, 2014], available from Thomson Reuters Healthcare Inc. at www.micromedexsolutions.com; Enoxaparin [Internet], Micromedex Healthcare Series, 2014 [cited September 10, 2014], available from Thomson Reuters Healthcare Inc. at www.micromedexsolutions.com; Tinzaparin [Internet], Micromedex Healthcare Series, 2014 [cited September 20, 2014], available from Thomson Reuters Healthcare Inc. at www.micromedexsolutions.com; Wittkowsky AK, *Pharmacotherapy*, 31(12), 1175, December 2011; DiPiro JT, *Pharmacotherapy: A Pathophysiologic Approach*, 8th ed., McGraw-Hill Medical, New York, 2011, pp. xxxii, 2668; Fragmin (dalteparin sodium), injection, solution, Pfizer, Kirkland, Quebec, Canada, 2014.

Abbreviations: ACS, acute coronary syndrome; DVT, deep vein thrombosis; PE, pulmonary embolus; hrs, hours; SC, subcutaneous; DIC, disseminated intravascular coagulation; IA, intra-arterial; IV, intravenous; N/A, not applicable.

[a] Therapeutic dosing only, no prophylactic dosing provided.

[b] Weight-based dosing in actual body weight.

[c] Intensity of anticoagulation varies depending on which clinical guideline is referenced (American College of Chest Physicians favours aPTT 1.5–2.5× control whereas American College of Cardiology favours aPTT 1.5–2× control).

[d] Specific dose adjustments are not provided in labeling; however, manufacturer suggests a dose reduction be considered as half-life is increased in renal insufficiency.

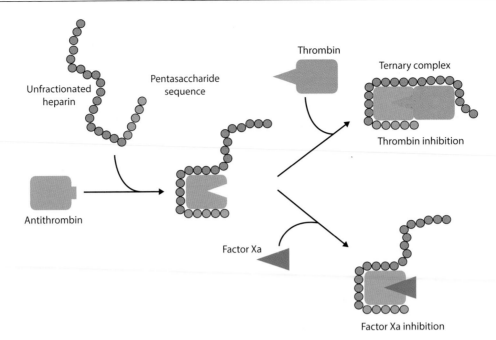

Figure 8.2 Mechanism of action of heparins.

LMWH over warfarin (Level 2, Grade B) and should receive extended therapy for unprovoked DVT/PE due to a higher risk of recurrence (Level 1, Grade B).[10]

Key points

Enoxaparin is superior to warfarin in cancer-related DVT/PE treatment and prophylaxis.

Important side effects

Bleeding is the most common complication of heparin therapy. Risk factors for bleeding complications include age > 65 years, recent surgery or trauma, concomitant antiplatelet therapy and alcohol abuse, among many others. As will be discussed in the section on monitoring, there are little data that routine monitoring of the activated partial thromboplastin time (aPTT) reduces the risk of bleeding or that a supratherapeutic aPTT predicts bleeding complications. Prolonged heparin therapy also has been associated with osteoporosis, potentially resulting in vertebral compression or long bone fractures. The mechanism for this is binding of UFH and LMWH to osteoblasts, triggering osteoclasts to break down bone matrix. LMWH is less likely to cause osteoporosis than UFH, due to the lower affinity of this shorter-chain heparin for osteoblasts.[20]

Heparins do not cross the placenta and therefore are the preferred medication (especially LMWH) for women requiring anticoagulation during pregnancy.[16] Heparin-induced thrombocytopenia (HIT) is a rare but life-threatening complication seen with UFH, and to a lesser degree with LMWH, and is addressed in greater detail later.

Monitoring and reversal

UFHs also bind with plasma proteins, resulting in variable pharmacokinetics. The aPTT is the primary test used to monitor UFH. The aPTT is readily available, easy to perform, inexpensive and familiar to most physicians. To achieve therapeutic anticoagulation, the aPTT should be prolonged 1.5–2.5-fold depending on the indication (Level 3). Because of sequestration of UFH by plasma proteins, monitoring is perhaps more important in the critically ill patient to avoid supratherapeutic levels of anticoagulation, which may result in bleeding complications, or subtherapeutic anticoagulation, which may cause recurrent thrombosis. LMWHs and fondaparinux have fewer interactions with plasma proteins, demonstrate more stable bioavailability and therefore do not require monitoring for most patients.

Surprisingly, limited evidence exists to support the common practice of scheduled aPTT draws and UFH dose adjustment. Furthermore, several studies and subgroup analyses have been unable to demonstrate an association between supratherapeutic aPTT and bleeding complications.[8,21–23] There are no randomized trials comparing monitored versus unmonitored UFH. Nonetheless, validated dose adjustment nomograms are used clinically to titrate UFH within the therapeutic range.[22,24] In patients with known or suspected AT deficiency or 'heparin resistance', anti-factor Xa levels should be measured rather than aPTT to determine appropriate dosing (Level 1, Grade A).

Generally, LMWH does not require monitoring, another advantage over UFH. If monitoring is necessary (patients with obesity, cachexia or renal dysfunction), newer assays measure peak anti-factor Xa levels to monitor the anticoagulation effect of LMWH and fondaparinux. These assays have not yet been standardized, are more expensive, are not widely available and are less familiar to physicians.[21] In light of the mechanism of action of LMWH, the aPTT is largely unaffected by this medication and therefore is not reliable.

> **Key point**
>
> If necessary, peak anti-factor Xa levels should be used for LMWH or fondaparinux.
> aPTT is not reliable for monitoring LMWH or fondaparinux.

UFH may be reversed with protamine sulphate. Protamine, first isolated from salmon sperm, causes rapid correction of the aPTT and anti-factor Xa levels. Roughly 1 mg of protamine will neutralize approximately 100 units of heparin. Protamine is administered IV. Slow administration (maximum of 50 mg over 10 minutes) and careful hemodynamic monitoring are recommended as hypotension or anaphylaxis may occur with administration (Micromedex). Anesthesia providers frequently will give a small test dose of protamine intraoperatively, to assess for hemodynamic changes before administering the full dosage needed for heparin reversal.

> **Key point**
>
> Approximately 100 units of UFH will neutralize in 1 mg of protamine.

Reversal of LMWH may be achieved by protamine administration and fresh frozen plasma (FFP). Depending on the timing of the last dose of LMWH, administer 0.5–1 mg protamine for every 1 mg of enoxaparin or 100 units of tinzaparin or dalteparin. However, protamine only will neutralize longer pentasaccharide chains within LMWH, inhibiting the anti-factor IIa effect, but having little impact on anti-factor Xa inhibition.

Pharmacology and effect of dialysis

All heparins are administered through a continuous infusion IV or by SC injection. UFH has a profoundly negative electrochemical charge owing to the many sulphur groups on the long, polysaccharide chains of the molecule. Therefore, it is rapidly bound to plasma proteins in addition to AT and to the endothelium. This results in a half-life that is dose dependent, ranging from approximately 45 to 90 minutes. Importantly, many of the heparin-binding proteins are acute phase reactants and their effect will vary depending upon the patient's physiologic status.[25]

The bioavailability of UFH is largely affected by the route of administration. SC injection requires a five-fold increase in dosage to achieve equipotent bioavailability.[26] Clearance is extrarenal with the breakdown of the polysaccharide by macrophages. Therefore, it is not cleared in dialysate and is almost entirely independent of renal function. Hence, no dosage adjustment is needed in patients with diminished glomerular filtration rate (GFR).

LMWH, on the other hand, is one-third the molecular weight of UFH. The length of the polysaccharide chains is considerably shorter, measuring on average only 16–18 polysaccharide units. Therefore, LMWH has fewer sulphur groups and is less negatively charged. This results in less sequestration of LMWH by plasma proteins or the endothelium, resulting in more reliable bioavailability, dose-independent clearance and a longer half-life. LMWHs are renally cleared and dosing should be adjusted for GFR. However, they are not removed by hemodialysis (HD).[27,28]

Special circumstance: AT deficiency, HIT and bridging

AT DEFICIENCY

The anticoagulant effect of UFH, LMWH and fondaparinux is largely dependent upon the presence of circulating AT. Acquired or congenital deficiencies in AT are well-described and termed 'heparin resistance'. Acquired AT deficiency may be seen in patients receiving UFH for longer than 4 hours, with AT levels falling as much as 33% with longer administration. This acquired decrease in AT is much less dramatic with LMWH. Patients with congenital AT deficiency will have even greater resistance to anticoagulation, but this subject is more fully discussed in Chapter 8.

HIT

HIT is the result of preformed IgG antibodies binding to a heparin–platelet factor 4 (PF4) complex, resulting in widespread platelet activation and aggregation. Thrombocytopenia results from the elimination of the antibody heparin–PF4 complex by splenic macrophages and the reticular endothelial system, as well as platelet consumption within diffuse thrombi. HIT can occur with any dose of UFH or LMWH or any administration route. Ultra-large heparin–PF4 complexes are more common with UFH and the incidence of HIT is more common in patients receiving UFH, when compared with LMWH.[29] Fondaparinux is not thought to cause HIT.[30] HIT causes thrombocytopenia, arterial and more commonly venous thrombosis, necrotizing skin lesions at heparin injection sites, and possibly anaphylactic reaction after IV injection and is associated with high mortality.[31] Patients with HIT should be treated with argatroban (Level 2) but direct thrombin inhibitors (DTIs) or factor Xa inhibitors also are acceptable. There are data reporting fondaparinux in lieu of DTIs for treatment of HIT but this is an off-label use.[32–34]

ANTICOAGULANT BRIDGING

The failure to properly manage anticoagulation around the time of surgery or other invasive procedure may result in elevated rates of post-procedural hemorrhage or thrombosis. The original indication for antithrombotic therapy (thrombosis risk) should be assessed and weighed against the magnitude of the invasive procedure (bleeding risk). The ACCP guidelines recommend stratification into high, moderate, and low risk for perioperative thromboembolism.[35,36]

Patients receiving chronic warfarin should discontinue therapy approximately 5 days prior to surgery (Level 1, Grade C). If the patient is at low risk for thromboembolism, then no bridging therapy is recommended (Level 2, Grade C). Patients who are at high risk for thromboembolism include those with mechanical mitral valves, atrial fibrillation with CHADS$_2$ score > 4 with recent cerebrovascular accident (CVA)/TIA and recent DVT/PE or severe thrombophilia. These patients generally should receive bridging antithrombotic therapy during interruption of the warfarin (Level 2, Grade C).[36] Options for bridging include IV UFH, generally administered on an inpatient basis. The UFH usually is discontinued 4–6 hours prior to the procedure (Level 2, Grade C). Another option for outpatient bridging includes therapeutic dosing with SC LMWH. The last dose of LMWH should be administered approximately 24 hours prior to surgery.

Postoperative resumption of anticoagulation should be tailored to the patients bleeding risk. For patients at high risk for bleeding, therapeutic doses of LMWH should be reinstituted no sooner than 48–72 hours postoperatively. Patients who are *not* at high risk for bleeding may reinitiate therapeutic LMWH approximately 24 hours after surgery (Level 2, Grade C).[35,37] Another option for postoperative bridging includes the use of prophylactic doses of LMWH. Although less well studied, we frequently utilize this regimen to balance the risk for hemorrhage in high-risk patients against the risk for venous or arterial thrombosis (Table 8.2).

Key point: HIT

Patients with HIT should be managed with argatroban.

WARFARIN

Warfarin is the most commonly prescribed oral anticoagulant for the treatment and prevention of thrombosis and thromboembolism. Warfarin initially was developed in the 1940s as a pesticide against rodents and later in 1954, as an FDA-approved anticoagulant for the prevention of thrombosis and thromboembolism in humans. Warfarin and other vitamin K antagonists inhibit hepatic synthesis of vitamin K–dependent clotting factors II, VII, IX and X. It also inhibits proteins C and S, two naturally occurring anticoagulant proteins. Since their development, vitamin K antagonists had remained the sole class of orally administered anticoagulants for over five decades. However, their use is now declining with the introduction of several novel oral agents.[38]

Mechanism of action

Each vitamin K–dependent clotting factor (II, VII, IX and X) shares a glutamic acid residue at the N-terminus of the protein. The gamma carbon of the glutamic acid residue receives a carboxyl group during post-translational modification. This process, termed gamma carboxylation, is dependent upon an oxidation–reduction reaction catalyzed by glutamyl carboxylase, in which reduced vitamin

Table 8.2 To bridge or not to bridge.

Risk	Mechanical valve	Atrial fibrillation	VTE	Bridging?
High	Any MVR Older aortic valve CVA or TIA < 6 mths	CHADS$_2$ = 5–6 CVA or TIA < 3 mths Rheumatic valvular disease	VTE < 3 mths Severe thrombophilia[a]	Yes (Grade 2C). Therapeutic SC LMWH or IV UFH.
Moderate	Bileaflet AVR and >1 of: AF, prior CVA or TIA, HTN, DM, CHF, age > 75 years	CHADS$_2$ = 3–4	VTE within 3–12 mths Non-severe thrombophilia[b] Recurrent VTE Active cancer < 6 mths	Weigh patient and surgical-specific factors. Therapeutic SC LMWH, SC UFH, IV UFH *OR* prophylactic dose SC LMWH.
Low	Bileaflet AVR wo AF or CVA risk factors	CHADS$_2$ = 0–2	VTE > 12 mths No other risk factors	No (Grade 2C)

Sources: Douketis JD et al., *Chest*, 141(2 Suppl.), e326S, February 2012; Whitlock RP et al., *Chest*, 141(2 Suppl.), e576S, February 2012.
Abbreviations: AF, atrial fibrillation; MVR, mitral valve replacement; CVA, cerebrovascular accident; TIA, transient ischemic attack; mths, months; CHADS$_2$, congestive heart failure, hypertension, age > 75 years, diabetes, stroke or transient ischemic attack; VTE, venous thromboembolism; SC, subcutaneous; IV, intravenous; UFH, unfractionated heparin; LMWH, low-molecular-weight heparin.
[a] Protein C deficiency, protein S deficiency, antiphospholipid antibody syndrome.
[b] Factor V Leiden, Prothrombin mutation.

K (vitamin K hydroquinone) donates the carboxyl group to the gamma carbon on the non-functional clotting factor, oxidizing vitamin K (becoming vitamin K epoxide) and producing a functional clotting factor.[39] Vitamin K epoxide reductase is a hepatic enzyme that recycles oxidized vitamin K epoxide back to reduced vitamin K hydroquinone, and warfarin interrupt this cycle. Inhibition of this enzyme prevents gamma carboxylation of the vitamin K–dependent clotting factors rendering the factors nonfunctional and ineffectual in clot formation.[40,41]

Initiation of warfarin therapy has no immediate effect on the concentration of functional gamma carboxylated vitamin K–dependent clotting factors already in circulation. These coagulation factors must degrade naturally, being slowly replaced by the inactive (non-carboxylated) forms. The relatively long half-life of some vitamin K–dependent factors (72 hours for factor II) is responsible for the delayed anticoagulant effect, taking as many as 5 days.[42] In fact, patients actually may become more hypercoagulable during initiation of warfarin, a result of a rapid decline in the vitamin K–dependent anticoagulants, protein C and S. Unlike the vitamin K–dependent clotting factors, the half-life of protein C is shorter, on the order of 6–8 hours.[43,44] Without concomitant parenteral anticoagulation, the balance of the coagulation cascade may shift towards thrombosis, potentially explaining one of the feared complications of warfarin-induced skin necrosis. The risk is potentially higher with larger starting doses of warfarin, as 10 mg reduces protein C and S faster than a 5 mg starting dose. However, an increased thrombosis risk with larger initiating doses has never been proved (Figure 8.3).[45]

> **Key point**
>
> Initiation of warfarin causes an early, transient hypercoagulable state as a result of inhibition of anticoagulants protein C and S.
> Bridging therapy is recommended.

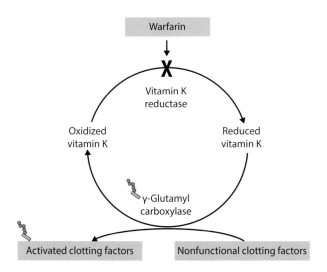

Figure 8.3 Warfarin mechanism of action.

FDA indications

Warfarin is approved in the United States for the prevention of stroke in patients with atrial fibrillation or artificial heart valves, treatment of DVT/PE and prevention of systemic embolism post-MI. Adjusted-dose warfarin is superior to fixed, low-dose warfarin plus antiplatelet agents in stroke prevention in patients with atrial fibrillation (Level 1).[46] The CHADS$_2$ (now the CHADS$_2$VASc) scoring system is used to calculate risk of thromboembolic stroke in patients with atrial fibrillation. The criteria used to calculate the CHADS$_2$VASc score include the presence of congestive heart failure, hypertension, age > 65 years, diabetes, prior stroke or transient ischemic attack, vascular disease and female sex. Warfarin is indicated for most patients with a score ≥2 (Level 1, Grade B) and is recommended over antiplatelet or dual antiplatelet therapy (Level 2, Grade B).[35,47] For most indications, parenteral anticoagulation *and* warfarin are initiated on the same day and continued for 5 days and until the international normalized ratio (INR) is within the therapeutic range (Level 1, Grade B). No bridging anticoagulation is required for atrial fibrillation, unless the patient is deemed high risk for thromboembolism (CHADS2 > 4 or CHADS2VASc > 5).[47]

Warfarin has a limited role in patients with peripheral arterial disease (PAD). When compared with aspirin alone, warfarin plus aspirin did not improve the overall of survival or rate of MI or CVA and was associated with higher bleeding complications. Therefore, ACCP guidelines recommend against warfarin plus aspirin for secondary prevention in patients with PAD or for primary patency of lower extremity bypass grafts (Level 1, Grade B).[11,48] Select patients with PAD, however, do have a proven benefit with warfarin. These include patients with high risk for failure lower extremity bypass grafts (poor outflow, suboptimal vein conduit or redo procedures) or patients with below-the-knee prosthetic bypass grafts (Level 3).[49–52]

Important side effects

There are several disadvantages to warfarin therapy, including the need for indefinite INR monitoring, numerous drug and dietary interactions, delayed onset and need for bridging, variable dosing and bleeding complications. Bleeding is more common during the first month of therapy, when warfarin is co-administered with antiplatelet agents such as aspirin, clopidogrel or non-steroidal anti-inflammatory agents, or when the INR is supratherapeutic (Level 2).[53–56] The incidence of major bleeding events (fatal hemorrhage, intracranial or retroperitoneal hemorrhage, bleeding requiring hospitalization or transfusion of two or more packed red blood cells) ranges from 0.4% to 7.2% per year,[57–60] and minor bleeding rates may be as high as 15% per year. The Atrial Fibrillation Follow-up Investigation of Rhythm Management trial of more than 4000 patients on warfarin demonstrated an annual major and minor bleeding rate of 2% and 18% per year respectively (Level 1).[61] Several meta-analyses also have compared bleeding complications of warfarin to the new oral anticoagulants. Overall major bleeding events were 2.8%–2.9% per year with warfarin versus 1.8%–2.4% per year for new oral agents, and rate of intracranial hemorrhage (ICH) was 0.52%–0.66% per year versus 0.19%–0.32% per year, respectively (Level 1).[62–64]

Warfarin is contraindicated during pregnancy and is associated with spontaneous abortion, neonatal death and fetal warfarin syndrome (a constellation of skeletal defects including nasal hypoplasia, vertebral and long bone calcification and brachydactyly). Administration of warfarin during the second and third trimester is associated with central nervous system problems such as seizure, developmental delay and spasticity.[65] Furthermore, warfarin crosses the placenta in an active form and may lead to ICH in utero or during delivery. It is therefore a category x drug in the United States. Pregnant patients requiring anticoagulation can be maintained on UFH, enoxaparin or fondaparinux which are safer during pregnancy. After delivery, breast-feeding patients may resume warfarin as it does not enter breast milk.

Warfarin-induced skin necrosis is a rare phenomenon which occurs during the initiation of therapy when the anticoagulants, proteins C and S, are depleted more rapidly than the vitamin K–dependent coagulation factors. This condition may manifest several days after starting warfarin and is more likely to occur in patients with protein C or S deficiency. However, only one-third of patients with warfarin-induced skin necrosis have underlying protein C deficiency.[66] Clinically, the characteristic sharp erythematous patches, usually on the trunk or extremities, progress to edematous lesions with central purpura and ultimately to necrosis. Skin biopsy demonstrates dermal and SC capillary microthrombi and endothelial damage. Treatment includes the discontinuation of warfarin, possible vitamin K repletion, protein C and S repletion with FFP and anticoagulation with therapeutic heparin.[67]

Lastly, warfarin has interactions with a variety of foods rich in vitamin K and numerous naturopathic and pharmaceutical agents. These alterations may occur through decreased absorption from the gastrointestinal (GI) tract, displacement of warfarin from albumin, an increase or decrease in warfarin metabolism by cytochrome (CYP) P450 in hepatocytes (primarily CYP 2C9), an increase or decrease in the plasma half-life of clotting factors or a decrease in the bioavailability of vitamin K. As with any medication, it is important to thoroughly review the patient's list of medications for potential interactions and educate about the associated risks and complications associated with warfarin.

Monitoring and reversal

Warfarin is monitored using the prothrombin time (PT) and is calculated by adding thromboplastin and calcium to citrated plasma. Since thromboplastins vary according to their ability to activate the external coagulation cascade, the PT is standardized against a laboratory normal value and is expressed as the INR. When initiating warfarin, the PT/INR should be monitored on a daily basis for 5 or more days until steady state is reached. Once the INR reaches the targeted therapeutic range, monitoring intervals may decrease to two or three times per week and eventually every 4 weeks, once the dosing remains stable. Bridging with UFH may occasionally prolong the PT/INR, depending on the type of thromboplastin reagent used. This is a result of the inhibition of factors IIa, IXa and Xa by AT. Patients on warfarin and antiplatelet agents also should have more frequent monitoring given their increased propensity for bleeding complications and potential drug interactions.[68]

The targeted INR for warfarin therapy is 2.0–3.0 for patients with DVT/PE, atrial fibrillation and most prosthetic heart valves (Level 2, Grade B). Mechanical mitral valves require a slightly higher target INR of 2.5–3.5.[69]

Treatment of minor bleeding complications may be as simple as omitting 1–2 doses of warfarin or supplementing with a low dose of vitamin K. Vitamin K may be given orally or intravenously, but a randomized trial demonstrated IV vitamin K to be superior to oral vitamin K for rapid correction (Level 1, Grade B).[70,71] Life-threatening hemorrhage requires aggressive and rapid correction of the coagulopathy. When available, prothrombin complex concentrates (PCCs), which contain high concentrations of vitamin K–dependent clotting factors or recombinant factor VIIa, are preferred to FFP (Level 3, Grade B). FFP carries an associated risk of transfusion-related acute lung injury, requires ABO compatibility, requires thawing and requires large volume transfusion to correct the INR.[45] PCC was FDA approved in 2013 for immediate warfarin reversal in patients with major hemorrhage or need for urgent surgery. They have consistently demonstrated an ability to more rapidly normalize INR compared to FFP or vitamin K; however, improved clinical outcome has not been convincingly demonstrated.[72–74] Table 8.3 delineates current guidelines for correction of INR.

Pharmacology and effect of dialysis

Once ingested, warfarin is completely absorbed and reaches maximum plasma concentration in approximately 120 hours. The half-life varies considerably but averages 36–40 hours. At therapeutic levels, warfarin is almost entirely (97%) bound to albumin. It is metabolized by hepatocytes by the CYP enzymes into water-soluble, inactive substrates that are almost entirely renally excreted.[56] Warfarin is not cleared by HD. Prolongation of the PT/INR is more dependent on the amount of dietary vitamin K, patient age, nutritional status and co-morbidities. Foods high in vitamin K such as broccoli, spinach, cabbage and yogurt will make warfarin less effective. On the contrary, warfarin administration will be potentiated in patients with hepatic and/or renal insufficiency, congestive heart failure, obstructive jaundice, malnutrition and patients receiving TPN without vitamin K supplementation.

Table 8.3 Guidelines for warfarin reversal.

INR and clinical status	Treatment
Single INR < 0.5	Continue current dose.
	Recheck INR 1–2 weeks.
INR 4.5–10 without bleeding	Omit 1–2 doses of warfarin.
	Close INR monitoring.
	Lower dose with INR therapeutic.
	(Suggest *against* routine vitamin K reversal.)
INR > 10 without bleeding	Oral vitamin K administration (2.5–5 mg).
	Close INR monitoring.
	Lower dose when INR therapeutic.
Any INR > 3 with major bleeding	PCC.
	FFP if PCC not available.
	IV vitamin K 5–10 mg.

Source: Adapted from Rosenberg RD and Lam L, *Proc Natl Acad Sci USA*, 76(3), 1218, 1979.

DIRECT THROMBIN INHIBITORS

Given the limitations and potential complications associated with heparin and warfarin therapy, pharmaceutical manufacturers have developed and studied newer classes of anticoagulants that are either FDA approved or in the advanced stages of clinical trials. DTIs and factor Xa inhibitors are relatively new anticoagulants now available in the United States and are the first oral anticoagulants to be introduced since warfarin in the 1950s. DTIs, available in an oral form (dabigatran) or parenteral forms (bivalirudin, desirudin and argatroban), are attractive to patients and clinicians alike because of a short onset of action and half-life and predictable pharmacokinetics. Dabigatran and desirudin do not require monitoring of coagulation. Generally, none of the newer oral anticoagulants require bridging on initiation or cessation of therapy. In addition, DTIs do not generate antiplatelet antibodies that cause HIT and are therefore the mainstay treatment for HIT. Another advantage of DTIs is that they have the ability to inactivate clot-bound thrombin unlike heparins or warfarin.[75]

The discovery of DTIs dates back to 1884 when John Haycraft observed that leeches secreted a potent anticoagulant from the salivary glands which he named 'hirudin'. The protein sequence and structure, however, was not elucidated until the 1950s and 1970s, respectively. Unfortunately, hirudin was difficult to extract in large quantities for clinical uses but the development of recombinant techniques made the production of large quantities of purified hirudin possible since several hirudin-based pharmaceuticals have been developed including bivalirudin, desirudin and lepirudin. Lepirudin was FDA approved for HIT, but the productions was discontinued in 2012 and it is no longer available (Table 8.4).[76]

Mechanism of action

DTIs exert their effects on thrombin (factor II), the final, common enzyme of the coagulation cascade that converts fibrinogen to fibrin resulting in cross-linking and thrombus formation. The 3D structure of thrombin is unique in that it has a deep groove in the centre of the protein which harbours the active site. There are two types of DTIs, *bivalent* and *univalent*. Univalent DTIs such as argatroban and dabigatran bind exclusively to the active site of thrombin resulting in inhibition. Bivalent DTIs including hirudin (no longer clinically available) and its analogs bivalirudin, desirudin and lepirudin exert inhibitory effects on thrombin via irreversible binding of the active site *and* an exosite (Figure 8.4). The exosite is involved in fibrin polymerization and cross-linking.[77]

Bivalirudin is approved for percutaneous coronary intervention (PCI) management of patients with acute coronary syndrome as well as for the treatment of HIT. It also is used (although not FDA approved) for patients undergoing coronary artery bypass grafting with proven or high risk for HIT.[78,79] American and European cardiology guidelines suggest that it is now one of the preferred drugs for patients undergoing PCI.[80–83] Bivalirudin is primarily cleared renally with minimal to no hepatic clearance. Dose adjustments should be made for patients with moderate to severe renal dysfunction and it can be only partially cleared by HD. All hirudins are immunogenic and anti-hirudin antibodies develop in 40%–76% of patients receiving hirudins for 4 days or longer.[84] Although most antibodies are clinically silent, fatal anaphylaxis from subsequent hirudin exposure has been reported, and it is recommended that a different anticoagulant be used for patients with prior exposure.[85,86]

Desirudin, also a bivalent DTI, is FDA approved for DVT/PE prevention following major joint arthroplasty. It has been studied against UFH and LMWH in DVT prophylaxis and against UFH for prevention of thrombotic complication after acute coronary syndrome and proved more efficacious for both but with higher bleeding rates.[87–90] Desirudin is available in SC and IV formulations. It has a half-life of 2–3 hours and peak effect is achieved within 1–3 hours of administration. Primary clearance is renal and it can be removed by HD.[90,91]

Argatroban, a univalent DTI, is available exclusively in parenteral form. It is FDA approved for PCI for patients with HIT and is the preferred treatment for prevention and treatment of DVT/PE in patients with HIT (Level 2, Grade C).[92] Clearance is primarily hepatic and is therefore the ideal DTI for patients with renal insufficiency but must be dose adjusted for patients with hepatic insufficiency. Argatroban is not immunogenic and a large prospective cohort study demonstrated lower bleeding events in patients on argatroban as compared to lepirudin.[88,92,93] In Japan argatroban is approved for patients with PAD.[94] Although not an approved FDA indication in the United States, patients undergoing surgery (elective or emergent) with a history of HIT can be managed with intraoperative argatroban as follows.

Table 8.4 Direct thrombin inhibitors.

	Desirudin (Iprivask®)	Bivalirudin (Angiomax®)	Argatroban (Acova®)	Dabigatran (Pradaxa®)
FDA-approved indications	1. DVT prophylaxis following hip replacement	1. UA/NSTEMI undergoing early invasive strategy 2. PCI wwo HIT	1. HIT 2. PCI	1. Non-valvular AF 2. DVT/PE treatment (including extended treatment)
Administration Route	IV or SC	IV or SC	IV	Oral
Peak effect (hrs)	1–3	1–3	1–3	1–3
Half-life (hrs)	2–3	0.42	0.5–0.85	14–17
Renal clearance	Primary route: 40%–50% unchanged	Primary route: 20% unchanged	22%–24% in urine, 16% as unchanged	80% excreted in urine
Dialyzable	Yes	Yes. 25% removed	Yes. 20% removed	Yes; 65% removed but re-equilibrates from tissues
Hepatic/other clearance	Minimal; <7% metabolized by carboxypeptidases	Minimal. Metabolized by blood proteases	Primary route; 65% via CYP	Partial via PGP; no CYP involvement
Dosing[a,b]	1. N/A	1. 0.75 mg/kg IV bolus, then 1.75 mg/kg/hr IV during procedure and up to 4 hrs post-procedure. If continued use desired, reduce to 0.25 mg/kg/hr IV for up to 72 hrs 2. Procedural and 4 hr post-procedure as described in #1. If continued use desired, reduce to 0.2 mg/kg/hr IV up to an additional 20 hrs	1. 2 mcg/kg/min IV 2. 350 mcg/kg IV bolus, then 25 mcg/kg/min IV If continued use is required, reduce to 2 mcg/kg/min IV	1. 150 mg orally every 12 hrs 2. Dosing as described in #1 (after 5–10 days of a parenteral anticoagulant)
Factors requiring dose adjustments	Renal	Renal	Hepatic	Renal, hepatic,[c] drug interactions

Sources: Hellwig T and Gulseth M, *Ann Pharmacother*, 47(11), 1478, November 2013; Nutescu EA, *Am J Health Syst Pharm*, 70(10 Suppl. 1), S1, May 15, 2013; Desirudin [Internet], Micromedex Healthcare Series, 2014 [cited September 1, 2014], available from Thomson Reuters Healthcare Inc. at www.micromedex.com; Wittkowsky AK, *Pharmacotherapy*, 31(12), 1175, December 2011; Heidbuchel H et al., *Europace*, 15(5), 625, May 2013; Bivalirudin [Internet], Micromedex Healthcare Series, 2014 [cited September 20, 2014], available from Thomson Reuters Healthcare Inc. at www.micromedex.com; Argatroban [Internet], Micromedex Healthcare Series, 2014 [cited September 20, 2014], available from Thomson Reuters Healthcare Inc. at www.micromedex.com; Dabigatran [Internet], Micromedex Healthcare Series, 2014 [cited September 20, 2014], available from Thomson Reuters Healthcare Inc. at www.micromedex.com.

Note: Lepirudin, another DTI, was discontinued in 2012 by the manufacturer.

Abbreviations: CYP, cytochrome P450; PGP, P-glycoprotein; HIT, heparin-induced thrombocytopenia; NSTEMI, non-ST elevation myocardial infarction; PCI, percutaneous coronary intervention; UA, unstable angina; AF, atrial fibrillation; N/A, not applicable; SC, subcutaneous; hrs, hours; min, minutes.

[a] Therapeutic dosing only, no prophylactic dosing provided.

[b] Weight-based dosing in actual body weight.

[c] No hepatic dose adjustments provided in US labeling, however, not recommended if enzymes >3× upper limit of normal per Canadian labelling.

Key point

Intraoperative anticoagulation in patients with HIT using argatroban

- Bolus 100 μg/kg IV
- Continuous 2 μg/kg/min IV
- 300 μg/kg IV bolus immediately prior to vascular clamping
- Surgical 'flushes': 10 mg in 1000 mL normal saline[33,95,96]

Dabigatran available in oral formulation is also a univalent DTI, approved in the United States in October 2010 for non-valvular atrial fibrillation and for DVT/PE treatment and prevention of recurrence. The main side effects of dabigatran are dyspepsia and gastroesophageal reflux occurring in 12%–33% of patients.[97] This effect is thought to be related to tartaric acid used in the formulation of the drug to improve bioavailability.[97] These are often severe enough

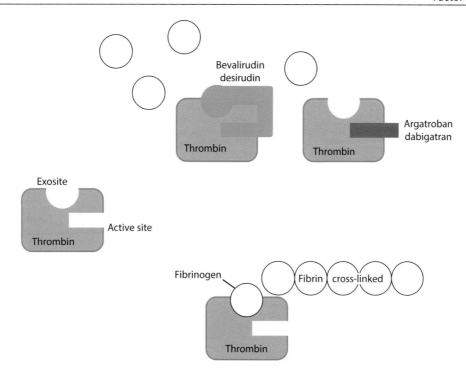

Figure 8.4 Direct thrombin inhibitor mechanism.

that patients elect to switch to a different anticoagulant. Also, GI bleeding is highest with dabigatran and rivaroxaban compared to warfarin and apixaban and it has a higher rate of MI compared to the other new oral anticoagulants. Additionally, there is a wide interindividual variability of GI drug absorption.[97] Its half-life is 14–17 hours and elimination is primarily renal after metabolism by P-glycoprotein (PGP) efflux transporter in the gut.[98] Drug–drug interactions exist as a result of PGP interactions. PGP inducers such as rifampin and prazosin will lower the plasma concentration, while PGP inhibitors such as amiodarone, ketoconazole, verapamil and clarithromycin may raise plasma levels. While clinically notable interactions are rare, dose adjustments should be made based on renal function and coadministration with PGP inhibitors. Of all the new oral anticoagulants, dabigatran is the most dependent upon renal function for elimination. It is contraindicated in severe renal impairment and is category C in pregnancy.[56]

Monitoring

Because of the relative predictable pharmacodynamics of DTIs, routine monitoring of coagulation is not required nor recommended. However, in certain patient scenarios such as active bleeding, progressive renal insufficiency, concern for over- or under-dosing or suspicion of non-adherence, it may be necessary to measure the anticoagulant effect. The most useful laboratory test is the ecarin clotting time (ECT) which directly measures thrombin generation. ECT is highly accurate; however, it is not widely available and not yet standardized. If ECT is not available, thrombin time (TT) can be measured which

tests the activity of thrombin against plasma. TT is more widely available, but it is less useful than ECT. Finally, aPTT is widely available, and although the dose–response curve is non-linear, it will detect the presence or absence of dabigatran and therefore may be of some utility in specific patient scenarios.[56] All of the DTIs will falsely elevate the INR especially argatroban. For example, patients on therapeutic argatroban will have an INR as high as 5–6. Measuring an INR in patients taking DTIs is of no benefit and will create confusion and is therefore not recommended.[56] For patients bridging from argatroban to warfarin therapy, chromogenic factor Xa levels should be monitored with a goal of 0.2–0.4 (UNITS). Alternatively, stopping the argatroban and checking an INR 4 hours after will allow sufficient time for the argatroban effect to dissipate.[99]

> **Key point**
>
> GI upset and twice-daily dosing are the most common patient-cited reasons to switch off dabigatran.

FACTOR Xa INHIBITORS

Factor Xa inhibitors are also new agents now commercially available in the United States. Similar to DTIs, factor Xa inhibitors are desirable alternatives to warfarin because of rapid onset of action, oral formulations and stable pharmacodynamics that don't require monitoring. Factor Xa inhibitors approved in the United States are rivaroxaban, apixaban and fondaparinux. Edoxaban is approved in Japan for DVT/PE prophylaxis following

Table 8.5 Factor Xa inhibitors.

	Fondaparinux (Arixtra®)	Rivaroxaban (Xarelto®)	Apixaban (Eliquis®)	Edoxaban (Savaysa®)
FDA-approved indications	1. DVT prophylaxis after hip/knee replacement or fracture or general surgery 2. DVT/PE treatment	1. DVT prophylaxis after hip/knee replacement 2. Non-valvular AF 3. DVT/PE (including extended treatment)	1. DVT prophylaxis after hip/knee replacement 2. Non-valvular AF 3. DVT/PE (including extended treatment)	TBD
Route of administration	SC	Oral	Oral	Oral
Peak effect (hrs)	2–3	2–4	1–3	1–3
Half-life (hrs)	17–21	5–9	8–15	9–11
Dosing	1. N/A 2. <50 kg = 5 mg, 50–100 kg = 7.5 mg and >100 kg = 10 mg SC q24 hrs	1. N/A 2. 20 mg orally q24 hrs 3. 15 mg orally q12 hrs for 21 days, then 20 mg orally q24 hrs	1. N/A 2. 5 mg orally q12 hrs 3. 10 mg orally q12 hrs for 7 days, then 5 mg orally q12 hrs; after 6 months, reducing to 2.5 mg orally q12 hrs	TBD – studies have evaluated 1. 60 mg orally q24 hrs 2. Dosing as described in #1 (after at least 5 days of parenteral anticoagulant)
Renal clearance	Primary: 77% unchanged	33%	25%	50%
Dialyzable	Yes; 20% removed, risk of accumulation, use contraindicated	No; not FDA approved, risk of accumulation, use not recommended	No; risk of accumulation, use not recommended	No; not FDA approved, risk of accumulation, use not recommended
Hepatic/other clearance	Not known	32% (mainly CYP)	15% (mainly CYP)	<4% (mainly CYP)
		Removed by PGP	Removed by PGP	Removed by PGP
Factors requiring dose adjustments	Renal	Renal, hepatic, drug interactions	Renal, hepatic, drug interactions, age, weight	TBD – suspect renal, hepatic, drug interactions, body weight

Sources: Hellwig T and Gulseth M, *Ann Pharmacother*, 47(11), 1478, November 2013; Nutescu EA, *Am J Health Syst Pharm*, 70(10 Suppl. 1), S1, May 15, 2013; Rivaroxaban [Internet], Micromedex Healthcare Series, 2014 [cited September 20, 2014], available from Thomson Reuters Healthcare Inc. at www.micromedex.com; Apixaban [Internet], Micromedex Healthcare Services, 2014 [cited September 10, 2014], available from Thomson Reuters Healthcare Inc. at www.micromedex.com; Wittkowsky AK, *Pharmacotherapy*, 31(12), 1175, December 2011; Heidbuchel H et al., *Europace*, 15(5), 625, May 2013; Eliquis (Apixaban) prescribing information, Bristol-Myers Squibb Company, Princeton, NJ, December 2012; Edoxaban [Internet], Micromedex Healthcare Series, 2014 [cited September 20, 2014], available from Thomson Reuters Healthcare Inc. www.micromedex.com.

Abbreviations: TBD, to be determined; SC, subcutaneous; CYP, cytochrome P450; PGP, P-glycoprotein; AF, atrial fibrillation; hrs, hours; q, every.

major orthopedic surgery, but approval in the United States is pending (Table 8.5).[100,101]

Mechanism of action

Factor Xa inhibitors are highly selective, reversible inhibitors of free factor Xa as well as factor Xa bound to prothrombinase complex.

Rivaroxaban was the first Xa inhibitor approved by the FDA. In 2011 it was approved for VTE prevention in patients undergoing knee or hip replacement after a phase 3 randomized, double-blind trial that demonstrated rivaroxaban at 10 mg daily was superior to enoxaparin at 40 mg daily in prevention of major VTE with similar safety profiles.[102] Later, it was FDA approved for stroke prevention in non-valvular atrial fibrillation and then DVT/PE treatment and prevention of recurrence (Level 1).[64]

Rivaroxaban has a high oral bioavailability, rapid onset of action, few drug–drug interactions and no active metabolites. These characteristics have important implications on the perioperative management of patients taking rivaroxaban (Table 8.6).

Apixaban is the newest target-specific oral anticoagulant to become available and was FDA approved in 2012 for DVT/PE prophylaxis following knee/hip replacement as well as for stroke prevention in non-valvular atrial fibrillation and lastly for DVT/PE treatment and prevention of recurrence. In a pooled meta-analysis of 10 randomized controlled trials, apixaban, rivaroxaban and dabigatran were compared against enoxaparin for prevention of DVT/PE after total hip or total knee arthroplasty, and all three new oral anticoagulants had a lower incidence of DVT/PE.[62,63]

When comparing the two available factor Xa inhibitors, apixaban and rivaroxaban, apixaban has a longer half-life.

Table 8.6 Recommendations for perioperative management of new anticoagulants.

Clinical scenario	Dabigatran	Rivaroxaban	Apixaban
Elective surgery[a]	Hold 24–48 hrs prior. No bridging or anticoag labs. Resume 24–48 hrs for low-risk bleeding and 48–72 hrs for high bleeding risk	Hold dose 24–48 hrs prior No bridging or anticoag labs Resume 24–48 hrs for low-risk bleeding and 48–72 hrs for high bleeding risk	Hold dose 24–48 hrs prior No bridging or anticoag labs Resume 24–48 hrs for low-risk bleeding and 48–72 hrs for high bleeding risk
Emergent surgery with hemorrhage	rfVIIa or FEIBA Exploration and hemostasis	PCC Exploration and hemostasis	Kcentra or Beriplex Exploration and hemostasis
Neuraxial anesthesia[a]	No data	Catheter removal at least 24 hrs from last dose Resume at least 6 hrs from catheter removal	No data
Converting FROM warfarin to	DC warfarin and initiate when INR < 2 (2.0–2.5 if higher bleeding risk) Stop checking INR	Same as dabigatran	Same as dabigatran
Converting to warfarin	DC after 3 days of warfarin[a]	Start warfarin concurrently[b] Check daily INR Stop when INR > 2.0	Start warfarin[b] Check daily INR Stop when INR > 2.0
Converting from UFH or LMWH to	Initiate <2 hrs prior to next dose of LMWH or at cessation of UFH infusion	Same as dabigatran	Same as dabigatran
Converting to LMWH or UFH	Initiate 12 hrs after last dabigatran dose[a]	Initiate 24 hrs after last rivaroxaban dose	Initiate 12 hours after last apixaban dose

Sources: Nutescu EA, *Am J Health Syst Pharm*, 70(10 Suppl. 1), S1, May 15, 2013; Patel MR et al., *N Engl J Med*, 365(10), 883, September 8, 2011; Turpie AG et al., *Thromb Haemost*, 108(5), 876, November 2012.

Abbreviations: UFH, unfractionated heparin; LMWH, low-molecular-weight heparin; hrs, hours; DC, discontinue; anticoag, anticoagulation; rfVIIa, recombinant factor VIIa; PCC, prothrombin complex concentrate; INR, international normalized ratio.

[a] Timing dependent on patients renal function especially for dabigatran.

[b] Rivaroxaban and apixaban may falsely prolong INR. Alternative is to stop rivaroxaban or apixaban and start warfarin. Bridging with a parenteral agent 24 hours after rivaroxaban or 12 hours after apixaban.

Furthermore, apixaban is administered twice daily while rivaroxaban is given once daily and so a greater peak and trough effect is noted with rivaroxaban. Plasma concentrations of rivaroxaban have been shown to fluctuate 75%–80% compared to less than 50% for apixaban levels.[98] Many physicians prefer rivaroxaban for younger patients who place higher value on once-daily dosing and may have a lower risk for GI bleeding, while apixaban is often preferred for older patients already taking other medications throughout the day and who are generally at higher risk for GI bleeding.

Rivaroxaban and apixaban undergo hepatic metabolism by CYP3A4 and PGP transporter, and therefore, caution regarding possible drug–drug interactions should be noted. Inhibitors of CYP3A4 and/or PGP will result in increased rivaroxaban and apixaban concentrations increasing bleeding risk. These agents include HIV protease inhibitors, ketoconazole and posaconazole as well as amiodarone, cimetidine, erythromycin, fluconazole, calcium channel blockers and grapefruit juice. Inducers of CYP3A4 and PGP, such as rifampin, St. John's wort and phenytoin, will result in subtherapeutic anticoagulation. It is recommended that rivaroxaban be avoided

if combined with a strong PGP or CYP 3A4 inducer or inhibitor and apixaban be dose adjusted in these circumstances. Rivaroxaban and apixaban are contraindicated in patients with a creatinine clearance (CrCl) <15 mL/min and Childs-Pugh class B or C and are category C and B, respectively, in pregnancy.[103,104]

Meta-analyses of all four new oral anticoagulants in the atrial fibrillation population are non-inferior to dose-adjusted warfarin. Dabigatran and apixaban are shown to be superior. The only agent to significantly reduce ischemic strokes was dabigatran. Mortality reduction was seen only with apixaban.[62]

Meta-analyses of all four new oral anticoagulants in the DVT/PE treatment population have demonstrated comparable efficacy to dose-adjusted warfarin in preventing recurrent DVT/PE or related death with no difference in overall mortality.[63]

Collectively, the new oral anticoagulants reduce most bleeding end points with the exception of GI bleeding. However, relative risk of bleeding is highly variable among the different agents. In the atrial fibrillation and DVT/PE data, the bleeding rate was reduced up to 31% with apixaban (ARISTOTLE trial), while rivaroxaban followed by dabigatran then warfarin had the highest incidence of bleeding complications (Level 1). Importantly the rate of ICH was significantly lower (~50%–60% relative risk reduction) with all agents compared to warfarin. However, dabigatran and rivaroxaban have an increased risk of GI bleeding.[105–107] Though the quick onset and offset of these newer agents are desirable, these same characteristics have also generated black box warnings on all agents that 'premature discontinuation places patients at risk for thrombotic events'. This highlights that patients with poor compliance are not candidates for these newer agents.

Fondaparinux, as described previously, is also a factor Xa inhibitor whose mechanisms originate from the pentasaccharide moiety common to UFH and LMWH. Unlike UFH and LMWH, its short pentasaccharide sequence does not participate in forming a ternary complex with AT and thrombin. Fondaparinux is a synthetic inhibitor of factor Xa that acts via AT inhibition which is distinct from the mechanisms of rivaroxaban and apixaban which bind and inhibit factor Xa directly. Because of its small size compared to UFH and LMWH, fondaparinux does not bind to PF4 and therefore does not cause formation of HIT antibodies. Small series have reported effective treatment of HIT with fondaparinux, but this is not an approved indication.[31,33] Fondaparinux only comes in a SC formulation; however, unlike enoxaparin and UFH, its half-life is sufficiently long (17–21 hours) such that only once-daily injection is required. Furthermore, because of its small size, there is negligible non-specific plasma protein-binding resulting in a predictable dose–response relationship.[108] Peak effect is achieved by 3 hours after administration and therefore no bridging therapy is required. Fondaparinux has been studied head to head with enoxaparin in several large randomized trials, and a risk reduction with fondaparinux from 26% to 55% has been consistently achieved with similar bleeding and overall mortality rates in patients undergoing joint arthroplasty.[109–112] Fondaparinux is FDA approved for DVT/PE treatment and prophylaxis for joint replacement and abdominal surgery. Clearance is primarily renal and dose adjustment is imperative. While it can be dialyzed, its use is not recommended in patients on dialysis due to risk of accumulation. There is no antidote for fondaparinux; however, recombinant factor VIIa at 90 mcg/kg is recommended.[20,27,113,114]

Key point

Dependence on renal function for elimination is dabigatran >> rivaroxaban > apixaban.

Apixaban and dabigatran are more effective at stroke prevention for atrial fibrillation, and all newer oral anticoagulants have a lower risk of ICH than warfarin.

Apixaban has the lowest bleeding risk of all new oral anticoagulants.

Monitoring

PT and aPTT are not useful to predict risk of bleeding events or thrombosis in patients on rivaroxaban and apixaban and are therefore not followed. However, in an emergent setting, a normal PT can reliably indicate that clinically significant effects from rivaroxaban or apixaban are unlikely.[115,116] Anti–factor Xa levels reliably correlate with rivaroxaban and apixaban concentrations and is the preferred method for measuring the degree of anticoagulation.[117] However, most healthcare settings currently lack a standardized chromogenic assay calibrated for these agents.

Reversal of DTIs and factor Xa inhibitors

While the advantages of many of the new oral anticoagulants such as DTIs and factor Xa inhibitors are attractive, traditional antidotes used for warfarin or UFH (vitamin K and/or factor replacement or protamine sulphate) are insufficient to reverse the effects of newer agents in cases of life-threatening hemorrhage or urgent surgery. This has raised concern among patients and physicians and has launched the development of new antidotes and new factor concentrates for reversal of anticoagulation. Currently, a dabigatran-specific antibody cleverly named 'idarucizumab' has proven effective in phase I studies. Nonetheless, it has been demonstrated that patients on dabigatran who suffer major bleeding have a significantly lower mortality, receive less plasma concentrate and have shorter ICU stays compared to patients with major bleeding on warfarin.[118]

PCC are plasma-derived products that contain high concentrations of several key clotting factors. Evidence supporting PCCs for the correction of anticoagulation with DTIs or factor Xa inhibitors is limited mainly to animal models, human in vitro studies, healthy human subjects and clinical case reports. There are few randomized clinical trials and a lack of well-designed, evidence-based recommendations on the management of bleeding in patients taking these agents.

PCCs come in several different commercial formulations with various components and concentrations of factors. rFVIIa (NovoSeven) contains concentrated factor VIIa only and is FDA approved for reversal of bleeding and perioperative management in acquired hemophilias. Three-factor PCC containing II, IX and X in an inactivated form is also available (Bebulin and Profilnine), both of which are FDA approved for bleeding in factors IX deficiency. Four-factor PCC contains factor VII plus II, IX and X in an inactivated form as well as protein C and S (Kcentra and Beriplex). Activated PCC (aPCC) contains activated factor VII (VIIa) plus inactive II, IX and X and is FDA approved for bleeding and perioperative management of hemophilias (FEIBA). The main difference between four-factor PCC and three-factor PCC products is the present of factor VII. Heparin is present in Bebulin

Table 8.7 Proposed selection criteria for oral anticoagulant.

Consider warfarin

Insurance issues

Prosthetic heart valves

Valvular AF

Arterial thrombosis

Venous thromboembolism in cancer patients

Inherited prothrombotic states

Renal insufficiency (CrCl < 30 mL/min)

Hepatic insufficiency

History of GI bleed

Consider new oral anticoagulant

Most situations for VTE/AF treatment, especially if

    History of ICH

    Variable INRs on warfarin

    Difficulty with follow-up for INR checks

    Warfarin stigmata

Apixaban preferred for

    AF

    History of bleeding complications

Dabigatran if[a]

    Recent ischemic CVA while anticoagulated

Abbreviations: CrCl, creatinine clearance; AF, atrial fibrillation; GI, gastrointestinal; ICH, intracranial hemorrhage; CVA, cerebrovascular accident; INR, international normalized ratio; VTE, venous thromboembolism.

[a] Avoid dabigatran in patients >75 years and/or with coronary artery disease.

and Kcentra and these agents are therefore contraindicated in patients with a history of HIT. All these agents carry a high risk of thrombotic complications which is well demonstrated in case series' and reports. NovoSeven (rfVIIa) or FEIBA (aPCC) should be used preferentially for patients on dabigatran with hemorrhage as improved outcomes have been noted[119–121] (Level 3). For emergent reversal of rivaroxaban or apixaban, Kcentra or Beriplex should be used[122] (Level 3).

Despite a lack of robust evidence, developing institutional management protocols guarding the use of PCCs and recombinant factors are important. A key component of our institutional protocol is early, rapid involvement of our hematology colleagues who serve as the gatekeepers to approve the use of these reversal agents. Given the high cost and potentially fatal thrombotic complications associated with these medications, it is imperative to require judicious use, strict patient selection criteria and monitoring (Table 8.7).

CONCLUSION

The management of anticoagulants requires an understanding of the coagulation cascade, mechanisms of action and their basic pharmacokinetics, routes of elimination and major side effects. Furthermore, several well-designed clinical trials have provided a wealth of evidence-based guidelines that the cardiovascular specialist and vascular surgeon should be familiar with. The advent of new oral anticoagulants likely will change clinical practice patterns and affect the practice of elective and emergent vascular surgical interventions.

DEFICIENCIES IN CURRENT KNOWLEDGE AND AREAS OF FUTURE RESEARCH

- Should therapeutic UFH be monitored?
- Does monitoring improve outcomes for UFH?
- What assays should be used to monitor effect of UFH?
- What is the role or benefit of the 'mini heparin drip' (500 U/h)?
- There is a lack of clinical trials evaluating the utility of various PCCs for management of severe hemorrhage in association with DTI or factor Xa inhibitor therapy.
- There were only few studies directly comparing one novel oral anticoagulant with another.
- What is the effect of novel oral anticoagulants on cancer-related thrombosis, relative to LMWH? Currently, these agents have been compared only with warfarin, which is known to be inferior to LMWH for cancer patients.
- What is the effect of the novel oral anticoagulants in arterial thrombosis for prothrombotic states?

KEY REFERENCES

1. Alonso-Coello P, Bellmunt S, McGorrian C et al. Antithrombotic therapy in peripheral artery disease: Antithrombotic Therapy and Prevention of Thrombosis, 9th ed: American College of Chest Physicians Evidence-Based Clinical Practice Guidelines. *Chest.* 2012 February;141(2 Suppl.):e669S–e690S.
2. Ruff CT, Giugliano RP, Braunwald E et al. Comparison of the efficacy and safety of new oral anticoagulants with warfarin in patients with atrial fibrillation: A meta-analysis of randomised trials. *Lancet.* 2014 March 15;383(9921):955–962.
3. Linkins LA, Dans AL, Moores LK et al. Treatment and prevention of heparin-induced thrombocytopenia: Antithrombotic Therapy and Prevention of Thrombosis, 9th ed: American College of Chest Physicians Evidence-Based Clinical Practice Guidelines. *Chest.* 2012 February;141(2 Suppl.):e495S–e530S.
4. Holbrook A, Schulman S, Witt DM et al. Evidence-based management of anticoagulant therapy: Antithrombotic Therapy and Prevention of Thrombosis, 9th ed: American College of Chest Physicians Evidence-Based Clinical Practice Guidelines. *Chest.* 2012 February;141(2 Suppl.):e152S–e184S.

5. Baumann Kreuziger LM, Keenan JC, Morton CT, Dries DJ. Management of the bleeding patient receiving new oral anticoagulants: A role for prothrombin complex concentrates. *Biomed Res Int.* 2014;2014:583794.

These references are listed as key as they provide consensus guidelines and thorough review of available primary data on topics most frequently encountered and relevant to vascular surgeons.

REFERENCES

1. Rosenberg RD, Lam L. Correlation between structure and function of heparin. *Proc Natl Acad Sci USA.* 1979 March;76(3):1218–1222.
2. Guyton AC, Hall JE. *Textbook of Medical Physiology,* 11 ed. Philadelphia, PA: Elsevier Saunders; 2006.
3. Andersson LO, Barrowcliffe TW, Holmer E, Johnson EA, Sims GE. Anticoagulant properties of heparin fractionated by affinity chromatography on matrix-bound antithrombin iii and by gel filtration. *Thromb Res.* 1976 December;9(6):575–583.
4. Casu B, Oreste P, Torri G et al. The structure of heparin oligosaccharide fragments with high anti-(factor Xa) activity containing the minimal antithrombin III-binding sequence: Chemical and 13C nuclear-magnetic-resonance studies. *Biochem J.* 1981 September 1;197(3):599–609.
5. Thomas DP. Heparin. *Clin Haematol.* 1981 June;10(2):443–458.
6. Lupu C, Poulsen E, Roquefeuil S, Westmuckett AD, Kakkar VV, Lupu F. Cellular effects of heparin on the production and release of tissue factor pathway inhibitor in human endothelial cells in culture. *Arterioscler Thromb Vasc Biol.* 1999 September;19(9):2251–2262.
7. Thyzel E, Kohli S, Siegling S, Prante C, Kleesiek K, Gotting C. Relative quantification of glycosaminoglycan-induced upregulation of TFPI-mRNA expression in vitro. *Thromb Res.* 2007;119(6):785–791.
8. Raschke RA, Reilly BM, Guidry JR, Fontana JR, Srinivas S. The weight-based heparin dosing nomogram compared with a 'standard care' nomogram: A randomized controlled trial. *Ann Int Med.* 1993 November 1;119(9):874–881.
9. Hull R, Delmore T, Carter C et al. Adjusted subcutaneous heparin versus warfarin sodium in the long-term treatment of venous thrombosis. *N Engl J Med.* 1982 January 28;306(4):189–194.
10. Kearon C, Ginsberg JS, Julian JA et al. Comparison of fixed-dose weight-adjusted unfractionated heparin and low-molecular-weight heparin for acute treatment of venous thromboembolism. *J Am Med Assoc.* 2006 August 23;296(8):935–942.
11. Alonso-Coello P, Bellmunt S, McGorrian C et al. Antithrombotic therapy in peripheral artery disease: Antithrombotic Therapy and Prevention of Thrombosis, 9th ed: American College of Chest Physicians Evidence-Based Clinical Practice Guidelines. *Chest.* 2012 February;141(2 Suppl.): e669S–e690S.
12. Momsen AH, Jensen MB, Norager CB, Madsen MR, Vestersgaard-Andersen T, Lindholt JS. Drug therapy for improving walking distance in intermittent claudication: A systematic review and meta-analysis of robust randomised controlled studies. *Eur J Vasc Endovasc Surg.* 2009 October;38(4):463–474.
13. Dalteparin [Internet]. Micromedes Healthcare Series. 2014 [cited September 20, 2014]. Available from: Thomson Reuters Healthcare Inc. at www.micromedexsolutions.com.
14. Enoxaparin [Internet]. Micromedex Healthcare Series. 2014 [cited September 10, 2014]. Available from: Thomson Reuters Healthcare Inc. at www.micromedexsolutions.com.
15. Tinzaparin [Internet]. Micromedex Healthcare Series. 2014 [cited September 20, 2014]. Available from: Thomson Reuters Healthcare Inc. at www.micromedexsolutions.com.
16. Heparin [Internet]. Micromedex Healthcare Series. 2014 [cited September 18, 2014]. Available from: Thomas Reuters Healthcare Inc. at www.micromedex.com.
17. Eikelboom JW, Anand SS, Malmberg K, Weitz JI, Ginsberg JS, Yusuf S. Unfractionated heparin and low-molecular-weight heparin in acute coronary syndrome without ST elevation: A meta-analysis. *Lancet.* 2000 June 3;355(9219):1936–1942.
18. Amsterdam EA, Wenger NK, Brindis RG et al. 2014 AHA/ACC guideline for the management of patients with non-ST-elevation acute coronary syndromes: Executive summary: A report of the American College of Cardiology/American Heart Association Task Force on Practice Guidelines. *Circulation.* 2014 December 23;130(25):2354–2394.
19. Lee AY, Rickles FR, Julian JA et al. Randomized comparison of low molecular weight heparin and coumarin derivatives on the survival of patients with cancer and venous thromboembolism. *J Clin Oncol.* 2005 April 1;23(10):2123–2129.
20. Rajgopal R, Bear M, Butcher MK, Shaughnessy SG. The effects of heparin and low molecular weight heparins on bone. *Thromb Res.* 2008;122(3):293–298.
21. Eikelboom JW, Hirsh J. Monitoring unfractionated heparin with the aPTT: Time for a fresh look. *Thromb Haemost.* 2006 November;96(5):547–552.
22. Hull RD, Raskob GE, Rosenbloom D et al. Optimal therapeutic level of heparin therapy in patients with venous thrombosis. *Arch Intern Med.* 1992 August;152(8):1589–1595.
23. Hull RD, Raskob GE, Hirsh J et al. Continuous intravenous heparin compared with intermittent subcutaneous heparin in the initial treatment of proximal-vein thrombosis. *N Engl J Med.* 1986 October 30;315(18):1109–1114.

24. Cruickshank MK, Levine MN, Hirsh J, Roberts R, Siguenza M. A standard heparin nomogram for the management of heparin therapy. *Arch Intern Med.* 1991 February;151(2):333–337.

25. Hirsh J, van Aken WG, Gallus AS, Dollery CT, Cade JF, Yung WL. Heparin kinetics in venous thrombosis and pulmonary embolism. *Circulation.* 1976 April;53(4):691–695.

26. Schran HF, Bitz DW, DiSerio FJ, Hirsh J. The pharmacokinetics and bioavailability of subcutaneously administered dihydroergotamine, heparin and the dihydroergotamine-heparin combination. *Thromb Res.* 1983 July 1;31(1):51–67.

27. Garcia DA, Baglin TP, Weitz JI, Samama MM, American College of Chest P. Parenteral anticoagulants: Antithrombotic Therapy and Prevention of Thrombosis, 9th ed: American College of Chest Physicians Evidence-Based Clinical Practice Guidelines. *Chest.* 2012 February;141(2 Suppl.):e24S–e43S.

28. Bailie GR, Mason NA. *Dialysis of Drug.* Saline, MI: Renal Pharmacy Consultants; 2013.

29. Linkins LA, Dans AL, Moores LK et al. Treatment and prevention of heparin-induced thrombocytopenia: Antithrombotic Therapy and Prevention of Thrombosis, 9th ed: American College of Chest Physicians Evidence-Based Clinical Practice Guidelines. *Chest.* 2012 February;141(2 Suppl.):e495S–e530S.

30. Warkentin TE, Cook RJ, Marder VJ et al. Antiplatelet factor 4/heparin antibodies in orthopedic surgery patients receiving antithrombotic prophylaxis with fondaparinux or enoxaparin. *Blood.* 2005 December 1;106(12):3791–3796.

31. Warkentin TE. Agents for the treatment of heparin-induced thrombocytopenia. *Hematol Oncol Clin North Am.* 2010 August;24(4):755–775, ix.

32. Kuo KH, Kovacs MJ. Fondaparinux: A potential new therapy for HIT. *Hematology.* 2005 August;10(4):271–275.

33. Warkentin TE. Heparin-induced thrombocytopenia and vascular surgery. *Acta Chir Belg.* 2004 June;104(3):257–265.

34. Harenberg J, Jorg I, Fenyvesi T. Treatment of heparin-induced thrombocytopenia with fondaparinux. *Haematologica.* 2004 August;89(8):1017–1018.

35. You JJ, Singer DE, Howard PA et al. Antithrombotic therapy for atrial fibrillation: Antithrombotic Therapy and Prevention of Thrombosis, 9th ed: American College of Chest Physicians Evidence-Based Clinical Practice Guidelines. *Chest.* 2012 February;141(2 Suppl.):e531S–e575S.

36. Douketis JD, Spyropoulos AC, Spencer FA et al. Perioperative management of antithrombotic therapy: Antithrombotic Therapy and Prevention of Thrombosis, 9th ed: American College of Chest Physicians Evidence-Based Clinical Practice Guidelines. *Chest.* 2012 February;141(2 Suppl.):e326S–e350S.

37. Hellwig T, Gulseth M. Pharmacokinetic and pharmacodynamic drug interactions with new oral anticoagulants: What do they mean for patients with atrial fibrillation? *Ann Pharmacother.* 2013 November;47(11):1478–1487.

38. Kirley K, Qato DM, Kornfield R, Stafford RS, Alexander GC. National trends in oral anticoagulant use in the United States, 2007 to 2011. *Circ Cardiovasc Qual Outcomes.* 2012 September 1;5(5):615–621.

39. Whitlon DS, Sadowski JA, Suttie JW. Mechanism of coumarin action: Significance of vitamin K epoxide reductase inhibition. *Biochemistry.* 1978 April 18;17(8):1371–1377.

40. Suttie JW. Warfarin and vitamin K. *Clin Cardiol.* 1990 April;13(4 Suppl. 6):VI16–VI18.

41. Hirsh J, Dalen J, Anderson DR et al. Oral anticoagulants: Mechanism of action, clinical effectiveness, and optimal therapeutic range. *Chest.* 2001 January;119(1 Suppl.):8S–21S.

42. Nutescu EA. Oral anticoagulant therapies: Balancing the risks. *Am J Health Syst Pharm.* 2013 May 15;70(10 Suppl. 1):S3–S11.

43. D'Angelo SV, Mazzola G, Della Valle P, Testa S, Pattarini E, D'Angelo A. Variable interference of activated protein C resistance in the measurement of protein S activity by commercial assays. *Thromb Res.* 1995 February 15;77(4):375–378.

44. Haines ST, Bussey HI. Thrombosis and the pharmacology of antithrombotic agents. *Ann Pharmacother.* 1995 September;29(9):892–905.

45. Holbrook A, Schulman S, Witt DM et al. Evidence-based management of anticoagulant therapy: Antithrombotic Therapy and Prevention of Thrombosis, 9th ed: American College of Chest Physicians Evidence-Based Clinical Practice Guidelines. *Chest.* 2012 February;141(2 Suppl.):e152S–e184S.

46. Adjusted-dose warfarin versus low-intensity, fixed-dose warfarin plus aspirin for high-risk patients with atrial fibrillation: Stroke Prevention in Atrial Fibrillation III randomised clinical trial. *Lancet.* 1996 September 7;348(9028):633–638.

47. January CT, Wann LS, Alpert JS et al. 2014 AHA/ACC/HRS guideline for the management of patients with atrial fibrillation: A report of the American College of Cardiology/American Heart Association Task Force on Practice Guidelines and the Heart Rhythm Society. *J Am Coll Cardiol.* 2014 December 2;130(23):2071–2104.

48. Johnson WC, Williford WO, Department of Veterans Affairs Cooperative S. Benefits, morbidity, and mortality associated with long-term administration of oral anticoagulant therapy to patients with peripheral arterial bypass procedures: A prospective randomized study. *J Vasc Surg.* 2002 March;35(3):413–421.

49. Kretschmer G, Wenzl E, Schemper M et al. Influence of postoperative anticoagulant treatment on patient survival after femoropopliteal vein bypass surgery. *Lancet.* 1988 April 9;1(8589):797–799.

50. Flinn WR, Rohrer MJ, Yao JS, McCarthy WJ 3rd, Fahey VA, Bergan JJ. Improved long-term patency of infragenicular polytetrafluoroethylene grafts. *J Vasc Surg*. 1988 May;7(5):685–690.

51. LeCroy CJ, Patterson MA, Taylor SM, Westfall AO, Jordan WD Jr. Effect of warfarin anticoagulation on below-knee polytetrafluoroethylene graft patency. *Ann Vasc Surg*. 2005 March;19(2):192–198.

52. Whayne TF. A review of the role of anticoagulation in the treatment of peripheral arterial disease. *Int J Angiol*. 2012 December;21(4):187–194.

53. Hart RG, Benavente O, Pearce LA. Increased risk of intracranial hemorrhage when aspirin is combined with warfarin: A meta-analysis and hypothesis. *Cerebrovasc Dis*. 1999 July–August;9(4):215–217.

54. Rothberg MB, Celestin C, Fiore LD, Lawler E, Cook JR. Warfarin plus aspirin after myocardial infarction or the acute coronary syndrome: Meta-analysis with estimates of risk and benefit. *Ann Intern Med*. 2005 August 16;143(4):241–250.

55. Battistella M, Mamdami MM, Juurlink DN, Rabeneck L, Laupacis A. Risk of upper gastrointestinal hemorrhage in warfarin users treated with nonselective NSAIDs or COX-2 inhibitors. *Arch Intern Med*. 2005 January 24;165(2):189–192.

56. Nutescu EA. New approaches to reversing oral anticoagulant therapy: Introduction. *Am J Health Syst Pharm*. 2013 May 15;70(10 Suppl. 1):S1–S2.

57. Holbrook AM, Pereira JA, Labiris R et al. Systematic overview of warfarin and its drug and food interactions. *Arch Intern Med*. 2005 May 23;165(10):1095–1106.

58. Lip GY. Bleeding risk assessment and management in atrial fibrillation patients. *Eur Heart J*. 2012 January;33(2):147–149.

59. Garcia DA, Lopes RD, Hylek EM. New-onset atrial fibrillation and warfarin initiation: High risk periods and implications for new antithrombotic drugs. *Thromb Haemost*. 2010 December;104(6):1099–1105.

60. DiMarco JP, Flaker G, Waldo AL et al. Factors affecting bleeding risk during anticoagulant therapy in patients with atrial fibrillation: Observations from the Atrial Fibrillation Follow-up Investigation of Rhythm Management (AFFIRM) study. *Am Heart J*. 2005 April;149(4):650–656.

61. Van Gelder IC, Hagens VE, Bosker HA et al. A comparison of rate control and rhythm control in patients with recurrent persistent atrial fibrillation. *N Engl J Med*. 2002 December 5;347(23):1834–1840.

62. Ruff CT, Giugliano RP, Braunwald E et al. Comparison of the efficacy and safety of new oral anticoagulants with warfarin in patients with atrial fibrillation: A meta-analysis of randomised trials. *Lancet*. 2014 March 15;383(9921):955–962.

63. van Es N, Coppens M, Schulman S, Middeldorp S, Buller HR. Direct oral anticoagulants compared with vitamin K antagonists for acute venous thromboembolism: Evidence from phase 3 trials. *Blood*. 2014 September 18;124(12):1968–1975.

64. Patel MR, Mahaffey KW, Garg J et al. Rivaroxaban versus warfarin in nonvalvular atrial fibrillation. *N Engl J Med*. 2011 September 8;365(10):883–891.

65. Warfarin [Internet]. Micromedex Healthcare Series. 2014 [cited September 1, 2014]. Available from: Thomson Reuters Healthcare Inc. at www.micromedex.com.

66. Broekmans AW, Bertina RM, Loeliger EA, Hofmann V, Klingemann HG. Protein C and the development of skin necrosis during anticoagulant therapy. *Thromb Haemost*. 1983 June 28;49(3):251.

67. Chan YC, Valenti D, Mansfield AO, Stansby G. Warfarin induced skin necrosis. *Br J Surg*. 2000 March;87(3):266–272.

68. Ageno W, Gallus AS, Wittkowsky A et al. Oral anticoagulant therapy: Antithrombotic Therapy and Prevention of Thrombosis, 9th ed: American College of Chest Physicians Evidence-Based Clinical Practice Guidelines. *Chest*. 2012 February;141(2 Suppl.):e44S–e488S.

69. Whitlock RP, Sun JC, Fremes SE, Rubens FD, Teoh KH, American College of Chest P. Antithrombotic and thrombolytic therapy for valvular disease: Antithrombotic Therapy and Prevention of Thrombosis, 9th ed: American College of Chest Physicians Evidence-Based Clinical Practice Guidelines. *Chest*. 2012 February;141(2 Suppl.):e576S–e600S.

70. Lubetsky A, Yonath H, Olchovsky D, Loebstein R, Halkin H, Ezra D. Comparison of oral vs intravenous phytonadione (vitamin K1) in patients with excessive anticoagulation: A prospective randomized controlled study. *Arch Intern Med*. 2003 November 10;163(20):2469–2473.

71. Ansell J, Hirsh J, Hylek E et al. Pharmacology and management of the vitamin K antagonists: American College of Chest Physicians Evidence-Based Clinical Practice Guidelines (8th Edition). *Chest*. 2008 June;133(6 Suppl.):160S–198S.

72. Yasaka M, Minematsu K, Naritomi H, Sakata T, Yamaguchi T. Predisposing factors for enlargement of intracerebral hemorrhage in patients treated with warfarin. *Thromb Haemost*. 2003 February;89(2):278–283.

73. Huttner HB, Schellinger PD, Hartmann M et al. Hematoma growth and outcome in treated neuro-critical care patients with intracerebral hemorrhage related to oral anticoagulant therapy: Comparison of acute treatment strategies using vitamin K, fresh frozen plasma, and prothrombin complex concentrates. *Stroke*. 2006 June;37(6):1465–1470.

74. Siddiq F, Jalil A, McDaniel C et al. Effectiveness of Factor IX complex concentrate in reversing warfarin associated coagulopathy for intracerebral hemorrhage. *Neurocrit Care*. 2008;8(1):36–41.

75. Weitz JI, Hudoba M, Massel D, Maraganore J, Hirsh J. Clot-bound thrombin is protected from inhibition by heparin-antithrombin III but is susceptible to inactivation by antithrombin III-independent inhibitors. *J Clin Invest*. 1990 August;86(2):385–391.

76. PL Detail-Document. Comparison of injectable anticoagulants. *Prescriber's Letter.* August 2012.

77. Di Nisio M, Middeldorp S, Buller HR. Direct thrombin inhibitors. *N Engl J Med.* 2005 September 8;353(10):1028–1040.

78. Koster A, Dyke CM, Aldea G et al. Bivalirudin during cardiopulmonary bypass in patients with previous or acute heparin-induced thrombocytopenia and heparin antibodies: Results of the CHOOSE-ON trial. *Ann Thorac Surg.* 2007 February;83(2):572–577.

79. Dyke CM, Aldea G, Koster A et al. Off-pump coronary artery bypass with bivalirudin for patients with heparin-induced thrombocytopenia or antiplatelet factor four/heparin antibodies. *Ann Thorac Surg.* 2007 September;84(3):836–839.

80. Levine GN, Bates ER, Blankenship JC et al. 2011 ACCF/AHA/SCAI guideline for percutaneous coronary intervention: A report of the American College of Cardiology Foundation/American Heart Association Task Force on Practice Guidelines and the Society for Cardiovascular Angiography and Interventions. *Circulation.* 2011 December 6;124(23):e574–e651.

81. Steg PG, James SK, Gersh BJ. 2012 ESC STEMI guidelines and reperfusion therapy: Evidence-based recommendations, ensuring optimal patient management. *Heart.* 2013 August;99(16):1156–1157.

82. Hamm CW, Bassand JP, Agewall S et al. ESC guidelines for the management of acute coronary syndromes in patients presenting without persistent ST-segment elevation. The Task Force for the management of acute coronary syndromes (ACS) in patients presenting without persistent ST-segment elevation of the European Society of Cardiology (ESC). *Giornale italiano di cardiologia.* 2012 March; 13(3):171–228.

83. Windecker S, Kolh P, Alfonso F et al. 2014 ESC/EACTS guidelines on myocardial revascularization: The Task Force on Myocardial Revascularization of the European Society of Cardiology (ESC) and the European Association for Cardio-Thoracic Surgery (EACTS) Developed with the special contribution of the European Association of Percutaneous Cardiovascular Interventions (EAPCI). *Eur J Cardiothorac Surg.* 2014 October;46(4):517–592.

84. Eichler P, Friesen HJ, Lubenow N, Jaeger B, Greinacher A. Antihirudin antibodies in patients with heparin-induced thrombocytopenia treated with lepirudin: Incidence, effects on aPTT, and clinical relevance. *Blood.* 2000 October 1;96(7):2373–2378.

85. Greinacher A, Lubenow N, Eichler P. Anaphylactic and anaphylactoid reactions associated with lepirudin in patients with heparin-induced thrombocytopenia. *Circulation.* 2003 October 28;108(17):2062–2065.

86. Warkentin TE, Greinacher A. Heparin-induced anaphylactic and anaphylactoid reactions: Two distinct but overlapping syndromes. *Expert Opin Drug Saf.* 2009 March;8(2):129–144.

87. Eriksson BI, Wille-Jorgensen P, Kalebo P et al. A comparison of recombinant hirudin with a low-molecular-weight heparin to prevent thromboembolic complications after total hip replacement. *N Engl J Med.* 1997 November 6;337(19):1329–1335.

88. Lubenow N, Eichler P, Lietz T, Farner B, Greinacher A. Lepirudin for prophylaxis of thrombosis in patients with acute isolated heparin-induced thrombocytopenia: An analysis of 3 prospective studies. *Blood.* 2004 November 15;104(10):3072–3077.

89. Matheson AJ, Goa KL. Desirudin: A review of its use in the management of thrombotic disorders. *Drugs.* 2000 September;60(3):679–700.

90. Graetz TJ, Tellor BR, Smith JR, Avidan MS. Desirudin: A review of the pharmacology and clinical application for the prevention of deep vein thrombosis. *Expert Rev Cardiovasc Ther.* 2011 September;9(9):1101–1109.

91. Desirudin [Internet]. Micromedex Healthcare Series. 2014 [cited September 1, 2014]. Available from: Thomson Reuters Healthcare Inc. at www.micromedex.com.

92. Lewis BE, Wallis DE, Leya F, Hursting MJ, Kelton JG, Argatroban I. Argatroban anticoagulation in patients with heparin-induced thrombocytopenia. *Arch Intern Med.* 2003 August 11–25;163(15):1849–1856.

93. Lewis BE, Wallis DE, Berkowitz SD et al. Argatroban anticoagulant therapy in patients with heparin-induced thrombocytopenia. *Circulation.* 2001 April 10;103(14):1838–1843.

94. Matsuo T, Kario K, Matsuda S, Yamaguchi N, Kakishita E. Effect of thrombin inhibition on patients with peripheral arterial obstructive disease: A multicenter clinical trial of argatroban. *J Thromb Thrombolysis.* 1995;2(2):131–136.

95. Ohteki H, Furukawa K, Ohnishi H, Narita Y, Sakai M, Doi K. Clinical experience of Argatroban for anticoagulation in cardiovascular surgery. *Jpn J Thorac Cardiovasc Surg.* 2000 January;48(1):39–46.

96. Mudaliar JH, Liem TK, Nichols WK, Spadone DP, Silver D. Lepirudin is a safe and effective anticoagulant for patients with heparin-associated antiplatelet antibodies. *J Vasc Surg.* 2001 July;34(1):17–20.

97. Connolly SJ, Ezekowitz MD, Yusuf S et al. Dabigatran versus warfarin in patients with atrial fibrillation. *N Engl J Med.* 2009 September 17;361(12):1139–1151.

98. Ufer M. Comparative efficacy and safety of the novel oral anticoagulants dabigatran, rivaroxaban and apixaban in preclinical and clinical development. *Thromb Haemost.* 2010 March;103(3):572–585.

99. Rosborough TK, Shepherd MF. Unreliability of international normalized ratio for monitoring warfarin therapy in patients with lupus anticoagulant. *Pharmacotherapy.* 2004 July;24(7):838–842.

100. Weitz JI, Connolly SJ, Patel I et al. Randomised, parallel-group, multicentre, multinational phase 2 study comparing edoxaban, an oral factor Xa inhibitor, with warfarin for stroke prevention in patients with atrial fibrillation. *Thromb Haemost.* 2010 September;104(3):633–641.

101. Raskob G, Cohen AT, Eriksson BI et al. Oral direct factor Xa inhibition with edoxaban for thromboprophylaxis after elective total hip replacement: A randomised double-blind dose-response study. *Thromb Haemost.* 2010 September;104(3):642–649.

102. Eriksson BI, Borris LC, Friedman RJ et al. Rivaroxaban versus enoxaparin for thromboprophylaxis after hip arthroplasty. *N Engl J Med.* 2008 June 26;358(26):2765–2775.

103. Rivaroxaban [Internet]. Micromedex Healthcare Series. 2014 [cited September 20, 2014]. Available from: Thomson Reuters Healthcare Inc. at www.micromedex.com.

104. Apixaban [Internet]. Micromedex Healthcare Services. 2014 [cited September 10, 2014]. Available from: Thomson Reuters Healthcare Inc. at www.micromedex.com.

105. Nieto JA, Espada NG, Merino RG, Gonzalez TC. Dabigatran, rivaroxaban and apixaban versus enoxaparin for thromboprophylaxis after total knee or hip arthroplasty: Pool-analysis of phase III randomized clinical trials. *Thromb Res.* 2012 August;130(2):183–191.

106. Delaney JA, Opatrny L, Brophy JM, Suissa S. Drug drug interactions between antithrombotic medications and the risk of gastrointestinal bleeding. *Can Med Assoc J.* 2007 August 14;177(4):347–351.

107. Granger CB, Alexander JH, McMurray JJ et al. Apixaban versus warfarin in patients with atrial fibrillation. *N Engl J Med.* 2011 September 15;365(11):981–992.

108. Donat F, Duret JP, Santoni A et al. The pharmacokinetics of fondaparinux sodium in healthy volunteers. *Clin Pharmacokinet.* 2002;41(Suppl 2.):1–9.

109. Turpie AG, Bauer KA, Eriksson BI, Lassen MR. Fondaparinux vs enoxaparin for the prevention of venous thromboembolism in major orthopedic surgery: A meta-analysis of 4 randomized double-blind studies. *Arch Intern Med.* 2002 September 9;162(16):1833–1840.

110. Turpie AG, Bauer KA, Eriksson BI, Lassen MR, Committee PSS. Postoperative fondaparinux versus postoperative enoxaparin for prevention of venous thromboembolism after elective hip-replacement surgery: A randomised double-blind trial. *Lancet.* 2002 May 18;359(9319):1721–1726.

111. Lassen MR, Bauer KA, Eriksson BI, Turpie AG, European Pentasaccharide Elective Surgery Study Steering C. Postoperative fondaparinux versus pre-operative enoxaparin for prevention of venous thromboembolism in elective hip-replacement surgery: A randomised double-blind comparison. *Lancet.* 2002 May 18;359(9319):1715–1720.

112. Bauer KA, Eriksson BI, Lassen MR, Turpie AG, Steering Committee of the Pentasaccharide in Major Knee Surgery S. Fondaparinux compared with enoxaparin for the prevention of venous thromboembolism after elective major knee surgery. *N Engl J Med.* 2001 November 1;345(18):1305–1310.

113. Nagler M, Fabbro T, Wuillemin WA. Prospective evaluation of the interobserver reliability of the 4Ts score in patients with suspected heparin-induced thrombocytopenia. *J Thromb Haemost.* 2012 January;10(1):151–152.

114. Bijsterveld NR, Moons AH, Boekholdt SM et al. Ability of recombinant factor VIIa to reverse the anticoagulant effect of the pentasaccharide fondaparinux in healthy volunteers. *Circulation.* 2002 November 12;106(20):2550–2554.

115. Samama MM, Guinet C. Laboratory assessment of new anticoagulants. *Clin Chem Lab Med.* 2011 May;49(5):761–772.

116. Koscielny J, Rutkauskaite E. Rivaroxaban and hemostasis in emergency care. *Emerg Med Int.* 2014;2014:935474.

117. Mani H, Rohde G, Stratmann G et al. Accurate determination of rivaroxaban levels requires different calibrator sets but not addition of antithrombin. *Thromb Haemost.* 2012 July;108(1):191–198.

118. Majeed A, Hwang HG, Connolly SJ et al. Management and outcomes of major bleeding during treatment with dabigatran or warfarin. *Circulation.* 2013 November 19;128(21):2325–2332.

119. Marlu R, Hodaj E, Paris A, Albaladejo P, Cracowski JL, Pernod G. Effect of non-specific reversal agents on anticoagulant activity of dabigatran and rivaroxaban: A randomised crossover ex vivo study in healthy volunteers. *Thromb Haemost.* 2012 August;108(2):217–224.

120. Eerenberg ES, Kamphuisen PW, Sijpkens MK, Meijers JC, Buller HR, Levi M. Reversal of rivaroxaban and dabigatran by prothrombin complex concentrate: A randomized, placebo-controlled, crossover study in healthy subjects. *Circulation.* 2011 October 4;124(14):1573–1579.

121. Baumann Kreuziger LM, Keenan JC, Morton CT, Dries DJ. Management of the bleeding patient receiving new oral anticoagulants: A role for prothrombin complex concentrates. *Biomed Res Int.* 2014;2014:583794.

122. Escolar G, Fernandez-Gallego V, Arellano-Rodrigo E et al. Reversal of apixaban induced alterations in hemostasis by different coagulation factor concentrates: Significance of studies in vitro with circulating human blood. *PLOS ONE.* 2013;8(11):e78696.

123. Wittkowsky AK. Novel oral anticoagulants and their role in clinical practice. *Pharmacotherapy.* 2011 December;31(12):1175–1191.

124. DiPiro JT. *Pharmacotherapy: A Pathophysiologic Approach*, 8th ed. New York: McGraw-Hill Medical; 2011, pp. xxxii, 2668.

125. Fragmin (dalteparin sodium), injection, solution. Kirkland, Quebec, Canada: Pfizer; 2014.

126. Heidbuchel H, Verhamme P, Alings M et al. European Heart Rhythm Association Practical Guide on the use of new oral anticoagulants in patients with non-valvular atrial fibrillation. *Europace*. 2013 May;15(5):625–651.

127. Bivalirudin [Internet]. Micromedex Healthcare Series. 2014 [cited September 20, 2014]. Available from: Thomson Reuters Healthcare Inc. at www.micromedex.com.

128. Argatroban [Internet]. Micromedex Healthcare Series. 2014 [cited September 20, 2014]. Available from: Thomson Reuters Healthcare Inc. at www.micromedex.com.

129. Dabigatran [Internet]. Micromedex Healthcare Series. 2014 [cited September 20, 2014]. Available from: Thomson Reuters Healthcare Inc. at www.micromedex.com.

130. Eliquis (Apixaban) prescribing information. Princeton, NJ: Bristol-Myers Squibb Company; December 2012.

131. Edoxaban [Internet]. Micromedex Healthcare Series. 2014 [cited September 20, 2014]. Available from: Thomson Reuters Healthcare Inc. at www.micromedex.com.

132. Turpie AG, Kreutz R, Llau J, Norrving B, Haas S. Management consensus guidance for the use of rivaroxaban – An oral, direct factor Xa inhibitor. *Thromb Haemost*. 2012 November;108(5):876–886.

9

Thrombolytic therapy

ELIZABETH L. CHOU and NII-KABU KABUTEY

CONTENTS

Thrombolysis describes the breakdown of blood clots through activation of fibrinolysis. Thrombolytic agents are proteins used to accelerate and facilitate the process of intravascular thrombi degradation by activating plasminogen, plasmin production and degradation of fibrin. These proteins have expanded the therapeutic options available for patients with arterial and venous occlusions. Therapy with thrombolytic agents may improve limb salvage, decrease morbidity and mortality, alleviate post-thrombotic symptoms and approach occlusions with minimally invasive techniques. The purpose of this chapter is to review the mechanisms of fibrinolysis, compare thrombolytic agents and overview current applications for thrombolysis therapy.

FIBRINOLYSIS

Fibrinolysis involves complex interactions between enzymes resulting in the breakdown of fibrin and dissolution of the fibrin network that supports thrombus structure. A key component to this process is plasminogen, an inactive proteolytic enzyme and a precursor to plasmin. Most fibrinolytic agents act indirectly through plasminogen. Plasminogen is synthesized in the liver prior to becoming a constituent of plasma, and the extracellular fluid.[1,2] Infancy, cirrhosis and disseminated intravascular coagulation are associated with low levels of plasminogen. Trauma, surgery and infectious processes are associated with an increase in circulating plasminogen, secondary to elevation of acute phase reactants.[3]

Human plasminogen is a single-chain glycoprotein with three kringle regions composed of disulfide bridges that function as independent domains. These domains exhibit homology with those found in lipoprotein a,

tissue plasminogen activator and prothromin.[4] The kringles are located on the heavy chain (NH_2 terminal) and have lysine-binding sites that bind to fibrin, plasminogen activators and plasminogen inhibitors such as α2-plasmin inhibitor. The catalytic site is located at the COOH terminus and is responsible for converting plasminogen to plasmin, an active serine protease. The light chain of plasmin is responsible for proteolytic activity and degrading active plasma proteins such as coagulation factors, complement, glucagon, ACTH growth hormone, fibrin and fibrinogen.[5] When cross-linked fibres are degraded by plasmin, several non-covalently bonded fragments are produced, including D-dimer,[6] which is a marker for true fibrin degradation.

The fibrinolytic system in humans can be activated by two mechanisms. The extrinsic pathway is mediated by the presence of plasminogen activators released from endothelial cells. These physiologic plasminogen activators include urokinase plasminogen activator (u-PA) and tissue plasminogen activator (t-PA). Other agents such as streptokinase and acetylated plasma streptokinase activator complex (APSAC) bind to plasminogen in equimolar complexes that subsequently become activators. Once activated, fibrinolysis is perpetuated through a positive feedback loop by plasmin. This process involves plasmin cleaving, an activation peptide on plasminogen to increase fibrin affinity and activity.[7,8] Furthermore, fibrin itself perpetuates the fibrinolytic cascade by enabling the fibrin-bound plasminogen molecules to incorporate into the clot and improves the availability of plasminogen for activation.

Plasmin is most active within the thrombus, where the concentration of its primary inhibitor, α2-antiplasmin, is low. Antiplasmin is present in plasma and platelets and can rapidly complex with plasmin.[9] Plasmin bound to fibrin is resistant to antiplasmin inhibition due to occupation of

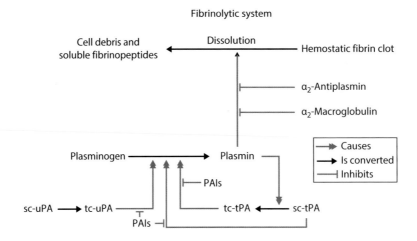

Figure 9.1 Schematic representation of the main components of the fibrinolytic system. (Adapted from Sherry S et al., *J Clin Invest.*, 38, 810, 1959.) *sc-tPA*, *tc-tPA* single-chain, two-chain tPA; *sc-uPA*, *tc-uPA* single-chain, two-chain uPA; *PAIs* plasminogen activator inhibitors.

binding sites. This allows fibrin degradation to occur with minimal systemic effects. When excess plasmin is present, however, α2-macroglobulin, a general protease inhibitor, may act as a plasmin inhibitor.[10]

Plasminogen may also be inhibited from conversion to plasmin by plasminogen activator inhibitor 1 (PAI-1), a glycoprotein present in endothelial cells, plasma and platelets. This inhibitor binds to fibrin thereby preventing t-PA and u-PA from activating plasminogen conversion. PAI-2 is only detectable during pregnancy, remains mostly intracellular and is produced by epithelial cells, monocytes, macrophages and keratinocytes. It may have a role in maintaining the placenta or in embryonic development and has influence on cell proliferation and differentiation, inhibition of apoptosis and gene expression (Figure 9.1).[10]

THROMBOLYTIC AGENTS

Thrombolytic agents are most commonly classified by their mechanism of action, but can also be classified by mode of production and fibrin specificity. Direct agents are enzymes that degrade fibrin without requiring intermediate plasminogen activation. The category includes plasmin and its derivatives, snake venom enzymes, Nattokinase (NK) and earthworm-derived enzymes.[11,12] Indirect agents are known as plasminogen activators because their enzymatic actions target plasminogen, the inactive zymogen of plasmin, and do not act upon the thrombus itself. Plasminogen activators such as streptokinase, urokinase and t-PA are the most commonly used agents in thrombolytic therapy due to their ability for systemic administration; however, they are expensive and have a risk for internal hemorrhage. These risks prompt further investigation of direct agents, which have the potential for lower bleeding risk due to neutralization by antiplasmin. Circulating antiplasmin, however, requires

catheter-directed delivery of direct agents. Furthermore, there are currently no definitive data comparing the effective use of direct and indirect thrombolytic agents.

Discussion of the agents in the following is organized by mechanism of action and subcategorized based on the origin of the parent compound. Direct agents discussed include plasmin, mini-plasmin, micro-plasmin, delta-plasmin, alfimeprase, NK and earthworm-derived enzymes. Indirect agents discussed include streptokinase, urokinase, tissue plasminogen activators and a miscellaneous group of novel agents.

Direct agents

PLASMIN AND DERIVATIVES

As discussed earlier in the chapter, plasmin is the active form of plasminogen and is the main proteolytic enzyme responsible for the fibrinolytic cascade. Direct agents have the potential benefit of direct fibrin proteolysis and a physiologic safety net due to plasma inhibitors (antiplasmin and macroglobulin) that can neutralize an administered dose. When compared to t-PA in animal and in vitro models, plasmin has been shown to have greater lytic activity and improved hemostatic safety.[13,14] These encouraging findings prompted evaluation of truncated derivatives of plasmin that retain fibrinolytic activity. These include mini-plasmin, micro-plasmin and delta-plasmin. Plasmin and micro-plasmin have been evaluated in clinical trials but have shown inconsistent results with regard to positive clinical end points.[12]

SNAKE VENOM ENZYMES

Fibrolase is a fibrinogenase isolated from the venom of the southern copperhead snake. It is a direct fibrinolytic agent that does not require plasminogen or other blood components for activation. Alfimeprase is a recombinant analogue of fibrolase that has been studied in animal models and found to be superior to urokinase and t-PA for recanalization.[15,16] Clinical trial results have been limited due to study design, cost and required catheter delivery.[12]

EARTHWORM ENZYMES

Several proteases have been isolated from the alimentary tract of earthworms. Due to their various living environments, proteases of different species have been independently studied. In general, however, these enzymes are suspected to directly hydrolyze thrombi and exhibit anti-platelet activity by attenuating calcium release and prompting platelet disaggregation.[11] Many studies continue to search for the potential clinical application of these enzymes but they have the potential to hydrolyze not only fibrinogen and fibrin, but also other proteins in vivo, thus further investigation is warranted.

NATTOKINASE

NK is an enzyme isolated from fermented boiled soybeans wrapped in straw, known as natto. Compared to UK, 50 g of natto has the same efficacy with lower cost and longer activity, lasting 2–12 hours.[17] Oral NK may also prevent conditions leading to blood clots, unlike t-PA, UK and SK which are only effective intravenously.[18] NK prevents coagulation and dissolves existing thrombi by cleaving cross-linked fibrin and activates production of t-PA. It also enhances fibrinolysis through cleavage and inactivation of PAI-1.[19] Furthermore, animal studies suggest that dietary supplementation of natto can suppress intimal thickening and modulate lysis of thrombi. Clinical trial data, however, remain limited. Preliminary findings show that 200 g of natto daily enhances ability to dissolve clots and improves fibrinolytic activity for 2–8 hours after administration.[20]

Indirect agents

STREPTOKINASE

Streptokinase (SK) is a single-chain polypeptide isolated from beta-hemolytic streptococci. It has no enzymatic activity by itself but forms an equimolar complex with plasminogen to function as a plasminogen activator and serine protease to convert plasminogen to plasmin. It also eventually forms an SK–plasmin complex, which also activates plasminogen.

Limitations of SK include immunogenicity and short half-life in circulation. SK is antigenic and antibodies are present in those with previous exposure. When bound to antibodies, SK activity is neutralized and its half-life is reduced from 90 to 18 minutes. Therefore, drug dosage must adjust for potentially circulating antibodies to establish therapeutic lysis. Some investigators recommend measurement of antibody titres before initiation of SK therapy.[21]

Human plasminogen complexed with SK, known as APSAC, was developed to extend the half-life of SK. It is an equimolar complex of SK and human Lys-plasminogen that has been acylated at its catalytic serine site, rendering the complex inactive. The greater fibrinolytic potential of APSAC is a result of its longer half-life, enhanced affinity of the Lys-plasminogen for fibrin, and protection from plasma inhibitors due to the acylated site. The agent can be given as a single bolus with a half-life of 90–105 minutes and therapeutic effect up to 6 hours. Therapy can be associated with adverse reactions similar to SK. Although the longer half-life of APSAC was thought to also reduce risk of rethrombosis, studies of the agent in coronary occlusion did not show any clinical benefit over SK or rt-PA. It is currently not employed in the setting of peripheral thrombolytic therapy.

The major complication associated with SK therapy is systemic bleeding. SK causes proteolytic depletion of coagulation factors such as fibrinogen, factor V and factor VIII, as demonstrated by prolonged prothrombin time, partial thromboplastin time (PTT) and thrombin time during therapy. SK-induced hyperplasminemia also causes nonspecific digestion of fibrin thrombi and increases fibrinogen degradation products which themselves worsen coagulopathy. Other complications of SK therapy include pyrexia and allergic reactions ranging from skin rashes (6%–9% reported)[1,2] to anaphylaxis and angioedema (incidence of 0.9%–2%).[2,21] Antihistamines, antipyretics and steroids have been used to treat adverse reactions during drug administration.

UROKINASE

Urokinase was isolated from human urine by MacFarlane and Pilling in 1946.[22] It is a serine protease composed of two polypeptide chains and exists in two forms that have similar activity: a high-molecular-weight entity (54 kDa) and a degradation product of the former called low-molecular-weight (32 kDa) urokinase. The high-molecular-weight form is the most common type isolated from urine, while the low-molecular-weight form is found from kidney cell culture.[23] Unlike SK, urokinase activates plasminogen directly without forming an activator complex and it is nonantigenic. Urokinase is degraded by the liver and has a half-life of approximately 15 minutes, which allows for rapid reversal after discontinuation of the agent.[24]

The most commonly used form of UK is from tissue culture of human neonatal kidney cells (Abbokinase, Abbott Laboratories, North Chicago, IL). A recombinant form, r-UK, has also been developed from a murine hybridoma cell line.[25] It has higher molecular weight than Abbokinase and a shorter half-life. The clinical effects are similar. Furthermore, a UK precursor called Prourokinase (ProUK) has been characterized and manufactured by recombinant technology using *Escherichia coli* (nonglycosylated) or mammalian cells (fully glycosylated). ProUK is an inert zymogen that is activated in the presence of fibrin clot. Once active, it can then activate plasminogen. Plasmin, or kallikrein, increases its plasminogen-activating capacity by converting ProUK to active UK, resulting in an amplification of the fibrinolytic progress. ProUK has the additional benefit of not reacting with inhibitors circulating in plasma, thus enhancing its ability to reach the clot intact, unlike urokinase. It also preferentially activates fibrin-bound plasminogen found in thrombus rather than free plasminogen for enhanced specificity. Non-selective activators such as SK and UK activate both free and bound plasminogen equally, resulting in systemic plasminemia, fibrinogenolysis and degradation of factors V and VII.

TISSUE PLASMINOGEN ACTIVATOR

Tissue plasminogen activator is a serine protease synthesized in endothelial cells. It is a single polypeptide chain (527 amino acids) with a molecular weight of 65 kDa. Plasmin converts t-PA to a single-chain and a double-chain form. Although the single-chain form has greater intrinsic plasminolytic activity, the activity of both forms is enhanced by fibrin without difference in activity levels. Unlike other agents, t-PA is both fibrin specific and has high fibrin affinity. Once bound to fibrin, t-PA enhances the conversion of plasminogen to plasmin and subsequent clot dissolution. The plasma half-life of t-PA is about 4 minutes due to metabolism by the liver. In addition to binding with plasminogen, PAI-1 can also bind with t-PA. The t-PAAPAI-1 complex can cause secondary vascular embolism thus prompting the development of new t-PAs that inhibit binding with PAI-1.[11]

The most common form of t-PA is from recombinant preparation (rt-PA).[26] It can also be isolated from cadaver perfusate, uterine tissue and human melanoma cells.[27]. Activase (Genetech), generic alteplase, is a single-chain form of rt-PA that has been extensively studied and approved for acute myocardial infarction and pulmonary embolism. The GUSTO-I study of 41,000 patients with acute myocardial infarction demonstrated better vascular patency with rt-PA compared to SK.[28] Overall mortality is lower with rt-PA despite a slightly greater risk of intracranial hemorrhage.[29] Intravenous alteplase has been approved for acute ischemic stroke in Europe for patients <80 years old with treatment within 4.5 hours to improve neurological recovery and reduce incidence of disability. It is usually initiated within 3 hours after onset stroke symptoms and after exclusion of intracranial hemorrhage.[11,30]

Efforts to increase the bioavailability of t-PA resulted in TNK-tPA (tenecteplase), which has four times slower clearance and 16-fold higher fibrin specificity than native t-PA. The drug can be administered as a single bolus rather than infusion. Its greater fibrin specificity than rt-PA also reduces risk of fibrinogen depletion. Furthermore, it has 80-fold greater resistance to inactivation by PAI-1, thereby decreasing thrombogenicity.[11,30] In acute coronary occlusion studies, TNK-tPA demonstrated equal efficacy and greater ease of administration than rt-PA.[31,32]

Similarly, reteplase (Centocor Malvern, PA) was also developed to address short half-life of native t-PA. It is produced in *E. coli* cells and is a nonglycosylated agent that demonstrates a lower fibrin-binding activity compared to alteplase and t-PA. The lower binding activity improves clot penetration and decreases risk of systemic bleeding complications. Reteplase also has diminished affinity to hepatocytes, thus extending its half-life to18 minutes. These factors assist in rapid reperfusion and low incidence of bleeding.[33] Reteplase has shown some benefit over rt-PA in the RAPID 1, RAPID 2 and GUSTO III coronary occlusion studies.[34,35]

NOVEL AGENTS

Staphylokinase is a by-product of *Staphylococcus aureus* that has been developed in recombinant form and studied in myocardial infarction,[36] peripheral arterial occlusion[37] and deep venous thrombosis. Like SK, it is antigenic and requires plasminogen binding for activation. Unlike SK, it is fibrin specific and thus spares circulating fibrinogen and plasminogen.

Desmoteplase (bat-PA) is cloned vampire bat plasminogen activator and derived from the saliva of the vampire bat *Desmodus rotundus* (DSPA alpha-1).[38,39] It is extremely fibrin specific and has a plasminogenolytic activity 100,000 times greater in the presence of fibrin.[40-42] The half-life of bat-PA is longer than that of rt-PA. Phase II trials DIAS and DEDAS showed that IV administration of bat-PA 3–9 hours after onset of ischemic stroke symptoms was associated with high rate of reperfusion and low rate of symptomatic intracranial hemorrhage at doses up to 125 μg/kg.[43-45] Like SK and other non-human proteins, bat-PA also has the potential for provoking an immune response, especially after repeated administration.

Saruplase is a single-chain recombinant (r-UK) converted by plasmin into an active, low-molecular-weight form of UK. The unconverted fraction activates plasminogen directly. It has a half-life of 7–8 minutes. Although it causes systemic plasminemia, as shown by decreases in α2-antiplasmin and fibrinogen and increases in fibrinogen degradation products, its systemic fibrinolytic activity is less than SK and greater than that of alteplase.[46] The safety and efficacy of saruplase was confirmed in the LIMITS study during which 20 mg bolus and 60 mg infusion over 60 minutes of saruplase was used with concomitant infusion of heparin and preliminary heparin bolus.[46] Current research seeks to modify and couple saruplase with t-PA to improve half-life. Other studies seek to cross-link saruplase with antifibrin and antiplatelet antibodies or Fab fragments to concentrate the compound at the thrombus. Cross-linking results in a 29-fold increase in thrombolytic potency in animal models compared with saruplase alone.[11]

CLINICAL APPLICATION OF THROMBOLYTIC AGENTS

Arterial thrombolysis

Thrombolytic agents have been experimentally used since the 1950s but intervention for ischemic limbs consisted primarily of amputation, surgical revascularization or balloon–catheter embolectomy.[47] Open surgical intervention is associated with a high rate of amputation and patient morbidity.[48–50] Thrombolytic agents used systemically or with minimally invasive delivery methods have the potential to restore arterial flow and preserve limb viability with decreased risk of morbidity compared to surgical intervention. The goal of arterial thrombolysis is to determine the etiologic mechanism of the occlusive event and limit the magnitude and morbidity of the subsequent interventions.

Peripheral arterial thrombolysis is most effective by a catheter-directed approach to directly deliver the agent to the thrombus – after a suitable lytic candidate is identified (Table 9.1). Good candidates for therapy are those with acute embolic of thrombotic occlusions (less than 14 days) of arteries inaccessible to mechanical thrombectomy. Charles Dotter first popularized the use of catheter-directed SK therapy and reported success rates greater than those achieved with systemic therapy.[51] Access for therapy is usually from the contralateral femoral artery. An antegrade (ipsilateral) approach may be used when the level of occlusion is sufficiently distal from the access site. When the occlusion and access site are in close proximity, antegrade access may be hampered by an inability to pass the catheter through the occluded graft or thrombus. There may also be an increased risk of bleeding. Multiple attempts for access can increase the risk of bleeding during thrombolytic therapy and are best avoided if possible. Ultrasound-guided access can be utilized to aid in accurate vessel puncture. Low-profile sheaths (5 French) and catheters can be used for delivery of the thrombolytic agent. Low-dose heparin therapy is concurrently administered to prevent pericatheter thrombus during prolonged thrombolytic therapy.

Complications of catheter-delivered thrombolysis are proportional to duration of infusion. Thus, recommended duration of drug administration is limited to 48 hours. If lysis has not been achieved after 48 hours, additional time is unlikely to be helpful.

There have been multiple established delivery techniques for pharmacological thrombolysis[52]:

1. *Regional intra-arterial infusion* includes selective and non-selective infusion. In the former, the catheter is placed within the proximal portion of the occlusion; in the latter, the catheter does not enter the occlusion.
2. *Intrathrombus infusion* is the most commonly used technique where the catheter tip is placed within the thrombus.
3. *Intrathrombus blousing or lacing* describes an initial bolus dose of concentrated thrombolytic agent within the thrombus to saturate the area of occlusion. As thrombolysis progresses, the catheter is slowly withdrawn to deliver the lytic agent along the thrombosed area.
4. *Stepwise infusion* also describes delivery of agent at the proximal portion of the thrombus, but as thrombolysis progresses, the catheter is advanced gradually towards the distal part of the occlusion.
5. *Continuous infusion* is enabled by catheter connection to a pump for constant drug delivery.
6. *Graded infusion* describes a time-dependent dose of drug delivery that is inversely proportional to the procedure time. Studies examining continuous versus periodic spray infusions have not shown statistically significant difference in treatment times.[53,54]
7. *Forced periodic infusion (pulse-spray technique)* is pressurized drug infusion designed to break the thrombus to create more surface area for drug delivery.

After catheter placement, the patient remains under monitoring throughout the infusion. Periodic angiograms are indicated every 12–20 hours to adjust the infusion rate as necessary or compensate for any catheter movement. Coagulation parameters (e.g. fibrinogen level) can be monitored, but their use remains controversial. Previous studies show that levels of coagulation factors do not predict risk of bleeding complications.[55] There have been other trials, however, that support an association between fibrinogen concentration, PTT and incidence of bleeding complications during thrombolytic procedures.[56]

In addition to catheter-directed delivery of thrombolytic agents, it should be mentioned that these agents are also used in percutaneous thrombectomy devices that combine both catheter delivery of agent and mechanical clot dissolution with hydrodynamic and ultrasonic force. These devices are reserved for peripheral applications due to risk of embolization. Some of the most commonly used percutaneous thrombectomy devices include the hydrolyzer, BSIC Oasis system, AngioJet, ThrombCat, Bacchus Trellis, OmniSonics Resolution Wire and the EKOS Lysus system.[52]

Table 9.1 Contraindications to thrombolytic therapy.

Absolute
1. Active internal bleeding
2. Recent cerebrovascular accident, trauma or intracranial pathology <12 months

Relative
Major
1. Recent surgery or trauma <10 days
2. Gastrointestinal or genitourinary bleeding
3. Uncontrolled hypertension (>200 systolic or >110 diastolic)
Minor
4. Pregnancy
5. Diabetic retinopathy with hemorrhage
6. Bleeding disorders
7. Left-sided cardiac thrombus
8. Bacterial endocarditis
9. Minor trauma or surgery

Results of thrombolysis in acute peripheral arterial occlusion

No randomized controlled studies were conducted to evaluate thrombolytic therapy prior to 1990. Previous retrospective studies failed to study limb salvage and morbidity.[57-59] Although there were multiple reports of successful thrombolysis in a large number of patients,[57,59] other studies found that thrombolysis did not mitigate the need for surgical intervention.[60,61]

The first randomized trial was conducted in Europe and compared rt-PA versus surgical thrombectomy, but it was limited to 20 patients.[62] The first randomized trial in the United States was performed in 1994 at the University of Rochester, comparing intra-arterial urokinase with surgical intervention.[63] One hundred fourteen patients with acute (less than 7 days duration) and limb-threatening ischemia were evaluated for primary end points of limb salvage and survival. Thrombolytic therapy was associated with a reduction in cardiopulmonary complications. This translated into an improved 12-month survival when compared to the primary operation group. Limb salvage was identical in both groups.

The Surgery or Thrombolysis for Ischemia of the Lower Extremity trial was published shortly after the Rochester report.[64] This multicentre randomized trial evaluated rt-PA, urokinase and surgical intervention in patients with ischemia of less than 6 months duration using a composite end point that included renal failure, wound complications and ongoing ischemia. The study found no difference in mortality or amputation rate. During the trial, it was noted that the thrombolysis group had a higher rate of continued ischemia compared to the surgical group, 54% versus 26%, respectively. Due to this difference, the trial was terminated. Further analysis of the rate of amputation suggested that patients with symptoms less than 2 weeks duration responded more favourably to thrombolysis compared to patients with chronic occlusions, who responded better to surgical intervention.

The Thrombolysis or Peripheral Arterial Surgery study[65] was a two-part study designed to compare recombinant urokinase and surgical intervention in peripheral arterial occlusions ≤14 days in duration. The first part of the trial evaluated the safety and efficacy of a 2000, 4000 or 6000 IU/min r-UK administration followed by 2000 IU/min for up to 48 hours. Result demonstrated the 4000 IU/min dose as the safest and most effective dose. Despite the intent to compare lytic intervention to surgical intervention, the Part I of the study was not adequately powered to evaluate the comparison. The second portion of the study randomized 544 patients to r-UK or surgery. It demonstrated that the efficacy of the r-UK was the same as surgery with respect to amputation and survival.[66] Patients were followed for 1 year after therapy and monitored for rate and magnitude of subsequent interventions. The thrombolysis group was noted to have a lower rate of invasive interventions (operative or endovascular) than the surgical group.

The Cochrane Peripheral Vascular Diseases Group conducted a comprehensive review to compare effectiveness of intra-arterial fibrinolytics for peripheral arterial ischemia. Five randomized controlled trials were analyzed, involving 687 participants. Analysis showed no significant difference in limb salvage at 30 days with urokinase or rt-PA or difference in hemorrhagic complications between intra-arterial UK and intra-arterial rt-PA. Overall, there was evidence suggesting that intra-arterial rt-PA is more effective than intra-arterial SK or intravenous rt-PA in improving vessel patency. The study remarked again, however, that each individual study was small, and larger studies are needed for definitive clinical guidance.[67]

Venous thrombolysis

Unlike arterial occlusions, venous occlusions often present with less acute and more subtle clinical signs and symptoms and less risk of tissue ischemia. As such, they are frequently treated with anticoagulation only. Acute deep venous thrombosis, however, remains a serious healthcare issue, with an estimated average population incidence of about 70–113 cases per 100,000 persons.[68] Furthermore, sequelae of acute deep venous thrombosis include pulmonary embolism and post-thrombotic syndrome. Up to 90% of patients initially diagnosed with deep venous thrombosis and treated by anticoagulation alone will go on to develop venous hypertension, 40% will have venous claudication and 15% will progress to venous ulceration.[69]

Thrombolysis of venous occlusions has the potential to prevent life-threatening and morbid sequelae by rapidly removing clot burden to preserve valvular function, re-establish luminal patency, and potentially minimize late developing complications that can occur due to post-thrombotic syndrome. There remains no consensus, however, of the exact indications for venous thrombolysis. General indications include younger patients with acute proximal thrombosis within the iliofemoral system, long life expectancy and few comorbidities. Limb-threatening thrombosis where venous occlusion threatens arterial flow such as phlegmasia alba or cerulea dolens may also benefit from thrombolysis. The most recent guidelines developed by the American College of Chest Physician Consensus Conference on Antithrombotic and Thrombolytic Therapy suggest that for selected patients, minimally invasive pharmacomechanical therapy may be considered for prevention of post-thrombotic syndrome.[70] This guideline is further supported by a Cochrane review of thrombolysis for acute deep vein thrombosis that analyzed 17 studies with 1103 participants.[71]

Compared to arterial thrombolysis, procedural protocol, catheter placement relative to thrombus, infusion techniques and equipment are similar. Direct infusion is achieved by accessing the contralateral femoral vein, right jugular vein or both. The ipsilateral femoral vein can be used as access when there is sufficient distance from the occlusion. Contralateral access, however, allows placement of a vena cava filter prior to infusion, if necessary. Acute venous occlusions of less than 2 weeks show an improved response to catheter-delivered thrombolysis.

REFERENCES

1. Alkjaersig N, Fletcher AP, Sherry S. The mechanism of clot dissolution by plasmin. *J Clin Invest.* 1959;38:1086–1095.

2. Sherry S, Lindemeyer RI, Fletcher AP, Alkjaersig N. Studies on enhanced fibrinolytic activity in man. *J Clin Invest.* 1959;38:810–822.

3. Sharma GV, Cella G, Parisi AF, Sasahara AA. Thrombolytic therapy. *N Engl J Med.* 1982;306:1268–1276.

4. Robbins KC. The plasminogen-plasmin enzyme system. In: Comerota AJ, ed. *Thrombolytic Therapy for Peripheral Vascular Disease.* New York: Lippincott; 1995, pp. 41–76.

5. Sherry S, Fletcher A, Alkjaersig N. Fibrinolysis and fibrinolytic activity in man. *Physiol Rev.* 1988;38:343–362.

6. Francis CW. The fibrinolytic system: Normal physiology and pathophysiology. In: Comerota AJ, ed. *Thrombolytic Therapy for Peripheral Vascular Disease.* New York: Lippincott; 1995, pp. 25–35.

7. Collen D, Zamarron C, Lijnen HR, Hoylaerts M. Activation of plasminogen by pro-urokinase. II. Kinetics. *J Biol Chem.* 1986;261:1259–1266.

8. Miles LA, Castellino FJ, Gong Y. Critical role for conversion of glu-plasminogen to Lys-plasminogen for optimal stimulation of plasminogen activation on cell surfaces. *Trends Cardiovasc Med.* 2003;13:21–30.

9. Henkin K, Marcotte P, Yang H. The plasminogen-plasmin system. *Prog Cardiovasc Dis.* 1991;34:135–162.

10. Schaller J, Gerber SS. The plasmin-antiplasmin system: Structural and functional aspects. *Cell Mol Life Sci.* 2011;68:785–801.

11. Kotb E. The biotechnological potential of fibrinolytic enzymes in the dissolution of endogenous blood thrombi. *Biotechnol Prog.* 2014;30:656–672.

12. Marder VJ, Novokhatny V. Direct fibrinolytic agents: Biochemical attributes, preclinical foundation and clinical potential. *J Thromb Haemost.* 2010;8:433–444.

13. Marder VJ. Pre-clinical studies of plasmin: Superior benefit-to-risk ratio of plasmin compared to tissue plasminogen activator. *Thromb Res.* 2008;122(Suppl. 3):S9–S15.

14. Novokhatny V, Taylor K, Zimmerman TP. Thrombolytic potency of acid-stabilized plasmin: Superiority over tissue-type plasminogen activator in an in vitro model of catheter-assisted thrombolysis. *J Thromb Haemost.* 2003;1:1034–1041.

15. Hong TT, Huang J, Lucchesi BR. Effect of thrombolysis on myocardial injury: Recombinant tissue plasminogen activator vs. alfimeprase. *Am J Physiol Heart Circ Physiol.* 2006;290:H959–H567.

16. Deitcher SR, Toombs CF. Non-clinical and clinical characterization of a novel acting thrombolytic: Alfimeprase. *Pathophysiol Haemost Thromb.* 2005;34:215–220.

17. Fujita M, Hong K, Ito Y, Fujii R, Kariya K, Nishimuro S. Thrombolytic effect of nattokinase on a chemically induced thrombosis model in rat. *Biol Pharm Bull.* 1995;18:1387–1391.

18. Sumi H, Hamada H, Tsushima H, Mihara H, Muraki H. A novel fibrinolytic enzyme (nattokinase) in the vegetable cheese Natto; a typical and popular soybean food in the Japanese diet. *Experientia.* 1987;43:1110–1111.

19. Urano T, Ihara H, Umemura K et al. The profibrinolytic enzyme subtilisin NAT purified from *Bacillus subtilis* cleaves and inactivates plasminogen activator inhibitor type 1. *J Biol Chem.* 2001;276:24690–24696.

20. Lee CK, Shin JS, Kim BS, Cho IH, Kim YS, Lee EB. Antithrombotic effects by oral administration of novel proteinase fraction from earthworm Eisenia andrei on venous thrombosis model in rats. *Arch Pharm Res.* 2007;30:475–480.

21. Marder VJ, Sherry S. Thrombolytic therapy: Current status (1). *N Engl J Med.* 1988;318:1512–1520.

22. Macfarlane RG, Pilling J. Observations on fibrinolysis; plasminogen, plasmin, and antiplasmin content of human blood. *Lancet.* 1946;2:562–565.

23. Bernik MB, Kwaan HC. Origin of fibrinolytic activity in cultures of the human kidney. *J Lab Clin Med.* 1967;70:650–661.

24. Ploug J, Kjeldgaard NO. Urokinase an activator of plasminogen from human urine. I. Isolation and properties. *Biochim Biophys Acta.* 1957;24:278–282.

25. Sherry S, Fletcher AP, Alkjaersig N. Developments in fibrinolytic therapy for thrombo-embolic disease. *Ann Intern Med.* 1959;50:560–570.

26. Froehlich J, Stump DL. Recombinant tissue plasminogen activator. In: Comerota AJ, ed. *Thrombolytic Therapy for Peripheral Vascular Disease.* New York: Lippincott; 1967, pp. 103–111.

27. Aasted B. Purification and characterization of human vascular plasminogen activator. *Biochim Biophys Acta.* 1980;621:241–254.

28. The GUSTO Investigators. An angiographic study within the global randomized trial of aggressive versus standard thrombolytic strategies in patients with acute myocardial infarction. *N Engl J Med.* 1993;329:1615.

29. The GUSTO Investigators. An international randomized trial comparing four thrombolytic therapies for acute myocardial infarction. *N Engl J Med.* 1993;329:673–682.

30. Wardlaw JM, Murray V, Berge E et al. Recombinant tissue plasminogen activator for acute ischaemic stroke: An updated systematic review and meta-analysis. *Lancet.* 2012;379:2364–2372.

31. Cannon CP, Gibson CM, McCabe CH et al. TNK-tissue plasminogen activator compared with front-loaded alteplase in acute myocardial infarction: Results of the TIMI 10B trial. Thrombolysis in Myocardial Infarction (TIMI) 10B Investigators. *Circulation.* 1998;98:2805–2814.

32. Cannon CP, McCabe CH, Gibson CM et al. TNK-tissue plasminogen activator in acute myocardial infarction. Results of the Thrombolysis in Myocardial Infarction (TIMI) 10A dose-ranging trial. *Circulation.* 1997;95:351–356.

33. Bode C, Smalling RW, Berg G et al. Randomized comparison of coronary thrombolysis achieved with double-bolus reteplase (recombinant plasminogen activator) and front-loaded, accelerated alteplase (recombinant tissue plasminogen activator) in patients with acute myocardial infarction. The RAPID II Investigators. *Circulation.* 1996;94:891–898.

34. The Global Use of Strategies to Open Occluded Coronary Arteries (GUSTO III) Investigators. A comparison of reteplase with alteplase for acute myocardial infarction. *N Engl J Med.* 1997;337:1118–1123.

35. Gurbel PA, Serebruany VL, Shustov AR et al. Effects of reteplase and alteplase on platelet aggregation and major receptor expression during the first 24 hours of acute myocardial infarction treatment. GUSTO-III Investigators. Global Use of Strategies to Open Occluded Coronary Arteries. *J Am Coll Cardiol.* 1998;31:1466–1473.

36. Vanderschueren S, Dens J, Kerdsinchai P et al. Randomized coronary patency trial of double-bolus recombinant staphylokinase versus front-loaded alteplase in acute myocardial infarction. *Am Heart J.* 1997;134:213–219.

37. Vanderschueren S, Stockx L, Wilms G et al. Thrombolytic therapy of peripheral arterial occlusion with recombinant staphylokinase. *Circulation.* 1995;92:2050–2057.

38. Gardell SJ, Duong LT, Diehl RE et al. Isolation, characterization, and cDNA cloning of a vampire bat salivary plasminogen activator. *J Biol Chem.* 1989;264:17947–17952.

39. Hawkey C. Plasminogen activator in saliva of the vampire bat *Desmodus rotundus. Nature.* 1966;211:434–435.

40. Mellott MJ, Stabilito II, Holahan MA et al. Vampire bat salivary plasminogen activator promotes rapid and sustained reperfusion without concomitant systemic plasminogen activation in a canine model of arterial thrombosis. *Arterioscler Thromb.* 1992;12:212–221.

41. Montoney M, Gardell SJ, Marder VJ. Comparison of the bleeding potential of vampire bat salivary plasminogen activator versus tissue plasminogen activator in an experimental rabbit model. *Circulation.* 1995;91:1540–1544.

42. Verstraete M, Lijnen HR, Collen D. Thrombolytic agents in development. *Drugs.* 1995;50:29–42.

43. Gulba DC, Bode C, Runge MS, Huber K. Thrombolytic agents – An overview. *Ann Hematol.* 1996;73(Suppl. 1):S9–S27.

44. Fiebach JB, Al-Rawi Y, Wintermark M et al. Vascular occlusion enables selecting acute ischemic stroke patients for treatment with desmoteplase. *Stroke.* 2012;43:1561–1566.

45. Schleuning WD, Bhargava A, Donner P. *Desmodus rotundus* (vampire bat) plasminogen activator DSPA-α1: A superior thrombolytic created by evolution. In: Loscalzo J, ed. *Sasahara Atomic Absorption: New Therapeutic Agents in Thrombosis and Thrombolysis.* New York: Marcel Dekker, Inc; 1997, pp. 603–623.

46. Tebbe U, Windeler J, Boesl I et al. Thrombolysis with recombinant unglycosylated single-chain urokinase-type plasminogen activator (saruplase) in acute myocardial infarction: Influence of heparin on early patency rate (LIMITS study). Liquemin in Myocardial Infarction During Thrombolysis With Saruplase. *J Am Coll Cardiol.* 1995;26:365–373.

47. Fogarty TJ, Cranley JJ, Krause RJ, Strasser ES, Hafner CD. A method for extraction of arterial emboli and thrombi. *Surg Gynecol Obstet.* 1963;116:241–244.

48. Blaisdell FW, Steele M, Allen RE. Management of acute lower extremity arterial ischemia due to embolism and thrombosis. *Surgery.* 1978;84:822–834.

49. Jivegard L, Holm J, Schersten T. Acute limb ischemia due to arterial embolism or thrombosis: Influence of limb ischemia versus pre-existing cardiac disease on postoperative mortality rate. *J Cardiovasc Surg.* 1988;29:32–36.

50. Yeager RA. Basic data related to cardiac testing and cardiac risk associated with vascular surgery. *Ann Vasc Surg.* 1990;4:193–197.

51. Dotter CT, Rosch J, Seaman AJ. Selective clot lysis with low-dose streptokinase. *Radiology.* 1974;111:31–37.

52. Karnabatidis D, Spiliopoulos S, Tsetis D, Siablis D. Quality improvement guidelines for percutaneous catheter-directed intra-arterial thrombolysis and mechanical thrombectomy for acute lower-limb ischemia. *Cardiovasc Intervent Radiol.* 2011;34:1123–1136.

53. Kandarpa K. Technical determinants of success in catheter-directed thrombolysis for peripheral arterial occlusions. *J Vasc Interv Radiol.* 1995;6:55S–61S.

54. Kandarpa K, Chopra PS, Aruny JE et al. Intraarterial thrombolysis of lower extremity occlusions: Prospective, randomized comparison of forced periodic infusion and conventional slow continuous infusion. *Radiology.* 1993;188:861–867.

55. Marder VJ. The use of thrombolytic agents: Choice of patient, drug administration, laboratory monitoring. *Ann Intern Med.* 1979;90:802–808.

56. Graor RA, Risius B, Young JR et al. Low-dose streptokinase for selective thrombolysis: Systemic effects and complications. *Radiology.* 1984;152:35–39.

57. Graor RA, Risius B, Lucas FV et al. Thrombolysis with recombinant human tissue-type plasminogen activator in patients with peripheral artery and bypass graft occlusions. *Circulation.* 1986;74:115–120.

58. Krings W, Roth FJ, Cappius G, Schmidtke I. Catheter-lysis: Indications and primary results. *Int Angiol.* 1985;4:117–123.

59. McNamara TO, Fischer JR. Thrombolysis of peripheral arterial and graft occlusions: Improved results using high-dose urokinase. *Am J Roentgenol.* 1985;144:769–775.

60. Ricotta J. Intra-arterial thrombolysis: A surgical view. *Circulation.* 1991;83:1120–1121.

61. Sicard GA, Schier JJ, Totty WG et al. Thrombolytic therapy for acute arterial occlusion. *J Vasc Surg.* 1985;2:65–78.

62. Nilsson L, Albrechtsson U, Jonung T et al. Surgical treatment versus thrombolysis in acute arterial occlusion: A randomised controlled study. *Eur J Vasc Surg.* 1992;6:189–193.

63. Ouriel K, Shortell CK, DeWeese JA et al. A comparison of thrombolytic therapy with operative revascularization in the initial treatment of acute peripheral arterial ischemia. *J Vasc Surg.* 1994;19:1021–1030.

64. Weaver FA, Comerota AJ, Youngblood M, Froehlich J, Hosking JD, Papanicolaou G. Surgical revascularization versus thrombolysis for nonembolic lower extremity native artery occlusions: Results of a prospective randomized trial. The STILE Investigators. Surgery versus Thrombolysis for Ischemia of the Lower Extremity. *J Vasc Surg.* 1996;24:513–521; discussion 21–23.

65. Ouriel K, Veith FJ, Sasahara AA. Thrombolysis or peripheral arterial surgery: Phase I results. TOPAS Investigators. *J Vasc Surg.* 1996;23:64–73; discussion 4–5.

66. Ouriel K, Veith FJ, Sasahara AA. A comparison of recombinant urokinase with vascular surgery as initial treatment for acute arterial occlusion of the legs. Thrombolysis or Peripheral Arterial Surgery (TOPAS) Investigators. *N Engl J Med.* 1998;338:1105–1111.

67. Robertson I, Kessel DO, Berridge DC. Fibrinolytic agents for peripheral arterial occlusion. *Cochrane Database Syst Rev.* 2013;12:CD001099.

68. White RH. The epidemiology of venous thromboembolism. *Circulation.* 2003;107:14–18.

69. Rutherford RB. *Vascular Surgery,* 6th ed. Philadelphia, PA: Saunders; 2005.

70. Kearon C, Kahn SR, Agnelli G et al. Antithrombotic therapy for venous thromboembolic disease: American College of Chest Physicians Evidence-Based Clinical Practice Guidelines (8th Edition). *Chest.* 2008;133:454S–545S.

71. Watson L, Broderick C, Armon MP. Thrombolysis for acute deep vein thrombosis. *Cochrane Database Syst Rev.* 2014;1:CD002783.

10

Antiplatelet therapy

IAN GORDON

CONTENTS

Platelets have long been appreciated as having a key role in hemostasis and thrombosis, but they also participate in the cellular and molecular events involved in inflammation, blood vessels remodelling, wound healing and atherosclerosis. Given the pivotal role platelets play in the pathologic processes that lead to cardiovascular disease, it is understandable that drugs that inhibit platelet function are effective in reducing the risk of stroke, myocardial infarction and death in high-risk patients. Antiplatelet therapy has also been shown to be beneficial in the setting of carotid surgery, lower-extremity bypass and endovascular interventions such as percutaneous transluminal angioplasty (PTA) and stenting. The focus of this review will be to review the pertinent aspects of platelet physiology that underlay the pharmacology of antiplatelet drugs and our understanding of how antiplatelet therapy is optimally employed in the management of common vascular problems.

To help put the role of antiplatelet therapy in a proper perspective, it should be noted that acetylsalicylic acid (ASA or aspirin) is the most commonly administered drug in the world (although this reflects in part aspirin's anti-inflammatory and analgesic properties). Over 40,000 tons of aspirin are manufactured worldwide each year; in the United States alone more than 50 million patients are on aspirin therapy for prevention of cardiovascular disease.[1]

Clinically, the most common setting in which antiplatelet therapy is employed is in secondary prevention of new cardiovascular events after previous TIA, stroke, myocardial infarction or coronary intervention. Antiplatelet therapy is routinely employed as an adjunct in the management of ST segment elevation MI (STEMI) and acute coronary syndrome (ACS) which includes unstable angina (UA) and non-ST segment elevation MI. Particularly when coronary angioplasty or stenting is performed, two antiplatelet drugs are combined to prevent stent thrombosis – usually dual therapy with aspirin combined with a $P2Y_{12}$ receptor antagonist, such as clopidogrel. Much of our understanding of the risks and benefits of antiplatelet therapy in general, and more specifically, the salient features of new drugs, is derived from the outcomes of prospective randomized trials of medical management and interventional therapy of coronary artery disease (CAD). Compared to trials evaluating outcomes of antiplatelet therapy for peripheral vascular problems such as infrainguinal bypass, peripheral stents, carotid surgery and dialysis access, the number of trials and subjects enrolled in trials related to CAD is far greater.

Antiplatelet therapy entails giving drugs that inhibit platelet function in the hope that this will reduce the magnitude of certain biologic processes and adverse health outcomes that are driven or influenced by platelet activity. The most obvious of these processes is coagulation, as platelets play a critical role in stopping hemorrhage and promoting thrombosis. They are the first line of defence in stopping hemorrhage because they rapidly adhere to damaged endothelium and initiate the clotting cascade. Many of the reactions in thrombosis occur on their membrane, and platelet activation leads to positive feedback in the coagulation cascade. Although beneficial in most settings, in vascular interventions, such as carotid surgery or coronary stenting, it can be disastrous. A surgeon's or interventionalist's perspective may not look beyond the immediate consequences afforded by platelet inhibition – prevention of periprocedural thrombosis without, hopefully, increased hazard of bleeding.

Just as important as the contribution of platelets to thrombosis, however, is their participation in atherogenesis and inflammation. It is increasingly appreciated that many of the stimuli that drive atherosclerotic plaque progression are a consequence of activated platelets and platelet–leukocyte aggregates binding to lesions and releasing inflammatory mediators. There likely is positive feedback in this process as platelets are activated by passing through areas of high shear generated by stenosis and by contact with plaque. Similarly, release of platelet factors into damaged intima is one of the key events driving intimal hyperplasia after revascularization. The ability of long-term platelet inhibition to ameliorate plaque progression and intimal hyperplasia is likely just as important as their immediate impact on thrombosis, but a detailed exposition of the role of platelets in the pathophysiology of atherosclerosis and intimal hyperplasia is beyond the scope of this essay. Instead, we will focus on the more practical aspects of how antiplatelet drugs inhibit platelet activation and the clinical impact of that inhibition.

PLATELET PHYSIOLOGY

Platelets are fragments of bone marrow megakaryocytes that lack a nucleus and, when inactivated, circulate as lens-shaped cells (Figure 10.1) approximately 1/5 the size of erythrocytes and approximately 5%–10% as numerous. Platelet counts normally are in the range of 150,000–400,000 per µL of the blood. Daily production is approximately 10[11] in health with an average life span of 8–9 days with aged platelets destroyed by phagocytes in the liver and spleen.[2] Although platelets have mitochondria, they lack a nucleus. Nonetheless, platelets synthesize proteins using ribosomes and mRNA derived from the parent megakaryocyte and transcription is sensitive to activation events.[3] The platelet cytoskeleton is highly specialized and contains an open canalicular system that is present throughout the cytoplasm and connected to the phospholipid bilayer plasma membrane through small pores. There is also a residual closed dense tubular system derived from the megakaryocyte smooth endoplasmic reticulum, which is the site of thromboxane A_2 (Tx A2) synthesis and is connected to the surface membrane to aid in Tx A2 release. The cytoskeleton is comprised of a spectrin-based membrane skeleton, actin and marginal coils of microtubules that maintain a discoid cell conformation that protects the cells from shear. The plasma membrane contains numerous surface receptors capable of stimulating or inhibiting platelet activation via binding a variety of ligands (Table 10.1). Although several types of cytoplasmic signal pathways are stimulated by binding of specific ligands to different surface membrane receptors, ligand occupation of G protein–coupled receptors (GPCRs) are particularly important. As illustrated in Figure 10.2, GPCRs have a seven-transmembrane α-helix structure that spans the plasma membrane with an external ligand binding site and a cytoplasmic linkage to a G protein comprised of α, β and γ subunits. Ligand binding to the external portion of a GPCR induces a conformational change

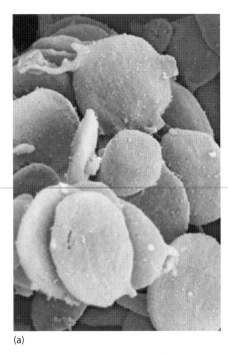

(a)

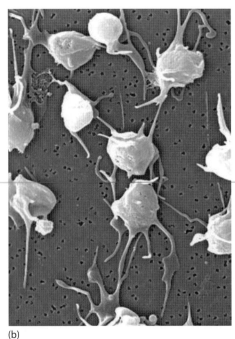

(b)

Figure 10.1 (a) Scanning electron micrograph showing disc-like morphology of quiescent platelets. (b) Scanning electron micrograph showing activated platelets which have become rounder in shape and expressing pseudopodia capable of binding to other platelets or damaged endothelium. ([a] From Pajnič M et al., *J Nanobiotechnology*, 13, 28, 2015.; [b] From Shani S et al., *ScientificWorldJournal*, Article ID 845293, 12, 2014.)

Table 10.1 Receptors and ligands.

Receptor	Family/type	Ligands
PECAM-1[a]	Ig superfamily	PECAM-1, collagen
PG$_{I2}$[a]	GPCRs	PGI$_2$ (prostacyclin)
GPIb-IX-V complex	Leucine-rich family	vWF, thrombin, FXI, FXIIP P-selectin, TSP-1
GPVI	Ig superfamily	Collagen, laminin
α$_2$β$_1$	Integrins	Collagen
α$_{IIIb}$β$_3$ (GPIIB/IIIa)	Integrins	Fibrinogen, fibrin, vWF
P2Y$_1$	GPCR	ADP
P2Y$_{12}$	GPCR	ADP
P2X$_1$	Ion channel	ATP
PAR-1	GPCR	Thrombin
PAR-4	GPCR	Thrombin
TPα	GPCR	Thromboxane A$_2$
Platelet-activating factor receptors	GPCR	Acetyl-glyceryl-ether-phosphorylcholine
5HT$_{2A}$ (serotonin receptor)	GPCR	Serotonin
PDGF receptor	Tyrosine kinase receptor	PDGF
P-selectin[b]	C-type lectin receptor family	gplb, tissue factor, PSGL-1

[a] Receptor occupation inhibits platelet activation.
[b] Source is α granules, after release inserts into platelet membrane.

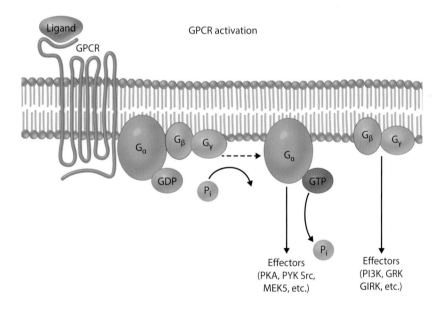

Figure 10.2 Schematic depiction of how binding agonist to the G protein–coupled receptor induces an exchange of GDP for GTP in the Gα subunit and dissociation of the Gα and Gβγ subunits. (From Belmonte SI et al., *Circ Res*, 109, 309, 2011.)

in the GPCR that activates the associated G protein via exchange of guanosine diphosphate (GDP) bound to the α subunit for guanosine triphosphate (GTP). This leads to dissociation of the activated α subunit and the Gβγ subunits from the GPCR G protein complex and subsequent interactions with secondary effector enzymes (typically a kinase, phospholipase or adenylate cyclase) whose activation further propagates the cytoplasmic signal associated with the plasma membrane receptor. For example, occupation of the surface prostacyclin receptor by prostacyclin leads to adenylate cyclase activation via interactions with

the GPCR-associated Gα subunit and subsequent downstream decrease in intracellular calcium – regulation of calcium being critical in the regulation of platelet activation.[4–6]

Platelets contain three types of granules which when activated rapidly release their contents into the canalicular system which facilitates release of granule outside the cell. Protein molecules bound to the granule membrane may reach the cell surface through a slower process entailing fusion of the granule to the plasma membrane. More than 300 distinct molecules released by platelets have been detected.[7] α granules are the largest (≈300 nm) and most abundant (50–60 per cell) and contain the majority of platelet factors involved in hemostasis and thrombosis. The contents of α granules include large proteins, such as thrombospondin and platelet factor 4, as well as coagulation factors (factors I, V, VIII, XI, XIII, von Willebrand factor [vWF]) and molecules involved in adhesion to blood vessels (fibronectin and vitronectin). The membranes of α granules also contain platelet surface receptors (glycoproteinVI [gpVI], gpIIa/IIIb, P-selectin). α granules also contain proteins involved in inflammation (e.g. TNF, MMP2, MMP9) and in wound healing and angiogenesis (e.g. platelet-derived growth factor [PDGF], vascular endothelial growth factor, transforming growth, factorβ1), as well as anti-angiogenic factors, such as angiostatin. Some of these proteins are produced by megakaryocytes and packaged into granules during platelet development. Other granule proteins (e.g. fibrinogen and Factor V) are thought to be captured by endocytosis by mature circulating platelets and then transported to granules.[8] It has been proposed that platelets differentially store and release their granular cargo in a thematic way, for example promoting angiogenesis by releasing VEGF from one granule subset under one circumstance and dampening angiogenesis in other circumstances via release of angiostatin from a different granule subset. The concept that platelets are 'smart' delivery systems in which mediator release varies with the specific situation is attractive but requires further substantiation.[9]

Dense granules (sometimes referred to as δ granules) are the smallest and appear dense in electron micrographs due to their high content of calcium and phosphate. They contain high concentrations of serotonin, ADP and ATP. Release of dense granules stimulates vasoconstriction (ATP and serotonin) and further platelet activation via ADP binding to surface receptors. One other type of platelet granule, γ granules, is present and contains contents similar to lysosomes (e.g. acid phosphatase and arylsulfatase) and is thought to participate in regulation of thrombus formation and remodelling of the extracellular matrix.

Normally, platelets circulate without significant adhesion to the intima. Inhibition of platelet activation is maintained by endothelial cell signals that act to keep calcium levels relatively low. When a vessel wall injury occurs, platelet activation is triggered by multiple signal pathways that lead to increased intracellular calcium, rapid degranulation and release of granule contents, deformation of the discoid platelet cell into more spherical shapes with pseudopodia and ultimately to aggregation of platelets into plugs that bind to and seal the injured intima, generate blood clot formation at the site of injury. Three distinct stages in the level of platelet activity that are present in the transition from *quiescence* to clot formation are discernable: *adhesion*, *activation* and *aggregation*. Most of the important events in this progression are driven by ligands binding to surface receptors whose occupation activates cytoplasmic signalling pathways that promote increased

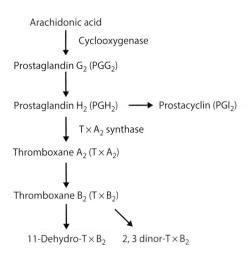

Prostaglandin synthesis pathway

Figure 10.3 Prostaglandin synthesis pathway. Arachidonic acid is converted to prostaglandin G2 by the action of cyclooxygenase as the first step. Prostacyclin (PGI$_2$) inhibits platelet activation by binding to the surface PGI$_2$ receptor. Thromboxane A$_2$ stimulates activation via binding to the surface TPα receptor. (From Ghoshal K and Bhattacharyya M, *ScientificWorldJournal*, Article ID 781857, 8, 2014.)

cytoplasmic calcium levels, release of granule contents and elaboration or release of other stimulatory factors, e.g. platelet-derived tissue factors transcribed de novo from mRNA.[10] Many of the mediators released from granules further stimulate activation via binding to the membrane of the activated significant overlap between phases. Although hundreds of interactions have been described as part of platelet physiology, the key features in the transition of resting platelets to aggregation and thrombosis are well established and not difficult to apprehend. Figure 10.3 shows the biochemical pathway for prostacyclin and Tx A2 synthesis; both of these prostaglandins play a pivotal role in regulation of platelet activity. Figure 10.4 is an overview of primary and secondary hemostasis. Platelets transition from quiescence through primary hemostasis (the initial platelet plug at the endothelial injury) to secondary hemostasis with a fibrin mesh trapping red cells and stabilizing the platelet plug.

Quiescence

Normally, platelet activation is inhibited by three different endothelium-dependent signals: endothelial elaboration of nitric oxide (NO), endothelial ADPase and endothelial prostacyclin (prostaglandin PGI$_2$) production. Resting platelets have relatively low intracellular calcium levels maintained by a cAMP-activated calcium pump which promotes calcium efflux to keep cytoplasmic calcium levels. NO released by endothelial cells diffuses into platelets and stimulates production of cyclic guanosine

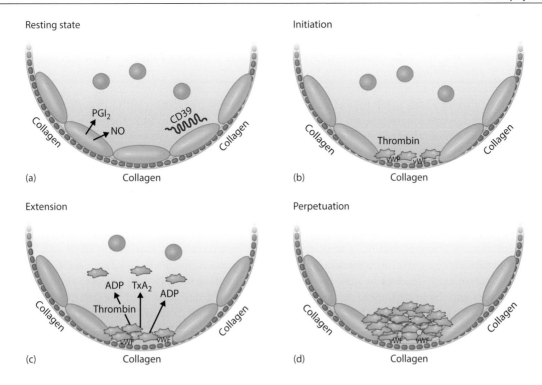

Figure 10.4 Stages in hemostasis. (a) Platelets are quiescent before vessel injury due to release of prostacyclin (PGI$_2$) and nitric oxide. (b) Initiation of platelet activation starts with binding to exposed subendothelial collagen and von Willebrand and activation of the signal pathways that lead to degranulation and initiation of the clotting cascade with generation of thrombin. (c) The platelet plug is extended as additional platelets are activated via the release of thromboxane A$_2$ (Tx A$_2$), ADP and other platelet agonists. Platelet-to-platelet aggregation is mediated primarily by activation of surface GP IIb/IIIa which binds fibrinogen. (d) A fibrin mesh perpetuates and stabilizes the platelet aggregate. (From Michelson AD, *Circulation*, 110, e489, 2004.)

monophosphate (cGMP) which regulates cGMP-dependent protein kinases, which in turn inactivate the Tx A2 receptor by phosphorylation, thus inhibiting the calcium mobilization that otherwise would be stimulated by Tx A2 binding.[11,12] Binding of endothelial prostacyclin to platelet prostacyclin receptor (a GPCR) stimulates increased cAMP production by the coupled G protein effect on adenylate cyclase and further calcium efflux via the cAMP-sensitive calcium pump. Endothelial cell ADPase enzymes degrade ADP which otherwise might bind to the purinergic platelet receptors P2Y$_{12}$ and P2Y$_1$ leading to platelet activation.

Adhesion

When the intimal of a vessel is disrupted and subendothelial collagen and vWF determinants are exposed, platelets rapidly bind to the damaged area via three different platelet receptors. The platelet receptor GP1b-IX-V complex binds to vWF; platelet GPVI and integrin α2β1 receptors bind to collagen. GPVI binding leads to activation of a tyrosine kinase cascade and calcium release. An important effect of GPVI binding to collagen is increased platelet production of Tx A2 and decreased production of inhibitory prostacyclin. The increase in Tx A2 is mediated through enzymes involved in prostaglandin synthesis

(see Figure 10.3) including cyclooxygenase (COX-1). Tx A2 produced in this early step is secreted and binds to platelet surface receptors (TPα) for Tx A2. Occupied TPα receptors are functionally coupled to a heterotrimeric Gq-protein, whose activation leads to activation of phospholipase C, calcium release and activation of protein kinase C (PKC). PLC activation and release of Ca^{++} from intracellular stores are the central events in Tx A2/TPα signalling.[13] Increased Tx A2 production and associated increases in intracellular Ca^{++} are the key early events leading to platelet activation.

Activation

The initial stimulatory signals induced by platelet adhesion trigger multiple further signal cascades that lead to the important events of platelet activation: (1) morphological changes in platelet shape, (2) release of the contents of α and dense granules, (3) rearrangement of plasma membrane phospholipids and (4) activation of GPIIb/IIIa receptors. Activation of GPIIb/IIIa is the final crucial event in platelet activation that leads to platelet aggregation and the formation of the initial platelet plug that causes primary hemostasis. The morphological changes in platelets from a discoid shape to a complex dendritic-type cell with pseudopodia involve mitochondrial hyperpolarization[14] and the increase in intracellular calcium, which stimulates interplay between microtubules and the actin filaments of the cytoskeleton. ADP released from dense granules binds to $P2Y_1$ and $P2Y_{12}$ receptors, leading to further elevation in intracellular Ca^{2+} through both inhibition of adenylate cyclase ($P2Y_{12}$) and activation of phospholipase C_β ($P2Y_1$). Dense granule serotonin binds to platelet surface serotonin receptors to provide further positive feedback. Release of α granule clotting factors also provides positive feedback via stimulation of coagulation and thrombin generation. The quiescent platelet has an asymmetric arrangement of phospholipids (phosphatidylserine and phosphatidylinositol) in the inner layer of the plasma membrane. During activation, the platelet surface exposes negatively charged aminophospholipids via floppases and scramlases[15] leading to avid binding of coagulation factors and the prothrombinase complex (FVa, FXa, FII and Ca^{2+}), which leads to thrombin generation and secondary hemostasis.[16]

Aggregation

There are an estimated 80,000 copies of GPIIb/IIIa receptors in resting platelets,[17] which are augmented via fusion with those in the α granule membrane during activation. In the resting platelet, the heterodimeric receptor is inactive in a curved conformation, with the extracellular head of the molecule containing the ligand binding site bent into a compact V shape and inaccessible. Elevation of intracellular calcium is the primary event[18] leading to a conformational change in the binding site with straightening of the head and exposure of the ligand binding site. GPIIb/IIIa binds to fibrinogen which, because fibrinogen has two ligands, one at each pole of the molecule leads to platelet aggregation. Binding of the first ligand leads to extension of the receptor molecule. Fibronectin, vWF and vitronectin are also ligands for GPIIb/IIIa; binding to vWF is important in achieving stable adhesion of platelet plugs to the damaged vessel wall. The formation of blood clot, incited by the activation of the coagulation cascade in parallel with platelet activation (in part due to release of platelet tissue factor and clotting factors stored in α granules), leads to generation of thrombin, which further stimulates platelet activation via activation of protease-activated receptors (PARs). Thrombin cleaves a portion of the extracellular domain of PAR 1 and PAR 4 to reveal a tethered ligand which occupies the receptors' binding sites leading to positive feedback signalling via GPLR pathways. Formation of fibrin monomer creates a self-assembled lattice which traps both erythrocytes and platelets into secondary aggregates ('red clot') and reinforces the initial platelet plug which becomes more stable as the coagulation cascade generates thrombin, which, acting on thrombin receptors, creates positive feedback for activation and further aggregation.

ANTIPLATELET DRUGS

Figure 10.5 is a schematic of the mechanisms of platelet activation and the sites where drugs can exert inhibition of activation either by blocking surface receptor occupation or by interfering with intracellular signal pathways. As shown in Table 10.2, there are 12 drugs that fall into 5 classes that are currently approved (United States Food and Drug Administration and/or European Medicines Agency) for management of cardiovascular diseases where platelet inhibition is beneficial. COX-1 inhibitors block the signal pathway triggered by adhesion to collagen via the GPVI receptor. Phosphodiesterase (PDE) inhibitors block elevation of intracellular calcium levels by increasing cytoplasmic levels of cAMP. Receptor antagonists for PAR-1, $P2Y_{12}$ and GPIIB/IIIa prevent stimulation mediated by receptor occupation. Although a detailed description of the pharmacologic features of each specific drug is beyond the scope of this review, each drug will be reviewed in reference to the underlying mechanism of action, accepted indications and salient features of clinical employment.

Cyclooxygenase inhibitors

ASPIRIN

ASA (aspirin) inhibits platelets by blocking prostaglandin synthesis via inactivation of COX-1. The inhibitory step is acetylation of the serine hydroxyl group of ser 529 located in the enzymatic active site near the N-terminus. This blocks arachidonic acid (AA) access to the active site of COX-1, and as platelets do not synthesize new COX-1, inhibition is irreversible. By inhibiting the first step in the conversion of AA to prostaglandins, Tx A2 synthesis is markedly reduced. Tx A2 is both an intense vasoconstrictor (it was originally identified as 'aortic rabbit aorta contracting substance'[19]) and stimulant of ADP release, which triggers platelet activation via binding to PY2 receptors. As endothelial cell production of prostacyclin, an inhibitor of platelet activation is also reduced by COX-1 inhibitors. The relatively high doses of aspirin appropriate for anti-inflammatory effects (e.g. 600 mg to treat headache) inhibit both platelet and endothelial COX-1, but the consequence of reducing endothelial production of prostacyclin is thought to diminish the cardiovascular protection afforded by aspirin. Multiple clinical trials indicate that doses above 600 mg/day are associated with higher risks for bleeding without greater protection from major adverse cardiovascular events (MACE – cardiovascular death, non-fatal MI and non-fatal ischemic stroke). That doses as low as 50–100 mg/day are clinically more effective is believed due to the ability of aspirin in the portal system to inhibit circulating platelets but not achieve systemic levels that affect endothelium elsewhere. This theory is supported by observations that low oral doses are as effective as larger IV doses for reducing platelet activity.[20] Current practice

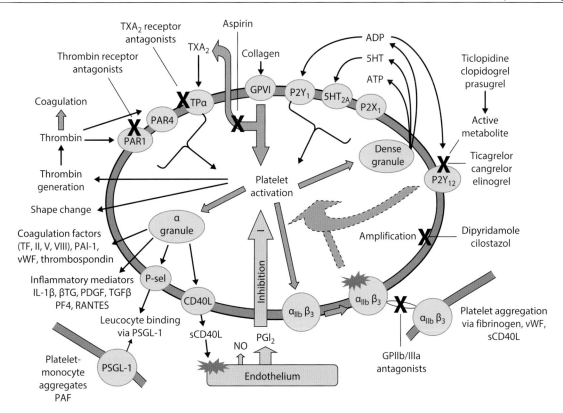

Figure 10.5 Overview of platelet activation and inhibitory drug mechanisms. Platelet activation occurs by multiple pathways and leads to shape changes, release of granules which contain ATP, serotonin (5HT) and the ADP which is particularly potent via its occupation of the purogenic receptors $P2Y_1$ and $P2Y_{12}$. Aspirin works by blocking the synthesis of thromboxane A_2 stimulated by GPVI binding to collagen and whose release outside the cell induces further stimulation via binding to the TPα receptor. Thienopyridines, ticagrelor and cangrelor block the $PY2_{12}$ receptor whose occupation by ADP leads to platelet activation. Phosphodiesterase inhibitors like dipyridamole and cilostazol prevent breakdown of cAMP which stimulates the intracellular calcium pump transport of calcium outside the cell, thus inhibiting signal amplification stimulated by other pathways. GPIIb/IIIa receptor antagonists prevent platelet aggregation induced by binding of fibrinogen and von Willebrand factor. Thrombin receptor antagonists block the stimulation induced by thrombin cleavage of the protease-activated receptors to release the receptors' internal ligand. (From Patrono C et al., *Eur Heart J*, 32, 2922, 2011.)

Table 10.2 Antiplatelet drugs.

Class	Antiplatelet drugs				
COX-1 inhibitors	ASA (aspirin)	Triflusal (Disgren)			
$P2Y_{12}$ (ADP) Receptor antagonists	Clopidogrel (Plavix)	Prasugrel (Efferent)	Ticagrelor (Brilliant)	Ticopidine (Ticlid)	Cangrelor (Kengreal)
Glycoprotein IIb/IIIa inhibitors	Abciximab (ReoPro)	Eptifibatide (Integrilin)	Tirofiban (Aggrastat)		
Phosphodiesterase inhibitors	Cilostazol (Pletal)	Dipyridamole (Persantin)			
PAR-1 antagonists	Vorapaxar (Zontivity)				

in the United States is generally to treat patients with 81 or 162 mg of ASA daily, and slightly lower doses, e.g. 75 mg, are commonly employed in other countries.

TRIFLUSAL

This COX-1 inhibitor is a salicylate compound but not a derivative of aspirin. It is not available in the United States but is available in 25 other countries in Europe, Asia and

Africa. In addition to blocking Tx A2 synthesis, it blocks PDE function thus increasing cAMP and lowers intracellular calcium levels to further inhibit activation. It is alleged to preserve endothelial prostacyclin synthesis, as well. It is recommended by the European Stroke Organization for secondary prevention of ischemic stroke in 2008.[21] Three clinical trials found triflusal to be equivalent to aspirin as secondary prevention after MI, TIA or non-disabling stroke, but with lower risk for all bleeding, as well as highly significant lower risk for intracranial hemorrhage (ICH).[22,23] A study of a vitamin K antagonist (VKA), acenocoumarol, used alone or in combination with triflusal for prevention of thromboembolic events in subjects with atrial fibrillation, found combined therapy to be superior than acenocoumarol alone, and in high-risk patients, the primary endpoint (vascular death, stroke or systemic embolism) was approximately 50% less with combined therapy.[24] A meta-analysis found that although aspirin and triflusal were comparable in efficacy, for secondary prevention in high-risk subjects, the frequency of non-hemorrhagic complications (abdominal pain, dyspepsia and peptic ulcer) was significantly higher with triflusal, but the incidence of all bleeding and intracranial bleeding was significantly lower.[25]

P2Y$_{12}$ ADP receptor antagonists

TICLOPIDINE

P2Y$_{12}$ receptors are GPCRs which bind ADP released from dense granules early in the platelet activation sequence. Via their linkage to cytoplasmic second messengers occupation leads to inactivation of adenyl cyclase (the enzyme that catalyzes synthesis of cAMP) causing intracellular calcium to rise. The first drug discovered that exerted inhibition by inactivating P2Y$_{12}$ receptors was ticlopidine (Ticlid®). Identified in 1972 during a search for new anti-inflammatory compounds, its ability to inhibit platelet aggregation was recognized soon after, but the mechanism of action was not elucidated until much later. It was initially approved in 1978 for prevention of thrombosis during extracorporeal circulation. Three trials in the 1980s showed ticlopidine to be superior to aspirin for secondary prevention after TIA and minor stroke,[26] superior to placebo for secondary prevention in patients with recent atherosclerotic stroke and superior for primary prevention of stroke and MI in subjects with intermittent claudication.[27]

Ticlopidine is a thienopyridine compound that by itself has no antiplatelet activity; platelet aggregation in vitro is not inhibited by ticlopidine. The activity of ticlopidine depends on liver metabolism and generation of a metabolite that irreversible binds to the PY$_{12}$ ADP receptor. Numerous metabolites of ticlopidine result from hepatic metabolism, but the specific metabolite responsible for inhibiting platelet aggregation has not been identified; available evidence suggests it has a short half-life and circulates at a low level.[28] In animal models of aggregation in vitro, three prior oral doses of ticlopidine are required to inhibit platelet responsiveness to ADP. The effect on platelets is irreversible as after washing platelets to remove external drug, inhibition is unchanged. The return to normal aggregation closely parallels the kinetics of bone marrow production of new platelets.[29] Although ticlopidine is a selective inhibitor of ADP-induced aggregation, it inhibits platelet activation stimulated by other agonists such as collagen and thrombin as the response to these agents

entails ADP release to amplify the effects of signals triggered by other platelet activation pathways.[30]

Ticlopidine had FDA approval to be used for secondary prevention of stroke and as adjunctive therapy with aspirin to reduce the risk of stent thrombosis and for coronary artery stents. In Canada, it is approved for reduction of risk of thrombotic stroke in patients who have experienced TIA or ischemic stroke but reserved for patients intolerant to aspirin due to its risks for life-threatening blood dyscrasias, including thrombotic thrombocytopenic purpura, neutropenia and aplastic anemia. Consequently, frequent monitoring of blood counts is advised. Ticlopidine is associated with a high risk for gastrointestinal side effects including diarrhea and nausea which occur in as many as 30% of patients. Although ticlopidine was found in many trials to be more effective than aspirin in preventing major adverse cardiovascular events (MACE), alone or in combination therapy, randomized trials have shown clopidogrel to be at least as effective and have fewer side effects.[31] Ticlopidine's use in many countries has been largely replaced by clopidogrel, but continues to be used in others due to lower cost. As of 2015, however, it is no longer sold in the United States.[32]

CLOPIDOGREL

Discovered in 1987, clopidogrel was first approved in 1997 for prevention of ischemic stroke, MI and vascular death in patients with symptomatic atherosclerosis based on the results of the landmark clopidogrel versus aspirin in patients at risk of ischemic events (CAPRIE).[33] A second, equally important trial in 2001, CURE, demonstrated that clopidogrel, in addition to aspirin, reduced atherothrombotic events in patients with ACS.[34] It is widely used either alone or in conjunction with aspirin in the management of many settings where antiplatelet therapy is indicated, including ACS, secondary prevention in patients at high risk for atherothrombotic events and after endovascular interventions.

Its pharmacologic properties are very similar to ticlopidine as it is a thienopyridine transformed by hepatic cytochrome P450 metabolism into an active metabolite which irreversibly binds to and inactivates the PY$_{12}$ receptor.[35] It is typically administered via a 300 mg loading dose followed by 75 mg daily. As opposed to ticlopidine, however, its onset of action is quicker – within 2–4 hours of a single dose inhibition of platelet activation is observed.[36] Further, although it has the associated risks for bleeding found with all antiplatelet agents, and like ticlopidine a small risk for thrombotic thrombocytopenic purpura, unlike ticlopidine, it does not induce bone marrow suppression or have significant gastrointestinal side effects.

Patients with decreased CYP2C19 hepatic enzyme activity may be poor responders and not get full benefit due to inadequate generation of the active clopidogrel metabolite. The estimated incidence of this deficiency is thought to be 2%–14% of the US population. Although increasing doses of clopidogrel may overcome this 'resistance' in heterozygotes, increased dosing in homozygotes is probably futile (see section 'Platelet function testing and drug resistance'). Genetic tests which can identify

CPY2C19 genotypes associated with decreased clopidogrel metabolism as well as increased metabolism (and thus increased risk for bleeding) are currently covered by many insurance providers in the United States including Medicare.[37] Proton pump inhibitors (e.g. omeprazole) and a few other drugs, which decrease CYP2C19 activity, should not be combined with clopidogrel. Due to its efficacy as a single agent compared to aspirin, clopidogrel is increasingly regarded as the gold standard to which new drugs are compared.

PRASUGREL

Prasugrel was approved in the United States in 2009 for reducing the risk of thrombotic cardiovascular events (including stent thrombosis) in patients with ACS undergoing percutaneous coronary intervention (PCI). Like clopidogrel, it is a thienopyridine prodrug whose active metabolite is generated by hepatic cytochrome metabolism, but prasugrel's effect on platelets is independent of CYP2C19-mediated metabolism, so far fewer patients have decreased responsiveness. Its onset of activity is faster than clopidogrel; after a 60 mg loading dose, approximately 90% of subjects demonstrate 50% inhibition of ADP-induced platelet aggregation within an hour. A mean steady-state inhibition of platelet aggregation of 70% is achieved when 10 mg daily dosing is employed after loading.

The TRITON–TIMI 38 trial compared prasugrel to clopidogrel in 16,608 subjects undergoing PCI. Subjects in both groups were loaded with the assigned ADP receptor antagonist no later than 1 hour after completing PCI and then maintained afterwards with either 75 mg clopidogrel or 10 mg prasugrel in conjunction with aspirin with follow-up for 6–15 months. MACE occurred in 12.1% of patients receiving clopidogrel versus 9.9% of patients receiving prasugrel (p < 0.001). Significant reductions were observed in the prasugrel group for rates of myocardial infarction (9.7% for clopidogrel vs. 7.4% for prasugrel, p < 0.001), urgent target-vessel revascularization (3.7% vs. 2.5%, p < 0.001) and stent thrombosis (2.4% vs. 1.1%, p < 0.001). Major bleeding, however, was observed in 2.4% of the prasugrel group compared to 1.8% of the clopidogrel group (odds ratio 1.32, p = 0.03). Life-threatening bleeding was also greater with prasugrel (1.4% vs. 0.9%) as was non-fatal bleeding (1.1%, p = 0.23) and fatal bleeding (0.4% vs. 0.1%, p = 0.002). ICH occurred in 3% of both groups. Although few patients overall underwent coronary artery bypass, in those who did perioperative bleeding was more severe with prasugrel. More patients treated with prasugrel discontinued treatment (2.5% vs. clopidogrel 1.4%). Death from combined cardiovascular causes and bleeding was virtually identical: 2.4% with clopidogrel and 2.2% with prasugrel. Other pertinent findings were that in subjects with a history of TIA or stroke <3 months before PCI, the overall risk for stroke with prasugrel was 6.5% of which 2.3% were due to ICH; in contrast only 1.2% treated with clopidogrel had strokes, none due to ICH. There was no increased risk for stroke or ICH in subjects without prior cerebrovascular symptoms. Diabetic subjects and those with a history of MI were two subgroups where prasugrel's better efficacy compared to clopidogrel was prominent.[38]

The TRILOGY ACS trial enrolled a total of 9326 subjects (77.3% <75 years old) with UA or non-ST elevation MI (NSTEMI) who were not candidates for revascularization. Subjects were randomized to be treated with either clopidogrel or prasugrel, both combined with low-dose aspirin. Prasugrel dosage was reduced to 5 mg daily in subjects >75 years of age or who weighed less than 60 kg. At a median follow-up of 17 months, the primary endpoint, MACE, for subjects under the age of 75 years occurred in 13.9% of the prasugrel group and 16.0% of the clopidogrel (odds ratio 0.91, p = 0.21). Rates of bleeding including severe and intracranial bleeding were similar in the two treatment groups. There was no significant between-group difference in the frequency of non-hemorrhagic serious adverse events. Although the overall 13% decrease in MACE associated with prasugrel therapy did not achieve statistical significance, the Kaplan–Meier plot showed divergence in favour of prasugrel therapy after 1 year in the number of events.[39]

Comparing the results of TRITON–TIMI 38 to TRILOGY ACS is a good illustration of how sometimes the paradigmatic problem in anticoagulation and antiplatelet therapy – more effective drugs have higher risks for bleeding – may sometimes be improved upon. When dosing was adjusted to 5 mg daily based on age and weight in TRILOGY ACS, bleeding risks decreased for prasugrel and were essentially identical to clopidogrel. Although the lower rate of MACE observed in TRILOGY ACS was not significant, if followed for longer the divergence in the incidence of MACE might have become statistically significant. The results of the TRILOGY TIMI 38 study led the FDA to advise in the package insert (black box warning) to not use prasugrel when urgent CABG is likely or in patients with a history of stroke or TIA. Although in TRITON–TIMI 38 a 6% reduction in risk for MACE was found in subjects ≥75 with prasugrel, the package insert states: *in patients ≥75 years of age prasugrel is generally not recommended, except in high-risk patients (diabetes or prior MI) where its use may be considered.*

TICAGRELOR

Ticagrelor was approved in 2010 in Europe and 2011 by the FDA for reducing the risk for thrombotic cardiovascular events and coronary stent thrombosis in the setting of ACS. The FDA package insert states: *maintenance doses of aspirin above 100 mg reduce the effectiveness … and should be avoided.* Ticagrelor is a nucleoside analog whose structure is similar to adenosine. Unlike thienopyridines, it binds reversible to a different location in the $PY2_{12}$ receptor and does not require metabolism to be active. Both ticagrelor and its main metabolite are equally effective. As it is rapidly absorbed and does not require metabolic activation, after a single dose maximum platelet inhibition is reached by 2 hours (much quicker than clopidogrel) and maintained for at least 8 hours. A loading dose of 180 mg followed by 90 mg twice daily dosing for maintenance is standard.

Despite a half-life of 7–12 hours for both ticagrelor and its main active metabolite, for unclear reasons (possibly high binding affinity), it still takes several days for platelet aggregation to return to normal after stopping ticagrelor.[40]

Ticgrelor's main side effects are different than the thienopyridines: dyspnea and bradycardic effects on heart rate. Dyspnea was reported in 12%–24% of subjects in clinical trials. The dyspnea tends to be mild and self-limiting, and the risk for dyspnea is not associated with congestive heart failure (CHF), obstructive pulmonary disease or asthma.[41] In an early study, 4.9% of subjects receiving 180 mg doses developed ventricular pauses longer than 2.5 seconds compared to 0.3% of subjects on clopidogrel. Both the development of dyspnea and ventricular pause have been attributed by some to blockage of erythrocyte uptake of adenosine, thus increasing circulating adenosine.[42] Adenosine infusions are known to induce SA nodal pauses. The effects of adenosine administration in canines and healthy volunteers are potentiated by ticagrelor and reversed with the adenosine inhibitor theophylline.[40,43]

The PLATO trial compared dual therapy with aspirin using ticagrelor (90 mg twice daily) or clopidogrel (75 mg daily) after loading doses to treat 13,408 subjects with ACS in whom PCI was planned before randomization, with follow-up for 1 year. MACE (including stent thrombosis) occurred in 9.0% of subjects treated with ticagrelor and 10.7 of the clopidogrel group (odds ratio 0.84, $p = 0.0025$). Major bleeding rates were nearly identical, 11.6% and 11.5%, but major bleeding when CABG was performed before hospital discharge was lower with ticagrelor. Similar results were observed when subjects who did not undergo PCI were added to the analysis. All-cause mortality was reduced 20% with ticagrelor representing a 1.1% absolute reduction in risk for death which was thought possibly to be a result of higher adenosine levels increasing microvascular cardiac perfusion. Dyspnea was noted in 13.9% of the ticagrelor group and 8% of the clopidogrel group – a problem discussed later in more detail. With the exception of subjects enrolled in North America who had a non-significant increased risk for MACE with ticagrelor (11.1% vs. 9.1%), MACE was lower with ticagrelor in all other subgroups except subjects without troponin 1 elevation. The higher rate of MACE in North American subjects was speculatively attributed to American tendencies to employ high (>100 mg) aspirin doses compared to the rest of the world, with possibly greater inhibition of endothelium release of prostacyclin compared to low doses of aspirin.[44]

In the Pegasus–TIMI 54 trial, 21,162 subjects with a history of previous MI 1–3 years before study enrollment were randomized to receive dual therapy with aspirin combined either with placebo, 60 mg ticagrelor twice daily or 90 mg ticagrelor twice daily.[45] The incidence of major bleeding was significantly higher ($p < 0.001$) with both doses of ticagrelor (2.3% and 2.6%) compared to placebo (1.06%). At 3 years, Kaplan–Meier rates of MACE were 7.85% with the 60 mg dose and 7.77% with 90 mg, compared to 9.04% with placebo ($p \leq 0.008$). Although major bleeding was higher in this study with ticagrelor,

it was compared to placebo plus aspirin, not clopidogrel plus aspirin. It appears from these two trials that when low-dose aspirin is employed in dual therapy, compared to clopidogrel, ticagrelor leads to a modest reduction in risk for MACE without an associated significant increase in major bleeding. Of note, a recent European trial compared in 405 subjects the risk for major bleeding when dual therapy with ticagrelor/aspirin or clopidogrel aspirin was stopped before CABG. When dual therapy was stopped 5 or more days in advance of CABG, major bleeding rates from surgery were very similar, but if stopped less than 24 hours before surgery, major bleeding was more frequent with ticagrelor (41.0% vs. 21.7%, $p = 0.063$).[46]

CANGRELOR

Cangrelor is currently the only intravenous PY212 receptor antagonist whose effect is achieved within 2 minutes of a bolus loading. It is a modified ATP derivative that reversibly binds to the ADP binding site without requiring metabolic activation. Platelet inhibition is gone within 1 hour of stopping infusion as cangrelor is rapidly deactivated by dephosphorylation to an inactive metabolite with an elimination half-life of 3–6 minutes. These pharmacodynamics features make cangrelor very attractive for antiplatelet therapy in the setting of acute MI and PCI interventions.

Based on the pivotal Champion Phoenix trial I[47] was approved by the US FDA in 2015 as *an adjunct to PCI for reducing the risk of periprocedural MI, repeat coronary revascularization and stent thrombosis who are not being treated with a P2Y$_{12}$ platelet inhibitor and are not being given a glycoprotein IIb/IIIa inhibitor.* Guidelines for administration recommend an initial 30 µg/kg IV bolus followed by 4 µg/kg/min infusion for at least 2 hours.

The Champion Phoenix trial enrolled 11,145 patients scheduled for PCI who were treated either with a loading dose of clopidogrel (300 or 600 mg per investigator's discretion) or bolus and infusion therapy with cangrelor. Fifty-six percent of the subjects had stable angina, not ACS. All subjects also received aspirin and an anticoagulant (unfractionated heparin [UH], fondaparinux, low-molecular-weight heparin or bivalirudin at the discretion of the investigator). Glycoprotein IIb/IIIa inhibitors were only allowed as rescue therapy. The primary efficacy endpoint was the composite of death, MI, stent thrombosis and ischemia-driven revascularization (IDR) (such as CABG) at 48 hours after randomization. The primary safety endpoint was severe bleeding at 48 hours. Those randomized to cangrelor were loaded with clopidogrel at the conclusion of the PCI procedure and maintained on clopidogrel for at least 48 hours. The incidence of the composite endpoint was 4.7% with cangrelor and 5.9% with clopidogrel (odds ratio 0.78, $p = 0.005$). Stent thrombosis was 0.8% with cangrelor and 1.4% with clopidogrel (odds ratio 0.62, $p = 0.01$). Overall bleeding was mostly minor in both groups with severe bleeding observed in 0.16% of the cangrelor group and 0.11% of the clopidogrel group (odds ratio 1.5, $p = 0.44$).[48] The trial design has been criticized on several grounds, the most important being the following: (1) the 300 mg clopidogrel loading dose employed in approximately one-fourth of the clopidogrel group is significantly inferior to 600 mg and inconsistent with current guidelines for PCI, and (2) 37% of the clopidogrel group were loaded during or after PCI, making the effects of clopidogrel suboptimal during PCI and and/or immediately afterwards. Of note, although two previous trials comparing cangrelor to clopidogrel as an adjunct to PCI failed to show superiority, they did show comparable efficacy. Cangrelor's rapid onset and rapid washout make it an attractive choice for periprocedural inhibition of platelet aggregation.

An increased incidence of dyspnea has been observed with the reversible $P2Y_{12}$ inhibitors compared to either placebo or clopidogrel. With ticagrelor the increase frequency of dyspnea in two larger trials ranged from 64% to 146%,[42,49] and in one small study with 200 subjects, dyspnea was reported in 10%–20% of patients depending on dose, but not at all in the clopidogrel arm. In the PLATO trial, dyspnea led to discontinuation in 0.9% of subjects on ticagrelor and 0.1% of the clopidogrel group.[41] Although dyspnea is less common with cangrelor, ranging from 1% to 1.9% in four reported trials, compared to controls, the incidence is two- to fourfold higher and statistically significant[48,50,51] compared to controls. Elinogrel is another reversible inhibitor of $P2Y_{12}$ whose development was stopped due to hepatotoxicity and dyspnea. Its structure is quite different from ticagrelor and cangrelor and is not an adenosine analog. It was observed to induce dyspnea in 12.3% of subjects compared to 3.8% of controls. Although the dyspnea observed in most subjects was not judged severe, it creates concern as many patients with atherosclerotic vascular disease have pulmonary disease. Dyspnea is seen an angina equivalent, particularly in diabetics, and its development may lead to additional investigations including coronary angiography. Although it has been proposed that dyspnea associated with ticagrelor was related to direct adenosine-like effects or possibly to inhibition of erythrocyte adenosine uptake, the observations with elinogrel make this unlikely. One speculation is that repeated reversible occupation of $P2Y_{12}$ stresses and destroys platelets leading to pulmonary sequestration and lung injury similar to transfusion-related acute lung injury.[49]

Glycoprotein IIb/IIIa inhibitors

In quiescent platelets, this heterodimeric receptor is incapable of binding to its ligands, fibrinogen, fibrin and vWF. Stimulation of the conformational change from inactive form to the active receptor capable of binding fibrinogen is the key event leading to platelet aggregation and secondary hemostasis. Agonists in the activation of GPIIb/IIIa include ADP, epinephrine, thrombin and collagen, making this receptor an obvious and attractive target for drug development. Development of GPIIb/IIIa inhibitors was facilitated by investigations of the rare autosomal recessive bleeding disorder Glanzmann's thrombasthenia, in which platelets lack GPIIb/IIIa receptors.[52]

The three currently available drugs, abciximab, eptifibatide and tirofiban, act to inhibit GPIIb/IIIa receptor–induced aggregation, specifically binding to the receptor. They are all administered intravenously and have many similarities in pharmacodynamics and are almost exclusively used in the setting of PCI. They have similar efficacy profiles and similar risks – hemorrhage and therapy-induced thrombocytopenia. Thrombocytopenia, although most common with abciximab, is found with all three and is thought to be related to exposure of neoantigens on the GPIIb/IIIa molecule after drug binding leads to induction of autoantibodies. Thrombocytopenia, when it does develop, resolves more rapidly in a few days with the reversible inhibitors but may persist for 2 weeks with abciximab. If thrombocytopenia develops with one GPIIb/IIIa inhibitor, another may be employed, but cross-reactivity may be as high as 15%.[53–57]

All three are given as an initial intravenous bolus or boluses, followed by infusion, and have a rapid onset of activity. Activity can be measured by ADP-stimulated platelet aggregation assays ex vivo or by prolongation of bleeding time. The clinical trials evaluating the three drugs use them as adjuncts to anticoagulants or other antiplatelet agents (usually both) in two settings: (1) medical management of patients with ACS including UA, NSTEMI and STEMI or (2) as adjuncts to periprocedural anticoagulation and antiplatelet therapy during PCIs such as percutaneous transluminal coronary angioplasty (PTCA) or stenting. As UA and NSTEMI are often indistinguishable at presentation, current guidelines have combined the two terms: NSTE-ACS. GPIIb/IIIa inhibitors are thought to be an effective adjunct in primary stenting for STEMI and NSTE-ACS and are widely used in North America and Europe in that setting.

In some trials, data for the outcomes in both situations – medical management or PCI – were gathered, as the trials enrolled NSTE-ACS subjects in whom coronary angiography was anticipated if the subject did not improve. In all these studies, the focus was on the ability of the chosen treatment regimen to reduce composite risk, MACE, including death, MI, stent thrombosis, ongoing ischemia, revascularization, repeat angiography and/or CABG. Although MACE endpoints were employed in virtually all studies, many minor variations in the exact combinations varied and are pointed out in the following discussion when appropriate.

In most of these large clinical trials, patients were administered anticoagulants and/or antiplatelet agents 'upstream' of anticipated angiography. Typically background aspirin and heparin anticoagulation was started before angiography, but when GPIIb/IIIa inhibitors were started varied between studies. Often subjects had GPIIb/IIIa inhibition started several hours or even days before angiography. In others, initiation of GPIIb/IIIa inhibition was started during angiography. GPIIb/IIIa receptor inhibition as an adjunct to medical management without

PCI tended to be limited to 2–4 days, but with PCI was continued for a few hours in some or ≥24 hours in others. In most studies, congruent with standard current practice, aspirin and/or clopidogrel therapy was administered on a long-term basis after PCI or hospital discharge. The timing with which clopidogrel was started in relation to PCI – before (upstream) of planned PCI or only after PCI and stopping GPIIb/IIIa inhibition (downstream) varied between studies. Upstream administration of clopidogrel before PCI combined with GPIIb/IIIa inhibitor therapy has only recently been studied in a small number of influential trials. The overall pattern of results in these studies is that when treatment arms containing a GPIIb/IIIa inhibitor demonstrated better efficacy in preventing MACE, bleeding events tended to be increased. A large proportion of the serious or major bleeding events in these trials were observed in the relatively small numbers of subjects requiring CABG; consequently in most trials, major or serious bleeding rates were small, and differences in overall bleeding rates were attributable mostly to differences in rates of minor hemorrhage.

ABCIXIMAB

Abciximab was the first GPIIb/IIa receptor inhibitor to be approved by the FDA (1997). It is the Fab fragment of a chimeric mouse–human monoclonal antibody which binds to the GPIIb/IIIa receptor and interferes with large molecules entering the binding site. It thus blocks the final event in platelet aggregation induced by fibrinogen binding to the GPIIb/IIIa receptor as well as adhesion to vWF and vitronectin receptors found on platelets and vessel wall endothelium. It also binds to Mac-1 receptors on monocytes and neutrophils, leading to impaired monocyte function in vitro. Like cangrelor and the two other GPIIb/IIIa inhibitors, abciximab is not a prodrug, so that administration via IV bolus loading and infusion leads to marked inhibition of platelet activity within minutes. Two hours after administration of high-dose boluses (e.g. 0.3 mg/kg), more than 80% of platelet GPIIb/IIIa receptors are blocked and bleeding time increases from 5 to over 30 minutes with almost complete abolition of ex vivo platelet aggregation induced by 20 µM ADP. After discontinuing infusion, bleeding time remains significantly prolonged for 24 hours or longer, and in vitro tests show inhibited platelet responses to ADP for up to 5 days. The persistent effect is a consequence of prolonged platelet receptor binding.

Based on several clinical trials, the FDA approved abciximab as an adjunct to PCI to prevent ischemic complications during and after PCI and to treat patients with UA when PCI is planned within 24 hours. In the FDA trials, both heparin and aspirin were employed for all PCI procedures with monitoring of heparin by activated partial thromboplastin time (aPTT) or activated clotting time (ACT) testing. The three key trials leading to approval were the EPIC, EPILOG and CAPTURE studies of patients undergoing PCI. In EPIC, subjects received either (1) bolus and infusion of placebo, (2) bolus of abciximab and infusion of placebo or (3) abciximab bolus and abciximab infusion. The primary endpoint was a 30-day composite of death from any cause, non-fatal MI, CABG, coronary stenting due to procedural failure or aortic balloon pump placement to manage cardiac ischemia. Compared to placebo bolus/infusion, abciximab bolus/infusion reduced the primary endpoint incidence 35% (from 12.8% to 8.3%, p = 0.008); abciximab bolus alone reduced the primary endpoint 10% (12.8% vs. 11.5%, p = 0.43). Major bleeding was more common in the group receiving both abciximab bolus and infusion (14%) than either the abciximab bolus alone (11%) or placebo (7%).[58] The EPILOG study had three treatment arms: (1) placebo bolus/infusion combined with standard heparin dosing (1000 units/kg loading dose plus repeated doses to keep ACT > 300 seconds), (2) abciximab bolus/infusion combined with standard heparin dosing and (3) abciximab bolus/infusion combined with low-dose heparin (700 units/kg loading dose + repeated doses to keep ACT > 200 seconds). The study was terminated early, as subjects in the placebo arm experienced an event rate of 11.7%, compared to 5.2% and 5.4% in the standard- and low-dose heparin groups. There was no significant difference in major bleeding between groups, although minor bleeding was more frequent in subjects receiving abciximab and standard-dose heparin.[59] The CAPTURE trial studied refractory UA patients randomized to receive either placebo bolus/infusion or bolus/infusion therapy with abciximab. It was stopped early due to a higher incidence of 30-day ischemic events in the placebo arm (15.9% vs. 11.3%, p = 0.012) with most of the difference due to lower MI rates before (2.1% vs. 0.6%, p = 0.029) and during the PCI procedure (2.6% vs. 5.5%, p = 0.009). Major bleeding occurred more often with abciximab than placebo (1.9% vs. 3.8%, p = 0.043). All three studies showed the same pattern, fewer periprocedural ischemic complications associated with an increased risk for bleeding with abciximab compared to placebo. The use of a low-dose heparin regimen compared to standard dosing of heparin decreased both minor and major bleeding in the EPILOG trial, but the effect of a lower heparin dose on major bleeding did not reach statistical significance.

TIROFIBAN

Tirofiban was approved by the FDA in 1998. It was one of the first drugs whose development can be traced to pharmacophore-based virtual screening in which libraries of small molecules have their binding affinity to a protein active assessed by purely computational methods. Unlike abciximab, it only binds to GPIIb/IIIa, but with lower affinity making it relatively short acting. Its plasma half-life is approximately 2 hours, but the platelet-binding half-life is very short, such that its effects on platelet function dissipate within 4–8 hours. When first employed in clinical trials, it was administered as a 0.4 µg/kg/min loading dose infused over 30 minutes (12 µg/kg total) followed by 0.1 µg/kg/min. The most important of the trials leading to FDA approval were the PRISM and PRISM-PLUS[60–62] trials. In PRISM-PLUS, 1915 subjects with NSTE-ACS were randomized to either tirofiban alone, tirofiban plus UH or UH alone on a background of daily aspirin. Infusions were started 48 hours upstream of planned angiography.

Approximately 90% of subjects underwent angiography and 30% had PTA or atherectomy. The tirofiban arm had a much lower incidence of MACE and was stopped early. At 7 days, the incidence of the composite MACE endpoint was significantly lower, with heparin plus tirofiban, compared to heparin alone (12.9% vs. 17.9%, p = 0.004) representing a 32% risk reduction, and similar benefit observed at 1 and 6 months. Major bleeding was 3.0% in the heparin group and 4.0% with heparin plus tirofiban (p = 0.34).

The FDA approved tirofiban in 1998 using the dose regimen employed in the PRISM-PLUS trial for medical management of ACS and for PTCA and coronary atherectomy. Subsequently, it was compared head to head with abciximab in the TARGET trial.[63] In this coronary stent trial, both aspirin and clopidogrel were administered upstream of angiography and stenting with the loading dose for tirofiban increased to 10 µg/kg and infusion rate increased to 0.15 µg/kg/min. The incidence of the composite endpoint was significantly higher with tirofiban than abciximab (6.9% and 5.4%, respectively, p = 0.04). Ex vivo measurement of platelet inhibition induced by the two drug regimens in the TARGET trial also showed tirofiban to be less effective than abciximab (62% vs. 92% inhibition of platelet aggregation). This led to a marked decrease in clinical use and the sale of the drug by Merck to another company and further changes in ownership through 2006, when it was acquired by Medicure.

Subsequently, three more trials (ACUITY, MULTI-STRATEGY and TENACITY) were carried out comparing a higher-dose tirofiban regimen (loading dose of 25 µg/kg then 0.15 µg/mL infusion) to either abciximab or eptifibatide in PCI – some of these studies included treatment arms with upstream administration of clopidogrel before PCI. The overall results showed equivalence to abciximab and eptifibatide, but with significantly higher rates of thrombocytopenia with abciximab. A recent meta-analysis of 31 trials with 20,006 patients showed similar efficacy for tirofiban compared to abciximab in management of ACS and as an adjunct to PCI.[64,65]

In 2013, the higher-dose loading regimen for tirofiban was approved by the FDA. Probably in response to the result of trials using the higher doses, the use of has increased and worldwide it has become the most commonly employed GPIIb/IIIa inhibitor.

EPTIFIBATIDE

Eptifibatide is a heptapeptide derived from a protein found in the venom of the pygmy rattle snake. It is approved by the FDA for medical management of ACS and as an adjunct during PCI. It binds reversibly to GP IIb/IIIa and has a plasma elimination half-life of approximately 2.5 hours. Recommended dosing is to initially load with two bolus doses (180 µg/kg) 10 minutes apart followed by infusion of 2 µg/kg/min. With this regimen, inhibition of ex vivo ADP-stimulated aggregation is >90% and bleeding time is increased more than fivefold. Inhibition of platelet aggregation falls to less than 50% 4 hours after stopping infusion; bleeding times remain elevated for more than 6 hours.[66]

With renal impairment (GFR < 50 mL/min), the infusion dose should be decreased to 1 µg/kg/min.

The multinational PURSUIT trial was the primary study leading to FDA approval. Enrolled subjects had NSTE-ACS and were treated on a background of aspirin (80–325 mg) and heparin, administered as a loading dose of 5000 units and then infused at rate adjusted to maintain the aPTT between 50–70 seconds. Initially, two dose regimens for eptifibatide after 180 µg/kg bolus administration (1.3 vs. 2.0 µg/kg/h) were compared to placebo, but the lower infusion dose after interim analysis showed no difference in bleeding and was discontinued early in the trial. Medically managed subjects could be treated for 72 hours, until hospital discharge or until CABG was performed, whichever occurred first. Subjects undergoing PCI could be treated up to 96 hours, but only approximately 25% of subjects had PCI and only half of PCI patients had stents implanted. The primary outcome was a composite of death and non-fatal MI in 30 days. A total of 10,948 patients were enrolled. The incidence of the primary endpoint was 14.2% in the eptifibatide group and 15.7% in the placebo group (p = 0.04). Men had greater risk reduction (odds ratio 0.8) compared to women (odds ratio 1.11). Overall bleeding was higher in the eptifibatide group, with moderate or severe bleeding occurring in 12.8% on eptifibatide versus 9.9% with placebo (p < 0.001), most of which was related to CABG.[67]

The ESPRIT trial employed the same dose regimen employed in PURSUIT but was aimed at 2064 patients undergoing PCI with intended stenting. Subjects were treated with aspirin and loaded with clopidogrel or ticlopidine prior to stenting. The primary composite outcome was incidence at 30 days of the death, MI, target vessel revascularization or bailout GPIIb/IIIa therapy within 48 hours of PCI. The study was stopped early for efficacy. The primary endpoint was 6.6% with eptifibatide and 10.5% with placebo (p = 0.0015; major bleeding was higher with eptifibatide, 1.3% vs. 0.4%, p = 0.027). Follow-up at 1 year showed maintenance of the benefit; the incidence of the composite endpoint was 22.1% with placebo and 17.5% with eptifibatide.[68]

CURRENT EMPLOYMENT OF GPIIb/IIa INHIBITORS

The 2012 American College of Cardiology/American Heart Association guidelines for UA/NSTEMI recommend that when initial conservative management is adopted but recurrent ischemia, heart failure or dangerous arrhythmia develops, either a $P2Y_{12}$ inhibitor or a GPIIb/IIIa inhibitor should be administered with aspirin. These are patients expected to undergo coronary catheterization and if feasible PCI. In that setting, eptifibatide or tirofiban may be started in advance of angiography, whereas the recommendation is for abciximab to be started only during PCI. All three drugs are equally recommended as they are regarded as similar in efficacy and the risks of bleeding.[69]

The guidelines regard GPIIb/IIIa inhibitors as effective adjuncts to primary PCI for STEMI or NSTE-ACS when UH has been started and regardless of whether pretreatment with clopidogrel has been instituted. When clopidogrel has not been started, the level of evidence supporting GPIIb/IIIa therapy is considered level A, as opposed to the level C designation of the evidence supporting the use of GPIIb/IIIa inhibitors when clopidogrel has been administered before PCI. The relative benefit of GPIIb/IIIa receptor blockade is greater when clopidogrel has not yet been started. In STEMI patients, both abciximab and eptifibatide provide similar outcomes. The presence of either a large clot burden or evidence for large anterior MI is thought to increase the benefit of adjunctive GPIIb/IIIa inhibition.[70-72]

The GPIIb/IIIa inhibitors have been used off label in North America to provide bridging antiplatelet inhibition during the 2–4 hour interval between loading an oral ADP inhibitor (e.g. clopidogrel or prasugrel) and achieving near-maximum ADP receptor blockade. The use of GPIIb/IIIa inhibitors for upstream management of SGTEMI patients is considered reasonable by current ACC/AHA guidelines, for example, during transport to an emergency department or PCI centre.[73]

Current American guidelines do not, however, recommend upstream GPIIb/IIIa inhibitors for NSTE-ACS in patients at low risk for ischemic events and at high risk for bleeding if already treated with aspirin and a $P2Y_{12}$ inhibitor. Current European guidelines for NSTE-ACS only recommend GPIIb/IIIa inhibitors as bailout therapy and not upstream of angiography. In STEMI patients, GPIIb/IIIa inhibition can be considered for upstream use for PCI in high-risk patients being transferred to PCI centres or as bailout when evidence for thrombotic complications is present.[74]

The use of GPIIIa/IIb inhibitors has declined in recent years due to several influences including (1) the results of the HORIZONS-AMI trial which showed that in STEMI, bivalirudin alone had better efficacy in reducing MACE and less bleeding than heparin plus a GPIIb/IIIa inhibitor[75] and (2) the newer $PY2_{12}$ inhibitors prasugrel and ticagrelor are more potent than clopidogrel and faster in onset. Thus, during or immediately after PCI, oral $P2Y_{12}$ inhibitors may be started without a bridge. The use of GPIIb/IIIa inhibitors is appropriate to bridge the interval (2–8 hours, depending on which $P2Y_{12}$ inhibitor is employed) between administration and achievement of maximum platelet inhibition. It is likely that cangrelor, the new intravenous $P2Y_{12}$ inhibitor, will increasingly impact the use of intravenous GPIIb/IIIa inhibitors, as it is just as fast in onset but more rapidly reversible than any of the other three drugs, and can also be used as a bridge until oral $P2Y_{12}$ inhibitors reach effective levels.

PAR-1 ANTAGONISTS

PAR receptor activators are proteases that cleave the receptor to expose a ligand moiety that binds to an active receptor that is part of the same molecule leading to signal transduction. The most important PAR on platelets is PAR-1. The signal pathway stimulated by PAR-1 cleavage by thrombin is downstream from the Tx A2, $P2Y_{12}$ and GPIIb/IIIa receptor signal pathways. There is a theoretical advantage to using PAR-1 receptor antagonism to prevent thrombotic complications as, if used without upstream

inhibitors like aspirin or thienopyridines, primary hemostasis via binding of platelets to the injured vessel wall is not necessarily inhibited, thus potentially decreasing the risk for bleeding. Only one antagonist, vorapaxar, has FDA approval to decrease the risk of thrombotic cardiovascular events in patients with a history of MI or with peripheral arterial disease (PAD). It is contraindicated in patients with a history of TIA or stroke due to increased risks for cerebral hemorrhage. It does not inhibit platelet aggregation induced by ADP, collagen or thromboxane. Another compound, atopaxar, has been evaluated in phase 2 clinical trials but is not approved.[76]

Zorapaxar is primarily metabolized by hepatic metabolism via CYP3A4-dependent pathways. Inhibitors of CYP3A4 (e.g. ketoconazole) increase exposure to the drug and should be avoided. Similarly, inducers (e.g. rifampin) of CYP3A4 lower plasma levels. With normal dosing of one 2.08 mg tablet daily, >80% inhibition of platelet activity of thrombin-induced aggregation in vitro is achieved within 1 week. Despite being a reversible antagonist, due to a prolonged effective half-life of 3–4 days and terminal half-life of 8 days, continued inhibition of thrombin-induced aggregation >50% is seen up to 4 weeks, making zorapaxar the longest-acting platelet inhibitor currently marketed.[76]

In the TRACER-ACS study, subjects with NSTE-ACS were randomized to receive aspirin and clopidogrel combined with either a placebo or zorapaxar. The composite endpoint was cardiovascular death, MI, CVA, recurrent ischemia and urgent revascularization. In both groups, 87% of subjects received aspirin and clopidogrel, 88% of each group had coronary angiography, and equivalent numbers underwent PCI. With a median follow-up of 502 days, life table analysis showed the risk of the primary endpoint at 2 years was 19.9% with placebo versus 18.5% with vorapaxar (p = 0.07); the risk for a composite endpoint of cardiovascular death, MI or stroke was 16.4% with placebo versus 14.7 with vorapaxar (p = 0.02). Almost all the differences in the rates of thrombotic complications were due to a decreased risk for MI, not the other endpoints. Moderate or severe bleeding occurred in 5.2% of the placebo group versus 7.2% in the vorapaxar group – ICH was markedly increased with vorapaxar compared to control: 1.1% versus 0.2% (p < 0.0001).[77]

The TRA 2P-TIMI 50 trial was a secondary prevention trial for subjects with a history of MI within 1 year of enrollment – subjects with a history of previous TIA or stroke were excluded. Its composite endpoint was cardiovascular death, MI or stroke. Subjects were allowed concomitant treatment with aspirin alone or a thienopyridine alone or both. Vorapaxar significantly reduced the composite endpoint when compared to placebo regardless of planned thienopyridine therapy (planned thienopyridine odds ratio 0.80, p < 0.001; no planned thienopyridine odds ratio 0.75, p = 0.011). Moderate or severe bleeding risk was increased with vorapaxar and was not significantly altered by planned thienopyridine use (odds ratio 1.50, p < 0.001; no planned HR 1.90, p = 0.009).[78]

Phosphodiesterase inhibitors

Inhibition of platelet aggregation can be mediated either by blockade of surface receptors (e.g. P2Y$_{12}$) or by interference with intracellular signalling pathway. While receptor antagonism may be more specific, interference with cytoplasmic signal pathways may induce broader effects that suppress activation independent of the initial stimulus. Cytoplasmic signal inhibition may result either from interference with second messengers or by augmenting the action of the physiologic inhibitors that act on adenylyl and guanylyl cyclases to increase intracellular cAMP and cGMP. Both cAMP and cGMP are critical second messengers regulating platelet physiology. Elevation of cyclic nucleotides blocks cytosol elevation of Ca^{++} and activates protein kinases whose phosphorylation of specific substrates interferes with the stimulatory signals generated by phospholipase C and PKC. Elevation of intracellular cyclic nucleotide levels interferes with all known platelet activation pathways and blocks cytoskeletal rearrangement, GPIIb/IIIa activation, degranulation and expression of proinflammatory mediators.[79,80]

PDEs catalyse hydrolysis of cAMP and cGMP and thus regulation of PDE directly affects the amplitude and duration of cyclic nucleotide signalling.[81] More than 60 isoforms of PDEs in mammalian tissues have been identified, grouped into 11 families (PDE1-PDE11) based on structure, kinetics, substrate specificity and sensitivity to inhibitors. The three isoforms found in platelets, PDE1, 2 and 3, have different substrate affinities. PDE2 degrades cAMP and GMP equally, PDE5 exclusively hydrolyses cGMP, and PDE3 is capable of hydrolyzing both cyclic nucleotides but has a much higher affinity for cGMP, so much so that cGMP may competitively inhibit cAMP breakdown by PDE3, thus drugs that activate guanylyl cyclase may indirectly inhibit platelets and thus potentiate the effects of adenylyl cyclase activation, e.g. adenosine.[82] Of note, the predominant PDE3 isoform, PDE3A, is highly expressed in both myocardium and vascular smooth muscle.[83]

DIPYRIDAMOLE

Dipyridamole was initially introduced into clinical practice as a treatment for angina in 1961, but its ability to inhibit thrombosis and platelet aggregation was recognized soon after based on animal studies of its impact on experimentally induced thrombosis.[84] It is an inhibitor of platelet activation via three biochemical effects: (1) inhibition of both PDE3 and PDE5 leading to increased cytoplasmic cAMP and cGMP and thus decreased intracellular levels of Ca^{++}; (2) its blockage of adenosine uptake by platelets, endothelial cells and erythrocytes increases local extracellular adenosine levels and thus occupancy of the platelet adenosine receptor (tPA) which increases cAMP levels and cGMP levels which suppress intracellular calcium mobilization and GPCR signal pathways involving kinases; and (3) due to its antioxidant activity (dipyridamole is more potent antioxidant than ascorbic acid or probucol), it scavenges free radicals that inactivate cyclooxygenase, thus enhancing prostacyclin synthesis.[85-87] Of the three effects, the first two are thought to be more significant and are responsible for dipyridamole's potent smooth muscle relaxant and vasodilator properties.

The effect of dipyridamole on adenosine may be as important as its inhibition of PDEs. Adenosine is released by tissues in the extracellular space due to breakdown of ATP during ischemia or by erythrocytes stressed by elevated shear forces. Erythrocytes also avidly take up adenosine to keep plasma levels low. Dipyridamole's inhibition of adenosine reuptake is concentration dependent, with near-complete inhibition of uptake achieved at 1 µM in whole blood, comparable to the levels achieved with standard oral regimens (0.5–0.6 µM).[88,89] Of note, dipyridamole inhibits platelet aggregation in whole blood based by aggregometry, but much less or not at all in in vitro or ex vivo; this difference is attributed to the influence of adenosine release from erythrocytes in whole blood.[90] It is currently employed in three ways: (1) for myocardial stress testing (intravenous infusion of high doses leads to both transient tachycardia and transient myocardial ischemia in areas perfused by coronary artery segments incapable of dilating due to fixed atherosclerotic stenosis; this leads to redistribution of myocardial perfusion (steal) to normal segments that appropriately dilate), (2) used in conjunction with VKAs (e.g. warfarin) to prevent thromboembolic complications after prosthetic heart valve surgery, and (3) used in conjunction with aspirin for secondary prevention of ischemic stroke.

After oral ingestion peak plasma levels are achieved in approximately 2 hours. The terminal half-life is about 10–12 hours and a wide variability in plasma levels has been observed at standard doses.[91] Plasma levels show a strong correlation with inhibition of platelet aggregation.[92] Timing of the peak ability to inhibit aggregation appears to parallel plasma concentrations, but the duration of platelet inhibition has not been extensively studied. Some reports indicate that standard oral dose regimens (100 mg four times daily or 200 mg extended release formulations twice daily) do not achieve adequate plasma levels to induce significant inhibit platelet function[93] although platelet survival is definitely prolonged in patients with prosthetic heart valves[94] indicating some degree of inhibition of platelet activation. Neither the degree of inhibition of platelet activity induced by dipyridamole nor the influence of the wide heterogeneity in plasma levels found with various dose regimens has been studied in relation to clinical outcomes.[95]

Adjunctive use of dipyridamole with warfarin or other VKAs after prosthetic heart valve surgery reduced thromboembolic events 62%–91% compared to vitamin K antagonism alone in three trials enrolling 854 subjects. The most common side effects were dizziness, which possibly is related to effects on blood pressure. Bleeding was no greater in frequency with warfarin plus dipyridamole than with warfarin alone. It is unclear, however, whether warfarin plus dipyridamole is better than warfarin plus aspirin.[96]

Although multiple studies of dipyridamole used in secondary prevention of ischemic stroke have been performed since 1961, two trials in particular demonstrated a beneficial effect. The first European Stroke Prevention Study showed that combined aspirin and dipyridamole compared to placebo reduced the risk for recurrent stroke after a first TIA or stroke. The subsequent European Stroke Prevention Study 2 followed 6302 subjects for 2 years assigned to one of four treatment arms: placebo, aspirin (25 mg twice daily), dipyridamole (extended release 200 mg twice daily) or combined aspirin and dipyridamole. Compared to placebo, the combined risk for stroke and death was reduced 13% with aspirin (p = 0.016), 15% with dipyridamole alone (p = 0.015) and 24% with the combination (p < 0.001). Most of the risk reduction was due to the effect on stroke. All-site bleeding and GI bleeding were increased with aspirin or the combination, but not dipyridamole alone. Headache was more common with dipyridamole and the primary cause of study discontinuation.[97]

The ESPRIT trial randomized 2739 subjects with recent TIA or minor stroke to receive either aspirin alone (median dose 75 mg, range 30–325 mg daily) or aspirin with dipyridamole (200 mg twice daily – most subjects received an extended release formulation). The mean follow-up was 3.5 ± 2.0 years. During the trial, 34% of the aspirin and dipyridamole group discontinued therapy due to adverse events or side effects (primarily headache) compared to 13% on aspirin alone. The primary outcome of MACE occurred in 13% of subjects on aspirin and dipyridamole versus 16% of those treated with aspirin alone. Major bleeding occurred more often with aspirin alone (3.9%) than with combination therapy (2.6%).[98]

CILOSTAZOL

Cilostazol was developed in the early 1980s in Japan to treat critical limb ischemia.[99] It is a strong and specific inhibitor of platelet and vascular smooth muscle PDE3 and like dipyridamole inhibits adenosine reuptake. The resulting increases in intracellular cAMP and cGMP lead to both platelet inhibition and vasodilation.[100–102] It has been shown to be effective in limiting the effects of ischemia in animal models, and both increases limb temperature and pedal artery diameters in humans with PAD,[103–108] and to improve walking distance in PAD patients with intermittent claudication.[109,110] It also has a favourable impact on lipid profiles, decreasing LDL and increasing HDL levels in patients with hyperlipidemia.[111] Although not approved by the FDA specifically for antiplatelet therapy, in vitro assays show it to inhibit aggregation induced by collagen, ADP, AA, adrenalin and shear stress[99,101] and to suppress the expression and release of molecules associated with intimal hyperplasia and atherosclerosis such as monocyte chemoattractant protein 1, P-selectin, PDGF and platelet factor 4.[102,112] Studies have shown cilostazol inhibits neointimal hyperplasia in animal models of PTA and stenting[113,114] and is now being studied as both an adjunct to PCI and for reduction of neointimal hyperplasia after endovascular intervention in the coronary, carotid and lower-extremity arteries.[115–117] It also has undergone extensive evaluation for secondary prevention of cerebral ischemia in conjunction with other antiplatelets.[118,119]

Based on eight treadmill performance trials, cilostazol was approved by the US FDA in 1999 to treat intermittent claudication with twice daily dosing with either 50 or 100 mg. The range of improvement in the maximum walking distance was 28%–100% compared to corresponding improvements in the placebo group of 10%–41%. Further studies have subsequently been performed with meta-analysis confirming the efficacy of cilostazol for increasing maximum walking distance in PAD.[120]

After ingestion, peak levels are achieved in about 2.4 hours. The drug is extensively metabolized by hepatic cytochromes with the resulting metabolites mostly excreted in urine.[121] The half-life for its principal metabolites is about 10 hours, and after stopping administration, platelet function returns to normal within 12–16 hours.[122] Compared to aspirin or clopidogrel, cilostazol does not prolong the bleeding time alone or in combination.[123] Due to its effect on the myocardium, its use is associated with an approximate increase of heart rate of 7 beats/min, an approximate 1% incidence of palpitations, and a modest increase in ventricular premature beats based on Holter monitoring. The most common side effect is mild headache, which usually subsides over a few weeks – in the FDA trials, 3.5% of subjects treated with 200 mg daily dosing discontinued taking drug. Other side effects include tachycardia and diarrhea, each of which occurred in 1.1% of subjects compared to 0.1% of controls.[124]

As other PDE3 inhibitors are associated with increased mortality in CHF patients, the United States approved package label warning against its use in heart failure patients although no study has ever shown that in fact cilostazol increases this risk – in the FDA trials, approximately 8% of the more than 2000 subjects enrolled had the diagnosis of CHF but no increased mortality was observed.[125] A recent computerized review (data mining) of the medical records of PAD patients with CHF treated with cilostazol showed no evidence for increased mortality in this high-risk group compared to other PAD patients.[126]

PREVENTION OF ADVERSE CARDIOVASCULAR EVENTS

Primary prevention

The question of whether antiplatelet therapy should be used to prevent cardiovascular events in low-risk patients remains controversial. Only aspirin has been subjected to rigorous clinical trials in large numbers of healthy subjects without cardiovascular disease, and other antiplatelet agents are not ordinarily being used for primary prevention. There is an enormous amount of data indicating that risks for MI and stroke are diminished with aspirin, but bleeding risks, including severe GI hemorrhage, intracranial bleeding and hemorrhagic stroke, are increased.

Further complicating assessment of the risk-to-benefit ratio for aspirin therapy is that risks for cancer, particularly colon cancer, may be diminished with long-term use of aspirin. As low dose (<600 mg/day) has become clearly preferable to higher doses in recent years, more recent trials using low doses (≤162 mg/day) more accurately reflect current practice patterns.

The Antithrombotic Trialists' Collaboration reporting in 2009 on aspirin for primary prevention reviewed 6 trials with 95,000 subjects at low average risk (660,000 patient-years) who experienced 3554 serious vascular events. Based on intention to treat, the meta-analysis showed aspirin to reduce the overall relative risk for MI, stroke and vascular death 12%–0.51% per year with aspirin versus 0.57% per year in controls (p = 0.0001). Most of the difference was attributable to a decrease in non-fatal MI (0.18% per year with aspirin vs. 0.23% per year in controls, p < 0.0001). No significant differences in the risk for all stroke (0.20 per year vs. 0.19 per year), hemorrhagic stroke (0.04% per year vs. 0.03% per year) or ischemic stroke (0.16% per year vs. 0.18% per year) were detected. Major gastrointestinal and extracranial bleeding was 0.10% per year with aspirin versus 0.07% per year in controls. If one combines the incidence of major bleeding with adverse cardiovascular events, 0.61% of subjects on aspirin would experience serious bleeding, MI, stroke or vascular death compared to 0.64% of controls – for every 100,000 patient-years, 30 fewer total events would be experienced by patients treated with aspirin due to its ability to reduce the absolute reduction of risk for this composite outcome of 0.03%. The number needed to treat to prevent one adverse outcome in a year would be 3300.[127]

The most recent meta-analysis of aspirin for primary prevention trials focused on trials reported between 2008 and 2012.[128] This review took into account the reduced risk for cancer associated with aspirin which was not assessed in the Antithrombotic Trialists' Collaboration review. Aspirin reduced the relative risk for all-cause mortality 6% and the risks for major cardiovascular events 10%. Death from cancer was reduced 9–24% depending on the length of follow-up (it appears to take 5 years of aspirin therapy to lead to an observable effect) and the dosing, as some studies used alternative day dosing, which has lower effects on both cancer and cardiovascular disease. Two large studies employing alternate day aspirin dosing showed essentially no cardiovascular benefit. The incidence of major bleeding was found to be increased 62%–64% consistent with the results of previous meta-analyses. The benefits and risks of aspirin therapy in primary prevention were rare, with magnitudes of tens of events per 100,000 patient-years. The reduction in adverse cardiovascular events was estimated as between 10 and 60 per 100,000 patient-years, compared to an increase in gastrointestinal bleeding of 68 to 117 per 100,000 patient-years. The data suggesting that aspirin reduces the risk for cancer were regarded with caution, as several large studies with follow-up at 10 years or longer showed no evidence for cancer protection.[129–133] The authors bemoaned the lack of standardization in dosing and the potential bias found in many studies: some of the core studies in primary prevention were conducted in health care providers potentially limiting their generalizability. The authors' final conclusion was that the benefit of regular aspirin use to prevent cardiovascular disease in healthy adults is modest and carries a significant risk for both hemorrhagic stroke and bleeding such that further study is required – essentially the same point of view that has surrounded this topic for decades.

Secondary prevention

As the potential benefit of first aspirin and then dipyridamole in preventing thrombotic cardiovascular events became appreciated in the 1960s and 1970s, efforts to delineate the relative benefits and risks of antiplatelet drug regimens for secondary prevention in patients with cardiovascular disease led to an explosion of clinical trials in Europe and North America with thousands of subjects enrolled in initially scores and then hundreds of studies. The first review of this topic by the Antiplatelet Trialists' Collaboration in 1988 reported on 31 studies with over 29,000 subjects enrolled. The second report in 1994 analyzed the results of 145 studies in 70,000 subjects, and the collaborative study of 2002 reported on 287 studies suitable for analysis involving 135,000 subjects.[117–119] The conclusion of the 2002 study was that in high-risk patients antiplatelet therapy reduced the risk for non-fatal MI by about one-third, the risk for non-fatal stroke by about one quarter and vascular mortality by one-sixth. Absolute reductions in the risk of having a serious vascular event were 36 ± 5 per 1000 treated for 2 years in subjects with previous MI and 22 ± 3 for subjects with PAD. Mortality immediately after acute MI or acute stroke was significantly reduced with aspirin started early. In every category, the absolute benefits outweighed the risks of major bleeding. The most common agent employed was aspirin and doses of 75–150 mg daily were found to be at least as effective as higher doses – addition of dipyridamole to aspirin therapy did not reduce risk further. Clopidogrel reduced serious vascular events by 10% compared to aspirin, comparable to a similar reduction of 12% observed with ticlopidine. The use of a second antiplatelet drug to aspirin was thought to possibly produce further benefit in some clinical circumstances, but the results of meta-analysis were not conclusive then and still are not conclusive for many situations.

The 1996 CAPRIE trial studied 75 mg of clopidogrel to 325 mg aspirin for reducing the composite risk of ischemic stroke, MI or vascular death in over 19,000 high-risk subjects (history of stroke, MI, claudication or intervention for PAD) with a mean follow-up of 1.91 years. Overall, the risk for the composite endpoint in all subjects was 5.32% with clopidogrel versus 5.83% with aspirin (p = 0.043). The overall safety profile of clopidogrel was regarded as being at least as good as aspirin. Of great interest and influence was the observation that the PAD subgroup experienced the greatest benefit from clopidogrel. The average event rate per year was 3.71% compared to 4.86% with aspirin (p = 0.0028) representing a relative risk reduction of 24% (Figure 10.6), which although is impressive, the absolute risk reduction of 1.5% indicates that 67 PAD patients would have to be treated with clopidogrel to prevent one event in 1 year.[134] No reduction for the risk of the composite outcome was observed in subjects with a history of MI and the benefit in stroke patients was less than that observed in PAD. Subsequently, the CHARISMA study looked at the long-term benefit of dual therapy comparing aspirin alone to aspirin plus clopidogrel. Over 15,000 high-risk patients were randomized to receive either low-dose aspirin (75–162 mg) with or without clopidogrel. PAD, defined as ankle brachial pressure index (ABI) < 0.85 or history of intervention for lower-extremity ischemia, was present in 23% of subjects. The primary outcome of MI, stroke or vascular death occurred in 6.8% of dual therapy subjects versus 7.3% of aspirin subjects (p = 0.22). The conclusion of the CHARISMA trial was that dual therapy was not significantly better than aspirin alone but a subgroup analysis for outcomes in PAD subjects was not carried out.[135] Looking at the CAPRIE and CHARISMA trials together creates doubt as to whether there is enough difference in secondary prevention outcomes to employ clopidogrel routinely over aspirin alone.

Although periprocedural dual and triple antiplatelet therapy with extended dual therapy has become commonplace with CAD patients, particularly after PCI, long-term multidrug antiplatelet therapy has not become standard practice in the management of most peripheral problems. In fact, it is clear from recent population surveys that many patients with either PAD or cerebrovascular disease are not receiving appropriate antiplatelet therapy. In the US National Health and Nutrition Examination Study looking at Americans with PAD during the interval 1999–2006, only 35.8% were taking aspirin or another antiplatelet drug[136] and failure to treat patients appropriately with antiplatelet drugs has been repeatedly documented as a problem, more in PAD than in cerebrovascular disease. An investigation found in 2012 that only about two-thirds of patients with PAD or carotid disease were prescribed both statins and antiplatelet medication after surgical or endovascular peripheral interventions, even though 5-year survival was significantly better with drug therapy. Patients treated with both statins and antiplatelet drugs at discharge had significantly better 5-year survival (79%) compared to patients discharged on just an antiplatelet drug (72%) or neither (61%).[137] Similar underutilization was observed in a recent Danish longitudinal study which found only 53% of PAD patients were receiving aspirin.[138] This is despite consensus guidelines from virtually all major societies and organizations involved with vascular disease (e.g. American Heart Association, American College of Chest Physicians, TransAtlantic Inter-Society Consensus[139–141]) strongly recommending antiplatelet therapy. The clinical trial data supporting the use of antiplatelet therapy are robust – the controversy is not whether to treat the typical patient with antiplatelet therapy; rather it is what antiplatelet regimen is best. Patients may have disease limited to a single territory (coronary, lower extremity or cerebrovascular) but more often have multiple manifestations: e.g. history of MI and stroke or stroke and PAD. No one therapy is best for all possible permutations, and PAD patients with a history of hemorrhagic stroke or peptic ulcer should not necessarily be treated the same as patients with PAD alone.

At this time, three specific regimens are most commonly employed for secondary prevention: monotherapy with either aspirin or clopidogrel or dual therapy with aspirin and clopidogrel. Multiple large studies of dual therapy (aspirin and clopidogrel or another P2Y$_{12}$ inhibitor) extended to 30 days after MI or PCI have shown a marked reduction in

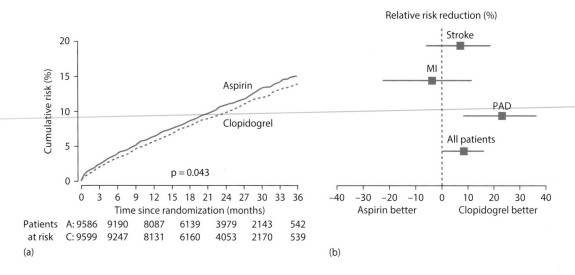

Figure 10.6 Results of the CAPRIE trial. (a) Life table analysis showing reduction of major adverse cardiovascular events in all patients for aspirin versus clopidogrel. (b) Subgroup analysis showing greater marked benefit in peripheral arterial disease and stroke patients. (From CAPRIE Steering Committee, *Lancet*, 348, 1329, 1996.)

risk for MACE.[142–146] Dual therapy after 30 days has also been shown to be superior to aspirin alone in the long-term management of PCI patients.[147] Current US guidelines for long-term antiplatelet therapy in patients with stable ischemic heart disease are to use aspirin alone or clopidogrel in patients with aspirin intolerance. Dual therapy with both is described as 'might be reasonable in certain high-risk patients with stable ischemic heart disease'.[148]

There are several clinical situations where vascular surgeons frequently have to choose between antithrombotic regimens to optimize long-term results after interventions: lower-extremity bypass, carotid bifurcation surgery, carotid stenting, carotid surgery and peripheral PTA and/or stenting. In this essay, we will concentrate on what is known regarding the efficacy and safety of antiplatelet regimens in the common peripheral interventions including lower-extremity bypass, carotid surgery, endovascular interventions and hemodialysis access. It should be appreciated that some of the common practices of PCI, e.g. intense combined anticoagulant and multidrug antiplatelet therapy started upstream of intervention, are not widely employed in lower-extremity interventions, where dual antiplatelet therapy is generally reserved for downstream management. Although PCI methods have heavily influenced peripheral endovascular therapy, whether the knowledge gained from experiences in the acute cardiac setting easily translates into the periphery is uncertain. Except for infrageniculate interventions, the calibre of the vessels being treated is not comparable. Further, in PCI detection of even small amounts of ischemic myonecrosis is feasible and standard practice, but interventions in the periphery do not have comparably sensitive measurements to measure immediate results – brain MRI could evaluate the impact of different antiplatelet regimens immediately after carotid surgery but would be much more costly than the ECG or troponin studies used to evaluate the immediate results of PCI.

Lower-extremity bypass

The earliest investigations into the effects of antiplatelet therapy for prolonging patency after lower-extremity bypass date to the late 1970s[149] and only one major prospective multicentre study (CASPAR) has been performed in the last decade.[150] The majority of clinical trials have employed aspirin or aspirin plus dipyridamole using aspirin doses of 325 mg or higher compared to placebo. A few studies have compared anticoagulant regimens employing VKAs alone or combined with aspirin (or another antiplatelet) to antiplatelet therapy alone. Several meta-analyses of these studies arrived at very comparable conclusions: (1) when both autologous and prosthetic graft types are combined, neither anticoagulation nor antiplatelet therapy provides significant patency improvement when compared to placebo; (2) when VKA anticoagulation is compared to placebo, subgroup analyses show patency of autologous vein grafts to be significantly better with anticoagulation but not prosthetic graft patency; (3) and when antiplatelet

therapy is compared to placebo, prosthetic graft patency is significantly better with antiplatelet therapy, but not vein graft patency.[151–154] In most studies, bleeding complications are higher with anticoagulation than with antiplatelet therapy. Most of the studies were done before lower doses of aspirin therapy (<162 mg/day) achieved their current popularity and employed doses ≥325 mg.

The largest recent study directly comparing aspirin to anticoagulation with a VKA was the Dutch Bypass Oral anticoagulants or Aspirin Study (BOA)[155] which enrolled 2690 subjects undergoing lower-extremity bypass (59% autologous vein, 41% prosthetic or composite). Subjects were randomized to be treated with either a VKA (phenprocoumon or acenocoumarol – target international normalized ratio (INR) of 3.0–4.5) or 100 mg daily carbasalate calcium (equivalent to 80 mg aspirin). The intention-to-treat analysis for all graft types found occlusion to occur in 23.2% of the VKA group versus 24.3% of the aspirin group (odds ratio 0.95, ns). A composite endpoint of vascular death, MI, stroke or amputation occurred in 18.7% of VKA subjects compared to 20.1% aspirin subjects (odds ratio 0.89, ns). Major bleeding was significantly higher with VKA therapy, 8.1% versus 4.2%. When analyzed by the type of conduit (Figure 10.7), patency outcomes

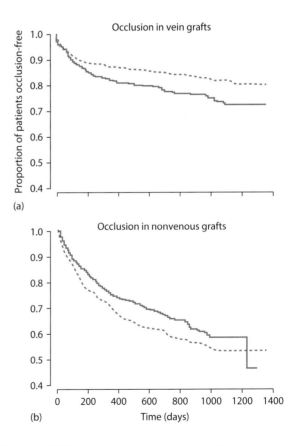

(a)

(b)

Figure 10.7 Results of the BOA study. Kaplan–Meier analysis of occlusion in lower-extremity bypass grafts with either vitamin K antagonist therapy (red line) or antiplatelet therapy (blue line) with an irreversible COX-1 inhibitor (carbasalate calcium) similar to aspirin. (a) Vein grafts. (b) Prosthetic grafts. (From BOA Study Group, *Lancet*, 355, 346, 2000.)

significantly differed – vein grafts showed better patency with VKA therapy and prosthetic grafts with antiplatelet therapy alone, consistent with the conclusions drawn from meta-analyses of earlier studies.[156]

The CASPAR study[150] was a multicentre, randomized, blinded trial to evaluate the effect of monotherapy with aspirin compared to dual therapy with clopidogrel and aspirin on outcomes after infrageniculate bypass. Aspirin (75–100 mg/day) plus placebo was compared to plus clopidogrel (75 mg/day) started 2–4 days after surgery. Prior to surgery, aspirin at any dose was encouraged but could be held for several days immediately prior to surgery. Postoperative prophylactic heparin or low molecular weight was also allowed. Subjects were followed for up to 2 years. The primary outcome was a composite of graft occlusion, revascularization, amputation and death. The overall outcome (independent of graft type) occurred in 149 of 425 subjects receiving placebo and 151 of 426 subjects on clopidogrel (odds ratio 0.98, ns). When the influence of graft type was analyzed (Figure 10.8), the primary endpoint was significantly reduced in patients with prosthetic grafts in the clopidogrel group compared to placebo (odds ratio 0.65, p = 0.25) but not in the venous grafts (odds ratio 1.25, ns). Although total bleeding was higher with clopidogrel, there were no significant differences in severe bleeding between clopidogrel and placebo (2.1% vs. 1.2%). The conclusion was that adding clopidogrel to aspirin did not improve autologous vein graft results but did confer benefit in patients receiving prosthetic grafts without significantly increasing major bleeding.

Does combining antiplatelet therapy with anticoagulation make a difference in bypass graft patency? Two recent studies looked at this issue. The first of these, US Veterans Affairs Cooperative Study #362,[156] looked at the effects of aspirin (325 mg/day) with or without VKA

(warfarin) therapy (INR 1.4–2.8) on bypass patency in 831 subjects undergoing bypass with a mean follow-up of 3 years. Other than increased major bleeding with aspirin plus anticoagulation compared to aspirin alone (8.4% vs. 3.6%, p = 0.02), no improvement in overall graft patency or vein graft patency was observed. When the results for just prosthetic grafts were assessed, no benefit was seen with 8 mm diameter grafts, but for 6 mm grafts, adding warfarin significantly increased assisted primary patency at 4 years (70% vs. 48%, p = 0.02). Overall, the patency for all prosthetic grafts combined was modestly better with warfarin plus aspirin than just aspirin alone (Figure 10.9) but was only borderline significant (p = 0.07). The failure of warfarin plus aspirin to induce better vein graft patency compared to aspirin alone was not congruent with earlier trial results, which the investigators attributed to a lower intensity of VKA therapy compared to other studies. More importantly, although a detailed subgroup analysis by graft position was not reported, it seems likely that infrainguinal bypass patency with 6 mm diameter prosthetic grafts was improved with combined therapy.

A more recent Italian study examined combined clopidogrel and oral anticoagulant therapy (C+OAT) compared to clopidogrel + aspirin (C+ASA).[157] The C+OAT group were treated with 75 mg/day clopidogrel and warfarin dosed to achieve a target INR between 2.0 and 2.5. The C+ASA group received clopidogrel and aspirin 100 mg/day. A total of 341 subjects undergoing femoropopliteal bypass were randomized 1:1 to each arm. Dacron collagen–impregnated prosthetic grafts were implanted for all above knee bypasses and reversed saphenous vein employed for all infrageniculate bypasses. Follow-up ranged from 4 to 9 years (mean 6.6 years). C+ASA and C+OAT were started on postoperative day 2 with the C+OAT group receiving low-molecular-weight heparin until a therapeutic INR was achieved. During the first 3 years of follow-up, freedom from adverse

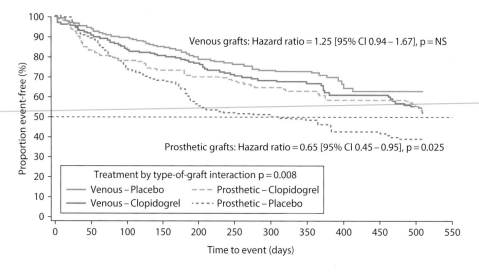

Figure 10.8 Results of the CASPAR trial. Kaplan–Meier analysis for the composite endpoint (graft occlusion, revascularization or replacement, above ankle amputation or death) by graft type and therapy (intention to treat). (From Belch JJ and Dormandy J, *J Vasc Surg*, 52, 825, 2010.)

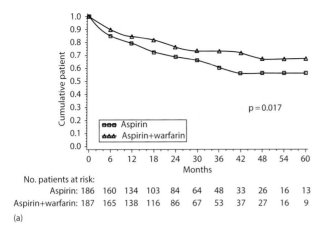

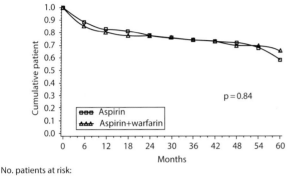

Figure 10.9 Results of Department of Veterans Affairs Cooperative Study #362, Kaplan–Meier analysis of assisted primary patency for prosthetic (a) and vein (b) bypass grafts. Patency was moderately better with combined vitamin K antagonist and aspirin compared to aspirin alone with all prosthetic grafts combined (axillofemoral, femorofemoral and femoropopliteal) (p = 0.07). (From Johnson WC and Williford WO, *J Vasc Surg*, 35, 413, 2002.)

events was remarkably similar in each group, including graft occlusion, MACE (cardiovascular death, MI, ACS or stroke) and amputation. After 3 years, the incidence of adverse events diverged modestly in favour of C+OAT compared to C+ASA with the differences in primary patency, amputation and MACE being statistically significant by Kaplan–Meier analysis. The investigators reported no influence of graft type (above knee prosthetic graft or below knee vein grafts) on the coprimary endpoints of secondary graft patency or occurrence of severe peripheral ischemia. Minor bleeding was significantly higher with C+OAT than C+ASA (2.9% per year vs. 1.4% per year, p = 0.03) but not bleeding requiring transfusion or hospitalization (1.8% per year vs. 1.6% per year, p = 0.7). Several factors were reported to significantly influence patency based on multivariate analysis, including ABI, urgent surgery, diabetes and poor tibial run-off, but the proportions of subjects with low ABI or needing urgent surgery (markers of CLI) were not reported, which is regrettable, as both CLI and the frequency of these surrogate markers are of great interest given the overall excellent patency and freedom form MACE and amputation reported. Figure 10.10 shows primary patency rates for all grafts combined based on the type of antithrombotic therapy. Despite uncertainty regarding the severity of disease treated, these results deserve attention and further studies to see if they can be replicated, as they indicate that dual antiplatelet therapy or warfarin plus clopidogrel should be routinely employed after infrainguinal bypass rather than monotherapy with clopidogrel, aspirin or a VKA.

The data from CASPAR also support the argument for using dual antiplatelet therapy for prosthetic grafts, and its consistency with previous studies of monotherapy makes its results more impressive. Whether combined anticoagulant/antiplatelet therapy is indicated for either venous or prosthetic grafts is not clearly supported by the available

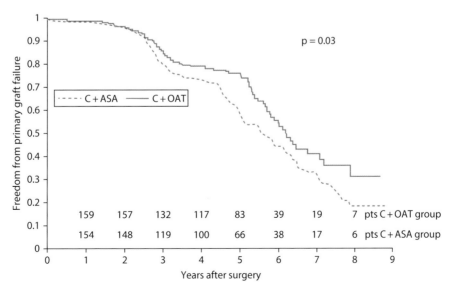

Figure 10.10 Lower-extremity bypass graft primary patency with antithrombotic therapy with clopidogrel and aspirin (C+ASA) compared to clopidogrel and oral anticoagulation with warfarin (C+OAT). Patency results for saphenous vein and prosthetic grafts are combined in each group with saphenous vein used for all infrageniculate grafts and prosthetic grafts for all suprageniculate bypasses. (From Monaco M et al., *J Vasc Surg*, 56, 96, 2012.)

data, but looking at the results of the recent Italian study as well as the VA cooperative trial suggests that this indeed may be true, such that further investigation is clearly warranted, perhaps with one of the new oral factor Xa inhibitors in lieu of warfarin.

Carotid endarterectomy

Antiplatelet therapy has been repeatedly demonstrated to reduce the risks of perioperative stroke and mortality in carotid bifurcation surgery. This is consistent with studies showing tagged platelets adherence to the freshly endarterectomized surface of the carotid artery to be significantly reduced by antiplatelet therapy.[158] Of note, monitoring patients immediately after surgery with transcranial Doppler shows that a relatively small number of patients have high rates of microemboli to the middle cerebral artery which is associated with markedly elevated risk for perioperative carotid thrombosis and embolic stroke.[159,160] Intuitively, this phenomenon seems likely to be sensitive to antithrombotic therapy.

Only a small number of well-designed randomized trials have looked at the ability of antiplatelet agents to reduce the risks of perioperative stroke as well as long-term outcomes in patients undergoing carotid endarterectomy. Nonetheless, careful review of the available evidence leads to a clear understanding of the benefit of antiplatelet therapy. A meta-analysis of five studies (total subjects = 907) of aspirin's effects on the risks for stroke and death in the perioperative period and during follow-up after carotid surgery showed a significant reduction in the risk for stroke when aspirin (at doses ≤325 mg/day) was compared to placebo (odds ratio 0.58, p = 0.04).[161] In this analysis, although there was a trend towards decreased mortality, the difference was modest (0.77) and not significant. If, however, the two studies in which aspirin was only administered after surgery are removed from analysis, the differences in observed mortality are clearly decreased with preoperative aspirin therapy – death occurred in 5.6% of subjects receiving aspirin before surgery compared to 13.1% with placebo (odds ratio 0.39, p = 0.0065). Similar significant differences in risk for stroke, or stroke and death combined, emerge when the two studies employing only postoperative aspirin are removed from meta-analysis. A recent retrospective study compared 267 patients taking aspirin before surgery to 273 patients who stopped aspirin 5 days before surgery. Preoperative therapy was associated with a marked reduction in MI (odds ratio 6.1, p = 0.012) and stroke (odds ratio 4.5, p = 0.036).[162]

The ASA and Carotid Endarterectomy study[163] compared outcomes in 2849 patients randomized to receive one of four doses of aspirin (81, 325, 650 or 1300 mg of aspirin daily) starting before surgery. The efficacy analysis excluded those who had been on >650 mg before randomization or randomized less than 2 days before surgery. The combined risk for stroke, MI and death in the two low-dose groups was compared to those receiving ≥325 mg. The risk for the combined outcome of stroke, MI or death was markedly lower

with the two lower-dose regimens: 4.2% versus 10.0% (odds ratio 0.40, p = 0.003). As expected, ICH rates were lower with the low doses (odds ratio 0.59, p = 0.191), but other bleeding complications were very similar.

A retrospective view employing multivariate regression analysis to assess risk factors for stroke and death in more than 10,000 Medicare patients undergoing carotid endarterectomy in the United States found that preoperative antiplatelet therapy (along with patching) was the most important factor associated with reduced risk. Antiplatelet therapy started before surgery led to a highly significant decrease in risk for death and stroke (odds ratio 0.73, p < 0.0001).[164] A similar finding was evident in analysis of 2714 patients undergoing carotid surgery in Northern New England: preoperative antiplatelet therapy was protective for both stroke and death (odds ratio 0.4, p = 0.02).[165]

Clopidogrel either alone or with aspirin has been used by some surgeons to reduce the risks of carotid surgery. The incidence of microembolism detected by transcranial Doppler immediately after carotid surgery in subjects already on aspirin is dramatically reduced by a single 75 mg dose of clopidogrel 12 hours before surgery,[159] but the clinical significance of this effect has not been assessed. It is very clear, however, that both bleeding and total operative time (thought to reflect more difficulty in achieving hemostasis) are increased by clopidogrel. Two retrospective analyses of risk factors for bleeding after endarterectomy found that preoperative clopidogrel was the most prominent factor associated with postoperative bleeding complications including neck hematoma and reoperation for bleeding. The risk for hematoma associated with clopidogrel in one study was overall 16% but increased to 35% when carotid patching was performed.[165,166]

There are no current data indicating that therapy with either clopidogrel alone or combined with aspirin leads to better outcomes with carotid surgery than aspirin alone. The evidence that starting or maintaining low-dose aspirin therapy before carotid surgery is particularly strong. The length of follow-up in the surgical trials is relatively brief compared to that found in secondary prevention trials for cerebrovascular disease. When data from the secondary prevention trials are incorporated into risk–benefit assessment, it seems clear that aspirin is a very important aspect of both perioperative and long-term management of patients requiring carotid surgery.

Hemodialysis access

Compared to arterial bypass grafts, the hemodynamics of arteriovenous fistulae and grafts have significant differences – high flow and turbulence due to the greater pressure gradients present between inflow and outflow vessels generate greater shear forces at the venous anastomoses that are thought to more intensely stimulate intimal hyperplasia. Greater compliance mismatch between relatively stiff prosthetic materials and native vein may also contribute to intimal hyperplasia[167] which, especially with prosthetic grafts, may develop rapidly and lead to early thrombosis. It is well appreciated that patency of AV fistulae and prosthetic grafts is poor: 2-year primary patency rates for prosthetic grafts are on the order of 30% and for arteriovenous fistulae which mature adequately to be suitable for access approximately 50%.[168,169]

Another factor that must be kept in perspective is the high incidence of qualitative platelet dysfunction in dialysis patients. Bleeding times are elevated in approximately 50% of dialysis patients and quantitatively related to the severity of uremia and the degree of impairment of platelet aggregation ex vivo.[170,171] This raises two issues, first, in patients who already have decreased platelet function, administration of inhibitors should, a priori, lead to less impact on the biology of events that lead to access failure such as intimal hyperplasia and thrombosis. Second, dialysis patients are already at higher risk for spontaneous bleeding, so antiplatelet therapy is potentially more dangerous. The concern that reasonably arises from these considerations explains why antiplatelet therapy is not routinely employed in hemodialysis patients. Surveys of dialysis centres in America, Europe and Japan show less than 30% of them are treated routinely with antiplatelet drugs,[172,173] far lower than in patients with the same morbidities not on dialysis. This pattern persists despite both the marked increased risk for cardiovascular disease in dialysis patients[174,175] and evidence from large retrospective studies showing that, at least with aspirin, access patency is better with antiplatelet therapy.[169,172,173,176] Another confounding factor in evaluating the role of antiplatelet therapy is that hemorrhage from initial attempts at placing catheters may lead to hematomas that compress the new access and possible lead to early failure (particularly in fistulae) creating further concern for the risks of antithrombotic agents.

A trial in 1974 of antiplatelet therapy to improve access patency looked at the effect of 500 mg aspirin started the day before surgery on fistula patency at 30 days. A marked difference was observed – thrombosis occurred in 11/47 subjects on placebo versus 2/45 on aspirin (OR 0.15, p = 0.019).[177] Regrettably, there have been subsequently only a few well-designed prospective studies to assess the impact of antiplatelet therapy on access patency. A recent Cochrane meta-analysis of all trials that evaluated the impact of medical therapy on access patency found only nine studies (total $n = 1548$) suitable for analysis; three looked at the early effect of ticlopidine on fistula patency.[178] The small number of studies, variability in whether the accesses were new or pre-existing and whether therapy was started before or after access surgery limits the import of this analysis. The issue of timing of antiplatelet therapy may be critical when viewed from the perspective of PCI and carotid trials. Platelet stimulation of intimal hyperplasia probably starts immediately after adherence to the damaged intima release of factors that induce smooth muscle cell proliferation. The longer the delay in starting antiplatelet therapy, the less likely it will limit intimal hyperplasia and possibly thrombus propagation which may be a factor in failure before 30 days.

Table 10.3 summarizes the major randomized trials of trials comparing patency with active therapy compared to placebo. In general, subjects with recent bleeding events, thrombocytopenia (platelet count < 100,000), known bleeding risks or receiving VKAs were excluded in these trials. Probably, this caution led to the low level of perioperative bleeding generally seen. Only one study, a 2003 study comparing aspirin combined with clopidogrel to placebo in patients with PTFE grafts, observed clinically significant increased bleeding,[179] but it was not perioperative. This study was unusual in that participants already had grafts implanted – half of which had previously thrombosed – that were already in use. The interval between initial surgery and study enrollment was not specified, but clearly the average onset was clearly many months after surgery. Although a modest benefit patency improvement was observed in subjects whose grafts had never thrombosed, the study was stopped due to a marked increase in risk for bleeding (odds ratio 1.98, p = 0.007).

Inspection of the table shows that compared to placebo, except for one study, Sreedhara[180], patency was better with antiplatelet therapy, although improvement tended to be modest. For example, the average increase in primary patency observed in Dixon was only 6 weeks.[181] It should be appreciated that with fistulae better early patency does not necessarily lead to increased suitability for dialysis, as found in the study by Dember.[182] Since then, adjunctive balloon-assisted maturation (BAM) has increasingly become employed to salvage fistulae that otherwise might be abandoned.[183] The consequence of increasing early patency with antiplatelet therapy (and clopidogrel may well be better in that regard than aspirin, but there are no trial data to confirm that speculation) is that small diameter fistulae, that might otherwise thrombose, can stay open until BAM is performed.

It should be appreciated that in many patients, pre-existing platelet dysfunction may obviate the impact of antiplatelet therapy; with platelet dysfunction, antiplatelet may only increase risks for bleeding and confer no benefit. At this time use of antiplatelet agents, even aspirin, to promote patency after access surgery is not standard practice. Of the agents that are associated with decreased intimal hyperplasia, cilostazol certainly deserves consideration, as it can be used safely in dialysis patients at daily doses of 50 and 100 mg. Until clinical trials distinguish between patients with and without platelet dysfunction, there will be gaps in our understanding of their significance. As we discuss in the following text, quantitative assessment of on platelet function may eventually help decide when to employ antiplatelet therapy and to monitor the results.

Endovascular therapy

The first randomized prospective trial evaluating the influence of antiplatelet therapy on long-term results of balloon angioplasty of lower-extremity arteries was reported by the University of Munich in 1985.[184] Inspired by the

Table 10.3 Randomized trials of antiplatelet therapy for hemodialysis access.

Author (year)	Drug regimen	Primary outcome	Treatment n/N	Treatment n/N	Odds ratio	p
Andrassy et al. (1974)[177]	ASA[a] 500 mg/day started pre-op	AVF[f] occlusion at 1 month	2/45	11/47	0.15	0.019
Harter et al. (1979)[218]	ASA 160/d started 30 days post-op	Scribner shunt thrombus	6/19	18/25	0.18	0.0098
Sreedhara et al. (1994)[180]	ASA 325 mg/day	Graft thrombosis	10/20	6/19	2.17	0.59
	DIP[b] 75 mg TID	"	4/23	"	0.46	0.11
	ASA 325 mg/day + DIP 75 mg TID, all started pre-op	"	5/22	"	0.64	0.16
Dixon et al. (2009)[181]	ASA 25 mg/day + DIP-ER[c] 200 mg BID started immediately post-op[d]	Loss of 1° graft patency at 1 year	256/321	274/321	0.78	0.21
Kaufman et al. (2003)[179]	ASA 325 mg/day + clopidogrel 75 mg/day started post-op[e]	1 year 1° graft patency	n = 321 0.53	n = 328 0.41	0.81	0.45
Dember et al. (2008)[182]	Clopidogrel 300 mg loading dose then 75 mg/day started day after surgery	AVF thrombosis at 6 weeks	53/441	84/436	0.54	0.0034
Ghorbani et al. (2009)[220]	Clopidogrel 75 mg started 7–10 days before surgery	AVF thrombosis at 8 weeks	2/46	10/47	0.17	0.027
Fiskerstrand et al. (1984)[221]	Ticlopidine 250 mg BID started 2 days pre-op continued for 30 days	AVF thrombosis at 1 month	2/8	5/10	0.33	0.04
Grontoft et al. (1985)[222]	Ticlopidine 250 mg BID started 2 days pre-op continued for 30 days	AVF thrombosis at 1 month	2/19	8/17	0.13	0.02
Grontoft et al. (1998)[223]	Ticlopidine 250 mg BID started 3–7 days pre-op continued for 30 days	AVF thrombosis at 1 month	16/144	25/141	0.58	0.3

[a] Acetylsalicylic acid.
[b] Dipyridamole.
[c] Extended release.
[d] Median 2.1 hours after surgery.
[e] Not specified, but only after dialysis had been successfully established.
[f] Arteriovenous fistula.

favourable results from studies of aspirin and dipyridamole on aortocoronary vein grafts, it examined the influence of high-dose aspirin (330 mg three times daily) with or without dipyridamole (75 mg three times daily) compared to placebo on restenosis after balloon angioplasty of the femoropopliteal arteries. Serial angiography 2 years after PTA demonstrated less progression of disease and restenosis with both aspirin regimens compared to placebo, with more of an effect with combination therapy. Since then, as shown in Table 10.4, only a few high-quality randomized trials have studied the influence of antiplatelet therapy on the results of endovascular treatment of arterial occlusive disease in the lower extremity. The results in general have found that when compared either to placebo or to prolonged anticoagulation with VKAs, antiplatelet therapy provides moderately better patency than either (and less risk for bleeding compared to anticoagulation) with both PTA and then stenting. The one exception, the Swedish Study Group trial of 1994,[185] failed to show a benefit for aspirin/dipyridamole, most likely a consequence of the very low doses employed (25/50 mg twice daily).

Based on PCI experiences, the use of $P2Y_{12}$ inhibitors became increasingly common in peripheral endovascular therapy. Current practice is to employ aspirin with clopidogrel or another $P2Y_{12}$ as routinely in all endovascular interventions, including stenting and catheter atherectomy. There are, however, a surprisingly low number of properly controlled trials that elucidate the optimal timing, dosing and duration. As a consequence, there is a wide variability in practice, at least in the United States[186]

Table 10.4 Randomized trials of antiplatelet therapy for lower extremity endovascular interventions.

Author (year)	Treatment	Control	Intervention	Primary outcome	Treatment n/N	Control n/N	Odds ratio	p
Hess et al. (1985)[184]	ASA 100 mg ASA/DIP 75 mg DIP TID ASA 330 mg/DIP 75 mg TID, started the same day after PTA	Placebo	PTA PTA	Patent at 6 months Patent at 6 months	28/57 35/57	21/63 21/63 "	1.93 3.18	0.42 0.002
Study Group (1994)[185]	ASA 25 mg/DIP 50 mg BID 1 day before surgery continued 90 days	Placebo	PTA	Patent at 12 months	50/100	59/108	0.83	0.5
Do and Mahler (1994)[224]	ASA 25 mg/DIP 200 mg BID, started 1 day before PTA continued 12 months	VKA	PTA	Patent at 12 months	54/79	43/81	1.91	0.049
Ansel et al. (2006)[225]	Abciximab bolus → 12-hour infusion, ASA and clopidogrel started day before and continued indefinitely (ASA) and 2 months (clopidogrel)	Abciximab placebo	Stent	Restenosis/ occlusion at 9 months	4/27	3/24	1.22	0.81
Tepe et al. (2012)[226]	Clopidogrel 300 mg/ASA 100 mg day before stenting and then clopidogrel 75 mg/ASA 100 mg daily	ASA + placebo	PTA ± stent 55% stent	6-month target vessel revascularization	2/40	8/40	0.21	0.04[a]
Iida et al. (2008)[227]	Cilostazol 100 mg BID + ASA 100 mg/day Started 7 days before	Ticlopidine 200 mg/day instead of cilostazol	Stent	3-year patency	46/63	33/64	1.42	0.013[a]
Soga et al. (2009)[228]	Cilostazol 100 mg BID started before + ASA 81–100 mg/ticlopidine 200 mg/day	No cilostazol	PTA ± stent 45% stent	2-year target vessel revascularization	6/39	15/39	0.29	0.04[a]
Iida et al. (2013)[117]	Cilostazol 100 mg BID + ASA 100 mg/day for 12 months	No cilostazol	PTA ± stent 89% stent	≥50% restenosis by angiography	15/75	38/77	0.26	0.002

[a] Log-rank statistics.

in relation to loading patients upstream or downstream with clopidogrel. In the United States, administration of clopidogrel upstream of lower-extremity intervention is not common; rather, loading doses are given soon after intervention. The duration of $P2Y_{12}$ inhibitor therapy is also highly variable. In the periphery, there are virtually no clinical trial data to guide judgement of how long dual therapy should be employed – even with coronary stents, the length of dual therapy is controversial, as the elevated costs of prolonged therapy and the risks of bleeding cloud the issue.[187] One common pattern is to employ aspirin prior to intervention and load with 300 or 600 mg of clopidogrel immediately after intervention, followed by aspirin therapy indefinitely, but with clopidogrel maintained for only 2 or 3 months.

The use of cilostazol in peripheral interventions has been studied in Japan, and three prospective randomized trials (see Table 10.4) and one retrospective analysis show that when used instead of a $P2Y_{12}$ inhibitor in dual therapy with aspirin, rates of restenosis, occlusion and target vessel revascularization are significantly better. Although cilostazol is a weak inhibitor of platelet aggregation, much of its benefit is attributed to a direct effect on smooth muscle proliferation. The data from Asia from studies of both coronary and peripheral interventions appear to strongly support the use of cilostazol, particularly angiographic data from a 2013 multicentre study reported by Iida[117] such that further trials are warranted. One problem with all the lower-extremity endovascular data is that most of it derives from trials of femoropopliteal intervention.

Although it is likely that the same patterns would be found in trials restricted to iliac or tibial vessels, in the absence of studies specific for these different anatomic segments, one can only hope that that is the case.

Carotid stenting

Compared to the situation with lower-extremity arterial stents, there are even less controlled clinical trial data (Table 10.5) regarding the optimal use of antiplatelet therapy in carotid artery stenting (CAS). There are only two prospective randomized trials and one retrospective cohort analysis comparing the impact of different antiplatelet regimens. McKivett et al. compared dual therapy with 75 mg aspirin combined with a loading dose of 300 mg clopidogrel 6–12 hours before stenting, to aspirin combined with a heparin drip maintained for 24 hours following stenting.[188] Dalainas et al. compared dual therapy with 325 mg aspirin and ticlopidine 250 mg twice daily to a 24 hour heparin infusion.[189] In both studies, the incidence of neurologic complications and bleeding was higher in group receiving aspirin only. Whether GPIIb/IIIa inhibitors may be beneficial when employed during CAS has been evaluated in one retrospective cohort analysis of the impact of abciximab combined with dual therapy with aspirin and clopidogrel on perioperative outcomes in patients deemed high risk

for CAS complications – no benefit was seen with additional abciximab and two hemorrhagic strokes occurred in the abciximab group compared to none with just dual therapy.[190]

Two Japanese retrospective studies analyzed the effect of cilostazol on CAS results. Takayama[191] reported used sonography or contrast imaging to assess with in-stent restenosis 6 months after CAS. Cilostazol (200 mg) and aspirin (100 mg/day) were employed in one group and aspirin and either ticlopidine (100 mg BID) or clopidogrel (75 mg/day) in the other group. Restenosis $\geq 50\%$ developed in 5 of 30 patients in the ticlopidine/clopidogrel group and none of 30 patients receiving cilostazol. A second study retrospectively evaluated the impact of cilostazol on the incidence of new ipsilateral cerebral ischemic lesions the day after CAS using diffusion-weighted MRI (DWI) in two cohorts of patients.[192] All patients received dual therapy with aspirin and clopidogrel started 4 weeks before CAS. All were tested for clopidogrel resistance with the VerifyNow assay (see later) to determine clopidogrel resistance (defined as $P2Y_{12}$ reaction units [PRUs] >240) 2 days before CAS. In the first cohort (group I), 12 of 28 patients (43%) were identified as clopidogrel resistant (group I), and in the second cohort (group II), 11 of 36 patients (36%) were found to be clopidogrel resistant. The 11 group II patients with clopidogrel resistance were started on adjunctive cilostazol (200 mg) therapy 2 days before CAS. Except for a higher proportion

Table 10.5 Randomized trials of antiplatelet therapy for carotid artery stenting.

Author (year)	Treatment	Control	Primary outcomes	Treatment n/N	Control n/N	Odds ratio	p
McKevitt et al. (2005)[188]	300 mg clopidogrel day before	After CAS 24 heparin infused 24 hours to maintain aPPT ratio > 1.5–2.5 ULN[b] aPTT	30-day occlusion	0/23	4/24	0.0997	0.125
	Clopidogrel 75 mg 2 hours after CAS			0/23	6/24	0.061	0.062
			Neurologic complications	2/23	4/24	0.48	0.42
	Clopidogrel 75 mg daily for 28 days	ASA 75 mg/day before and after	Bleeding				
	ASA 75 mg/day before and after						
Dalainas et al. (2006)[189]	Ticlopidine 250 mg BID starting 7 days before CAS	24-hour post-op heparin infusion	30-day occlusion	0/50	1//50	0.32	0.50
		ASA 325 mg/day before and after[b]		0/50	8/50	0.495	0.041
	Ticlopidine continued for 30 days after		Neurologic complications	1/50	2/50	0.49	0.57
	ASA 325 mg/day before and after		Bleeding				
Qureshi et al. (2002)[190,d]	Abciximab bolus → 12 hour infusion	No abciximab	Transient ischemia[c]	9/37	1/34	10.3	0.032
	ASA + P2Y$_{12}$ inhibitior[a] started 3 days before heparin bolus and infusion during procedure	ASA + clopidogrel started 3 days before heparin bolus and infusion during procedure	Ischemic stroke	1/37	4/33	0.21	0.16
			Hemorrhagic stroke	2/37	0/33	4.72	0.32
			Major bleeding	4/37	4/33	0.88	0.86

[a] Clopidogrel 75 mg daily or ticlopidine 250 BID.
[b] Upper limit of normal.
[c] Neurologic symptoms resolved $\leq$ 24 hours.
[d] Retrospective cohort study.

of open cell stents employed in group II (43% vs. 25%), the CAS techniques employed were identical. DWI identified new ischemic lesions in 2/36 of group II subjects compared to 7/28 of group I patients (odds ratio 0.18, p = 0.049). No significant bleeding or neurologic events were identified in either group. Although the results of this second study support using triple antiplatelet therapy with cilostazol in CAS, the import of these findings is weakened as the number of new DWI lesions occurring in clopidogrel-resistant and clopidogrel-sensitive patients was not described.

Fatal strokes have resulted when only aspirin or no platelet therapy was employed in CAS.[191] In 2007, five US societies released a guideline, Consensus Document on Carotid Stenting,[192] recommending that dual therapy with aspirin and clopidogrel be started 4 days before stenting when possible, or at least 24 hours beforehand, and that clopidogrel be continued a minimum of 30 days and aspirin indefinitely. Virtually identical guidelines were issued in 2011 by the American College of Cardiology in conjunction with the American Stroke Association and the American College of Neurology, such that dual therapy starting before CAS and continuing for at least 30 days after has become standard therapy.[193]

PLATELET FUNCTION TESTING AND DRUG RESISTANCE

What was once a widely used test of platelet function, bleeding time, has been found to be of little value in the modern era for evaluating platelet function and has been essentially abandoned, as it is non-specific, insensitive and highly operator dependent and may leave scars. There are now more sophisticated tests for platelet function which can demonstrate increased activity in ACS and during PCI with test results showing correlations with risk for adverse cardiovascular events. These methods include point-of-care devices that measure platelet plug formation in vitro in response to shear, flow cytometric measurement of platelet surface P-selectin, detection of circulating platelet–monocyte aggregate levels and determination of plasma CD40L. These tests have not been validated by large clinical trials as sufficiently predictive to become accepted as standard practice.[194]

The current clinical focus of tests of platelet function aims at identifying patients in whom platelet inhibition is either too high or too low during prolonged therapy after a procedure or for secondary prevention. Almost all investigations with this intention have studied aspirin and $P2Y_{12}$ inhibitors. With each drug, too much inhibition has been repeatedly associated with bleeding and too little inhibition associated with increased hazard for stent thrombosis, MI, stroke or death. The underlying goal is to achieve personalized antiplatelet therapy where the dose or regimen employed achieves an optimal balance between therapeutic effect (prevention of MACE) and risks for bleeding. Ironically, given the public health impact of antiplatelet

therapy and unlike the ability to monitor most therapies employed in cardiovascular medicine (INR testing with VKAs or measurement of plasma lipids with statins) with antiplatelet therapy, a 'one-size-fits-all' strategy dominates – testing the effects of antiplatelet drugs on individual patient responses is not part of standard practice. Given the importance of antiplatelet therapy in managing atherosclerotic disease in the developed world, this is a remarkable and deplorable state of affairs.

There are several reasons for this situation. First, there are a wide variety of platelet function tests such as light transmission aggregometry (LTA), flow cytometry, measurement of urine and plasma levels of substances released by activated platelets and point-of-care devices that measure platelet aggregation or adhesion, as well as genetic tests for polymorphisms that affect drug metabolism. Further, the agonists (e.g. shear, epinephrine, collagen, AA, ADP) used in test procedures and concentrations vary (e.g. 5 μmol/L vs. 20 μmol/L ADP to test inhibition of $P2Y_{12}$ receptor activity). The marked heterogeneity of available test procedures demonstrates a lack of consensus regarding what constitutes optimal testing of platelet reactivity – the market for tests is unsettled and should be regarded as in a very early stage of development. Further complicating the situation are uncertainties or controversies regarding testing platelet function. These include the following: (1) What are the best tests of platelet function? (2) With any given test, what are the thresholds that define too little or too much inhibition? (3) Is aspirin resistance clinically significant? (4) Although clopidogrel resistance is generally regarded as real, what is the definition? (5) Does adjusting antiplatelet therapy based on platelet function tests lead to improved outcomes?

These questions are all related, with uncertainty regarding the best test procedures and their thresholds the biggest problems. Further complicating the situation is that although tests of platelet reactivity have been shown in certain circumstances to predict risk for MACE, all the tests have low ability to predict for any given patient a poor outcome (i.e. low positive predictive value) because in general poor outcomes are uncommon. Further, most of the information regarding the relations between function test results, bleeding and MACE come from studies of patients with CAD undergoing PCI with modest contributions from secondary prevention trials, and little or no information derived from peripheral occlusive disease or cerebrovascular disease studies. This lowers the confidence with which inferences from the available data can be generalized.

Table 10.6 is a partial list of existing tests for platelet function. LTA measures platelet reactivity by adding agonists such as AA or ADP to platelet enriched plasma and measuring the increase in light transmitted through a photometer cuvette as the platelets aggregate. LTA is time consuming and not generally available in most community hospitals or clinics.[194] The definition of high platelet reactivity (HPR) while on therapy for aspirin varies depending

Table 10.6 Platelet function tests.

Test basis	Name	Advantages	Disadvantages	Reported to predict clinical outcomes	Monitors aspirin	Monitors thienopyridines	Monitors GP IIb/IIIa antagonists
Shear-induced platelet plug formation	PFA-100	Low sample size, no sample prep whole blood	Depends on vWF hematocrit	Yes	Yes	Not recommended	Not recommended
Platelet-to-platelet aggregation	Aggregometry (light transmission)	Historical gold standard	Poor reproducibility, high sample volume, time-consuming sample preparation	Yes	Yes with arachidonic acid and ADP	Yes with ADP	Yes
	Aggregometry impedance	Whole blood assay	High sample size, time consuming, expensive	Yes	Yes with arachidonic acid and ADP	Yes with ADP	Yes
	VerifyNow	Low sample size point-of-care whole blood	No instrument adjustment	Yes	Yes with arachidonic acid cartridge	Yes with ADP cartridge	Yes with TRAP cartridge
Activation-induced changes in platelet surface	Surface P-selectin	Small sample size whole blood	Expensive sample prep, flow cytometry needs experienced tech	Yes	Yes with arachidonic acid	Yes with ADP	Yes
Adhesion-dependent signalling	VASP phosphorylation state	Depends on $P2Y_{12}$ low sample size whole blood	Expensive sample prep, flow cytometry needs experienced tech	No	No	Yes	No
Activation dependent release from	Platelet-derived microparticles	Low sample size whole blood	Expensive sample prep, flow cytometry needs experienced tech	Yes	No	No	No
	Urinary 11-dehydrothromboxane	Directly depends on COX-1 activity	Indirect measure not platelet specific	No	Yes	No	No
	Plasma CD40L	Most plasma CD40L is platelet derived	Sample preparation may activate platelets leading to artifact	Yes	No	No	No

Source: After Michelson AD, *Circulation*, 110, e489, 2004.

on what agonist is employed. For example, $\geq 70\%$ residual aggregation is the threshold when 10 μmol ADP is used, but $\geq 20\%$ residual platelet aggregation is the threshold when 0.5 mg/mL AA stimulation is employed.[195] AA is generally regarded as a more suitable agonist as reactivity to ADP or other agonists induce aggregation through pathways less dependent on thromboxaneA_2.[196]

Measurement of platelet plug formation in the PFA-100 system uses a narrow artificial vessel that mimics resistance in a small artery with a membrane containing a biologically active coating (collagen and ADP or collagen and epinephrine) and an aperture that stimulates platelet plug formation at the aperture. The time required to occlude the aperture is the measure of platelet reactivity.[196]

The VerifyNow system is a point-of-care light transmission aggregometer using anticoagulated whole blood inserted into a small machine that uses cartridges specific for aspirin, $P2Y_{12}$ receptor antagonists or GPIIb/IIIa antagonists. Results are reported as arbitrary reaction units (for aspirin as ARU and for $P2Y_{12}$ inhibitors, PRU) so when sensitivity to clopidogrel is measured, the system reports PRU.[197] The system recently has been the mostly commonly employed method for detecting high on-treatment platelet reactivity (HPR) in clinical trials due to its rapidity, ease of use and low sample size requirement. HPR is defined as PRU results above a designated threshold, which, unfortunately, has not been standardized. The definition of HPR on clopidogrel has variously been defined as >272 PRU,[198] >235 PRU,[199] >230 PRU,[200] >208 PRU[201] or >170 PRU.[202] The lack of agreement regarding what PRU value should be the threshold for defining HPR for clopidogrel perfectly reflects current uncertainty.

Urinary levels of the thromboxaneA_2 metabolite 11-dehydrothromboxane can be measured using mass spectroscopy to assess COX-1 activity, but other factors that increase thromboxane include increased COX-2 activity in mononuclear leukocytes in inflammatory states and non-COX-dependent production of thromboxane due to lipid peroxidation catalyzed by oxygen free radicals – both are confounding factors. The latter pathway is associated with smoking, diabetes and hyperlipidemia[196] and may lead to increased urinary levels even when aspirin effectively inhibits platelet COX-1 due to systemic inflammation. There is no agreed upon value for the urinary metabolite level that represents a threshold value for platelet resistance, although elevated urinary 11-dehydro-thromboxane B2/creatinine ratios have been found to be associated with increased risk for MACE in one secondary prevention trial.[203]

Flow cytometry has been used to detect increased expression of platelet surface markers of activation such as P-selectin,[204] cytoplasmic markers of activation such as phosphorylated vasodilator stimulated phosphoprotein (VASP-P) which is specific for $P2Y_{12}$ receptor inhibition[205] and the density of platelet microparticles in the blood.[206] All of these tests are sensitive to platelet activation and have the potential to define the degree of platelet inhibition by drugs. Flow cytometry, due to its cost and technical complexity, is still primarily a research tool and has had little or no impact on current practice. Similarly, quantification of serum levels of molecules released by activated platelets such as soluble CD40 and P-selectin could be employed as markers of platelet activity, but these techniques also are not employed in current practice and require standardization.

The question of whether aspirin resistance exists and is clinically relevant has to be appreciated in light of observations that the most common reason for HPR in patients on aspirin is that they actually are not taking it. One study found patients thought to be taking aspirin whose tests showed resistance, i.e. no inhibition of reactivity, were in fact actually not taking aspirin[207] – if retested after documented ingestion, the expected levels of inhibition are found in most cases. As many as 37% of patients with angina are non-compliant with taking aspirin.[208]

Other factors which may cause tests to indicate decreased responsiveness to aspirin include concomitant therapy with NSAIDs like ibuprofen that interfere with aspirin inhibition of COX-1, impaired gastrointestinal absorption and stress-related accelerated platelet production during the 24 hours before testing.[196] Investigations into polymorphisms in COX-1 gene have demonstrated polymorphisms which correlate with platelet function testing but have not been shown to correlate with risk for cardiovascular events, undermining speculation that genetic variability may be a cause of clinically significant aspirin resistance.[209] Despite the likelihood that true aspirin resistance due to metabolic or genetic diversity is uncommon, several studies have shown a correlation between HPR for aspirin therapy and subsequent MACE, but with few exceptions, these studies have not measured aspirin or thromboxane metabolite levels. Figure 10.11 shows the result of a study looking at MACE in patients with known CAD or history of stroke. Aspirin resistance was defined by LTA using AA and ADP as agonists and was present in 5.2% of all subject believed to be on aspirin based on interview – confirmation of aspirin ingestion was not performed in most cases, but an unspecified number of subjects were noted to have reported ingestion within 1 hour of blood collection for LTA.[195]

Critics of the argument for routine testing of platelet function with aspirin therapy point to the lack of standardization of testing, the failure of studies to confirm patient compliance and the use of ADP and other agonists which may not be as reliable as AA for detecting a hyperreactive platelet phenotype. Given the routine use of dual therapy in most cardiology patients, even if true aspirin resistance is present, MACE outcomes are not necessarily going to be increased to the degree represented in monotherapy trials. The overall consequence is that current opinion holds that routine testing for aspirin resistance in PCI patients is not warranted.[210–212]

Clopidogrel activity entails a two-step metabolic conversion by hepatic enzymes to produce the active metabolite which inhibits $P2Y_{12}$ receptor activity. The CYP2C19 enzyme has many polymorphisms, with the CYP2C19*1

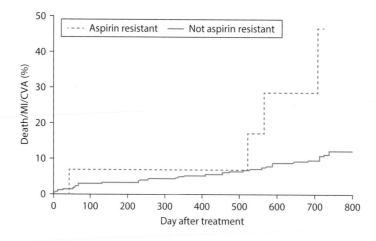

Figure 10.11 Major adverse events (MACE) in subjects with aspirin resistance versus responders – all subjects were reported as taking aspirin. The difference in the time-to-event curves was significant (p = 0.03). (From Gum PA et al., *Am J Cardiol*, 41, 961, 2003.)

allele, the most common. Patients carrying one copy of the CYP2C19*2 allele, known as the loss of function (LOF) allele, have reduced metabolism demonstrated by function tests employing ADP when on 75 mg; but increasing the dose to 150 mg leads to more inhibition of platelet activity. Patients homozygous for CYP2C19*2 have very poor metabolism and have very little or no inhibition induced by clopidogrel even when doses are double or tripled. Another allele, CYP2C19*17, causes ultrarapid metabolism and has been associated with increased risk for bleeding.[213–215] There is good evidence that the LOF allele for clopidogrel metabolism correlates with two- to fourfold increased risk for MAC,[202] and expert opinion and guidelines suggest routine genetic testing for the CYP2C19*2 allele in high-risk patients. Currently, in the United States, genetic testing for the CYP2C19*2 allele is supported by Medicare and many insurance companies, so that detection of poor responders to clopidogrel is feasible. The use of prasugrel or ticagrelor in lieu of clopidogrel is recommended when the LOF allele is identified.

As opposed to genetic testing for poor metabolism, which is one of the few issues not disputed, the value of testing for HPR with clopidogrel therapy is very controversial. Ignoring the influence of genotype, it is estimated that about 20%–30% of patients on clopidogrel have continued high levels of platelet reactivity, although this estimate varies widely depending on the type of platelet function assay employed. Of major importance are the results of the two recent multicentre prospective trials evaluating therapy tailored to platelet function testing. The first was the GRAVITAS trial.[201] In it, the VerifyNow system was used to measure clopidogrel HPR with an ADP aggregation assay immediately after drug eluting coronary stent deployment. All subjects had already been started on conventional dual therapy with aspirin and clopidogrel prior to stenting, testing and randomization. Based on PRU > 230, 2214 patients with HPR for clopidogrel were enrolled – 40% of screened patients met this criterion. HPR subjects were entered into one of two treatment arms: conventional therapy with standard 75 mg

clopidogrel dosing and a high-dose clopidogrel group who on the day of stenting received more clopidogrel for a total dose of 600 mg followed by 150 mg maintenance dosing for 6 months. A control group with normal levels of inhibition (PRU ≤ 230) was also treated with standard clopidogrel dosing. At 6 months, the incidence of MACE was exactly the same (2.3%) in both HPR groups, even though platelet reactivity was significantly diminished 22% in the high-dose clopidogrel group (p < 0.001). Bleeding events were actually less common in the high-dose HPR group than the conventional therapy HPR group (odds ratio 0.59, p = 0.10). Not unexpectedly, the incidence of MACE at 6 months was lower in the group with PRU ≤ 230 (p = 0.2).

Despite the failure of the GRAVITAS study to support efficacy for platelet function monitoring to guide clopidogrel therapy, supporters of individualized therapy point out that identification of LOF in the HPR patients was not carried out and that increased dosing has little effect on LOF heterozygotes and no effect on homozygotes.[202] Forty percent of HPR subjects in the GRAVITAS study remained HPR despite dose increases supporting this criticism.[205] It is also argued that the chosen threshold of 230 PRU was too high, as subsequent ad hoc analysis showed that when adjusted for other factors, HPR subjects in the high clopidogrel dose arm who achieved a PRU ≤ 208 had a marked decrease in MACE that bordered on significance (odds ratio, 0.54, p = 0.065).[201]

A subsequent multicentre trial, ARCTIC,[216] compared tailored dual therapy (aspirin combined with either clopidogrel or prasugrel) in 2440 subjects undergoing drug-eluting coronary stent deployment. The VerifyNow system was employed using AA and ADP agonists to measure sensitivity to aspirin and P2Y_{12} inhibitor therapy. Subjects were randomized prior to stenting. Half received conventional therapy and the other half had therapy tailored to test results performed before stenting and 2–4 weeks after hospital discharge. Subjects in the monitored group had adjustment of P2Y_{12} antagonist dosing based on an algorithm. Subjects with HPR on clopidogrel were either switched to prasugrel or had increases in clopidogrel dosing; those with very low thienopyridine reactivity (>90% inhibition) had dose reductions. After hospital discharge, HPR for aspirin and HPR for thienopyridines were detected in 3.9% and 15.6% of subjects in the monitored group. In the monitored group, 11.2% of subjects had dose reductions in thienopyridine dosing and 10.8% had increases in thienopyridine dosing. Based on aspirin reaction unit measurements after discharge, aspirin dosing was increased in 3.4% and decreased in 3.1%. Antiplatelet therapy in the control arm was based on investigator discretion. The primary outcome of MACE at 1 year occurred in 8.6% of the monitored arm and 7.9% in the conventional arm (OR 1.105 p = 0.48. Major bleeding occurred in 1.8% of the monitored group and 2.8% of controls (p = 0.11). The conclusion was that platelet hyperreactivity could not be considered a risk factor requiring intervention for secondary prevention after PCI.

Just like the situation with aspirin, there is no clear consensus that monitoring platelet activity with the currently available tests is indicated – even though true resistance may be found in as many as 5% of compliant patients. The argument for personalized therapy is based on the reasonable hope that eventually studies will show that monitoring treatment will achieve better results: fewer thrombotic complications and less bleeding. There are critical gaps in our current understanding and employment of antiplatelet therapy: some as simple as knowing whether using venous or arterial blood for the measurement of platelet function makes a difference as recent exposure to arterial shear or plaque may influence test results.[217] The various tests available do not have a high level of concordance and there is no consensus on the appropriate test thresholds that should lead to treatment modification. The one point that experts agree upon is that further research is warranted to assess the reliability of functional tests and their impact on outcomes when used for monitoring therapy.

FUTURE PROSPECTS

Clopidogrel remains the mainstay of dual or monotherapy in high-risk patients. Despite evidence that high reactivity on therapy is associated with more cardiovascular events, it is not clear how to manage non-responders – should it be a switch to prasugrel or ticagrelor despite their higher costs and risks for hemorrhage, or should the next step be triple therapy with cilostazol? This remains an important issue and demands more investigation. Except for carotid stenting, upstream therapy with P2Y$_{12}$ inhibitors or GP IIb/IIIa inhibitors is not standard practice in peripheral interventions, except in carotid stenting – particularly so in bypass surgery, dialysis access and peripheral endovascular interventions. These last three interventions are clearly situations where current results are far from satisfactory, especially in critical limb ischemia and hemodialysis access. Intensification of antiplatelet therapy during these procedures could lead to better outcomes. Preventing platelet activation of inflammation in the traumatized

vessel wall during and immediately after surgery may turn out to be as important as preventing periprocedural thrombosis with antithrombotic drugs. By analogy with PCI methods, in the periphery periprocedural antithrombotic therapy combining heparin (or bivalirudin) and short-acting intravenous P2Y$_{12}$ inhibition with cangrelor might be very helpful. The methodology for monitoring cangrelor with point-of-care methods might be easily achieved with minimal modifications of available platelet function tests.

It seems likely that increasing attention will be focused on the promise of cilostazol as an agent for improving outcomes after peripheral bypass, hemodialysis access and endovascular interventions.

Although pharmaceutical companies undoubtedly will continue to invest large sums of money to develop better antiplatelet agents, what probably is more important now is investment in monitoring tests that are practical and have reliable thresholds, available in both the operating room and community clinics and that are comparable to INR, aPTT and ACT in predictive power. The currently available technologies and the present understanding of platelet physiology should be adequate to meet these goals. The real issue is how to generate a public commitment to provide the resources necessary for clinical investigations leading to effective monitoring regimens and improvement of clinical outcomes with optimal antiplatelet therapy.

REFERENCES

1. Fuster V, Sweeny J. Aspirin: A historic and contemporary therapeutic overview. *Circulation.* 2011;123:768–778.
2. Harker LA, Roskos LK, Marzec UM et al. Effects of megakaryocyte growth and development factor on platelet production, platelet lifespan, and platelet function in healthy human volunteers. *Blood.* 2000;95:2514–2522.
3. Flaumenhaft R. Platelets get the message. *Blood.* 2011;118:1712–1714.
4. Belmonte S, Blaxall B. G protein coupled receptor kinase as therapeutic targets in cardiovascular disease. *Circ Res.* 2011;109:309–319.
5. Gutkind JS. The pathways connecting G protein-coupled receptors to the nucleus through divergent mitogen-activated protein. *J Biol Chem.* 1998;273:1839–1842.
6. Ting HJ, Murad JP, Espinosa EV et al. Thromboxane A2 receptor: Biology and function of a peculiar receptor that remains resistant for therapeutic targeting. *J Cardiovasc Pharmacol Ther.* 2012;17:248–259.
7. Coppinger JA, Cageny G, Toomey S et al. Characterization of the proteins released from activated platelet leads to localization of novel platelet proteins in human astherosclerotic regions. *Blood.* 2004;103;2096–2104.

8. Heijnen HF, Debili N, Vainchencker W et al. Multivesicular bodies are an intermediate stage in the formation of platelet alpha-granules. *Blood.* 1998;91:2313–2325.

9. Whiteheart S. Platelet granules: Surprise packages. *Blood.* 2011;118:1190–1191.

10. Schwertz H, Tolley ND, Foulks JM et al. Signal-dependent splicing of tissue factor pre-mRNA modulates the thrombogenicity of human platelets. *J Exp Med.* 2006;203:2433–2440.

11. Yip J, Shen Y, Berndt MC et al. Primary platelet adhesion receptors. *IUBMB Life.* 2005;57:103–108.

12. Wang G, Zhu Y, Haluska PV et al. Mechanism of platelet inhibition by nitric oxide: In vivo phosphorylation of thromboxane receptor by cyclic GMP-dependent protein kinase. *Proc Natl Acad Sci USA.* 1998;95:4888–4893.

13. Dorn GW, Becker MW. Thromboxane A2 stimulated signal transduction in vascular smooth muscle. *J Pharmacol Exp Therapeut.* 1993;265:447–456.

14. Matarrese P, Straface E, Palumbo G et al. Mitochondria regulate platelet metamorphosis induced by opsonized zymosan A-activation and long-term commitment to cell death. *FEBS J.* 2009;276:845–856.

15. Heemskerk JW, Bevers EM, Lindhout T. Platelet activation and blood coagulation. *Thromb Haemost.* 2002;88:186–193.

16. Thomas S. Platelet membrane glycoproteins in haemostasis. *Clin Lab.* 2002;48:247–262.

17. Wagner CL, Mascalli MA, Neblock DS et al. Analysis of GPIIb/IIIa receptor number by quantification of 7E3 binding to human platelets. *Blood.* 1996;88:907–914.

18. Calvette JJ. On the structure and function of platelet integrin alpha IIb beta 3, the fibrinogen receptor. *Proc Soc Exp Biol Med.* 1995;4:346–360.

19. Piper PJ, Vane JR. Release of additional factors in anaphylaxis and its antagonism by anti-inflammatory drugs. *Nature.* 1969;223:29–35.

20. Roth G, Calverley C. Aspirin, platelets, and thrombosis: Theory and practice. *Blood.* 1994;83:885–898.

21. Anninos H, Andrikopoulos G, Pastromas S et al. Triflusal: An old drug in modern antiplatelet therapy: Review of its action, use, safety and effectiveness. *Hellenic J Cardiol.* 2009;50:199–207.

22. Matias-Guiu J, Ferro JM, Alvarez-Sabin J et al. Randomized comparison trial of triflusal and aspirin following acute myocardial infarction. *Eur Heart J.* 2000;21:457–465.

23. Culebras A, Rotta-Escalante R, Vila J et al. Triflusal vs. aspirin for prevention of cerebral infarction: A randomized stroke study. *Neurology.* 2004;62:1073–1080.

24. Perez-Gomez F, ALegria E, Berjon J et al. Comparative effects of antiplatelet, anticoagulant or combined therapy in patients with valvular and nonvalvular atrial fibrillation: A randomized multicenter study. *J Am Coll Cardiol.* 2004;44:1557–1566.

25. Costa J, Ferro JM, Maatias-Guiu J et al. Triflusal for preventing serious vascular events in people at high risk. *Cochrane Database Syst Rev.* 2005;3:CD004296.

26. Gent M, Blakeley JA, Easton JD et al. The Canadian American ticlopidine study (CATS) in thromboembolic stroke. *Lancet.* 1989;1:1215–1220.

27. Janzon L, Bergqvist D, Boberg J et al. Prevention of myocardial infarction and stroke in patients with intermittent claudication; effects of ticlopidine: Results from STIMS, the Swedish ticlopidine multicenter study. *J Intern Med.* 1990;227:301–308.

28. Savi P, Herbet J. Clopidogrel and ticlopidine: P2Y12 adenosine diphosphate-receptor antagonists for the prevention of atherothrombosis. *Semin Thromb Hemost.* 2005;32(2):174–183.

29. Di Perri T, Pasini FL, Frigerio C et al. Pharmacodynamics of ticlopidine in man in relation to plasma and blood cell concentration. *Eur J Clin Pharmacol.* 1991;41:429–434.

30. Wagner WR, Hubbell JA. ADP receptor antagonists converting enzyme systems reduce platelet deposition onto collagen. *Thromb Haemost.* 1992;67:461–467.

31. Moussa I, Oetgen M, Roubin S et al. Effectiveness of clopidogrel and aspirin versus ticlopidine and aspirin in preventing stent thrombosis after coronary stent implantation. *Circulation.* 1999;99:2363–2366.

32. Ticlopidine Tablets. *Resolved Shortages Bulletin.* American Society of Health-System Pharmacists. Accessed April 1, 2015 at aspashp.org/menu/Drug Shortages/ResolvedShortages?Bulletin.aspx?Source =Resolved&Type=Rss&Id=661.

33. CAPRIE Steering Committee. A randomised, blinded, trial of clopidogrel versus aspirin in patients at risk of ischaemic events (CAPRIE). *Lancet.* 1996;348:1329–1339.

34. Yusuf S, Zhao F, Mehta SR et al. Effects of clopidogrel in addition to aspirin in patients with acute coronary syndromes without ST-segment elevation. *N Engl J Med.* 2001;345;494–502.

35. Savi P, Herbert JM, Pflieger AM et al. Importance of hepatic metabolism in the antiaggregating activity of the thienopyridine clopidogrel. *Biochem Pharmacol.* 1992;44:527–532.

36. Denninger MH, Necciari J, Serre-Lacroix E, Sissmann J. Clopidogrel antiplatelet activity is independent of age and presence of atherosclerosis. *Semin Thromb Hemost.* 1999;25:41–45.

37. Lala A, Berger JS, Sharma G et al. Genetic testing in patients with acute coronary syndrome undergoing percutaneous coronary intervention: a cost-effectiveness analysis. *J Thromb Haemost.* 2013;11:81–91.

38. Wiviott, SD, Braunwald E, McCabe CH et al. Prasugrel versus clopidogrel in patients with acute coronary syndromes. *N Engl J Med.* 2007;357:2001–2015.

39. Roe TM, Armstrong PW, Fox KAA et al. Prasugrel versus clopidogrel for acute coronary syndromes without revascularization. *N Engl J Med.* 2012;367:1297–1309.

40. Dobesh P, Oestreich J. Ticagrelor: Pharmacokinetics, pharmacodynamics, clinical efficacy, and safety. *Pharmacotherapy.* 2014;34(10):1077–1090.

41. Storey RF, Becker RC, Harrington RA et al. Characterization of dyspnoea in PLATO study patients treated with ticagrelor or clopidogrel and its association with clinical outcomes. *Eur Heart J.* 2011;32:2945–2953.

42. Cannon CP, Husted S, Harrington RA et al. Safety, tolerability, and initial efficacy of AZD6140, the first reversible oral adenosine diphosphate receptor antagonist, compared with clopidogrel, in patients with non-ST-segment elevation acute coronary syndrome: Primary results of the DISPERSE-2 trial. *J Am Coll Cardiol.* 2007;50:1844–1851.

43. Björkman J-A, Kirk I, van Giezen JJ. AZD6140 inhibits adenosine uptake into erythrocytes and enhances coronary blood flow after local ischemia or intracoronary adenosine infusion. *Circulation.* 2007;116:11–28.

44. Cannon C, Harrington R, Stefan J et al. Comparison of ticagrelor with clopidogrel in patients with a planned invasive strategy for acute coronary syndromes (PLATO): A randomized double-blind study. *Lancet.* 2010;375:283–293.

45. Bonaca MP, Bhatt DL, Cohen M et al. Long-term use of ticagrelor in patients with prior myocardial infarction. *N Engl J Med.* 2015;372:1791–1800.

46. Hansson EC, Rexius H, Deiliborg M et al. Coronary artery bypass grafting-related bleeding complications in real-life acute coronary syndrome patients treated with clopidogrel or ticagrelor. *Eur J Caridothorac Surg.* 2014;46:699–705.

47. Bhatt Deepak L, Stone Gregg W, Mahaffey Kenneth W et al. Effect of platelet inhibition with cangrelor during PCI on ischemic events. *N Engl J Med.* 2013;368:1303–1313.

48. Lange RA, Hillis LD. The duel between dual antiplatelet therapies. *N Engl J Med.* 2013;368(14):1356–1357.

49. Serebruany VL, Sibbing D, DiNicolantonio JJ et al. Dyspnea and reversibility of antiplatelet agents: Ticagrelor, elinogrel, cangrelor, and beyond. *Cardiology.* 2014;127:20–24.

50. Angiolillo DJ, Firstenberg MS, Price MJ et al. Bridging antiplatelet therapy with cangrelor in patients undergoing cardiac surgery: A randomized controlled trial. *J Am Med Assoc.* 2012;307:265–274.

51. Harrington RA, Stone GW, McNulty S et al. Platelet inhibition with cangrelor in patients undergoing PCI. *N Engl J Med.* 2009;361–2318–2329.

52. Seligsohn U. Glanzmann thrombasthenia: A model disease which paved the way to powerful therapeutic agents. *Pathophysiol Haemost Thromb.* 2002;32:216–217.

53. Berkowitz SD, Harrington RA, Rund M, Tcheng JE. Acute profound thrombocytopenia after C7E3 Fab (abciximab) therapy. *Circulation.* 1997;95:809–813.

54. King S, Short M, Harmon C. Glycoprotein IIb/IIIa inhibitors: The resurgence of tirofiban. *Vascul Pharmacol.* 2016 March;78:10–16.

55. Bougie PR, Wilker ED, Wuitschick ED et al. Acute thrombocytopenia after treatment with tirofiban or eptifibatide is associated with antibodies specific for ligand-occupied GPIIb/IIIa. *Blood.* 2002;100:2071–2076.

56. Paradiso-Hardy FL, Madan M, Radhakrishnan S et al. Severe thrombocytopenia possibly related to readministration of eptifibatide. *Catheter Cardiovasc Interv.* 2001;54:63–67.

57. Epic Investigators. Use of a monoclonal antibody directed against the platelet glycoprotein IIb/IIIa receptor in high-risk coronary angioplasty. *N Engl J Med.* 1994;330:956–961.

58. Epilog Investigators. Platelet glycoprotein IIb/IIIa receptor blockade and low-dose heparin during percutaneous coronary revascularization. *N Engl J Med.* 1997;336:1689–1696.

59. Capture Investigators. Randomised placebo-controlled trial of abciximab before and during coronary intervention in refractory unstable angina: The Capture study. *Lancet.* 1997;349:1429–1435.

60. The Prism Study Investigators. A comparison of aspirin plus tirofiban with aspirin plus heparin for unstable angina. *N Eng J Med.* 1998;338:1498–1505.

61. The Prism-Plus Study Investigators. Inhibition of the platelet glycoprotein IIb/IIIa receptor with tirofiban in unstable angina and non-Q-wave myocardial infarction. Platelet receptor inhibition in ischemic syndrome management in patients limited by unstable signs and symptoms. *N Engl J Med.* 1998;338:1488–1497.

62. Topol EJ, Moliterno DJ, Herrmann HC et al. Comparison of two platelet glycoprotein IIb/IIIa inhibitors, tirofiban and abciximab, for the prevention of ischemic events with percutaneous coronary revascularization. *N Engl J Med.* 2001;244:1888–1894.

63. Nazif TM, Mehran R, Lee EA et al. Comparative effectiveness of upstream glycoprotein IIb/IIIa inhibitors in patients with moderate-and high-risk acute coronary syndromes: An acute catheterization and urgent intervention triage strategy ACUITY substudy. *Am Heart J.* 2014;167:43–50.

64. Valgimigli M, Campo G, Percoco G et al. Comparison of angioplasty with infusion of tirofiban or abciximab and with implantation of sirolimus-eluting or uncoated stents for acute myocardial infarction: The Multistrategy randomized trial. *J Am Med Assoc.* 2008;299:1788–1799.

65. The PURSUIT trial investigators. Inhibition of platelet glycoprotein IIb/IIIa with eptifibatide in patients with acute coronary syndromes: Platelet glycoprotein IIb/IIIa in unstable angina: Receptor suppression using integrilin therapy. *N Engl J Med.* 1998;339:436–444.

66. Patrono C, Andreotti F, Arnesen H et al. Antiplatelet agents for the treatment and prevention of athero-thrombosis. *Eur Heart J.* 2011;32:2922–2932.

67. PURSUIT Trial Investigators. Inhibition of platelet glycoprotein IIb/IIIa with eptifibatide in patients with acute coronary syndromes. *N Engl J Med.* 1998;339:436–443.

68. ESPRIT Investigators. Novel dosing regimen of eptifibatide in planned coronary stent implantation (ESPRIT): A randomized, placebo-controlled trial. *Lancet.* 2000;356:2037–2044.

69. Amsterdam EA, Wenger NK, Brindis RG et al. 2014 AHA/ACC guideline for the management of patients with non-ST-elevation acute coronary syndromes: Executive summary: A report of the American College of Cardiology/American Heart Association Task Force on Practice Guidelines. *Circulation.* 2014;130:2354–2394.

70. De Luca G, Ucci G, Cassetti E et al. Benefits from small molecule administration as compared with abciximab among patients with ST-segment eleva-tion myocardial infarction treated with primary angioplasty: A meta-analysis. *J Am Coll Cardiol.* 2009;53:1668–1673.

71. Gurm HS, Smith DE, Collins JS et al. The relative safety and efficacy of abciximab and eptifibatide in patients undergoing primary percutaneous coronary intervention: Insights from a large regional registry of contemporary percutaneous coronary interven-tion. *J Am Coll Cardiol.* 2008;51:529–535.

72. Zeymer U, Margenet A, Haude M et al. Randomized comparison of eptifibatide versus abciximab in primary percutaneous coronary intervention in patients with acute ST-segment elevation myocardial infarction: Results of the EVA-AMI Trial. *J Am Coll Cardiol.* 2010;56:463–469.

73. O'Gara PT, Kushner FG, Ascheim DD et al. 2013 ACCF/AHA guideline for the management of ST-elevation myocardial infarction: Executive summary: A report of the American College of Cardiology Foundation/American Heart Association Task Force on Practice Guidelines. *Circulation.* 2013;127:529–555.

74. Windecker S, Kolh P, Alfonso F et al. 2014 ESC/EACTS Guidelines on myocardial revascularization: The Task Force on Myocardial Revascularization of the European Society of Cardiology (ESC) and the European Association for Cardio-Thoracic Surgery (EACTS)Developed with the special contribution of the European Association of Percutaneous Cardiovascular Interventions. *Eur Heart J.* 2014;35:2541–2619.

75. Stone GW, Witzenbichler B, Guagliumi G et al. Bivalirudin during primary PCI in acute myocardial infarction. *N Engl J Med.* 2008;358:2218–2230.

76. Capodanno AD, Bhatt DL, Goto M et al. Safety and efficacy of protease-activated receptor-1 antago-nists in patients with coronary artery disease: A meta-analysis of randomized clinical trials. *J Thomb Haemost.* 2012;10:2006–2015.

77. Tricoci P, Huang Z, Held C et al. Thrombin-receptor antagonist vorapaxar in acute coronary syndromes. *N Engl J Med.* 2012;366:20–33.

78. Bohula WA, Aylward PE, Bobaca MP et al. The effi-cacy and safety of vorapaxar with and without a thienopyridine for secondary prevention in patients with prior myocardial infarction and no history of stroke or TIA: Results from TRA 2°P-TIMI 50. *Circulation.* 2015;132(20):1871–1879.

79. Gresele P, Momi S, Falcinelli E. Anti-platelet therapy: Phosphodiesterase inhibitors. *Br J Clin Pharmacol.* 2011;72:634–646.

80. Daniel JL, Ashby B, Pulcinelli F. Platelet signal-ing: cAMP and cGMP. In: Gresele P, ed. *Platelets in Thrombotic and Non-Thrombotic Disorders.* Cambridge, UK: Cambridge University Press; 2002, pp. 290–304.

81. Bender AT, Beavo JA. Cyclic nucleotide phospho-diesterases: Molecular regulation to clinical use. *Pharmacol Rev.* 2006;58:488–520.

82. Maurice DH, Haslam RJ. Molecular basis of the synergistic inhibition of platelet function by nitro-vasodilators and activators of adenylate cyclase: Inhibition of cyclic AMP breakdown by cyclic GMP. *Mol Pharmacol.* 1990;37:671–681.

83. Sun B, Li H, Shakur Y et al. Role of phosphodiester-ase type 3A and 3B in regulating platelet and cardiac function using subtype-selective knockout mice. *Cell Signal.* 2007;19:1765–1771.

84. Emmons PR. Postoperative changes in platelet-clumping activity. *Lancet.* 1965;71:255–257.

85. Iuliano L, Colavita AR, Camastra P et al. Protection of low density lipoprotein oxidation at chemical and cellular level by the antioxidant drug dipyridamole. *Br J Pharmacol.* 1996;119:1438–1443.

86. Pascual C, Romay C. Effect of antioxidant and che-miluminescence produced by reactive oxygen spe-cies. *J Biolumin Chemilumin.* 1992;7:123–132.

87. Ghoshal K Bhattacharyya M. Overview of platelet physiology: Its hemostatic and nonhemostatic role in disease pathogenesis. *ScientificWorldJournal.* 2014;Article ID 781857:8.

88. Wang G-R, Zhu Y, Halushka P et al. Mechanism of platelet inhibition by nitric oxide: In vivo phosphor-ylation of thromboxane receptor by cyclic GMP-dependent protein kinase. *Proc Natl Acad Sci USA.* 1998;95:4888–4893.

89. Gresele P, Zoja C, Deckmyn H et al. Dipyridamole inhibits platelet aggregation in whole blood. *Thromb Haemost.* 1983;30:852–856.

90. Muller TH, Su CA, Weisemberg H et al. Dipyridamole alone or combined with low-dose acetylsalicylic acid inhibits platelet aggregation in human whole blood ex vivo. *Br J Clin Pharmacol.* 1990;30:179–186.

91. Bjornsson TD, Mahony C. Clinical pharmacokinetics of dipyridamole. *Thomb Res Suppl.* 1983; 4:93–104.

92. Fitzgerald GA. Dipyridamole. *N Engl J Med.* 1987;316: 1247–1257.

93. Lutomski DM, Harker LA, Hirsh J et al. Critical evaluation of platelet-inhibition drugs in thrombotic disease. *Prog Hematol.* 1975;9:225–254.

94. Verstreta M, Kienast J. Pharmacology of the interaction between platelets and vessel wall. *Clin Haematol.* 1986;15:493–508.

95. Lutomski DM, Bottorff M, Sangha K. Pharmacokinetic optimisation of the treatment embolic disorders. *Clin Pharmacokinet.* 1995; 28:67–92.

96. Stein PD, Alpert JS, Bussey HI et al. Antithrombotic therapy in patients with mechanical and biological prosthetic heart valves. *Chest.* 2001;119:220S–227S.

97. Diener H C, Cunha L, Forbes C et al. European Stroke Prevention Study 2. Dipyridamole and acetylsalicylic acid in the secondary prevention of stroke. *J Neurol Sci.* 1996;143:1–13.

98. The Espirit Study Group. Aspirin plus dipyridamole versus aspirin alone after cerebral ischaemia of arterial origin (ESPRIT): Randomized controlled trial. *Lancet.* 2006;367:1665–1673.

99. Kimura Y, Tani T, Kanbe T et al. Effect of cilostazol on platelet aggregation and experimental thrombosis. *Arzneimittelforschung.* 1985;35:1144–1149.

100. Yasunaga K, Mase K. Antiaggregatory effect of oral cilostazol and recovery of platelet aggregability in patients with cerebrovascular disease. *Arzneimittelforschung.* 1985;35:1189–1192.

101. Minami N, Suzuki Y, Yamamoto M et al. Inhibition of shear stress-induced platelet aggregation by cilostazol, a specific inhibitor of cGMP-inhibited phosphodiesterase, in vitro and ex vivo. *Life Sci.* 1997;61:383–389.

102. Kariyazono H, Nakamura K, Shinkawa T et al. Inhibition of platelet aggregation and the release of P-selectin from platelets by cilostazol. *Thromb Res.* 2001;101:445–453.

103. Miyashita Y, Saito S, Lida O et al. Cilostazol increases skin perfusion pressure in severely ischemic limbs. *Angiology.* 2011;62:15–17.

104. O'Donnell ME, Badger SA, Sharif MA et al. The vascular and biochemical effects of cilostazol in patients with peripheral arterial disease. *J Vasc Surg.* 2009;49:1226–1234.

105. Mohler ER 3rd, Beebe HG, Salles-Cuhna S et al. Effects of cilostazol on resting ankle pressures and exercise-induced ischemia in patients with intermittent claudication. *Vasc Med.* 2001;6:151–156.

106. Okuda Y, Mizutani M, Ikegami T et al. Hemodynamic effects of cilostazol on peripheral artery in patients with diabetic neuropathy. *Arzneimittelforschung.* 1992;42:540–542.

107. Kamiya T, Sakaguchi S. Hemodynamic effects of the antithrombotic drug cilostazol in chronic arterial occlusion in the extremities. *Arzneimittelforschung.* 1985;35:1201–1203.

108. Ohashi S, Iwatani M, Hyakuna Y et al. Thermographic evaluation of the hemodynamic effect of the antithrombotic drug cilostazol in peripheral arterial occlusion. *Arzneimittelforschung.* 1985;35:1203–1208.

109. Money SR, Herd JA, Isaacsohn JL et al. Effect of cilostazol on walking distances in patients with intermittent claudication caused by peripheral vascular disease. *J Vasc Surg.* 1998;27:267–274.

110. Dawson DL, Cutler BS, Hiatt WR et al. A comparison of cilostazol and pentoxifylline for treating intermittent claudication. *Am J Med.* 2000;109:523–530.

111. Elam MB, Heckman J, Crouse JR et al. Effect of the novel antiplatelet agent Cilostazol on plasma lipoproteins in patients with intermittent claudication. *Arterioscler Thromb Vasc Biol.* 1998;18:1942–1947.

112. Nishio Y, Kashiwagi A, Takahara N et al. Cilostazol, a cAMP phosphodiesterase inhibitor, attenuates the production of monocyte chemoattractant protein-1 in response to tumor necrosis factor-alpha in vascular endothelial cells. *Horm Metab Res.* 1997;29: 491–495.

113. Tsai CS, Lin FY, Chen YH et al. Cilostazol attenuates MCP-1 and MMP-9 expression in vivo in LPS-administrated balloon-injured rabbit aorta and in vitro in LPS-treated monocytic THP-1 cells. *J Cell Biochem.* 2008;103:54–66.

114. Kubota Y, Kichikawa K, Uchida H et al. Pharmacologic treatment of intimal hyperplasia after metallic stent placement in the peripheral arteries: An experimental study. *Invest Radiol.* 1995;9:532–537.

115. Weintraub WS, Foster J, Culler SD et al. Cilostazol for RESTenosis trial. Cilostazol for RESTenosis trial: Methods for the economic and quality of life supplement to the cilostazol for RESTenosis. *J Invasive Cardiol.* 2004;16:257–259.

116. Yamagami H, Sakai N, Matsumaru Y et al. Periprocedural cilostazol treatment and restenosis after carotid artery stenting: The retrospective study of in-stent restenosis after carotid artery stenting (ReSISteR-CAS). *J Stroke Cerebrovasc Dis.* 2010;21:193–199.

117. Iida O, Yokoi H, Soga Y et al. Cilostazol reduces angiographic restenosis after endovascular therapy for femoropopliteal lesions in the Sufficient Treatment of Peripheral Intervention by Cilostazol study. *Circulation.* 2013;127:2307–2315.

118. Gotoh F, Tohgi H, Hirai S et al. Stroke Prevention Study: A placebo-controlled double-blind trial for secondary prevention of cerebral infarction. *J Stroke Cerebrovasc Dis.* 2000;9:147–157.

119. Shinohara Y, Katayama Y, Uchiyama S et al. Cilostazol for prevention of secondary stroke (CSPS 2): An aspirin-controlled, double-blind, randomised non-inferiority trial. *Lancet Neurol.* 2010;90:959–968.

120. Stewart M, Bedenis R, Cleanthis M et al. Cilostazol for intermittent claudication. *Cochrane Database Syst Rev.* 2014 October 31;10:CD003748.

121. Bramer SL, Forbes WP, Mallikaarjun S. Cilostazol pharmacokinetics after single and multiple oral doses in healthy males and patients with intermittent claudication resulting from peripheral arterial disease. *Clin Pharmacokinet.* 1999;37:1–11.

122. Iwamoto T, Kin K, Miyazaki K et al. Recovery of platelet function after withdrawal of cilostazol administered orally for a long period. *J Atheroscler Thromb.* 2003;10:348–354.

123. Tamai Y, Takami H, Nakahata R et al. Comparison of the effects of acetylsalicylic acid, ticlopidine and cilostazol on primary hemostasis using a quantitative bleeding time test apparatus. *Haemostasis.* 1999;29:269–276.

124. Pletal. http://www.accessdata.fda.gov/drugsatfda_docs/label//2007/020863s021lbl.pdf. Accessed August 21, 2016.

125. Drug Approval Package. http://www.accessdata.fda.gov/drugsatfda_docs/nda/99/20863.cfm. Accessed August 21, 2016.

126. Leeper N, Mehren A, Iyer S et al. Practice-based evidence: profiling the safety of cilostazol by text-mining of clinical notes. *PLOS ONE.* 2013 May 23;8(5):e63499.

127. Antithrombotic Trialists' (ATT) Collaboration. Aspirin in the primary and secondary prevention of vascular disease: Collaborative meta-analysis of individual participant data from randomised trials. *Lancet.* 2009;373:1849–1860.

128. Sutcliffe P, Connock M, Gurung T et al. Aspirin for prophylactic use in the primary prevention of cardiovascular disease and cancer: A systematic review and overview of reviews. *Health Technol Assess.* 2013;17(43):1–253.

129. Ridker PM, Cook NR, Lee IM et al. A randomized trial of low-dose aspirin in the primary prevention of cardiovascular disease in women. *N Engl J Med.* 2005;352(13):1293–1304.

130. Final report on the aspirin component of the ongoing Physicians' Health Study. Steering Committee of the Physicians' Health Study Research Group. *N Engl J Med.* 1989;321:129–135.

131. Antiplatelet Trialists' Collaboration. Secondary prevention of vascular disease by prolonged antiplatelet treatment. *Br Med J.* 1998;296:320–331.

132. Antiplatelet Trialists' Collaboration. Collaborative overview of randomised trials of antiplatelet therapy-I: Prevention of death, myocardial infarction, and stroke by prolonged antiplatelet therapy in various categories of patients. *Br Med J.* 1994;30:81–106.

133. Antithrombotic Trialists' Collaboration. Collaborative metaanalysis of randomised trials of antiplatelet therapy for prevention of death, myocardial infarction, and stroke in high risk patients. *Br Med J.* 2002;324:71–86.

134. Shani S, Ahman RE, Naveen SV et al. Platelet rich concentrate promotes early cellular proliferation and multiple lineage differentiation of human mesenchymal stromal cells in vitro. *ScientificWorldJournal* 2014;2014:845293.

135. Bhatt DL, Fox KAA, Hacke W et al. Clopidogrel and aspirin versus aspirin alone for the prevention of atherothrombotic events. *N Engl J Med.* 2006;354:1706–1717.

136. Pande RL, Perlstein TS, Beckman JA et al. Secondary prevention and mortality in peripheral artery disease. *Circulation.* 2011;124:17–23.

137. De Martino RR, Eldrup-Jorgensen J, Nolan BW et al. Perioperative management with antiplatelet and statin medication is associated with reduced mortality following vascular surgery. *J Vasc Surg.* 2014 June;59:1615–1621.

138. Subherwal S, Patel MR, Kober L et al. Missed opportunities: Despite improvement in use of cardioprotective medications among patients with lower-extremity peripheral artery disease, underuse remains. *Circulation.* 2012;126:1345–1354.

139. Brott TG, Halperin JL, Abbara S et al. ASA/ACCF/AHA/AANN/AANS/ACR/ASNR/CNS/SAIP/SCAI/SIR/SNIS/SVM/SVS guideline on the management of patients with extracranial carotid and vertebral artery disease: Executive summary. A report of the American College of Cardiology Foundation/American Heart Association Task Force on Practice Guidelines, and the American Stroke Association, American Association of Neuroscience Nurses, American Association of Neurological Surgeons, American College of Radiology, American Society of Neuroradiology, Congress of Neurological Surgeons, Society of Atherosclerosis Imaging and Prevention, Society for Cardiovascular Angiography and Interventions, Society of Interventional Radiology, Society of Neuro-Interventional Surgery, Society for Vascular Medicine, and Society for Vascular Surgery. *Circulation.* 2011;124:489–532.

140. Rooke TW, Hirsch AT, Misra S et al. 2011 ACCF/AHA focused update of the guideline for the management of patients with peripheral artery disease (updating the 2005 guideline): A report of the American College of Cardiology Foundation/American Heart Association Task Force on Practice Guidelines: Developed in collaboration with the Society for Cardiovascular Angiography and Interventions, Society of Interventional Radiology, Society for Vascular Medicine, and Society for Vascular Surgery. *J Vasc Surg.* 2011;54:32–58.

141. Sobel M, Verhaeghe R. Antithrombotic therapy for peripheral artery occlusive disease: American College of Chest Physicians Evidence-Based Clinical Practice Guidelines. *Chest.* 2008;133:815S–843S.

142. Yusuf S, Phil D, Zhao F et al. Effects of clopidogrel in addition to aspirin in patients with acute coronary syndromes without ST-segment elevation. *N Engl J Med.* 2001;345:495–502.

143. Xiao-Fang T, Jing-Yao F, Jing M et al. Impact of new oral or intravenous P2Y12 inhibitors and clopidogrel on major ischemic and bleeding events in patients with coronary artery disease: A meta-analysis of randomized trials. *Atherosclerosis.* 2014;233:568–578.

144. Yusuf S, Zhao F, Mehta SR, Chrolavicius S, Tognoni G, Fox KK. Effects of clopidogrel in addition to aspirin in patients with acute coronary syndromes without ST-segment elevation. *N Engl J Med.* 2001;345:494–502.

145. Steinhubl SR, Berger PB, Mann JT 3rd et al. Early and sustained dual oral antiplatelet therapy following percutaneous coronary intervention: A randomized controlled trial. *J Am Med Assoc*. 2002;288:2411–2420.

146. Chen ZM, Jiang LX, Chen YP et al. Addition of clopidogrel to aspirin in 45,852 patients with acute myocardial infarction: Randomised placebo-controlled trial. *Lancet*. 2005;366:1607–1621.

147. Mehta SR, Yusuf S, Peters RJG et al. Effects of pretreatment with clopidogrel and aspirin followed by long-term therapy in patients undergoing percutaneous coronary intervention: The PCI-CURE study. *Lancet*. 2001;358:527–533.

148. Fihn SD, Gardin JM, Abrams J et al. 2012 ACCF/AHA/ACP/AATS/PCNA/SCAI/STS Guideline for the diagnosis and management of patients with stable ischemic heart disease. *Circulation*. 2012;126:354–471.

149. Ehersmann U, Alemany J, Loew D. Use of acetylsalicylic acid in the prevention of reocclusion following revascularization interventions: Results of a double blind long term study. *Medizinische Welt*. 1977;28:1157–1162.

150. Belch JJ, Dormandy J. Results of the randomized, placebo-controlled clopidogrel and acetylsalicylic acid in bypass surgery for peripheral arterial disease (CASPAR) trial. *J Vasc Surg*. 2010;52:825–833.

151. Geraghty AJ, Welch K, Alistair J. Antithrombotic agents for preventing thrombosis after infrainguinal arterial bypass surgery. *Cochrane Database Syst Rev*. 2011;6:1–97.

152. Bedenis R, Lethaby A, Maxwell H et al. Antiplatelet agents for preventing thrombosis after peripheral arterial bypass surgery. *Cochrane Database Syst Rev*. 2015;3:1–90.

152. WAVE Investigators. The effects of oral anticoagulants in patients with peripheral arterial disease: Rationale, design, and baseline characteristics of the Warfarin and Antiplatelet Vascular Evaluation (WAVE) trial, including a meta-analysis of trials. *Am Heart J*. 2006;151:1–9.

153. Brown J, Lethaby A, Maxwell H et al. Antiplatelet agents for preventing thrombosis after peripheral arterial bypass surgery. *Cochrane Database Syst Rev*. 2011;3:1–32.

154. Watson H, Skene AM, Belcher G. Graft material and results of platelet inhibitor trials in peripheral arterial reconstructions: Reappraisal of results from a meta-analysis. *Br J Clin Pharmacol*. 2000;49:479–483.

155. BOA Study Group. Efficacy of oral anticoagulants compared with aspirin after infrainguinal bypass surgery (The Dutch Bypass Oral anticoagulants or Aspirin study): A randomised trial. *Lancet*. 2000;355:346–351.

156. Johnson WC, Williford WO. Benefits, morbidity, and mortality associated with long-term administration of oral anticoagulant therapy to patients with peripheral arterial bypass procedures. A prospective randomized study. *J Vasc Surg*. 2002;35:413–421.

157. Monaco M, Di Tommaso L, Battista Pinna G et al. Combination therapy with warfarin plus clopidogrel improves outcomes in femoropopliteal bypass surgery patients. *J Vasc Surg*. 2012;56:96–105.

158. Stratton JR, Zierler RE, Kazmers A. Platelet deposition at carotid endarterectomy sites in humans. *Stroke*. 1987;18:722–727.

159. Payne DA, Jones CI, Hayes PD et al. Beneficial effects of clopidogrel combined with aspirin in reducing cerebral emboli in patients undergoing carotid endarterectomy. *Circulation*. 2004;109:1476–1481.

160. Naylor AR, Sayers RD, McCarthy MJ et al. Closing the loop: A 21-year audit of strategies for preventing stroke and death following carotid endarterectomy. *Eur Soc Vasc Surg*. 2013;46:162–170.

161. Engelter S, Lyrer P. Antiplatelet therapy for preventing stroke and other vascular events after carotid endarterectomy. *Stroke*. 2004;35:1227–1228.

162. Schoenfeld E, Donas K, Radicke A et al. Perioperative use of aspirin for patients undergoing carotid endarterectomy. *Vasa*. 2012;41:282–287.

163. Taylor DW, Barnett HJ, Haynes R et al. Low-dose and high-dose acetylsalicylic acid for patients undergoing carotid endarterectomy: A randomized trial. *Lancet*. 1999;353:2179–2184.

164. Kresowik TF, Bratzler DW, Kresowik RA et al. Multistate improvement in process and outcomes of carotid endarterectomy. *J Vasc Surg*. 2004;39:372–380.

165. Rosenbaum A, Rizvi AZ, Alden PB et al. Outcomes related to antiplatelet or anticoagulation use in patients undergoing carotid endarterectomy. *Ann Vasc Surg*. 2011;25:25–31.

166. Morales Gisbert SM, Sala Almonacil VA, Zaragoza García JM et al. Predictors of cervical bleeding after carotid endarterectomy. *Ann Vasc Surg*. 2014;28:366–374.

167. Gordon IL, Arefi M. Physiology of the arteriovenous fistula. In: Wilson SE, ed. *Vascular Access*, 4 ed. St. Louis, MO: Mosby; 2002, Chapter 5, pp. 33–47.

168. Cinat ME, Hopkins J, Wilson SE. A prospective evaluation of PTFE graft patency and surveillance techniques in hemodialysis access. *Ann Vasc Surg*. 1999;13:191–198.

169. Jackson RS, Sidawy AN, Amdur RL et al. Angiotensin receptor blockers and antiplatelet agents are associated with improved primary patency after arteriovenous hemodialysis access placement. *J Vasc Surg*. 2011;54:1706–1712.

170. Castillo R, Lozano T, Esscolar G et al. Defective platelet adhesion on vessel subendothelium in uremic patients. *Blood*. 1986;68:337–342.

171. Mezzano D, Tagle R, Panes O et al. Hemostatic disorder of uremia: The platelet defect, main determinant of the prolonged bleeding time, is correlated with indices of activation of coagulation and fibrinolysis. *Thromb Haemost*. 1996;3:312–321.

172. Hasegawa T, Elder SJ, Bragg-Gresham JL et al. Consistent aspirin use associated with improved arteriovenous fistula survival among incident hemodialysis patients in the dialysis outcomes and practice patterns study. *Clin J Am Soc Nephrol.* 2008;3:1373–1378.

173. Saran R, Dykstra DM, Wolfe RA et al. Association between vascular access failure and the use of specific drugs: The dialysis outcomes and practice patterns study (DOPPS). *Am J Kidney Dis.* 2002;40:1255–1263.

174. Foley RN, Parfrey PS, Sarnak MJ. Epidemiology of cardiovascular disease in chronic renal disease. *J Am Soc Nephrol.* 1998;9(12 Suppl.):S16–S23.

175. Soubassi LP, Chiras TC, Papadakis ED et al. Incidence and risk factors of coronary heart disease in elderly patients on chronic hemodialysis. *Int Urol Nephrol.* 2006;38:795–800.

176. Mousa AY, Patterson W, Abu-Halimah S et al. Patency in arteriovenous grafts in hemodialysis patients. *Vasc Endovasc Surg.* 2013;47:438–443.

177. Andrassy K, Malluche H, Bornefeld H et al. Prevention of p.o. clotting of av. ciminofistulae with acetylsalicyl acid: Results of a prospective double blind study. *Klinische Wochenschrift.* 1974;52:348–349.

178. Tanner NC, Da Silva A. Medical adjuvant treatment to increase patency of arteriovenous fistulae and grafts (Review). *Cochrane Database Syst Rev.* 2015; July 16;7:CD002786.

179. Kaufman JS, O'Connor TZ, Zhang JH et al. Randomized controlled trial of clopidogrel plus aspirin to prevent hemodialysis access graft thrombosis. *J Am Soc Nephrol.* 2003;14:2313–2321.

180. Sreedhara R, Himmelfarb J, Lazarus M et al. Antiplatelet therapy in graft thrombosis: Results of a prospective, randomized, double-blind study. *Kidney Int.* 1994;45:1477–1483.

181. Dixon BS, Beck GJ, Vazquez MA et al. Effect of dipyridamole plus aspirin on hemodialysis graft patency. *N Engl J Med.* 2009;360:2191–2201.

182. Dember LM, Beck GJ, Allon M et al. Effect of clopidogrel on early failure of arteriovenous fistulas for hemodialysis. *J Am Med Assoc.* 2008;299:2164–2171.

183. Roy-Chaudhury P, Lee T, Woodle B et al. Balloon assisted maturation (BAM) of the arteriovenous fistula: The good, the bad and the ugly! *Semin Nephrol.* 2012;32:558–563.

184. Hess H, Mietaschkg A, Deichsel G. Drug-induced inhibition of platelet function delays progression of peripheral occlusive arterial disease. *Lancet.* 1985;2:415–419.

185. Study Group 1994. Platelet inhibition with ASA/dipyridamole after percutaneous balloon angioplasty in patients with symptomatic lower limb arterial disease. A prospective double-blind trial. Study group on pharmacological treatment after PTA. *Eur J Vasc Surg.* 1994;1:83–88.

186. Allemang MT, Rajani RR, Peter R. Nelson PR et al. Prescribing patterns of antiplatelet agents are highly variable after lower extremity endovascular procedures. *Ann Vasc Surg.* 2013;27:62–67.

187. Becker RC, Helmy T. Are at least 12 months of dual antiplatelet therapy needed for all patients with drug-eluting stents? *Circulation.* 2015;131:2010–2019.

188. McKevitt FM, Randall MS, Cleveland TJ et al. The benefits of combined anti-platelet treatment in carotid artery stenting. *Eur J Vasc Endovasc Surg.* 2005;29:522–527.

189. Dalainas I, Nano G, Bianchi P et al. Dual antiplatelet regime versus acetyl-acetic acid for carotid artery stenting. *Cardiovasc Intervent Radiol.* 2006;29:519–521.

190. Qureshi AI, Suri MFK, Ali Z et al. Carotid angioplasty and stent placement: A prospective analysis of perioperative complications and impact of intravenously administered abciximab. *Neurosurgery.* 2002;50:466–475.

191. Takayama K, Taoka T, Nakagawa H et al. Effect of cilostazol in preventing restenosis after carotid artery stenting using the carotid wallstent: A multicenter retrospective study. *Am J Neuroradiol.* 2012;33:2167–2170.

190. Nakagawa I, Wada T, Park HS et al. Platelet inhibition by adjunctive cilostazol suppresses the frequency of cerebral ischemic lesions after carotid artery stenting in patients with carotid artery stenosis. *J Vasc Surg.* 2014;3:761–767.

191. Chaturvedi S, Sohrab S, Tselis A. Carotid stent thrombosis: Report of 2 fatal cases. *Stroke.* 2001;32:2700–2702.

192. Bates ER, Babb JD, Casey DE Jr. et al. American College of Cardiology Foundation Task Force, American Society of Interventional and Therapeutic Neuroradiology, Society for Cardiovascular Angiography and Interventions, Society for Vascular Medicine and Biology, Society for Interventional Radiology: ACCF/SCAI/SVMB/SIR/ASITN 2007 clinical expert consensus document on carotid stenting. *Vasc Med.* 2007;12:35–83.

193. AHA ACC ASA. Guideline on the management of patients with extracranial carotid and vertebral artery disease. , Washington, DC: American College of Cardiology Foundation; 2011, pp. 1–51.

194. Michelson AD. Platelet function testing in cardiovascular diseases. *Circulation.* 2004;110:e489–e493.

195. Gum PA, Kottke-Marchant K, Welsch PA et al. A prospective, blinded determination of the natural history of aspirin resistance among stable patients with cardiovascular disease. *Am J Cardiol.* 2003;41:961–965.

197. Buonamici P, Marcucci R, Migliorini A et al. Impact of platelet reactivity after clopidogrel administration on drug-eluting stent thrombosis. *J Am Coll Cardiol.* 2007;49:2312–2317.

198. Ahn SG, Lee SH, Yoon JH et al. Different prognostic significance of high on-treatment platelet reactivity as assessed by the VerifyNow P2Y12 assay after coronary stenting in patients with and without acute myocardial infarction. *J Am Coll Cardiol Interv.* 2012;5:259–267.

199. Park DW, Ahn JM, Song HG et al. Differential prognostic impact of high on-treatment platelet reactivity among patients with acute coronary syndromes versus stable coronary artery disease undergoing percutaneous coronary intervention. *Am Heart J.* 2013;165:34–42.

200. Price JM, Berger PB, Teirstein PS et al. Standard- vs high-dose clopidogrel based on platelet function testing after percutaneous coronary intervention. *J Am Med Assoc.* 2011;305:1097–1105.

201. Price MJ, Angiolillo DJ, Teirstein PS et al. Platelet reactivity and cardiovascular outcomes after percutaneous coronary intervention: A time-dependent analysis of the Gauging Responsiveness with a VerifyNow P2Y12 assay: Impact on Thrombosis and Safety (GRAVITAS) trial. *Circulation.* 2011;124:1132–1137.

202. Gurbel PA, Tantry US. Do platelet function testing and genotyping improve outcome in patients treated with antithrombotic agents? *Circulation.* 2012;125:1276–1287.

203. Eikelboom JW, Hirsh J, White JI et al. Aspirin resistant thromboxane biosynthesis and the risk of myocardial infarction, stroke or cardiovascular death in patients at risk of high for cardiovascular event. *Circulation.* 2002;105:1650–1655.

204. Cha JK, Jeong MH, Jang JY et al. Serial measurement of surface expressions of CD63, P-selectin and CD40 ligand on platelets in atherosclerotic ischemic stroke. A possible role of CD40 ligand on platelets in atherosclerotic ischemic stroke. *Cerebrovasc Dis.* 2003;16:376–382.

205. Leunissen T, De Borst G, Janssen P et al. The role of perioperative antiplatelet therapy and platelet. *J Cardiovasc Surg.* 2015;56:165–175.

206. Vajen T, Mause SF, Koenen RR. Microvesicles from platelets: Novel drivers of vascular inflammation. *Thromb Haemost.* 2015;114:228–236.

207. Cotter G, Shemesh E, Zehavi M et al. Lack of aspirin effect: Aspirin resistance or resistance to taking aspirin? *Am Heart J.* 2004;147:293–300.

208. Carney RM, Freedland KE, Eisen SA et al. Adherence to a prophylactic medication regimen in patients with symptomatic versus asymptomatic ischemic heart disease. *Behav Med.* 1998;24:35–39.

209. Ross S, Nejat S. Pare G. Use of genetic data to guide therapy in arterial disease. *J Thromb Haemost.* 2015;13:S281–S289.

210. Aradil D, Storey RF, Komócsi A et al. Expert position paper on the role of platelet function testing in patients undergoing percutaneous coronary intervention. *Eur Heart J.* 2014;35:209–215.

211. Dretzke J, Riley RD, Lordkipanidzé M et al. The prognostic utility of tests of platelet function for the detection of 'aspirin resistance' in patients with established cardiovascular or cerebrovascular disease: A systematic review and economic evaluation. *Health Technol Assess.* 2015;19:1–365.

212. Krishna V, Diamond GA, Sanjay Kaul S. The role of platelet reactivity and genotype testing in the prevention of atherothrombotic cardiovascular events remains unproven. *Circulation.* 2012;125:1288–1303.

213. Sibbing D, Koch W, Gebhard D et al. Cytochrome 2C19*17 allelic variant, platelet aggregation, bleeding events, and stent thrombosis in clopidogrel-treated patients with coronary stent placement. *Circulation.* 2010;121:512–518.

214. Tantry US, Bliden KP, Wei C et al. First analysis of the relation between CYP2C19 genotype and pharmacodynamics in patients treated with ticagrelor versus clopidogrel: The ONSET/OFFSET and RESPOND genotype studies. *Circ Cardiovasc Genet.* 2010;3:556–566.

215. Patti G, Pasceri V, Vizzi V et al. Usefulness of platelet response to clopidogrel by point-of-care testing to predict bleeding outcomes in patients undergoing percutaneous coronary intervention (from the Antiplatelet Therapy for Reduction of Myocardial Damage During Angioplasty-Bleeding Study). *Am J Cardiol.* 2011;107:995–1000.

216. Monalescot G, Range G, Silvain J et al. High-on-treatment platelet reactivity as a risk factor for secondary prevention after coronary stent revascularization a landmark analysis of the ARTIC study. *Circulation.* 2014;129:2136–2143.

217. Hu YF, Lu TM, Wu CH et al. Differences in high-on-treatment platelet reactivity between intracoronary and peripheral blood after dual anti platelet agents in patients with coronary artery disease. *Thromb Haemost.* 2013;110:124–130.

218. Harter HR, Burch JW, Majerus PW et al. Prevention of thrombosis in patients on hemodialysis. *N Engl J Med.* 1979; 301:577–579.

219. Belmonte SI, Blaxall BC, Rockman H. G protein coupled receptor kinases as therapeutic targets in cardiovascular disease. *Circ Res.* 2011;109:309–319.

220. Ghorbani A, Aalamshah M, Shahbazian H et al. Randomized controlled trial of clopidogrel to prevent primary arteriovenous fistula failure in hemodialysis patients. *Indian J Nephrol.* 2009;19(2):57–61.

221. Fiskerstrand CE, Thompson IW, Burnet ME et al. Double-blind randomized trial of the effect of ticlopidine in arteriovenous fistulas for hemodialysis. *Artif Organs.* 1984;9:61–63.

222. Grontoft KC, Mulec H, Gutierrez A et al. Thromboprophylactic effect of ticlopidine in arteriovenous fistulas for haemodialysis. *Scan J Urol Nephrol.* 1985;1:55–57.

223. Grontoft KC, Larsson R, Mulec H et al. Effects of ticlopidine in AV-fistula surgery in uremia. *Scand J Urol Nephrol.* 1998;32:276–283.

224. Do DD, Mahler F. Low-dose aspirin combined with dipyridamole versus anticoagulants after femoropopliteal percutaneous transluminal angioplasty. *Radiology.* 1994;193:567–571.

225. Ansel GM, Silver MJ, Botti CF et al. Functional and clinical outcomes of nitinol stenting with and without Abciximab for complex superficial femoral artery disease: A randomized trial. *Catheter Cardiovasc Interv.* 2006;67:288–297.

226. Tepe G, Bantleon R, Brechtel K et al. Management of peripheral arterial interventions with mono or dual antiplatelet therapy – The MIRROR study: A randomised and double-blinded clinical trial. *Eur Soc Radiol.* 2012;22:1998–2006.

227. Iida O, Nanto S, Uematsu M et al. Cilostazol reduces restenosis after endovascular therapy in patients with femoropopliteal lesions. *J Vasc Surg.* 2008;48:144–149.

228. Soga Y, Yokoi H, Kawasaki T et al. Efficacy of cilostazol after endovascular therapy for femoropopliteal artery disease in patients with intermittent claudication. *J Am Coll Cardiol.* 2009; 53:48–53.

229. Pajnič M, Drasler B, Sustar V et al. Effect of carbon black nanomaterial on biological membranes revealed by shape of human erythrocytes, platelets, and phospholipid vesicles. *J Nanobiotechnology.* 2015;13:28.

230. Shani S, Ahman RE, Naveen SV et al. Platelet rich concentrate promotes early cellular proliferation and multiple lineage differentiation of human mesenchymal stromal cells in vitro. *ScientificWorldJournal* 2014;Article ID 845293:12.

231. Ghoshal K Bhattacharyya M. Overview of platelet physiology: Its hemostatic and nonhemostatic role in disease pathogenesis. *ScientificWorldJournal.* 2014;Article ID 781857:8.

232. Patrono C, Andreotti F, Arnesen H et al. Antiplatelet agents for the treatment and prevention of atherothrombosis. *Eur Heart J.* 2011;32:2922–2932.

233. Belmonte SI, Blaxall BC, Rockman H. G Protein coupled receptor kinases as therapeutic targets in cardiovascular disease. *Circ Res.* 2011;109:309–319.

11

Vasoactive pharmaceuticals for treatment of peripheral arterial disease

CRISTINE S. VELAZCO, MARK E. O'DONNELL and SAMUEL R. MONEY

CONTENTS

INTRODUCTION

Peripheral arterial disease (PAD) is defined by the presence of significant narrowing of arteries distal to the arch of the aorta, most often due to atherosclerosis. PAD of the lower limb occurs when narrowing of arteries occurs distal to the aortic bifurcation and remains one of the major manifestations of atherosclerosis.[1,2] PAD is usually asymptomatic in the initial stages. Disease progression to intermittent claudication (IC) is defined as a reproducible lower extremity muscular pain induced by exercise and relieved by short periods of rest. A resting ankle-brachial index of ≤0.90 indicates a hemodynamically significant arterial stenosis and is most often used to define PAD.[1] Further deterioration to critical limb ischemia, which potentially threatens the viability of the limb, may be defined as a persistent rest pain for a period greater than 2 weeks' duration requiring regular analgesia, with or without associated tissue ulceration or gangrene.[3]

Accurate epidemiological prevalence is compromised by subjective differences in patient assessment, lack of uniformity in PAD definition, study design and investigative modality variances as well as incomplete symptomatic expression whereby only 10%–30% of patients diagnosed with PAD based on the ankle-brachial index will have classic symptoms of IC.[4] Hankey et al.[5] reported that PAD affects approximately 20% of adults older than 55 years with an estimated total of 27 million people suffering PAD in North America and Europe. This peak incidence equates to 60 new cases per 10,000 persons per year with between 5 and 8 million people affected with PAD in the United States, more so in Medicare and Medicaid patients.[6,7]

Atherosclerosis is a progressive process with multiple contributory risk factors including hypertension, hypercholesterolemia and diabetes which all warrant pharmacological optimization and incorporation of antiplatelet and lipid-lowering strategies to reduce longer-term cardiovascular morbidity as well as lower limb disease progression.

Although there are no previously reported clinical trials assessing the effect of smoking cessation in PAD patients, previous researchers have described a reduction in claudication severity and risk of developing critical rest pain with smoking cessation.[8,9] Exercise significantly improves maximum walking time and overall walking ability.[10] The absolute or peak walking distance (PWD) can be improved by more than 100% with greater effect seen in hospital-based programmes of more than 2 months' duration.[11,12] Gardner and Poehlman[13] documented that exercise was more effective than angioplasty or antiplatelet therapy for improving walking time and quality of life, but was similar to surgical treatment. Claudication symptomatology may be further ameliorated through prescription of vasoactive pharmacotherapies which will be discussed in this chapter.

CILOSTAZOL (PLETAL)

Mechanism of action

Cilostazol is a 2-oxo-quinolone derivative which is a reversible, selective inhibitor of phosphodiesterase-3A (PDE-3A) with antiplatelet, antithrombotic, vasodilatory, antimitogenic, cardiogenic and lipid-lowering properties.[14-16]

Clinical use

Cilostazol has been marketed as a therapeutic agent for PAD since 1988 in Japan, 1999 in the United States and 2002 in the United Kingdom. Cilostazol is available in 50 mg or 100 mg tablets to be taken twice a day. A 2008 Cochrane review assessed multiple outcomes from seven randomized controlled trials involving over 1500 stable IC patients randomized to cilostazol, pentoxifylline or placebo for 12–24 weeks.[17] Twice daily 100 mg oral cilostazol produced a weighed mean improvement of 31.1 m (95% CI 21.3–40.9 m) for initial claudication distance and 49.7 m (95% CI 24.2–75.2 m) for absolute claudication distance (ACD). A more recent meta-analysis by Stevens et al.[18] reported that cilostazol had a 25% and 13% improvement from baseline for maximal walking (MWD) and pain-free walking (PFWD) distance when compared to placebo (Level 1). Combination antiplatelet and cilostazol therapies have also improved patency, limb-related outcomes including amputation-free survival, limb salvage and freedom from target lesion revascularization following peripheral endovascular interventions while restenosis and occlusion rates were reduced.[19]

Cilostazol is contraindicated in congestive heart failure due to its classification as a PDE-3A inhibitor and should not be administered in patients with severe hepatic or renal failure.[14] Cilostazol is associated with side effects, particularly headache, as a result of its vasodilatory properties, occurring in up to 32% of patients.[20,21] Discontinuation of cilostazol due to headache was seen in 3.7% and 1.3% of patients taking twice daily 100 mg and

50 mg, respectively.[17] Diarrhea, abnormal stools, palpitations, rhinitis, pharyngitis, peripheral edema and nausea also occurred in 5% of patients. Lee and Nelson[22] observed real-world compliance of cilostazol with encouraging results, where 58% of all patients and 72% of fully compliant patients reported subjective walking improvement after 3 months despite only 4% reporting smoking cessation and 7% incorporating an exercise regimen.[22]

Further long-term analysis of serious cilostazol-related adverse events from the CASTLE study (*Cilostazol: A Study in Long-Term Effects*) (n = 1439) demonstrated that there was no significant difference between cilostazol and placebo-treated groups in rates of myocardial infarction, stroke or cardiovascular death during follow-up.[20,23] However, the study was discontinued early as less than half of the anticipated number of deaths had occurred and study dropout rate was high.[23] The rates of bleeding events were similar in patients who used aspirin, aspirin plus clopidogrel or anticoagulants at any time during the course of the study.[23]

Recommendations

Cilostazol has been demonstrated to be a safe treatment for IC in patients without congestive heart failure. We recommend cilostazol as a first-line pharmaceutical treatment in patients with IC in the United States (Grade A).

NAFTIDROFURYL (DUSODRIL)

Mechanism

After vascular injury, serotonin stimulates 5-hydroxytryptamine type-2 (5-HT$_2$) receptors in smooth muscle cells of the vascular media resulting in vasoconstriction. Additional activation of platelets, via 5-HT$_2$ receptors, causes platelet aggregation and thrombus formation. Naftidrofuryl, a 5-HT$_2$ antagonist derived from lidocaine, improves tissue oxygenation and muscle metabolism through an increase in intracellular adenosine triphosphate which leads to vasodilatory and antithrombotic effects, reductions in erythrocyte/platelet aggregation, lactic acid production and vascular permeability as well as an inhibition of 5-HT-induced smooth muscle cell proliferation.[24]

Clinical use

Since 1972, naftidrofuryl has been the first-line agent for IC in the United Kingdom and Europe. However, it has never been approved for clinical use in the United States by the Food and Drug Administration (FDA). The recommended dose is 200 milligrams orally three times per day. An updated Cochrane review by de Backer et al.[25] reported a mean gain of 48.4 m (95% CI 35.94, 60.95) in PFWD with naftidrofuryl compared to placebo from clinical trials completed between 1984 and 2001.[25] Additional walking improvements were also reported in Stevens et al.'s[18] network meta-analysis comparing naftidrofuryl, cilostazol and pentoxifylline in PAD patients. Naftidrofuryl was the most effective IC therapy with a 60% (9%–138%) increase in MWD compared to placebo and the highest increase 49% (23%–81%) in PFWD relative to placebo after 24 weeks from all three assessed pharmacotherapeutic agents (Level 1).[18] Patients with IC and a poor quality of life may be considered for treatment with naftidrofuryl.[1]

Serious adverse events from naftidrofuryl therapy include liver injury, calcium oxalate crystalluria with nephrolithiasis, cardiac rhythm and conduction abnormalities.[26] Non-serious side effects include gastrointestinal dysmotility, headache and dry mouth. de Backer and colleagues[25] found that there was only a higher incidence of gastrointestinal disorders when compared to placebo.[25]

Cost effectiveness analyses performed by Meng et al.[27] identified higher treatment costs with cilostazol compared with naftidrofuryl with a total cilostazol cost of £964 for a 0.019 increase in quality-adjusted life year (QALY) and a total naftidrofuryl cost of £298 for a 0.049 increase in QALY when either therapy was compared to placebo. These authors suggested that cilostazol was not cost-beneficial when naftidrofuryl was available as an alternative.[27]

Recommendations

Although naftidrofuryl has been demonstrated to be a safe and efficacious treatment in the United Kingdom and Europe (Grade A), the lack of FDA approval precludes its use in the United States which remains unlikely to change due to the lack of perceived future financial gain.[24]

PENTOXIFYLLINE (TRENTAL)

Mechanism

Pentoxifylline is a trisubstituted xanthine derivative which inhibits phosphodiesterase and potentiates endogenous prostacyclin producing dose-related hemorrheologic effects including possible reductions in blood viscosity and improvements in erythrocyte flexibility and microcirculatory flow.[28] Further research into its actual mechanism of action is warranted as more recent research suggests alternative pharmacotherapeutic pathways than previously reported (Level 1).[28]

Clinical use

Approved by the FDA in 1984, pentoxifylline is dosed at 400 mg orally three times daily. Creager (2008) reported a 13.9% improvement (p = 0.039) in ACD with pentoxifylline compared to placebo.[29] However, Stevens et al.[18] found pentoxifylline to be the least effective treatment for IC when compared to cilostazol and naftidrofuryl with an 11% and 9% improvement in MWD and PFWD, respectively. Despite study design limitations during the evaluation of pentoxifylline efficacy from Salhiyyah et al.'s[30] meta-analysis, 1 of 11 studies included reported a 20% improvement (p < 0.0001) in PFWD compared to placebo (Level 1).[30] In contrast to cilostazol, walking distance does not deteriorate following withdrawal of pentoxifylline therapy.[31]

Overall, pentoxifylline is well tolerated with mainly gastrointestinal side effects reported including nausea, vomiting, dyspepsia, bloating, pharyngitis and dizziness.[30,32] Unlike cilostazol, pentoxifylline is not contraindicated in heart disease. However, it should be closely monitored in patients with liver and renal disease.[32]

Recommendations

Pentoxifylline treatment provides modest improvements in PAD symptomatology. We recommend pentoxifylline as a second-line agent for use in PAD patients with a contraindication to cilostazol therapy (Grade A).

CARNITINE

Mechanism

During metabolic stress, incomplete utilization of acyl-coenzyme A intermediates in the Krebs cycle leads to accumulation of acylcarnitine particularly in affected muscles of PAD patients. Carnitine acts as a buffer to acyl-CoA by forming acylcarnitines. Propionyl-L-carnitine (PLC) may help restore total carnitine and acylcarnitine in patients with severe PAD leading to potential improvements in phosphocreatine synthesis, endothelial function, respiratory exchange and muscle strength.[33]

Clinical use

Carnitine is not approved for use by the FDA. However, multiple European clinical studies have reported improvements in walking ability and quality of life with 1 g of PLC orally twice daily. When combined with exercise, PLC showed a 75.2% increase in peak walking time compared to 64.4% increase in placebo. However, no significant difference on claudication time was demonstrated at 6 months (p = 0.154).[34] Luo et al.[35] reported a statistically significant improvement on peak walking and claudication times with PLC compared to placebo at 1.33 minutes or 70.5 m longer and suggested such an improvement may be related to improvements in muscle tolerance to ischemia. Brass et al.[36] further reported a statistically significant improvement of 35 m (95% CI, 13–57 m, standardized effect size 0.22) in PWD with PLC from their systematic meta-analysis derived from 13 studies including 6 phase III clinical trials[36] (Level 1).

PLC side effects include nausea, diarrhea, bronchitis and possible hyperglycemia.[34,35]

Recommendations

Despite promising therapeutic results, carnitine and its analogues will require further larger clinical trials prior to consideration for FDA approval (Grade A).

PROSTANOIDS

Mechanism of action

Although prostanoids' most important actions on IC patients relate to vasodilatation, antiplatelet activity and advantageous peripheral blood flow, additional broader effects also include inhibition of neutrophil activation and subsequent release of oxygen radicals, antiproliferative activity on vascular smooth muscle, reduction of vascular cholesterol content and an increase erythrocyte deformability.[37]

Clinical use

Prostaglandin E_1 (PGE$_1$) and prostacyclin (PGI$_2$) have been used worldwide for over 20 years. PGE$_1$ may be administered intravenously at 60 µg once or 40 µg twice daily. As PGI$_2$ is not stable chemically, some of its more stable intravenous analogues, such as beraprost and iloprost, are therefore used clinically. Iloprost has been dosed as 50, 100 or 150 µg twice daily. Beraprost is dosed at 120 µg.[37]

A meta-analysis by Amendt[38] reported significant increases in walking distance after administration of PGE$_1$ (107% PFWD and 97% MWD, p < 0.001) from 9 out of 13 studies assessed (n = 344). Further beneficial effects with other prostaglandins (beraprost, iloprost, AS-013) (n = 402) were also identified with a significant increase of 42% for both PFWD and MWD when compared to placebo. Overall, PGE$_1$ therapy provided the maximal walking benefits when compared to placebo (Level 1).[38] A more recent Cochrane review, using stricter study inclusion criteria, identified only 3 out of 18 studies which demonstrated significant PFWD and MWD improvements of 40 m (p = 0.003) and 56 m (p = 0.002), respectively, with PGE$_1$ therapy. As these authors described significant variation in the quality of included studies and compounding data pooling difficulties, they recommended that current evidence remains insufficient to recommend PGE$_1$ for routine use in patients with IC.[37]

Creager et al.[29] reported improvements in PFWD of 7.7%, 8.8% and 25.7% and in MWD of 3.2%, 7.1% and 13.7% in the 50, 100 or 150 µg iloprost treatment groups compared to 3.3% and 3.2% in the placebo group (p > 0.05). Robertson and Andras[37] also identified possible beneficial effects of beraprost in PAD patients with one study reviewed showing non-significant improvements in PFWD (mean difference 56%, 95% confidence interval −13% to 126%) and MWD (mean difference 38%, 95% CI −23% to 99%) (p > 0.05). However, a second study reviewed by these authors suggested that beraprost did not improve walking distances.

Overall, PGE$_1$ is the best tolerated of the prostaglandins, but infusion site side effects are commonly reported including erythema, pain and swelling. Other systemic side effects include headache, flushing, nausea and diarrhea.[38] Other prostaglandins (beraprost, iloprost, AS-013) had a higher rate of similar side effects to PGE$_1$ (27.6% vs. about 4%) with a 3.2% risk of significant cardiovascular events.

Recommendations

Current evidence does not support the recommendation of prostanoids for use in patients with PAD (Grade A). Although larger clinical trials are warranted before FDA approval could be obtained, logistical issues are also likely to complicate routine administration due to the requirement for intravenous infusion.

GINKGO BILOBA

Mechanism of action

Ginkgo biloba extract is naturally derived from its dried leaves. Advantageous microcirculatory and vasodilatory effects are mediated through antioxidant properties and free radical scavenging combined with increases in endothelial-derived relaxing factor. Other researchers have also demonstrated antiplatelet-activating factor properties leading to decreases in platelet aggregation, neutrophil degranulation and free radical production.[39]

Clinical use

Ginkgo biloba has been used for centuries in Asian medicine. There is no standardized dosage. Clinical trials have assessed the effects of between 120 mg and 320 mg daily.[40,41] Although a meta-analysis of 11 clinical trials (n = 477) assessing ginkgo biloba in PAD patients demonstrated a non-statistically significant increase in walking distance of 64.5 m, extended treatment to 24 weeks from 6 of the clinical trials assessed (n = 321) reported significant increases in ACD of 85.3 m (p = 0.0002).[39] In contrast, Wang and colleagues[40] attributed beneficial walking distances from their small ginkgo biloba versus placebo study (n = 17) to an optimized exercise programme rather than the pharmacological treatment.

Generally, ginkgo biloba is well tolerated with only minor side effects including headache, skin reactions and gastrointestinal complaints as well as a small increase in bleeding risk.[39]

Recommendations

Based on current clinical evidence, we do not recommend ginkgo biloba for treatment of PAD (Grade A).

VERAPAMIL (ISOPTIN)

Mechanism of action

Verapamil is a calcium ion influx inhibitor (channel blocker) which selectively inhibits the transmembrane influx of ionic calcium into arterial smooth muscle and myocardial cells. Potential advantageous effects in PAD patients relate to its vasodilatory properties and its ability to increase oxygen extraction in both coronary and peripheral arterial systems.[42]

Clinical use

Verapamil has been approved in the United States since 1982 and is indicated for treatment of hypertension and cardiac arrhythmias. Bagger and colleagues[42] reported positive effects on both MWD (49%, p < 0.001) and mean PFWD (29%, p < 0.01) with verapamil doses titrated to individual levels ranging from 120 to 480 mg per day to facilitate the longest MWD.

Common side effects include dizziness, headache and constipation.

Recommendations

Despite widespread usage of verapamil in cardiovascular disease, clinical evidence for recommendation in PAD is somewhat outdated and certainly lacking in the advent of best medical therapy. More studies are needed to demonstrate its benefit, and if such beneficial effects are dose dependent, integration in clinical practice may be challenging (Grade A).

INOSITOL NICOTINATE (HEXOPAL)

Mechanism of action

Inositol nicotinate is a peripheral vasodilator which is thought to act through slowing the release of nicotinic acid.[43]

Clinical use

Inositol nicotinate is currently approved in the United Kingdom for the symptomatic relief of IC. Dosage ranges from 1 g orally three times a day up to a total of 4 g daily. Squires et al.'s[43] systematic review of three studies reported variable improvements in walking capacity when inositol nicotinate was compared to placebo. One study demonstrated a significant improvement (p < 0.05) in pain-free walking paces at 12 weeks and another identified a significant improvement in claudication time for patients with moderately severe PAD with inositol nicotinate (p < 0.001). The third study did not show any difference in MWD between treatment groups with a 65.4 and 102.8 m change for inositol nicotinate and placebo, respectively[43] (Level 1).

Frequently reported side effects are mainly gastrointestinal or secondary to difficulty swallowing tablets.

Recommendations

Currently, inositol nicotinate is not recommended for the treatment of IC due to the small number of clinical trials and lack of sufficient evidence demonstrating proof of therapeutic efficacy (Grade A).

BUFLOMEDIL (LOFTYL)

Mechanism of action

Buflomedil is a vasodilator which also inhibits platelet aggregation, improves red cell deformity and reduces plasma fibrinogen leading to reductions in blood viscosity.[44] It also has weak non-specific calcium antagonist effects.[45]

Clinical use

Although used in Europe, buflomedil is currently not approved for PAD by the FDA. Daily dosage is 300 mg orally twice daily. de Backer and Vander Stichele's[44] Cochrane review based on two studies reported a statistically significant increase in PFWD (p < 0.001) and MWD (p < 0.01) in the buflomedil group after 84 days of treatment.[46] Diamantopoulos[47] also reported significant increases in PFWD (52.8 m vs. 8.6%, p = 0.018) and MWD (81.1 m vs. 8.8 m, p = 0.022) for buflomedil therapy when compared to placebo after 3 months. Although treatment effect for MWD continued at 6 months (191.9 m vs. 20.5 m, p = 0.011), no significant improvements were identified in PFWD (112.2 m vs. 31.6 m, p = 0.05) for this time period (Level 1).

Although generalized side effects include headache, vertigo, dizziness, flushing, nausea and vomiting, safety of buflomedil therapy has raised significant concerns with neurological (epileptic) and cardiovascular (arrhythmias) toxicity after overdoses at levels as low as 3 g with fatality at doses as small as 6 g especially in those with renal insufficiency. France has now withdrawn the 300 mg dosage from the market.[44]

Recommendations

Due to the lack of larger randomized clinical trials and recent concerns for toxicity at relatively low levels, we do not recommend buflomedil as a treatment for PAD (Grade A).

GENE THERAPY

Mechanism of action

Gene and stem cell therapy may be the future of treatment for IC. Hypoxia-inducible factor-1α (HIF-1α) is a heterodimeric transcription factor that regulates oxygen homeostasis and metabolism through pathways that mediate angiogenesis, cell survival and metabolism. Preclinical trials showed increased collateral blood vessels, capillary density and regional blood flow in rabbits.[48]

Clinical use

Creager et al.[48] evaluated the effects of 20 separate HIF-1α injections to each leg in PAD patients where no significant improvement in peak walking time compared with placebo was identified during the 52-week follow-up when compared to placebo.

Side effects were similar when compared to placebo, with injection-site pain and hematoma occurring most frequently. However, there was a slight increase of stroke in the treatment groups (Level 1).

Recommendations

Gene therapy is an exciting future direction for drug therapy for IC and PAD. However, more studies are warranted to determine which therapies are safest and efficacious. At this time, we do not recommend gene therapy for treatment of PAD (Grade A).

STEM CELL THERAPY

Mechanism of action

Current stem cell therapy research for PAD has involved the administration of bone marrow mononuclear cells (BM-MNCs) to increase collateral vessel formation and granulocyte-macrophage colony-stimulating factor (GM-CSF) to stimulate mobilization of hematopoietic and other progenitor cells (PC) from bone marrow.[49,50] GM-CSF has also been shown to increase capillary density and arteriogenesis in murine models and help with neo-endothelialization of denuded arteries while promoting proliferation and differentiation of hematopoietic cells.[50]

Clinical use

The first stem cell research for PAD patients was the Therapeutic Angiogenesis using Cell Transplantation study involving the intramuscular administration of autologous BM-MNCs.[49] Significant improvements in PFWT were demonstrated in PAD patients with both unilateral and bilateral limb ischemia (Unilateral IC: 3 min and Bilateral IC: 1 min, p < 0.0001) when compared with saline placebo with continued benefit at both 6 months (p < 0.001) and 1 year post-treatment[51] (Level 1). Poole et al.[50] evaluated the self-administration of 500 μg of GM-CSF three times a week combined with walking exercise encouragement of at least three exercise periods per day. Both treatment and placebo groups showed significant increases in PWT (109 vs. 56 seconds, p < 0.01) at 3 months. Although there was no difference in PWT between treatment groups at 3 months, post hoc per protocol analyses reported significant PWT increases from baseline in the GM-CSF group compared to placebo at 3 months (113 vs. 44 seconds, p = 0.02) and 6 months (122 vs. 57 seconds, p = 0.02). The authors did comment that their study protocol exercise regimen may have been a possible confounding factor.

Serious side effect rates were similar in both groups including headache, fatigue and gastrointestinal symptoms and a slightly increased rate of injection-site rash in the GM-CSF group[50] (Level 1).

Recommendations

Stem cell therapy is a promising new area of research. However, due to the limited data available on various cell line therapies, we do not recommend current use until further research can be completed (Grade A).

OTHER DRUGS NOT IN ACTIVE USE

Ketanserin, a 5-HT$_2$ agonist, has also been used historically for the treatment of IC with marked variations in walking efficacy. It is no longer used for PAD in current practice.[52] Cinnarizine is a vasoconstrictive antagonist not currently recommended for use in IC due to poor evidence proving benefit.[53]

VENOACTIVE DRUGS

Mechanism of action

Venoactive, also known as phlebotonic, drugs (VAD) have been used to treat chronic venous disease (CVD). The main classes of VADs include alpha-benzopyrones (coumarin), gamma-benzopyrones (flavonoids), saponins, synthetic products (calcium dobesilate) and plant extracts.[54] Horse chestnut seed extract (HCSE) is also commonly used.[55] VAD are postulated to increase venous tone related to the noradrenaline pathway leading to an increase in capillary resistance and decrease in capillary filtration, improvements in lymphatic flow and reduction in edema.[56] VADs also have hemorrheologic effects including a reduction in blood viscosity, increased red cell velocity and amelioration of red cell aggregation. HCSE is thought to inhibit capillary protein permeability.[57]

Clinical use

Flavonoids have been used for CVD since the 1960s with reported clinical reductions in peripheral edema when combined with compression hosiery in patients with chronic venous hypertension. They have also been shown to accelerate the healing of venous ulcers.[54] Unfortunately, there have been few long-term randomized controlled trials to assess their efficacy. The most recent Cochrane review by Martinez et al.[58] evaluated 44 VAD clinical trials where rutosides (flavonoid) demonstrated an improvement in lower limb edema while calcium dobesilate improved cramps and restless legs.[58] HCSE has been shown to significantly improve leg pain, edema and pruritus in some studies for CVD.[55]

Pentoxifylline has also been used to treat CVD. It has been shown to improve ulcer healing and local inflammation.[59]

Side effects of VADs most commonly include gastrointestinal complaints.[58] HCSE may cause dizziness, nausea, headache and pruritus.[55]

Recommendations

Currently, there is insufficient evidence to support the broad use of VADs in PAD[58] (Grade A). However, these agents remain an exciting prospect for future arterial research.

BEST CLINICAL PRACTICE TEXT BOX

- Best medical therapy, optimization of cardiovascular risk factors and exercise regimens should be encouraged in all PAD patients.
- Cilostazol should be prescribed as first-line treatment in the US market.
- Naftidrofuryl is a safe and cheaper alternative to first-line treatment in non-US markets.
- Pentoxifylline may be used as a second-line treatment or in those patients with CHF.

Key points

- Cilostazol is the most widely studied of the vasoactive pharmaceuticals and remains a safe and efficacious treatment for IC.
- Naftidrofuryl should be prescribed in non-US markets as an alternative to cilostazol. However, it is currently unlikely to be approved in the United States.
- Pentoxifylline remains a second-line agent.
- Carnitine and verapamil show promising results but more studies are needed prior to consideration of FDA approval for treatment of PAD.
- Ginkgo biloba is not an effective treatment.
- Gene and stem cell therapy are an exciting future prospect and may warrant multimodal agent administration for clinical benefit.

DEFICIENCIES IN CURRENT KNOWLEDGE AND AREAS FOR FUTURE RESEARCH

- More clinical trial data are needed for approval of promising drugs.
- Future research directions include continuing pursuit of gene and stem therapy and potential application of venoactive therapies in the arterial system.

KEY REFERENCES

1. de Backer TL, Vander Stichele R, Lehert P, Van Bortel L. Naftidrofuryl for intermittent claudication. *Cochrane Database Syst Rev.* 2012;12:CD001368.
2. Hiatt WR, Money SR, Brass EP. Long-term safety of cilostazol in patients with peripheral artery disease: The castle study (Cilostazol: A Study in Long-Term Effects). *J Vasc Surg.* 2008 February;47(2):330–336.
3. Robless P, Mikhailidis DP, Stansby GP. Cilostazol for peripheral arterial disease. *Cochrane Database Syst Rev.* 2008;1:CD003748.
4. Salhiyyah K, Senanayake E, Abdel-Hadi M, Booth A, Michaels JA. Pentoxifylline for intermittent claudication. *Cochrane Database Syst Rev.* 2012;1:CD005262.
5. Stevens JW, Simpson E, Harnan S, Squires H, Meng Y, Thomas S, Michaels J, Stansby G. Systematic review of the efficacy of cilostazol, naftidrofuryl oxalate and pentoxifylline for the treatment of intermittent claudication. *Br J Surg.* 2012 December;99(12):1630–1638.

REFERENCES

1. Norgren L, Hiatt WR, Dormandy JA et al. Intersociety consensus for the management of peripheral arterial disease (Tasc II). *Eur J Vasc Endovasc Surg.* 2007;33(Suppl. 1):S1–S75.
2. Sigvant B, Wiberg-Hedman K, Bergqvist D, Rolandsson O, Andersson B, Persson E, Wahlberg E. A population-based study of peripheral arterial disease prevalence with special focus on critical limb ischemia and sex differences. *J Vasc Surg.* 2007 June;45(6):1185–1191.
3. Second European Consensus Document on chronic critical leg ischemia. *Eur J Vasc Surg.* 1992 May;6(Suppl. A):1–32.
4. McDermott MM. The magnitude of the problem of peripheral arterial disease: Epidemiology and clinical significance. *Cleve Clin J Med.* 2006 October;73(Suppl. 4):S2–S7.
5. Hankey GJ, Norman PE, Eikelboom JW. Medical treatment of peripheral arterial disease. *J Am Med Assoc.* 2006 February 1;295(5):547–553.
6. Hiatt WR, Nehler MR. Peripheral arterial disease. *Adv Intern Med.* 2001;47:89–110.

7. Selvin E, Erlinger TP. Prevalence of and risk factors for peripheral arterial disease in the United States: Results from the National Health and Nutrition Examination Survey, 1999–2000. *Circulation*. 2004 August 10;110(6):738–743.

8. Girolami B, Bernardi E, Prins MH, Ten Cate JW, Hettiarachchi R, Prandoni P, Girolami A, Buller HR. Treatment of intermittent claudication with physical training, smoking cessation, pentoxifylline, or nafronyl: A meta-analysis. *Arch Intern Med*. 1999 February 22;159(4):337–345.

9. Jonason T, Bergstrom R. Cessation of smoking in patients with intermittent claudication: Effects on the risk of peripheral vascular complications, myocardial infarction and mortality. *Acta Med Scand*. 1987;221(3):253–260.

10. Leng GC, Fowler B, Ernst E. Exercise for intermittent claudication. *Cochrane Database Syst Rev*. 2000;2:CD000990.

11. Ernst E, Fialka V. A review of the clinical effectiveness of exercise therapy for intermittent claudication. *Arch Intern Med*. 1993 October 25;153(20):2357–2360.

12. Housley E. Treating claudication in five words. *Br Med J*. 1988 May 28;296(6635):1483–1484.

13. Gardner AW, Poehlman ET. Exercise rehabilitation programs for the treatment of claudication pain: A meta-analysis. *J Am Med Assoc*. 1995 September 27;274(12):975–980.

14. Chapman TM, Goa KL. Cilostazol: A review of its use in intermittent claudication. *Am J Cardiovasc Drugs*. 2003;3(2):117–138.

15. Schrör K. The pharmacology of cilostazol. *Diabetes Obes Metab*. 2002 March;4(Suppl. 2):S14–S19.

16. O'Donnell ME, Badger SA, Sharif MA, Young IS, Lee B, Soong CV. The vascular and biochemical effects of cilostazol in patients with peripheral arterial disease. *J Vasc Surg*. 2009 March;49(5):1226–1234.

17. Robless P, Mikhailidis DP, Stansby GP. Cilostazol for peripheral arterial disease. *Cochrane Database Syst Rev*. 2008;1:CD003748.

18. Stevens JW, Simpson E, Harnan S, Squires H, Meng Y, Thomas S, Michaels J, Stansby G. Systematic review of the efficacy of cilostazol, naftidrofuryl oxalate and pentoxifylline for the treatment of intermittent claudication. *Br J Surg*. 2012 December;99(12):1630–1638.

19. Warner CJ, Greaves SW, Larson RJ, Stone DH, Powell RJ, Walsh DB, Goodney PP. Cilostazol is associated with improved outcomes after peripheral endovascular interventions. *J Vasc Surg*. 2014 June;59(6):1607–1614.

20. Hiatt WR. The US experience with cilostazol in treating intermittent claudication. *Atheroscler Suppl*. 2005 December 15;6(4):21–31.

21. Pratt CM. Analysis of the cilostazol safety database. *Am J Cardiol*. 2001 June 28;87(12A):28D–33D.

22. Lee C, Nelson PR. Effect of cilostazol prescribed in a pragmatic treatment program for intermittent claudication. *Vasc Endovascular Surg*. 2014 April;48(3):224–229.

23. Hiatt WR, Money SR, Brass EP. Long-term safety of cilostazol in patients with peripheral artery disease: The castle study (Cilostazol: A Study in Long-Term Effects). *J Vasc Surg*. 2008 February;47(2):330–336.

24. Hong H, Mackey WC. The limits of evidence in drug approval and availability: A case study of cilostazol and naftidrofuryl for the treatment of intermittent claudication. *Clin Ther*. 2014 August 1;36(8):1290–1301.

25. de Backer TL, Vander Stichele R, Lehert P, Van Bortel L. Naftidrofuryl for intermittent claudication. *Cochrane Database Syst Rev*. 2012;12:CD001368.

26. de Backer T, Vander Stichele R, Lehert P, Van Bortel L. Naftidrofuryl for intermittent claudication: Meta-analysis based on individual patient data. *Br Med J*. 2009;338:b603.

27. Meng Y, Squires H, Stevens JW, Simpson E, Harnan S, Thomas S, Michaels J, Stansby G, O'Donnell ME. Cost-effectiveness of cilostazol, naftidrofuryl oxalate, and pentoxifylline for the treatment of intermittent claudication in people with peripheral arterial disease. *Angiology*. 2014 March;65(3):190–197.

28. Dawson DL, Zheng Q, Worthy SA, Charles B, Bradley DV Jr. Failure of pentoxifylline or cilostazol to improve blood and plasma viscosity, fibrinogen, and erythrocyte deformability in claudication. *Angiology*. 2002 September–October;53(5):509–520.

29. Creager MA, Pande RL, Hiatt WR. A randomized trial of iloprost in patients with intermittent claudication. *Vasc Med*. 2008 February;13(1):5–13.

30. Salhiyyah K, Senanayake E, Abdel-Hadi M, Booth A, Michaels JA. Pentoxifylline for intermittent claudication. *Cochrane Database Syst Rev*. 2012;1:CD005262.

31. Dawson DL, DeMaioribus CA, Hagino RT, Light JT, Bradley DV Jr., Britt KE, Charles BE. The effect of withdrawal of drugs treating intermittent claudication. *Am J Surg*. 1999 August;178(2):141–146.

32. Aviado DM, Porter JM. Pentoxifylline: A new drug for the treatment of intermittent claudication: Mechanism of action, pharmacokinetics, clinical efficacy and adverse effects. *Pharmacotherapy*. 1984 November–December;4(6):297–307.

33. Hiatt WR. Carnitine and peripheral arterial disease. *Ann N Y Acad Sci*. 2004 November;1033:92–98.

34. Hiatt WR, Creager MA, Amato A, Brass EP. Effect of propionyl-L-carnitine on a background of monitored exercise in patients with claudication secondary to peripheral artery disease. *J Cardiopulm Rehabil Prev*. 2011 March–April;31(2):125–132.

35. Luo T, Li J, Li L et al. A Study on the efficacy and safety assessment of propionyl-L-carnitine tablets in treatment of intermittent claudication. *Thromb Res*. 2013 October;132(4):427–432.

36. Brass EP, Koster D, Hiatt WR, Amato A. A systematic review and meta-analysis of propionyl-L-carnitine effects on exercise performance in patients with claudication. *Vasc Med*. 2013 February;18(1):3–12.

37. Robertson L, Andras A. Prostanoids for intermittent claudication. *Cochrane Database Syst Rev.* 2013;4:CD000986.

38. Amendt K. PGE1 and other prostaglandins in the treatment of intermittent claudication: A meta-analysis. *Angiology.* 2005 July–August;56(4):409–415.

39. Nicolai SP, Kruidenier LM, Bendermacher BL, Prins MH, Stokmans RA, Broos PP, Teijink JA. Ginkgo biloba for intermittent claudication. *Cochrane Database Syst Rev.* 2013;6:CD006888.

40. Wang J, Zhou S, Bronks R, Graham J, Myers S. Supervised exercise training combined with ginkgo biloba treatment for patients with peripheral arterial disease. *Clin Rehabil.* 2007 July;21(7):579–586.

41. Gardner CD, Taylor-Piliae RE, Kiazand A, Nicholus J, Rigby AJ, Farquhar JW. Effect of ginkgo biloba (Egb 761) on treadmill walking time among adults with peripheral artery disease: A randomized clinical trial. *J Cardiopulm Rehabil Prev.* 2008 July–August;28(4):258–265.

42. Bagger JP, Helligsoe P, Randsbaek F, Kimose HH, Jensen BS. Effect of verapamil in intermittent claudication a randomized, double-blind, placebo-controlled, cross-over study after individual dose-response assessment. *Circulation.* 1997 January 21;95(2):411–414.

43. Squires H, Simpson E, Meng Y, Harnan S, Stevens J, Wong R, Thomas S, Michaels J, Stansby G. A systematic review and economic evaluation of cilostazol, naftidrofuryl oxalate, pentoxifylline and inositol nicotinate for the treatment of intermittent claudication in people with peripheral arterial disease. *Health Technol Assess.* 2011 December;15(40):1–210.

44. de Backer TL, Vander Stichele R. Buflomedil for intermittent claudication. *Cochrane Database Syst Rev.* 2013;3:CD000988.

45. Clissold SP, Lynch S, Sorkin EM, Buflomedil. A review of its pharmacodynamic and pharmacokinetic properties, and therapeutic efficacy in peripheral and cerebral vascular diseases. *Drugs.* 1987 May;33(5):430–460.

46. Trubestein G, Balzer K, Bisler H, Kluken N, Muller-Wiefel H, Unkel B, Mahfoud Y, Ziegler W. Buflomedil in arterial occlusive disease: results of a controlled multicenter study. *Angiology.* 1984 August;35(8):500–505.

47. Diamantopoulos EJ, Grigoriadou M, Ifanti G, Raptis SA. Clinical and hemorheological effects of buflomedil in diabetic subjects with intermittent claudication. *Int Angiol.* 2001 December;20(4):337–344.

48. Creager MA, Olin JW, Belch JJ, Moneta GL, Henry TD, Rajagopalan S, Annex BH, Hiatt WR. Effect of hypoxia-inducible factor-1alpha gene therapy on walking performance in patients with intermittent claudication. *Circulation.* 2011 October 18;124(16):1765–1773.

49. Tateishi-Yuyama E, Matsubara H, Murohara T et al. Therapeutic angiogenesis for patients with limb ischaemia by autologous transplantation of bone-marrow cells: A pilot study and a randomised controlled trial. *Lancet.* 2002 August 10;360(9331):427–435.

50. Poole J, Mavromatis K, Binongo JN et al. Effect of progenitor cell mobilization with granulocyte-macrophage colony-stimulating factor in patients with peripheral artery disease: A randomized clinical trial. *J Am Med Assoc.* 2013 December 25;310(24):2631–2639.

51. Matoba S, Tatsumi T, Murohara T et al. Long-term clinical outcome after intramuscular implantation of bone marrow mononuclear cells (Therapeutic Angiogenesis by Cell Transplantation [Tact] trial) in patients with chronic limb ischemia. *Am Heart J.* 2008 November;156(5):1010–1018.

52. Bounameaux H, Holditch T, Hellemans H, Berent A, Verhaeghe R. Placebo-controlled, double-blind, two-centre trial of ketanserin in intermittent claudication. *Lancet.* 1985 December 7;2(8467):1268–1271.

53. O'Donnell ME, Reid JA, Lau LL, Hannon RJ, Lee B. Optimal management of peripheral arterial disease for the non-specialist. *Ulster Med J.* 2011 January;80(1):33–41.

54. Rabe E, Guex JJ, Morrison N, Ramelet AA, Schuller-Petrovic S, Scuderi A, Staelens I, Pannier F. Treatment of chronic venous disease with flavonoids: Recommendations for treatment and further studies. *Phlebology.* 2013 September;28(6):308–319.

55. Pittler MH, Ernst E. Horse chestnut seed extract for chronic venous insufficiency. *Cochrane Database Syst Rev.* 2012;11:CD003230.

56. Perrin M, Ramelet AA. Pharmacological treatment of primary chronic venous disease: Rationale, results and unanswered questions. *Eur J Vasc Endovasc Surg.* 2011 January;41(1):117–125.

57. Diehm C, Trampisch HJ, Lange S, Schmidt C. Comparison of leg compression stocking and oral horse-chestnut seed extract therapy in patients with chronic venous insufficiency. *Lancet.* 1996;347:292–294.

58. Martinez MJ, Bonfill X, Moreno RM, Vargas E, Capella D. Phlebotonics for venous insufficiency. *Cochrane Database Syst Rev.* 2005;3:CD003229.

59. Wollina W, Abdel-Naser MB, Mani R. A review of the microcirculation in skin in patients with chronic venous insufficiency: The problem and the evidence available for therapeutic options. *Int J Low Extrem Wounds.* 2006 September;5(3):169–180.

12

Perioperative evaluation and management of cardiac risk in vascular surgery

NARIMAN NASSIRI, JERRY J. KIM and CHRISTIAN DE VIRGILIO

CONTENTS

INTRODUCTION

Cardiac complications are among the most common causes of perioperative morbidity and mortality after vascular surgery (Level 1).[1] Studies have shown that such risk is not limited to the perioperative period. As an example, long-term cardiovascular risk has been shown to be greater in patients undergoing intervention for peripheral arterial disease (PAD), abdominal aortic aneurysm (AAA) and carotid artery stenosis than for patients undergoing first-time coronary angioplasty for coronary artery disease (CAD) (Level 2).[2] The reasons for the increased cardiac risk are varied. Major arterial procedures often involve lengthy anesthetic times and can be associated with substantial hemodynamic stress including fluctuations in heart rate, systemic vascular resistance, intra- and extravascular fluid volume and blood pressure. Due to the similarity of risk factors between PAD and CAD (e.g. diabetes mellitus, dyslipidemia, smoking), patients with PAD inevitably have concomitant CAD. Up to 70% of patients with PAD have been shown to have concomitant CAD which increases the risk of perioperative myocardial ischemia, arrhythmia, congestive heart failure and cardiac death (Level 1).[3] Finally, many vascular patients

with severe CAD may not have overt cardiac symptoms due to functionally limiting claudication.

> Patients undergoing vascular surgery are at high risk for perioperative cardiac morbidity and mortality.

Therefore, it is essential for patients undergoing vascular interventions to receive perioperative assessment and optimization (Grade A).[4–9] Failure to do so has been shown to result in significant increases of peri- and postoperative morbidity and mortality (Level 1).[6–10]

AIMS AND GOALS

It's important to note that preoperative evaluation should be considered an assessment of risk and a not 'clearance' for surgery, as there is no way to guarantee an event-free outcome. Thus, the primary goals of perioperative cardiac risk evaluation are (1) to risk stratify patients and procedures as being low, moderate or high risk of adverse perioperative as well as long-term cardiac events and (2) to determine if these risks can be mitigated via preoperative optimization.

Patients deemed to be low risk can proceed to the operating room without further intervention, thus avoiding unnecessary delays (Grade A).[4–7] On the other hand, patients with moderate or high risk require a more detailed assessment and potential interventions in order to reduce peri-interventional risk (Grade A).[4–7]

Preoperative cardiac risk assessment should not only be 'clearance' for surgery. The goal should be:

1. Risk stratification of patients and procedures as being low, moderate or high risk.
2. Recommendations on preoperative optimization.

As previously mentioned, an appropriate cardiac risk evaluation should not grant medical clearance. Too often, routine cardiology consultations are obtained simply to 'clear' the patient. Such routine evaluations add unnecessary delays given that up to 40% of preoperative cardiology consultations contain no specific recommendations other than 'proceed with case', 'cleared for surgery' or 'continue current medications (Level 3)'.[11,12] Such consultations do little to guide perioperative management in a high-risk population, add costs and delay surgical care.[11,12]

GENERAL ASSESSMENT: THE AMERICAN COLLEGE OF CARDIOLOGY/AMERICAN HEART ASSOCIATION GUIDELINE FOR PERIOPERATIVE CARDIAC RISK EVALUATION

The American College of Cardiology/American Heart Association (ACC/AHA) guideline is an evidence-based algorithm for the assessment and management of cardiac risks before non-cardiac surgery.[4–8] The guideline takes a stepwise approach taking into account the urgency of the surgery, the type of surgery and its risk level; the patient's functional capacity and cardiac risk factors and the presence or absence of active cardiac conditions.[4–8] It should provide a basis for informed clinical decision-making during the perioperative period for both the anesthesiologist and the surgeon.[5]

Steps of the ACC/AHA guideline for perioperative cardiac risk evaluation include

1. Urgency of the surgery
2. Type of surgery and its risk level
3. Presence or absence of active cardiac conditions
4. Patient's functional capacity
5. Patient's cardiac risk factors

Urgency of surgery

The first step in the ACC/AHA guideline is determining the urgency of the surgical procedure (Grade A).[6,7] The guidelines start by determining if the case is emergent or non-emergent. For emergent cases (e.g. ruptured AAA, acute limb ischemia), there is no opportunity for cardiac evaluation. Per guidelines, a non-emergent case permits a more measured approach, in which additional consultations and testing can be considered. This creates a potential pitfall, in our opinion, as the guidelines do not take into consideration a third category: the urgent vascular procedures. This category includes such cases as a symptomatic AAA, a very large (>8 cm) AAA, severe ischemic rest pain, high-grade carotid stenosis with a recent stroke or crescendo transient ischemic attacks, and recent amputation for wet gangrene that requires revascularization. Although these cases are not emergent, the clinician may lose sight of the fact that significant delays to surgery in urgent cases may result in another stroke or loss of life or limb (Level 1).[13] The risks of such delays in such situations are not accounted for in the ACC/AHA guidelines.

Thus, close communication between the surgeon and anesthesiologist is needed to plan an approach to cardiac assessment that is appropriate for the individual patient, the underlying disease, and the urgency of the situation. In urgent cases, the consultant (e.g. cardiologist or internist) should provide recommendations for perioperative medical management and surveillance without delaying urgent treatment (Grade A).[5]

Assessment of procedure-related risk

Independent of patient-related factors, the planned operation carries inherent risks to the patient. Based on the ACC/AHA guideline, surgical procedures are categorized into low, intermediate and high risk with regard to cardiac risk.[6,7] The majority of vascular surgical procedures, partly due to the high degree of anticipated perioperative hemodynamic stress, are classified as intermediate (1%–5% 30-day myocardial infarction [MI] or mortality) to high (>5%) risk. Carotid procedures fall under the intermediate category while all other major vascular and peripheral vascular procedures are classified as high risk.

However, these guidelines do not factor in the lower anticipated cardiac morbidity and mortality associated with endovascular procedures as compared to open ones.

Assessment of patient-related risk

Assessment of patient-related cardiac risk begins with a comprehensive history and physical examination. There are three components of the patient-related cardiac risk evaluation: assessment for active cardiac conditions, functional capacity and clinical cardiac risk factors.[6,7] It is important to note that the vascular surgeon should take an active role in this initial assessment of patient-related risk and not simply defer this to other specialists. In that way, the vascular surgeon will be empowered to become an active partner in the process.

> Vascular surgeons should take an active role in perioperative assessment of patient-related cardiac risk.

ASSESSMENT OF ACTIVE CARDIAC CONDITIONS THAT CONFER MAJOR RISK

The most important part of this assessment is to determine at the outset whether the patient has active cardiac conditions that require immediate cardiology evaluation and would therefore preclude surgery. It is imperative that the presence of four conditions, termed *major* cardiac risk factors, be ruled out (Level 1).[6,7] These include:

1. *Unstable coronary syndromes*, such as
   a. Unstable or severe angina
   b. Recent MI (within 30 days)
   The high cardiac risk of a recent MI is highlighted in a study by Livhits et al. (Level 3).[14] The authors found that the 30-day rate of MI and death in the setting of recent MI (within 30 days) was an alarming 37.9% for AAA repair and 17.2% for major amputation, respectively.[14] The study also demonstrated that a 30-day waiting period after an MI may not be sufficient to perform elective surgery, as the high cardiac risk persisted even up to 60 days after an MI.[14]
2. *Decompensated heart failure*, which includes New York Heart Association functional class IV disease, worsening heart failure and new-onset heart failure
3. *Significant arrhythmias*, which include
   a. High-grade or Mobitz II atrioventricular heart block
   b. Third-degree atrioventricular heart block
   c. Symptomatic ventricular arrhythmias
   d. Supraventricular arrhythmias with uncontrolled ventricular rate
   e. Symptomatic bradycardia
   f. Newly recognized ventricular tachycardia
4. *Severe valvular disease*, which includes
   a. Severe aortic stenosis (i.e. mean pressure gradient >40 mmHg, area <1 cm^2 or symptomatic)
   b. Symptomatic mitral stenosis

AORTIC STENOSIS

Severe aortic stenosis has the greatest cardiac risk during non-cardiac surgery (Level 1).[15] The rate of cardiac events in patients with undiagnosed severe aortic stenosis undergoing non-cardiac surgery is estimated to be 10%–30% (Level 1).[15] In the presence of a systolic murmur suggestive of aortic stenosis, transthoracic echocardiography should be performed to evaluate the severity of stenosis and left ventricular systolic function (Grade A).[15] If significant aortic stenosis is confirmed, the patient should be evaluated for the presence of concurrent CAD (Grade A).[15] Patients with severe uncorrected aortic stenosis poorly tolerate the hemodynamic effects of anesthesia. Systemic hypotension and tachycardia may lead to decreased coronary perfusion pressure, arrhythmias, myocardial ischemia,

cardiac failure and death. Aortic valve replacement is suggested in patients with symptomatic severe aortic stenosis and should be performed before the vascular procedure to avoid intraoperative and postoperative hemodynamic instability (Grade A).[6,7,15] If a patient is not a candidate for aortic valve replacement, percutaneous balloon aortic valvuloplasty may be reasonable as a bridge (Grade A).[6,7,15]

> Patients with symptomatic severe aortic stenosis should be evaluated for aortic valve replacement or percutaneous balloon aortic valvuloplasty prior to vascular procedure.

ASSESSMENT OF FUNCTIONAL CAPACITY

Functional capacity is an important predictor of perioperative and long-term cardiac events (Level 1).[6,7] It is measured in metabolic equivalents (METs) and can be assessed by exercise testing or instruments such as the Duke Activity Status Index, a questionnaire based on common daily activities.[16] The Duke Index is correlated well with the maximum oxygen uptake on treadmill testing.[17] Functional capacity is classified as excellent (>10 METs), good (7–10 METs), moderate (4–6 METs), poor (<4 METs) or unknown (Table 12.1).[6,7] On assessment, patients with <4 METS (i.e. unable to walk four blocks or climb two flights of stairs) are at relatively high risk for perioperative

Table 12.1 Average metabolic equivalent levels for common activities.

Activity	METs[a]
Getting dressed	1.0
Walking indoors	1.5
Walking at 2.0 mph	2.5
Walking at 3.0 mph	3.5
Golf (with cart)	2.5
Golf (without cart)	4.9
Light work around the house	3.9
Calisthenics (no weights)	4.0
Climbing a flight of stairs	4.0
Gardening	4.4
Cycling (leisurely)	4.0
Cycling (moderately)	5.7
Swimming (slowly)	4.5
Swimming (fast)	7.0
Climbing hills	
No load	6.9
With 5 kg load	7.5
Tennis (doubles)	6.0
Tennis (singles)	7.5
Running (l0 min/mile)	10.2
Running (7.5 min/mile)	13.2

a Functional capacity can be expressed in metabolic equivalent (MET) levels; the oxygen consumption (VO2) of a 70 kg, 40-year-old man in a resting state is 3.5 mL/kg/min, or 1 MET, i.e. 3 MET represents an exercise intensity three times the metabolic rate at rest.

cardiac events,[18] while patients with >10 METS are at very low risk.[5] Patients with 4–10 METs are considered to have fair functional capacity and are generally considered low risk for perioperative events.[6,7]

A potential pitfall may occur if functional capacity is not assessed preoperatively, leading to an unnecessary cardiology consultation. For instance, a patient who is able to climb two flights of stairs has acceptable functional capacity and thus a predicted low risk of a cardiac event. Such a patient should be able to proceed to surgery without further workup, even if intermediate cardiac risk factors are identified. The value of this simple test has previously been demonstrated.[6,7,19] Yet, patients with good exercise tolerance are often still referred to cardiology for 'clearance'.

> If a patient is able to climb two flights of stairs, this demonstrates acceptable functional capacity and obviates the need for additional cardiac testing.

Table 12.2 Clinical predictors of the Revised Cardiac Risk Index.

Intraperitoneal, intrathoracic or suprainguinal vascular surgery
Ischemic heart disease
History of congestive heart failure
History of cerebrovascular disease
Diabetes mellitus with preoperative insulin use
Renal insufficiency with serum creatinine level >2 mg/dL

Source: Lee TH et al., *Circulation*, 100, 1043, 1999.

ASSESSMENT OF CLINICAL CARDIAC RISK FACTORS

In the absence of any of the four major cardiac risk factors described earlier, the next step is to calculate the patient's cardiac risk using one of several available scoring systems.[20–23] Among these, the Revised Cardiac Risk Index (RCRI)[22] and the Vascular Study Group of New England Cardiac Risk Index (VSG-CRI)[23] are most commonly used in patients undergoing vascular surgery. Both are easily calculated in clinical practice, and elevated scores are associated with an increased risk of perioperative cardiovascular complications (Table 12.2; Figure 12.1). Currently, only the RCRI has been incorporated into both the American (i.e. ACC/AHA)[6,7] and European[9] guidelines for perioperative cardiac risk assessment. The RCRI model stratifies patients into low-, intermediate-, and high-risk groups before elective, non-cardiac surgery. All clinical predictors (Table 12.2) contribute equally to the index (1 point each), with scores of 0, 1, 2 and ≥3 points corresponding to estimated risk of major cardiac complications of 0.4%, 0.9%, 7% and 11%, respectively.[6,7] Low-risk patients have an RCRI score of 0, intermediate-risk patients have a score of 1 or 2, and high-risk patients have a score of 3 or more.

The VSG-CRI is more specific to vascular surgery patients, as the RCRI was developed from a heterogeneous patient population with only a small subset of vascular surgery patients.[24,25] The VSG-CRI places a greater emphasis on age because of its strong correlation with cardiovascular co-morbidities (Figure 12.1).[26] The developers of the VSG-CRI have reported considerable underestimation of in-hospital

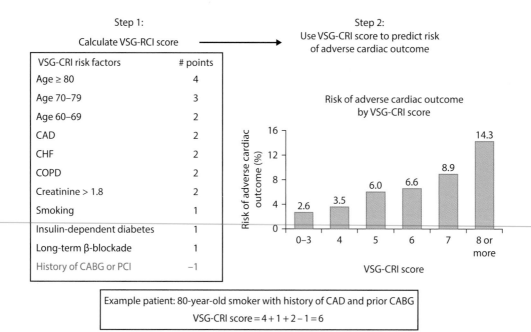

Figure 12.1 Vascular Surgery Group Cardiac Risk Index scoring system and predicted risk of adverse cardiac events. *Legend:* CAD, coronary artery disease; CHF, congestive heart failure; COPD, chronic obstructive pulmonary disease; CABG, coronary artery bypass grafting; PCI, percutaneous coronary intervention. (Reprinted *Journal of Vascular Surgery*, Volume 52, Bertges DJ, Goodney PP, Zhao Y et al. The Vascular Study Group of New England Cardiac Risk Index (VSG-CRI) predicts cardiac complications more accurately than the Revised Cardiac Risk Index in vascular surgery patients, 674–683, 2010, with permission from Elsevier.)

cardiac complications by the RCRI in patients undergoing elective or urgent vascular surgery, especially after lower extremity bypass, endovascular and open AAA repair.[23]

ADDITIONAL TESTING

A common misstep among practitioners is to routinely perform additional testing prior to vascular surgery. This is done either (1) to reassure oneself that the patient's cardiac risk is low, (2) to assuage the anesthesiologist and prevent any potential roadblocks to the operation, (3) as a routine or (4) in the belief that severe asymptomatic CAD will be detected and corrected prior to vascular surgery so as to decrease risk. The logic behind this approach is faulty for several reasons, which will be expanded upon later. Per ACC/AHA guidelines, additional cardiac testing should only be considered if the RCRI is three or more and only if the patient has poor exercise tolerance (Grade A).[6,7] Thus, there are other potential areas for pitfalls. Other patients are sent for cardiac stress testing because their exercise tolerance is poor, without factoring in the RCRI. If the RCRI is low (<3), stress testing is not necessary, as the predicted cardiac risk will be sufficiently low. In other circumstances, the patient will be sent for stress testing because the RCRI is high (3 or more), yet the patient is able to climb two flights of stairs, which per guidelines renders such testing unnecessary. The premise that stress testing identifies patients at higher risk for a perioperative cardiac event is also questionable at best, as will be explained later. Finally, prophylactic preoperative coronary revascularization has not been shown to reduce cardiac risk of subsequent vascular procedures (see the succeeding text as well).

> Per ACC/AHA guidelines, additional cardiac testing should only be considered if the RCRI is three or more and only if the patient has poor exercise tolerance.

Non-invasive stress testing

Non-invasive stress testing includes exercise ECG and pharmacologic cardiac stress imaging (dobutamine stress echocardiography and dipyridamole sestamibi/thallium). Exercise ECG is preferred in those who can tolerate walking. As mentioned previously, there is no role for stress testing in emergency procedures or in patients with excellent functional capacity. For most urgent cases, stress testing similarly should be avoided in our opinion (this situation is not directly addressed in the ACC/AHA guidelines). Stress testing leads to significant delays and such delays while awaiting urgent vascular surgery can lead to limb loss, recurrent embolic stroke or a ruptured AAA.

Pharmacologic cardiac stress imaging can be performed by echocardiography with intravenous dobutamine (the dobutamine simulates exercise as it increases myocardial oxygen demand). Other options include myocardial perfusion imaging with thallium-201 or technetium-99 m with pharmacologic agents such as intravenous dipyridamole/adenosine (which again simulate exercise by causing coronary artery vasodilation). These methods can detect areas of myocardium that are at risk for ischemia. Studies have shown that dobutamine echocardiography in particular has a very high negative predictive value for perioperative cardiac complications (97%–100%), and thus negative results should be reassuring.[26] However, the value of a positive stress test for predicting whether a patient will have an adverse perioperative cardiac event is relatively low (10%–45%).[26] Numerous studies have found no predictive value for dipyridamole thallium or sestamibi.[27,28] In fact, in one prospective blinded study, the rate of adverse cardiac events was the same for a positive and negative dipyridamole sestamibi/thallium.[28] Thus, it is our opinion these latter studies should be avoided in the preoperative assessment, as little clinical information is provided to guide decision-making. Dipyridamole is contraindicated in patients treated with theophylline, those with severe obstructive pulmonary disease and patients with critical carotid stenosis. Dobutamine should be avoided in patients with severe hypertension, significant arrhythmias or poor echocardiographic images.

Resting echocardiogram

Resting echocardiogram is not considered useful as a supplemental test for routine preoperative cardiac assessment.[6,7] Its preoperative use should be limited to patients suspected of having severe valvular disease or active heart failure, based on history and physical examination (Grade A).[29] Echocardiography has little value in patients lacking clinical features of heart failure or valvular heart disease and has poor ability to accurately predict perioperative cardiovascular events (Level 1).[29] A population-based retrospective cohort study of over 250,000 patients has shown that there is no benefit in survival or hospital length of stay by performing resting echocardiogram within 6 months prior to major elective non-cardiac surgery (Level 3).[30]

Computed tomography coronary angiography

Currently, computed tomography coronary angiography (CTCA) has not been incorporated into the ACC/AHA guidelines. One study has shown that CTCA may provide additive value to the RCRI in assessing patients undergoing intermediate-risk non-cardiac surgery (Level 2).[31] The authors found that the presence of significant coronary artery stenosis (≥50%) correlated with postoperative cardiac events.[31] However, there are little data on its usefulness in patients undergoing vascular interventions, and thus we do not recommend it at this time.

Coronary artery revascularization with percutaneous coronary intervention or coronary artery bypass grafting

Coronary artery revascularization (CAR) via percutaneous coronary intervention or coronary artery bypass grafting is indicated before non-cardiac surgery in patients with unstable coronary syndromes (those with unstable angina, recent MI or ventricular arrhythmias) with significant left main or three-vessel (or two-vessel if this includes the proximal left anterior descending artery) CAD (Grade A).[6,7] In the absence of these indications, the role of prophylactic coronary CAR prior to elective vascular surgery is controversial and in most instances is not indicated.[6,7] Intuitively, one would expect that identifying and correcting severe CAD before vascular surgery would lower the cardiac risk of the subsequent procedure. However, postoperative MI occurs by two mechanisms.[32] Type 1 occurs when an unstable or vulnerable plaque undergoes spontaneous rupture or erosion, leading to acute coronary thrombosis, ischemia and infarctions, whereas type 2 is due to prolonged myocardial oxygen supply–demand imbalance in the presence of stable CAD. Triggers of type 2 postoperative MI, which are the most common cause of postoperative MI, include prolonged tachycardia, hypoxia and anemia.[32] Typically, the cardiologist would not have recommended preoperative coronary intervention in such patients with stable CAD. In addition, patients who undergo prophylactic CAR followed by vascular surgery incur the risk of two major operations. Thus, prophylactic CAR (i.e. for asymptomatic CAD uncovered via stress testing) prior to vascular surgery, in our opinion, is not indicated as it has not been shown to benefit patients and leads to significant delays. This is supported by the CAR prophylaxis trial, in which patients with documented significant CAD were randomized to CAR versus no CAR prior to vascular surgery (Level 1).[33] Median time from randomization to vascular surgery was 54 days in CAR patients versus 18 days in patients who did not undergo CAR. At a 30-day follow-up, there was no difference in mortality between the CAR and no CAR groups (3.1% vs. 3.4%, respectively; p = 0.87). The incidence of perioperative MI was similar in the CAR than the non-CAR group (11.6% vs. 14.3%, p = 0.37).[33] It should be noted, however, that patients with left main disease or ejection fraction <20% were excluded from the study.

> Prophylactic CAR before non-cardiac surgery in the absence of unstable angina, recent MI or ventricular arrhythmias has not been shown to be beneficial.

MEDICAL OPTIMIZATION

In patients with known CAD or those at high risk for CAD (which includes most vascular patients), a strategy of medical optimization should be implemented. In general, patients should continue medications that are already receiving for CAD throughout the perioperative period in the absence of specific contraindications.

Beta-blockers

There has recently been a significant shift in the approach to perioperative beta-blockade.[34] Most prominently, the POISE trial reported that perioperative beta-blockers significantly reduced the incidence of MI (4.2% vs. 5.7%, 0.73, 0.60–0.89; p = 0·0017) (Level 1).[35] However, there were more deaths (3.1% vs. 2.3%; 1.33, 1.03–1.74; p = 0.0317) and more strokes (1.0% vs. 0.5%; 2.17, 1.26–3.74; p = 0.0053) in the metoprolol group than in the placebo group.[35] The POISE trial has been criticized for some aspects of the study design.[35] For instance, elderly patients who were beta-blocker naïve were included.[34] Such patients were given a high dose of slow-release metoprolol, and it was given just before surgery without any preoperative titration.[34] Thus, current recommendations are to continue beta-blockade in patients who have received it long term. Otherwise, beta-blockade should be considered only in high-risk patients undergoing high-risk or possibly intermediate-risk surgery.[34,36] Since most vascular patients fit this risk profile, it is reasonable to consider beta-blockade, particularly if the patient has hypertension. Our opinion is that initiation of beta-blockade is reasonable in many vascular patients preoperatively. However, it should be slowly titrated (to a heart rate between 60 and 70 beats/min) over several days or weeks before surgery and not started on the day of surgery.[37] In fact, using such an approach, de Virgilio et al. observed no deaths, MI or stroke in 100 consecutive patients followed prospectively (Level 2).[37] They did, however, observe an increased risk of intraoperative hypotension.[37]

Metoprolol (beta1-selective receptor antagonists) 25–50 mg daily without intrinsic activity is preferable (Grade A).[38] Perioperative beta-blocker withdrawal should be avoided unless necessary,[39] as it is associated with an increased risk of MI and chest pain.[40]

> Beta-blockade is recommended only in high-risk patients undergoing high-risk or possibly intermediate-risk surgery. It should be slowly titrated over days or weeks and not be administered for the first time immediately preoperatively.

Statins

Several studies have shown benefit of statin therapy in lowering cardiac morbidity and mortality in patients undergoing non-cardiac surgery, particularly in vascular surgery patients.[41] Statins improve endothelial function, reduce vascular inflammation and stabilize atherosclerotic plaque. The ACC/AHA recommendations[6,7] state that statin therapy is reasonable for patients undergoing vascular surgery with or without clinical risk factors.

Our approach is to routinely administer statins in vascular patients in the absence of contraindications. The timing and duration of therapy are still not well defined.[6,7]

> Statin therapy is *reasonable* for patients undergoing vascular surgery with or without clinical risk factors.

Alpha-2 agonists

Alpha-2 agonists reduce morbidity (i.e. MI) and mortality in patients undergoing vascular surgery. Current ACC/AHA recommendations state that alpha-2 agonists for perioperative control of hypertension may be considered for patients with known CAD or at least one clinical risk factor who are undergoing surgery.[6,7] Our practice is not to routinely add this medication preoperatively.

Calcium channel blockers

Although there are data to support the perioperative use of calcium channel blockers, the current ACC/AHA guidelines[6,7] do not make recommendations for their use.

Angiotensin-converting enzyme inhibitors or angiotensin receptor blockers

Angiotensin-converting enzyme inhibitors and angiotensin receptor blockers have not been associated with improvement of outcomes in the absence of left ventricular systolic dysfunction.[24,42] These drugs increase the risk of severe intraoperative hypotension, particularly if they are combined with beta-blockers or diuretics. This may result in increased 30-day mortality in patients undergoing major vascular surgery.[43] There is debate about whether these agents should be withheld one half-life prior to anesthesia induction or if they can be continued in adequately hydrated patients.[44] Further trials are needed to elucidate the efficacy and safety of perioperative use of these agents.

Aspirin

Aspirin irreversibly inhibits the cyclooxygenase enzyme system and prevents platelet aggregation, which decreases risk of coronary thrombosis and increases risk of perioperative bleeding. When aspirin is held preoperatively, the aspirin withdrawal syndrome may significantly increase the risk of major thromboembolic complications. In patients with known CAD, excluding those with recent coronary artery stent insertion, risk of subsequent MI or death is increased two- to threefold if aspirin is ceased preoperatively (Level 1).[45] While the reduced likelihood

of major postoperative bleeding may offset this cardiac risk for some procedures, a meta-analysis of 41 studies including almost 50,000 surgical patients showed that, overall, the cardiac risk exceeded bleeding risk for most surgical patients with known CAD when aspirin is withheld (Level 1).[46] Furthermore, in a randomized, double-blind, placebo-controlled trial including 220 patients, Oscarsson et al. showed that the perioperative use of low-dose aspirin (75 mg) initiated 7 days before non-cardiac surgery (i.e. abdominal, urology, orthopedics, gynecology) and continued 3 days after surgery reduced the risk of major adverse cardiac events without increasing bleeding complications in high-risk patients (Level 1).[47] However, the study did not include patients undergoing vascular procedures.[47] The result of POISE-2 study has recently shown that administration of aspirin before surgery and throughout the early postsurgical period (started at a dose of 200 mg and continued at a dose of 100 mg) had no significant effect on the rate of cardiac morbidity and mortality but increased the risk of major bleeding (Level 1).[48] However, since only 6% of patients had vascular procedures, the results may not be applicable to this population. In fact, it has been shown that there is a benefit of aspirin in terms of a reduction of perioperative stroke in patients undergoing carotid endarterectomy (Level 2).[49] Thus, in the majority of vascular patients, we recommend continuation of aspirin.

> In the majority of patients undergoing vascular surgery, aspirin should be administered and continued perioperatively.

HYPERTENSION

Since hypertension is common in vascular patients, the perioperative evaluation is a unique opportunity to initiate appropriate therapy. Preoperative elevated blood pressure in a patient with previously undiagnosed or untreated hypertension has been associated with labile blood pressure under anesthesia.[50] Hypertension makes hemodynamic control during anesthesia more difficult, increases the risk of intra- and postoperative cardiovascular events (e.g. myocardial ischemia) and makes postoperative blood pressure control challenging. Therefore, preoperative control of blood pressure can facilitate smoother intra- and postoperative hemodynamic management.[50]

An important question that arises is whether surgery should be delayed to better control hypertension, so as to mitigate cardiac risk. If the hypertension is mild or moderate and there is no associated metabolic or cardiovascular abnormality, there is no evidence that it is beneficial to delay surgery (Level 1).[6,7,51] In patients with stage 3 hypertension (systolic blood pressure ≥180 mmHg and diastolic blood pressure ≥110 mmHg), the potential benefits of delaying the procedure to optimize the effects of antihypertensive agents should be weighed against the risk of delaying the surgery (Grade A).[6,7,51] At least one study has shown that patients without significant cardiovascular co-morbidities can proceed with surgical intervention without a significant increased rate of postoperative complications in spite of increased blood pressure on the day of operation (Level 1).[52] This issue needs to be further studied. Blood pressure can usually be controlled within a few hours with rapidly acting intravenous anti-hypertensive agents. Nevertheless, poorly controlled hypertension has been shown to increase the risk of complications following carotid endarterectomy (Level 1).[53] So our recommendations are to delay surgery in these patients, particularly if the patient has asymptomatic carotid stenosis.

> In patients with stage 3 hypertension (systolic blood pressure ≥180 mmHg and diastolic blood pressure ≥110 mmHg), the potential benefits of delaying the procedure to optimize the effects of anti-hypertensive agents should be weighed against the risk of delaying the surgery.

BLOOD GLUCOSE

Hyperglycemia is an independent risk factor for cardiovascular complications, particularly in older patients. Management of blood glucose in the perioperative period can be challenging and is best managed with adjusted doses and infusions of short-acting insulin based on frequent blood sugar determinations.[6,7,54] Although the ideal intra- and postoperative glycemic target level for cardiovascular benefit is not completely clear, results of regression analyses suggest that maintaining blood glucose concentrations below 150 mg/dL in the perioperative period may improve outcome and reduce the risk of severe hypoglycemia in anesthetized patients (Level 1).[6,7,54] The American College of Endocrinology recommends a preprandial glucose level below 140 mg/dL, with maximal glucose not to exceed 180 mg/dL in hospitalized patients (Grade A).[55] The benefits of strict control of blood glucose concentration (i.e. less than 150 mg/dL) during the perioperative period is outweighed by the detrimental effects of inadvertent hypoglycemia.

> In hospitalized patients, a preprandial glucose level below 140 mg/dL, with maximal glucose not to exceed 180 mg/dL is recommended.

ANEMIA

Perioperative anemia is stressful to the cardiovascular system and can aggravate myocardial ischemia and worsen heart failure. On the other hand, polycythemia and thrombocytosis increase viscosity and hypercoagulability and are associated with an increased risk of thromboembolism. It has been shown that hematocrit less than 28% is associated with an increased risk of perioperative ischemia and postoperative adverse events in patients undergoing vascular surgery.[56] The adjusted risk of 30-day postoperative

mortality and cardiac morbidity begins to rise when hematocrit levels decrease to less than 39% or exceed 51%.[57] Appropriate steps to reduce these risks should be considered and tailored to the individual patient's particular circumstances. Some studies have shown that perioperative transfusion in severely anemic patients with advanced CAD and/or heart failure may reduce perioperative cardiac events (Levels 2 and 3).[58,59] However, one study has recently shown that perioperative transfusion in vascular surgical patients is an independent predictor for increased 30-day morbidity and mortality (Level 2).[60] The current ACC/AHA guidelines[6,7] do not make any recommendation on the threshold of perioperative hemoglobin at which blood transfusion should be performed. This necessitates future studies to define perioperative transfusion threshold in vascular surgery patients.[61,62] The American Society of Anesthesiologists guidelines state that blood transfusion in the perioperative setting is usually indicated in otherwise healthy patients with hemoglobin <6 g/dL and rarely indicated with hemoglobin >10 g/dL (Grade A).[61,62] In patients with hemoglobin 6–10 g/dL, other factors should be considered to direct transfusion decisions, including evidence of organ ischemia, rate and amount of bleeding, intravascular volume status and risk factors for complications of inadequate oxygenation (e.g. low cardiopulmonary reserve).[61] Given that vascular patients are more vulnerable to type 2 postoperative MI (myocardial oxygen supply–demand imbalance), the optimal threshold for transfusion in vascular patients is likely somewhere between 6 and 10 g/dL.

> Preoperative blood transfusion is indicated in otherwise healthy patients with hemoglobin <6 g/dL and rarely in those with hemoglobin >10 g/dL.

SUMMARY

The following summarizes our approach to cardiac assessment:

1. The vast majority of vascular patients can safely proceed to surgery without an extensive preoperative cardiac workup.
2. Patients with emergent vascular surgical procedures should proceed directly to surgery.
3. For non-emergent procedures, it is imperative to identify those who have major cardiac risk factors (unstable coronary syndromes, decompensated CHF, significant arrhythmias, severe valvular disease), as surgery should be delayed to address these issues.
4. Patients with excellent exercise tolerance (4 or more METs) do not need additional evaluation and can proceed to surgery without any further workup. Good communication between the anesthesiologist and the surgeon can avoid unnecessary cardiology consult in this setting.
5. For remaining patients (urgent or elective surgery, absence of major cardiac predictors and poor exercise

tolerance), cardiac risk should be calculated using the RCRI or VSG-CRI.

6. An RCRI of three or more (per AHA guidelines), or a VSG of seven or more, should alert the vascular surgeon to a significantly increased cardiac risk.

7. For urgent cases (symptomatic AAA, very large AAA, severe ischemic rest pain, etc.), proceeding with surgery regardless of the RCRI is the most expeditious option in the majority of patients.

8. For elective cases with an RCRI of two, or less, one can proceed to surgery.

9. For elective cases with an RCRI of three or more, there are several options: (a) cancel the surgery completely (for instance, an endarterectomy in an asymptomatic patient or an aortobifemoral bypass for claudication), (b) postpone surgery to perform stress testing, (c) modify the operation to a less stressful one or (d) other modifications (involve additional specialists in the perioperative care, modify intraoperative or postoperative monitoring).

10. Stress testing has poor predictive value for perioperative cardiac events.

11. The use of stress testing has not been shown to lower perioperative cardiac events.

12. Resting echocardiography is not beneficial.

13. Prophylactic coronary revascularization prior to vascular surgery has not been shown to reduce the risk of postoperative MI or death.

14. The benefit of beta-blockade is unclear. If instituted preoperatively for blood pressure control, it should be done gradually and titrated. Stopping beta-blockers should be avoided.

15. Aspirin and statins should be continued perioperatively.

16. Postoperative MI are divided into two types: type 1 is due to rupture of a coronary artery plaque, whereas type 2 (more common) is due to an imbalance between myocardial supply and demand.

DEFICIENCIES IN CURRENT KNOWLEDGE AND AREAS FOR FUTURE RESEARCH

1. Is targeted and slowly titrated beta-blockade beneficial in reducing cardiac risk in vascular patients?

2. Is perioperative aspirin beneficial in reducing cardiac events in vascular patients?

3. Should vascular surgery be delayed to optimize blood pressure? To optimize hemoglobin A1C?

4. What is the optimal threshold for transfusion in vascular patients?

CONFLICT OF INTEREST

This is to certify that the authors did not receive any financial support from any public or private sources. The authors have no financial or proprietary interest in a product, method or material described herein.

REFERENCES

1. Kertai MD, Klein J, van Urk H, Bax JJ, Poldermans D. Cardiac complications after elective major vascular surgery. *Acta Anaesthesiol Scand.* 2003;47(6):643–654.

2. Welten GM, Schouten O, Hoeks SE et al. Long-term prognosis of patients with peripheral arterial disease: A comparison in patients with coronary artery disease. *J Am Coll Cardiol.* 2008;51:1588–1596.

3. Norgren L, Hiatt WR, Dormandy JA, Nehler MR, Harris KA, Fowkes FG. Inter-society consensus for the management of peripheral arterial disease (TASC II). *J Vasc Surg.* 2007;45(Suppl. S):S5–S67.

4. Hirsch AT, Haskal ZJ, Hertzer NR et al.; American Association for Vascular Surgery; Society for Vascular Surgery; Society for Cardiovascular Angiography and Interventions; Society for Vascular Medicine and Biology; Society of Interventional Radiology; ACC/AHA Task Force on Practice Guidelines Writing Committee to Develop Guidelines for the Management of Patients With Peripheral Arterial Disease; American Association of Cardiovascular and Pulmonary Rehabilitation; National Heart, Lung, and Blood Institute; Society for Vascular Nursing; TransAtlantic Inter-Society Consensus; Vascular Disease Foundation. ACC/AHA 2005 Practice Guidelines for the management of patients with peripheral arterial disease (lower extremity, renal, mesenteric, and abdominal aortic): A collaborative report from the American Association for Vascular Surgery/Society for Vascular Surgery, Society for Cardiovascular Angiography and Interventions, Society for Vascular Medicine and Biology, Society of Interventional Radiology, and the ACC/AHA Task Force on Practice Guidelines (Writing Committee to Develop Guidelines for the Management of Patients With Peripheral Arterial Disease): Endorsed by the American Association of Cardiovascular and Pulmonary Rehabilitation; National Heart, Lung, and Blood Institute; Society for Vascular Nursing; TransAtlantic Inter-Society Consensus; and Vascular Disease Foundation. *Circulation.* 2006;113(11):e463–e654.

5. Fleisher LA; American College of Cardiology/American Heart Association. Cardiac risk stratification for noncardiac surgery: Update from the American College of Cardiology/American Heart Association 2007 guidelines. *Cleve Clin J Med.* 2009;76(Suppl. 4):S9–S15.

6. Fleisher LA, Beckman JA, Brown KA et al.; American College of Cardiology/American Heart Association Task Force on Practice Guidelines (Writing Committee to Revise the 2002 Guidelines on Perioperative Cardiovascular Evaluation for Noncardiac Surgery); American Society of Echocardiography; American Society of Nuclear Cardiology; Heart Rhythm Society; Society of Cardiovascular Anesthesiologists; Society for Cardiovascular Angiography and Interventions;

Society for Vascular Medicine and Biology; Society for Vascular Surgery. ACC/AHA 2007 guidelines on perioperative cardiovascular evaluation and care for noncardiac surgery: A report of the American College of Cardiology/American Heart Association Task Force on Practice Guidelines (Writing Committee to Revise the 2002 Guidelines on Perioperative Cardiovascular Evaluation for Noncardiac Surgery): Developed in collaboration with the American Society of Echocardiography, American Society of Nuclear Cardiology, Heart Rhythm Society, Society of Cardiovascular Anesthesiologists, Society for Cardiovascular Angiography and Interventions, Society for Vascular Medicine and Biology, and Society for Vascular Surgery. *Circulation.* 2007;116:e418–e499.

7. Fleisher LA, Beckman JA, Brown KA et al.; 2009 ACCF/AHA focused update on perioperative beta blockade incorporated into the ACC/AHA 2007 guidelines on perioperative cardiovascular evaluation and care for noncardiac surgery. American College of Cardiology Foundation/American Heart Association Task Force on Practice Guidelines; American Society of Echocardiography; American Society of Nuclear Cardiology; Heart Rhythm Society; Society of Cardiovascular Anesthesiologists; Society for Cardiovascular Angiography and Interventions; Society for Vascular Medicine; Society for Vascular Surgery. *J Am Coll Cardiol.* 2009;54(22):e13–e118.

8. Eagle KA, Berger PB, Calkins H et al.; American College of Cardiology/American Heart Association Task Force on Practice Guidelines (Committee to Update the 1996 Guidelines on Perioperative Cardiovascular Evaluation for Noncardiac Surgery). ACC/AHA guideline update for perioperative cardiovascular evaluation for noncardiac surgery – Executive summary a report of the American College of Cardiology/American Heart Association Task Force on Practice Guidelines (Committee to Update the 1996 Guidelines on Perioperative Cardiovascular Evaluation for Noncardiac Surgery). *Circulation.* 2002;105:1257–1267.

9. European Stroke Organisation, Tendera M, Aboyans V et al.; ESC Committee for Practice Guidelines. ESC Guidelines on the diagnosis and treatment of peripheral artery diseases: Document covering atherosclerotic disease of extracranial carotid and vertebral, mesenteric, renal, upper and lower extremity arteries: The Task Force on the Diagnosis and Treatment of Peripheral Artery Diseases of the European Society of Cardiology (ESC). *Eur Heart J.* 2011;32(22):2851–2906.

10. Fleisher LA, Pasternak LR, Herbert R, Anderson GF. Inpatient hospital admission and death after outpatient surgery in elderly patients: Importance of patient and system characteristics and location of care. *Arch Surg.* 2004;139:67–72.

11. Katz RI, Barnhart JM, Ho G et al. A survey on the intended purposes and perceived utility of preoperative cardiology consultations. *Anesth Analg.* 1998;87:830–836.

12. Katz RI, Cimino L, Vitkun SA. Preoperative medical consultations: Impact on perioperative management and surgical outcome. *Can J Anaesth.* 2005;52:697–702.

13. Rooke TW, Hirsch AT, Misra S et al.; Society for Cardiovascular Angiography and Interventions; Society of Interventional Radiology; Society for Vascular Medicine; Society for Vascular Surgery. 2011 ACCF/AHA Focused Update of the Guideline for the Management of Patients With Peripheral Artery Disease (updating the 2005 guideline): A report of the American College of Cardiology Foundation/American Heart Association Task Force on Practice Guidelines. *J Am Coll Cardiol.* 2011;58(19):2020–2045.

14. Livhits M, Ko CY, Leonardi MJ, Zingmond DS, Gibbons MM, de Virgilio C. Risk of surgery following recent myocardial infarction. *Ann Surg.* 2011;253(5):857–864.

15. Nishimura RA, Otto CM, Bonow RO et al.; American College of Cardiology; American College of Cardiology/American Heart Association; American Heart Association. 2014 AHA/ACC guideline for the management of patients with valvular heart disease: A report of the American College of Cardiology/American Heart Association Task Force on Practice Guidelines. *J Thorac Cardiovasc Surg.* 2014;148(1):e1–e132.

16. Nelson CL, Herndon JE, Mark DB et al. Relation of clinical and angiographic factors to functional capacity as measured by the Duke Activity Status Index. *Am J Cardiol.* 1991;68:973–975.

17. Hlatky MA, Boineau RE, Higginbotham MB et al. A brief self-administered questionnaire to determine functional capacity (the Duke Activity Status Index). *Am J Cardiol.* 1989;64(10):651–654.

18. Reilly DF, McNeely MJ, Doerner D et al. Self-reported exercise tolerance and the risk of serious perioperative complications. *Arch Intern Med.* 1999;159:2185–2192.

19. Biccard BM. Relationship between the inability to climb two flights of stairs and outcome after major non-cardiac surgery: Implications for the pre-operative assessment of functional capacity. *Anaesthesia.* 2005;60(6):588–593.

20. L'Italien GJ, Paul SD, Hendel RC et al. Development and validation of a Bayesian model for perioperative cardiac risk assessment in a cohort of 1,081 vascular surgical candidates. *J Am Coll Cardiol.* 1996;27:779–786.

21. Kertai MD, Boersma E, Klein J, van Urk H, Poldermans D. Optimizing the prediction of perioperative mortality in vascular surgery by using a customized probability model. *Arch Intern Med.* 2005;165:898–904.

22. Lee TH, Marcantonio ER, Mangione CM et al. Derivation and prospective validation of a simple index for prediction of cardiac risk of major noncardiac surgery. *Circulation.* 1999;100:1043–1049.

23. Bertges DJ, Goodney PP, Zhao Y et al. The Vascular Study Group of New England Cardiac Risk Index (VSG-CRI) predicts cardiac complications more accurately than the Revised Cardiac Risk Index in vascular surgery patients. *J Vasc Surg.* 2010;52:674–683.

24. Scott IA, Shohag HA, Kam PC, Jelinek MV, Khadem GM. Preoperative cardiac evaluation and management of patients undergoing elective non-cardiac surgery. *Med J Aust.* 2013;199(10):667–673.

25. Ford MK, Beattie WS, Wijeysundera DN. Systematic review: Prediction of perioperative cardiac complications and mortality by the Revised Cardiac Risk Index. *Ann Intern Med.* 2010;152:26–35.

26. Mahlmann A, Rodionov RN, Ludwig S, Neidel J, Weiss N. How to asses and improve cardiopulmonary risk prior to vascular surgery? *Vasa.* 2013;42(5):323–330.

27. de Virgilio C, Wall DB, Ephraim L et al. An abnormal dipyridamole thallium/sestamibi fails to predict long-term cardiac events in vascular surgery patients. *Ann Vasc Surg.* 2001;15(2):267–271.

28. de Virgilio C, Toosie K, Elbassir M et al. Dipyridamole-thallium/sestamibi before vascular surgery: A prospective blinded study in moderate-risk patients. *J Vasc Surg.* 2000;32(1):77–89.

29. Douglas PS, Garcia MJ, Haines DE et al. ACCF/ASE/AHA/ASNC/HFSA/HRS/SCAI/SCCM/SCCT/SCMR 2011. Appropriate use criteria for echocardiography. *J Am Coll Cardiol.* 2011;57:1126–1166.

30. Wijeysundera DN, Beattie WS, Karkouti K et al. Association of echocardiography before major elective non-cardiac surgery with postoperative survival and length of hospital stay: Population based cohort study. *Br Med J.* 2011;342:d3695.

31. Ahn JH, Park JR, Min JH et al. Risk stratification using computed tomography coronary angiography in patients undergoing intermediate-risk noncardiac surgery. *Am Coll Cardiol.* 2013;61(6):661–668.

32. Landesberg G, Beattie WS, Mosseri M, Jaffe AS, Alpert JS. Perioperative myocardial infarction. *Circulation.* 2009;119(22):2936–2944.

33. Santilli SM. The Coronary Artery Revascularization Prophylaxis (CARP) Trial: Results and remaining controversies. *Perspect Vasc Surg Endovasc Ther.* 2006;18(4):282–285.

34. POISE Study Group, Devereaux PJ, Yang H et al. Effects of extended-release metoprolol succinate in patients undergoing non-cardiac surgery (POISE trial): A randomised controlled trial. *Lancet.* 2008;371(9627):1839–1847.

35. Sanfilippo F, Santonocito C, Foëx P. Use of beta-blockers in non-cardiac surgery: An open debate. *Minerva Anestesiol.* 2014;80(4):482–494.

36. Koniari I, Hahalis G. Perioperative B-blockers in non-cardiac surgery: Actual situation. *Curr Pharm Des.* 2013;19(22):3946–3962.

37. de Virgilio C, Yaghoubian A, Nguyen A et al. Peripheral vascular surgery using targeted beta blockade reduces perioperative cardiac event rate. *J Am Coll Surg.* 2009;208(1):14–20.

38. London MJ, Zaugg M, Schaub MC, Spahn DR. Perioperative beta-adrenergic receptor blockade: Physiologic foundations and clinical controversies. *Anesthesiology.* 2004;100:170–175.

39. Psaty BM, Koepsell TD, Wagner EH et al. The relative risk of incident coronary heart disease associated with recently stopping the use of beta-blockers. *J Am Med Assoc.* 1990;263:1653–1657.

40. Hoeks SE, Scholte Op Reimer WJ, van Urk H et al. Increase of 1-year mortality after perioperative beta-blocker withdrawal in endovascular and vascular surgery patients. *Eur J Vasc Endovasc Surg.* 2006;33:13–19.

41. Sanders RD, Nicholson A, Lewis SR, Smith AF, Alderson P. Perioperative statin therapy for improving outcomes during and after noncardiac vascular surgery. *Cochrane Database Syst Rev.* 2013;7:CD009971.

42. Lau WC, Froehlich JB, Jewell ES et al. Impact of adding aspirin to beta-blocker and statin in high-risk patients undergoing major vascular surgery. *Ann Vasc Surg.* 2013;27(4):537–545.

43. Railton CJ, Wolpin J, Lam-McCulloch J, Belo SE. Renin-angiotensin blockade is associated with increased mortality after vascular surgery. *Can J Anaesth.* 2010;57:736–744.

44. Auron M, Harte B, Kumar A, Michota F. Renin-angiotensin system antagonists in the perioperative setting: Clinical consequences and recommendations for practice. *Postgrad Med J.* 2011;87:472–481.

45. Burger W, Chemnitius JM, Kneissl GD, Rücker G. Low-dose aspirin for secondary cardiovascular prevention – Cardiovascular risks after its perioperative withdrawal versus bleeding risks with its continuation – Review and meta-analysis. *J Intern Med.* 2005;257:399–414.

46. Biondi-Zoccai GG, Lotrionte M, Agostoni P et al. A systematic review and meta-analysis on the hazards of discontinuing or not adhering to aspirin among 50,279 patients at risk for coronary artery disease. *Eur Heart J.* 2006;27:2667–2674.

47. Oscarsson A, Gupta A, Fredrikson M et al. To continue or discontinue aspirin in the perioperative period: A randomized, controlled clinical trial. *Br J Anaesth.* 2010;104(3):305–312.

48. Devereaux PJ, Mrkobrada M, Sessler DI et al.; POISE-2 Investigators. Aspirin in patients undergoing noncardiac surgery. *N Engl J Med.* 2014;370(16):1494–1503.

49. Schoenefeld E, Donas K, Radicke A, Osada N, Austermann M, Torsello G. Perioperative use of aspirin for patients undergoing carotid endarterectomy. *VASA.* 2012;41(4):282–287.

50. The fifth report of the Joint National Committee on Detection, Evaluation, and Treatment of High Blood Pressure (JNC V). *Arch Intern Med.* 1993;153:154–183.

51. James PA, Oparil S, Carter BL et al. 2014 evidence-based guideline for the management of high blood pressure in adults: Report from the panel members appointed to the Eighth Joint National Committee (JNC 8). *J Am Med Assoc.* 2014;311(5):507–520.

52. Weksler N, Klein M, Szendro G et al. The dilemma of immediate preoperative hypertension: To treat and operate, or to postpone surgery? *J Clin Anesth.* 2003;15:179–183.

53. Rostamzadeh A, Zumbrunn T, Jongen LM et al.; ICSS-MRI Substudy Investigators. Predictors of acute and persisting ischemic brain lesions in patients randomized to carotid stenting or endarterectomy. *Stroke.* 2014 February;45(2):591–594.

54. Garber AJ, Moghissi ES, Bransome EDJ et al. American College of Endocrinology position statement on inpatient diabetes and metabolic control. *Endocr Pract.* 2004;10:77–82.

55. Umpierrez GE, Hellman R, Korytkowski MT et al.; Endocrine Society. Management of hyperglycemia in hospitalized patients in non-critical care setting: An endocrine society clinical practice guideline. *J Clin Endocrinol Metab.* 2012;97(1):16–38.

56. Nelson AH, Fleisher LA, Rosenbaum SH. Relationship between postoperative anemia and cardiac morbidity in high-risk vascular patients in the intensive care unit. *Crit Care Med.* 1993;21:860–866.

57. Wu WC, Schifftner TL, Henderson WG et al. Preoperative hematocrit levels and postoperative outcomes in older patients undergoing noncardiac surgery. *J Am Med Assoc.* 2007;297:2481–2488.

58. Wu WC, Smith TS, Henderson WG et al. Operative blood loss, blood transfusion, and 30-day mortality in older patients after major noncardiac surgery. *Ann Surg.* 2010;252:11–17.

59. Wu WC, Trivedi A, Friedmann PD et al. Association between hospital intraoperative blood transfusion practices for surgical blood loss and hospital surgical mortality rates. *Ann Surg.* 2012;255:708–714.

60. Obi AT, Park YJ, Bove P, Cuff R, Kazmers A, Gurm HS, Grossman PM, Henke PK. The association of perioperative transfusion with 30-day morbidity and mortality in patients undergoing major vascular surgery. *J Vasc Surg.* 2015 April;61(4):1000–1009.e1.

61. Shander A, Gross I, Hill S, Javidroozi M, Sledge S; College of American Pathologists; American Society of Anesthesiologists; Society of Thoracic Surgeons and Society of Cardiovascular Anesthesiologists; Society of Critical Care Medicine; Italian Society of Transfusion Medicine and Immunohaematology; American Association of Blood Banks. A new perspective on best transfusion practices. *Blood Transfus.* 2013;11(2):193–202.

62. American Society of Anesthesiologists Task Force on Perioperative Blood Transfusion and Adjuvant Therapies. Practice guidelines for perioperative blood transfusion and adjuvant therapies: An updated report by the American Society of Anesthesiologists Task Force on Perioperative Blood Transfusion and Adjuvant Therapies. *Anesthesiology.* 2006;105:198–208.

13

The biology of restenosis and neointimal hyperplasia

ADAM M. GWOZDZ, MOSTAFA ALBAYATI and BIJAN MODARAI

CONTENTS

INTRODUCTION

Definition

Handling an artery by clamping, performing anastomoses or balloon angioplasty/stenting can promote a pathologic healing process that can lead to luminal narrowing. Despite advances in open vascular surgery and endovascular techniques over the past half-century, restenosis remains one of the most important determinants of long-term arterial patency and the ultimate success of interventions.

The term neointima is used to describe the pathologic intima that forms in response to vessel wall injury.[1] The physiologic response to injury, which produces the neointima, comprises the process of smooth muscle migration/proliferation and extracellular matrix deposition and is called neointimal hyperplasia. Neointimal hyperplasia represents an attempt to heal the injured arterial wall and is analogous to wound-healing responses in other areas of the body.

Restenosis is the narrowing or occlusion of a vessel that was previously stenotic and has undergone a therapeutic procedure to open it. Restenosis comprises two main processes – neointimal hyperplasia and vessel remodelling. This term is often inappropriately used when a stenosis develops after the injury of a normal artery in an animal model. The mechanisms that control neointimal hyperplasia are redundant and are governed by multiple factors, including numerous cell types, growth factors and hormones. The molecular basis of this enhanced proliferative response has been the focus of pharmacological prevention of restenosis and led to the development of drug-eluting balloons and stents.

Clinical significance

Atherosclerosis is the leading cause of morbidity and mortality in the western world. Consequently, a large number of procedures have been devised to treat disease. Balloon angioplasty was a common procedure used to treat the stenosis caused by atherosclerotic lesions in both the heart and periphery. Bare metal stent was a major advancement over balloon angioplasty as it prevented restenosis by attenuating early arterial recoil and contraction, both commonly seen after balloon angioplasty. Unfortunately, restenosis at 1 year remained relatively high (10%–20%), often due to excessive neointimal growth[2] (Figure 13.1). Drug-eluting stents (DESs) promise to reduce the relatively high rate of restenosis, and some clinical trials have confirmed a reduction of as much as 50%–70% in target lesion revascularization using DES as opposed to bare metal stents.[3,4] Neointimal hyperplasia is also the leading cause of vein graft failure 3 months to 2 years after bypass surgery.[5–7] The failure rate for lower extremity vein grafts averages 20%–30% in long-term follow-up.[8] The problem of neointimal hyperplasia is even worse with prosthetic grafts. Restenosis is also seen

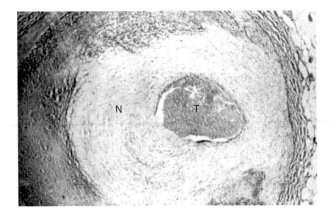

Figure 13.1 Thrombosed coronary artery with intimal hyperplasia after percutaneous transluminal coronary angioplasty. N, neointima; T, thrombus.

after surgical endarterectomy. As many as 20% of patients undergoing carotid endarterectomy will develop a haemodynamically significant neointimal lesion.[9] Fortunately, few of these become symptomatic.

EMBRYOLOGY/HISTOLOGY

The arterial wall is comprised of three concentric layers of cells and connective tissue (Figure 13.2). The innermost layer is the intima, which is formed by a thin layer of endothelial cells on the basement membrane, a variable amount of subendothelial connective tissue and the internal elastic lamina.

Between the internal and external elastic laminae is the arterial media. This layer is made up of smooth muscle cells (SMCs) and extracellular matrix made up of primarily elastin and collagen. The exact composition of the media depends on the size and location of the artery. Arterioles responsible for the control of systemic vascular resistance have relatively more SMCs than larger arteries like the aorta.

The outer layer of the arterial wall is the adventitia. This layer is primarily made up of loose connective tissue, some

SMCs and fibroblasts. The adventitia is supplied with tiny blood vessels of its own, vasa vasorum, which also nourish the outer layers of the media.

At birth, the intima of human arteries consists solely of endothelial cells lining the internal elastic lamina.[10] Two notable exceptions include the ductus arteriosus and the origin of the left main coronary artery, which have SMCs in the intima at this time.[11] In the first few years of life, however, SMCs begin to appear in the space between the endothelial cells and the internal elastic lamina in the aorta and other large muscular arteries. The areas of SMC accumulation are called intimal cushions; these represent areas prone to future development of atherosclerotic plaques.

INJURY RESPONSE

Models

Much of our understanding of the cellular and molecular biology of neointimal hyperplasia has been gained from studies performed in animal models such as balloon denudation, angioplasty, endarterectomy and the insertion of vein or prosthetic grafts,[12,13] which allow for controlled environments and less complex injury responses.

Many of the earlier studies of the mechanisms of neointimal hyperplasia were undertaken in the rat and rabbit carotid arteries.[14,15] The rat carotid artery is a relatively simple artery, comprising a single layer of endothelium lining, the internal elastic lamina.[16] For experimental purposes, it has fairly easy access via the external carotid artery, and the common carotid artery is devoid of braches, limiting the origin of re-endothelialization to the proximal and distal artery. The response of the rat carotid to injury has been studied extensively and occurs without an inflammatory response or fibrin deposition (Figure 13.3).[14,17] The simplicity of this model allows for a close examination of the basic mechanisms of the response to injury, but it may not be directly applicable to the much more complex environment of an injured atherosclerotic human artery.

Mouse models have been very useful for genetic studies due to the development of transgenic and knockout mice.[18] For this reason and other advantages when compared to other animal models, including their small size and ease of husbandry, there are nearly 10 different mouse models for studying all types of neointimal lesions.[19] Several methods, including carotid artery ligation,[16,17] wire injury and external electrocautery,[20] have been devised to provide an easier and more reproducible method of arterial injury. Several mouse models manifesting lesions resembling neointimal hyperplasia of human vein grafts have been developed to address specific interventional issues. Activation or dysfunction of the grafted venous endothelium by the arterial blood pressure and by traumatic and ischaemic injury may play a role in the induction of SMC responses and neointimal thickening of the graft.[20]

Rabbits have the advantage of being very responsive to atherogenic diets, developing hypercholesterolaemia,

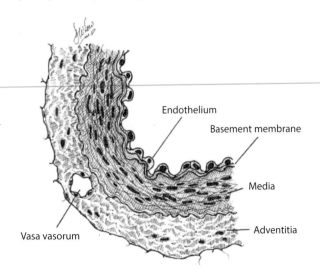

Figure 13.2 Arterial wall histology. (From David Low.)

Endothelium

Basement membrane

Media

Adventitia

Vasa vasorum

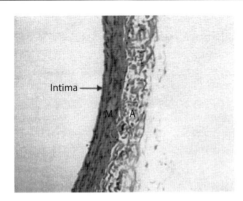
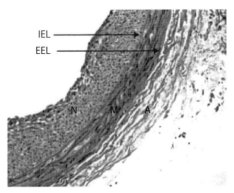

Figure 13.3 Hotomicrograph of rat carotid before and 2 weeks after balloon injury. M, media; A, adventitia; N, neointima; IEL, internal elastic lamina; EEL, external elastic lamina.

which makes it possible to investigate the combined effects of mechanical injury and dyslipidaemia in a physiologic milieu more complex than the rat and more closely approximating human disease.

Pig models of balloon angioplasty are widely used to study the effects of coronary angioplasty and stenting. The pig responds to arterial injury with a thrombotic process similar to that seen in humans. They also develop arterial wall calcifications akin to those in human disease. This model is frequently used to study new endovascular techniques and devices. Although swine, canine and non-human primate are animal models that are more relevant to clinical neointimal hyperplasia, the high cost and limited genetic information and molecular reagents are major hurdles in using these models.

A neointimal injury response can be induced by a number of methods. The most commonly used method is the balloon catheter technique: The catheter is inserted into the artery, the balloon inflated, and the catheter withdrawn, with or without twisting. Other methods of injury include using a small guidewire for denudement of the artery, electrocoagulation of the exterior of the artery, distal ligation of the artery, placement of a perivascular collar and chemic injury to the vessel wall. There are also vein graft models in mice, rats and rabbits. Each method has strengths and weaknesses as a model of the neointimal response in humans. Each of the injury methods produces a different set of responses, including varying degrees of endothelial damage, medial damage, thrombosis and flow modification. By carefully choosing the animal model (with specific genetic and metabolic characteristics, such a hyperlipidemia) and the method of injury, one can focus the experiment on a specific vascular wall process or a particular aspect of the injury response.

Cellular response to injury

ENDOTHELIUM

The endothelium is a confluent monolayer of thin, flattened, rhomboid-shaped cells lining the intimal surface of all blood vessels. Endothelial integrity is essential for maintaining vascular homeostasis, and endothelial denudation results in neointimal thickening. Endothelial cell products inhibit platelet function and thrombosis, control vessel wall permeability[21] and bind and inactivate mitogens, thereby inhibiting SMC growth.[22]

After experimental vascular injury, re-endothelialization begins within 24 hours, starting from the leading edge of the denuded area and the ostea of branch arteries.[14] It has been shown that after mild injury, consisting of a gentle endothelial denudation, complete re-endothelialization can occur.[23] However, after more severe injury involving disruption of the basement membrane and the deeper layers of the media, endothelial dysfunction persists even if the regrowth is complete.[23,24] After vascular injury and endothelial regrowth, vasodilators which work via an endothelium-dependent mechanism show a decreased effect, whilst the ability of the underlying SMCs to relax or contract is unchanged. This may be due to decreased levels of nitric oxide (NO) synthesis in the endothelial cells.[25]

Endothelial dysfunction may persist for >3 months after vascular injury and is more pronounced after bare metal stent implantation as compared with balloon angioplasty.[26] Experimental evidence from animal models suggests that the anti-proliferative properties of paclitaxel, one of the agents that have been used in drug-eluting balloon and stent technologies, may limit endothelial cell regrowth.[27] Analysis of human coronary arteries treated with sirolimus-eluting stents, however, confirms extensive (>80%) re-endothelialization of stents at 16 months post-implantation.[28] The functional status of the endothelial cells covering the DES is not known. Reassuringly, the incidence of stent thrombosis, which can be a clinical consequence of abnormal healing and re-endothelialization, can be prevented after implantation of a DES using dual antiplatelet therapy.[29]

PLATELETS

Platelets are propelled to the vessel edge by blood flow, which positions them near the surface of the endothelium, allowing them to detect and respond to vascular damage rapidly.[30] Platelet adhesion and activation are mediated primarily by their interactions with the subendothelial proteins von Willebrand factor (vWF) and collagen. Platelets bind to subendothelial vWF via the platelet membrane glycoprotein (GP) Ib-IX-V complex and to collagen via the integrin α2β1 and GPVI. Platelet adherence to collagen via GPVI triggers the intracellular signalling events that result in their activation. Stimulated platelets develop a procoagulant surface and degranulate, releasing several factors, including platelet-derived growth factor (PDGF) and transforming growth factor-β (TGF-β), an essential step in haemostasis. PDGF is an important factor in initiating migration of SMCs from the media to the intima.

SMCs

Resting vascular SMCs are spindle shaped, with single, elongated nuclei, resembling fibroblasts. The contractile function of SMCs is mediated by cytoplasmic filaments that contain actin and myosin. Vascular SMCs are capable of many functions, including vasoconstriction and dilation in response to normal or pharmacologic stimuli; synthesis of collagen, elastin and proteoglycans; elaboration of growth factors and cytokines; and migration to the intima and proliferation.

The migratory and proliferative activity of SMCs is physiologically regulated by growth promoters and inhibitors. One of the earliest indicators of SMC activation is the expression of proto-oncogenes (e.g. c-myc, c-myb, c-jun and c-fos), which are associated with the events proceeding DNA replication. These have been detected as early as 30 minutes after injury.[31] Indeed, prevention of proto-oncogene expression using antisense oligonucleotides has reduced the neointimal response in animal models.[32]

The first consequence of SMC activation is proliferation. Under normal circumstances, there is very little turnover in the SMC population, only 0.06% per day in the adult rat.[14] In response to hypertension or direct injury,[14] however, there is a dramatic increase in the proliferation rate of medial SMCs. This is followed by the migration of SMCs to the intima and the deposition of extracellular matrix.

SMC PROLIFERATION AND MIGRATION

Vascular injury stimulates SMC growth by disrupting the physiologic balance between inhibition and stimulation. The formation of a neointima involves SMC migration from the media to the intima, proliferation of intimal cells and synthesis and deposition of extracellular matrix. SMCs migrating from the media to the intima lose the capacity to contract, gain the capacity to divide and increase the synthesis of ECM. Consequently, a great deal of attention has been focused on the role of the SMC in the arterial response to injury.

INCREASED RESPONSE OF SMCs TO MITOGENS

A fourth phase in SMC response has been proposed with the observation that proliferating intimal SMCs in a previously injured artery have an increased responsiveness to re-stimulation with mitogens. The factors that determine mediation of this response are poorly understood.

INFLAMMATION

Adhesive interactions between cells within and around the vessel play important roles in orchestrating the inflammatory response. Recruitment of circulating leukocytes to vascular endothelium requires multistep adhesive and signalling events that result in the infiltration of inflammatory cells into the blood vessel wall.[33] Leukocyte recruitment and infiltration occur at sites of vascular injury where the lining endothelial cells have been denuded and platelets and fibrin have been deposited. Experimental observations support a causal relationship between inflammation and experimental restenosis. Antibody-mediated blockade[34] or selective absence of Mac-1[35] reduces leukocyte accumulation and limits neointimal thickening after experimental angioplasty or stent implantation.

Mediators

GROWTH FACTORS

The importance of growth factors to the arterial response to injury cannot be understated.[36,37] One of the most closely studied of these is basic fibroblast growth factor (bFGF). This 18 kDa protein is a member of the heparin-binding growth factor family and is a potent SMC and endothelial cell mitogen. It is located within preformed granules in the quiescent medial SMC and does not contain a secretory domain. Its action, therefore, depends on its release from injured or dead SMCs into the extracellular matrix. At the time of SMC injury, bFGF is released and stimulates the initial phase of SMC proliferation. If antibodies to bFGF are given at the time of injury, the initial wave of SMC proliferation is reduced by 80%, but the final degree of neointimal thickening is not affected.[36] This is due in part to the ongoing production of bFGF in the activated SMCs and to the presence of other mediators that stimulate neointimal thickening.

PDGF is another important regulator of the arterial response to injury. It is a basic dimeric protein with a molecular weight of about 30 kDa, with the two isoforms of the monomers being PDGF-A and PDGF-B. It is present in the α-granules of platelets, primarily as PDGF-AB, and is released during degranulation. PDGF can also be expressed by several other cell types, including endothelium, SMCs[38] and leukocytes. As mentioned before, PDGF does not significantly induce replication among medial SMCs in vivo, but is a potent factor in stimulating their migration to the intima.[39] In vitro, however, it does have some mitogenic effect.

TGF-β is a potent stimulator of SMC collagen production and matrix deposition. In vitro, TGF has anti-proliferative effects on SMCs that vary with the growth rate.[40] In rat carotid injury models, however, antibodies to TGF-β given at the time of injury reduce neointimal formation.[41]

Nitric oxide, a molecule central to the regulation of vascular tone, is also an important regulator of medial SMC activation and neointimal formation after injury. NO has been found to be a potent inhibitor of SMC proliferation and migration.[42] In animal studies, adenoviral gene transfer of nitric oxide synthase (NOS) to injured arteries reduced the subsequent neointimal hyperplasia.[43,44]

HORMONAL FACTORS

The renin–angiotensin system, long known to be important in the pathogenesis of hypertension, has also been found to play a role in the neointimal response.[45] In the classic description of this system, the juxtaglomerular apparatus in the kidney produces renin in response to haemodynamic and electrolyte stimuli. Circulating renin then cleaves angiotensinogen (produced by the liver) to produce angiotensin I, which is physiologically inactive. Circulating angiotensin I is then cleaved to produce angiotensin II by the angiotensin-converting enzyme (ACE), which is expressed on endothelial cells throughout the body, especially in the lungs. Angiotensin II is a potent vasoconstrictor and is the mediator of the neointimal response. This classic description has been expanded by the observation that rennin[46] and angiotensinogen[47] are produced in vascular endothelial cells and SMCs. Thus, with the ACE present, the complete system is contained within the vascular wall. The significance of this tissue renin–angiotensin system is still unclear.

The exact mechanism underlying the effect of angiotensin II on neointimal hyperplasia is not known, but it is believed to stimulate the production of other growth factors, such as PDGF, and mitogens, including the proto-oncogenes c-fos, c-jun and c-myc. Angiotensin II has been shown to be a potent mitogen of SMCs in vitro[48] and in vivo.[45] Additionally, angiotensinogen gene expression is increased in arterial wall after injury, providing a higher concentration of substrate for local ACE.[49]

ACE inhibitors such as captopril and enalapril block the conversion of angiotensin I to angiotensin II. The use of ACE inhibitors has been shown to reduce the amount of neointimal hyperplasia in a dose-dependent fashion in the rat model of arterial injury.[50] This response has also been shown in the rabbit model.[51] In addition, treatment with ACE inhibitors was shown to reduce the biosynthesis of PDGF-AB[52] and bFGF[53] in the arterial wall after injury. These results were promising and led to the study of the effects of ACE inhibitors in higher animals. Unfortunately, experiments using baboons were not able to replicate the beneficial effects seen in rodents.[54] Likewise, clinical trials in humans have failed to show any ability to prevent restenosis,[55] although medication doses for humans were less aggressive than those for the experimental animals.

In addition to blocking the production of angiotensin II, investigators have studied the effects of blocking the angiotensin receptor. Angiotensin II receptors have been classified into two types, angiotensin II type 1 (AT_1) and AT_2. The AT_1 receptor mediates vasoconstriction and is the predominant type on SMCs. It has been shown that neointimal tissue possesses up to four times the number of AT_1 receptors compared to the normal arterial wall, perhaps augmenting the responsiveness of the neointima to angiotensin II stimulation.[56] In the rat model, blockade of the AT receptor was shown to reduce neointima formation after balloon arterial injury. The receptor blockade was also shown to suppress several cell proliferation proto-oncogenes, which likely contributed to the histologic effect.[57,58]

MECHANICAL FACTORS

Changes in haemodynamics within the artery and turbulent pressure/flow patterns can promote restenosis in the arterial wall. These forces can influence the development of a pathologic neointima after arterial injury and play a particularly important role after vein and prosthetic bypass grafting.

Arterial flow within a vein graft causes repetitive stretch injuries that can lead to thickening of the graft wall. Equally, grafts with lower blood velocities, and subsequently lower shear stress, have a more pronounced neointimal response.[59]

Both endothelial cells and SMCs have been shown to respond to changes in shear forces. Changes in the shear force can also affect an existing neointima. Experiments in baboons using PTFE grafts have shown that the thick neointima that forms in a low shear stress graft can be reduced by increasing the flow/shear stress in the graft using an arterial–venous fistula.[60] The loss in neointimal mass appears to result from a reduction in its SMC and extracellular matrix content.

Extracellular matrix

In the injured rat artery, up to 80% of the intimal mass consists of extracellular matrix,[61] which is produced for up to 3 months after injury.[62] The matrix contains elastic microfibrils (elastin, fibrilins), collagens (mainly types I, III, IV, V and VI), matricellular proteins (fibronectin, tenascin and thrombospondin), growth factors and proteases sequestered in matrix and proteoglycans.[63] When the artery enters a phase of remodelling, there is a shift to fewer cellular elements and greater production of matrix. Not only does the matrix provide a scaffold for the SMCs of the neointima, it also helps to facilitate the migration of activated SMCs by interacting with specific integrin receptors expressed by these cells.[64]

In order for the medial SMCs to migrate to the neointima, they must be able to digest the surrounding matrix. Several proteases are activated by arterial injury and are important to neointimal formation. Plasminogen activators[65] and matrix metalloproteinases (MMPs)[66] have been shown to increase after injury in animal models. Both urokinase and tissue type plasminogen activators are stimulated by arterial injury and remain active for about 2 weeks.

The proteolytic enzymes MMP2 and MMP9 have been shown to be important in the SMC migration process after arterial injury.[66] In fact, the use of an MMP inhibitor prevents SMC migration.[67] It has also been shown that knockout mice deficient in the urokinase plasminogen activator show a delayed and reduced neointimal response after arterial injury.[20] In arterial balloon angioplasty, reorganization of the matrix, replacing hydrated molecules by collagen, may lead to shrinkage of the entire artery and negative remodelling. In the stented artery, this phase has less impact because of minimal negative remodelling.

In addition to the structural importance of the matrix, it also functions as a repository for growth factors, especially bFGF. As SMCs die, they release bFGF into the surrounding matrix, where it adheres to the heparin sulphate proteoglycans.[68] As the matrix is degraded by proteases, the bound bFGF is released and can stimulate adjacent SMCs.

Thrombosis

In animal models more complex than the rat, thrombosis appears to play a key role in the restenosis process. This is well established in porcine stent models.[69] Thrombin stimulates SMC proliferation in vitro,[70] and antibodies against the thrombin receptor reduce injury-induced neointimal thickening in vivo.[71]

Recently, 2 MMPs have been discovered to have agonist activity for protease-activated receptor-1, a G protein-coupled receptor that is classically activated through cleavage of the N-terminal exodomain by the serine protease thrombin. The BRILLIANT-EU study examined whether DESs coated with the broad-spectrum MMP inhibitor, batimastat, would prevent in-stent restenosis in patients without affecting re-endothelialization.[72,73] The study, recruiting 550 patients, concluded that batimastat-coated stents were safe but that there was no difference in primary (major adverse cardiac events) or secondary (binary restenosis, subacute thrombosis, angiography) endpoints compared with non-drug-eluting technology.[74]

ATHEROSCLEROSIS AND HUMAN ANGIOPLASTY

The pathophysiology of restenosis in a human atherosclerotic artery is likely to be more complex than the arterial response to injury in animal models. Human atherosclerotic lesions, unlike the uninjured rat carotid artery, are populated with SMCs.[1] In addition, there is some evidence to suggest that smooth muscle replication may not be as important a factor in human restenosis as in experimental models.[75] Since most of the experimental models use initially normal vessels, the process of stenosis that occurs after injury may be very different from that in a stenosed, atherosclerotic artery.

Three mechanisms are known to be responsible for affecting the patency of an artery after balloon angioplasty. The first is elastic recoil of the artery, which occurs shortly after the procedure. Second, there is remodelling of the artery, which results in the change of the total vessel area and the last factor is intimal thickening. The relative contribution of these three processes determines the degree of restenosis that can occur[76] (Figure 13.4). Elastic recoil

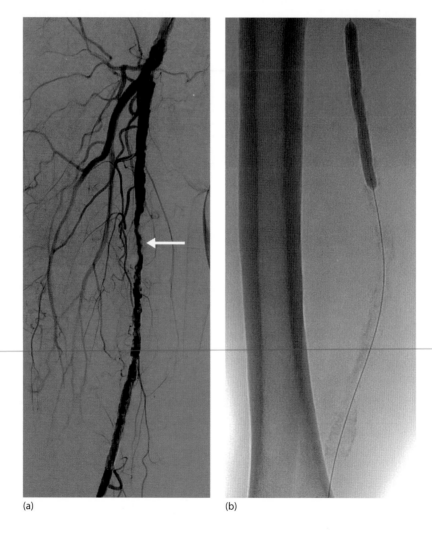

(a)   (b)

Figure 13.4 Lower limb angiogram of a 62-year-old male undergoing percutaneous balloon angioplasty for stenosis (white arrow) of the right superficial femoral artery (SFA). (a) Pre-intervention angiogram; (b) balloon positioning.   (*Continued*)

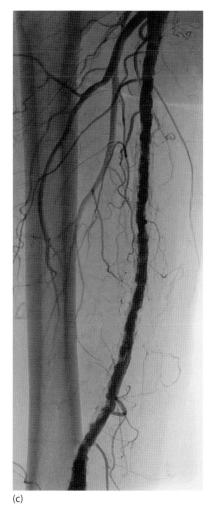
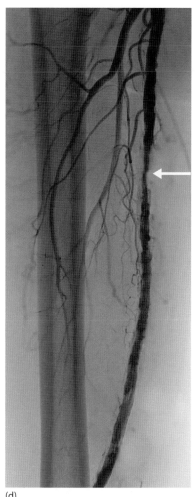

(c)   (d)

Figure 13.4 (*Continued*) Lower limb angiogram of a 62-year-old male undergoing percutaneous balloon angioplasty for stenosis of the right superficial femoral artery (SFA). (c) recanalization of SFA; and (d) restenosis (white arrow) at 9 months.

has become less important with increasing use of stents designed to hold the arterial wall in place. Remodelling and neointimal hyperplasia, however, remain as major areas of interest.

Human vessels can compensate for increased luminal mass by dilation and remodelling.[77] Vessels can maintain constant levels of blood flow until the lesion mass exceeds approximately 40% of the area encompassed by the internal elastic lamina. Indeed, in the hypercholesterolaemic rabbit model, it has been shown that compensatory enlargement occurs after experimental angioplasty, compensating for about 60% of the luminal area lost to neointimal hyperplasia.[78] The mechanisms underlying the remodelling process are not well understood, but possibly include responses to increased flow and wall stress resulting in altered extracellular matrix metabolism.[77] It appears that the endothelium plays a role in the remodelling process, likely regulated by the response to changes in shear stress.[79] In the absence of functional endothelium, or with dysfunctional regenerated endothelium, the compensatory enlargement is prevented.

Chronic inflammation has been found to occur in injured arteries.[80] Increased expression of TGF-β and tissue inhibitors of metalloproteinases may cause an increase in matrix deposition and a decrease in matrix digestion, resulting in the inability to remodel outwardly.

NEOINTIMAL HYPERPLASIA IN VEIN BYPASS GRAFTS

The use of autologous vein for the bypass of arterial lesions is a staple for cardiac and peripheral vascular surgery. One of the main factors contributing to the failure of these grafts is stenosis due to neointimal thickening, which occurs by a process that is similar to that which leads to neointimal hyperplasia after angioplasty. An injury response, modulated by growth factors such as bFGF, PDGF and TGF-β, causes SMC proliferation and matrix deposition. The difference, however, is that the injury response in vein grafts is initially one of healthy adaptation, which in some grafts progresses to a pathologic state.

The insertion of a vein into the high-pressure, high-flow environment of the arterial system subjects it to stresses to which it is unaccustomed and results in the thickening of its wall. This process is driven by the repetitive injury caused by the arterial pressures. Other factors also contribute to graft injury early on, including rough handling during harvest, hypotonic irrigation fluids and overzealous distention during testing and preparation of the graft.[81]

The thickening of the vein wall serves to reduce the tangential stress applied to it by arterial pressures. According to LaPlace's law, the tangential stress (τ) in the wall of a sphere is proportional to the pressure (P) and the radius (r) and inversely proportional to the wall thickness (δ):

$$\tau = Pr/\delta$$

Thus, by increasing the wall thickness the stress in the wall is reduced. In an experimental rabbit model, reducing the stress exerted on a vein graft by placing a rigid cuff around the graft was shown to decrease the intimal thickening.[82]

The shear stress (s), exerted longitudinally on the vessel wall, is a function of the blood flow (Q), vessel radius (r) and blood viscosity (η). Assuming laminar flow

$$S = 4\eta Q/\pi r^3$$

With the high flow rate of the arterial system, the shear stress is increased in vein grafts and is important in the regulation of neointimal hyperplasia. It is well known that high-flow grafts develop less intimal thickening than low-flow systems.[83] One hypothesis for this phenomenon is that in high-flow systems, it is more difficult for circulating cells to adhere to the vessel wall. Adherent platelets and leukocytes secrete growth factors that can stimulate SMC proliferation and matrix deposition. It has also been shown that increased shear stress induces endothelial cells to produce nitric oxide,[84] a potent inhibitor of SMC proliferation. Shear stress is probably more important in the development of neointimal thickening in prosthetic grafts, as described later.

The kinetics of the adaptation of a vein graft to the arterial environment has been studied in the rabbit model.[85] Early events include platelet aggregation and microthrombi at areas of endothelial denudation around the anastomoses. By 2 weeks, the denuded areas have been re-endothelialized and the vein wall starts to thicken. For the first 4 weeks, proliferating SMCs provide the bulk of the neointima, followed by the progressive deposition of ECM. This process reaches a maximum at 12 weeks, by which time the ratio of wall thickness to vessel diameter is the same in the vein graft as in the artery. At this point, the wall tension in the vein graft is equal to that of the artery.

Unlike neointimal hyperplasia that occurs after the angioplasty of an atherosclerotic lesion, the SMC proliferation that occurs in the vein graft takes place under an intact endothelium. Clearly, the normally anti-proliferative influences of the endothelium seen in the arterial system are not present in the vein graft. It has been shown that vein graft endothelium produces less nitric oxide,[86] a potent SMC proliferation inhibitor. Restoration of nitric oxide to the vein graft reduces neointimal hyperplasia.[87,88]

Stenoses are frequently seen at the anastomoses of vein grafts. The turbulent flow and compliance mismatch between the vein and artery produce additional stresses that cause local endothelial disruption and persistent intimal proliferation.[83,89] In fact, the geometry of the anastomosis may contribute to the development of neointimal hyperplasia. Biomechanical analyses have shown that the suture line stress generated by compliance mismatch is greater in end-to-side anastomoses compared to end-to-end.[90] It has also been shown that the shear stress at an anastomosis is dependent on the angle of the anastomosis, with larger angles producing more shear stress.[91,92]

NEOINTIMAL HYPERPLASIA IN PROSTHETIC BYPASS GRAFTS

Prosthetic grafts are used frequently for the replacement of larger arteries and when autogenous vein is not available for arterial reconstruction. Prosthetic grafts are affected by neointimal hyperplasia and, particularly in the peripheral circulation, have a lower patency rate than their autogenous counterpart.

Work in animal models has shown that porous grafts, such as ePTFE, become lined with a neointima composed of SMCs and endothelial cells which populate the graft from capillary ingrowth through the pores of the graft.[93] Endothelialization is complete by 3 weeks, but the SMCs continue to proliferate and deposit matrix for several months.[94,95] The neointima in the prosthetic graft is metabolically active and produces several growth factors that stimulate SMC proliferation,[96,97] including PDGF[98] and TGF-β.[97]

As in vein grafts, the stresses induced by the arterial system play a central role in the development of prosthetic graft neointimal thickening. Unlike vein grafts, however, the prosthetic grafts are rigid and can support the tangential stress easily. The neointima responds primarily to the shear stress caused by the flowing arterial blood. This has been studied extensively in baboon models, where high-flow grafts were found to have less neointimal hyperplasia than normal-flow grafts.[99] It has also been shown that exposing a graft with a mature neointima to high-flow conditions (by creating a distal arteriovenous fistula) can cause the regression of the neointima.[60] Closure of the AV fistula results in an increase in neointimal thickness. As in vein grafts, it has been postulated that shear stress induces the production of nitric oxide, which inhibits SMCs proliferation. Indeed, NOS was shown to be induced in the neointima of high-flow grafts.[60]

Compliance mismatch between graft and artery is a greater concern when a stiff prosthetic graft is used. A Dacron graft in the end-to-side configuration has been shown to have a 40% greater suture line strain than an autologous graft.[90] The geometry of the anastomosis also plays an important role. In the end-to-end position, the Dacron graft was associated with only a 5% increase in suture line stress compared to an arterial graft.[90]

The combination of decreased flow velocities (and thus shear force) and increased suture line stress of prosthetic grafts likely contributes to the poor performance of below-knee prosthetic bypass grafts compared to autologous vein grafts. A great deal of effort is being directed towards finding ways to increase the long-term patency of these grafts for patients without adequate autologous conduit.

RESTENOSIS AFTER ENDARTERECTOMY

Since its introduction by Dos Santos[100] in 1947, the technique of endarterectomy has been an important part of vascular surgery. A natural cleavage plane tends to develop in the outer region of the media in older, atherosclerotic arteries. The careful dissection of this cleavage plane allows for the removal of the diseased intima and inner media. The result is a relatively clean surface comprised of SMCs and extracellular matrix.

Endarterectomy has been used in almost every part of the vascular system with variable success. The limiting factor is generally restenosis due to neointimal hyperplasia. Results for long-term patency of endarterectomized arteries vary by location, with more proximal arteries having better results. The carotid artery system is a special case.

Recurrent restenosis to greater than 50% of luminal diameter develops in 16%–22% of patients.[9] It generally develops within the first year and becomes stable thereafter; about 10% of lesions will eventually regress.[9] These lesions are quite different from the atherosclerotic lesions seen in primary operations. The neointima is smooth and white and rarely ulcerates. In addition, they do not frequently produce symptoms, with only 3%–4% of patients suffering recurrent transient ischaemic events or strokes.[9] Recurrent atherosclerotic stenosis usually takes many years to develop, making control of atherosclerosis risk factors critically important.

The aetiology of neointimal hyperplasia after endarterectomy is similar to that seen in other forms of arterial injury. SMCs become activated, proliferate and produce extracellular matrix. The basic mechanisms have not been as clearly defined as in the angioplasty model, but strong parallels are evident. The endothelium is removed by the procedure, and the loss of the endothelial inhibition on SMCs likely contributes to the process. The endarterectomized artery is quite thrombogenic, and the exposed media provides a rich scaffold for platelet adhesion and activation. Growth factors are also important in the development of the neointima. Infusing bFGF locally to endarterectomized carotid arteries in a canine model has been shown to increase the degree of neointimal thickening by 72% and increase the SMC proliferation rate by 73%.[101] The inflammatory response likely also plays a role. Administration of an antibody to block very late antigen-4, which is important to monocyte adhesion and migration, has been shown to reduce neointimal hyperplasia in a primate carotid endarterectomy model.[102] Mechanical stresses have also been implicated in the development of neointimal hyperplasia. Patients who were found to have residual flow disturbances by duplex scanning after carotid endarterectomy were found to have a 22% incidence restenosis compared to 9% in patients without residual flow defects.[103]

Preventive strategies

As the understanding of the mechanisms of restenosis has increased, efforts are being concentrated on attempts to counteract the process. Methods being studied include pharmacological intervention, different mechanisms for drug delivery and newer biological agent strategies such as gene therapy and endovascular irradiation.

HEPARIN

Heparin is well known to reduce the amount of neointimal hyperplasia in animals.[104] Thrombosis is an important event in the development of restenosis in humans and larger animal models, but not rat models. Although heparin is a potent anticoagulant, its ability to reduce neointimal hyperplasia is not entirely due to its anticoagulant properties.

Potential mechanisms, clearly independent of its anticoagulant activity, include direct inhibition of the first phase of SMC activation, i.e. proliferation and the start of SMC migration to the intima. If heparin therapy is initiated more than 4 days after the experimental injury, there is no effect on neointimal hyperplasia. The inhibition of SMC activation is due, at least partly, to the ability of heparin to bind a range of growth factors, collectively called the heparin-binding growth factors. The most important of these growth factors is bFGF, which has already been shown to be a key regulator of early SMC activation. This ability of heparin to bind certain growth factors is not related to its antithrombotic effects. In fact, several heparin analogues have been developed which also bind growth factors avidly,[105] yet have no antithrombotic effects. These compounds have also been shown to reduce neointimal hyperplasia.[106] Heparin also has been shown to prevent SMC activation by other pathways, such as inhibition of mitogen-activated protein kinase activation,[107] which is important in cell proliferation and migration as well as its response to thrombin and angiotensin II stimulation.

The usefulness of heparin in reducing restenosis in humans remains unproven.[108] The anticoagulant effects of heparin limit the dosage and duration of therapy that can be used in human trials; bleeding is a significant concern.

The doses of heparin and length of therapy that successfully reduce neointimal hyperplasia in animal models are generally not safe to use in humans. Technological modifications, which include coating the graft fabric with heparin thereby allowing localized delivery, may offer some improvement in patency and outcomes; however, definitive data are still pending.[109]

Low molecular weight heparin (LMWH) has also been used to try to prevent neointimal hyperplasia. Because of easier dosing and administration and a lower risk of severe bleeding complications compared to unfractionated heparin, LMWH is preferred to unfractionated heparin in clinical practice and would be a better choice in human trials. Indeed, studies have shown a reduction in neointimal hyperplasia in rabbits treated with LMWH.[110] Unfortunately, human trials have not been able to match these results, even when therapy is started before treatment and continued for several weeks afterwards.[111–113] However, some trials suggest that the effectiveness of LMWH on graft patency is related to the severity of peripheral arterial disease; higher rates of long-term patency following femoropopliteal bypass grafting are reported in patients with critical limb ischaemia.[114,115] The biological explanation for this is unclear.

ANGIOTENSIN-CONVERTING ENZYME INHIBITORS

The success of ACE inhibitors in the prevention of neointimal hyperplasia in animal models spurred the organization of several large clinical trials of human restenosis. Follow-up studies in these models showed that the favourable effects of ACE inhibition could be attributed, in part, to the bradykinin/endothelial NO synthase pathway and/or oxidative stress/NAD(P)H pathway.[116]

However, in large clinical trials, low antihypertensive doses of cilazapril did not prevent restenosis nor had favourable effects on overall clinical outcome after percutaneous transluminal coronary angioplasty (PTCA).[9,117] Several explanations for the inability of ACE inhibitors to prevent restenosis have been postulated. One difference is that the doses used to treat experimental animals greatly exceed the doses used to treat hypertension in humans. In addition, several other vasoactive peptides are inactivated by ACE, including bradykinin and the enkephalins.[118] Bradykinin is a potent vasodilator and stimulator of constitutive NOS. The prevention of bradykinin degradation by ACE inhibitors may contribute to the effect on neointimal hyperplasia.[119] Differences between human and rodent metabolism of bradykinin may contribute to the different outcomes of ACE inhibitor treatment.

In conclusion, ACE inhibition is not effective in reducing restenosis in patients after PTCA and the results of clinical trials do not advocate its use in these patients. However, this does not exclude the important role of angiotensin II in the development of restenosis. Experimental studies have shown that the AT1 receptor and downstream pathways are involved in neointima formation; moreover, selective angiotensin receptor blockade may be effective in preventing restenosis in patients with complex lesions.[120]

In the Val-PREST trial, it was shown that restenosis was only 19% in valsartan-treated patients, compared with 39% in the control group.[121]

LIPID-LOWERING AGENTS

Lipids play a central role in atherogenesis and are important in the development of restenosis after angioplasty. Patients who have low high-density lipoprotein levels have been shown to have a higher risk for restenosis.[122] Lovastatin, an HMG–CoA reductase inhibitor, has been shown to reduce neointimal hyperplasia in both normocholesterolaemic[123] and hypercholesterolaemic[62] rabbit arterial injury models, suggesting other cholesterol-independent effects of lipid-lowering agents. In the same animal models, simvastatin decreases in-stent restenosis and neointimal thickness. Although the exact mechanism remains unclear, this may be achieved by downregulation of pathways promoting vascular SMC proliferation and migration.[124] These findings from pre-clinical models have stimulated the development of statin-coated stents (discussed later) as a potential option for reducing restenosis. In humans, however, the results have been less than impressive in clinical trials with lovastatin,[125] luvastatin[126] and pravastatin.[127]

PHOTODYNAMIC THERAPY

Photodynamic therapy (PDT) has been used for many years in experimental cancer therapy. It involves the administration of a non-toxic photosensitizing dye, which is taken up preferentially by proliferating cells. The area of interest is then exposed to a specific wavelength and intensity of laser light, which causes the dye to produce highly reactive oxygen radicals. These radicals denature cellular proteins and lipids, resulting in cell death.

The preferential uptake of the photosensitizers by proliferating cells spurred interest in its ability to prevent neointimal hyperplasia. It has been shown that intimal hyperplastic tissue accumulates photosensitizing dye more avidly than normal arterial tissue and retains it longer.[128] PDT has been shown to prevent neointimal hyperplasia in rat[129] and rabbit[130] models of arterial injury. Histologically, the treated artery is found to contain an acellular media with little signs of inflammation. The endothelium was shown to regenerate by 4 weeks in the rat model, but the media remained barren.[128] The anti-intimal hyperplastic effects of PDT have been reported to last up to 25 weeks[131]; however, longer-term effects of this phenotype remain unclear.

A great deal of research still needs to be done before PDT can be applied to human restenosis, but the early results of endovascular lasers in treating in-stent restenosis demonstrate favourable outcomes. Early clinical trials of excimer laser arthrectomy combined with percutaneous transluminal angioplasty (PTA) versus PTA alone in the treatment of infra-inguinal in-stent restenosis support the safety of laser arthrectomy combined with PTA and demonstrate superiority at 6 months, particularly in treating longer segments of restenosis.[132] Based on these results, the US Food and Drug Administration (FDA) has recently approved a labelling indication for excimer laser devices in the treatment of infra-inguinal in-stent restenosis. However, the Inter-Society Consensus for the Management of Peripheral Arterial Disease (TASC II) does not routinely recommend the use of laser therapy until the results from larger, well-controlled registries are available.[133]

GENE THERAPY

Vascular gene therapy can potentially control cellular growth-related restenosis by modifying gene expression. Viral or plasmid technology can be used to overexpress endogenous cell cycle inhibitory proteins or novel cell cycle inhibitory proteins. It has been shown that transduction of cells with a gene encoding for a nonphosphorylatable, constitutively active form of the pRb gene product significantly inhibited neointimal hyperplasia.[134] Additionally, expression of cell cycle inhibitors, such as p21 and p27 by an adenoviral technology or p53 by a naked plasmid vector, significantly reduced neointimal hyperplasia in several animal models.[135–137] Inhibiting cell proliferation and migration by arresting vascular SMCs in the G0/G1 phase of the cell cycle has also been a common approach using cell cycle regulatory proteins, particularly the E2F transcription factor.[138]

Many pre-clinical studies have been performed and aimed at targeting the aforementioned mechanisms, using several different vector approaches in multiple diverse animal models. Only a few however have progressed to clinical trials. In the first trial (PREVENT I), ex vivo delivery of E2F decoy to grafts demonstrated fewer graft stenosis at 12 months. In the PREVENT II trial, involving 200 patients undergoing CABG, the same dose of E2F transcription factor was tested versus control, again demonstrating favourable effects on graft remodelling. Unfortunately, PREVENT III results showed no difference between E2F and placebo on vein graft restenosis.[139] Potential reasons for the lack of efficacy include the possibility that the dose of E2F decoy was too low or duration of exposure of the vascular graft too short to allow efficient transfection. As well as investigating optimal doses required, finding the optimal method of delivery to target tissue remains a future challenge. Vein grafts can be accessed ex vivo allowing incubation with a chosen vector; however, for endovascular interventions, this remains more difficult. Intuitively, 'gene-eluting' stents may serve as an alternative vector in future.

RADIATION

Radiation therapy is used extensively to kill proliferating cancer cells. Cellular proliferation is also important in the development of neointimal hyperplasia, prompting investigators to study use of locally delivered radiation for preventing restenosis.

Several animal models have been used to study the effects of radiation on neointimal hyperplasia. In a porcine balloon injury model, the use of intravascular beta irradiation (14–56 Gy) was shown to inhibit neointimal

thickening in a dose-dependent manner.[140] Similarly, in a rat carotid injury model of intravascular ^{192}Ir radiation, doses as low as 5 Gy were found to significantly inhibit neointimal hyperplasia.[141]

Due to the success in animal models, several clinical trials have been organized to see if radiation therapy can reduce neointimal hyperplasia in humans. The Scripps Coronary Radiation to Inhibit Proliferation Post Stenting trial[142] used a gamma-emitting ^{192}Ir ribbon compared to placebo in 55 patients undergoing angioplasty and stenting. At 6 months, the mean stenosis in the radiated group was 17% compared to 37% in controls. Additionally, only 11.5% of patients in the treated group required revascularization of the target lesion by 12 months, compared to 44.8% of patients in the control group. A 2-year follow-up of these patients showed that the reduced need for revascularization of the target lesion remained reduced in the radiated group (15.4%) compared to controls (44.8%).[142]

The results of radiation therapy for prevention of restenosis are promising; however, when compared to DESs, the TAXUS V ISR and SISR trials demonstrated significantly better outcomes for in-stent restenosis with DESs compared to intracoronary radiation.[143,144] Use of radiation therapy for the treatment of in-stent restenosis has therefore fallen out of favour. There is also some concern regarding the long-term effects of irradiating arteries. Radiation exposure to arteries as a consequence of treating cancers causes several pathologic changes including aneurysm formation, occlusion, intimal/medial fibrosis, occlusion of the vasa vasora, plaque formation and peri-arterial fibrosis causing extrinsic arterial constriction.

IN SITU DRUG DELIVERY METHODS

Contemporary catheter-based technologies have been developed that aim to deliver preventive agents to the treated arterial segment. These include DES and DEB devices, bioresorbable stents and more recently nanoparticle-based delivery solutions.

These solutions capitalize on the central role that cell proliferation has in the development of neointimal hyperplasia, delivering high concentrations of immunosuppressive or anti-tumour agents into the vessel wall.

The first generation of DES was approved by the FDA in 2003 for use in the coronary circulation and is now in routine use. These stents are coated with sirolimus, an immunosuppressant drug that directly inhibits the mTOR/70 pathway which regulates vascular SMC differentiation.[145] It has been shown to reduce neointimal thickening leading to coronary restenosis in clinical trials comparing it to both bare metal stent and polymer-coated stent.[3]

The aforementioned technology has more recently been evaluated in the peripheral circulation. The SIROCCO trials were randomized, double-blinded studies designed to assess the efficacy of the sirolimus-eluting SMART stent (Cordis Corporation) with its BMS counterpart for the treatment of long superficial femoral artery (SFA) lesions.[146] The STRIDES trial (Abbott Vascular) utilized a novel everolimus-DES designed with a higher drug load (225 µg/cm²) and longer elution profile (80% elution over 90 days) for the treatment of SFA and popliteal lesions.[147] This is compared to approximately 140 µg/cm² sirolimus dose released over 30 days in coronary DES. In both of these trials, however, there were similar long-term restenosis rates between the drug eluting and BMS suggesting that either the elution kinetics, drug type or concentrations used were ineffective.

The Zilver PTX stent (Cook Medical), however, has demonstrated more favourable outcomes in a multi-centre, randomized trial assessing patency of short SFA lesions after treatment. The Zilver PTX stent is coated on its outer surface with paclitaxel, a highly lipophilic drug that alters microtubule formation and inhibits SMC migration and proliferation.[148] Paclitaxel has a narrow therapeutic range and, at higher concentrations, can disrupt the internal elastic lamina.[149] The primary patency at 12, 24 and 48 months was significantly better in the Zilver PTX group compared with just balloon angioplasty or bare metal stent.[150–152] Some criticisms of the trial were that the lesions treated were relatively short and not typical of those seen in clinical practice. However, subsequent registry data from diabetic patients with longer, more complex lesions also demonstrated higher primary patency rates following Zilver PTX stent implantation.[153] Currently, the Zilver PTX is the only FDA-approved DES for use in infra-inguinal arterial disease.

The patterns of in-stent restenosis with DES appear to be specific for each type of device. Restenosis after sirolimus-eluting stents is mostly focal and usually located at the stent edges,[154] whereas diffuse intimal proliferation or total occlusion accounts for ~50% of the restenosis cases after paclitaxel-eluting stent implantation.[155]

The ability to deliver drugs locally using a coated angioplasty balloon is an attractive option, particularly as part of re-intervention for restenosis where the placement of a second stent can limit luminal gain and create an unfavourable haemodynamics. Initial feasibility of pacli-taxel-coated balloon catheters has been promising,[156] and a meta-analysis of randomized trials comparing drug-eluting versus standard balloons demonstrates superiority of DEB for late lumen loss, restenosis and target lesion revascularization.[157]

DES and DEB technologies are also being extended to treat infrapopliteal arterial disease, which remains challenging due to the longer length of lesions and small-diameter vessels in this region. There is now strong evidence from four randomized trials[158–160] demonstrating the significant benefit of paclitaxel and sirolimus-eluting stents over both BMS and PTA for primary patency and re-intervention for restenosis, supporting their use as a primary option in anatomically suitable infrapopliteal lesions.[133] The clinical data available on below-knee applications of DEB are currently limited. It is therefore too early to

recommend their use in infrapopliteal lesions, particularly given the superior comparative results of the DES.

Bioresorbable stent devices are another promising development since they can provide temporary architectural support for the vessel wall and can be engineered to elute drugs. Their potential advantages include (1) avoidance of a permanent foreign body, which may diminish the inflammatory response of the arterial wall to stent implantation, and (2) temporary rigidity of the arterial wall, allowing the vessel to revert to normal physiological vasomotor tone.[161] Clinical evaluation of these latest DES platforms is currently under way in the coronary circulation. The ABSORB I trial (Abbott Vascular), which evaluated an everolimus-eluting bioresorbable stent in a small cohort with single de novo coronary lesions, found that the stents had completely resorbed at 2 years with no restenosis.[162] However, interim 12-month results of the larger ABSORB II trial comparing the Absorb stent to the Xience Prime everolimus-DES demonstrate a smaller lumen gain in the Absorb stent cohort.[163] Longer-term results are needed to verify that this technology is indeed an advance over DES and DEB. Their feasibility and initial evaluation have also been tested in the peripheral circulation. Although immediate angiographic results are comparable to those of metal stents, the restenosis rate at 12 months was high (68%).[164] Modifications to stent characteristics with the goal to reduce the restenosis rate during the reabsorption period are yet to be achieved.

FUTURE DIRECTIONS

Much has been learnt about the biology of the vessel wall, but restenosis and neointimal hyperplasia remain a significant clinical problem. Development of agents that directly target cellular and molecular pathways involved in this phenomenon has been a major advance. Drug-eluting balloons and stents are a particularly promising area, but their full potential can only be assessed by large, well-designed clinical trials.

As well as improving device characteristics, there is also a need to develop platforms that sustain a local delivery of high concentrations of the drug of choice whilst avoiding systemic effects. New methods of targeted drug delivery using nanoparticles binding to specific proteins within the injured arterial wall are currently being evaluated in animals. The site-specific delivery of substances using nanoparticles could provide a safe and effective treatment of restenosis that does not require a direct intra- or extraluminal intervention.[165]

These new techniques not only provide potential treatments for neointimal hyperplasia but allow important insights into the genetic and molecular control of this complex pathologic process. The multifaceted nature of the arterial response to injury may require a combination of several strategies for successful control of neointimal hyperplasia.

REFERENCES

1. Schwartz SM, deBlois D, O'Brien ER. The intima: Soil for atherosclerosis and restenosis. *Circ Res.* 1995;77:445–465.

2. Cutlip DE, Chauhan MS, Baim DS, Ho KK, Popma JJ, Carrozza JP, Cohen DJ, Kuntz RE. Clinical restenosis after coronary stenting: Perspectives from multicenter clinical trials. *J Am Coll Cardiol.* 2002;40:2082–2089.

3. Moses JW, Leon MB, Popma JJ et al. Sirolimus-eluting stents versus standard stents in patients with stenosis in a native coronary artery. *N Engl J Med.* 2003;349:1315–1323.

4. Stone GW, Ellis SG, Cox DA et al. A polymer-based, paclitaxel-eluting stent in patients with coronary artery disease. *N Engl J Med.* 2004;350:221–231.

5. Ip JH, Fuster V, Badimon L, Badimon J, Taubman MB, Chesebro JH. Syndromes of accelerated atherosclerosis: Role of vascular injury and smooth muscle cell proliferation. *J Am Coll Cardiol.* 1990;15:1667–1687.

6. Lawrie GM, Lie JT, Morris GC Jr., Beazley HL. Vein graft patency and intimal proliferation after aortocoronary bypass: Early and long-term angiopathologic correlations. *Am J Cardiol.* 1976;38:856–862.

7. Whittemore AD, Donaldson MC, Polak JF, Mannick JA. Limitations of balloon angioplasty for vein graft stenosis. *J Vasc Surg.* 1991;14:340–345.

8. Taylor LM Jr., Edwards JM, Porter JM. Present status of reversed vein bypass grafting: Five-year results of a modern series. *J Vasc Surg.* 1990;11:193–205; discussion 205–206.

9. Healy DA, Zierler RE, Nicholls SC, Clowes AW, Primozich JF, Bergelin RO, Strandness DE Jr. Long-term follow-up and clinical outcome of carotid restenosis. *J Vasc Surg.* 1989;10:662–668; discussion 668–669.

10. Stary HC, Blankenhorn DH, Chandler AB et al. A definition of the intima of human arteries and of its atherosclerosis-prone regions: A report from the committee on vascular lesions of the council on arteriosclerosis, american heart association. *Circulation.* 1992;85:391–405.

11. Gittenberger-de Groot AC, van Ertbruggen I, Moulaert AJ, Harinck E. The ductus arteriosus in the preterm infant: Histologic and clinical observations. *J Pediatr.* 1980;96:88–93.

12. Ferns GA, Avades TY. The mechanisms of coronary restenosis: Insights from experimental models. *Int J Exp Pathol.* 2000;81:63–88.

13. Reidy MA, Clowes AW, Schwartz SM. Endothelial regeneration. V. Inhibition of endothelial regrowth in arteries of rat and rabbit. *Lab Invest.* 1983;49:569–575.

14. Clowes AW, Reidy MA, Clowes MM. Kinetics of cellular proliferation after arterial injury. I. Smooth muscle growth in the absence of endothelium. *Lab Invest.* 1983;49:327–333.

15. Richardson M, Kinlough-Rathbone RL, Groves HM, Jorgensen L, Mustard JF, Moore S. Ultrastructural changes in re-endothelialized and non-endothelialized rabbit aortic neo-intima following re-injury with a balloon catheter. *Br J Exp Pathol.* 1984;65:597–611.

16. Schwartz SM, Reidy MA, de Blois D. Factors important in arterial narrowing. *J Hypertens Suppl.* 1996;14:S71–S81.

17. Clowes AW, Reidy MA, Clowes MM. Mechanisms of stenosis after arterial injury. *Lab Invest.* 1983;49:208–215.

18. Allayee H, Ghazalpour A, Lusis AJ. Using mice to dissect genetic factors in atherosclerosis. *Arterioscler Thromb Vasc Biol.* 2003;23:1501–1509.

19. Wang X, Chai H, Lin PH, Lumsden AB, Yao Q, Chen C. Mouse models of neointimal hyperplasia: Techniques and applications. *Med Sci Monit.* 2006;12:RA177–RA185.

20. Carmeliet P, Moons L, Stassen JM, De Mol M, Bouche A, van den Oord JJ, Kockx M, Collen D. Vascular wound healing and neointima formation induced by perivascular electric injury in mice. *Am J Pathol.* 1997;150:761–776.

21. Castellot JJ Jr., Addonizio ML, Rosenberg R, Karnovsky MJ. Cultured endothelial cells produce a heparinlike inhibitor of smooth muscle cell growth. *J Cell Biol.* 1981;90:372–379.

22. Edelman ER, Nugent MA, Karnovsky MJ. Perivascular and intravenous administration of basic fibroblast growth factor: Vascular and solid organ deposition. *Proc Natl Acad Sci USA.* 1993;90:1513–1517.

23. Lindner V, Reidy MA, Fingerle J. Regrowth of arterial endothelium. Denudation with minimal trauma leads to complete endothelial cell regrowth. *Lab Invest.* 1989;61:556–563.

24. Weidinger FF, McLenachan JM, Cybulsky MI, Gordon JB, Rennke HG, Hollenberg NK, Fallon JT, Ganz P, Cooke JP. Persistent dysfunction of regenerated endothelium after balloon angioplasty of rabbit iliac artery. *Circulation.* 1990;81:1667–1679.

25. Saroyan RM, Roberts MP, Light JT Jr. et al. Differential recovery of prostacyclin and endothelium-derived relaxing factor after vascular injury. *Am J Physiol.* 1992;262:H1449–H1457.

26. van Beusekom HM, Whelan DM, Hofma SH, Krabbendam SC, van Hinsbergh VW, Verdouw PD, van der Giessen WJ. Long-term endothelial dysfunction is more pronounced after stenting than after balloon angioplasty in porcine coronary arteries. *J Am Coll Cardiol.* 1998;32:1109–1117.

27. Drachman DE, Edelman ER, Seifert P, Groothuis AR, Bornstein DA, Kamath KR, Palasis M, Yang D, Nott SH, Rogers C. Neointimal thickening after stent delivery of paclitaxel: Change in composition and arrest of growth over six months. *J Am Coll Cardiol.* 2000;36:2325–2332.

28. Guagliumi G, Farb A, Musumeci G, Valsecchi O, Tespili M, Motta T, Virmani R. Images in cardiovascular medicine. Sirolimus-eluting stent implanted in human coronary artery for 16 months: Pathological findings. *Circulation*. 2003;107:1340–1341.

29. Jeremias A, Sylvia B, Bridges J et al. Stent thrombosis after successful sirolimus-eluting stent implantation. *Circulation*. 2004;109:1930–1932.

30. Ruggeri ZM. Platelets in atherothrombosis. *Nat Med*. 2002;8:1227–1234.

31. Bauters C, de Groote P, Adamantidis M, Delcayre C, Hamon M, Lablanche JM, Bertrand ME, Dupuis B, Swynghedauw B. Proto-oncogene expression in rabbit aorta after wall injury: First marker of the cellular process leading to restenosis after angioplasty? *Eur Heart J*. 1992;13:556–559.

32. Bennett MR, Anglin S, McEwan JR, Jagoe R, Newby AC, Evan GI. Inhibition of vascular smooth muscle cell proliferation in vitro and in vivo by c-myc antisense oligodeoxynucleotides. *J Clin Invest*. 1994;93:820–828.

33. Springer TA. Traffic signals for lymphocyte recirculation and leukocyte emigration: The multistep paradigm. *Cell*. 1994;76:301–314.

34. Rogers C, Edelman ER, Simon DI. A mab to the beta2-leukocyte integrin mac-1 (cd11b/cd18) reduces intimal thickening after angioplasty or stent implantation in rabbits. *Proc Natl Acad Sci USA*. 1998;95:10134–10139.

35. Simon DI, Dhen Z, Seifert P, Edelman ER, Ballantyne CM, Rogers C. Decreased neointimal formation in Mac-1(−/−) mice reveals a role for inflammation in vascular repair after angioplasty. *J Clin Invest*. 2000;105:293–300.

36. Lindner V, Reidy MA. Proliferation of smooth muscle cells after vascular injury is inhibited by an antibody against basic fibroblast growth factor. *Proc Natl Acad Sci USA*. 1991;88:3739–3743.

37. Olson NE, Chao S, Lindner V, Reidy MA. Intimal smooth muscle cell proliferation after balloon catheter injury. The role of basic fibroblast growth factor. *Am J Pathol*. 1992;140:1017–1023.

38. Lindner V, Giachelli CM, Schwartz SM, Reidy MA. A subpopulation of smooth muscle cells in injured rat arteries expresses platelet-derived growth factor-b chain mrna. *Circ Res*. 1995;76:951–957.

39. Jawien A, Bowen-Pope DF, Lindner V, Schwartz SM, Clowes AW. Platelet-derived growth factor promotes smooth muscle migration and intimal thickening in a rat model of balloon angioplasty. *J Clin Invest*. 1992;89:507–511.

40. Halloran BG, Prorok GD, So BJ, Baxter BT. Transforming growth factor-beta 1 inhibits human arterial smooth-muscle cell proliferation in a growth-rate-dependent manner. *Am J Surg*. 1995;170:193–197.

41. Wolf YG, Rasmussen LM, Ruoslahti E. Antibodies against transforming growth factor-beta 1 suppress intimal hyperplasia in a rat model. *J Clin Invest*. 1994;93:1172–1178.

42. Sarkar R, Meinberg EG, Stanley JC, Gordon D, Webb RC. Nitric oxide reversibly inhibits the migration of cultured vascular smooth muscle cells. *Circ Res*. 1996;78:225–230.

43. Janssens S, Flaherty D, Nong Z, Varenne O, van Pelt N, Haustermans C, Zoldhelyi P, Gerard R, Collen D. Human endothelial nitric oxide synthase gene transfer inhibits vascular smooth muscle cell proliferation and neointima formation after balloon injury in rats. *Circulation*. 1998;97:1274–1281.

44. Varenne O, Pislaru S, Gillijns H, Van Pelt N, Gerard RD, Zoldhelyi P, Van de Werf F, Collen D, Janssens SP. Local adenovirus-mediated transfer of human endothelial nitric oxide synthase reduces luminal narrowing after coronary angioplasty in pigs. *Circulation*. 1998;98:919–926.

45. Daemen MJ, Lombardi DM, Bosman FT, Schwartz SM. Angiotensin II induces smooth muscle cell proliferation in the normal and injured rat arterial wall. *Circ Res*. 1991;68:450–456.

46. Re R, Fallon JT, Dzau V, Ouay SC, Haber E. Renin synthesis by canine aortic smooth muscle cells in culture. *Life Sci*. 1982;30:99–106.

47. Campbell DJ, Habener JF. Angiotensinogen gene is expressed and differentially regulated in multiple tissues of the rat. *J Clin Invest*. 1986;78:31–39.

48. Campbell-Boswell M, Robertson AL Jr. Effects of angiotensin II and vasopressin on human smooth muscle cells in vitro. *Exp Mol Pathol*. 1981;35:265–276.

49. Rakugi H, Jacob HJ, Krieger JE, Ingelfinger JR, Pratt RE. Vascular injury induces angiotensinogen gene expression in the media and neointima. *Circulation*. 1993;87:283–290.

50. Petrik PV, Law MM, Moore WS, Colburn MD, Quinones-Baldrich W, Gelabert HA. Pharmacologic suppression of intimal hyperplasia: A dose-response suppression by enalapril. *Am Surg*. 1995;61:851–855.

51. Law MM, Colburn MD, Hajjar GE, Gelabert HA, Quinones-Baldrich WJ, Moore WS. Suppression of intimal hyperplasia in a rabbit model of arterial balloon injury by enalaprilat but not dimethyl sulfoxide. *Ann Vasc Surg*. 1994;8:158–165.

52. Wong J, Rauhoft C, Dilley RJ, Agrotis A, Jennings GL, Bobik A. Angiotensin-converting enzyme inhibition abolishes medial smooth muscle PDGF-AB biosynthesis and attenuates cell proliferation in injured carotid arteries: Relationships to neointima formation. *Circulation*. 1997;96:1631–1640.

53. Iwata A, Masago A, Yamada K. Angiotensin-converting enzyme inhibitor cilazapril suppresses expression of basic fibroblast growth factor messenger ribonucleic acid and protein in endothelial and intimal smooth muscle cells in a vascular injury model of spontaneous hypertensive rats. *Neurol Med Chir*. 1998;38:257–264; discussion 264–265.

54. Hanson SR, Powell JS, Dodson T, Lumsden A, Kelly AB, Anderson JS, Clowes AW, Harker LA. Effects of angiotensin converting enzyme inhibition with cilazapril on intimal hyperplasia in injured arteries and vascular grafts in the baboon. *Hypertension.* 1991;18:II70–II76.

55. Does the new angiotensin converting enzyme inhibitor cilazapril prevent restenosis after percutaneous transluminal coronary angioplasty? Results of the mercator study: A multicenter, randomized, double-blind placebo-controlled trial. Multicenter european research trial with cilazapril after angioplasty to prevent transluminal coronary obstruction and restenosis (mercator) study group. *Circulation.* 1992;86:100–110.

56. Viswanathan M, Stromberg C, Seltzer A, Saavedra JM. Balloon angioplasty enhances the expression of angiotensin ii at1 receptors in neointima of rat aorta. *J Clin Invest.* 1992;90:1707–1712.

57. Van Belle E, Bauters C, Wernert N, Delcayre C, McFadden EP, Dupuis B, Lablanche JM, Bertrand ME, Swynghedauw B. Angiotensin converting enzyme inhibition prevents proto-oncogene expression in the vascular wall after injury. *J Hypertens.* 1995;13:105–112.

58. Kim S, Kawamura M, Wanibuchi H, Ohta K, Hamaguchi A, Omura T, Yukimura T, Miura K, Iwao H. Angiotensin ii type 1 receptor blockade inhibits the expression of immediate-early genes and fibronectin in rat injured artery. *Circulation.* 1995;92:88–95.

59. Kohler TR, Jawien A. Flow affects development of intimal hyperplasia after arterial injury in rats. *Arterioscler Thromb.* 1992;12:963–971.

60. Mattsson EJ, Kohler TR, Vergel SM, Clowes AW. Increased blood flow induces regression of intimal hyperplasia. *Arterioscler Thromb Vasc Biol.* 1997;17:2245–2249.

61. Snow AD, Bolender RP, Wight TN, Clowes AW. Heparin modulates the composition of the extracellular matrix domain surrounding arterial smooth muscle cells. *Am J Pathol.* 1990;137:313–330.

62. Gellman J, Ezekowitz MD, Sarembock IJ, Azrin MA, Nochomowitz LE, Lerner E, Haudenschild CC. Effect of lovastatin on intimal hyperplasia after balloon angioplasty: A study in an atherosclerotic hypercholesterolemic rabbit. *J Am Coll Cardiol.* 1991;17:251–259.

63. Ponticos M, Smith BD. Extracellular matrix synthesis in vascular disease: Hypertension, and atherosclerosis. *J Biomed Res.* 2014;28:25–39.

64. Clark RA, Tonnesen MG, Gailit J, Cheresh DA. Transient functional expression of alphavbeta 3 on vascular cells during wound repair. *Am J Pathol.* 1996;148:1407–1421.

65. Reidy MA, Irvin C, Lindner V. Migration of arterial wall cells: Expression of plasminogen activators and inhibitors in injured rat arteries. *Circ Res.* 1996;78:405–414.

66. Bendeck MP, Zempo N, Clowes AW, Galardy RE, Reidy MA. Smooth muscle cell migration and matrix metalloproteinase expression after arterial injury in the rat. *Circ Res.* 1994;75:539–545.

67. Bendeck MP, Irvin C, Reidy MA. Inhibition of matrix metalloproteinase activity inhibits smooth muscle cell migration but not neointimal thickening after arterial injury. *Circ Res.* 1996;78:38–43.

68. Vlodavsky I, Folkman J, Sullivan R, Fridman R, Ishai-Michaeli R, Sasse J, Klagsbrun M. Endothelial cell-derived basic fibroblast growth factor: Synthesis and deposition into subendothelial extracellular matrix. *Proc Natl Acad Sci USA.* 1987;84:2292–2296.

69. Schwartz RS, Edwards WD, Huber KC, Antoniades LC, Bailey KR, Camrud AR, Jorgenson MA, Holmes DR Jr. Coronary restenosis: Prospects for solution and new perspectives from a porcine model. *Mayo Clin Proc.* 1993;68:54–62.

70. McNamara CA, Sarembock IJ, Gimple LW, Fenton JW 2nd, Coughlin SR, Owens GK. Thrombin stimulates proliferation of cultured rat aortic smooth muscle cells by a proteolytically activated receptor. *J Clin Invest.* 1993;91:94–98.

71. Takada M, Tanaka H, Yamada T et al. Antibody to thrombin receptor inhibits neointimal smooth muscle cell accumulation without causing inhibition of platelet aggregation or altering hemostatic parameters after angioplasty in rat. *Circ Res.* 1998;82:980–987.

72. Margolin L, Fishbein I, Banai S, Golomb G, Reich R, Perez LS, Gertz SD. Metalloproteinase inhibitor attenuates neointima formation and constrictive remodeling after angioplasty in rats: Augmentative effect of alpha(v)beta(3) receptor blockade. *Atherosclerosis.* 2002;163:269–277.

73. Fingleton B. Matrix metalloproteinases as valid clinical targets. *Curr Pharmaceut Des.* 2007;13:333–346.

74. Peterson JT. The importance of estimating the therapeutic index in the development of matrix metalloproteinase inhibitors. *Cardiovasc Res.* 2006;69:677–687.

75. O'Brien ER, Alpers CE, Stewart DK, Ferguson M, Tran N, Gordon D, Benditt EP, Hinohara T, Simpson JB, Schwartz SM. Proliferation in primary and restenotic coronary atherectomy tissue. Implications for antiproliferative therapy. *Circ Res.* 1993;73:223–231.

76. Currier JW, Faxon DP. Restenosis after percutaneous transluminal coronary angioplasty: Have we been aiming at the wrong target? *J Am Coll Cardiol.* 1995;25:516–520.

77. Glagov S, Weisenberg E, Zarins CK, Stankunavicius R, Kolettis GJ. Compensatory enlargement of human atherosclerotic coronary arteries. *N Engl J Med.* 1987;316:1371–1375.

78. Kakuta T, Currier JW, Haudenschild CC, Ryan TJ, Faxon DP. Differences in compensatory vessel enlargement, not intimal formation, account for restenosis after angioplasty in the hypercholesterolemic rabbit model. *Circulation.* 1994;89:2809–2815.

79. Langille BL, O'Donnell F. Reductions in arterial diameter produced by chronic decreases in blood flow are endothelium-dependent. *Science.* 1986;231:405–407.

80. Tanaka H, Sukhova GK, Swanson SJ, Clinton SK, Ganz P, Cybulsky MI, Libby P. Sustained activation of vascular cells and leukocytes in the rabbit aorta after balloon injury. *Circulation*. 1993;88:1788–1803.

81. Cox JL, Chiasson DA, Gotlieb AI. Stranger in a strange land: The pathogenesis of saphenous vein graft stenosis with emphasis on structural and functional differences between veins and arteries. *Progr Cardiovasc Dis*. 1991;34:45–68.

82. Kohler TR, Kirkman TR, Clowes AW. The effect of rigid external support on vein graft adaptation to the arterial circulation. *J Vasc Surg*. 1989;9:277–285.

83. Rittgers SE, Karayannacos PE, Guy JF, Nerem RM, Shaw GM, Hostetler JR, Vasko JS. Velocity distribution and intimal proliferation in autologous vein grafts in dogs. *Circ Res*. 1978;42:792–801.

84. Noris M, Morigi M, Donadelli R, Aiello S, Foppolo M, Todeschini M, Orisio S, Remuzzi G, Remuzzi A. Nitric oxide synthesis by cultured endothelial cells is modulated by flow conditions. *Circ Res*. 1995;76:536–543.

85. Zwolak RM, Adams MC, Clowes AW. Kinetics of vein graft hyperplasia: Association with tangential stress. *J Vasc Surg*. 1987;5:126–136.

86. Luscher TF, Diederich D, Siebenmann R et al. Difference between endothelium-dependent relaxation in arterial and in venous coronary bypass grafts. *N Engl J Med*. 1988;319:462–467.

87. Chaux A, Ruan XM, Fishbein MC, Ouyang Y, Kaul S, Pass JA, Matloff JM. Perivascular delivery of a nitric oxide donor inhibits neointimal hyperplasia in vein grafts implanted in the arterial circulation. *J Thorac Cardiovasc Surg*. 1998;115:604–612; discussion 612–614.

88. Davies MG, Kim JH, Dalen H, Makhoul RG, Svendsen E, Hagen PO. Reduction of experimental vein graft intimal hyperplasia and preservation of nitric oxide-mediated relaxation by the nitric oxide precursor l-arginine. *Surgery*. 1994;116:557–568.

89. Bassiouny HS, White S, Glagov S, Choi E, Giddens DP, Zarins CK. Anastomotic intimal hyperplasia: Mechanical injury or flow induced. *J Vasc Surg*. 1992;15:708–716; discussion 716–717.

90. Ballyk PD, Walsh C, Butany J, Ojha M. Compliance mismatch may promote graft-artery intimal hyperplasia by altering suture-line stresses. *J Biomech*. 1998;31:229–237.

91. Fei DY, Thomas JD, Rittgers SE. The effect of angle and flow rate upon hemodynamics in distal vascular graft anastomoses: A numerical model study. *J Biomech Eng*. 1994;116:331–336.

92. Ojha M, Cobbold RS, Johnston KW. Influence of angle on wall shear stress distribution for an end-to-side anastomosis. *J Vasc Surg*. 1994;19:1067–1073.

93. Golden MA, Hanson SR, Kirkman TR, Schneider PA, Clowes AW. Healing of polytetrafluoroethylene arterial grafts is influenced by graft porosity. *J Vasc Surg*. 1990;11:838–844; discussion 845.

94. Clowes AW, Kirkman TR, Reidy MA. Mechanisms of arterial graft healing. Rapid transmural capillary ingrowth provides a source of intimal endothelium and smooth muscle in porous ptfe prostheses. *Am J Pathol*. 1986;123:220–230.

95. Clowes AW, Gown AM, Hanson SR, Reidy MA. Mechanisms of arterial graft failure. 1. Role of cellular proliferation in early healing of ptfe prostheses. *Am J Pathol*. 1985;118:43–54.

96. Zacharias RK, Kirkman TR, Kenagy RD, Bowen-Pope DF, Clowes AW. Growth factor production by polytetrafluoroethylene vascular grafts. *J Vasc Surg*. 1988;7:606–610.

97. Golden MA, Au YP, Kenagy RD, Clowes AW. Growth factor gene expression by intimal cells in healing polytetrafluoroethylene grafts. *J Vasc Surg*. 1990;11:580–585.

98. Golden MA, Au YP, Kirkman TR, Wilcox JN, Raines EW, Ross R, Clowes AW. Platelet-derived growth factor activity and mrna expression in healing vascular grafts in baboons: Association in vivo of platelet-derived growth factor mrna and protein with cellular proliferation. *J Clin Invest*. 1991;87:406–414.

99. Kohler TR, Kirkman TR, Kraiss LW, Zierler BK, Clowes AW. Increased blood flow inhibits neointimal hyperplasia in endothelialized vascular grafts. *Circ Res*. 1991;69:1557–1565.

100. Dos Santos JD. Sur la desobstruction des thromboses arterielles anciennes. *Mem Acad Chir*. 1947;73:409–411.

101. Chen C, Li J, Mattar SG, Pierce GF, Aukerman L, Hanson SR, Lumsden AB. Boundary layer infusion of basic fibroblast growth factor accelerates intimal hyperplasia in endarterectomized canine artery. *J Surg Res*. 1997;69:300–306.

102. Lumsden AB, Chen C, Hughes JD, Kelly AB, Hanson SR, Harker LA. Anti-vla-4 antibody reduces intimal hyperplasia in the endarterectomized carotid artery in nonhuman primates. *J Vasc Surg*. 1997;26:87–93.

103. Bandyk DF, Kaebnick HW, Adams MB, Towne JB. Turbulence occurring after carotid bifurcation endarterectomy: A harbinger of residual and recurrent carotid stenosis. *J Vasc Surg*. 1988;7:261–274.

104. Clowes AW, Karnowsky MJ. Suppression by heparin of smooth muscle cell proliferation in injured arteries. *Nature*. 1977;265:625–626.

105. Weisz PB, Joullie MM, Hunter CM, Kumor KM, Zhang Z, Levine E, Macarak E, Weiner D, Barnathan ES. A basic compositional requirement of agents having heparin-like cell-modulating activities. *Biochem Pharmacol*. 1997;54:149–157.

106. Bachinsky WB, Barnathan ES, Liu H et al. Sustained inhibition of intimal thickening. In vitro and in vivo effects of polymeric beta-cyclodextrin sulfate. *J Clin Invest*. 1995;96:2583–2592.

107. Hedin U, Daum G, Clowes AW. Heparin inhibits thrombin-induced mitogen-activated protein kinase signaling in arterial smooth muscle cells. *J Vasc Surg.* 1998;27:512–520.

108. Ellis SG, Roubin GS, Wilentz J, Douglas JS Jr., King SB 3rd. Effect of 18- to 24-hour heparin administration for prevention of restenosis after uncomplicated coronary angioplasty. *Am Heart J.* 1989;117:777–782.

109. Saxon RR, Chervu A, Jones PA et al. Heparin-bonded, expanded polytetrafluoroethylene-lined stent graft in the treatment of femoropopliteal artery disease: 1-year results of the viper (viabahn endoprosthesis with heparin bioactive surface in the treatment of superficial femoral artery obstructive disease) trial. *J Vasc Interv Radiol.* 2013;24:165–173; quiz 174.

110. Wilson NV, Salisbury JR, Kakkar VV. Effect of low molecular weight heparin on intimal hyperplasia. *Br J Surg.* 1991;78:1381–1383.

111. Lablanche JM, McFadden EP, Meneveau N et al. Effect of nadroparin, a low-molecular-weight heparin, on clinical and angiographic restenosis after coronary balloon angioplasty: The fact study. Fraxiparine angioplastie coronaire transluminale. *Circulation.* 1997;96:3396–3402.

112. Cairns JA, Gill J, Morton B et al. Fish oils and low-molecular-weight heparin for the reduction of restenosis after percutaneous transluminal coronary angioplasty: The empar study. *Circulation.* 1996;94:1553–1560.

113. Karsch KR, Preisack MB, Baildon R et al. Low molecular weight heparin (reviparin) in percutaneous transluminal coronary angioplasty. Results of a randomized, double-blind, unfractionated heparin and placebo-controlled, multicenter trial (reduce trial). Reduction of restenosis after ptca, early administration of reviparin in a double-blind unfractionated heparin and placebo-controlled evaluation. *J Am Coll Cardiol.* 1996;28:1437–1443.

114. Edmondson RA, Cohen AT, Das SK, Wagner MB, Kakkar VV. Low-molecular weight heparin versus aspirin and dipyridamole after femoropopliteal bypass grafting. *Lancet.* 1994;344:914–918.

115. Koppensteiner R, Spring S, Amann-Vesti BR, Meier T, Pfammatter T, Rousson V, Banyai M, van der Loo B. Low-molecular-weight heparin for prevention of restenosis after femoropopliteal percutaneous transluminal angioplasty: A randomized controlled trial. *J Vasc Surg.* 2006;44:1247–1253.

116. Kobayashi N, Honda T, Yoshida K, Nakano S, Ohno T, Tsubokou Y, Matsuoka H. Critical role of bradykinin-eNOS and oxidative stress-LOX-1 pathway in cardiovascular remodeling under chronic angiotensin-converting enzyme inhibition. *Atherosclerosis.* 2006;187:92–100.

117. Faxon DP. Effect of high dose angiotensin-converting enzyme inhibition on restenosis: Final results of the marcator study, a multicenter, double-blind, placebo-controlled trial of cilazapril. The multicenter american research trial with cilazapril after angioplasty to prevent transluminal coronary obstruction and restenosis (marcator) study group. *J Am Coll Cardiol.* 1995;25:362–369.

118. Campbell DJ. Circulating and tissue angiotensin systems. *J Clin Invest.* 1987;79:1–6.

119. Farhy RD, Carretero OA, Ho KL, Scicli AG. Role of kinins and nitric oxide in the effects of angiotensin converting enzyme inhibitors on neointima formation. *Circ Res.* 1993;72:1202–1210.

120. Igase M, Kohara K, Nagai T, Miki T, Ferrario CM. Increased expression of angiotensin converting enzyme 2 in conjunction with reduction of neointima by angiotensin ii type 1 receptor blockade. *Hypertens Res.* 2008;31:553–559.

121. Peters S, Gotting B, Trummel M, Rust H, Brattstrom A. Valsartan for prevention of restenosis after stenting of type b2/c lesions: The val-prest trial. *J Invasive Cardiol.* 2001;13:93–97.

122. Shah PK, Amin J. Low high density lipoprotein level is associated with increased restenosis rate after coronary angioplasty. *Circulation.* 1992;85:1279–1285.

123. Soma MR, Donetti E, Parolini C, Mazzini G, Ferrari C, Fumagalli R, Paoletti R. Hmg coa reductase inhibitors. In vivo effects on carotid intimal thickening in normocholesterolemic rabbits. *Arterioscler Thromb.* 1993;13:571–578.

124. Gao C, Xu W, Xiao W, Yu J, Li M. Simvastatin decreases stent-induced in-stent restenosis rate via downregulating the expression of pcna and upregulating that of p27kip1. *J Interv Cardiol.* 2013;26:384–391.

125. Weintraub WS, Boccuzzi SJ, Klein JL et al. Lack of effect of lovastatin on restenosis after coronary angioplasty. Lovastatin restenosis trial study group. *N Engl J Med.* 1994;331:1331–1337.

126. Serruys PW, Foley DP, Jackson G et al. A randomized placebo-controlled trial of fluvastatin for prevention of restenosis after successful coronary balloon angioplasty; final results of the fluvastatin angiographic restenosis (flare) trial. *Eur Heart J.* 1999;20:58–69.

127. Bertrand ME, McFadden EP, Fruchart JC et al. Effect of pravastatin on angiographic restenosis after coronary balloon angioplasty. The predict trial investigators. Prevention of restenosis by elisor after transluminal coronary angioplasty. *J Am Coll Cardiol.* 1997;30:863–869.

128. LaMuraglia GM, Ortu P, Flotte TJ, Roberts WG, Schomacker KT, ChandraSekar NR, Hasan T. Chloroaluminum sulfonated phthalocyanine partitioning in normal and intimal hyperplastic artery in the rat: Implications for photodynamic therapy. *Am J Pathol.* 1993;142:1898–1905.

129. Ortu P, LaMuraglia GM, Roberts WG, Flotte TJ, Hasan T. Photodynamic therapy of arteries: A novel approach for treatment of experimental intimal hyperplasia. *Circulation.* 1992;85:1189–1196.

130. Eton D, Colburn MD, Shim V, Panek W, Lee D, Moore WS, Ahn SS. Inhibition of intimal hyperplasia by photodynamic therapy using photofrin. *J Surg Res.* 1992;53:558–562.

131. Wakamatsu T, Saito T, Hayashi J, Takeichi T, Kitamoto K, Aizawa K. Long-term inhibition of intimal hyperplasia using vascular photodynamic therapy in balloon-injured carotid arteries. *Med Mol Morphol.* 2005;38:225–232.

132. Dippel EJ, Makam P, Kovach R et al. Randomized controlled study of excimer laser atherectomy for treatment of femoropopliteal in-stent restenosis: Initial results from the excite isr trial (excimer laser randomized controlled study for treatment of femoropopliteal in-stent restenosis). *JACC Cardiovasc Interv.* 2015;8:92–101.

133. Committee TS, Jaff MR, White CJ, Hiatt WR, Fowkes GR, Dormandy J, Razavi M, Reekers J, Norgren L. An update on methods for revascularization and expansion of the tasc lesion classification to include below-the-knee arteries: A supplement to the inter-society consensus for the management of peripheral arterial disease (TASC II). *J Endovasc Ther.* 2015 October;22(5):663–677.

134. Chang MW, Barr E, Seltzer J, Jiang YQ, Nabel GJ, Nabel EG, Parmacek MS, Leiden JM. Cytostatic gene therapy for vascular proliferative disorders with a constitutively active form of the retinoblastoma gene product. *Science.* 1995;267:518–522.

135. Chen D, Krasinski K, Sylvester A, Chen J, Nisen PD, Andres V. Downregulation of cyclin-dependent kinase 2 activity and cyclin a promoter activity in vascular smooth muscle cells by p27(KIP1), an inhibitor of neointima formation in the rat carotid artery. *J Clin Invest.* 1997;99:2334–2341.

136. Yonemitsu Y, Kaneda Y, Tanaka S, Nakashima Y, Komori K, Sugimachi K, Sueishi K. Transfer of wild-type p53 gene effectively inhibits vascular smooth muscle cell proliferation in vitro and in vivo. *Circ Res.* 1998;82:147–156.

137. Maillard L, Van Belle E, Tio FO, Rivard A, Kearney M, Branellec D, Steg PG, Isner JM, Walsh K. Effect of percutaneous adenovirus-mediated gax gene delivery to the arterial wall in double-injured atheromatous stented rabbit iliac arteries. *Gene Ther.* 2000;7:1353–1361.

138. Robertson KE, McDonald RA, Oldroyd KG, Nicklin SA, Baker AH. Prevention of coronary in-stent restenosis and vein graft failure: Does vascular gene therapy have a role? *Pharmacol Therapeut.* 2012;136:23–34.

139. Conte MS, Bandyk DF, Clowes AW et al. Results of prevent III: A multicenter, randomized trial of edifoligide for the prevention of vein graft failure in lower extremity bypass surgery. *J Vasc Surg.* 2006;43:742–7751; discussion 751.

140. Waksman R, Robinson KA, Crocker IR, Wang C, Gravanis MB, Cipolla GD, Hillstead RA, King SB 3rd. Intracoronary low-dose beta-irradiation inhibits neointima formation after coronary artery balloon injury in the swine restenosis model. *Circulation.* 1995;92:3025–3031.

141. Sarac TP, Riggs PN, Williams JP, Feins RH, Baggs R, Rubin P, Green RM. The effects of low-dose radiation on neointimal hyperplasia. *J Vasc Surg.* 1995;22:17–24.

142. Teirstein PS, Massullo V, Jani S et al. Two-year follow-up after catheter-based radiotherapy to inhibit coronary restenosis. *Circulation.* 1999;99:243–247.

143. Waksman R, Ajani AE, White RL et al. Two-year follow-up after beta and gamma intracoronary radiation therapy for patients with diffuse in-stent restenosis. *Am J Cardiol.* 2001;88:425–428.

144. Stone GW, Ellis SG, O'Shaughnessy CD et al. Paclitaxel-eluting stents vs vascular brachytherapy for in-stent restenosis within bare-metal stents: The taxus v isr randomized trial. *J Am Med Assoc.* 2006;295:1253–1263.

145. Martin KA, Rzucidlo EM, Merenick BL, Fingar DC, Brown DJ, Wagner RJ, Powell RJ. The mTOR/p70 S6K1 pathway regulates vascular smooth muscle cell differentiation. *Am J Physiol Cell Physiol.* 2004;286:C507–C517.

146. Duda SH, Bosiers M, Lammer J et al. Drug-eluting and bare nitinol stents for the treatment of atherosclerotic lesions in the superficial femoral artery: Long-term results from the sirocco trial. *J Endovasc Ther.* 2006;13:701–710.

147. Lammer J, Bosiers M, Zeller T, Schillinger M, Boone E, Zaugg MJ, Verta P, Peng L, Gao X, Schwartz LB. First clinical trial of nitinol self-expanding everolimus-eluting stent implantation for peripheral arterial occlusive disease. *J Vasc Surg.* 2011;54:394–401.

148. Axel DI, Kunert W, Goggelmann C et al. Paclitaxel inhibits arterial smooth muscle cell proliferation and migration in vitro and in vivo using local drug delivery. *Circulation.* 1997;96:636–645.

149. Pires NM, Eefting D, de Vries MR, Quax PH, Jukema JW. Sirolimus and paclitaxel provoke different vascular pathological responses after local delivery in a murine model for restenosis on underlying atherosclerotic arteries. *Heart.* 2007;93:922–927.

150. Dake MD, Ansel GM, Jaff MR et al. Paclitaxel-eluting stents show superiority to balloon angioplasty and bare metal stents in femoropopliteal disease: Twelve-month Zilver PTX randomized study results. *Circ Cardiovasc Interv.* 2011;4:495–504.

151. Dake MD, Ansel GM, Jaff MR et al. Sustained safety and effectiveness of paclitaxel-eluting stents for femoropopliteal lesions: 2-year follow-up from the Zilver PTX randomized and single-arm clinical studies. *J Am Coll Cardiol.* 2013;61:2417–2427.

152. Ansel G. Zilver PTX randomized trial of paclitaxel-eluting stents for femoropopliteal artery disease: 4-year results. *Vascular Interventional Advances*, Las Vegas, NV, 2013.

153. Zeller T, Dake MD, Tepe G, Brechtel K, Noory E, Beschorner U, Kultgen PL, Rastan A. Treatment of femoropopliteal in-stent restenosis with paclitaxel-eluting stents. *JACC Cardiovasc Interv*. 2013;6:274–281.

154. Colombo A, Orlic D, Stankovic G et al. Preliminary observations regarding angiographic pattern of restenosis after rapamycin-eluting stent implantation. *Circulation*. 2003;107:2178–2180.

155. Costa MA, Simon DI. Molecular basis of restenosis and drug-eluting stents. *Circulation*. 2005;111:2257–2273.

156. Rosenfield K, Jaff MR, White CJ et al. Trial of a paclitaxel-coated balloon for femoropopliteal artery disease. *N Engl J Med*. 2015;373:145–153.

157. Baerlocher MO, Kennedy SA, Rajebi MR, Baerlocher FJ, Misra S, Liu D, Nikolic B. Meta-analysis of drug-eluting balloon angioplasty and drug-eluting stent placement for infrainguinal peripheral arterial disease. *J Vasc Interv Radiol*. 2015;26:459–473.e454; quiz 474.

158. Rastan A, Brechtel K, Krankenberg H et al. Sirolimus-eluting stents for treatment of infrapopliteal arteries reduce clinical event rate compared to bare-metal stents: Long-term results from a randomized trial. *J Am Coll Cardiol*. 2012;60:587–591.

159. Rastan A, Tepe G, Krankenberg H et al. Sirolimus-eluting stents vs. Bare-metal stents for treatment of focal lesions in infrapopliteal arteries: A double-blind, multi-centre, randomized clinical trial. *Eur Heart J*. 2011;32:2274–2281.

160. Scheinert D, Katsanos K, Zeller T et al. A prospective randomized multicenter comparison of balloon angioplasty and infrapopliteal stenting with the sirolimus-eluting stent in patients with ischemic peripheral arterial disease: 1-year results from the achilles trial. *J Am Coll Cardiol*. 2012;60:2290–2295.

161. Seedial SM, Ghosh S, Saunders RS, Suwanabol PA, Shi X, Liu B, Kent KC. Local drug delivery to prevent restenosis. *J Vasc Surg*. 2013;57:1403–1414.

162. Serruys PW, Ormiston JA, Onuma Y et al. A bioabsorbable everolimus-eluting coronary stent system (absorb): 2-year outcomes and results from multiple imaging methods. *Lancet*. 2009;373:897–910.

163. Serruys PW, Chevalier B, Dudek D et al. A bioresorbable everolimus-eluting scaffold versus a metallic everolimus-eluting stent for ischaemic heart disease caused by de-novo native coronary artery lesions (absorb II): An interim 1-year analysis of clinical and procedural secondary outcomes from a randomised controlled trial. *Lancet*. 2015;385:43–54.

164. Werner M, Micari A, Cioppa A, Vadala G, Schmidt A, Sievert H, Rubino P, Angelini A, Scheinert D, Biamino G. Evaluation of the biodegradable peripheral igaki-tamai stent in the treatment of de novo lesions in the superficial femoral artery: The gaia study. *JACC Cardiovasc Interv*. 2014;7:305–312.

165. Chan JM, Rhee JW, Drum CL, Bronson RT, Golomb G, Langer R, Farokhzad OC. In vivo prevention of arterial restenosis with paclitaxel-encapsulated targeted lipid-polymeric nanoparticles. *Proc Natl Acad Sci USA*. 2011;108:19347–19352.

SECTION III

Peripheral Occlusive Disease

14

Acute arterial insufficiency

MARK M. ARCHIE and JANE K. YANG

CONTENTS

Whenever the motion of the blood in the arteries is impeded, by compression, by infarction, or by interception, there is less pulsation distally, since the beat of the arteries is nothing else than the impulse of blood in these vessels.

William Harvey

Acute arterial insufficiency remains a morbid disease; 30-day mortality remains nearly 15% with an amputation rate of 10%–30%.[1] There has, however, been marked improvement in the treatment options, decreasing the morbidity and mortality that the treatment itself brings. The most significant progress in limb salvage for acute arterial ischemia came about with two developments in the twentieth century. First, heparin anticoagulation has made it possible to limit the propagation of clot distal to the point of occlusion and to reduce the incidence of recurrent embolus and thrombosis. Second, the Fogarty balloon catheter, introduced in 1963, made it possible to extract emboli and thrombi from arteries, with a device far better suited for this purpose than the devices used in the past such as corkscrew wires or suction catheters.[2] Furthermore, the expanding array of endovascular techniques and their successes in chronic peripheral arterial disease have created increasing minimally invasive options for acute arterial insufficiency as well. This chapter describes the etiology, pathophysiology, diagnosis and current procedures for treatment of acute arterial insufficiency.

ETIOLOGY

Acute arterial ischemia is caused by one of three general etiologies: acute thrombosis, emboli or trauma (Table 14.1). Acute thrombosis is currently the most common cause of acute arterial insufficiency, cited at up to 60% of acute ischemic episodes reported. Thrombosis usually occurs at a point of narrowing in a progressively atherosclerotic vessel, particularly in association with a flow-related disorder, such as congestive heart failure, shock, dehydration or polycythemia. Hemorrhage within a ruptured atheromatous plaque can cause acute occlusion, as can dissection and hypercoagulability.

Anticoagulation for these cardiac diseases has dropped emboli from the most common to the second most common cause of acute arterial insufficiency. Emboli can be of cardiac or non-cardiac origin. In the past, approximately

Table 14.1 Etiology of acute arterial occlusion.

Embolic
Cardiac
Atrial fibrillation
Valvular heart disease (rheumatic heart disease or endocarditis)
Myocardial infarction (with or without ventricular aneurysm)
Prosthetic heart valves
Left atrial myxoma
Paradoxical embolus
Congestive cardiomyopathy
Hypertrophic cardiomyopathy
Mitral annulus calcification
Mitral valve prolapse
Peripheral
Ulcerating atherosclerotic lesions
Aneurysms (aortic, iliac, femoral, popliteal, subclavian, axillary)
Arterial catheterization complications
Thrombotic
Narrowed atherosclerotic segment (with or without
　a flow-related disorder)
Intraplaque hemorrhage
Drugs of abuse

75%–80% of all emboli originated from the heart, the majority of those being of left atrial origin in patients with rheumatic heart disease and atrial fibrillation. With the decreased incidence of rheumatic heart disease, the most common cardiac source of an embolus is seen in the diseased myocardium, due to hypokinesis and stasis of blood, with atrial fibrillation being most commonly caused by coronary artery disease.[3] The most common non-cardiac sources of arterial emboli include debris from ulcerating atheromatous plaques in the aorta and common iliac arteries. These lesions may be associated with aneurysmal disease of the proximal circulation, as well as more distal vessels, such as the popliteal artery. Other sources or causes of emboli are listed in Table 14.1 and include atrial myxoma, endocarditis, prosthetic heart valves, complications of arterial catheterization and paradoxical embolization. In approximately 25% of cases of acute ischemia caused by embolism, no source for the embolus can be identified. These cases may be due to small ulcerative lesions not demonstrated angiographically or may be caused by paradoxical emboli in which a septal defect cannot be identified.

Trauma-induced arterial insufficiency will be discussed in a later chapter.

PATHOPHYSIOLOGY

The source of emboli, more often than not, dictates which arteries are affected and subsequently, the deficits encountered. Occlusions found at the bifurcations of large arteries are mainly of cardiac origin, while those of more distal, smaller vessels can be attributed to atheroemboli from atherosclerotic plaques (cholesterol embolization syndrome). The size of the obstructed vessel then can help in differentiating between emboli that originate from the heart and emboli that originate from the aorta or common iliac arteries. For example, an embolus that lodges in the common femoral artery, a medium-sized artery, is usually of cardiac origin. An embolus that leads to ischemia of an isolated toe most likely originates from the distal aorta or common iliac arteries. Thrombosis will often present with milder limb ischemia than emboli because of the chronic nature of the underlying atherosclerotic lesions. Patients with longstanding arteriosclerosis often have a complex collateral circulation in place.

Once an embolus or thrombus occludes an artery, the distal vasculature goes into spasm. Extension of the thromboembolus then forms proximal to the site of occlusion, back to the point of adequate collateralization. The distal spasm lasts for approximately 8 hours and then subsides. At this point, clot forms in the arterial system distal to the site of obstruction and propagates downward, obstructing any residual collateral flow, resulting in worsening of the ischemia. As a result, the skin usually becomes patchy, blue and mottled. Skeletal muscle and peripheral nerves withstand acute ischemia for some 8 hours without permanent damage; skin can withstand severe ischemia for as long as 24 hours. The extent of the ischemic necrosis depends on the adequacy of collateral circulation, the patient's underlying cardiovascular function, viscosity of the blood, oxygen-carrying capacity of the blood, propagation of clot into the microvasculature and effectiveness and promptness of treatment.

If muscle ischemia progresses to necrosis, the muscle becomes paralyzed and acquires a firm, spastic consistency. When peripheral nerves become ischemic, they cease to function, and the affected parts become anesthetized. As the skin undergoes profound ischemia, maximum oxygen extraction results in a cyanotic, blotchy appearance. When these blotchy, cyanotic areas no longer blanch with pressure, the skin is gangrenous and the ischemia is no longer reversible.[4]

The reperfusion of ischemic muscle poses a threat to other organ systems.[5,6] Anaerobic metabolism produces unbuffered acid, dead cells release potassium and myoglobin, microthrombi form in the areas of stasis and acidosis, and procoagulants and inflammatory products accumulate. With reperfusion, oxygen radicals, leukotrienes and many other inflammatory mediators are generated, and all of these products are released into the systemic circulation. Here they produce systemic vascular permeability, extravasation of plasma into the interstitium and damage to remote organs. The lungs receive the initial insult, with further damage occurring in the heart and kidneys.[7] A mortality rate of 85% when a limb with advanced ischemia is revascularized has been documented. The degree of insult to the body as a whole depends upon the mass of ischemic tissue, the duration of the ischemia and the underlying condition of the remote organs.

DIAGNOSIS

In most cases, the history and physical examination allow identification of the level of obstruction, the probable cause and the degree of ischemia (Tables 14.2 and 14.3). This information usually dictates the extent and mode of therapy.

The history should review the duration and progression of the symptoms and should document prior cardiac or vascular disease that might complicate the treatment. A history of claudication indicates prior atherosclerotic disease and points towards superimposed thrombosis as the culprit. In a nonsmoker, aortoiliac occlusive disease is unlikely. A history of heart disease, particularly one

Table 14.2 Signs of ischemia.

Acute ischemia
Pale extremity at resting position
Temperature change, with sharp line of demarcation
Pain and paresthesias
Decreased sensation
Mottled cyanotic colour that blanches with pressure
Mottled cyanotic colour that does not blanch
Paresis progressing to paralysis
Firm, spastic musculature
Chronic ischemia
Atrophic musculature
Decreased hair
Hypertrophic nails
Pulse deficits
Temperature
Venous troughing[a]
Slow capillary refill
Prolonged pallor with elevation
Dependent rubor

[a] Collapse of the superficial veins of the foot.

Table 14.3 Patient evaluation.

Cardiac evaluation	Vascular evaluation
History	
Myocardial infarction	Transient ischemic attack
Arrhythmias – syncope	Amaurosis fugax
Angina	Claudication
Palpitations	Impotence
Medications	Intestinal angina
Congestive heart failure	Prior surgery
Physical examination	
Rate and rhythm	Absent pulses
Murmurs and gallops	Aneurysmal vessels
Blood pressure	Bruits
Cardiomegaly	Acute ischemia
Peripheral edema	Chronic ischemia
Jugular venous distension	Dehydration

associated with arrhythmias, makes the possibility of embolization from the heart likely.

The physical examination may give information regarding any cardiac disease and the likelihood that the heart is the source of an embolus. Signs of chronic ischemia in the lower extremities, hypertrophic nails, atrophic skin and hair loss indicate chronic obstructive disease.

The presence of acute arterial insufficiency is usually manifested by an abrupt temperature change in an extremity distal to the level of the obstruction (Figure 14.1). The ability to dorsiflex and plantarflex the toes indicates the viability of the musculature in the calves; the inability to move the toes indicates impending necrosis of a muscle group. Development of firm, spastic musculature, especially if the contralateral side is normal, indicates extensive necrosis or impending acute compartment syndrome (ACS).

Paresthesias and anesthesia indicate that the nerves have undergone ischemic changes. Waxy, white skin is characteristic of active arteriolar spasm and indicates viability of arterioles to the skin. Blotchy cyanosis that does not blanch with pressure indicates thrombosed capillaries in the subcuticular areas and skin necrosis.

Laboratory tests are aimed at evaluating fluid balance, oxygen-carrying capacity of the blood, renal function, cardiac function and muscular damage (Table 14.4). A chest x-ray shows the size of the heart and may identify thoracic aortic disease. A hematocrit can make a diagnosis of polycythemia. A urinalysis that shows protein and pigment suggests the presence of myoglobin in the urine. The determination of creatinine phosphokinase with isoenzymes can give information about muscle necrosis. An electrocardiogram defines arrhythmias and gives information about the status of the heart. Two-dimensional echocardiography identifies the cardiac chamber size, estimates the ejection fraction, studies the valvular pathology, evaluates the wall motion and sometimes identifies intracardiac thrombus or tumor.[8,9] Echocardiography may also detect a potentially patent atrial septal defect, which may be involved in a paroxysmal embolus. Echocardiography is not helpful acutely in deciding whether to operate, anticoagulate, or amputate.[10] It is of value in discovering underlying cardiac disease that requires attention after successful management of the acute ischemic event. The most important imaging modalities, however, include computed tomographic angiography with intravenous contrast as well as a Duplex ultrasonography of the vessels of the extremity. An ultrasound examination of the abdomen may reveal an abdominal aortic aneurysm.

Unless a therapeutic decision hangs in the balance, we do not obtain arteriograms initially. However, when an arteriogram is obtained intraoperatively, it can give useful information. An arteriogram sometimes shows a sharp cut-off of a proximally normal artery, indicating an embolus. It may also show pre-existing underlying atherosclerotic occlusive disease. Abdominal aortic aneurysms or atheromatous disease involving the distal aorta and common iliac arteries may be demonstrated.

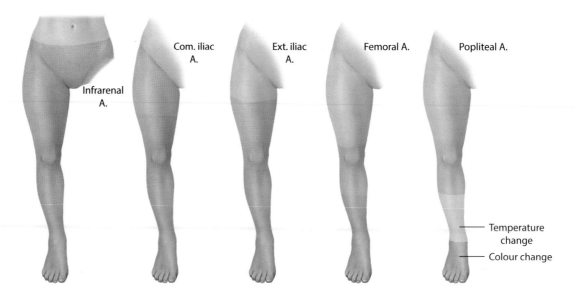

Figure 14.1 Level of temperature and colour change with occlusion of different arteries.

Table 14.4 Laboratory assessment.

Hematocrit, PT/PTT, platelets
Electrolytes, BUN, creatinine, glucose
Urinalysis – test for myoglobinuria
CPK with isoenzymes
Chest radiograph
Electrocardiogram
2D echocardiogram
Arteriogram

TREATMENT

With the advent of increased options for revascularization of an acutely ischemic limb, choosing the appropriate treatment modality has become more difficult. To a large extent, it is the presentation itself that should dictate what treatment is chosen. As the incidence of peripheral thrombotic occlusion has increased compared to embolic arterial occlusion, patients increasingly present with less severe limb ischemia because many of them have already developed collateral circulation from their chronic peripheral vascular disease. To aid the decision making is the most commonly used classification scheme, created by Rutherford and adopted by the Inter-Society Consensus for the Management of Peripheral Arterial Disease Workgroup. As demonstrated in Table 14.5, the viability of the limb is determined by the extent of sensory loss, motor loss and arterial and venous Doppler signal.

Level I ischemia patients can be treated with therapeutic anticoagulation. Level III indicates an advanced level of ischemia where the exam suggests *irreversible* ischemic changes with profound sensory loss and paralysis with no audible Doppler arterial or venous signals. Despite this, these patients occasionally may have a functional limb if revascularization occurs immediately, depending on their history and time of onset of symptoms. Cases of embolic arterial occlusion will often present with such severe exams but also can be surgically resolved very quickly. Unfortunately, it is more common for limbs at this ischemic level to be unsalvageable with revascularization attempts causing more harm to the patient due to myoglobinemia and chronic pain from a non-functional limb. The history is integral in determining whether to attempt

Table 14.5 Clinical categories of acute limb ischemia.

Category	Findings			Doppler signals	
	Description/prognosis	Sensory loss	Muscle weakness	Arterial	Venous
I. Viable	Not imminently threatened	None	None	Audible	Audible
II. Threatened					
A. Marginally	Salvageable if promptly treated	Minimal (toes) or none	None	Inaudible	Audible
B. Immediately	Salvageable with immediate revascularization	More than toes, associated with rest pain	Mild, moderate	Inaudible	Audible
III. Irreversible	Major tissue loss or permanent nerve damage inevitable	Profound, anesthetic	Profound, paralysis (rigor)	Inaudible	Inaudible

Source: Rutherford RB, *Semin Vasc Surg*, 22(1), 5, 2009.

revascularization or to proceed to a primary amputation of these advanced ischemia limbs.

Previously, the division between level IIA and IIB limbs indicated the division between those who could undergo endovascular and those who should undergo surgical revascularization. It was based on the time needed for revascularization, but this is no longer true with the increased endovascular capabilities. Though endovascular interventions are expected to require more time to restore full patency, there is significant improvement in limb perfusion before complete removal of the clot burden.

Regardless of which category the patient presents with, all patients should be immediately started on therapeutic systemic anticoagulation. While there are a number of new drugs in this class, heparin remains the drug of choice due to its fast onset, rapid metabolism and reversibility with protamine sulphate. In patients with heparin-induced thrombocytopenia (HIT), an argatroban infusion may be used as a substitute. Many surgeons use conventional dosages of heparin (100–200 USP units/kg bolus, followed by 15–30 USP units/kg/h by constant infusion). We strongly advise higher dosages and prefer a bolus of 300 USP units/kg, followed by 60–70 USP units/kg/h.[11]

An activated clotting time (ACT) or activated partial thromboplastin time (aPTT) should be obtained to determine response to anticoagulation (whether heparin or argatroban). These tests, however, are not used to gauge the adequacy of the heparin dose. The degree of anticoagulation distal to an obstruction is theoretically not equivalent to the anticoagulation of blood taken from a peripheral vein, as is used for the measurement of ACT or aPTT. Higher doses of heparin are used to achieve adequate anticoagulation in areas of ischemia. The clinical response, and not the degree of anticoagulation per laboratory values, is what determines the success of anticoagulation.[12] Active thrombosis results in the release of pro-inflammatory mediators that further produce vasospasm. While this is helpful in limiting clot propagation distal to an obstruction, this interferes with collateral flow. Full anticoagulation may decrease the extent of vasospasm, thereby decreasing the level of ischemia and pain in the extremity. If the limb is viable at initiation of anticoagulation, viability will improve with adequate anticoagulation, and revascularization, if necessary, may be carried out electively.

The onset of symptoms is important to note in the history. If the patient is seen within 4–6 hours of onset of ischemia and viability of the limb is in question – as manifest by pain, paralysis or paresthesia – immediate operative or endovascular intervention is indicated. In the patient with probable thrombosis superimposed on pre-existing vascular disease who has an ischemic but viable limb, revascularization is delayed until anticoagulation has resulted in improved collateralization and stabilization of the level of ischemia. An extensive early reconstructive procedure compromises the ability to administer full heparin therapy postoperatively because of a prohibitively high rate of hemorrhage. Emergent operations on patients who present

with ischemia of longer than 8 hours duration is currently not indicated. If the ischemic insult is severe enough to result in muscle necrosis, the necrosis will already be established within 8 hours. Revascularization after this period of time salvages no more muscle beyond that salvaged by anticoagulation, a treatment associated with a lower mortality. As a result, the rate of limb amputation rises following 6–8 hours after the onset of ischemic symptoms. Before the decision to revascularize a patient is made, they must be medically optimized based on their current co-morbidities. Revascularization of ischemic tissue washes products of ischemia into the central circulation, where such by-products can cause multi-organ failure.

Improvement of the patient's symptoms is gauged by progression of the line of temperature demarcation distally along the leg, recovery of sensation in the extremity, maintenance or recovery of skeletal muscle function in the extremity and the appearance of the skin. Skin blanching with pressure is proof of skin perfusion. However, when the skin develops blotchy, cyanotic areas that do not blanch with pressure, the tissue involved is beyond salvage.

Hemorrhage is the major complication of anticoagulation with heparin.[13] Patients without surgical wounds and without underlying bleeding dyscrasias seldom bleed on heparin, even high-dose heparin, for the first several days of therapy. Bleeding becomes more common on about the fifth day, when HIT can contribute to the anticoagulant effect of the heparin itself. Fortunately, most patients receive most of the benefit from heparin anticoagulation within the first few days of treatment. This permits a gradual reduction of heparin dosage, over the next 3–4 days, to more conventional levels. Failure to maintain therapeutic benefit on these lower doses, however, requires raising the level of anticoagulation. If bleeding should develop on the fifth day or later, the heparin can usually be stopped at that time, and in most instances, therapeutic benefit will be maintained.

A treatment plan that emphasizes early anticoagulation results in low mortality and salvages extremities as well as those treatment regimens that emphasize immediate revascularization in all patients, both low risk and high risk.[11] Early surgical or endovascular interventions, whether thrombectomy or thrombolysis, in patients who are seen shortly after the onset of symptoms are appropriate. In the remaining patients who present with ischemic but viable limbs, revascularization can be performed at a time of election if anticoagulation is given in adequate dosages to prevent thrombus propagation. In these patients with ischemic skin necrosis or dead muscle, initial anticoagulation followed later by amputation is the treatment of choice.

Patients presenting with a viable extremity (Level I) more than 48 hours after the onset of symptoms can be managed like patients with chronic severe obstructive disease. High-dose heparin therapy is of limited value, as these extremities have already survived the initial ischemic insult by developing collateral flow. An angiogram to evaluate the vasculature should be obtained. Many of these patients will require surgical or endovascular revascularization. Chronic anticoagulant therapy with warfarin (Coumadin) or subcutaneous heparin is subsequently indicated in many of these patients.

Interventional treatments include fibrinolytic therapy and embolectomy, which is often all that is needed for acute limb ischemia caused by emboli. In cases of thrombosis or trauma, these techniques usually need to be combined with surgical bypasses or endovascular recanalization.

FIBRINOLYTIC THERAPY

In patients with acute or subacute thromboembolism without advanced stages of ischemia, thrombolytic therapy may be instituted for revascularization and limb salvage. Previously, systemic thrombolysis was used to achieve patency of the occluded vessel. However, the hemorrhagic consequences, such as stroke, rendered this option dangerous. The three main types of plasminogen activators are streptokinase, urokinase and recombinant tissue plasminogen activator (tPA). tPAs are now being selectively infused proximal to the site of the occlusion.

Streptokinase is a non-enzymatic protein product of group C beta-hemolytic streptococci that combines with plasminogen to form an active enzymatic complex capable of converting plasminogen to plasmin. The low-dose intra-arterial regimen provides for 5,000–10,000 IU/h to be selectively infused for 12–48 hours with the therapeutic effect monitored by physical examination or by serial arteriography. The low-grade fever at times accompanying the treatment is thought to be caused by the antigen – antibody interaction of streptokinase with preformed streptococcal antibodies.

Urokinase is harvested from human renal cells in tissue culture and is not antigenic. It is a trypsin-like protease that directly converts plasminogen to plasmin. Low-dose urokinase at 20,000 IU/h, selectively infused, has been effective in restoring vessel patency.

With the use of recombinant DNA technology, recombinant tPA has been produced for thrombolysis. Advances in selective catheterization of acute occlusions have led to the development of ultrasound-accelerated thrombolysis (EKOS), with the aim of early onset of uninterrupted flow. The Dutch study, DUET, studied the onset of return of flow in two randomized groups. They concluded that those in the ultrasound-accelerated group achieved patency earlier than those with just selective thrombolysis.

Ideally, fibrinolytic therapy would be most useful for fresh thrombosis prior to clot organization, propagation or vessel wall damage. In contrast to heparin, which only inhibits propagation of already formed thrombus, the streptokinase actively lyses clot and therefore may potentially accelerate the return of circulation. Heparin can be given systemically and, by preventing clot formation, allows collateral circulation to develop while the patient's fibrinolytic system slowly lyses the existent thrombus.

Table 14.6 Complications of fibrinolytic therapy.

Intracranial hemorrhage
Arterial site hematomas
Distal embolization
Extravasation of blood through graft interstices – lysis of pseudointima of Dacron prosthesis
Retroperitoneal hemorrhage
Mild allergic reaction

Fibrinolytic therapy is especially ideal in patients who present with limb ischemia due to acute thrombosis. Thrombolysis has been combined with percutaneous transluminal angioplasty to achieve better long-term patency by revealing the underlying chronic lesion, which can then be treated with endovascular means. It has also been successful in restoring patency in vessels occluded for several weeks. The appropriateness of chronic anticoagulation in both of these groups of patients should be determined on an individual basis.

The advent of selective thrombolysis has not completely eradicated systemic complications. Thrombin time, fibrinogen levels, prothrombin times, partial thromboplastin time, platelet counts, hematocrit and fibrin split products should be monitored to prevent complications associated with fibrinolytic therapy (Table 14.6). Post-treatment anticoagulation should be monitored because patients have an increased susceptibility to bleeding complications.

EMBOLECTOMY

In low-risk patients who present with ischemia of less than 6–8 hours duration, an embolectomy may be performed if it is likely that the acute event is caused by an embolus. With the patient under local or regional anesthesia, thrombus or embolus can frequently be easily removed via a peripheral incision.[14] A Fogarty balloon catheter is passed through the clot or embolus, the balloon inflated gently, and the catheter withdrawn. There are several important aspects to the application of this technique. Proximal and distal control of the vessel should be ensured before arteriotomy. The common femoral, popliteal and brachial arteries allow access to most vessels. Catheter-related complications can be kept to a minimum by continually modifying the amount of fluid in the balloon while the catheter is being withdrawn to prevent overinflation at plaque sites and consequent vessel damage. Back-bleeding, as well as distal pulsation, do not guarantee adequate clot extraction. Therefore, an angiogram should be obtained after the removal of the embolus to confirm adequate vessel patency.

The nature of the operation is subsequently dictated by the arteriographic and operative findings. Most acute thromboemboli can be removed completely through the groin. However, if the occlusion is atherosclerotic or is

Table 14.7 Complications of revascularization.

Hemorrhage
Thrombosis
Recurrent emboli
Pulmonary embolus
Microembolic acute respiratory distress syndrome
Extremity edema
Acute renal failure
Cardiac dysfunction – myocardial infarction, arrhythmias
Mesenteric infarction

distal to the distal superficial femoral artery, clearing the occlusion may be difficult or impossible. In such cases, the arteriotomy is better performed in the distal popliteal artery or in the tibioperoneal trunk opposite the origin of the anterior tibial artery. Balloon catheter embolectomy of the tibial arteries can then be performed gently and accurately. In some cases, with arteriosclerotic or aneurysmal changes, a bypass operation must be performed with or without extraction of the proximal thrombus or embolus.

There are four primary complications associated with the use of the balloon catheter: rupture, perforation, intimal injury and fragmentation of clot resulting in inadequate removal and distal embolization. These complications serve to emphasize another reason for obtaining an angiogram after an embolus extraction. If the angiogram demonstrates an intimal injury compromising circulation, repair is necessary. If there is extravasation of contrast material but good distal perfusion without signs of ongoing hemorrhage, repair may or may not be necessary. These patients can often be followed clinically and studied later with arteriograms to confirm the resolution of the problem.

For at least 24 hours after surgery, the patient should be placed in an intensive care unit so that the distal circulation can be monitored. Frequent pulse check with the use of Doppler is standard to ensure maintained distal pulses. If evidence of re-thrombosis or recurrent embolus is identified, the patient should be returned to the operating room immediately. Pulmonary, cardiac and renal complications should be treated in standard fashion as they present. Common complications of revascularization are noted in Table 14.7.

THROMBOLYTIC THERAPY VERSUS SURGICAL INTERVENTION FOR ACUTE ARTERIAL INSUFFICIENCY

It had previously been believed that patients who presented with neurologic deficit should undergo open surgical revascularization because of the temporal necessity for emergent revascularization. However, though it may take more time to completely remove the clot burden with thrombolysis, frequently, decreasing the clot burden is enough to resolve the neurologic deficits before they are permanent. Newer techniques, such as percutaneous mechanical thrombectomy, have decreased the amount of time to reperfusion as compared with using just thrombolysis, allowing for endovascular techniques to be a viable option for more patients. Furthermore, in cases of thrombosis or when the clot extends throughout the leg with no outflow vessel visible on angiogram, it is extremely advantageous to use thrombolysis to reveal an outflow, or *target* vessel.

In the STILE and TOPAS trials, thrombolysis required greater than 24 hours to re-establish flow. This time delay limits the patients who can avoid open surgery as those who present with category IIB limbs are unable to tolerate the wait. Clots may be concentrated with platelets and plasminogen activation inhibitor 1, making them more resistant to thrombolysis. Some systemic circulation of catheter-directed thrombolysis is inevitable, delivering with it an increased risk of hemorrhage. Percutaneous mechanical thrombectomy has become an additional option, combining the benefits of endovascular access with a more immediate relief of clot burden. There are now multiple types of mechanical thrombectomy devices available. The first was a simple monorail aspiration catheter which has proven ineffective for the significant clot burden that patients usually present with. Many, including the widely used AngioJet, use active aspiration, while the increasingly popular EKOS catheter, among others, makes use of sound waves to mechanically fragment clots and augment fibrinolysis.

In a recent Cochrane review, five randomized trials, with a total of 1283 patients, have compared the benefits and risks of thrombolysis versus surgical revascularization in patients presenting with acute limb ischemia. There was no significant difference in limb salvage or death at 30 days, 6 months and 1 year. Thrombolysis incurred an increased risk of stroke and major hemorrhage at 30 days. Also, 12.3% of the thrombolysis patients evidenced distal embolization while there were no such events in those who underwent open surgery. The difficulty in this meta-analysis lies in the heterogeneity of the patients included. The criteria for thrombolysis were variable and, in some studies, unclear, with there still being no known temporal cutoff. This review suggests that both methods are effective in acute arterial insufficiency, but that specific patient factors need to be taken into consideration. For example, the STILE trial was aborted before inclusion of 600 patients due to the excess of complications in the thrombolysis group. Issues with proper catheter placement in this trial were significant, though this may reflect *real-world* scenarios.[15]

In addition, hybrid procedures combining the use of both open and endovascular surgery has been increasingly utilized. Schrijver et al. performed a literature review of papers from 2000 to 2010 analyzing outcomes of hybrid procedures for peripheral obstructive disease. In mixed hybrid procedures, the primary patency ranged from 53% to 79% at 12 months.[16] Dosluogo's retrospective paper of

108 patients treated with hybrid procedures treated a combination of both inflow and outflow arterial occlusions and demonstrated patency and limb salvage rates to open surgery.[17] This is a fortunate era in which the endovascular techniques available continue to expand, allowing the surgeon to combine open and minimally invasive techniques to build optimal treatment plans. The difficulty is in extrapolating data from these heterogeneous patients and therapies to determine which is the most efficacious, though it increasingly seems that the treatment detail must be individualized for optimal results.

POST-OPERATIVE ANTICOAGULATION

Post-operatively, patients should remain on anticoagulation with heparin (or argatroban if HIT), with bridging to Coumadin or one of the newer oral anticoagulants if an embolic source was the culprit. Hemorrhage is the most common complication in patients receiving heparin following an operation or intervention. Postoperative bleeding can be minor, as indicated by melena, hematuria, ecchymosis or hematomas, in which case the heparin therapy can be continued with monitoring of the hematocrit, platelet count and partial thromboplastin time. The conversion to oral anticoagulation therapy should be accomplished as soon as possible. Major bleeding can be defined as that requiring transfusion, cerebrovascular accidents, pulmonary infarction and large wound hematomas. Such bleeds may prompt heparin reversal with protamine sulphate. Further anticoagulation therapy should then await the stabilization of the patient and re-evaluation.

Acutely, heparin is used in the postoperative period to prevent recurrent embolus or thrombosis and is associated with lower mortality.[18] The trade-off is a 20% incidence of wound complications, including an 8% incidence of hematomas requiring drainage.[19]

FASCIOTOMY

Not infrequent are reperfusion injuries following revascularization of acute occlusions. Following limb revascularization, it is common for reperfusion to cause edema and, therefore, ACS. When the subfascial compartments become tense and, in particular, when compartment pressures exceed 30–40 mmHg, many surgeons feel that four-compartment fasciotomy is indicated to preserve circulation and enhance muscle viability.[20]

When the increased compartment pressure is due to direct tissue injury, hemorrhage or venous obstruction, fasciotomy is noncontroversial. However, when increased compartment pressure is due to swelling of ischemic muscle, fasciotomy that exposes this muscle will not necessarily reverse the damage, which is often irreversible necrosis. Exposed ischemic or dead muscle is vulnerable to infection, and when infection occurs above the knee, amputation is usually the necessary. Limbs are lost only when the skin is non-viable. Necrotic muscle, protected from infection, atrophies and resorbs. Lower leg muscles, which are the ones most commonly involved, affect ankle function, but a partially paralyzed limb is still functional. Moreover, a below-knee amputation, should this be required, is associated with much less disability than is amputation above the knee. Finally, the decision for or against fasciotomy is a judgement in which the risk/benefit ratio must be weighed. Fasciotomy is rarely necessary when the ischemic limb is revascularized within the period of muscle tolerance (6–8 hours of profound ischemia) or when the muscle is still functional.[20] However, once this time period has passed and revascularization is performed, a fasciotomy should be routinely considered, if not performed.

PEDIATRIC POPULATION

Management of acute limb ischemia in the pediatric population is especially difficult because of the patient's difficulty in verbalizing their symptoms, as well as the extremely small size of the vasculature involved. Acute arterial insufficiency in the pediatric population can be managed with anticoagulation, likely because of their enhanced ability to form collaterals, but also because of differences in their physiology and pharmacologic responses to anticoagulation. Current guidelines recommend therapeutic anticoagulation for a 5–7-day course with unfractionated heparin or LMWH in the pediatric population with acute femoral arterial thrombosis. The guidelines are limited, however, and do not provide recommendation in patients who improve but continue to demonstrate a clot burden on imaging, hypercoagulable patients or patients who also demonstrate venous thrombosis. Because of the paucity of specific guidelines for surgical intervention, even in the setting of traumatic injury, in pediatric patients, protocols are group and institution specific. However, the recurrence rate and risk of chronic vascular damage is significantly high. Surgical intervention is reserved for those with the threat of immediate limb loss. Risks of this include the risks of compartment syndrome and limb length discrepancies.[21]

UPPER EXTREMITY ISCHEMIA

Upper extremity ischemia is far less common than lower extremity ischemia, with an incidence of only 0.86–1.3 cases per 100,000 per year. Risk factors include advancing age and male sex, and possible etiologies include all of those previously mentioned for lower limb ischemia. In addition, thoracic outlet obstructions in the distal third of the subclavian artery can result in intimal damage, aneurysmal or poststenotic dilatation and subsequent atheroemboli or thrombosis.[22]

The presentation and treatment of arterial insufficiency in the upper extremity follow the same principles as in the lower extremity. The key factors to remember include the inherent risk of embolectomy in the comparatively diminutive size of the arteries in the upper extremity as well as the danger of dislodging thrombus into the carotid or vertebral arteries. Still, the mortality of upper extremity ischemia is lower and the rate of limb salvage higher, compared with lower extremity ischemia, presumably because of the increased collateralization. This collateralization also makes nonsurgical treatment with therapeutic anticoagulation more often effective than when used as the sole treatment modality in lower extremity ischemia.[23]

CEREBRAL ISCHEMIA

Embolism is responsible for approximately 20%–30% of all strokes, with the incidence of stroke being five times greater in patients with atrial fibrillation than in the general population.[24] Because the risk of recurrent stroke in these patients is approximately 20% per year, the treatment is directed at controlling cardiac arrhythmias and at preventing further cerebral infarctions with oral anticoagulants.[25]

VISCERAL ISCHEMIA

Most acute visceral ischemia occurs when the superior mesenteric artery is occluded by an embolus or by thrombosis. Abdominal catastrophe associated with cardiac disease is the classic setting. Traditionally, mortality has been extremely high, over 50%, and treatment has focused on resection of necrotic bowel rather than revascularization. However, revascularization by aorto-mesenteric bypass, trans-aortic endarterectomy or embolectomy may rarely be successful in the acute case. More recently, a combination of revascularization followed by resection of necrotic bowel has been advocated to improve mortality.[26] A second-look procedure may be indicated and is of particular value when marginal bowel has been left behind at the initial operation.

REFERENCES

1. Patel NH, Krishnamurthy VN, Kim S, Saad WE, Ganguli S, Walker TG, Nikolic B. Quality improvement guidelines for percutaneous management of acute lower-extremity ischemia. *J Vasc Interv Radiol.* 2013;24(1):3–15.
2. Abbot WM, Maloney RD, McCabe CC et al. Arterial embolism: A 44 year perspective. *Am J Surg.* 1982;143:460.
3. Lyaker MR, Tulman DB, Dimitrova GT et al. Arterial embolism. *Int J Crit Illn Inj Sci.* 2013 January–March;3(1):77–87.
4. Jivegard L, Holm J, Schersten T. Acute limb ischemia due to arterial embolism of thrombosis: Influence of limb ischemia versus pre-existing cardiac disease on postoperative mortality rate. *J Cardiovasc Surg.* 1988;29:32.
5. Blaisdell FW, Lim RG, Amberg JR et al. Pulmonary microembolism: A cause of morbidity and death after vascular surgery. *Arch Surg.* 1966;93:776.
6. Stallone RJ, Blaisdell FW, Cafferata HT, Levin SM. Analysis of morbidity and mortality from arterial embolectomy. *Surgery.* 1969;65:207.
7. Haimovici, H. Metabolic complications of acute arterial occlusions. *J Cardiovasc Surg.* 1979;20:349.
8. Nishide M, Irino T, Gotoh M et al. Cardiac abnormalities in ischemic cerebrovascular disease studied by two-dimensional echocardiography. *Stroke.* 1983;14:541.
9. Caplan LR, Hier DB, D'Cruz I. Cerebral embolism in the Michael Reese stroke registry. *Stroke.* 1983;14:530.
10. Robbins JA, Sagar KB, French M, Smith PJ. Influence of echocardiography on management of patients with systemic emboli. *Stroke.* 1983;14:546.
11. Blaisdell FW, Steele M, Allen RE. Management of acute lower extremity arterial ischemia due to embolism and thrombosis. *Surgery.* 1978;84:822.
12. Blaisdell FW. Use of anticoagulants in the ischemic lower extremity. In: Kempzczinkski RF, ed. *Management of Lower Extremity Ischemia.* Chicago, IL: Year Book; 1989.
13. Walker AM, Jick J. Predictors of bleeding during heparin therapy. *J Am Med Assoc.* 1980;244:1209.
14. Fogarty TJ, Cranley JJ, Krause RJ et al. A method for extraction of arterial emboli and thrombi. *Surg Gynecol Obstet.* 1963;116:241.
15. Berridge DC, Kessel DO, Robertson I. Surgery versus thrombolysis for initial management of acute limb ischaemia. *Cochrane Database Syst Rev.* 2013;6:CD002784.
16. Schrijver AM, Moll FL, De Vries JP. Hybrid procedures for peripheral obstructive disease. *J Cardiovasc Surg.* 2010;51(6):833–843.
17. Dosluoglu HH, Lall P, Cherr GS, Harris LM, Dryjski ML. Role of simple and complex hybrid revascularization procedures for symptomatic lower extremity occlusive disease. *J Vasc Surg.* 2010 June;51(6):1425–1435.
18. Holm J, Schersten T. Anticoagulant treatment during and after embolectomy. *Acta Chir Scand.* 1972;138:683.
19. Tawes RL, Beare JP, Scribner RG et al. Value of postoperative heparin therapy in peripheral arterial thromboembolism. *Am J Surg.* 1983;146:213.
20. Patman RD, Thompson JE. Fasciotomy in peripheral vascular surgery. *Arch Surg.* 1970;101:663.
21. Kayssi A, Shaikh F, Roche-Nagle G, Brandao LR, Williams SA, Rubin BB. Management of acute limb ischemia in the pediatric population. *J Vasc Surg.* 2014 July;60(1):106–110.
22. Haimovici H. Arterial thromboembolism of the upper extremity associated with thoracic outlet syndrome. *J Cardiovasc Surg.* 1982;23:214.

23. Coskun S, Soylu L, Coskun P, Bayazıt M. Short series of upper limb acute arterial occlusions in 4 different etiologies and review of literature. *Am J Emerg Med.* 2013 December;31(12):1719.e1-4.

24. Sage JI, Van Uitert RL. Risk of recurrent stroke in patients with atrial fibrillation and non-valvular heart disease. *Stroke.* 1983;14:537.

25. Easton JD, Sherman DG. Management of cerebral embolism of cardiac origin. *Stroke.* 1980;11:433.

26. Bergan JJ, Dean RH, Conn J, Yao JST. Revascularization in treatment of mesenteric infarction. *Ann Surg.* 1975;182:430.

27. Rutherford RB. Clinical staging of acute limb ischemia as the basis for choice of revascularization method: When and how to intervene. *Semin Vasc Surg.* 2009;22(1):5–9.

15

The pathophysiology of skeletal muscle reperfusion

DARIN J. SALTZMAN and DMITRI V. GELFAND

CONTENTS

INTRODUCTION

Rapid restoration of blood flow to the ischemic tissue is essential to minimize irreversible parenchymal damage. When obstruction times are minimal (<1.5 hours), full functional recovery of the tissue can be expected. Periods of 2–3 hours of ischemia followed by reperfusion will result in histological damage to a minority of fibres within the muscle; however, return of normal function is anticipated. Perfusion following a 4-hour ischemic period results in both functional and histologic damage, while return of blood supply after 6-hour ischemia will result in a significant functional deficit.[1] As such, it is generally agreed that ischemic times over 6 hours is detrimental to skeletal tissue in both traumatic and elective occlusions.

Although it is accepted that immediate release of obstruction is mandatory for tissue recovery, restoration of blood flow may elicit cell damage in what would otherwise appear as healthy tissue. Harman et al. commented that structural changes following reperfusion were not observed 'in muscles with unrelieved ischemia' and only 'occurred exclusively in ischemic muscles to which blood supply was readmitted'.[1] More recently Burkhardt et al. noted that reperfusion in a porcine limb rendered ischemic by 6-hour iliac artery ligation resulted in a significantly decreased functional recovery when compared to the recovery of a permanently ischemic limb without reperfusion (Figure 15.1). From this the authors concluded that uncontrolled reperfusion following prolonged ischemia had a 'negative impact' on the otherwise healthy tissue.[2] The sequela of reperfusion injury, therefore, appears to be most significant between 4 and 6 hours of ischemia. Skeletal tissue recovery for ischemic times less than 4 hours may be expected to regain function with little to no deficit, whereas ischemic times greater than 6 hours will result in considerable permanent damage.

The main goal of reperfusion is to replenish diminished nutrients (e.g. oxygen, glucose) and remove waste products. Following this immediate need, the repair of ischemic tissue damage ensues. This process is marked by the inflammatory reaction that can be roughly broken down into two components: the release of cytokines to initiate inflammation and the reactive phase often characterized by whole blood cellular components (e.g. neutrophils, macrophages) charged with breaking down and removing damage and necrotic tissue. Under normal conditions, these systems are tightly regulated; however, in extreme circumstance, such as prolonged ischemia, the ensuing inflammation may undergo an unfavourable imbalance that results in continued injury to the surrounding tissue.

The 'reflow paradox' is considered an accumulation of injurious free radicals in the ischemic limb that are

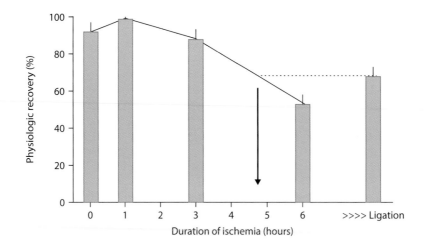

Figure 15.1 Functional muscle recovery for ischemic times (shown in hours) followed by 14 days of reperfusion. The bar labelled 'ligation' denotes permanent occlusion without reperfusion. Extrapolating the curve between 3 and 6 hours of ischemia demonstrates that an ischemic period of 4.7 hours would lead to a similar functional recovery to that of permanent occlusion. Ischemia followed by flow restoration for time periods greater than this would theoretically lead to a poorer recovery when compared to permanent ligation. (Adapted from Burkhardt GE et al., *J Vasc Surg*, 53, 165, 2011.)

generated in abundance during reperfusion and has been implicated in initiating an uncontrolled inflammatory response.[3] This may be due to an excess generation of these toxic metabolites and/or an inability to scavenge these molecules. In either case, the result is progressive damage during blood flow restoration to tissue. It is believed that if the production of these radicals were halted or kept to a minimum, a significant degree of organ injury could be circumvented. The 'no-reflow phenomenon'[4] is an event that is characterized by the continued impairment to restored blood flow despite the removal of the obstructing source (Figure 15.2). This persistent obstruction may be an independent inflammatory event or may be exacerbated by and/or a result of generated oxygen radicals (reflow paradox) during reperfusion.

To minimize reperfusion damage, investigations by either pharmacologic or mechanical means are underway. These studies are looking at ways to lessen injury during the ischemic period (predominately in elective cases) and during the initial minutes of reperfusion.

CLINICAL MANIFESTATIONS OF REPERFUSION INJURY

Edema

Clinical manifestations of reperfusion injury may occur independently or in combination. At the macro level, tissue edema as a result of increased capillary permeability and microcirculatory dysfunction is the first indication of

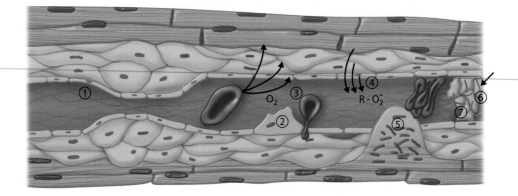

Figure 15.2 Theoretical mechanisms involved in the 'no-reflow' phenomenon. Continued microvascular obstruction during reperfusion has been observed despite a patent flowing feed artery. Mechanisms include smooth muscle vasoconstriction, endothelial and muscle cell swelling and protrusion into the capillary, red blood cell (RBC) and platelet aggregation and neutrophil plugging secondary to an inflammatory response. These may be a response to or independent of the pathology resulting from toxic oxygen radical formations. (1) Smooth muscle vasoconstriction. (2) Endothelial Δ's (swelling, protrusion). (3) Leukocyte adherence. (4) Oxygen radical formation. (5) Parenchymal Δ's (swelling, blebs). (6) RBC stasis. (7) Platelet aggregation.

muscle compromise during reperfusion. If not sufficient to cause deleterious events, this edema in itself will often resolve without any residual effects. In extreme cases, however, this edema especially in closed compartments can result in increased tissue pressures that will result in obstruction to capillary and venous blood flow. If not addressed (e.g. by fasciotomy), a pressure increase will continue leading to arteriole occlusion and nerve pathology followed by persistent ischemia with resultant tissue death and necrosis.

Artery and vein vasospasm

Changes to the macrocirculation with reperfusion with longer ischemic times are evident by the presence of large vessel vasospasm. This may be severe enough that persistent oxygen deprivation continues. The cause for this vasospasm, either a pathologic result of reperfusion or an unrestrained compensatory effect to control perfusion following ischemia, remains unclear.

Microvascular thrombosis and obstruction

Reperfusion injuries with ischemic times indicative of complex transplantation procedures may manifests itself by the gradual reduction of tissue perfusion despite a widely patent feeding artery. This is often characterized by a reduction or obstruction in venous outflow as a result of microvascular and/or venous thrombosis.

Multi-organ failure

Reperfusion of large volumes of ischemic tissue incurs compensatory modifications and damage to distant organs, such as the cardiopulmonary, renal, hepatobiliary and gastrointestinal systems. Washout of the toxic metabolites causes a significant rise in systemic lactate and hydrogen ions affecting the acid–base balance and can trigger a systemic inflammatory response. Cardiac arrhythmias are often the first sign of systemic ion shifts. The pulmonary system secondary to release of injurious cytokines can become compromised within 24–72 resulting in acute respiratory distress.[5] Rhabdomyolysis secondary to a large release of myoglobin often precipitates acute renal damage.[6] Multi-organ failure is a devastating consequence of remote reperfusion injury and is associated with high mortality rates.[7]

MICROVASCULAR ARTERIOLE AND VENULE ANATOMY

To appreciate events that occur in the parenchyma during ischemia and reperfusion, it is important to understand the basic anatomic structure and physiology of the microcirculation.[8] Skeletal muscle microcirculation (Figure 15.3), consisting of arterioles, capillaries and venules, will undergo significant functional and structural adjustments during ischemia. Microvascular derangement can be exacerbated by rapid metabolic and ionic alterations

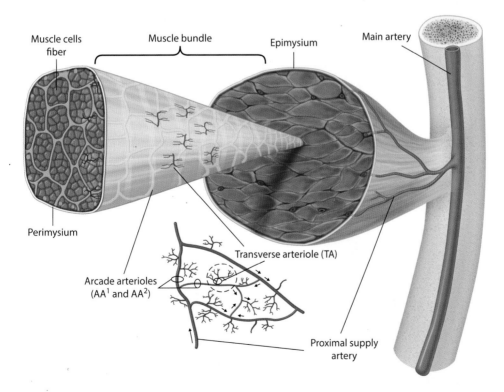

Figure 15.3 Schematic representation of skeletal muscle microcirculation observed in human and animal studies. Feeding arteries (long arrows) provide blood to the arcade 'mesh-like' network. Blood flow (short arrows) in arcade arterioles (AA[1] and AA[2]) can shift depending on the needs of tissue. Transition of multidirectional to unidirectional flow occurs at the transverse arteriole (TA). The TA delivers blood to a unit of tissue via the capillary bed.

during reperfusion, which in turn may further compromise the surrounding tissue.

The arteriolar network in skeletal muscle is dominated by arcades located in the fascial planes of the perimysium (Figure 15.4a and b) that give rise to an array of transverse arterioles[9] that provide the conduits from the arcading system to the capillary network. The arcade arteriolar network allows for a uniform pressure along the entry points along the transverse arterioles,[10] and depending on the tissue demand, small rapid pressure gradient changes in the arcade arterioles will allow for bidirectional flow to shunt red blood cells (RBCs) to the tissue sections in need of perfusion.[9]

The majority of arcade vessels have one or two layers of smooth muscle cells in their media, whereas the majority of transverse arterioles have only a single smooth muscle layer.[11] The adrenergic innervation of these small arteries and arterioles is limited to the layer between the adventitia and the smooth muscle.[12] Small arterioles tend to display a high density of innervation with the highest innervation at the root of the transverse arteriole when compared to arteries (Figure 15.5).[13] The correlation between sympathetic function and innervation density[14] has been supported by previous studies that have demonstrated that arterioles with diameters <25 μm exhibit a striking vasoconstrictor response to both electrical and chemical stimuli.[15]

In skeletal muscle, the largest pressure drop occurs across the transverse arterioles[10] and these vessels have

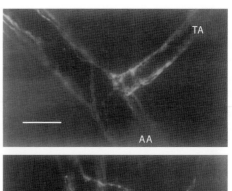

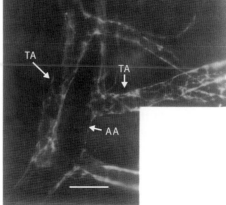

Figure 15.5 Adrenergic density in the arcade arteriole (AA) and transverse arteriole (TA). The TA root has the highest length of adrenergic nerve fibre per area of smooth muscle when compared to the larger AAs and the smaller precapillary arterioles. Capillaries were devoid of innervation.

the greatest tone along the arteriole network. The location of these transverse arterioles, their tone, degree of innervation and responsiveness to sympathetic stimulation are compatible with a microvascular design in which flow in a capillary bundle is regulated by the inflow from this vessel (Figure 15.3). Furthermore, these transverse arterioles appear to be in a strategic position to control RBC oxygen supply to the capillary network (Figure 15.6) and as a consequence may dictate survival in pathological conditions such as hemorrhagic or septic shock.[16] A similar control mechanism has also been reported to exist in cat sartorius muscle.[17]

PATHOPHYSIOLOGY OF REPERFUSION

The recent decades has brought on an explosion of reperfusion injury research. Investigations expand from the exploration of reactive radical molecules and DNA to whole organ responses to perfusion perturbations (Figure 15.7). Tremendous amount of work has been done to uncover the inciting events with the hope of providing a therapy to circumvent or minimize collateral injury associated with reperfusion. Whether one primary episode or the accumulation of multiple occurrences exists is still under question.

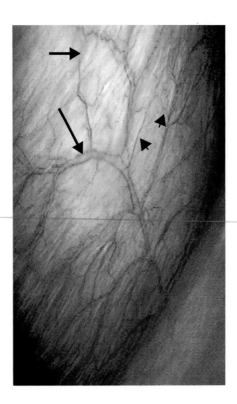

Figure 15.4 The arcade arteriole in the fascial planes with branching transverse arterioles. The larger arrows and arrowheads mark the boundaries of the arcade loop.

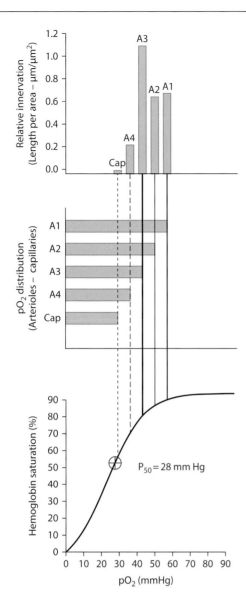

Figure 15.6 Oxygen distribution in arcade arterioles (A1 and A2), transverse arterioles (A3), precapillary arterioles (A4) and capillaries (Cap). The transverse arteriole has an oxygen tension (pO$_2$) that corresponds to the 'knee' position of the of the oxygen dissociation curve for hemoglobin. These arterioles also have the highest degree of innervation (length of nerve per area of smooth muscle). The location, anatomy and physiology of these vessels suggest that these vessels are instrumental in regulating oxygen supply to a unit of tissue. (Adapted from Intaglietta M et al., *Cardiovasc Res*, 32, 632, 1996.)

Generation and scavenging of oxygen free radicals (reflow paradox)

Reactive oxygen species (ROS) sometimes referred to as oxygen radicals are ubiquitous and are involved in many biochemical reactions: electron transport chain, cell signalling, destruction of foreign pathogens and bodies, etc. These molecules are highly reactive and under normal conditions are kept under tight regulatory control.

In adverse conditions of hypoxia, the depletion of oxygen, the natural sequester of these radicals, causes a disturbance in the regulatory pathways resulting in an accumulation of free radical intermediates[18] that damage surrounding cellular components such as cellular and mitochondrial membranes, proteins and DNA.[19]

During reperfusion, the ischemic tissue becomes re-oxygenated and a burst of oxygen radicals dependent upon the ischemic time occurs[3] producing significant damage to the surrounding muscle.[20] Mitochondria and xanthine oxidase, an enzyme involved in the catabolism of purines, are considered to be the predominant pathways of oxygen radical formation. Xanthine oxidase, an enzyme involved in the catabolism of purines, is considered to be the predominate pathway of oxygen radical formation (Figure 15.8).[21] The formation of these radicals can 'attack' nearby fatty acids and start a chain reaction of lipid peroxidation that further destabilizes the membrane allowing ions to leak through. These radicals, in addition, can damage membrane proteins interrupting receptor recognition and signal transduction.[22] The body's defence is to remove these radicals via antioxidant enzymes. Proteins that have been identified with antioxidant properties include superoxide dismutase (SOD), catalase and glutathione peroxidase (GSHPX).[22]

THERAPY: ANTIOXIDANTS

There have been numerous animal studies demonstrating beneficial outcomes of antioxidants in skeletal muscle reperfusion injury.[23] Clinical trials utilizing recombinant human superoxide dismutase (h-SOD) and edaravone (a potent antioxidant) in cardiac muscle to scavenge oxygen radicals, however, have been generally disappointing.[24] Allopurinol, an inhibitor of xanthine oxidase, in some human trials has shown some beneficial result against cardiac reperfusion injury;[25] however, the data are limited. A decrease in skeletal muscle injury, similarly, was demonstrated when acute limb ischemic patients were revascularized utilizing a controlled perfusate containing allopurinol.[26] Unfortunately, a randomized multicentre trial implementing the same protocol did not exhibit improved outcomes when compared to immediate reperfusion by conventional treatment thromboembolectomy.[27]

Mannitol, a sugar and an isomer of sorbitol, has been investigated as an oxygen radical scavenger[28] and used clinically for limb salvage revascularization.[29] Animal investigations, however, have casted doubt on its usefulness,[30] and in a human investigation, mannitol given during and after release of the tourniquet did not influence the oxidative stress seen during reperfusion.[31] Mannitol is routinely used as an adjunct to minimize renal injury, and in a randomized clinical double-blinded trial in patients with off pump cardiac surgery, it was shown to improve intravascular oxygenation and a reduction in creatine kinase MB compared to control.[32] This protective effect, however, may be more attributed to its hyperosmolality rather than its antioxidant properties. Randomized clinical trials are needed to test the efficacy of mannitol in skeletal reperfusion injury.

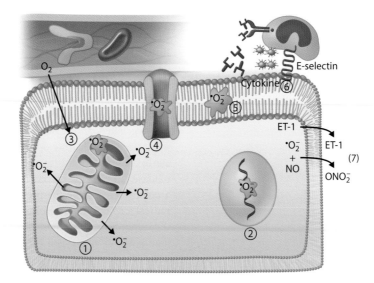

Figure 15.7 Reperfusion injury has been shown to generate (1) toxic oxygen radicals injure (2) DNA, (3) mitochondria, (4) cell membrane proteins and (5) cytoskeleton and cause (6) inflammatory and ion changes and (7) alterations in endothelial function. Endothelin 1 (ET-1), Nitric Oxide (NO), Peroxynitrite (ONO_2^-).

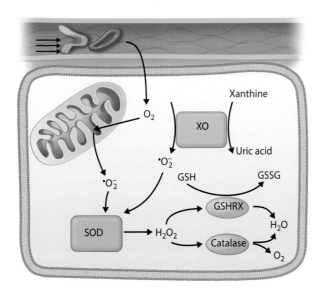

Figure 15.8 Reperfusion following significant ischemia results in the generation of oxygen radicals by mitochondria and the enzyme xanthine oxidase (XO), which is involved in the catabolism of purines. These toxic molecules are scavenged by superoxide dismutase (SOD), catalase and glutathione peroxidase (GSHPX) an enzyme that converts reduced glutathione (GSH) to its oxidized form (GSSG).

Numerous animal investigations of shock, sepsis and ischemia–reperfusion injury have demonstrated beneficial outcomes of ethyl pyruvate in a ringer's solution.[33] Ethyl pyruvate, an alpha-keto acid, has the ability to scavenge both H_2O_2 and hydroxyl radicals.[34] However, a double-blind placebo-controlled study in patients undergoing cardiac surgery did not show any benefit compared to the placebo.[35] Ongoing investigations, nevertheless, continue despite these discouraging findings.

N-acetylcysteine (NAC; Mucomyst) works as an anti-oxidant by replenishing glutathione stores and has shown promise in animal trials in minimizing skeletal reperfusion injury.[36] Interestingly, in a randomized clinical trial investigating cardiac reperfusion injury, NAC was shown to reduce oxidative stress in patients undergoing primary angioplasty following acute myocardial infarction; however, this did not translate into an improvement of myocardial reperfusion injury.[37] Looking at skeletal muscle, a randomized trail investigating reperfusion injury following tourniquet ischemia, similarly, yielded a protective effect against oxidative injury when patients were given NAC 30 minutes prior to the tourniquet application.[38] Functional recovery, however, was not addressed so how these results translate to a clinical improvement remains uncertain.

Despite many studies that have investigated therapeutic antioxidants, the variability in experimental protocols and therapeutic approaches have lead to questions regarding their efficacy in ischemia–reperfusion injury. 'Tightening' the scientific design will hopefully provide a clear picture and conclusive role of these promising agents.[39,40]

Nucleotide dysfunction

ROS generated during reperfusion have deleterious effects on DNA. Restoration of these strands accounts for a significant depletion of adenosine triphosphate (ATP). The main role of polyadenosine diphosphate-ribose polymerase (PARP), found in the cell's nucleus, is detection and repair of DNA damage. The consequence, however, appears to be at the expense of depleting pivotal energy needed for other essential structural and biologic cell functions.[41]

In addition, cell injury secondary to hypoxia and reactive radicals during reperfusion causes the cell to express toll-like receptors (TLRs). These receptors are involved in a number of singling pathways to release cytokines, chemokines and interferons that are involved in inflammatory pathways. After ischemia–reperfusion injury, these TLRs respond to both endogenous and exogenous signals resulting in the activation of numerous inflammatory mediators that can exacerbate cell damage and induce apoptosis.[42]

THERAPY: PARP INHIBITOR

Animal studies investigating PARP inhibitors in cardiac, cerebral and pulmonary reperfusion injuries have shown promising results.[43–45] In animals treated with PARP inhibitors and in PARP-1 knockout mice muscle viability during reperfusion following 3 hours of tourniquet ischemia was increased, when compared to untreated mice.[46] Human clinical trials involving skeletal reperfusion injury involving PARP inhibitors have not been reported yet, but these new classes of agents may provide a novel therapeutic approach.

THERAPY: TLR ANTAGONIST

The role of TLR antagonist is to block the cascade that leads to the activation of transcriptions factors that release pro-inflammatory cytokines with the goal of minimizing reperfusion injury. In support of this, studies in mutant TLR4 mice involving hindlimb reperfusion damage have demonstrated significantly reduced injury when compared to wild type mice.[47]

There are limited numbers of TLR antagonist available for therapeutic interventions in skeletal muscle reperfusion injury; however, of the few in existence, promising results have been shown in clinical trials. Eritoran tetrasodium (E5564) inhibits Lipopolysaccharides (LPS)-induced inflammation by blocking TLR 4 and has been shown to provide some benefit in patients with sepsis.[48,49]

Mitochondrial dysfunction

Mitochondria are the main source of ATP used to carry out the cell's biologic function. In human tissues, the mitochondrial electron transport chain generates 80%–90% of the cell's ATP.[50] The mitochondrial membrane, when not stressed, is impermeable in order to maintain the membrane potential essential for generation of ATP via oxidative phosphorylation. The mitochondria are also the largest producers of ROS. During ischemia and the period followed by reperfusion, ATP production, which is essential for repair mechanisms and functional recovery of the cell, is blunted. This occurs when overproduction of ROS causes pathologic mitochondrial membrane swelling and rupture.[51] In addition, cardiolipin, a phospholipid composed mainly of linoleic acid, involved in terminal enzyme complex of the mitochondrial respiratory chain, is adversely affected by ischemia–reperfusion injury. As a result the mitochondrial inner membrane is disrupted thereby altering the physiologic function.[52] Integrity of the outer mitochondrial membrane, similarly, may be compromised. Hexokinase II, an outer mitochondrial membrane protein, has been shown to protect skeletal muscle from ischemia–reperfusion injury.

Stabilization or upregulation of this protein may offer potential means to reduce reperfusion damage.[53]

THERAPY: AICA-RIBOSE

Acadesine (AICA-riboside) is a purine nucleoside analogue that has been shown to provide therapeutic benefit in cardiac reperfusion injury. Although the therapeutic benefits were thought to come from being an intermediate for ATP generation, it is now believed that the benefits may be related to the activation of AMP-activated protein kinase (AMPK). AMPKs have been shown to be important regulators of energetic stress pathways, some of which in skeletal muscle include, vasodilation via nitric oxide (NO) pathway,[54] increase glucose uptake[55] and mitochondrial biogenesis.[56] Although clinical applications for myocardial ischemia–reperfusion injury have yielded mixed results,[57] this class of compounds may hold some promise for skeletal muscle reperfusion.

THERAPY: EXOGENOUS ADENOSINE

The use of exogenous adenosine has been studied extensively in cardiac ischemia–reperfusion injury.[58] Reduction in reperfusion injury has been shown in cardiac and skeletal muscle, however, the mechanism for that protection is still under debate.[59] Exogenous adenosine not only increases intracellular ATP, but also, by increasing microvascular vasodilation and by enhancing glucose transport to increase energy protection, provides a protective effect by limiting ROS.[58]

THERAPY: DIPYRIDAMOLE

Endogenous adenosine, similarly, protects against reperfusion injury by inhibiting inflammation and platelet aggregation.[60] Dipyridamole given to human control subjects twice daily over a week prior to an elective ischemic insult (as would be seen in some orthopedic cases) was shown to limit ischemia–reperfusion injury in human muscle.

This was achieved by dipyridamole's ability to increase extracellular adenosine concentrations by inhibiting adenosine cellular uptake into erythrocytes, platelets and endothelial cells.[61] The protection mechanism is assumed that by the limiting ADP uptake by microvessel RBCs, the concentration gradient between the parenchymal tissues (the predominate source of ADP) and intravascular plasma is significantly reduced, thereby minimizing muscle release of endogenous ADP.[62] Clinical trials are needed to confirm this protection.

THERAPY: SS-31

The acute insult from ischemia followed by reperfusion on the mitochondria will result with a swollen organelle and loss of the crista membrane. Szeto-Schiller (SS) peptides have been shown to minimize peroxidation injury to cardiolipin, a key structural component of the mitochondrial membrane.[63] These specific mitochondrial inner membrane SS peptides have been shown to reduce mitochondrial injury by oxygen radicals in mice skeletal muscle.[64] Phase II clinical trials investigating Bendavia (SS-31) for cardiac reperfusion injury are underway.[65]

Mitochondrial and cell membrane ionic shifts

During the ischemic period, mitochondria adjust their biochemistry to adapt to the changing hypoxic environment by switching to the glycolysis pathway (Figure 15.9). This produces an increase in intracellular H^+ ions.[66] To protect against this increased acidity, the Na^+-H^+ exchange pump is activated and an increase in intracellular $[Na^+]$ occurs. In a normal physiologic environment, the Na^+-K^+ ATPase exchange pump would react to bring $[Na^+]$ back to appropriate levels; however, because of the hypoxic environment, the energy needed for this exchange is not available. An increased intracellular $[Na^+]$ will also influence the Na^+/Ca^{2+} gradient and consequently minimize Ca^{2+} extrusion via the Na^+-Ca^{2+} exchanger. The result is an increased intracellular $[Ca^{2+}]$. During reperfusion, a rapid washout of extracellular H^+ causes an increase in the Na^+-H^+ exchanger to maintain the cellular pH environment further increasing intracellular sodium, leading to a further $[Ca^{2+}]$ increase.[67] This intracellular calcium overload will lead to non-specific mitochondrial inner membrane pores to open creating mitochondrial membrane changes that will eventually lead to irreversible damage. A decrease in respiratory chain and ATPase activity with a concomitant decrease in adenine nucleoside content will follow.[68]

THERAPY: CYCLOSPORIN

Cyclosporin has been suggested to block the mitochondrial membrane pore opening thereby minimizing energy loss that occurs with reperfusion injury.[69] This has been supported by the pretreatment with a single-dose of cyclosporin to improve tissue oxygenation and minimize mitochondrial damage in rabbit skeletal muscle subjected to 4 hours of ischemia followed by 2 hours of reperfusion.

THERAPY: Na/H INHIBITION

Cariporide, a Na^+-H^+ exchange inhibitor, when given 10 minutes before 4 hour ischemia or at the onset of reperfusion significantly minimized skeletal tissue infarction in porcine latissimus dorsi muscle flaps.[70] Inhibition of the Na^+-H^+ exchange is believed to minimize the intracellular $[Na^+]$. This in turn maintains the Na^+/Ca^{2+} gradient needed for proper functioning of the Na^+-Ca^{2+} exchanger thereby minimizing mitochondrial $[Ca^{2+}]$ overload.[70] Although results observed in clinical studies of cardiac reperfusion injury have been discouraging, some trials have shown beneficial results in minimizing reperfusion necrosis in controlled conditions given prior to cardiac ischemia.[71] Clinical trials are needed to determine if these findings, observed in elective cardiac operations, translate to elective vascular and orthopedic procedures.

THERAPY: CALCIUM CHANNEL BLOCKERS

Earlier clinical studies of verapamil to treat myocardial 'no-reflow' seen in cardiac reperfusion injury demonstrated positive results by increasing microvascular flow. The mechanism of these pharmacologic therapies was believed to alleviate vasospasm during reperfusion and allow the much needed flow to the otherwise non-perfused tissue.[72,73] In animal models, skeletal muscle injury was minimized with the use of calcium channel blockers, although there was no difference in microvascular flow between treated and non-treated animals.[74] In a more recent randomized phase III clinical trial, the use of a purinergic receptor antagonist, which had been shown to prevent calcium overload and minimize cardiac injury in a prior clinical phase II study,[75] did not reduce the rate of myocardial infarction or cardiovascular death compared to placebo.[76] The use of calcium channel blockers is still under debate and more clinical investigations are needed to prove their efficacy.

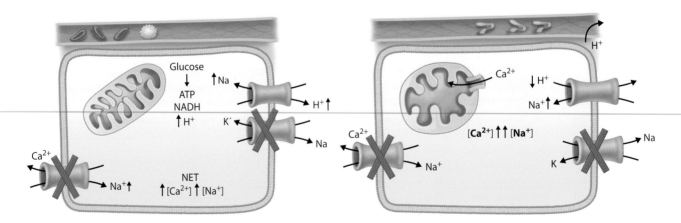

Figure 15.9 During ischemia the cell reverts to glycolysis and an intracellular increase in hydrogen atoms occurs. The sodium–hydrogen (Na^+-H^+) exchange pump is activated to minimize the intracellular acidic environment. Since there is a decrease of ATP, the sodium–potassium (Na^+-K^+) ATPase pump is hampered which causes an increase in intracellular sodium. This increase in $[Na^+]$ causes a shift in the gradient that is needed for the sodium–calcium (Ca^{2+}-Na^+) exchanger to function. The result is a rise of intracellular $[Ca^{2+}]$. During reperfusion a rapid washout of the hydrogen atoms causes a further increase in intracellular $[Na^+]$ leading to a further increase in intracellular $[Ca^{2+}]$. Intracellular calcium overload is thought to result in the mitochondrial pores to open leading to irreversible mitochondrial membrane damage.

Cell membrane and cytoskeleton dysfunction

Oxidative injury to skeletal muscle and its microvasculature will initiate degradation of cellular components that can be exacerbated by reperfusion.[3,77] Ion changes during reperfusion can precipitate a net water cytosol influx, cell gap junction dysfunction, enzyme and membrane alterations and a Ca^{2+} cytosol overload that will lead to uncontrolled myofibril contraction and eventual irreversible cell injury.[67] This in turn can lead to increased capillary permeability, leakage of cytosolic enzymes, intracellular edema and blebs that can lead to microvascular obstruction and cell death (Figure 15.10).[78]

THERAPY: MEMBRANE REPAIR – MG53 PROTEIN

A recently discovered protein, Mitsugumin 53 (MG53), has been shown to be involved in acute membrane repair of skeletal and cardiac muscle, intracellular vesicle trafficking and myogenesis.[79] Consequently, MG53 is believed to be vital in the protective effects of ischemic pre- and postconditioning against cardiac ischemia–reperfusion injury[80] as well as skeletal muscle damage repair induced by exercise injury.[81] These studies point to potential therapeutic promise in skeletal muscle reperfusion injury; however, a recent study involving rat skeletal muscle ischemia–reperfusion damage has cast some concerns in its effectiveness.[82] Nevertheless, this is an exciting new field that is being aggressively investigated. Its benefit in skeletal reperfusion injury will undoubtedly be explored in great detail.

THERAPY: POLOXAMER 188

Compartment syndrome as previously mentioned is a deleterious outcome of muscle edema. Efforts to minimize this acute injury by membrane repair utilizing poloxamer 188 (P-188) have shown promising results in ischemia–reperfusion injury in animal studies.[83,84] P-188 is a surfactant that has been demonstrated to seal damaged membranes during reperfusion and, in addition, has been observed to inhibit inflammatory reactions of neutrophils.[85,86] Although human randomized clinical trials in cardiac reperfusion injury demonstrated beneficial results,[87] clinical trials for skeletal reperfusion injury are needed to explore the potential of this novel therapy.

Endothelial dysfunction

An increasing number of investigations have pointed to the endothelial cell as 'ground zero' of reperfusion injury. During ischemia and early reperfusion, endothelium alterations 'trigger' a sequence of events that result in tissue and microvascular damage.[88] It has been well known that these cells have a unique influence on the vascular reactivity via mechanism of paracrine signalling through nitric oxide or endothelin.[89]

A number of reports have demonstrated arteriole vasoconstriction during reperfusion,[90,91] and it has been suggested to occur in human cardiac microvessels following percutaneous coronary intervention.[92] Its contribution to the 'no-reflow' phenomenon, however, is largely unknown. A robust response to physiologic shifts in the surrounding environment is facilitated by the intimate contact and communication between the endothelium and vascular smooth muscle. As a consequence, alterations in the endothelium or smooth muscle may lead to a pathologic vasoreactivity.[93]

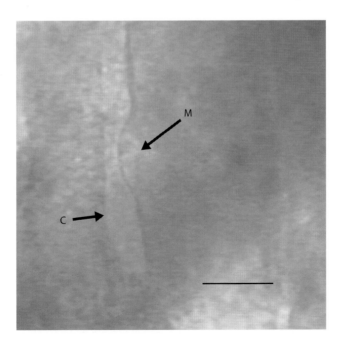

Figure 15.10 During ischemia and subsequent reperfusion, the cellular cytoskeleton can be damaged, leading to muscle cell swelling and blebs of the membrane (M) that can protrude into and increase the microhemodynamic resistance of surrounding capillaries (C).

Mast cell degranulation mediated by adenosine may also play a prominent role in arteriole vasoconstriction during reperfusion.[94]

Nitric oxide is involved in a number of cell functions including vasorelaxation of smooth muscle, capillary permeability and membrane expression of cell adhesion molecules (CAMs). During ischemia, nitric oxide levels decrease in the endothelial cells leading to vessel smooth muscle contraction and during reperfusion will lead to vasospasm that may contribute and prolong the no-reflow condition.[95] Decreased levels of nitric oxide, in addition to causing an increased microvascular permeability, may lead to increased P-selectin membrane expression resulting in increase neutrophil and platelet aggregation.[96] The destructive effects of neutrophil activation coupled with the increased permeability are thought to be a major contributing factor to the increased tissue damage during reperfusion.[88]

Endothelin is a peptide produced in endothelium that produces vascular smooth muscle contraction.[97] Hypoxia induces release of endothelin[98] and peak levels can be observed during reperfusion.[89] It is probable that NO and endothelin are both active in healthy vessel endothelium to allow for a homeostatic balance that can adjust depending on the tissue's needs. Ischemia followed by reperfusion appears to adversely affect this balance perpetuating a pathologic vasoconstriction.[99]

THERAPY: NITRIC OXIDE

Exogenous sources of NO such as sodium nitroprusside (SNP) and nicorandil used in cardiac clinical trials have proven beneficial in minimizing reperfusion injury.[100,101] Although there is a lack of clinical trials utilizing NO donors in skeletal muscle reperfusion injury, there has been a suggestion that the beneficial effects of AICA-riboside (see earlier text) in human studies are mediated by NO-dependent mechanism.[54] The mechanisms of these positive outcomes via vasodilation and/or anti-inflammatory properties have generated numerous investigations.[90,102]

THERAPY: ENDOTHELIN BLOCKER

Much of the current human studies involving endothelin inhibition involve studies of forearm blood flow.[99] Clinical trials involving short-term endothelin A receptor blockade for on-pump CABG patients are currently underway (Clinical Trial Number: NCT01658410). Although these studies are supported by the positive results of animal investigations, there has been a lack of clinical investigations with regard to skeletal muscle reperfusion injury.[89] Despite this, these new pharmacologic therapies may prove promising and warrant further investigation.

THERAPY: INFLAMMATORY INHIBITORS

The past two decades has generated numerous interest and investigations into adhesion molecules and their contribution to ischemia–reperfusion damage.[103] Clinical trials in cardiac reperfusion injury utilizing monoclonal antibodies against P-selectin have yielded beneficial outcomes.[104] Other trials, however, blocking integrin receptors CD11/CD18 and complement pathway have not yielded positive results[105,106] despite the encouraging findings from animal investigations.[107] Further clinical trials are needed to determine the benefits associated with blocking these inflammatory mediators.

Microvascular obstruction during reperfusion (no-reflow phenomenon)

During ischemia, capillary endothelium swells and undergoes structural changes[108] that protrude into the capillary lumen thereby increasing vessel resistance (Figure 15.11). These structural changes can be exacerbated during reperfusion dramatically increasing the resistance in the terminal arterioles.[109] This may result in the entrapment of white blood cells[110] and create an environment that creates blood stagnation resulting in the beginning events of thrombosis.[111] Platelet activation can result in increased platelet clumping and secretion of cytokines. This in turn will impact vessel vasoreactivity and increase recruitment

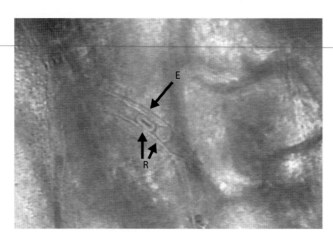

Figure 15.11 Changes in the endothelium (E) cytoskeleton or endothelial swelling may impede capillary flow by protruding into the capillary and trapping or compressing red (R) or white blood cells.

of other cellular and complement components that are deleterious to the surrounding tissue.[112] This is also believed to be indicative of hyperacute allograft rejection.[113]

THERAPY: ANTI-NEUTROPHILS

There is an abundance of evidence that supports neutrophil depletion or receptor blockade reduces cardiac reperfusion injury in experimental models.[114] Clinical trials, however, have failed to show beneficial outcomes with regard to reperfusion injury in acute stroke[115,116] and acute myocardial infarction.[105] Studies have demonstrated that parenchymal injury may occur prior to leukocyte plugging and suggested that neutrophil trapping may be a *result* of tissue injury and not an initiator of reperfusion damage.[117] The limited success of these clinical studies also brings into question if the microvascular permeability associated with injury is actually attributed to the interaction between the endothelium and the leukocyte.[118] Investigations are needed to determine if the mechanisms leading to leukocyte adhesion and plugging are distinct (or the same) from those mechanisms that trigger the harmful oxidative burst attributed to neutrophil activation.[118]

THERAPY: ANTI-THROMBOSIS

Antiplatelets such as clopidogrel are a mainstay therapy following thrombolysis or thrombectomy. These agents are used with the intent to prevent platelet activation, aggregation and adhesion in the compromised or damaged vessels during the reperfusion period. The role of coagulation pathology in microvessels and its contribution to the no-reflow phenomenon, however, are still under debate.[119,120] Nevertheless, clinical trials involving these drug classes of $P2Y_{12}$ platelet inhibitors have shown beneficial results in improving cardiovascular outcomes following reperfusion.[121] Newer $P2Y_{12}$ antiplatelet therapies are currently in clinical trials to investigate the influence of these drugs on microvascular flow.[122]

OTHER THERAPEUTIC INTERVENTIONS

Controlled perfusion

Initial clinical trials that controlled the perfusate content and perfusion pressure demonstrated promising results.[26] The belief was that by controlling the perfusion pressure, the degree and burst of metabolic waste washout into the systemic vasculature could be regulated in a manner that it would not create a shock to the circulatory system.[123] Adding substrates to the perfusion media to provide antioxidants, ATP and glucose replenishment and a buffer to minimize effects of systemic acidosis and calcium overload was shown to minimize reperfusion injury.[124] Despite promising results, randomized clinical trials have failed to show a significant difference between controlled and conventional treatment following acute limb ischemia.[27] Technical limitations and protocol violations may have attributed

to the lack of significance. Future research in optimizing and refining controlled perfusion therapy may validate the positive outcomes seen in the previous studies.

Preconditioning/postconditioning/remote pre- and postconditioning

Reimer et al., when investigating the lethality of 40 minutes continuous versus 40 minutes of intermittent coronary occlusion, determined that brief episodes of ischemia improved tissue survivability when faced with a subsequent longer periods of blood flow obstruction.[125] This phenomenon was later coined as 'preconditioning', and since these initial studies, numerous clinical trials subjecting patients to brief periods of ischemia prior to cardiac surgery have demonstrated some beneficial results.[126] Events that lead to an unplanned acute ischemic event, however, may not benefit from this intervention, and therefore, investigations to look at intermittent periods of controlled ischemia during reperfusion (postconditioning) were explored with the hope that this therapy may take advantage of the physiologic protection mechanisms observed in preconditioning.[127] Although smaller clinical trials investigating postconditioning have demonstrated similar promising results in limiting reperfusion damage in cardiac tissue, a recent meta-analysis has questioned the efficacy of this modality.[128] These pre- and postconditioning trials, however, have led to further studies that apply a pressure cuff to an uninvolved limb during a myocardial insult to produce intermittent ischemic periods termed 'remote conditioning' and can be applied to the patient in transit.[129] Randomized clinical trials have demonstrated positive results with this mode of cardioprotection against reperfusion injury.[130]

Although much of this work has been pioneered in subjects with cardiac pathology, numerous animal experiments have demonstrated similar positive outcomes in minimizing skeletal muscle reperfusion injury.[131] The protection mechanism is thought to involve the preservation of the mitochondrial respiratory chain by stabilizing the membrane potential thus preserving the mitochondrial pore function (see earlier text).[132] The ability to produce this protective effect during reperfusion without the use of a pharmacologic agent in addition to it being relatively safe has made this new approach an attractive and compelling therapy. Investigational findings have produced encouraging results and therefore have prompted a call to randomized clinical trials of 'remote pre- and postconditioning' in major vascular procedures.[126,133]

Hypothermia

Hypothermia during elective cardiac surgery and following an ischemic cardiac event is done routinely to minimize neurologic and myocardial ischemia–reperfusion injury. Recent randomized controlled trials and reviews, however, have questioned the efficacy of this adjunct therapy.[134-136] The rational for hypothermia is to minimize the inflammatory process and preserve ATP. This practice has been implemented to preserve an amputated limb prior to re-implantation and yet has not been used in elective or emergent revascularization procedures. Animal studies have shown that local hypothermia to the ischemic limb minimizes the inflammatory process during reperfusion,[137] but unfortunately the authors could not comment on functional recovery. Concern for microvascular vasoconstriction and contribution to multiorgan failure in the trauma patient[138] has subdued the excitement for this modality to minimize reperfusion injury in limb revascularization.

Therapeutic angiogenesis

Interventions that focus on the repair process by increasing collateral flow to the ischemic tissue via angiogenesis have undergone intensive investigation.[139] The hypoxic environment causes an upregulation of hematopoietic and vascular modulators that regulate genes aimed at increasing and remodelling the microvasculature of the effected tissue. Some of the genes targeted include vascular endothelial growth factor, erythropoietin and nitric oxide which are involved in angiogenesis, hematopoiesis and vasodilation, respectively.

Encouraging results from animal investigations, however, have not been reproduced in large clinical trials.[140] The lack of positive outcomes with regard to therapeutic arteriogenesis (remodelling of existing arterioles) and angiogenesis is believed to be an oversimplification of the trial design.[139] Trials that include combination of more than one growth factor may provide superior results when compared to monotherapy trials.[140]

CONCLUSION

Reperfusion injury remains a significant concern that has generated decades of research. Our understanding of the mechanisms continues to evolve and may explain the lack of efficacy in recent clinical trials aimed at minimizing this unwarranted consequence of flow restoration to an ischemic organ. Therapeutic intervention to injurious oxygen radical formation during ischemia and reperfusion (reflow paradox) has generated excitement in the preclinical stage, but as of yet has not yielded significant protection in clinical trials. This is similarly true for attempts to interfere with the inflammatory process of reperfusion. Immediate restoration of blood flow to an ischemic tissue with adjunct antiplatelet therapy, therefore, is still considered the mainstay approach to minimize organ damage. Much of the current research focuses on the protection of cellular organelles such as the mitochondria, maintenance of ion gradients that have been compromised secondary to membrane disruption, and energy preservation/supplementation to heal and maintain cellular physiology. 'Conditioning' the tissue with planned ischemic insults so that the tissue may be better prepared to handle future and more severe ischemic events has shown promise. The mechanism of protection, however, is still under investigation. Insight into this may lead to a pharmacologic equivalent. What has been repeatedly proven is that collateral damage to otherwise healthy tissue during reperfusion does indeed occur and that attempts to minimize this will significantly benefit the patient. For this reason, the scientific community will continue diligently to investigate therapies to minimize reperfusion injury.

REFERENCES

1. Harman JW, Gwinn RP. The recovery of skeletal muscle fibers from acute ischemia as determined by histologic and chemical methods. *Am J Pathol.* 1949;25:741–755.
2. Burkhardt GE, Gifford SM, Propper B, Spencer JR, Williams K, Jones L, Sumner N, Cowart J, Rasmussen TE. The impact of ischemic intervals on neuromuscular recovery in a porcine (*Sus scrofa*) survival model of extremity vascular injury. *J Vasc Surg.* 2011;53:165–173.
3. McCord JM. Oxygen-derived free radicals in postischemic tissue injury. *N Engl J Med.* 1985;312:159–163.
4. Ames A III, Wright RL, Kowada M, Thurston JM, Majno G. Cerebral ischemia. II. The no-reflow phenomenon. *Am J Pathol.* 1968;52:437–453.
5. Seekamp A, Mulligan MS, Till GO, Ward PA. Requirements for neutrophil products and L-arginine in ischemia–reperfusion injury. *Am J Pathol.* 1993;142:1217–1226.
6. Warren JD, Blumbergs PC, Thompson PD. Rhabdomyolysis: A review. *Muscle Nerve.* 2002;25:332–347.
7. Collard CD, Gelman S. Pathophysiology, clinical manifestations, and prevention of ischemia–reperfusion injury. *Anesthesiology* 2001;94:1133–1138.
8. Kusza K, Siemionow M. Is the knowledge on tissue microcirculation important for microsurgeon? *Microsurgery.* 2011;31:572–579.
9. Engelson ET, Skalak TC, Schmid-Schonbein GW. The microvasculature in skeletal muscle. I. Arteriolar network in rat spinotrapezius muscle. *Microvasc Res.* 1985;30:29–44.
10. Zweifach BW, Kovalcheck S, De Lano F, Chen P. Micropressure-flow relationships in a skeletal muscle of spontaneously hypertensive rats. *Hypertension.* 1981;3:601–614.
11. Schmid-Schonbein GW, Delano FA, Chu S, Zweifach BW. Wall structure of arteries and arterioles feeding the spinotrapezius muscle of normotensive and spontaneously hypertensive rats. *Int J Microcirc Clin Exp.* 1990;9:47–66.

12. Cowen T, Burnstock G. Quantitative analysis of the density and pattern of adrenergic innervation of blood vessels. A new method. *Histochemistry.* 1980;66:19–34.

13. Saltzman D, DeLano FA, Schmid-Schonbein GW. The microvasculature in skeletal muscle. VI. Adrenergic innervation of arterioles in normotensive and spontaneously hypertensive rats. *Microvasc Res.* 1992;44:263–273.

14. Griffith SG, Crowe R, Lincoln J, Haven AJ, Burnstock G. Regional differences in the density of perivascular nerves and varicosities, noradrenaline content and responses to nerve stimulation in the rabbit ear artery. *Blood Vessels.* 1982;19:41–52.

15. Marshall JM. The influence of the sympathetic nervous system on individual vessels of the microcirculation of skeletal muscle of the rat. *J Physiol.* 1982;332:169–186.

16. Intaglietta M, Johnson PC, Winslow RM. Microvascular and tissue oxygen distribution. *Cardiovasc Res.* 1996;32:632–643.

17. Dodd LR, Johnson PC. Diameter changes in arteriolar networks of contracting skeletal muscle. *Am J Physiol.* 1991;260:H662–H670.

18. Flamm ES, Demopoulos HB, Seligman ML, Poser RG, Ransohoff J. Free radicals in cerebral ischemia. *Stroke.* 1978;9:445–447.

19. Hunter FE Jr., Scott A, Hoffsten PE, Gebicki JM, Weinstein J, Schneider A. Studies on the mechanism of swelling, lysis, and disintegration of isolated liver mitochondria exposed to mixtures of oxidized and reduced glutathione. *J Biol Chem.* 1964;239:614–621.

20. Presta M, Ragnotti G. Quantification of damage to striated muscle after normothermic or hypothermic ischemia. *Clin Chem.* 1981;27:297–302.

21. Parks DA, Granger DN. Ischemia-induced vascular changes: Role of xanthine oxidase and hydroxyl radicals. *Am J Physiol.* 1983;245:G285–G289.

22. Halliwell B. Free radicals, antioxidants, and human disease: Curiosity, cause, or consequence? *Lancet.* 1994;344:721–724.

23. Wang WZ, Baynosa RC, Zamboni WA. Therapeutic interventions against reperfusion injury in skeletal muscle. *J Surg Res.* 2011;171:175–182.

24. Dirksen MT, Laarman GJ, Simoons ML, Duncker DJ. Reperfusion injury in humans: A review of clinical trials on reperfusion injury inhibitory strategies. *Cardiovasc Res.* 2007;74:343–355.

25. Rentoukas E, Tsarouhas K, Tsitsimpikou C, Lazaros G, Deftereos S, Vavetsi S. The prognostic impact of allopurinol in patients with acute myocardial infarction undergoing primary percutaneous coronary intervention. *Int J Cardiol.* 2010;145:257–258.

26. Wilhelm MP, Schlensak C, Hoh A, Knipping L, Mangold G, Dallmeier Rojas D, Beyersdorf F. Controlled reperfusion using a simplified perfusion system preserves function after acute and persistent limb ischemia: A preliminary study. *J Vasc Surg.* 2005;42:690–694.

27. Heilmann C, Schmoor C, Siepe M, Schlensak C, Hoh A, Fraedrich G, Beyersdorf F. Controlled reperfusion versus conventional treatment of the acutely ischemic limb: Results of a randomized, open-label, multicenter trial. *Circ Cardiovasc Interv.* 2013;6:417–427.

28. Goldstein S, Czapski G. Mannitol as an OH. scavenger in aqueous solutions and in biological systems. *Int J Radiat Biol Relat Stud Phys Chem Med.* 1984;46:725–729.

29. Shah DM, Bock DE, Darling RC III, Chang BB, Kupinski AM, Leather RP. Beneficial effects of hypertonic mannitol in acute ischemia – Reperfusion injuries in humans. *Cardiovasc Surg.* 1996;4:97–100.

30. Schlag MG, Clarke S, Carson MW, Harris KA, Potter RF. The effect of mannitol versus dimethyl thiourea at attenuating ischemia/reperfusion-induced injury to skeletal muscle. *J Vasc Surg.* 1999;29:511–521.

31. Westman B, Weidenhielm L, Rooyackers O, Fredriksson K, Wernerman J, Hammarqvist F. Knee replacement surgery as a human clinical model of the effects of ischaemia/reperfusion upon skeletal muscle. *Clin Sci.* 2007;113:313–318.

32. Shim JK, Choi SH, Oh YJ, Kim CS, Yoo KJ, Kwak YL. The effect of mannitol on oxygenation and creatine kinase MB release in patients undergoing multivessel off-pump coronary artery bypass surgery. *J Thorac Cardiovasc Surg.* 2007;133:704–709.

33. Fink MP. Ringer's ethyl pyruvate solution: A novel resuscitation fluid for the treatment of hemorrhagic shock and sepsis. *J Trauma.* 2003;54:S141–S143.

34. Dobsak P, Courderot-Masuyer C, Zeller M, Vergely C, Laubriet A, Assem M, Eicher JC, Teyssier JR, Wolf JE, Rochette L. Antioxidative properties of pyruvate and protection of the ischemic rat heart during cardioplegia. *J Cardiovasc Pharmacol.* 1999;34:651–659.

35. Bennett-Guerrero E, Swaminathan M, Grigore AM, Roach GW, Aberle LG, Johnston JM, Fink MP. A phase II multicenter double-blind placebo-controlled study of ethyl pyruvate in high-risk patients undergoing cardiac surgery with cardiopulmonary bypass. *J Cardiothorac Vasc Anesth.* 2009;23:324–329.

36. Koksal C, Bozkurt AK, Cangel U, Ustundag N, Konukoglu D, Musellim B, Sayin AG. Attenuation of ischemia/reperfusion injury by N-acetylcysteine in a rat hind limb model. *J Surg Res.* 2003;111:236–239.

37. Thiele H, Hildebrand L, Schirdewahn C et al. Impact of high-dose N-acetylcysteine versus placebo on contrast-induced nephropathy and myocardial reperfusion injury in unselected patients with ST-segment elevation myocardial infarction undergoing primary percutaneous coronary intervention. The LIPSIA-N-ACC (Prospective, Single-Blind, Placebo-Controlled, Randomized Leipzig Immediate Percutaneous Coronary Intervention Acute Myocardial Infarction N-ACC) Trial. *J Am Coll Cardiol.* 2010;55:2201–2209.

38. Koca K, Yurttas Y, Cayci T et al. The role of pre-conditioning and N-acetylcysteine on oxidative stress resulting from tourniquet-induced ischemia-reperfusion in arthroscopic knee surgery. *J Trauma.* 2011;70:717–723.

39. Greenwald RA. Superoxide dismutase and catalase as therapeutic agents for human diseases: A critical review. *Free Radic Biol Med.* 1990;8:201–209.

40. Halladin NL, Zahle FV, Rosenberg J, Gogenur I. Interventions to reduce tourniquet-related ischaemic damage in orthopaedic surgery: A qualitative systematic review of randomised trials. *Anaesthesia.* 2014;69:1033–1050.

41. Schraufstatter IU, Hinshaw DB, Hyslop PA, Spragg RG, Cochrane CG. Oxidant injury of cells: DNA strand-breaks activate polyadenosine diphosphate-ribose polymerase and lead to depletion of nicotinamide adenine dinucleotide. *J Clin Invest.* 1986;77:1312–1320.

42. Patel H, Shaw SG, Shi-Wen X, Abraham D, Baker DM, Tsui JC. Toll-like receptors in ischaemia and its potential role in the pathophysiology of muscle damage in critical limb ischaemia. *Cardiol Res Pract.* 2012;2012:121237.

43. Virag L, Szabo C. The therapeutic potential of poly(ADP-ribose) polymerase inhibitors. *Pharmacol Rev.* 2002;54:375–429.

44. Szabo G, Bahrle S, Stumpf N et al. Poly(ADP-Ribose) polymerase inhibition reduces reperfusion injury after heart transplantation. *Circ Res.* 2002;90:100–106.

45. Hatachi G, Tsuchiya T, Miyazaki T, Matsumoto K, Yamasaki N, Okita N, Nanashima A, Higami Y, Nagayasu T. The poly(adenosine diphosphate-ribose) polymerase inhibitor PJ34 reduces pulmonary ischemia–reperfusion injury in rats. *Transplantation.* 2014;98:618–624.

46. Hua HT, Albadawi H, Entabi F, Conrad M, Stoner MC, Meriam BT, Sroufe R, Houser S, Lamuraglia GM, Watkins MT. Polyadenosine diphosphate-ribose polymerase inhibition modulates skeletal muscle injury following ischemia reperfusion. *Arch Surg.* 2005;140:344–351; discussion 351–352.

47. Oklu R, Albadawi H, Jones JE, Yoo HJ, Watkins MT. Reduced hind limb ischemia-reperfusion injury in Toll-like receptor-4 mutant mice is associated with decreased neutrophil extracellular traps. *J Vasc Surg.* 2013;58:1627–1636.

48. Mullarkey M, Rose JR, Bristol J et al. Inhibition of endotoxin response by e5564, a novel Toll-like receptor 4-directed endotoxin antagonist. *J Pharmacol Exp Ther.* 2003;304:1093–1102.

49. Barochia A, Solomon S, Cui X, Natanson C, Eichacker PQ. Eritoran tetrasodium (E5564) treatment for sepsis: Review of preclinical and clinical studies. *Expert Opin Drug Metab Toxicol.* 2011;7:479–494.

50. Szeto HH, Birk AV. Serendipity and the discovery of novel compounds that restore mitochondrial plasticity. *Clin Pharmacol Ther.* 2014;96:672–683.

51. Bosetti F, Baracca A, Lenaz G, Solaini G. Increased state 4 mitochondrial respiration and swelling in early post-ischemic reperfusion of rat heart. *FEBS Lett.* 2004;563:161–164.

52. Szeto HH. First-in-class cardiolipin-protective compound as a therapeutic agent to restore mitochondrial bioenergetics. *Br J Pharmacol.* 2014;171:2029–2050.

53. Nederlof R, Eerbeek O, Hollmann MW, Southworth R, Zuurbier CJ. Targeting hexokinase II to mitochondria to modulate energy metabolism and reduce ischaemia-reperfusion injury in heart. *Br J Pharmacol.* 2014;171:2067–2079.

54. Bosselaar M, Boon H, van Loon LJ, van den Broek PH, Smits P, Tack CJ. Intra-arterial AICA-riboside administration induces NO-dependent vasodilation in vivo in human skeletal muscle. *Am J Physiol Endocrinol Metab.* 2009;297:E759–E766.

55. Fryer LG, Foufelle F, Barnes K, Baldwin SA, Woods A, Carling D. Characterization of the role of the AMP-activated protein kinase in the stimulation of glucose transport in skeletal muscle cells. *Biochem J.* 2002;363:167–174.

56. Bergeron R, Ren JM, Cadman KS, Moore IK, Perret P, Pypaert M, Young LH, Semenkovich CF, Shulman GI. Chronic activation of AMP kinase results in NRF-1 activation and mitochondrial biogenesis. *Am J Physiol Endocrinol Metab.* 2001;281:E1340–E1346.

57. Alkhulaifi AM, Pugsley WB. Role of acadesine in clinical myocardial protection. *Br Heart J.* 1995;73:304–305.

58. Ely SW, Berne RM. Protective effects of adenosine in myocardial ischemia. *Circulation.* 1992;85:893–904.

59. Maldonado C, Pushpakumar SB, Perez-Abadia G, Arumugam S, Lane AN. Administration of exogenous adenosine triphosphate to ischemic skeletal muscle induces an energy-sparing effect: Role of adenosine receptors. *J Surg Res.* 2013;181:e15–e22.

60. Akinosoglou K, Alexopoulos D. Use of antiplatelet agents in sepsis: A glimpse into the future. *Thromb Res.* 2014;133:131–138.

61. Riksen NP, Oyen WJ, Ramakers BP, Van den Broek PH, Engbersen R, Boerman OC, Smits P, Rongen GA. Oral therapy with dipyridamole limits ischemia–reperfusion injury in humans. *Clin Pharmacol Ther.* 2005;78:52–59.

62. Moser GH, Schrader J, Deussen A. Turnover of adenosine in plasma of human and dog blood. *Am J Physiol.* 1989;256:C799–C806.

63. Birk AV, Liu S, Soong Y, Mills W, Singh P, Warren JD, Seshan SV, Pardee JD, Szeto HH. The mitochondrial-targeted compound SS-31 re-energizes ischemic mitochondria by interacting with cardiolipin. *J Am Soc Nephrol.* 2013;24:1250–1261.

64. Lee HY, Kaneki M, Andreas J, Tompkins RG, Martyn JA. Novel mitochondria-targeted antioxidant peptide ameliorates burn-induced apoptosis and endoplasmic reticulum stress in the skeletal muscle of mice. *Shock.* 2011;36:580–585.

65. Chakrabarti AK, Feeney K, Abueg C et al. Rationale and design of the EMBRACE STEMI study: A phase 2a, randomized, double-blind, placebo-controlled trial to evaluate the safety, tolerability and efficacy of intravenous Bendavia on reperfusion injury in patients treated with standard therapy including primary percutaneous coronary intervention and stenting for ST-segment elevation myocardial infarction. *Am Heart J.* 2013;165:509–514.e7.

66. Dennis SC, Gevers W, Opie LH. Protons in ischemia: Where do they come from; where do they go to? *J Mol Cell Cardiol.* 1991;23:1077–1086.

67. Piper HM, Abdallah Y, Kasseckert S, Schluter KD. Sarcoplasmic reticulum–mitochondrial interaction in the mechanism of acute reperfusion injury: Viewpoint. *Cardiovasc Res.* 2008;77:234–236.

68. Griffiths EJ, Halestrap AP. Mitochondrial non-specific pores remain closed during cardiac ischaemia, but open upon reperfusion. *Biochem J.* 1995;307 (Pt 1):93–98.

69. Troitzsch D, Moosdorf R, Hasenkam JM, Nygaard H, Vogt S. Effects of cyclosporine pretreatment on tissue oxygen levels and cytochrome oxidase in skeletal muscle ischemia and reperfusion. *Shock.* 2013;39:220–226.

70. McAllister SE, Moses MA, Jindal K, Ashrafpour H, Cahoon NJ, Huang N, Neligan PC, Forrest CR, Lipa JE, Pang CY. Na$^+$/H$^+$ exchange inhibitor cariporide attenuates skeletal muscle infarction when administered before ischemia or reperfusion. *J Appl Physiol.* 2009;106:20–28.

71. Chaitman BR. A review of the GUARDIAN trial results: Clinical implications and the significance of elevated perioperative CK-MB on 6-month survival. *J Card Surg.* 2003;18(Suppl. 1):13–20.

72. Taniyama Y, Ito H, Iwakura K, Masuyama T, Hori M, Takiuchi S, Nishikawa N, Higashino Y, Fujii K, Minamino T. Beneficial effect of intracoronary verapamil on microvascular and myocardial salvage in patients with acute myocardial infarction. *J Am Coll Cardiol.* 1997;30:1193–1199.

73. Umemura S, Nakamura S, Sugiura T, Tsuka Y, Fujitaka K, Yoshida S, Baden M, Iwasaka T. The effect of verapamil on the restoration of myocardial perfusion and functional recovery in patients with angiographic no-reflow after primary percutaneous coronary intervention. *Nucl Med Commun.* 2006;27:247–254.

74. Zavitsanos G, Huang L, Panza W, Serafin D, Klitzman B. Limiting impairment of muscle function following ischemia and reperfusion in rabbits. *J Reconstr Microsurg.* 1996;12:183–187.

75. Kandzari DE, Labinaz M, Cantor WJ et al. Reduction of myocardial ischemic injury following coronary intervention (the MC-1 to Eliminate Necrosis and Damage trial). *Am J Cardiol.* 2003;92:660–664.

76. Alexander JH, Emery RW Jr., Carrier M et al. Efficacy and safety of pyridoxal 5′-phosphate (MC-1) in high-risk patients undergoing coronary artery bypass graft surgery: The MEND-CABG II randomized clinical trial. *J Am Med Assoc.* 2008;299:1777–1787.

77. Wolff SP, Dean RT. Fragmentation of proteins by free radicals and its effect on their susceptibility to enzymatic hydrolysis. *Biochem J.* 1986;234:399–403.

78. Grisotto PC, dos Santos AC, Coutinho-Netto J, Cherri J, Piccinato CE. Indicators of oxidative injury and alterations of the cell membrane in the skeletal muscle of rats submitted to ischemia and reperfusion. *J Surg Res.* 2000;92:1–6.

79. Cai C, Masumiya H, Weisleder N et al. MG53 nucleates assembly of cell membrane repair machinery. *Nat Cell Biol.* 2009;11:56–64.

80. Zhang Y, Lv F, Jin L, Peng W, Song R, Ma J, Cao CM, Xiao RP. MG53 participates in ischaemic postconditioning through the RISK signalling pathway. *Cardiovasc Res.* 2011;91:108–115.

81. Weisleder N, Takizawa N, Lin P et al. Recombinant MG53 protein modulates therapeutic cell membrane repair in treatment of muscular dystrophy. *Sci Transl Med.* 2012;4:139ra85.

82. Corona BT, Garg K, Roe JL, Zhu H, Park KH, Ma J, Walters TJ. Effect of recombinant human MG53 protein on tourniquet-induced ischemia–reperfusion injury in rat muscle. *Muscle Nerve.* 2014;49:919–921.

83. Murphy AD, McCormack MC, Bichara DA, Nguyen JT, Randolph MA, Watkins MT, Lee RC, Austen WG Jr. Poloxamer 188 protects against ischemia-reperfusion injury in a murine hind-limb model. *Plast Reconstr Surg.* 2010;125:1651–1660.

84. Walters TJ, Mase VJ Jr., Roe JL, Dubick MA, Christy RJ. Poloxamer-188 reduces muscular edema after tourniquet-induced ischemia–reperfusion injury in rats. *J Trauma.* 2011;70:1192–1197.

85. Justicz AG, Farnsworth WV, Soberman MS, Tuvlin MB, Bonner GD, Hunter RL, Martino-Saltzman D, Sink JD, Austin GE. Reduction of myocardial infarct size by poloxamer 188 and mannitol in a canine model. *Am Heart J.* 1991;122:671–680.

86. Hunter RL, Luo AZ, Zhang R, Kozar RA, Moore FA. Poloxamer 188 inhibition of ischemia/reperfusion injury: Evidence for a novel anti-adhesive mechanism. *Ann Clin Lab Sci.* 2010;40:115–125.

87. Schaer GL, Spaccavento LJ, Browne KF et al. Beneficial effects of RheothRx injection in patients receiving thrombolytic therapy for acute myocardial infarction: Results of a randomized, double-blind, placebo-controlled trial. *Circulation.* 1996;94:298–307.

88. Lefer AM, Lefer DJ. The role of nitric oxide and cell adhesion molecules on the microcirculation in ischaemia-reperfusion. *Cardiovasc Res.* 1996;32:743–751.

89. Herbert KJ, Hickey MJ, Lepore DA, Knight KR, Morrison WA, Stewart AG. Effects of the endothelin receptor antagonist Bosentan on ischaemia/reperfusion injury in rat skeletal muscle. *Eur J Pharmacol.* 2001;424:59–67.

90. Pemberton M, Anderson G, Barker J. In vivo microscopy of microcirculatory injury in skeletal muscle following ischemia/reperfusion. *Microsurgery.* 1994;15:374–382.

91. Saltzman DJ, Kerger H, Jimenez JC, Farzan D, Wilson JM, Thompson JE, Intaglietta M. Microvascular changes following four-hour single arteriole occlusion. *Microsurgery.* 2013;33:207–215.

92. Piana RN, Paik GY, Moscucci M, Cohen DJ, Gibson CM, Kugelmass AD, Carrozza JP Jr., Kuntz RE, Baim DS. Incidence and treatment of 'no-reflow' after percutaneous coronary intervention. *Circulation.* 1994;89:2514–2518.

93. Louie EK, Hariman RJ, Wang Y, Hwang MH, Loeb HS, Scanlon PJ. Impairment of myocardial vascular responsiveness after transient myocardial ischemia and reperfusion. *Am Heart J.* 1994;128:1084–1091.

94. Keller MW. Arteriolar constriction in skeletal muscle during vascular stunning: Role of mast cells. *Am J Physiol.* 1997;272:H2154–H2163.

95. Wang WZ, Anderson G, Fleming JT, Peter FW, Franken RJ, Acland RD, Barker J. Lack of nitric oxide contributes to vasospasm during ischemia/reperfusion injury. *Plast Reconstr Surg.* 1997;99:1099–1108.

96. Kuo YR, Wang FS, Jeng SF, Huang HC, Wei FC, Yang KD. Nitrosoglutathione modulation of platelet activation and nitric oxide synthase expression in promotion of flap survival after ischemia/reperfusion injury. *J Surg Res.* 2004;119:92–99.

97. Rubanyi GM, Polokoff MA. Endothelins: Molecular biology, biochemistry, pharmacology, physiology, and pathophysiology. *Pharmacol Rev.* 1994;46:325–415.

98. Rubanyi GM, Vanhoutte PM. Hypoxia releases a vasoconstrictor substance from the canine vascular endothelium. *J Physiol.* 1985;364:45–56.

99. Bohm F, Pernow J. The importance of endothelin-1 for vascular dysfunction in cardiovascular disease. *Cardiovasc Res.* 2007;76:8–18.

100. Ono H, Osanai T, Ishizaka H, Hanada H, Kamada T, Onodera H, Fujita N, Sasaki S, Matsunaga T, Okumura K. Nicorandil improves cardiac function and clinical outcome in patients with acute myocardial infarction undergoing primary percutaneous coronary intervention: Role of inhibitory effect on reactive oxygen species formation. *Am Heart J.* 2004;148:E15.

101. Nazir SA, Khan JN, Mahmoud IZ et al. The REFLO-STEMI trial comparing intracoronary adenosine, sodium nitroprusside and standard therapy for the attenuation of infarct size and microvascular obstruction during primary percutaneous coronary intervention: Study protocol for a randomised controlled trial. *Trials.* 2104;15:371.

102. Cahoon NJ, Naparus A, Ashrafpour H, Hofer SO, Huang N, Lipa JE, Forrest CR, Pang CY. Pharmacologic prophylactic treatment for perioperative protection of skeletal muscle from ischemia-reperfusion injury in reconstructive surgery. *Plast Reconstr Surg.* 2013;131:473–485.

103. Krieglstein CF, Granger DN. Adhesion molecules and their role in vascular disease. *Am J Hypertens.* 2001;14:44S–54S.

104. Tardif JC, Tanguay JF, Wright SS et al. Effects of the P-selectin antagonist inclacumab on myocardial damage after percutaneous coronary intervention for non-ST-segment elevation myocardial infarction: Results of the SELECT-ACS trial. *J Am Coll Cardiol.* 2013;61:2048–2055.

105. Faxon DP, Gibbons RJ, Chronos NA, Gurbel PA, Sheehan F. The effect of blockade of the CD11/CD18 integrin receptor on infarct size in patients with acute myocardial infarction treated with direct angioplasty: The results of the HALT-MI study. *J Am Coll Cardiol.* 2002;40:1199–1204.

106. Armstrong PW, Granger CB, Adams PX, Hamm C, Holmes D Jr., O'Neill WW, Todaro TG, Vahanian A, Van de Werf F. Pexelizumab for acute ST-elevation myocardial infarction in patients undergoing primary percutaneous coronary intervention: A randomized controlled trial. *J Am Med Assoc.* 2007;297:43–51.

107. Walker PM. Ischemia/reperfusion injury in skeletal muscle. *Ann Vasc Surg.* 1991;5:399–402.

118. Strock PE, Majno G. Microvascular changes in acutely ischemic rat muscle. *Surg Gynecol Obstet.* 1969;129:1213–1224.

109. Menger MD, Steiner D, Messmer K. Microvascular ischemia-reperfusion injury in striated muscle: Significance of "no reflow". *Am J Physiol.* 1992;263:H1892–H1900.

110. Schmid-Schonbein GW. Capillary plugging by granulocytes and the no-reflow phenomenon in the microcirculation. *Fed Proc.* 1987;46:2397–2401.

111. Quinones-Baldrich WJ, Chervu A, Hernandez JJ, Colburn M, Moore WS. Skeletal muscle function after ischemia: "No reflow" versus reperfusion injury. *J Surg Res.* 1991;51:5–12.

112. Kharbanda RK, Peters M, Walton B, Kattenhorn M, Mullen M, Klein N, Vallance P, Deanfield J, MacAllister R. Ischemic preconditioning prevents endothelial injury and systemic neutrophil activation during ischemia-reperfusion in humans in vivo. *Circulation.* 2001;103:1624–1630.

113. Busch GJ, Martins AC, Hollenberg NK, Wilson RE, Colman RW. A primate model of hyperacute renal allograft rejection. *Am J Pathol.* 1975;79:31–56.

114. Jordan JE, Zhao ZQ, Vinten-Johansen J. The role of neutrophils in myocardial ischemia-reperfusion injury. *Cardiovasc Res.* 1999;43:860–878.

115. Investigators EAST. Use of anti-ICAM-1 therapy in ischemic stroke: Results of the Enlimomab Acute Stroke Trial. *Neurology.* 2001;57:1428–1434.

116. Becker KJ. Anti-leukocyte antibodies: LeukArrest (Hu23F2G) and Enlimomab (R6.5) in acute stroke. *Curr Med Res Opin.* 2002;18(Suppl. 2):s18–s22.

117. Suematsu M, DeLano FA, Poole D, Engler RL, Miyasaka M, Zweifach BW, Schmid-Schonbein GW. Spatial and temporal correlation between leukocyte behavior and cell injury in postischemic rat skeletal muscle microcirculation. *Lab Invest.* 1994;70:684–695.

118. He P. Leucocyte/endothelium interactions and microvessel permeability: Coupled or uncoupled? *Cardiovasc Res.* 2010;87:281–290.

119. Reffelmann T, Kloner RA. The no-reflow phenomenon: A basic mechanism of myocardial ischemia and reperfusion. *Basic Res Cardiol.* 2006;101:359–372.

120. Yang XM, Liu Y, Cui L, Yang X, Liu Y, Tandon N, Kambayashi J, Downey JM, Cohen MV. Platelet P2Y(1)(2) blockers confer direct postconditioning-like protection in reperfused rabbit hearts. *J Cardiovasc Pharmacol Ther.* 2013;18:251–262.

121. Yusuf S, Zhao F, Mehta SR, Chrolavicius S, Tognoni G, Fox KK. Effects of clopidogrel in addition to aspirin in patients with acute coronary syndromes without ST-segment elevation. *N Engl J Med.* 2001;345:494–502.

122. Park SD, Baek YS, Woo SI, Kim SH, Shin SH, Kim DH, Kwan J, Park KS. Comparing the effect of clopidogrel versus ticagrelor on coronary microvascular dysfunction in acute coronary syndrome patients (TIME trial): Study protocol for a randomized controlled trial. *Trials.* 2014;15:151.

123. Dick F, Li J, Giraud MN, Kalka C, Schmidli J, Tevaearai H. Basic control of reperfusion effectively protects against reperfusion injury in a realistic rodent model of acute limb ischemia. *Circulation.* 2008;118:1920–1928.

124. Beyersdorf F, Matheis G, Kruger S, Hanselmann A, Freisleben HG, Zimmer G, Satter P. Avoiding reperfusion injury after limb revascularization: Experimental observations and recommendations for clinical application. *J Vasc Surg.* 1989;9:757–766.

125. Reimer KA, Murry CE, Yamasawa I, Hill ML, Jennings RB. Four brief periods of myocardial ischemia cause no cumulative ATP loss or necrosis. *Am J Physiol.* 1986;251:H1306–H1315.

126. Walsh SR, Tang TY, Kullar P, Jenkins DP, Dutka DP, Gaunt ME. Ischaemic preconditioning during cardiac surgery: Systematic review and meta-analysis of perioperative outcomes in randomised clinical trials. *Eur J Cardiothorac Surg.* 2008;34:985–994.

127. Zhao ZQ, Corvera JS, Halkos ME, Kerendi F, Wang NP, Guyton RA, Vinten-Johansen J. Inhibition of myocardial injury by ischemic postconditioning during reperfusion: Comparison with ischemic preconditioning. *Am J Physiol Heart Circ Physiol.* 2003;285:H579–H588.

128. Abdelnoor M, Sandven I, Limalanathan S, Eritsland J. Postconditioning in ST-elevation myocardial infarction: A systematic review, critical appraisal, and meta-analysis of randomized clinical trials. *Vasc Health Risk Manag.* 2014;10:477–491.

129. Loukogeorgakis SP, Williams R, Panagiotidou AT, Kolvekar SK, Donald A, Cole TJ, Yellon DM, Deanfield JE, MacAllister RJ. Transient limb ischemia induces remote preconditioning and remote postconditioning in humans by a K(ATP)-channel dependent mechanism. *Circulation.* 2007;116:1386–1395.

130. Crimi G, Pica S, Raineri C et al. Remote ischemic post-conditioning of the lower limb during primary percutaneous coronary intervention safely reduces enzymatic infarct size in anterior myocardial infarction: A randomized controlled trial. *JACC Cardiovasc Interv.* 2013;6:1055–1063.

131. Wang WZ. Investigation of reperfusion injury and ischemic preconditioning in microsurgery. *Microsurgery.* 2009;29:72–79.

132. Argaud L, Gateau-Roesch O, Raisky O, Loufouat J, Robert D, Ovize M. Postconditioning inhibits mitochondrial permeability transition. *Circulation.* 2005;111:194–197.

133. Lim SY, Hausenloy DJ. Remote ischemic conditioning: From bench to bedside. *Front Physiol.* 2012;3:27.

134. Rees K, Beranek-Stanley M, Burke M, Ebrahim S. Hypothermia to reduce neurological damage following coronary artery bypass surgery. *Cochrane Database Syst Rev.* 2001;1:CD002138.

135. Alassar A, Bazerbashi S, Moawad N, Marchbank A. What is the value of topical cooling as an adjunct to myocardial protection? *Interact Cardiovasc Thorac Surg.* 2014;19:856–860.

136. Kim F, Nichol G, Maynard C et al. Effect of prehospital induction of mild hypothermia on survival and neurological status among adults with cardiac arrest: A randomized clinical trial. *J Am Med Assoc.* 2014;311:45–52.

137. Mowlavi A, Neumeister MW, Wilhelmi BJ, Song YH, Suchy H, Russell RC. Local hypothermia during early reperfusion protects skeletal muscle from ischemia-reperfusion injury. *Plast Reconstr Surg.* 2003;111:242–250.

138. Seekamp A, Ziegler M, Van Griensven M, Grotz M and Regel G. The role of hypothermia in trauma patients. *Eur J Emerg Med.* 1995;2(1):28–32.

139. Cao Y. Therapeutic angiogenesis for ischemic disorders: What is missing for clinical benefits? *Discov Med.* 2010;9:179–184.

140. Simons M, Bonow RO, Chronos NA et al. Clinical trials in coronary angiogenesis: Issues, problems, consensus: An expert panel summary. *Circulation.* 2000;102:E73–E86.

141. Yamamoto Y, Matsuura T, Narazaki G, Sugitani M, Tanaka K, Maeda A, Shiota G, Sato K, Yoshida A, Hisatome I. Synergistic effects of autologous cell and hepatocyte growth factor gene therapy for neovascularization in a murine model of hindlimb ischemia. *Am J Physiol Heart Circ Physiol.* 2009;297:H1329–H1336.

16

Aortoiliac occlusive disease
Endovascular and surgical therapies

MADHUKAR S. PATEL, JUAN CARLOS JIMENEZ and SAMUEL ERIC WILSON

CONTENTS

OUTLINE

The purpose of this chapter is to review the endovascular and surgical therapy for aortoiliac occlusive disease (AIOD) with attention to the historical aspects, pathophysiology, diagnosis, management and treatment.

HISTORICAL ASPECTS

The possibility for surgical correction of aortoiliac obstruction was suggested by Leriche[1] in 1940, when he described the syndrome of bilateral claudication, sexual impotence and absent common femoral pulses. Thromboendarterectomy was introduced by Dos Santos[2] in 1947 and first described for the aortoiliac segment by Wylie[3] in 1952 and later by Barker and Carmon[4] in 1953. Resection of the obstructed segment and replacement with an arterial allograft was described by Oudot[5] in 1951, Julian et al.[6] in 1952 and DeBakey et al.[7] in 1954. The allografts were cumbersome to obtain and were complicated by the development of late aneurysms. Following the description by Voorhees et al.[8] of a fabric arterial prosthesis in 1952, durable grafts made of Teflon or Dacron were introduced by Edwards[9] and DeBakey and Crawford[10] in 1957. Throughout

the 1960s, bypass grafting from the aorta to the external iliac arteries increased in popularity. Moore et al.[11] in 1968 and Perdue et al.[12] in 1970 suggested that superior long-term results followed anastomoses to the common femoral rather than the external iliac level, and this was confirmed by Baird et al.[13] in 1977. At present, operations are selected that correct the entire aortobifemoral occlusive segment as well as the frequently associated disease involving the profunda femoris. The current focus is on the durability of the procedure and the prevention of complications.

In the past decade, the most common operation for correction of AIOD, an aortobifemoral bypass, has been performed less commonly because of the impact of endovascular therapy and the recognition that claudication is generally a benign disease.[14]

PATHOPHYSIOLOGY

Chronic atherosclerosis

Atherosclerosis may produce partial or complete occlusion of the distal aorta and one or both common iliac arteries, and it frequently extends into the proximal portion of the external and/or internal iliac arteries. Usually the plaque is more extensive on the posterior wall; thus, the distal lumbar and median sacral arteries are occluded at an early stage.

Immediately distal to the renal arteries, the aorta is usually free of disease or minimally involved, and the periarterial surgical planes are well preserved. These features are exploited in the surgical repair: the upper clamp is placed immediately below the renal arteries and the upper anastomosis is performed about 2 cm distally. In some cases, the disease process extends proximally and involves the orifices of the renal arteries. In these cases, clamps must be placed at a higher level and care taken to ensure that the arterial supply to the kidneys is not compromised by embolization of atherosclerotic debris or inadequate removal of the obstructive material. Of note, the origin of the inferior mesenteric artery may be occluded, and the status of this vessel influences the design of the operation.

With chronic AIOD, collateral vessels enlarge and compensate to some degree. The potential for collateral flow is higher with aortoiliac than with femoral, popliteal or tibial artery obstruction. Important collateral pathways include internal mammary to inferior epigastric, superior mesenteric to inferior mesenteric and internal iliac, intercostals and lumbars to circumflex iliac and internal iliac, inferior mesenteric to internal iliac and internal iliac to profunda femoris.

Patients with isolated aortoiliac disease generally present with complaints of intermittent claudication and/or sexual impotence. By the time symptoms are noted, half the patients also have occlusive disease in the femoral popliteal and/or tibial arteries. By comparison to the patients with only aortoiliac involvement, those with multilevel disease present at an earlier age, and the viability of the leg may be threatened.[13,15,16]

Occlusive mild-aneurysmal disease

Although patients with abdominal aortic aneurysms rarely have claudication, symptoms from occlusive disease may be associated with aortoiliac aneurysms if there is significant coexisting atherosclerotic occlusive disease, embolic occlusion from the mural thrombus or kinking of the arteries.

Hypoplastic aorta

The hypoplastic aortoiliac syndrome almost always occurs in women with a history of significant, long-standing cigarette smoking. Characteristic features include a high aortic bifurcation, acute angle of the aortic bifurcation, straight iliac arteries without the normal lateral bowing, an aortic diameter less than 14 mm (or less than one-quarter of the diameter of the lumbar vertebrae) and a common iliac diameter less than 7 mm.[17] Collaterals are poorly developed and the femoral and distal vessels are also small.

Symptoms of claudication are more severe than expected from the angiographic pattern.[18]

Recognition of this syndrome is important because the operative procedures are technically difficult and the long-term results of bypass surgery are often poor.[17,19] If conservative treatment fails, aortoiliac endarterectomy with patch grafting or percutaneous transluminal angioplasty is recommended for those with localized disease. For patients with extensive occlusive disease, an aortofemoral bypass graft is indicated, using a small prosthesis (12 × 6 mm in diameter) with a proximal end-to-side anastomosis to minimize the size discrepancy.[17] Burke et al.[20] noted improved results with a PTFE prosthesis. In a group of 24 women less than 50 years of age with AIOD, Gagne et al. found a high incidence of coagulation abnormalities, particularly antiphospholipid antibody, and encouraged further investigation and aggressive anticoagulant management of this group.[21]

Acute obstruction

Acute aortoiliac occlusion may result from an embolus originating in the heart or from an aortic aneurysm. Other causes include an aortic dissection, blunt or penetrating trauma, or iatrogenic injury (e.g. diagnostic catheters, intra-aortic balloons or percutaneous transluminal dilatation). Since collateral channels are poorly developed in these cases, severe ischemia and the risk of tissue loss is relatively high.

CLINICAL DIAGNOSIS

Typically, patients with isolated aortoiliac disease are male cigarette smokers who present with buttock, thigh and calf claudication, and often have some degree of sexual impotence. Complaints of rest pain or ischemic night pain are usually absent unless multilevel disease is present or the occlusion extends up to the renal arteries, thereby interfering with collateral pathways. On physical examination, one or both femoral pulses are reduced and iliac or femoral bruits are audible. The feet usually appear warm and well perfused, without nutritional changes.

An accurate clinical diagnosis of AIOD is usually straightforward; however, one-quarter of the patients with isolated aortoiliac disease complain only of calf claudication rather than thigh or buttock pain. Conversely, one-quarter of the patients with normal aortoiliac segments and isolated femoral popliteal disease have low thigh as well as calf claudication.[22] Femoral bruits are present in only two-thirds of the patients with symptomatic isolated aortoiliac obstruction.

The differential diagnosis must identify patients complaining of buttock and thigh pain of neurogenic or musculogenic origin. The symptoms from spinal stenosis may be difficult to distinguish; however, these patients usually complain of leg pain or 'weakness' on standing or on walking very short or variable distances, and relief is achieved only by sitting or lying down for prolonged periods or after adequate analgesics. Numbness and tingling are common and are usually localized in the distribution of one or more nerve roots.

An uncommon clinical presentation of aortoiliac disease is the blue toe syndrome.[23] These patients present with an ischemic blue and tender toes in the setting of palpable peripherial pulses. Arteriography may demonstrate an ulcerating plaque, but occasionally a high-resolution computed tomographic arteriography (CTA) scan is necessary to demonstrate the ulcerating atherosclerotic lesion.

OBJECTIVE DIAGNOSIS

Conventional arteriography

Conventional arteriography is obtained only when the history indicates that the symptoms are sufficiently disabling to warrant a consideration of endovascular therapy or surgery. Although arteriography remains the most important method for evaluating the severity of aortoiliac disease, standard anterior–posterior views may underestimate the severity of the occlusive disease[24] in which case biplane views will be necessary. Digital subtraction angiography (DSA) allows for better visualization of blood vessels and newer techniques have led to higher image resolution and reconstruction with three-dimensional DSA (Figure 16.1). Further, the use of carbon dioxide DSA when imaging the aortoiliac system allows for imaging of

patients with impairments in kidney function and minimizes the use of iodinated contrast in these individuals. As conventional arteriography mandates arterial puncture, access related complications including distal embolization, dissection, pseudoaneurysm formation and local bleeding or hematoma formation remain inherent procedural risks which can be minimized by removing sheaths as soon as possible and choosing sheaths of the smallest necessary diameter.

When the severity of AIOD is difficult to determine from the arteriogram, the best method for assessing the hemodynamic significance of an aortoiliac lesion is to directly measure the transstenotic pressure gradient at rest or after reactive hyperemia has been induced. This pressure difference is measured from pressure recordings that are made as the angiographic catheter is withdrawn from the aorta. A mean pressure gradient of more than 5 mmHg at rest is considered to be hemodynamically significant. Alternatively, a transstenotic pressure difference of greater than 10–15 mmHg after intra-arterial injection of papaverine is also noted to be significant as normally pressure does not fall substantially after vasodilator administration.

Computed tomographic arteriography

Multislice CTA allows for excellent visualization of aortoiliac segments when evaluating for AOID. The modality uses an intravenously delivered bolus of iodinated contrast which is timed so that image acquisition can be performed to achieve optimal arterial contrast enhancement in the vessels of concern. CTA allows for depiction of luminal abnormalities, mural calcifications, collateral vessels and vascular false lumens better than conventional arteriography and is without the associated arterial puncture related complications. As CTA requires iodinated contrast, however, it is often challenging to obtain in patients with inadequate renal function.

Contrast-enhanced magnetic resonance angiography

Contrast-enhanced magnetic resonance angiography (MRA) is another non-invasive method for imaging. This method differs from conventional arteriography and CTA in that it performed without the use of radiation. In order to acquire images, contrast-enhanced MRA uses a precisely timed bolus of a paramagnetic gadolinium-based agent. Contrast-enhanced MRA images can easily be distorted by patient movement or metallic interference from implants or previously placed stents. Further, gadolinium-induced contrast nephropathy has been known to occur in patients with renal failure and limit use of this modality in this patient population. Despite these drawbacks, contrast-enhanced MRA has been noted in

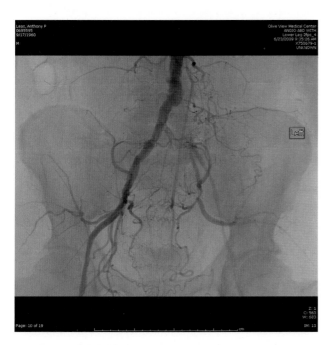

Figure 16.1 Conventional angiography demonstrating a chronic left common iliac artery occlusion.

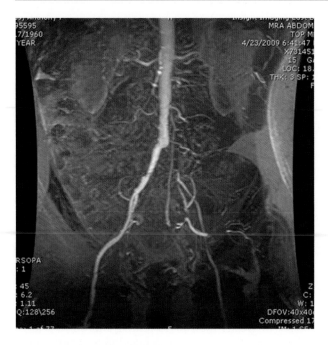

Figure 16.2 Magnetic resonance angiography in a patient with a chronic iliac artery occlusion.

meta-analysis to have a pooled sensitivity of 97.5% and a pool specificity of 96.2% when evaluating patients with peripheral artery disease[25] (Figure 16.2).

Non-invasive assessment

Non-invasive tests augment clinical and arteriographic assessment and in general have a role in determining the severity of arterial occlusive disease, localizing the site of involvement and clarifying the differential diagnosis. Several non-invasive methods are potentially useful for assessing the severity of aortoiliac disease.[22] Although the thigh systolic blood pressure can be measured, it is not sufficiently accurate for assessing the aortoiliac segment, particularly in patients with combined aortoiliac and femoral popliteal disease. It is not possible to place the pressure cuff high enough on the thigh to measure a pressure equivalent to that in the common femoral artery and thus, accurately assess the severity of the iliac disease. Hemodynamically, significant aortoiliac disease can be detected through analysis of Doppler recordings of blood-flow velocity from the common femoral artery using duplex Doppler equipment.[26] The Doppler waveform is normally triphasic, with a large initial forward component followed by a reverse and then a second smaller forward flow component. If the waveform is dampened (i.e. monophasic or a reverse flow lost), significant iliac disease is likely to be present. The waveforms are usually analyzed by subjective evaluation or quantified by the calculation of pulsatility index[27] or other measurements. Alternatively, peak velocity measurements can be made along the length of the aortoiliac segment. A stenosis greater than 50% is diagnosed if the peak velocity is at least two times greater than the velocity in an adjacent normal arterial segment, the waveform becomes monophasic, and spectral broadening is present.[28]

MANAGEMENT

Conservative therapy

Mild intermittent claudication from aortoiliac disease causes minimal disability and its natural history is usually favourable.[29] After the discovery of significant atherosclerosis, steps should be taken to identify and control risk factors and patients with AIOD should be medically optimized with regard to dietary habits, smoking cessation, diabetes management and medication therapy (antihypertensives, antiplatelets and statins). In addition to optimal medical therapy, it has been shown that a supervised exercise programme has led to improved treadmill walking performance in patients with claudication from AIOD and has been shown to be superior to primary stent revascularization with regard to reaching this endpoint.[30] Vasodilators, megavitamins and most pharmacologic products are unproved or of little benefit.

TREATMENT

Considerations for choosing a revascularization approach

If after a trial of conservative therapy and supervised exercise the patient continues to suffer from symptoms that significantly threaten their employment and enjoyment of life, they should be assessed for endovascular, open or hybrid intervention. In brief, endovascular therapies for AIOD include iliac angioplasty as well as aortic and iliac artery stent grafting. Open surgical approaches can be classified as either direct anatomic (aortobifemoral bypass, aortounifemoral bypass, aortoiliac endarterectomy, descending thoracic aorta to femoral bypass, ascending aorta to femoral bypass and iliofemoral bypass) or extra-anatomic bypass (axillofemoral bypass and femorofemoral bypass). Finally, hybrid approaches involve a combination of open and endovascular intervention.

In a recent meta-analysis by Indes et al. of 5383 patients undergoing direct open bypass or endovascular treatment for AIOD, 29 open bypass studies and 28 endovascular studies were analyzed.[31] The pooled 5-year primary patency rate was found to be significantly greater in the open bypass group (82.7% vs. 71.4%) as was the pooled 5-year secondary patency rate (91% vs. 82.5%). It should be mentioned, however, that the open bypass strategy was associated with significantly longer length of stay as well as significantly increased morbidity (18.0% vs. 13.4%) and 30-day mortality (2.6% vs. 0.7%). Factoring in these results with a persistent lack of adequate randomized clinical trial data, endovascular therapy for AIOD is nonetheless increasing due to advances in device design. Thus, considerations for choosing a revascularization approach should include patient anatomy, patient co-morbidities, technical factors, surgical experience and resources and patient preference.

PATIENT ANATOMY

In 2007, the Trans-Atlantic Inter-Society Consensus (TASC) for the Management of peripheral artery disease published its most current recommendations, the TASC II guidelines.[32] Within these guidelines, the committee classified aortoiliac lesions by anatomic location and extent (Figure 16.3) in order to provide management recommendations.[32] Conventionally, in this classification scheme, the TASC II committee suggested that TASC A lesions are those in which endovascular therapy is the treatment of choice and TASC D lesions are those in which surgery is the treatment of choice (Grade D).[32] For TASC B lesions, endovascular therapy was felt to be preferred, and for TASC C lesions, open revascularization was recommended; however, these decisions were felt to be more contingent upon the patient's co-morbidities and preference as well as the expertise of the operator than those made for TASC A and TASC D lesions (Grade D).[32] Further, regardless of the TASC classification

Type A lesions
• Unilateral or bilateral stenoses of CIA
• Unilateral or bilateral single short (≤3 cm) stenosis of EIA

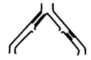

Type B lesions
• Short (≤3 cm) stenosis of infrarenal aorta
• Unilateral CIA occlusion
• Single or multiple stenosis totaling 3–10 cm involving the EIA not extending into the CFA
• Unilateral EIA occlusion not involving the origins of internal iliac or CFA

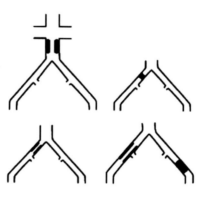

Type C lesions
• Bilateral CIA occlusions
• Bilateral EIA stenoses 3–10 cm long not extending into the CFA
• Unilateral EIA stenosis extending into the CFA
• Unilateral EIA occlusion that involves the origins of internal iliac and/or CFA
• Heavily calcified unilateral EIA occlusion with or without involvement of origins of internal iliac and/or CFA

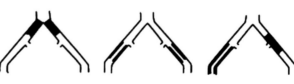

Type D lesions
• Infrarenal aortoiliac occlusion
• Diffuse disease involving the aorta and both iliac arteries requiring treatment
• Diffuse multiple stenoses involving the unilateral CIA, EIA and CFA
• Unilateral occlusions of both CIA and EIA
• Bilateral occlusions of EIA
• Iliac stenoses in patients with AAA requiring treatment and not amenable to endograft placement or other lesions requiring open aortic or iliac surgery

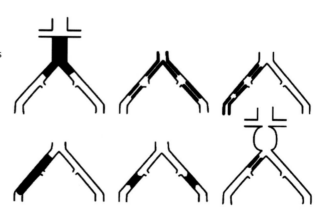

Figure 16.3 Trans-Atlantic Inter-Society Consensus (TASC) classification of aortoiliac lesions. (From Norgren L et al., *J Vasc Surg*, 45(Suppl. S), S5, January 2007.) CIA, common iliac artery; EIA, external iliac artery; CFA, common femoral artery; AAA, abdominal aortic aneurysm.

for a particular lesion, the presence or absence of concurrent lesions either proximal, distal or contralateral to the aortoiliac lesion of concern should be factored into the management strategy which is ultimately decided upon. It should be noted that subsequent to the publication of these guidelines, endovascular therapies have evolved and lesions originally thought to be better managed through an open approach (TASC C and TASC D) have now been successfully treated endovascularly (see the section "Results of endovascular therapy").

PATIENT CO-MORBIDITIES

Open direct anatomic revascularization strategies are the most invasive procedures for management of AIOD and thus often carry high morbidity and mortality rates as well as require longer recovery times when compared to open extra-anatomic bypass, endovascular therapies or hybrid approaches. Thus, for lesions that may seem to be best managed via an open surgical approach, patient co-morbidities must be carefully accounted for as those who are at high risk for repair may be better served with endovascular therapy despite need for secondary intervention given their overall co-morbid condition.

TECHNICAL FACTORS

Technical factors should be considered prior to deciding on a revascularization strategy. Patients with AIOD extending to or associated with significant stenosis of the common femoral artery will most likely warrant either a hybrid approach with a direct endarterectomy and patch repair of the common femoral artery with concurrent iliac artery angioplasty and stenting or a direct open repair. Additionally, patients with small external iliac arteries, high-risk lesions for embolization (e.g. ulcerated plaques) or failed endovascular therapy may benefit from open repair.

SURGICAL EXPERIENCE AND RESOURCES

Aside from the operator's personal experience with open, endovascular and hybrid techniques, it is important to consider facility resources and limitations when planning a revascularization strategy for the AOID patient. Access to high quality angiographic facilities with hybrid capabilities increases the scope of options available, assuming the operator is substantially trained and experienced with these techniques. Even though this may not be available at the centre in which the patient is first evaluated, available options (as well as their associated benefits and risks) should be discussed with patients before commitment to a specific revascularization strategy is made.

PATIENT PREFERENCE

During the informed consent process, it is important that the surgeon elicit the patient's preference of therapeutic approach. This is important as the data on therapeutic options for AOID are not absolute and the potential risks as well as benefits for patients undergoing intervention for this disease must be individualized. In addition to

morbidity and mortality, factors such as increased hospital length of stay and time of recovery for direct open procedures may play into a patient's decision to choose a less invasive approach with the understanding that repeat interventions may be more likely.

ADDITIONAL CONSIDERATIONS

Additional considerations such as the presence of acute critical limb ischemia and the patient's overall life expectancy are important in deciding upon a treatment algorithm. Patients presenting with acute onset symptoms who are not able to obtain an appropriate preoperative medical evaluation and those without significant life expectancy due to age and overall health are less likely to benefit from the increased patency rates of a direct anatomic open procedure and may be best managed with a less invasive approach.

ENDOVACULAR THERAPY

Technique of percutaneous arterial angioplasty with and without stenting

ACCESS

An ipsilateral retrograde femoral approach is typically used for interventions in AOID, although a contralateral femoral puncture with a retrograde over-the-top approach may be employed if necessary. In situations where lower extremity access poses challenge, upper extremity access can be considered but carries increased access site morbidity due to the need for larger arteriotomies in smaller vessels in order to accommodate sheaths and devices for angioplasty and/or stenting.

APPROACH

After adequate arterial access is obtained, conventional catheters and guidewire technique is used to navigate across the lesion of concern. It is critical to traverse the entire lesion. If difficulty is encountered, use of different catheter/guidewire combinations such as those that are angled and hydrophilic is recommended in addition to consideration of choosing a different access site if necessary.

Upon traversing the lesion of concern, a decision of whether to use transluminal angioplasty alone versus transluminal angioplasty with stenting for technical failure versus primary stenting alone is made. Transluminal balloon angioplasty is often primarily used but has been associated with failure resulting from creation of flow-limiting dissections and inadequate dilation due to elastic recoil from atherosclerotic plaques. In these scenarios, subsequent deployment of a stent serves to cover the created dissection plane and oppose the inherent recoil in the newly dilated segment.

With regard to stenting, further decisions involve whether to use balloon expandable or self-expanding stents as well as whether to use bare metal stents or covered stents. Stent choice is often based on operator preference and availability, and no one stent has demonstrated superiority. Currently, the DISCOVER (Dutch Iliac Stent Trial: COVERed balloon-expandable vs. uncovered balloon-expandable stent) trial is randomizing patients with aims to answer whether there is an advantage of one type of stent in decreasing restenosis.[33] It should be mentioned that in patients with AOID involving the aortic bifurcation, kissing stents are often used. Numerous modifications to the kissing stent position have been made in efforts to reduce the difference between the stented lumen and the aortic lumen in order to minimize radial mismatch. Recently, in vitro studies supporting the use of the Covered Endovascular Reconstruction of the Aortic Bifurcation technique, in which the two iliac limbs are placed inside the tapered portion of the aortic cuff, were found to be beneficial in maximally reducing radial mismatch.[34] General complications of stent placement to be considered involve recurrent stentosis from intimal hyperplasia as well as sizing error that can result in either vessel injury or inadequate dilation.

Finally, for either balloon angioplasty or stenting, sizing is determined so that balloon or stent diameter is 10%–15% greater in diameter compared to the adjacent normal artery. The appropriate length of the balloon or stent is chosen so that the entire lesion of concern is traversed while minimizing the amount of adjacent normal artery covered.

ASSESSMENT OF INTERVENTION

After balloon angioplasty and/or stenting, multiplane completion arteriography, intravascular ultrasound or blood pressure gradient measurements should be performed to assess the intervention. A persistent diameter reduction of more than 30% is considered to be inadequate as is a mean blood pressure gradient greater than 5 mmHg. Using both radiographic methods of assessment in conjunction with direct blood pressure gradient measurement allows for assessing the anatomic and hemodynamic impact of the endovascular intervention performed.

Results of endovascular therapy

In 1998, the Dutch Iliac Stent Trial Study Group released results of their randomized comparison of primary stent placement versus primary angioplasty followed by selective stent placement in patients with iliac artery occlusive disease.[35] Results from this study which randomized 279 patients into two groups based on either primary stent placement versus angioplasty with stenting performed for patients with a residual mean pressure gradient of 10 mmHg or higher demonstrated no substantial difference in clinical outcomes of the two revascularization strategies in both the short term and follow-up.[35] Specifically, as only 43% of patients undergoing angioplasty ultimately needed selective stent placement, it was ultimately recommended that this strategy may be less expensive than primary stent placement and is thus preferred.[35]

With advancements in endovascular technique continuing to progress, the scope of endovascular therapy has successfully been expanded. Specifically, in a systematic review of endovascular treatment of extensive AIOD (TASC C and TASC D lesions), 19 non-randomized cohort studies representing 1711 patients were analyzed.[36] Results from this study included technical success in 86%–100% of patients with 4 or 5 year primary patency rates of 60%–86% and secondary patency rates of 80%–98%.[36] These results suggest that despite primary patency rates being lower than those reported for open surgical revascularization, with percutaneous re-intervention, secondary patency is comparable to open surgical repair, and thus, endovascular treatment can be performed by experienced operators for these lesions once felt to be primarily managed through an open approach.[36]

SURGICAL TREATMENT

The surgical repair of atherosclerotic AIOD is achieved by direct anatomic revascularization (aortoiliac endarterectomy or an anatomic bypass graft) or extra-anatomical bypass graft (axillofemoral or femorofemoral bypass graft).

Aortoiliac endarterectomy

Endarterectomy still has a role in the management of aortoiliac disease, but its place has diminished greatly since the 1960s (Figure 16.4). The procedure usually involves an open endarterectomy of the distal aorta and either an open or semi-closed endarterectomy of one or both common iliac segments down to the level of the external iliac arteries. Extensive aortoiliac femoral endarterectomy has been abandoned. Closed endarterectomy using the LeVeen 'plaque cracker' was popularized in Europe and permits extensive retroperitoneal endarterectomy of the aorta, iliac and femoral segments.[37,38] In general, the long-term results of endarterectomy for localized disease are excellent and are comparable to those of bypass grafting; however, the results

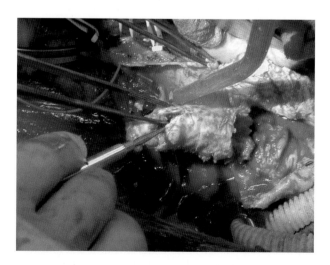

Figure 16.4 Open aortic endarterectomy demonstrating the presence of a 'coral-reef'-like plaque.

of extensive endarterectomy are poor.[15] By comparison to bypass grafting, endarterectomy is more tedious, time-consuming and technically demanding and is associated with a greater blood loss. The procedure should be considered in young patients with localized AIOD that does not involve the external iliac artery, since involvement of this site is often associated with recurrence of symptoms necessitating reoperation.[39] Many patients with this distribution of localized disease can now be treated quite satisfactorily by endovascular therapy. If the risk of infection is high, endarterectomy is preferable to prosthetic bypass grafting. In selected cases, aortoiliac endarterectomy is useful as a salvage procedure for the treatment of an infected aortofemoral bypass graft. After removal of the infected prosthesis, the arterial channel to the leg can be reconstituted by endarterectomy of the native vessels and patching with autogenous material.[40] In spite of its limited application at the present time, every vascular surgeon should be aware of and competent in the techniques of aortoiliac endarterectomy.

Anatomical bypass grafts

Over the past three decades, bypass grafting has become the standard operative method for aortoiliac repair. An iliofemoral bypass graft is a durable procedure for managing external iliac occlusive disease that is not amenable to endovascular therapy, especially when it extends down to the level of the common femoral artery or is the result of iatrogenic occlusion following arterial catheterization.[41] A unilateral aortofemoral bypass graft is rarely indicated.

The standard open operation for aortoiliac disease is an aortobifemoral bypass. This operation is indicated for good-risk patients with bilateral AIOD. Although we advocate a unilateral reconstruction of iliac occlusive disease if feasible, others prefer an aortobifemoral bypass for the management of unilateral disease, especially if the superficial femoral artery is also occluded.[42]

GENERAL PRINCIPLES OF AORTOBIFEMORAL BYPASS

The aortic anastomosis can be made either end-to-side or end-to-end. End-to-side anastomosis is indicated in the following circumstances: if a large aberrant renal artery that supplies a significant amount of renal parenchyma is present; if a large inferior mesenteric artery is present, especially if pelvic flow is reduced because of associated severe iliac disease; if the patient is a male who is concerned about his sexual potency and there is a significant occlusive disease involving both external iliac arteries, therefore compromising retrograde flow to the internals after aortobifemoral bypass; or if the aorta is hypoplastic. End-to-end anastomosis is indicated in patients with coexisting aortic aneurysmal disease or a complete aortic occlusion extending up to the renal arteries. Melliere et al.[43] could not find any difference between the results of end-to-end and end-to-side anastomoses and suggested choosing the simplest procedure that maintains adequate pelvic and colonic flow according to the angiographic findings.

The distal anastomosis is usually made to the common femoral artery. If the distal anastomosis is made to the external iliac artery, there is an increased chance that a subsequent downstream repair will be required unless the external iliac artery is completely free of disease. If the superficial femoral artery is occluded or severely stenosed and any narrowing of the profunda femoris artery is present, the toe of the graft should be extended onto the profunda as far as necessary beyond palpable disease.

TECHNIQUE OF AORTOBIFEMORAL BYPASS

Preoperatively, bowel preparation is achieved by a fluid diet for 24 hours and administering enemas until clear the evening prior to surgery. Prophylactic antibiotics, usually a cephalosporin, are administered preoperatively. The electrocardiogram, arterial blood pressure and central venous pressures are monitored routinely.

Once in the operating room, the patient is positioned in the supine position and draped so that the groins and legs are exposed and the feet are visible in transparent plastic 'bowel' bags.[13] Longitudinal groin incisions are made to expose the common femoral artery from the inguinal ligament to the bifurcation. If the superficial femoral artery is occluded, the first 1–2 cm of the profunda femoris artery is also exposed and is carefully palpated to confirm the absence of disease at its origin. The anterior 3–4 mm of the inguinal ligament is cut and the incision carried posteriorly to divide the posterior layer as well. Gentle blunt dissection is used to create a tunnel into the retroperitoneal space anterior to the iliac artery and the lateral circumflex iliac vein. The groin wounds are loosely packed with a moist sponge and the self-retaining retractors removed.

Next, the abdomen is opened through a midline incision from the xiphoid to midway between the umbilicus and pubis. Laparotomy is performed and a large fixed abdominal retractor is positioned. The transverse colon is elevated, and the small bowel is gathered to the right (either inside or outside the abdomen depending on body habitus) and protected by moist towels. A retroperitoneal incision to expose the aorta may be a good alternative to the standard transperitoneal incision.[44] It can be carried out without endotracheal intubation and general anaesthetic and may be of advantage in high-risk patients.

The surgeon identifies the duodenum on the right and the inferior mesenteric vein on the left and dissects between them directly down to the anterior wall of the aorta. The origin of the inferior mesenteric artery is noted but is not dissected. The anterior and lateral walls of the aorta are exposed up to the level of the renal vein. No attempt is made to divide lumbar arteries or to encircle the aorta. In the male, post-operative sexual dysfunction can be minimized by preserving the pre-aortic autonomic nerves and dissecting the pre-aortic tissue longitudinally and towards the right side and by not dividing the tissue in the region of the inferior mesenteric artery or near the aortic bifurcation.[45,46]

Heparin (75–100 units/kg, usually approximately 5000 units) is administered by the anaesthetist. Before the aorta is cross-clamped, the anaesthetist is given appropriate warning so that pharmacologic intervention is possible as required to reduce the cardiac afterload if necessary.

Knitted Dacron, rather than woven, is preferred because of its greater ease of handling, improved healing properties and ease of appropriate fashioning for distal anastomoses without fraying of edges. However, the type of Dacron prosthesis implanted does not appear to be of great importance for outcome. There is no significant difference in early or late thrombogenicity between knitted and woven Dacron prostheses as assessed by ^{111}In-labeled platelet deposition studies,[47] nor is there a difference in the early or late patency rates.[48] Collagen- or gelatin-coated grafts are commonly used because they eliminate the necessity for preclotting and reduce blood loss. Since current Dacron grafts usually exhibit an initial dilatation upon exposure to arterial blood pressure and 10%–25% diameter dilatation over the first year,[49] we prefer a 14 × 7 mm graft rather than a larger prosthesis. When the graft was selected to match the size of the native arteries, there was no difference in long-term patency between small (12 or 14 mm) and large (16 or 18 mm) grafts.[50]

For an end-to-end anastomosis, the proximal clamp is placed just below the renal arteries and the distal clamp approximately 3 cm distally. The clamps are placed from an anterior position and no attempt is made to dissect behind the aorta. The aorta is divided 1 cm proximal to the distal clamp, with great care being taken to avoid entering posterior lumbar veins. The removal of a small wedge of the anterior wall of the distal aorta often allows the surgeon to visualize the posterior aortic wall more clearly prior to dividing it.

The distal stump of aorta is oversewn with a 2-0 or 3-0 monofilament polypropylene suture, starting at the posterior wall and coming anteriorly with both needles in two layers so that only one knot is required. The lower clamp is removed as this suture is pulled tight and tied, so that the aortic tissue comes together snugly.

Debris in the proximal aortic trunk is carefully removed. The graft is cut so that the aortic trunk is about 3–3.5 cm long. It is sewn to the end of aorta with a double-ended 2-0 or 3-0 monofilament polypropylene suture which is started on the left lateral wall and continued across the back wall to the right lateral wall with a 'parachute' technique in which the end of the prosthesis is held about 4–5 cm from the aorta. Great care is taken not to exert caudad traction on the aortic stump. The suture is moistened with saline, pulled down into place and tightened. A nerve hook is used to tighten any loose strands and the final traction is exerted in the plane parallel to the posterior wall of the aorta. The left limb of the suture is then fixed in a taut position and held in place by a rubber-shod clamp. The right side is continued to the midline of the graft, where it is then held tautly while the left suture is continued to meet it.

The clamp is temporarily released and hemostasis is confirmed by inspecting the circumference of the anastomosis. Any leaks are repaired with interrupted sutures. A long curved clamp is then passed from each groin to grasp the limbs of the prosthesis and draw them into

the femoral incisions. Care is taken to make each tunnel behind the ureter if possible and, on the left, behind the sigmoid arterial and venous branches.

In performing an end-to-side anastomosis, the proximal aorta is clamped just distal to the renal arteries and this distal clamp is positioned just above or below the inferior mesenteric artery and clamped in an oblique direction so that patent lumbar arteries are occluded. An arteriotomy 3.5–5 cm in length is made. Atheromatous debris is removed, the arteriotomy is flushed with saline and the clamps are released temporarily to expel loose debris. The graft is suitably beveled and anastomosed using a single running monofilament suture starting at the base.

The design of each lower anastomosis is determined by the severity of disease in the infrainguinal arteries. If the superficial and profunda femoris arteries are normal, the anastomosis is made to the common femoral artery. Narrowing at the origin of the superficial or profunda femoris arteries is corrected by appropriate arterioplasties. Good-quality preoperative angiograms with oblique views are helpful in detecting stenosis at the origin of the profunda femoris artery, but the final decision about a stenosis involving this artery is made in the operating room. If there is any doubt, the common femoral arteriotomy is continued into the profunda. The profunda femoris artery is often quite fragile and thin walled; great care is taken to avoid injury to it or its branches, and extensive endarterectomies are avoided.[51-58] The groin anastomoses can be performed simultaneously if two experienced surgeons are available. The anastomoses are made with 5-0 or 6-0 monofilament polypropylene sutures, starting and finishing on one side of the heel and using a one-knot technique. Before the anastomoses are completed, adequate flushing of all the vessels is necessary, including the native superficial femoral, profunda femoris and common femoral arteries as well as the graft.

The anaesthetist is given 5–10 minutes warning before the graft is opened. The surgeon controls the flow through the new conduit until the blood pressure has stabilized. The heparin is then reversed with protamine. Hemostasis is checked, the colour of the sigmoid colon is noted and the retroperitoneal space is closed. All blood is removed from the abdomen, a careful sponge and instrument count is completed and the abdominal incision is closed with a single-layer continuous 1-0 monofilament polypropylene suture.

Before the groin incisions are closed, the femoral pulses are checked and the feet inspected to ensure that the peripheral flow is adequate. If there is any concern, intraoperative angiograms should be obtained or the anastomoses reopened and a Fogarty catheter passed. Groin closure is important and should be done in two to three layers to minimize dead space and avoid a lymphatic leak. Skin closure is with metallic skin clips.

Post-operatively, the patient is monitored for hemodynamic stability, respiratory function, renal function and the status of the circulation to both legs. In most cases, the patient can be extubated in the operating room or shortly after surgery. If the patient is hemodynamically stable, observation in a step-down unit, rather than an intensive care unit, is adequate. Ambulation begins on the first or second day and most patients are ready for discharge between the fifth to seventh post-operative day. Before discharge, they are evaluated in the non-invasive vascular laboratory to provide an objective baseline for follow-up studies.

EXTRA-ANATOMICAL BYPASS GRAFTS

When indicated, femorofemoral and axillobifemoral bypasses are good alternatives for aortoiliac revascularization. Femorofemoral graft is the procedure of choice if a normal donor artery is available to bypass extensive unilateral iliac disease[59,60] (Figure 16.5a and b). Axillobifemoral bypass is justified in high-risk patients, especially those in whom a transabdominal approach is contraindicated.[61]

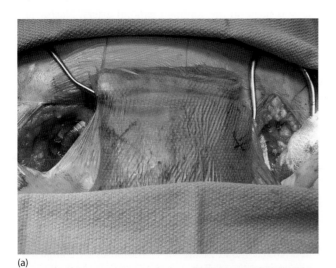

(a)

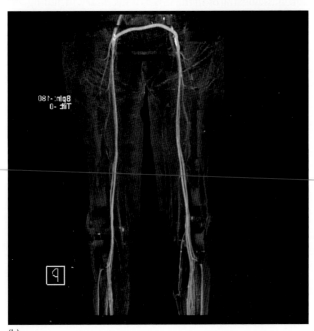

(b)

Figure 16.5 (a) Femoral to femoral bypass with ringed PTFE and (b) subsequent MRA demonstrating patency of the graft with run-off.

There are certain low-risk patients in whom a transabdominal approach is contraindicated but who should be considered for a more durable procedure than axillobifemoral bypass. Baird et al.[62] described the technique of using the ascending aorta as an inflow source for revascularization to the level of the femoral arteries and have reported excellent, durable results. Alternatively, the descending thoracic aorta can be used as the inflow site.[63–68] The choice between these two procedures is largely dependent on personal preference. The advantage of using the descending aorta is that it is a shorter bypass, is less susceptible to kinking and does not interfere with future abdominal or coronary surgery. However, a lateral thoracotomy is more painful than a sternotomy.

Results of open bypass surgery

In a meta-analysis of 23 studies, de Vries and Hunink reported a mortality rate of 3.3% for studies that started after 1975.[69] In the hands of very experienced surgeons, the perioperative mortality for aortobifemoral reconstruction is now between 2% and 3%.[13,70,71] Perioperative myocardial infarction accounts for half the deaths, and stroke, respiratory failure or renal failure for the remainder.[71] Five years post-operatively, 25% will be dead, and 10 years post-operatively, 50%.[71,72]

There is general agreement that the expected long-term patency rates of aortofemoral bypasses are excellent. From their meta-analysis, de Vries and Hunink reported that limb-based patency rates for patients with claudication were 91.0% and 86.8% at 5 and 10 years, respectively, as compared with 87.5% and 81.8% for patients with severe ischemia.[69,73–78] Thus, patency rates are lower if the indication for the operation is ischemic rest pain or ulceration but also the results are less satisfactory if coexisting femoropopliteal occlusive disease is present.[41]

Other surgical options for management of AIOD

LAPAROSCOPIC AORTOFEMORAL BYPASS

Early experimental and human studies demonstrated the feasibility of performing an aortobifemoral bypass using laparoscopic methods, with the first report of laparoscopic aortobifemoral bypass being in 1993 by Dion et al.[79] Techniques used in laparoscopic aortic surgery can be totally laparoscopic or laparoscopic-assisted with either hand-assisted laparoscopy or laparoscopic dissection followed by a mini-laparotomy to facilitate a conventional vascular anastomosis. Since the time it was first described, there have only been a limited number of studies on evaluating laparoscopic vascular surgery. In a systematic review of the literature from 1966 to 2006, Nio et al. identified only 30 studies on laparoscopic vascular surgery, the majority of which were descriptive in nature.[80] Theoretical benefits of the laparoscopic approach include decreased hospital stay, post-operative pain and recovery time while maintaining outcomes typically seen after open revascularization. Unfortunately, however, the mastery of laparoscopic aortic surgery has a significantly long learning curve and has yet to demonstrate substantial advantage over conventional therapies. With most studies being descriptive and having an element of patient selection bias,[80] current experience is still limited and the advantage of the laparoscopic approach over an open technique will have to be demonstrated in a carefully controlled comparative study prior to more widespread implementation.

ROBOTIC AORTOFEMORAL BYPASS

Robotic-assisted aortoiliac surgery first surfaced in 2002 in a report of two cases by Wisselink et al. who used robotic technology in two laparoscopic aortobifemoral bypass cases.[81] In a subsequent report by Stadler et al., a series of 100 robotic-assisted aortoiliac reconstructions for aneurysm and occlusive disease was presented demonstrating a 3% conversion rate, median operating time of 235 minutes, median anastomosis time of 29 minutes, median hospital stay of 5.1 days and a 30-day survival of 100% with non-lethal post-operative complications noted in 3% of patients.[82] Although these results are impressive and improve upon the prolonged aortic cross clamp and anastomotic times often noted in laparoscopic vascular surgery, the substantial learning curve and capital investment as well as the availability and expanded use of less invasive endovascular approaches has staggered the wide adoption of this technology in vascular surgery.

CONCLUSION

AIOD is generally benign and is often successfully managed with optimal medical therapy and participation in a supervised exercise programme. In patients with progressive symptoms or acute presentation, however, revascularization via endovascular or surgical therapy may be necessary. Despite the lack of established randomized clinical trial data, endovascular techniques are becoming increasingly utilized and have been successful for even extensive aortoiliac lesions. Until more absolute recommendations are available on the basis of ongoing studies, strategies for revascularization should be individualized based on patient factors, technical considerations and operator expertise. With proper selection of a management approach, gratifying long-term results can be achieved.

REFERENCES

1. Leriche R. De la resection du carrefour aorto-iliaque avec double sympathectomie lombaire pour thrombose artéritique de l'aorte: Le syndrome de l'oblitération terminoaortique par artérite. *Presse Med.* 1940;48:601–604.
2. Dos Santos JD. Sur la Desobstruction des Thromboses Arterielles Anciennes. *Mem Acad Chir.* 1947;73:409–411.
3. Wylie EJ. Thromboendarterectomy for arteriosclerotic thrombosis of major arteries. *Surgery.* 1952 August;32(2):275–292.
4. Barker WF, Cannon JA. An evaluation of endarterectomy. *AMA Arch Surg.* 1953 April;66(4):488–495.
5. Oudot J. La Greffe Vasculaire dans les thromboses du Carrefour Aortique. *Presse Med.* 1951;59:234–236.
6. Julian OC, Dye WS, Olwin JH, Jordan PH. Direct surgery of arteriosclerosis. *Ann Surg.* 1952 September;136(3):459–474.
7. Debakey ME, Creech O Jr., Cooley DA. Occlusive disease of the aorta and its treatment by resection and homograft replacement. *Ann Surg.* 1954 September;140(3):290–310.
8. Voorhees AB Jr., Jaretzki A III, Blakemore AH. The use of tubes constructed from vinyon "N" cloth in bridging arterial defects. *Ann Surg.* 1952 March;135(3):332–336.
9. Edwards WS. *Plastic Arterial Grafts.* Springfield, IL: Charles C. Thomas, Publisher; 1957.
10. De Bakey ME, Stanley E, Crawford ES. Vascular prostheses. *Transplant Bull.* 1957 January;4(1):2–4.
11. Moore WS, Cafferata HT, Hall AD, Blaisdell FW. In defense of grafts across the inguinal ligament: An evaluation of early and late results of aorto-femoral bypass grafts. *Ann Surg.* 1968 August;168(2):207–214.
12. Perdue GD, Long WD, Smith RB III. Perspective concerning aorto-femoral arterial reconstruction. *Ann Surg.* 1971 June;173(6):940–944.
13. Baird RJ, Feldman P, Miles JT, Madras PM, Gurry JF. Subsequent downstream repair after aorta-iliac and aorta-femoral bypass operations. *Surgery.* 1977 December;82(6):785–793.
14. Whiteley MS, Ray-Chaudhuri SB, Galland RB. Changing patterns in aortoiliac reconstruction: A 7-year audit. *Br J Surg.* 1996 October;83(10):1367–1369.
15. Brewster DC, Darling RC. Optimal methods of aortoiliac reconstruction. *Surgery.* 1978 December;84(6):739–748.
16. Imparato AM, Sanoudos G, Epstein HY, Abrams RM, Beranbaum ER. Results in 96 aortoiliac reconstructive procedures: Preoperative angiographic and functional classifications used as prognostic guides. *Surgery.* 1970 October;68(4):610–616.
17. Jernigan WR, Fallat ME, Hatfield DR. Hypoplastic aortoiliac syndrome: An entity peculiar to women. *Surgery.* 1983 November;94(5):752–757.
18. DeLaurentis DA, Friedman P, Wolferth CC Jr., Wilson A, Naide D. Atherosclerosis and the hypoplastic aortoiliac system. *Surgery.* 1978 January;83(1):27–37.
19. Ameli FM, Hoy F. Preoperative diagnosis and management of the hypoplastic vessel syndrome. *J Cardiovasc Surg.* 1983 November–December;24(6):654–657.
20. Burke PM Jr., Herrmann JB, Cutler BS. Optimal grafting methods for the small abdominal aorta. *J Cardiovasc Surg.* 1987 July–August;28(4):420–426.
21. Gagne PJ, Vitti MJ, Fink LM et al. Young women with advanced aortoiliac occlusive disease: New insights. *Ann Vasc Surg.* 1996 November;10(6):546–557.

22. Johnston KW, Demorais D, Colapinto RF. Difficulty in assessing the severity of aorto-iliac disease by clinical and arteriographic methods. *Angiology*. 1981 September;32(9):609–614.

23. Karmody AM, Powers SR, Monaco VJ, Leather RP. "Blue toe" syndrome: An indication for limb salvage surgery. *Arch Surg*. 1976 November;111(11):1263–1268.

24. Brewster DC, Waltman AC, O'Hara PJ, Darling RC. Femoral artery pressure measurement during aortography. *Circulation*. 1979 August;60(2 Pt 2):120–124.

25. Visser K, Hunink MG. Peripheral arterial disease: Gadolinium-enhanced MR angiography versus color-guided duplex US – A meta-analysis. *Radiology*. 2000 July;216(1):67–77.

26. Strandness DE Jr. An overview of research in peripheral vascular disease, 1986. *J Vasc Surg*. 1987 April;5(4):635–644.

27. Johnston KW, Kassam M, Cobbold RS. Relationship between Doppler pulsatility index and direct femoral pressure measurements in the diagnosis of aortoiliac occlusive disease. *Ultrasound Med Biol*. 1983 May–June;9(3):271–281.

28. Kohler TR, Nance DR, Cramer MM, Vandenburghe N, Strandness DE Jr. Duplex scanning for diagnosis of aortoiliac and femoropopliteal disease: A prospective study. *Circulation*. 1987 November;76(5):1074–1080.

29. McDaniel MD, Cronenwett JL. Basic data related to the natural history of intermittent claudication. *Ann Vasc Surg*. 1989 July;3(3):273–277.

30. Murphy TP, Cutlip DE, Regensteiner JG et al. Supervised exercise versus primary stenting for claudication resulting from aortoiliac peripheral artery disease: Six-month outcomes from the claudication: Exercise versus endoluminal revascularization (CLEVER) study. *Circulation*. 2012 January 3;125(1):130–139.

31. Indes JE, Pfaff MJ, Farrokhyar F et al. Clinical outcomes of 5358 patients undergoing direct open bypass or endovascular treatment for aortoiliac occlusive disease: A systematic review and meta-analysis. *J Endovasc Ther*. 2013 August;20(4):443–455.

32. Norgren L, Hiatt WR, Dormandy JA et al. Inter-Society Consensus for the Management of Peripheral Arterial Disease (TASC II). *J Vasc Surg*. 2007 January;45(Suppl. S):S5–S67.

33. Bekken JA, Vos JA, Aarts RA, de Vries JP, Fioole B. DISCOVER: Dutch Iliac Stent trial: COVERed balloon-expandable versus uncovered balloon-expandable stents in the common iliac artery: Study protocol for a randomized controlled trial. *Trials*. 2012;13:215.

34. Groot Jebbink E, Grimme FA, Goverde PC, van Oostayen JA, Slump CH, Reijnen MM. Geometrical consequences of kissing stents and the Covered Endovascular Reconstruction of the Aortic Bifurcation configuration in an in vitro model for endovascular reconstruction of aortic bifurcation. *J Vasc Surg*. 2015 May;61(5):1306–1311.

35. Tetteroo E, van der Graaf Y, Bosch JL et al. Randomised comparison of primary stent placement versus primary angioplasty followed by selective stent placement in patients with iliac-artery occlusive disease: Dutch Iliac Stent Trial Study Group. *Lancet*. 1998 April 18;351(9110):1153–1159.

36. Jongkind V, Akkersdijk GJ, Yeung KK, Wisselink W. A systematic review of endovascular treatment of extensive aortoiliac occlusive disease. *J Vasc Surg*. 2010 November;52(5):1376–1383.

37. Willekens FG, Wever J, Nevelsteen A et al. Extensive disobliteration of the aorto-iliac and common femoral arteries using the LeVeen plaque cracker. *Eur J Vasc Surg*. 1987 December;1(6):391–395.

38. Widdershoven RM, LeVeen HH. Closed endarterectomy: Preferred operation for aortoiliac occlusive disease. *Arch Surg*. 1989 August;124(8):986–990.

39. Naylor AR, Ah-See AK, Engeset J. Aortoiliac endarterectomy: An 11-year review. *Br J Surg*. 1990 February;77(2):190–193.

40. Ehrenfeld WK, Wilbur BG, Olcott CN, Stoney RJ. Autogenous tissue reconstruction in the management of infected prosthetic grafts. *Surgery*. 1979 January;85(1):82–92.

41. Kalman PG, Hosang M, Johnston KW, Walker PM. Unilateral iliac disease: The role of iliofemoral bypass. *J Vasc Surg*. 1987 August;6(2):139–143.

42. Piotrowski JJ, Pearce WH, Jones DN et al. Aortobifemoral bypass: The operation of choice for unilateral iliac occlusion? *J Vasc Surg*. 1988 September;8(3):211–218.

43. Melliere D, Labastie J, Becquemin JP, Kassab M, Paris E. Proximal anastomosis in aortobifemoral bypass: End-to-end or end-to-side? *J Cardiovasc Surg*. 1990 January–February;31(1):77–80.

44. Rosenbaum GJ, Arroyo PJ, Sivina M. Retroperitoneal approach used exclusively with epidural anesthesia for infrarenal aortic disease. *Am J Surg*. 1994 August;168(2):136–139.

45. DePalma RG, Levine SB, Feldman S. Preservation of erectile function after aortoiliac reconstruction. *Arch Surg*. 1978 August;113(8):958–962.

46. Flanigan DP, Schuler JJ, Keifer T, Schwartz JA, Lim LT. Elimination of iatrogenic impotence and improvement of sexual function after aortoiliac revascularization. *Arch Surg*. 1982 May;117(5):544–550.

47. Robicsek F, Duncan GD, Anderson CE et al. Indium 111-labeled platelet deposition in woven and knitted Dacron bifurcated aortic grafts with the same patient as a clinical model. *J Vasc Surg*. 1987 June;5(6):833–837.

48. Robicsek F, Daugherty HK, Cook JC et al. Patency rate of bifurcated aortic grafts: Comparative analysis of woven versus knitted prostheses in the same patient. *Ann Thorac Surg*. 1985 August;40(2):172–174.

49. Blumenberg RM, Gelfand ML, Barton EA, Bowers CA, Gittleman DA. Clinical significance of aortic graft dilation. *J Vasc Surg.* 1991 August;14(2):175–180.

50. Schneider JR, Zwolak RM, Walsh DB, McDaniel MD, Cronenwett JL. Lack of diameter effect on short-term patency of size-matched Dacron aortobifemoral grafts. *J Vasc Surg.* 1991 June;13(6):785–790; discussion 790–781.

51. Sterpetti AV, Feldhaus RJ, Schultz RD. Combined aortofemoral and extended deep femoral artery reconstruction. Functional results and predictors of need for distal bypass. *Arch Surg.* 1988 October;123(10):1269–1273.

52. Pearce WH, Kempczinski RF. Extended autogenous profundaplasty and aortofemoral grafting: An alternative to synchronous distal bypass. *J Vasc Surg.* 1984 May;1(3):455–458.

53. Nevelsteen A, Beyens G, Smet G, Suy R. Aortofemoral reconstruction for multilevel disease: A prospective hemodynamic study. *Acta Chir Belg.* 1989 July–August;89(4):179–184.

54. Sladen JG, Gerein AN, Maxwell TM, Wong R. Reoperation within 2 years of aortofemoral bypass. *Can J Surg.* 1988 July;31(4):224–227.

55. Brewster DC, Perler BA, Robison JG, Darling RC. Aortofemoral graft for multilevel occlusive disease: Predictors of success and need for distal bypass. *Arch Surg.* 1982 December;117(12):1593–1600.

56. Kalman PG, Johnston KW, Walker PM. Is aortoprofunda bypass a successful operation for multilevel occlusive disease? *Vasc Endovascular Surg.* 1989;23:265–271.

57. Eidt J, Charlesworth D. Combined aortobifemoral and femoropopliteal bypass in the management of patients with extensive atherosclerosis. *Ann Vasc Surg.* 1987 May;1(4):453–460.

58. Harris PL, Bigley DJ, McSweeney L. Aortofemoral bypass and the role of concomitant femorodistal reconstruction. *Br J Surg.* 1985 April;72(4):317–320.

59. Kalman PG, Hosang M, Johnston KW, Walker PM. The current role for femorofemoral bypass. *J Vasc Surg.* 1987 July;6(1):71–76.

60. Fahal AH, McDonald AM, Marston A. Femorofemoral bypass in unilateral iliac artery occlusion. *Br J Surg.* 1989 January;76(1):22–25.

61. Kalman PG, Hosang M, Cina C et al. Current indications for axillounifemoral and axillobifemoral bypass grafts. *J Vasc Surg.* 1987 June;5(6):828–832.

62. Baird RJ, Ropchan GV, Oates TK, Weisel RD, Provan JL. Ascending aorta to bifemoral bypass – A ventral aorta. *J Vasc Surg.* 1986 March;3(3):405–410.

63. McCarthy WJ, Rubin JR, Flinn WR, Williams LR, Bergan JJ, Yao JS. Descending thoracic aorta-to-femoral artery bypass. *Arch Surg.* 1986 June;121(6):681–688.

64. Schellack J, Fulenwider JT, Smith RB III. Descending thoracic aortofemoral-femoral bypass: A remedial alternative for the failed aortobifemoral bypass. *J Cardiovasc Surg.* 1988 March–April;29(2):201–204.

65. Schultz RD, Sterpetti AV, Feldhaus RJ. Thoracic aorta as source of inflow in reoperation for occluded aortoiliac reconstruction. *Surgery.* 1986 October;100(4):635–645.

66. Bowes DE, Keagy BA, Benoit CH, Pharr WF. Descending thoracic aortobifemoral bypass for occluded abdominal aorta: Retroperitoneal route without an abdominal incision. *J Cardiovasc Surg.* 1985 January–February;26(1):41–45.

67. Kalman PG. Thoracic aorta to femoral bypass: A useful expedient. *Semin Vasc Surg.* 1994 March;7(1):54–59.

68. Kalman PG, Johnston KW, Walker PM. Descending thoracic aortofemoral bypass as an alternative for aortoiliac revascularization. *J Cardiovasc Surg.* 1991 July–August;32(4):443–446.

69. de Vries SO, Hunink MG. Results of aortic bifurcation grafts for aortoiliac occlusive disease: A meta-analysis. *J Vasc Surg.* 1997 October;26(4):558–569.

70. Baird RJ. Techniques and results of arterial prosthetic bypass for aortoiliac occlusive disease. *Can J Surg.* 1982 September;25(5):476–478.

71. Crawford ES, Bomberger RA, Glaeser DH, Saleh SA, Russell WL. Aortoiliac occlusive disease: Factors influencing survival and function following reconstructive operation over a twenty-five-year period. *Surgery.* 1981 December;90(6):1055–1067.

72. Szilagyi DE, Elliott JP Jr., Smith RF, Reddy DJ, McPharlin M. A thirty-year survey of the reconstructive surgical treatment of aortoiliac occlusive disease. *J Vasc Surg.* 1986 March;3(3):421–436.

73. Malone JM, Moore WS, Goldstone J. The natural history of bilateral aortofemoral bypass grafts for ischemia of the lower extremities. *Arch Surg.* 1975 November;110(11):1300–1306.

74. Martinez BD, Hertzer NR, Beven EG. Influence of distal arterial occlusive disease on prognosis following aortobifemoral bypass. *Surgery.* 1980 December;88(6):795–805.

75. Naylor AR, Ah-See AK, Engeset J. Graft occlusion following aortofemoral bypass for peripheral ischaemia. *Br J Surg.* 1989 June;76(6):572–575.

76. Sladen JG, Gilmour JL, Wong RW. Cumulative patency and actual palliation in patients with claudication after aortofemoral bypass: Prospective long-term follow-up of 100 patients. *Am J Surg.* 1986 August;152(2):190–195.

77. Hertzer NR, Avellone JC, Farrell CJ et al. The risk of vascular surgery in a metropolitan community: With observations on surgeon experience and hospital size. *J Vasc Surg.* 1984 January;1(1):13–21.

78. Rutherford RB, Jones DN, Martin MS, Kempczinski RF, Gordon RD. Serial hemodynamic assessment of aortobifemoral bypass. *J Vasc Surg.* 1986 November;4(5):428–435.

79. Dion YM, Katkhouda N, Rouleau C, Aucoin A. Laparoscopy-assisted aortobifemoral bypass. *Surg Laparosc Endosc.* 1993 October;3(5):425–429.

80. Nio D, Diks J, Bemelman WA, Wisselink W, Legemate DA. Laparoscopic vascular surgery: A systematic review. *Eur J Vasc Endovasc Surg.* 2007 March;33(3):263–271.

81. Wisselink W, Cuesta MA, Gracia C, Rauwerda JA. Robot-assisted laparoscopic aortobifemoral bypass for aortoiliac occlusive disease: A report of two cases. *J Vasc Surg.* 2002 November;36(5):1079–1082.

82. Stadler P, Dvoracek L, Vitasek P, Matous P. Is robotic surgery appropriate for vascular procedures? Report of 100 aortoiliac cases. *Eur J Vasc Endovasc Surg.* 2008 October;36(4):401–404.

17

Femoral–popliteal–tibial occlusive disease

Open surgical therapy

FRANK J. VEITH, NEAL S. CAYNE, EVAN C. LIPSITZ, GREGG S. LANDIS,
NICHOLAS J. GARGIULO III and ENRICO ASCHER

CONTENTS

In this chapter we will discuss open surgical procedures for femoral, popliteal and tibial arterial occlusive diseases. Although some of these procedures may occasionally be performed for disabling intermittent claudication, the majority should only be performed for critical lower limb ischemia (CLI). This may be defined as sufficiently poor arterial blood supply to pose a threat to the viability of the lower extremity. Manifestations of CLI are true ischemic rest pain, ulceration and gangrene. These manifestations typically occur because of arteriosclerotic occlusive disease of large-, medium- and/or small-sized arteries, although other aetiologies may produce or contribute to these conditions. For example, many non-vascular causes may cause limb pain at rest, infection may cause or contribute to gangrene, and trauma and decreased sensation may produce ulceration. Although thromboembolism and other aetiologies can produce acute CLI, this chapter will only deal with chronic lower extremity ischemia due to obliterative arteriosclerosis. Over the last three decades, it has become increasingly apparent that limbs that are threatened by this process almost always have multilevel occlusive disease which often includes occlusions of arteries in the thigh, leg and foot.[1]

Open surgical procedures for chronic CLI include local amputations of toes and other portions of the foot, a variety of debriding procedures including open amputations of portions of the foot to control infection and a variety of traditional open surgical revascularization procedures primarily vein and prosthetic arterial bypasses above or below the inguinal ligament. These may, on occasion, be supplemented with localized endarterectomies with or without patch angioplasties. Except for an occasional patient with common femoral artery (CFA) and deep femoral artery (DFA) lesions, these operations alone are rarely enough alone to save a severely ischemic limb.

TOE AND FOOT AMPUTATIONS, DEBRIDEMENTS AND CONSERVATIVE TREATMENT

A detailed description of these procedures is beyond the scope of this chapter. However, certain principles should be emphasized. Gangrenous and infected toes can be successfully amputated by closed or open techniques in patients with good circulation as manifest by pedal pulses. Extensive debridements and partial foot amputations will also usually heal in such patients if all infected and necrotic tissue is excised. These procedures will usually result in patients regaining an effective walking status. Amputation of one or more gangrenous or ulcerated toes or limited debridements may also sometimes result in a healed foot in patients without distal pulses and substantial arterial occlusive disease (e.g. an occluded superficial femoral artery [SFA]) with good collaterals. Determination of moderately good collateral circulation by ankle–brachial indices or pulse volume recordings may be helpful in predicting such healing. However, sometimes in patients with borderline circulation, a trial of such local procedures is warranted before proceeding with a major revascularization. If prompt evidence of healing does not result, revascularization is then justified and should be performed without delay.

Furthermore, some patients with critical ischemia as manifest by mild ischemic rest pain and/or limited gangrene or ulceration can be successfully managed conservatively with good foot care, antibiotics, analgesics and limited ambulation.[2] A trial of such conservative treatment is particularly indicated in patients who might not tolerate revascularization procedures because of major co-morbidities. Long periods of palliation and occasional healing of small ulcerations or gangrenous patches may take place in a few such patients with critical ischemia.[2]

AGGRESSIVE APPROACH TO LIMB SALVAGE IN PATIENTS WITH CRITICAL ISCHEMIA DUE TO INFRAINGUINAL ARTERIOSCLEROSIS: A HISTORY AND THE EVOLUTION OF THE RELATIONSHIP BETWEEN OPEN BYPASS SURGERY AND ANGIOGRAPHIC TECHNIQUES AND ENDOVASCULAR TREATMENTS

In the 1960s and 1970s, major below-knee or above-knee amputation was regarded as the safest and best treatment for gangrene and ulceration from arteriosclerotic occlusive disease below the inguinal ligament,[3] despite the effectiveness of reconstructive arterial surgery (bypass and endarterectomy) for aortoiliac occlusive disease and despite some occasional positive results from femoropopliteal and even femorotibial bypasses. Because we had access to unusually good arteriography which visualized all the arteries in the leg and foot, we developed and promoted an aggressive approach to salvage threatened limbs including those with extensive gangrene.[4] Over 96% of patients with threatened limbs were subjected to an effort to save the limb. Only 4%, those with severe dementia or gangrene extending beyond the mid-foot were excluded. Only 6% of all patients with threatened

limbs, when examined by this extensive arteriography, had no patent artery in the leg or foot which could serve as an outflow site for a bypass.[4] With improvements in technique which we and others developed, this proportion of patients with arteries unsuitable for a bypass fell to 1%–2%.[1,5–11] Successful foot salvage was achieved in 81%–95% of patients in whom bypasses were performed for the period that they lived up to 5 years.[1,4] However, 52% of these limb salvage patients had many medical co-morbidities and died, usually from cardiac causes, within the first 5 years after their initial bypass.[4] More than two-thirds of the patients who lived beyond 5 years retained a useable limb and were able to ambulate beyond the 5-year time point.[4] However, to maintain limb salvage, many of these patients required some form of reoperation or reintervention because they developed a failed (thrombosed) or failing (threatened but patent) graft from a lesion in their graft or its inflow or outflow tracts.[1,4,5] These worthwhile limb salvage results were in part achieved because of a myriad of improvements in the surgical techniques,[1,4–11] because of the development of methods to facilitate the many reoperations these patients required,[12–14] and importantly because of improved anaesthetic and intensive care management of these limb salvage patients who often had advanced cardiorespiratory disease, poor kidney function and diabetes. Collectively, these improvements made possible attempts at limb salvage in almost all patients with a threatened limb and intact brain functions,[1,4,9] and many vascular centres throughout the world adopted these policies and were able to achieve equally good results.

EARLY COMBINATION OF ENDOVASCULAR TECHNIQUES (ANGIOPLASTY AND STENTING) WITH BYPASS SURGERY

In the mid-1970s, we and some other centres embraced the use of percutaneous transluminal angioplasty (PTA) to treat these elderly, debilitated patients with threatened lower limbs.[4] At the outset, PTA was used to correct hemodynamically significant iliac artery stenosis. In most instances, this was combined with some form of infrainguinal bypass. However, as PTA techniques improved, balloon angioplasty was used to treat short iliac occlusions and some SFA lesions as well. In this early experience, approximately 19% of patients with a threatened limb could be treated by PTA alone without an adjunctive bypass, while another 14% required some form of open surgical revascularization along with their PTA.[1] These percentages increased and results improved with the introduction of iliac stents. As technical improvements in endovascular technology were developed, our group was one of the first to use popliteal, infrapopliteal and tibial PTA to facilitate the treatment of these limb salvage patients, to manage them less invasively and to avoid some of the systemic and local complications of the lengthy and sometimes difficult distal operations in these complex patients.[15–17] We also used and advocated these endovascular techniques, where possible, to help in the treatment of patients with failed or failing bypasses, since reoperative procedures were often more difficult than primary bypass operations.[1,4,18,19] Sometimes (in approximately 20% of patients) PTA eliminated the need for a secondary bypass; more often it made the secondary bypass simpler. In addition, we developed a number of unusual approaches to lower extremity arteries to facilitate reoperations by eliminating the need to re-dissect previously dissected arteries.[12–14,20]

PRESENT AND FUTURE RELATIONSHIP BETWEEN ENDOVASCULAR TREATMENTS AND OPEN BYPASS SURGERY

Recent improvements in catheter, guidewire, stent and stent-graft technology have transformed the treatment of lower limb ischemia from a primarily open surgical (bypass) modality supplemented by some catheter-based treatments to a primarily endovascular modality. Most clinicians who treat critical ischemia today regard endovascular treatments as the first option to treat chronic obstructive arteriosclerosis at all levels including disease in the leg and foot, and other chapters in this text discuss improved endovascular techniques for doing so. In fact, there are some endovascular enthusiasts who mistakenly maintain that if a limb cannot be salvaged by endovascular treatment, the next option should be a major amputation.

While we are endovascular enthusiasts and while we also believe that endovascular treatment should be the first therapeutic option to revascularize a critically ischemic limb in most patients, we still believe that some patients whose leg and foot cannot be saved by some form of endovascular treatment can undergo an open surgical bypass procedure or a partially open removal of a resistant clot with a successful salvage of the foot.

Although almost all experts will agree that there are still some indications for open surgical bypasses for limb threatening ischemia, there is wide variation in opinions about the proportion of patients with critical ischemia that will require an open bypass or thrombectomy at some point in their disease process. We currently believe that at least 20%–35% of patients with critical ischemia will require an open surgical procedure at some point in the course of their disease, although we acknowledge that endovascular techniques continue to improve so that this proportion may decrease in the future. We also believe that such procedures will usually be indicated after failures of one, or usually more, endovascular treatments, although there are some patients with extensive foot gangrene, very long occlusions, limited target outflow arteries and a good greater saphenous vein in whom a bypass should be considered as the best initial treatment option.[21,22] To some extent, such an option will depend on many factors such as the age and health of the patient, the pattern of disease and the skills of the involved interventionalist and surgeon. One real concern is that as fewer bypasses will be required, fewer surgeons will be skilled in these demanding bypass techniques, particularly in the difficult circumstances in which they will be needed. Perhaps referral centres for such bypasses should be established for the same reasons that such centres have been recommended for the few patients who require open thoraco-abdominal aneurysm repair.

It has been recognized for many years that repetitive or redo procedures are an important component of care for patients with critical ischemia.[1,4,5] This will continue. Endovascular procedures may be used to salvage limbs after failed or failing open surgical bypasses.[1,18,19] This tendency will increase as technology improves. Similarly, bypass operations or partially open thrombectomy will be required after early or late failure of endovascular treatment or prior bypasses in patients in whom no further endovascular options are available. We believe most of the 20%–35% of critical ischemia patients who will require an open surgical bypass or thrombectomy will require it in such a setting.

There are certain principles and precautions that those performing endovascular interventions for limb ischemia should observe. These interventions should be used in a way that preserves at least one good target outflow artery, thereby leaving the option of an open surgical rescue if the intervention fails. In addition, care must be taken not to render initially patent arterial segments unusable, thereby necessitating a more distal bypass than would have been required prior to the endovascular procedure. Moreover, key collateral vessels should be preserved so that the patient will not be worse than he originally was if the intervention fails. This is particularly important to avoid the need for some reinterventions if ulcerated or gangrenous lesions have healed. These lesions may remain healed solely on the basis of preserved collateral pathways.

SPECIFIC OPEN SURGICAL REVASCULARIZATION PROCEDURES

These fall under two major headings: bypass procedures and revision of failed (thrombosed) prior bypasses that cannot be rescued by endovascular means. The latter circumstance is usually associated with an organized fibrinous plug that cannot be lysed, dilated or removed at either the proximal or distal anastomosis of a prosthetic bypass.

Superficial femoral artery and above-knee popliteal occlusive disease

With the introduction of improved techniques for crossing total occlusions, subintimal or intraluminal PTA with standard or drug coated balloons can be used to treat most occlusions of the SFA and above-knee popliteal artery. Nitinol self-expanding stents and stent grafts (Viabahn) can be used as adjuncts to these procedures.[23–25] When performing these procedures, care must be taken not to violate the principles and precautions outlined earlier and to preserve important collateral vessels, like the profunda femoris artery. In the unusual instance when these endovascular interventions fail and cannot be restored to patency or when technical difficulty is encountered, a femoropopliteal bypass can be performed to the below-knee popliteal artery or tibioperoneal trunk via standard medial approaches.[26] This is best performed with a reversed greater saphenous vein harvested via skip incisions, although endoscopic vein harvest has been described.[27] However, this technique requires special equipment and technical expertise. In situ vein bypass offers no advantage in the femoropopliteal position. If the groin is heavily scarred or infected, the distal two-thirds of the DFA can be accessed directly in the thigh and used for bypass inflow (or outflow if a bypass ends in the groin).[13] In circumstances in which the medial approaches to the popliteal artery are rendered difficult or impossible because of scarring or infection, both the above-knee and the below-knee popliteal arteries can be accessed via lateral approaches and used for bypass outflow.[14] If this is done, the graft can be tunnelled laterally in a subcutaneous plane. If patients do not have a saphenous vein or arm vein or if their veins are too small (<3.5 mm in distended diameter) or involved with pre-existing disease[28] and they require a femoropopliteal bypass, a 6 mm PTFE conduit may be used.[29] If this is done or even if a vein is used, duplex surveillance is warranted and reintervention is justified for a failing (threatened) graft. However, if the graft has failed (thrombosed), reintervention is only indicated if the failure results in renewed critical ischemia, which only occurs in about 65% of cases in whom the original bypass was performed for critical ischemia.[12]

Tibial and peroneal artery bypasses

These may be indicated after multiple failures of endovascular treatments. Some also believe they are sometimes also indicated when long segments of all three crural vessels and the below-knee popliteal or tibioperoneal trunk are occluded, especially if extensive foot necrosis is present. However, even in this circumstance some believe long segment tibial PTA is effective.[30,31]

For tibial and peroneal bypasses, autologous vein is the graft of choice provided it is disease-free.[28] The source of the superficial vein can be from any limb or site, and the vein can be used in either the reversed or in situ configuration. Our own randomized comparison of reversed and in situ vein grafts to crural arteries demonstrated no significant patency or limb salvage differences except for veins <3.0 mm in distended diameter.[32] In this circumstance in situ grafts performed better but the difference was not statistically significant. To facilitate the use of vein as the conduit, the grafts should be as short as possible and the SFA, the popliteal and even tibial arteries have proven to be effective sites of origin for these distal bypasses when there is no important proximal disease.[6–8,10] If there is, it can often be treated by PTA enabling a distal short vein graft without compromising patency.[33] Moreover, if there is a patent popliteal blind or isolated segment (without tibial or peroneal outflow) and limited lengths of autologous vein, a composite sequential bypass may be performed with the distal component being a vein graft from the isolated popliteal to a patent tibial artery and the proximal component being a PTFE graft from a femoral artery to the proximal end of the vein graft.[34] If a critical ischemia patient is faced with an imminent amputation and is totally without satisfactory autologous vein, a PTFE tibial bypass is in our opinion an acceptable option, and over the years we have obtained good secondary patency and limb salvage results (43% for a 5-year secondary patency and 66% for a 5-year limb salvage) in this setting.[29,35] Although some advocate use of a distal vein patch or cuff to improve patency,[36] we have not been convinced that any of these adjunctive procedures improve patency results more than a carefully constructed distal PTFE graft anastomosis. We have also reviewed our recent experience with PTFE bypasses to leg arteries and are convinced that they have a role in achieving and maintaining limb salvage when other options are not available.[37] The graft must, however, be implanted into a leg artery which has luminal continuity to its normal terminal branches and preferably richly supplies the foot, and the surgeon must be willing to do a secondary or redo prosthetic tibial bypass if the original graft fails.[37] We also acknowledge that many groups have not been able to duplicate our results although others have.[38,39]

Bypasses to foot arteries and their branches

In the late 1970s and early 1980s, we realized that many patients who were thought to have patterns of arteriosclerosis totally unsuited for revascularization actually had patent named arteries in their foot that could be used as outflow sites for distal bypasses.[1,4,7,10] By performing bypasses to these vessels, we could substantially increase the number of critical ischemia patients that could have their threatened limb saved.[1,7,10] Many other groups subsequently confirmed our initial results.

These very distal grafts can only be performed with vein as a conduit. However, many of these very distal grafts can originate from the below-knee popliteal artery or even from patent proximal tibial arteries.[1,6,7,10] As with all infrainguinal bypass grafts, and especially those to crural or pedal arteries, the procedures must be performed with care and technical perfection. Any technical error in graft preparation, tunnelling or anastomotic construction will result in failure. Good lighting (headlight), a dry field and patience are essential. Magnification and micro-surgical instruments are often required, and care must be taken to treat outflow arteries atraumatically and to preserve all outflow branches even those small ones that are unnamed. Completion arteriography is also essential, as with all infrapopliteal bypasses to assure good anastomotic configuration and bypass flow rates. If spasm or decreased flow is noted, vasodilators (nitroglycerin, papaverine) may be helpful.[40] Further technical details and illustrations are provided in a chapter in the previous edition of this text.[26]

Although these foot artery procedures were developed before endovascular approaches existed to revascularize these very distal arteries, these foot artery bypasses still have a limited role today. The use of 014″ guidewire-based systems, coronary balloons and stents and drug eluting balloons are now being used to revascularize patent arteries in the lower leg and even the foot. These techniques can work well in the short term, but more long-term results are needed. Also exactly how the results of these newer endovascular treatments will compare to those of bypass operations in comparable patients needs to be determined. We embrace and use these newer less invasive techniques and are optimistic that they will work. However, that remains to be proven, and we believe there will always be a role for these very distal bypasses when an endovascular option is not available – provided there are surgeons trained and willing to do them.

NEWER TECHNIQUES FOR REDO PROCEDURES AFTER FAILED BYPASSES: THROMBECTOMY AND TOTAL OR PARTIAL RESCUE OF A FAILED PTFE BYPASS OR TOTALLY NEW BYPASSES

It is well known that infrainguinal revascularization procedures, both endovascular and open surgical, are associated with a progressively increasing failure rate, with a diminished luminal calibre followed by thrombosis. This is due to both intimal hyperplasia, largely a reaction to vascular injury and progression of the arteriosclerotic process. When bypasses or PTAs that have been performed for critical ischemia fail after a patency interval of 6 months or longer, the originally threatened limb is only rethreatened in about 65% of patients. This may be due to healing of the original gangrenous or ulcerated lesion and the fact that greater blood flow is required to achieve healing than to maintain it. Alternatively, the maintenance of a healed foot after a revascularization failure may be due to improved collateral blood flow or absence of the trauma or infection which contributed to the gangrene or ulceration in the first place.

Whatever the reason, management strategies for patients with failed revascularization procedures should be influenced by the fact that critical ischemia may not recur. Only if it does, should a secondary intervention be undertaken since such secondary procedures are generally more difficult and have worse results than primary procedures. Thus, redo procedures are not indicated to prevent CLI from developing. The one exception is when a primary procedure is determined by physical examination, symptoms or noninvasive testing to be in the *failing state*, i.e. threatened by the development of a new or recurrent lesion which reduces flow but without thrombosis of the revascularization.

A full description of all possible redo procedures that are indicated when a primary bypass, with vein or prosthetic, fails is beyond the scope of this chapter and is available elsewhere.[12] Nevertheless, some principles, in addition to those already mentioned, deserve emphasis. First, endovascular interventions should always be considered the first option in patients requiring a redo procedure even if the original revascularization was a bypass. Improved technology that was previously unavailable may be effective and may provide sufficient increased blood flow to maintain foot viability.

Second, redissection of previously dissected arteries, particularly in the groin, should be avoided since they are difficult and prone to a fivefold increased risk of infection. If a totally new bypass is required, as is usually the case when a failed vein graft cannot be freed of clot, alternate or new approaches to patent arteries should be used and these have been well described.[12–14,20]

Third, complete pre-procedural arteriography should precede any reoperative attempt. Planning can only be optimized when the surgeon or interventionalist is fully aware of the location and extent of all occlusive and stenotic arterial disease throughout the iliac system and the entire lower extremity.

Fourth, if the failed bypass is a prosthetic conduit, an effort should be made to restore patency percutaneously using mechanical thrombectomy devices and lytic agents. This is often facilitated if the proximal anastomotic hood of the original graft can be seen angiographically to facilitate guidewire passage. Only if interventional procedures fail should reoperation be undertaken. This is generally required when the proximal or distal organized thrombotic plug cannot be lysed or removed by percutaneous means. In this circumstance the PTFE graft is approached at its most accessible mid-portion, usually in a subcutaneous position and remote from any anastomosis. The graft is opened longitudinally and the liquified clot gently removed with balloon catheters. Then, using fluoroscopic guidance, guidewires and catheters are gently used to traverse the anastomosis. Fluoroscopy with contrast injections is used to identify any inflow or anastomotic lesions and similarly any outflow lesions. A double lumen balloon catheter is then passed over the guidewire across the anastomosis, the balloon is inflated with dilute contrast and under fluoroscopic control the balloon is gently withdrawn to remove free clot. By observing the distortion of the balloon, hyperplastic and arteriosclerotic lesions can be observed and corrected by PTA without or with stent placement.[41,42] Balloon distortion within the proximal graft indicates the presence of an organized gelatinous or fibrinous plug which cannot usually be removed with a balloon catheter.[42] In that case and because loose clot has been removed, there may often be some flow in the opened graft presenting a problem with hemostasis. If so, a 9 Fr hemostatic sheath is placed into the graft and bleeding around the sheath is controlled with doubled vessel loops. The sheath and its dilator are passed over the wire across the anastomosis. The dilator is removed and an adherent clot removal catheter can be passed within the sheath under fluoroscopic control. The sheath is retracted and the wires of the clot removal catheter are deployed only within the graft under fluoroscopic control to engage the adherent plug and remove it without injuring the adjacent artery.[42] Angiography is used to demonstrate absence of residual luminal defects. A similar procedure is then carried out distally. If unobstructed distal flow cannot be obtained after PTA and stent placement, the proximal graft now with unobstructed inflow is transected and used as the origin for a partially new bypass to another patent distal artery accessed via a virginal approach.[12,14,20] Completion contrast fluoroscopy should be used to confirm an adequate lumen without defects and unimpeded flow through the graft and into the outflow tract.

Multiple redo procedures

Some patients are subject to repetitive failure of lower extremity revascularization procedures including bypasses. Some believe that patients who have failure of two or more bypasses in the same lower extremity should, if they redevelop critical ischemia, undergo a major amputation. We do not agree with this concept and have recently demonstrated the value of repetitive redo bypasses, usually performed over several years (up to 15), in preserving the limb and lifestyle of these patients.[43] We observed the duration of patency following more than three bypasses was substantial and resulted in more than 3 years of extended limb salvage in more than 50% of the patients who would otherwise have required an amputation.[43] These beneficial results were only obtained when the repetitive bypasses were performed according to the principles already outlined. Moreover, these repetitive bypasses should only be performed when the patient would otherwise require an immediate major amputation.

FINAL REMARKS

The bottom line of all these treatment efforts for critical ischemia is that everything possible should be done to salvage the threatened foot in these elderly, sick patients who do not walk well after one major amputation and certainly

do not do so after bilateral amputations, which 25% of this population may otherwise require at some point in their course. Although the methods needed to save limbs initially and maintain this salvage may be time consuming and technically demanding and although they require continuing commitment on the part of the vascular surgeon or vascular specialist, they are gratifying to those that carry them out effectively and are rewarding in maintaining an acceptable lifestyle in this group of patients with advanced atherosclerosis.

REFERENCES

1. Veith FJ, Gupta SK, Wengerter KR, Goldsmith J, Rivers SP, Bakal C, Sprayregen S, Gliedman ML. Changing arteriosclerotic disease patterns and management strategies in lower limb threatening ischemia. *Ann Surg.* 1990;212:402–414.

2. Rivers SP, Veith FJ, Ascer EE, Gupta SK. Successful conservative therapy of severe limb threatening ischemia: The value of nonsympathectomy. *Surgery.* 1986;99:759–763.

3. Stoney RJ. Ultimate salvage for the patient with limb-threatening ischemia – Realistic goals and surgical considerations. *Am J Surg.* 1978;136:228–233.

4. Veith, FJ, Gupta SK, Samson RH et al. Progress in limb salvage by reconstructive arterial surgery combined with new or improved adjunctive procedures. *Ann Surg.* 1981;194:386–401.

5. Veith, FJ, Weiser RF, Gupta SK, Scher LA, Samson RH, Ascer E, Flores SW, Sprayregen S. Diagnosis and management of failing lower extremity arterial reconstructions prior to graft occlusion. *J Cardiovasc Surg.* 1984;25:381–384.

6. Veith, FJ, Gupta SK, Samson RH, White-Flores S, Janko G, Scher LA. The superficial femoral and popliteal arteries as inflow sites for distal bypasses. *Surgery.* 1981;90:980–991.

7. Ascer E, Veith FJ, Gupta SK. Bypasses to plantar arteries and other tibial branches: An extended approach to limb salvage. *J Vasc Surg.* 1988;8:434–441.

8. Ascer, E, Veith FJ, Gupta SK, White S, Bakal C, Wengerter KR, Sprayregen S. Short vein grafts: A superior option for arterial reconstruction to poor or compromised outflow tracts. *J Vasc Surg.* 1988;7:370–377.

9. Leather RP, Shah DM, Chang BB, Leather RP. Resurrection of the in situ vein bypass: 1000 Cases later. *Ann Surg.* 1988;208(4):435–442.

10. Veith, FJ, Ascher E, Gupta SK, White-Flores S, Sprayregen S, Scher LA, Samson RH. Tibiotibial vein bypass grafts: A new operation for limb salvage. *J Vasc Surg.* 1985;2:552–557.

11. Ascer E, Veith FJ, White-Flores S. Infrapopliteal bypasses to heavily calcified rock-like arteries: Management and results. *Am J Surg.* 1986;152:220–223.

12. Veith FJ, Gupta SK, Ascer E, Rivers SP, Wengerter KP. Improved strategies for secondary operations on infrainguinal arteries. *Ann Vasc Surg.* 1990;4:85–93.

13. Veith FJ, Nunez A, Gupta SK, Wengerter KR, White-Flores S, Skopetos M. Direct approaches to the middle and distal portions of the deep femoral artery for use as sites of origin or termination for secondary bypasses. *Perspect Vasc Surg.* 1988;1:94–102.

14. Veith FJ, Ascer E, Gupta SK, Wengerter KR. Lateral approach to the popliteal artery. *J Vasc Surg.* 1987;6:119–123.

15. Sprayregen S, Sniderman HW, Sos TA, Vieux U, Singer A, Veith FJ. Popliteal artery branches: Percutaneous transluminal angioplasty. *Am J Roentgenol.* 1980;135:945–951.

16. Bakal CW, Sprayregen S, Scheinbaum K, Cynamon J, Veith FJ. Percutaneous transluminal angioplasty of the infrapopliteal arteries: Results in 53 patients. *Am J Roentgenol.* 1990;154:171–174.

17. Veith FJ, Gupta SK, Wengerter KR, Rivers SP, Bakal C. Impact of nonoperative therapy on the clinical management of peripheral arterial disease. *Circulation.* 1991;83:137–142.

18. Sanchez L, Gupta SK, Veith FJ et al. A ten-year experience with one hundred fifty failing or threatened vein and polytetrafluoroethylene arterial bypass grafts. *J Vasc Surg.* 1991;14:729–738.

19. Sanchez LA, Suggs WD, Marin ML, Panetta TF, Wengerter KR, Veith FJ. Is percutaneous balloon angioplasty appropriate in the treatment of graft and anastomotic lesions responsible for failing vein bypasses. *Am J Surg.* 1994;168:97–101.

20. Dardik H, Dardik I, Veith FJ. Exposure of the tibial-peroneal arteries by a single lateral approach. *Surgery.* 1974;75:337.

21. Conte MS. Bypass versus angioplasty in severe ischaemia of the leg (BASIL) and the (hoped for) dawn of evidence-based treatment for advanced limb ischemia. *J Vasc Surg.* 2010;51(Suppl. 5):69S–75S.

22. Neville RF. Open surgical revascularization for wound healing: past performance and future directions. *Plast Reconstr Surg.* 2011;127(Suppl. 1): 154S–162S.

23. Martin S, Sabeti S, Loewe C, Dick P, Amighi J, Mlekusch W, Schlager O, Cejna M, Lammer J, Minar E. Balloon angioplasty versus implantation of nitonol stents in the superficial femoral artery. *N Engl J Med.* 2006;354:1879–1888.

24. Johannes L, Dake MD, Bleyn J, Katzen BT, Cejn M, Piquet P, Becker GJ, Settlage RA. Peripheral arterial obstruction: prospective study of treatment with a transluminally placed self-expanding stent graft. *Radiology.* 2000;217:95–104.

25. Fischer M, Schwabe C, Schulte K-L. Value of the hemobahn/viabahn endoprosthesis in the treatment of long chronic lesions of the superficial femoral artery: 6 Years of experience. *J Endovasc Ther.* 2006;13:281–290.

26. Veith FJ, Lipsitz EC. Femoral-popliteal-tibial occlusive disease. In: Hobson RW, Wilson SE, Veith FJ, eds. *Vascular Surgery: Principles and Practice.* New York: Marcel Dekker, Inc.; 2004, pp. 455–484.

27. Jordan WD, Alcocer F, Voellinger DC, Wirthlin DJ. The durability of endoscopic saphenous vein grafts: A 5-year observational study. *J Vasc Surg.* 2001;34:434–439.

28. Panetta TF, Marin ML, Veith FJ, Goldsmith J, Gordon RE, Jones AM, Schwartz ML, Gupta SK, Wengerter KR. Unsuspected pre-existing saphenous vein disease: An unrecognized cause of vein bypass failure. *J Vasc Surg.* 1992;15:102–112.

29. Veith FJ, Gupta SK, Ascer E et al. Six year prospective multicenter randomized comparison of autologous saphenous vein and expanded polytetrafluoroethylene grafts in infrainguinal arterial reconstructions. *J Vasc Surg.* 1986;3:104–115.

30. Bolia A. Subintimal angioplasty in lower limb ischaemia. *J Cardiovasc Surg.* 2005;46(4):385–394.

31. Lipsitz EC, Ohki T, Veith FJ, Suggs WD, Wain RA, Cynamon J, Mehta M, Cayne N, Gargiulo N. Does subintimal angioplasty have a role in the treatment of severe lower extremity ischemia? *J Vasc Surg.* 2003;37:386–391.

32. Harris PL, Veith FJ, Shanik GD, Nott D, Wengerter KR, Moore DJ. Prospective randomized comparison of in-situ and reversed infrapopliteal vein grafts. *Br J Surg.* 1993;80:173–176.

33. Wengerter KR, Yang PM, Veith FJ, Gupta SK, Panetta TF. A twelve-year experience with the popliteal-to-distal artery bypass: The significance and management of proximal disease. *J Vasc Surg.* 1992;15:143–151.

34. Gargiulo NJ, Veith FJ, O'Connor DJ, Lipsitz EC, Suggs WD, Scher LA. Experience with a modified composite sequential bypass technique for limb threatening ischemia. *Ann Vasc Surg.* 2010;24:1000–1004.

35. Parsons RE, Suggs WD, Veith FJ, Sanchez LA, Lyon RT, Marin ML, Goldsmith J, Faries PL, Wengerter KR, Schwartz ML. Polytetrafluoroethylene bypasses to infrapopliteal arteries without cuffs or patches: A better option than amputation in patients without autologous vein. *J Vasc Surg.* 1996;23:347–456.

36. Neville RF, Tempesta B, Sidaway A. Tibial bypass for limb salvage using polytetrafluoroethylene and a distal vein patch. *J Vasc Surg.* 2001;33(2):266–271.

37. Landis GS, Gargiulo NJ, Veith FJ et al. Polytetrafluoroethylene bypasses to infrapopliteal arteries without cuffs, patches or other adjunctive procedures: A 25-year experience. Manuscript in preparation.

38. Schweiger H, Klein P, Lang W. Tibial bypass grafting for limb salvage with ringed polytetrafluoroethylene prostheses: Results of primary and secondary procedures. *J Vasc Surg.* 1993;18(5):867–874.

39. Klinkert P, Van Dijk PJ, Breslau PJ. Polytetrafluoroethylene femorotibial bypass grafting: 5-Year patency and limb savage. *Ann Vasc Surg.* 2003;17(5):486–491.

40. Gargiulo NJ, Veith FJ, Lipsitz EC, Cayne NS, Landis GS. Pseudodefects in completion arteriography and their management by less invasive means. Manuscript in preparation.

41. Parsons RE, Marin ML, Veith FJ, Sanchez LA, Lyon RT, Suggs WD, Faries PL, Schwartz ML. Fluoroscopically assisted thromboembolectomy: An improved method for treating acute arterial occlusions. *Ann Vasc Surg.* 1996;10:201–210.

42. Cayne NS, Veith FJ. Operative thrombectomy for acute thrombosis of lower extremity bypass grafts. In: Stanley JC, Veith SJ, Wakefield TW, eds. *Current Therapy in Vascular and Endovascular Surgery,* 5th ed. Philadelphia, PA: Elsevier; 2014, pp. 584–587.

43. Lipsitz EC, Veith FJ, Cayne NS, Harvey J, Rhee S. Repetitive bypass and revisions with extensions for limb salvage after multiple previous failures. *Vascular.* 2013;21:63–68.

18

Results of endovascular therapy for femoral, popliteal and tibial disease

ADAM Z. OSKOWITZ and BRIAN G. DERUBERTIS

CONTENTS

INTRODUCTION

The treatment of infrainguinal arterial disease has changed significantly in the last 20 years, with the introduction of many new devices. There are now numerous options to restore flow through the infrainguinal arterial system and provide adequate perfusion to the leg. Endovascular treatment includes percutaneous transluminal angioplasty (PTA), stenting and atherectomy. These modalities can be used alone or in combination, depending on the severity of the disease and the preference of the surgeon. Each technique is further characterized by the particular devices used for treatment. Angioplasty can be performed with balloons that vary in size and compliance. Balloons coated with antimyoproliferative drugs have recently become commercially available in the United States and have been advocated to reduce restenosis. Several atherectomy tools are also available for use, including excisional, orbital and laser atherectomy devices. Stents currently used include self-expanding laser-cut nitinol bare-metal stents (BMSs), stents composed of helical interwoven nitinol wires, drug-coated stents and polytetrafluoroethylene-covered stents.

In this chapter, we will review the relevant literature for all of these treatment modalities, with a focus on the patency rates and freedom from amputation in patients with critical limb ischemia (CLI). The analysis is further subdivided into treatment of femoropopliteal disease and infrapopliteal disease, as the results between these groups are often discordant. When evaluating these treatment paradigms, it is important to realize that the risk of re-intervention following endovascular treatment is relatively high compared to open surgical reconstruction, and therefore, any treatment modality that does not impair further therapeutic possibilities has increased value. For example, while stenting may offer improved primary patency compared to PTA or atherectomy alone, indwelling stents in the femoral or popliteal arteries can limit treatment options and therefore should be used prudently.

Technique: General principles of endovascular revascularization

All types of percutaneous infrainguinal revascularization strategies employ similar basic principles. Standard arterial access and angiography techniques are required to delineate the culprit lesions requiring treatment, and then following initial angiography, the operator must cross the lesion and regain true-luminal position within the non-diseased or reconstituted artery distally. In the case of stenotic lesions, every effort is made to remain in the true lumen of the vessel while crossing the lesion, and this can be accomplished by using steerable guidewires and angled catheters to direct the tip of the wire around the areas of disease. In the case of total occlusions, however, one must advance the tip of the wire through the occlusion, either within the *true-luminal* position or by proceeding into the subintimal plane, whereby the wire traverses between the medial and intimal layers of the vessel wall. Upon using a subintimal approach, the operator must redirect the tip of the wire back into the reconstituted vessel distally and confirm luminal position before bringing the treatment device into the vessel.

Once the lesion has been crossed and wire access has been established across the lesion and into the outflow vessel, a device can be selected to treat the lesion based on the lesion characteristics and operator preference. If a distal embolic protection device (EPD) is thought to be necessary to prevent against distal embolization, then the EPD is brought in over the wire at this time and deployed beyond the lesion, using caution to select a landing zone for the EPD that is distal enough to allow working room for the treatment device between the end of the lesion and the EPD. At this point, the treatment device can be brought into position and used to treat the lesion.

As noted earlier, there are a number of devices available for treating infrainguinal occlusive disease, and these devices can be delivered via sheath access ranging from 5 to 8F and over 0.014, 0.018 and 0.035 in. wire platforms. Individual devices and techniques are described further in the following sections.

Following treatment of the target lesions, it is imperative to evaluate not only the treated region but also the distal runoff to ensure the absence of embolic complications. Completion angiography should therefore include both anteroposterior and lateral foot views of the lower leg and anteroposterior views of the tibial trifurcation, and these images are then compared to the preoperative views. Any evidence of worsening of runoff vessels or other embolic issues must be dealt with through various rescue techniques to avoid worsening the patient's clinical scenario, and operators performing endovascular infrainguinal interventions should therefore be familiar with these rescue manoeuvres.

PERCUTANEOUS TRANSLUMINAL ANGIOPLASTY

Percutaneous balloon angioplasty has been available for more than 30 years with several large trials and meta-analysis characterizing technical success and patency rates across a variety of different patients and lesions. Multiple manufacturers have developed a range of PTA balloons in diameters and lengths appropriate for lower extremity interventions. Most manufactures produce devices in 0.014, 0.018 and 0.035 in. wire platforms, and these devices vary in their crossing profile and trackability (both between manufacturers and most importantly between wire platforms).

Technique: Percutaneous transluminal angioplasty

Once the lesion has been crossed and wire access has been established, the angioplasty balloon is brought across the lesion and the balloon is inflated to its nominal diameter as directed by the balloon's respective compliance chart. Most balloons have rated nominal and burst pressures, at which the balloon achieves its nominal diameter and is at risk of rupturing with increased inflation pressure, respectively. Modern angioplasty balloons are relatively non-compliant, meaning that the balloon diameter will change very little with increased inflation pressures beyond the nominally rated pressure.

While inflation times vary by operator preference, there is some evidence that prolonged inflation times (2–3 minute inflations) and lower inflation pressures may result in improved lumen gain and decreased rates of intimal dissections.[1] Zorger and colleagues demonstrated a significant reduction in dissections and a trend towards reduced degree of residual stenosis following 180 second inflation times compared to 30 second inflations. Additionally, recent trials evaluating the use of drug-coated balloons (DCBs) have demonstrated surprisingly low bailout stent rates compared to traditional trials of PTA with selective stenting, and some have hypothesized that this was due to the protocol-driven 180 second balloon inflation times.[17]

RESULTS OF PERCUTANEOUS TRANSLUMINAL ANGIOPLASTY

Femoropopliteal disease

A review of PTA for femoropopliteal disease over 20 years identified the immediate technical success rate was 90% with a 4% procedural complication rate. The 1- and 5-year primary patency rates were 61% and 48%, respectively.[2] Multiple variables affect the outcomes of PTA including degree of stenosis, clinical stage (claudication vs. limb threat), lesion length and runoff. Two meta-analyses of femoral–popliteal PTA have been performed, reporting patency rates based on treatment indications for both occlusive and stenotic lesions.[3,4] Patency at 1 year ranged from 26% to 52% for occlusive lesions to 62%–79% in patients with stenotic lesions. At 5 years, the patency ranges dropped to 12%–47% and 35%–68%, respectively. In these analyses, patency rates were lower in patients with limb threat compared to claudication across all time frames. The length of the lesion also has a significant effect on patency, with focal lesions responding most favourably to PTA as a stand-alone treatment. Currie and colleagues reported that 22 of 23 patients with severe limb ischemia treated with PTA for occlusions greater than 5 cm had re-occluded at 6 months, and Jean and colleagues found similar results for lesions greater than 5 cm.[3,5,6] While angioplasty alone can be used on focal lesions of the superficial femoral artery (SFA) <4 cm long, most SFA lesions are associated with more complex and extensive disease than a single short stenosis.[7] In these situations, PTA should not be used as stand-alone treatment (Recommendation Grade A Level of Evidence 1).

Recommendations
Grade A Recommendations with Level 1 Evidence

- PTA alone can be used on focal femoropopliteal lesions <4 cm long but not lesions that represent more complex and extensive disease than a single short stenosis.
  - PTA for lesions longer than 4 cm has significantly reduced patency than shorter lesions.
- PTA of infrapopliteal disease appears safe and effective in preventing limb loss.
  - The more infrapopliteal vessels that are patent, the higher the limb salvage rates.
- DCB can be used safely in the treatment of femoropopliteal disease.
  - PTA with DCB has improved patency compared to PTA with standard balloons; however, longer-term follow-up is still needed.
- Treatment of infrapopliteal disease with DCB should be avoided.
  - Infrapopliteal PTA with DCB has not shown consistent benefit in clinical trials and may be harmful.
- BMS can be used effectively in femoropopliteal disease.
  - BMS appear to be effective in the treatment of femoropopliteal disease with improved short-term primary patency compared to PTA alone.
- Drug-eluting stent (DES) may show patency benefit over standard BMSs in femoropopliteal disease.
  - RCT show improved patency although data on the various devices can be conflicting.
- When stents are used in the treatment of infrapopliteal lesions, we recommend the use of DES.
  - For infrapopliteal lesions, the primary patency at 1 year is significantly higher in patients treated with DES compared to patients treated with either BMS or PTA.

Grade B Recommendations with Level 2 Evidence

- Excisional atherectomy can be used safely and effectively in treating femoropopliteal disease.
  - Prospective trials show higher patency than other published patency rates for PTA in femoropopliteal disease.
- When stenting is used for femoropopliteal lesions, we recommend the use of stents made of helical interwoven nitinol wires in a closed cell geometry.
  - Initial data show patency rates that are higher than published BMS patency rates.

Grade C Recommendations with Level 3 Evidence

- We recommend caution when using excisional atherectomy below the knee.
  - Large prospective studies and RCT studies are not yet available.

Infrapopliteal disease

Balloon angioplasty of the infrapopliteal segments has also been studied, though not commonly in a rigorously controlled fashion. The vast majority of patients requiring infra-geniculate intervention are suffering from CLI and thus outcomes often focus on limb salvage in addition to patency rates. Romiti and colleagues performed a systematic review of infrapopliteal PTA including 30 studies over a 16-year period. Immediate technical success was achieved in 89% of patients.[8] One- and three-year primary patency was 58% and 48%, respectively. Limb salvage was achieved in 86% and 82% of patients at 1 and 3 years. Two recent meta-analyses comparing PTA and stenting in infrapopliteal disease provide useful data on outcomes based on current PTA.[9,10] In one analysis, primary patency was 73% at 6 months and 57% at 12 months with a 12-month limb salvage rate of 93% in patients undergoing only PTA. The second analysis of over 16 trials (Yang et al.) identified that a 1-year primary patency was 57% with a limb salvage rate of 88% at 1 year. Predictors of long-term success in infrapopliteal PTA are similar to femoropopliteal interventions, as patients with stenosis (rather than occlusions) and focal disease show improved primary patency rates compared to more complex disease.[11] Interestingly, Giles et al. additionally found treatment of multilevel disease to improve outcomes, and other authors have also demonstrated improved outcomes with multilevel interventions, possibly related to improved runoff compared to patients undergoing single-level intervention.[12] In a review of over 1200 patients, Peregrin and colleagues found that the limb salvage rate at 1 year was improved in patients with more patent tibial vessels (83 vs. 56% in pts with 3 vs. 0 patent tibial vessels).[13] Based on these data, PTA of infrapopliteal disease appears safe and effective in preventing limb loss (Recommendation Grade A Level of Evidence 1).

Technique: Subintimal recanalization in conjunction with balloon angioplasty

Subintimal dissection typically involves the use of a hydrophilic guidewire that is looped in the patent portion of the vessel and then advanced into the area of occlusion in conjunction with a support catheter. This allows the wire to traverse into the subintimal plane where it can often pass with little resistance until reaching the reconstituted vessel, at which point the wire is then redirected into the true lumen of the vessel using either standard catheter techniques or re-entry devices. While this approach is often faster than attempting to remain within the true lumen of the occluded vessel, it also has the theoretical advantage of excluding much of the plaque and intraluminal thrombus contained within the occlusion from the newly recanalized lumen. When standard catheter and wire techniques do allow for return to the true lumen of the reconstituted vessel, the use of a specialized re-entry device can facilitate this process. These devices generally employ the use of a catheter or modified balloon placed over a 0.014 in. wire platform which then directs an obliquely oriented needed or angled guidewire towards the true lumen of the vessel. These devices generally work best when the dissection plane created by the subintimal dissection technique is in close proximity to the lumen of the reconstituted vessel, so if one intends to use one of these devices, it is advisable to utilize the device before multiple attempts at catheter-based re-entry has created a large false lumen. Commonly used re-entry catheters include the Pioneer Catheter (Volcano Corporation, San Diego, CA) and the Outback Re-Entry Catheter (Cordis, Freemont, CA) for above-knee re-entry and the Enteer Catheter (Medtronic, Minneapolis, MN) which can be used for both above-knee and below-knee re-entry.

SUBINTIMAL RECANALIZATION IN CONJUNCTION WITH BALLOON ANGIOPLASTY

Subintimal recanalization deserves special consideration as patients treated with this technique typically have long occlusive lesions and sometimes require specialized devices for re-entry into the true lumen of the vessel. While the exclusion of the plaque and thrombus burden from the neo-lumen could have a positive impact on patency rates, this is a hypothetical advantage that has not been demonstrated in the literature, in part because one can never be sure whether the guidewire is within a true-luminal or subintimal plane. Results in which predominantly subintimal techniques have been utilized appear to be similar to other series on percutaneous lower extremity angioplasty. One study showed patency of 71% and 58% at 1 and 3 years, respectively.[14] In tibial disease, one study of 46 patients showed a primary patency of 46% at 12 months with an 87% limb salvage rate at 1 year.[15] While the use of specialized re-entry devices can facilitate return to the true lumen and allow for faster and more consistent interventional success, there is no evidence that they improve patency outcomes.

DRUG-COATED BALLOON ANGIOPLASTY

Antimyoproliferative DCBs have been evaluated for the treatment of SFA and popliteal disease in patients with peripheral arterial occlusive disease, and these devices have been available in Europe and other countries for several years and in the United States more recently. There are currently two DCBs available for use in the United States, including the Lutonix (Bard, Covington, GA) and the IN.PACT Admiral 035 (Medtronic) DCBs, and each has randomized controlled trial (RCT) data comparing the efficacy of these balloons to plain balloon angioplasty alone. Both balloons combined paclitaxel with an excipient to facilitate drug delivery and are available in diameters and lengths appropriate for the treatment of the SFA and popliteal artery.

Technique: Transluminal angioplasty with drug-coated balloons

Angioplasty technique with DCBs differs from standard balloon angioplasty due to concerns regarding drug loss during balloon transit and regarding drug transfer during inflation. During preparation and flushing of the DCB on the cath lab back table, care should be used to avoid wetting the balloon surface, and the balloon should be advanced to the target lesion expediently after opening the packaging and prepping the balloon. Lesions should be pre-dilated with plain balloon angioplasty (using a balloon diameter 1 mm smaller than the estimated target vessel diameter) prior to use of the DCB. To avoid 'geographic miss', the DCB length should be 2 cm longer than the initial pre-dilation balloon such that the DCB extends beyond the treated artery 1 cm proximally and distally, and the DCB diameter should be sized in a 1:1 manner to the target vessel. Most of the clinically relevant drug transfer to the vessel wall occurs during the first 60 seconds of balloon inflation, but general recommendations for the use of DCBs are to perform a 180 second inflation.

RESULTS OF DRUG-COATED BALLOON ANGIOPLASTY
Femoropopliteal disease

The THUNDER trial evaluated patients treated with paclitaxel-coated balloons and standard balloons.[16] At 6 months, 66% of patients were free from angiographic restenosis (similar to primary patency) in the control group compared to 83% in the DCB arm. There was also a significantly reduced need to re-intervene at 24 months after initial PTA with a DCB compared to PTA with a standard balloon (15% vs. 52%). The FEMPAC trial showed similar results with only 13% of patients treated with DCB requiring re-intervention at 18 months.[17]

Two randomized controlled clinical trials led to FDA approval for the DCB devices that are currently available in the United States, including the LEVANT trial (Bard Lutonix Balloon) and the IN.PACT SFA trial (Medtronic IN.PACT Admiral Balloon). The study design was similar in both of these trials and included 2:1 randomization to the DCB or plain angioplasty balloon only after the target lesion was crossed and treated with an initial trial of balloon angioplasty. Provided an angiographically acceptable result was attained with the initial (plain) balloon inflation, the patient was then randomized to a second inflation either with the DCB or plain balloon again. Based on the initial publication of the European LEVANT I trial, reduced levels of restenosis after PTA with DCB were seen compared to standard PTA.[18] This effect persisted for 24 months; however, primary patency was still only 57% at 24 months. Updated results of the LEVANT trial as included in the FDA submission for device approval demonstrated a 390-day primary patency with the Lutonix DCB of 65% versus 53% for the plain angioplasty arm (p < 0.05)

Table 18.1 Randomized control trials examining outcomes using drug-coated balloons in femoropopliteal disease.

Authors	Time	Year	Patients	Primary patency		Freedom from TLR	
				DCB (%)	Control (%)	DCB (%)	Control (%)
Scheinert et al.[18]	1 year	2014	101	67	55	29	33
Werk et al.[17]	6 months	2008	87	81[a]	53	93[a]	67
Tepe et al.[16]	6 months	2008	102	83[a]	66	96[a]	63
Tepe et al.[20]	1 year	2014	331	82[a]	52	97[a]	79

Note: Control is traditional PTA: time from treatment until data collection.
[a] Statistical significance compared to control ($p < 0.05$).

and a freedom from target vessel revascularization (TLR) of 87.7% versus 83.2% ($p > 0.05$, not significant), respectively.[19] The results of the IN.PACT SFA trial were more promising with significantly improved primary patency at 1 year compared to traditional PTA (82% vs. 52%).[20] Two-year data from these trials are forthcoming. Based on these trials, DCB appears safe for use in femoropopliteal disease with improved patency compared to PTA with standard balloons. (Recommendation Grade A Level of Evidence 1). However, limitations in these trials include considerable selection bias due to inclusion criteria and trial design, resulting in patients who are primarily claudicants (Rutherford category 2–3) and whose lesion characteristics include short simple lesions (primarily non-calcified, stenotic lesions of 6.2 and 8.9 cm in LEVANT and IN.PACT SFA, respectively). Studies with longer follow-up and inclusion of more complex patient and lesion characteristics are necessary to more fully evaluate this therapy in the SFA and popliteal circulation (Table 18.1).

Infrapopliteal disease

The DEBELLUM trial evaluated treatment of multilevel disease with DCB versus conventional PTA.[21] In a subset of these patients, there was reduced late luminal loss at 1 year for lesions below the knee; however, this included only 30 total patients. However, the IN.PACTDEEP evaluated infrapopliteal revascularization with DCB and PTA in patients with CLI and found no difference in 12-month patency and a trend towards increased amputation rate in the DCB arm.[22] Thus, treatment of infrapopliteal with DCB has not shown any benefit in clinical trial and may be harmful. We recommend against this treatment until further study confirms these findings (Recommendation Grade A Level of Evidence 1) (Table 18.2).

ATHERECTOMY

Percutaneous atherectomy, utilizing either directional, orbital, laser or rotational devices, can allow for treatment of occlusive or stenotic lesions of the femoropopliteal and tibial circulation with minimal requirement for adjunctive stent implantation. Each of these different types of atherectomy devices has advantages and disadvantages that vary according to lesion location, composition and other patient-related factors.

Technique: Percutaneous atherectomy

Directional excisional atherectomy (SilverHawk and TurboHawk Plaque Excision System, Medtronic-Covidien Inc., Minneapolis, Minnesota) uses a rotating blade which is oriented to one side of a monorail catheter to excise plaque from the lumen of the diseased vessel. The device then packs the plaque into the nose cone of the catheter until it is full, at which point the device is removed from the patient for cleaning. Laser atherectomy (Turbo-Elite Laser Atherectomy Catheter, Spectranetics, Colorado Springs, CO) uses 308 nm wavelength laser energy to achieve photoablation of the intraluminal plaque and is the only atherectomy catheter currently indicated for in-stent restenosis in addition to de novo lesions. Orbital atherectomy (Diamondback 360, CSI Systems, St. Paul, MN) utilizes an eccentrically positioned diamond covered bur to grind down plaque into particles sufficiently small enough to pass through the capillary circulation. With increased orbital speeds, the device's centripetal force achieves a wider rotational diameter and thus increasing lumen diameters. Rotational atherectomy (Jetstream Pathway and Rotablator atherectomy systems, Boston Scientific, Marlborough, MA;

Table 18.2 Randomized control trials examining outcomes using drug-eluting stent versus bare-metal stent for infrapopliteal lesions.

Author	Year	Number of patients	Drug coating	1-year primary patency		Freedom from TVR		Freedom from amputation	
				BMS (%)	DES (%)	BMS (%)	DES (%)	BMS (%)	Control (%)
Bosiers et al.[43]	2012	140	Everolimus	85[a]	54	91[a]	66	98	97
Rastan et al.[41]	2012	161	Sirolimus	80[a]	55	91	80	97[a]	87

Abbreviations: DES, drug-eluting stent; BMS, bare-metal stent; TVR, target vessel revascularization.
[a] Reached significance compared to BMS population.

Phoenix Atherectomy System, Volcano Corp, San Diego, CA) uses front-end blades or burs on rotating catheter tips to cut or grind down plaque from the lumen, in some cases combining these modalities with active aspiration through the catheters. Each of these atherectomy systems have devices of varying sizes, requiring sheaths that vary from 5 to 8Fr, to treat a range of vessel diameters. These devices are passed over 0.014 guidewire systems in either over-the-wire or monorail fashion. Like all other treatment modalities, these devices require lesion crossing and true-luminal re-entry before passing the device, and generally the devices are passed at slow speeds to reduce embolization risk.

RESULTS OF DIRECTIONAL ATHERECTOMY

Femoropopliteal disease

In general, there are limited data comparing the effectiveness of atherectomy to other therapeutic modalities with the majority of information coming from large registries. The multicentre DEFINITIVE LE trial evaluated the safety and effectiveness of directional atherectomy for all infrainguinal lesions in 800 patients, and this prospective core-lab adjudicated registry is the largest series of data validating the use of atherectomy to date.[23] Although not randomized, the study was stratified by symptoms (claudication vs. CLI) and lesion location. The overall 1-year primary patency was 78% in claudicants and 71% in patients with CLI. Freedom from major amputation at 1 year in the CLI group was 95%. Directional atherectomy, using the SilverHawk device, was evaluated by Zeller and colleagues. One year after treatment, primary patency was 84% for new native vessel lesions and 54% for treatment of restenosis including in-stent restenosis. Another large cohort trial of 579 patients showed 18-month primary patency rates of 50% and 58% for claudicants and patients with CLI, respectively.[24] A meta-analysis published in 2014 of four randomized studies compared atherectomy to angioplasty and concluded there was no superiority of atherectomy, compared to PTA, for any outcomes studied including primary patency at 6 and 12 months.[25] Thus, excisional atherectomy appears safe and effective in treating femoropopliteal disease but has not shown any proven benefit compared to PTA (Recommendation Grade B Level of Evidence 2).

Infrapopliteal disease

Data regarding tibial vessel atherectomy are even more limited. The DEFINITIVE LE trial described earlier included a cohort of infrapopliteal patients.[19] The 1-year primary patency of infrapopliteal lesions was 90% for claudicants and 78% for patients with CLI. The study did not report on limb salvage rates specifically for infrapopliteal lesions. We recommend caution when using excisional atherectomy below the knee, as focused RCT studies are not yet available (Recommendation Grade C Level of Evidence 3).

RESULTS OF LASER ATHERECTOMY

Laser atherectomy has been reported to be effective in treating patients with CLI who were poor surgical candidates.[26] However, when evaluated as an adjunct to PTA in claudicants, laser atherectomy did not improve 12-month patency rates.[27] Another study evaluated the use of the excimer laser to treat patients who had recently failed PTA attempts. In 40 patients with a mean lesion length or 17.5 cm, the primary patency rate at 1 year was 59%.[28] Stent placement was required in 10% of the treated patients.

RESULTS OF ORBITAL AND ROTATIONAL ATHERECTOMY

Data for orbital and rotational atherectomy are limited to registries focusing on the safety of specific devices and small, randomized trials. As such, it is difficult to assess the efficacy of these devices. The multicentre Pathway PVD trial evaluated the safety of rotational atherectomy in 172 patients. The procedural complication rate was 1%. At 1 year, 38.2% of the patients had evidence of vessel restenosis, and 26% of the patients required repeat target lesion revascularization.[29] The CONFIRM registry collected data on 3135 patients undergoing orbital atherectomy demonstrating the technique safety with a low rate of provisional stenting (3.8%–5.8%).[30] The CALCIUM 360° trial was RCT of orbital atherectomy with PTA versus PTA alone in 50 patients with Rutherford class 4–6 disease. The primary patency rate in the orbital atherectomy with PTA arm was 93% compared to 82% in the PTA-only group.[31]

SELF-EXPANDING NITINOL STENTS

Self-expanding stents are widely used in the treatment of infrainguinal disease and are available from a variety of different manufacturers. These stents vary in diameter, length, conformability and delivery mechanisms. They are overall easy to use and provide an efficient mechanism to treat complex peripheral arterial disease. These devices can be used alone or in combination with other treatment modalities. Since these devices are implantable, they continue to provide treatment after deployment but also alter the anatomy and physiology of the vessel being treated.

Technique: Stenting of the SFA and popliteal arteries

Stent selection is based on the size of the native vessel and the characteristics of the target lesion. Ideally, the stent will return the area being treated to the diameter of the native vessel. Significant oversizing can cause perforations or an uneven surface after deployment. Care must be taken to avoid undersizing as this can result in stent dislodgment and migration. Use of a stent requires wire access across the target lesion. Pre-dilation of the target lesion with a balloon may be required depending on the ability of the stent to track across a lesion. The stent should be selected and placed such that it crosses the entire lesion and comes into contact with a portion of health artery on both sides of the lesion to avoid edge stenosis. The stent is deployed based on the specific design of the device being used. Post-balloon dilation of self-expanding stents is not required but is often performed to help facilitate full stent expansion.

RESULTS OF SELF-EXPANDING BARE-METAL STENTS
Femoropopliteal disease

The use of a self-expanding nitinol BMSs has been reported to improve patency of SFA lesions, compared to PTA alone. These stents have also proven effective in treating acute complications of PTA. The RESILIENT study compared bare-metal nitinol stents to angioplasty; the observed patency at 1 year was 81.3% and 36.7%, respectively.[6] Freedom from target lesion revascularization was significantly higher at 3 years in patients treated with a primary stent, compared to PTA.[32] A meta-analysis of stenting in the treatment of femoral and popliteal occlusive disease found a 63%–66% patency rate at 3 years for stenting depending on lesion type and symptoms with 3-year patency of PTA being more variable, ranging from 30% to 61%.[3] A more recent Cochrane review published in 2014 found that primary patency was improved in patients treated with BMS compared to PTA alone at 12 months, but this difference was not longer evident at 24 months.[33] BMS appear to be effective in the treatment of femoropopliteal disease with improved short-term primary patency compared to PTA alone (Recommendation Grade A Level of Evidence 1).

Infrapopliteal disease

Bosiers and colleagues prospectively evaluated the treatment of infrapopliteal disease in patients with CLI using PTA or PTA with stenting in 443 patients.[34] One-year primary patency was 68% and 75%, respectively. The limb salvage rate was over 95% in both groups. A systematic review of 16 studies showed a primary patency rate of 61% at 1 year in patients treated with BMS; this did not differ significantly from those treated with PTA alone[9] (see 'DES' section for recommendations).

RESULTS OF DRUG-COATED AND DRUG-ELUTING STENTS
Femoropopliteal disease

The Zilver PTX trial showed improved patency for a sirolimus DES compared to PTA at 1 year (83% vs. 32%).[35] It also compared BMS to DES in a subset of patients requiring stent placement for immediate PTA failure who were then secondarily randomized to BMS or DES. This provisional subgroup has been followed but no data on lesion characteristics are available to ensure appropriate comparisons. At 1 year, patency was significantly better for DES compared to BMS (89.9% vs. 73%).[36] A follow-up of the entire Zilver study group at 2 years showed a persistent improvement in primary patency compared to PTA (75% vs. 26.5%). The provisional group also showed improved primary patency in the DES group compared to the BMS group (83% vs. 64%). Two previous studies did not show improved outcomes for sirolimus DES compared to BMSs.[37,38] A study using everolimus DES showed only 68% primary patency rates at 12 months.[39] Based on these

data, it can be argued that the patency of DES in femoropopliteal disease generally exceeds that of standard laser-cut bare-metal nitinol stents and should be considered over these standard BMSs (Recommendation Grade A Level of Evidence 1).

Infrapopliteal disease

Treatment of infrapopliteal disease has been evaluated using DES designed for coronary intervention. The multicentre randomized ACHILLES trial compared PTA with sirolimus DES in the treatment of infrapopliteal lesions in 200 patients.[40] Primary patency was 75% in the DES group, significantly higher than the 57% primary patency in patients undergoing PTA. In the DES group, 13% of the patients required amputation compared to 20% in the PTA group, a non-statistically significant difference. Another multicentre randomized trial compared sirolimus DES to BMS in the treatment of infrapopliteal lesions.[41] At 1 year, the primary patency rate of patients treated with DES was 80% compared to 55% in the BMS cohort. In a long-term follow-up at almost 3 years, freedom from amputation was significantly higher in the DES group.[42] Another RCT evaluated found similar results at 1 year.[43] A systematic review including 16 trials compared DES to BMS and to PTA in the treatment of infrapopliteal lesions.[9] The primary patency at 1 year was significantly higher in the DES group compared to both the BMS and PTA groups. Based on these data when stents are used in the treatment of infrapopliteal lesions, we recommend the use of DES (Recommendation Grade A Level of Evidence 1).

RESULTS OF INTERWOVEN NITINOL STENTS

Novel stent designs have recently demonstrated promise for improved outcomes. Stents made of helical interwoven nitinol wires in a closed cell geometry provide increased radial strength. SUPERA peripheral stent system (Abbott Laboratories, Abbott Park, IL) utilizes this technology and was evaluated in a European study of over 500 patients with femoropopliteal disease including 277 patients with infrainguinal occlusive disease.[44] The primary patency in this cohort study was 83% at 1 year and 72% at 2 years. Early studies in the United States have shown similar primary patency rates at 12 months.[45,46] SUPERA stents have also shown promise in treating patients with long lesions. Brescia and colleagues evaluated the use of SUPERA stents in 48 patients with an average lesion length of 24.5 cm. All patients were evaluated at least once post-procedure. Kaplan–Meier analysis of these patients estimated primary patency rates of 86%, 83% and 77% at 1, 2 and 3 years, respectively.[47] All of these studies have shown remarkable consistency in primary patency rates indicating that these stents can be used to treat a broad range of lesions. When stenting is used for femoropopliteal lesions, we recommend the use of stents with this novel design (Recommendation Grade B Level of Evidence 2).

COVERED STENTS

Covered stent grafts have been approved for use in the SFA and have been studied in both native SFA occlusive disease and in-stent restenosis. The theoretical advantage of covered stents is the prevention of myointimal ingrowth into the arterial lumen because of the covered nature of these devices. The primary disadvantage of these stent grafts is the obligatory loss of collaterals that occurs with their use, and users have noted 'edge stenosis' that can occur at the proximal and distal aspect of these grafts, ultimately leading to device failure. Occlusion of these grafts can lead to acute ischemia anecdotally, though studies on the use of these grafts do not tend to show inordinately high rates of acute ischemia.

Technique: Use of covered stents in the SFA and popliteal arteries

The use of covered stents in the femoropopliteal circulation requires careful attention to vessel diameter, as oversizing can lead to stent infolding and this is thought to predispose to stent graft thrombosis. Use of intravascular ultrasound or 'sizing-balloon' angioplasty is generally used to assess the actual target vessel diameter, and then stent grafts are chosen for 1:1 sizing with the target vessel. Generally accepted practice is to cover all diseases and place stents from healthy inflow artery to healthy outflow, but caution should be used to avoid unnecessary coverage of large collaterals. Post-dilatation is generally recommended to expand any areas of infolding or irregularity. Patients are kept on lifelong dual antiplatelet therapy, and intolerance to antiplatelet therapy is considered a contraindication to use of covered stent grafts in the infrainguinal circulation.

RESULTS OF COVERED STENTS

Studies evaluating covered self-expanding stents have not shown improved outcomes over BMS.[48,49] The VIASTAR trial evaluated Viabahn stents (Gore, Flagstaff, AZ) compared to uncovered BMSs in the treatment of femoropopliteal lesions. At 12 months, patients treated with Viabahn stents had a primary patency of 70% compared to 55% in the BMS group. This difference did not reach clinical significance. In the subgroup of patients with lesions longer than 20 cm, there was an improved primary patency rate in patients treated with Viabahn stents compared to BMS (71% vs. 37%).[48] The VIBRANT trial evaluated 148 patients with TASC C and D lesions. The study also failed to show any significant difference in primary patency when comparing patients treated with covered stents or BMS.[49] Covered stents also have the potential to increase acute ischemic events after reconstruction, due to initial coverage of collateral vessels (Figure 18.1).[50]

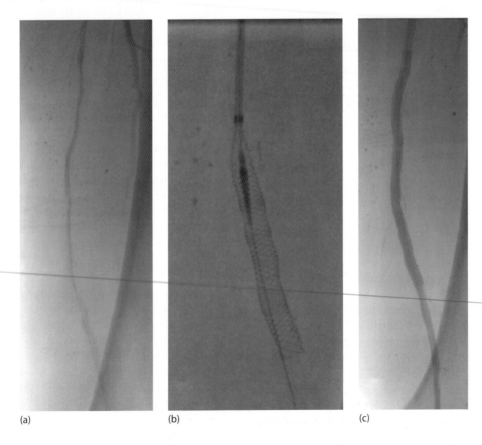

(a)   (b)   (c)

Figure 18.1 Deployment of self-expanding stent comprised of woven nitionol wires into the SFA after balloon angioplasty. Treatment of a long occlusion with balloon angioplasty resulted in significant recoil and residual stenosis (a), and therefore this vessel was treated with deployment of a self-expanding nitinol scaffold (b), with an excellent result (c).

BIORESORBABLE VASCULAR SCAFFOLD

Bioresorbable vascular scaffolds (BVSs) have been evaluated and will soon be released for use in the coronary circulation in the United States, though these devices do not currently have an indication for use in the peripheral circulation. Despite this, these devices are worth mentioning as the preliminary data from small trials applying this technology to the periphery suggest they may fill an important need in the future. These scaffolds can be engineered to include anti-myoproliferative drugs, and after implantation the scaffold biodegrades over a period of months while it elutes the antiproliferative drug. The design has the theoretical benefit of providing radial support after the initial treatment of a lesion, while allowing anti-myoproliferative medications to be eluted as the vessel regains its native structure and function. While peer-reviewed published data evaluating these devices are limited, preliminary data suggest favourable results in short lesions.[51,52] One group reported on 22 patients with Rutherford category 3–6 disease treated with BVS in the infra-geniculate circulation. In this group, 12-month primary patency was 94%, with a 100% secondary patency rate after one patient (who was not on antiplatelet therapy) underwent re-intervention for early post-op stent thrombosis.

REFERENCES

1. Zorger N, Manke C, Lenhart M et al. Peripheral arterial balloon angioplasty: Effect of short versus long balloon inflation times on the morphologic results. *J Vasc Interv Radiol*. 2002;13:355–359.
2. Dormandy JA, Rutherford RB. Management of peripheral arterial disease (PAD). TASC Working Group. TransAtlantic Inter-Society Consensus (TASC). *J Vasc Surg*. 2000;31(1):S1–S296.
3. Hunink MGM, Wong JB, Donaldson MC, Meyerovitz MF, Harrington DP. Patency results of percutaneous and surgical revascularization for femoropopliteal arterial disease. *Med Decis Making*. 1994;14(1):71–81.
4. Muradin GS, Bosch JL, Stijnen T, Hunink MG. Balloon dilation and stent implantation for treatment of femoropopliteal arterial disease: Meta-analysis. *Radiology*. 2001;221:137–145.
5. Jeans WD, Armstrong S, Cole SE, Horrocks M, Baird RN. Fate of patients undergoing transluminal angioplasty for lower-limb ischemia. *Radiology*. 1990;177(2):559–564.
6. Murray JG, Apthorp LA, Wilkins RA: Long-segment (≥10 cm) femoropopliteal angioplasty: Improved technical success and long-term patency. *Radiology*. 1995;195:158–162.
7. Laird JR, Katzen BT, Scheinert D et al. Nitinol stent implantation versus balloon angioplasty for lesions in the superficial femoral artery and proximal popliteal artery: Twelve-month results from the RESILIENT randomized trial. *Circ Cardiovasc Interv*. 2010;3(3):267–276.
8. Romiti M, Albers M, Brochado-Neto FC, Durasso AE, Pereira CA, De Luccia N. Meta-analysis of infrapopliteal angioplasty for chronic critical limb ischemia. *J Vasc Surg*. 2008;47(5):975–981.
9. Wu R, Yao C, Wang S, Xu X, Wang M, Li Z, Wang S. Percutaneous transluminal angioplasty versus primary stenting in infrapopliteal arterial disease: A meta-analysis of randomized trials. *J Vasc Surg*. 2014;59(6):1711–1720.
10. Yang X, Lu X, Ye K, Li X, Qin J, Jiang M. Systematic review and meta-analysis of balloon angioplasty versus primary stenting in the infrapopliteal disease. *Vasc Endovasc Surg*. 2014;48(1):18–26.
11. Giles KA, Pomposelli FB, Spence TL, Hamdan AD, Blattman SB, Panossian H, Schermerhorn ML. Infrapopliteal angioplasty for critical limb ischemia: Relation of TransAtlantic InterSociety Consensus class to outcome in 176 limbs. *J Vasc Surg*. 2008;48(1):126–136.
12. Sadek M, Ellozy S, Turnbull I, Lookstein R, Marin M, Faries P. Improved outcomes are associated with multilevel endovascular intervention involving the tibial vessels compared with isolated tibial intervention. *J Vasc Surg*. 2009;49(3):638–644.
13. Peregrin JH, Koznar B, Kovac J, Lastovickova J, Novotny J, Vedlich D, Skibova J. PTA of infrapopliteal arteries: Long-term clinical follow-up and analysis of factors influencing clinical outcome. *Cardiovasc Intervent Radiol*. 2010;33(4):720–725.
14. London NJ, Srinivasan R, Naylor AR, Hartshome T, Ratliff DA, Bell PR, Bolia A. Subintimal angioplasty of femoropopliteal artery occlusions: The long-term results. *Eur J Vasc Surg*. 1994;8(2):148–155.
15. Vraux H, Bertoncello N. Subintimal angioplasty of tibial vessel occlusions in critical limb ischaemia: A good opportunity? *Eur J Vasc Endovasc Surg*. 2006;32(6):663–667.
16. Tepe G, Zeller T, Albrecht T et al. Local delivery of paclitaxel to inhibit restenosis during angioplasty of the leg. *N Engl J Med*. 2008;358(7):689–699.
17. Werk M, Langner S, Reinkensmeier B et al. Inhibition of restenosis in femoropopliteal arteries. *Circulation*. 2008;118:1358–1365.
18. Scheinert D, Duda S, Zeller T et al. The LEVANT I (Lutonix paclitaxel-coated balloon for the prevention of femoropopliteal restenosis) trial for femoropopliteal revascularization: First-in-human randomized trial of low-dose drug-coated balloon versus uncoated balloon angioplasty. *JACC Cardiovasc Interv*. 2014;7(1):10–19.
19. FDA Executive Summary, Bard LUTONIX 035 Drug Coated Balloon PTA Catheter, 12 June 2014.
20. Tepe G, Laird J, Schneider P, Brodman M, Krishnan P, Micari A. Drug-coated balloon versus standard percutaneous transluminal angioplasty for the

treatment of femoral and/or popliteal peripheral artery disease: 12-Month results from the IN.PACT SFA randomized trial. *Circulation*. 2015 February 3;131(5):495–502.

21. Fanelli F, Cannavale A, Corona M, Lucatelli P, Wlderk A, Salvatori FM. The "DEBELLUM" – Lower limb multilevel treatment with drug eluting balloon – Randomized trial: 1-year results. *J Cardiovasc Surg*. 2014;55(2):207–216.

22. Zeller T, Baumgartner I, Scheinert D et al. Drug-eluting balloon versus standard balloon angioplasty for infrapopliteal arterial revascularization in critical limb ischemia: 12-month results from the IN.PACT DEEP randomized trial. *J Am Coll Cardiol*. 2014;64(15):1568–1576.

23. McKinsey JF, Zeller T, Rocha-Singh KJ, Jaff MR, Carcia LA. Lower extremity revascularization using directional atherectomy: 12-Month prospective results of the DEFINITIVE LE study. *JACC Cardiovasc Interv*. 2014;7(8):923–933.

24. McKinsey JF, Goldstein L, Khan HU et al. Novel treatment of patients with lower extremity ischemia: Use of percutaneous atherectomy in 579 lesions. *Ann Surg*. 2008;248(4):519–528.

25. Ambler GK, Radwan R, Hayes PD, Twine CP. Atherectomy for peripheral arterial disease. *Cochrane Database Syst Rev*. 2014;3:CD006680.

26. Laird JR, Zeller T, Gray BH et al. Limb salvage following laser-assisted angioplasty for critical limb ischemia: Results of the LACI multicenter trial. *J Endovasc Ther*. 2006;13(1):1–11.

27. Laird J. PELA trial: Peripheral excimer laser angioplasty. Data presented at *Transcatheter Therapeutics (TCT) Annual Meeting*, Washington, DC, 24–28 September 2002.

28. Wissgott C, Kamusella P, Ludtke C, Andressen R. Excimer laser atherectomy after unsuccessful angioplasty of TASC C and D lesions in femoropopliteal arteries. *J Cardiovasc Surg*. 2013;54(3):359–365.

29. Zeller T, Krankenberg H, Steinkamp H. One-year outcome of percutaneous rotational atherectomy with aspiration in infrainguinal peripheral arterial occlusive disease: The multicenter pathway PVD trial. *J Endovasc Ther*. 2009;16(6):653–662.

30. Das T, Mustapha J, Indes J. Technique optimization of orbital atherectomy in calcified peripheral lesions of the lower extremities: The CONFIRM series, a prospective multicenter registry. *Catheter Cardiovasc Interv*. 2014 January 1;83(1):115–122.

31. Shammas NW, Lam R, Mustapha J. Comparison of orbital atherectomy plus balloon angioplasty vs. balloon angioplasty alone in patients with critical limb ischemia: Results of the CALCIUM 360 randomized pilot trial. *J Endovasc Ther*. 2012;19(4):480–488.

32. Laird JR, Katzen BT, Scheinert D et al. Nitinol stent implantation vs. balloon angioplasty for lesions in the superficial femoral and proximal popliteal arteries of patients with claudication: Three-year follow-up from the RESILIENT randomized trial. *J Endovasc Ther*. 2012;19(1):1–9.

33. Chowdhury MM, McLain AD, Twine CP. Angioplasty versus bare metal stenting for superficial femoral artery lesions. *Cochrane Database Syst Rev*. 2014;6:CD006767.

34. Bosiers M, Hart JP, Deloose K, Verbist JJ, Peeters P. Endovascular therapy as the primary approach for limb salvage in patients with critical limb ischemia: Experience with 443 infrapopliteal procedures. *Vascular*. 2006;14(2):63–69.

35. Drake MD, Ansel GM, Jaff MR et al. Paclitaxel-eluting stents show superiority to balloon angioplasty and bare metal stents in femoropopliteal disease: Twelve-month Zilver PTX randomized study results. *Circ Cardiovasc Interv*. 2011;4(5):495–504.

36. Drake MD, Ansel GM, Jaff MR et al. Sustained safety and effectiveness of paclitaxel-eluting stents for femoropopliteal lesions: 2-year follow-up from the Zilver PTX randomized and single-arm clinical studies. *J Am Coll Cardiol*. 2013;61(24):2417–2427.

37. Duda SH, Bosiers M, Lammer J et al. Drug-eluting and bare nitinol stents for the treatment of atherosclerotic lesions in the superficial femoral artery: Long-term results from the SIROCCO trial. *J Endovasc Ther*. 2006 December;13(6):701–710.

38. Duda SH, Bosiers M, Lammer J et al. Sirolimus-eluting versus bare nitinol stent for obstructive superficial femoral artery disease: The SIROCCO II trial. *J Vasc Interv Radiol*. 2005;16(3):331–338.

39. Lammer J, Bosiers M, Zeller T et al. First clinical trial of nitinol self-expanding everolimus-eluting stent implantation for peripheral arterial occlusive disease. *J Vasc Surg*. 2011;54(2):394–401.

40. Scheinert D, Katsanos K, Zeller T et al. A prospective randomized multicenter comparison of balloon angioplasty and infrapopliteal stenting with the sirolimus-eluting stent in patients with ischemic peripheral arterial disease: 1-year results from the ACHILLES trial. *J Am Coll Cardiol*. 2012;60(22):2290–2295.

41. Rastan A, Tepe G, Krankenberg H et al. Sirolimus-eluting stents vs. bare-metal stents for treatment of focal lesions in infrapopliteal arteries: A double-blind, multi-centre, randomized clinical trial. *Eur Heart J*. 2011;32(18):2274–2281.

42. Rastan A, Brechtel K, Krankenberg H et al. Sirolimus-eluting stents for treatment of infrapopliteal arteries reduce clinical event rate compared to bare-metal stents: Long-term results from a randomized trial. *J Am Coll Cardiol*. 2012;60(7):587–591.

43. Bosiers M, Scheinert D, Peeters P et al. Randomized comparison of everolimus-eluting versus bare-metal stents in patients with critical limb ischemia and infrapopliteal arterial occlusive disease. *J Vasc Surg.* 2012;55(2):390–398.

44. Werner M, Paetzold A, Banning-Eichenseer U et al. Treatment of complex atherosclerotic femoropopliteal artery disease with a self-expanding interwoven nitinol stent: Midterm results from the Leipzig SUPERA 500 registry. *EuroIntervention.* 2014 November;10(7):861–868.

45. Leon JR Jr., Dieter RS, Gadd CL et al. Preliminary results of the initial United States experience with the Supera woven nitinol stent in the popliteal artery. *J Vasc Surg.* 2013;57(4):1014–1022.

46. Chan YC, Cheng SW, Ting AC, Cheung GC. Primary stenting of femoropopliteal atherosclerotic lesions using new helical interwoven nitinol stents. *J Vasc Surg.* 2014;59(2):384–391.

47. Brescia A, Wickers B, Correa JC, Smeds M, Jacobs D. Stenting of femoropopliteal lesions using interwoven nitinol stents. *J Vasc Surg.* 2015 June;61(6):1472–1478.

48. Lammer J, Zeller T, Gschwendtern M et al. Heparin-bonded covered stents versus bare-metal stents for complex femoropopliteal artery lesions: The randomized VIASTAR trial (Viabahn endoprosthesis with PROPATEN bioactive surface [VIA] versus bare nitinol stent in the treatment of long lesions in superficial femoral artery occlusive disease). *J Am Coll Cardiol.* 2013;62(15):1320–1327.

49. Geraghty PJ, Mewissen MW, Jaff MR, Ansel GM. Three-year results of the VIBRANT trial of VIABAHN endoprosthesis versus bare nitinol stent implantation for complex superficial femoral artery occlusive disease. *J Vasc Surg.* 2013;58(2):386–395.

50. Johnston PC, Vartanian SM, Runge SJ et al. Risk factors for clinical failure after stent graft treatment for femoropopliteal occlusive disease. *J Vasc Surg.* 2012;56(4):998–1007.

51. Varcoe RL, Schouten O, Thomas SD, Lennox AF. Initial experience with the absorb bioresorbable vascular scaffold below the knee: Six-month clinical and imaging outcomes. *J Endovasc Ther.* 2015 April;22(2):226–232.

52. Varcoe RL. Initial experience with drug-eluting bioresorbable scaffolds below the knee. Presented at the *Leipzig Interventional Course*, Leipzig, Germany, January 2015.

19

In situ saphenous vein arterial bypass

DHIRAJ M. SHAH, R. CLEMENT DARLING III, BENJAMIN B. CHANG and PAUL B. KREIENBERG

CONTENTS

INTRODUCTION

The removal of a venous conduit from its bed subjects it to the cumulative injurious effects of surgical manipulation, transmural warm ischemia, contact with nonhemic solutions and hydrostatic dilatation.[1] With the rapid increase in aortocoronary and infrainguinal vein grafting as the stimulus for the evaluation of these injuries,[2,3] it has now been shown that there is widespread destruction of the endothelium with alterations in normal prostacyclin and thromboxane production, thus producing a relatively thrombogenic surface. Furthermore, the rate of degeneration in such veins appears to be inversely related to the subsequent rate of flow.[4]

All these factors may contribute to the initial failure rate of these bypass conduits, particularly when the outflow tracts are limited.[5] Although the most recent methods of preparing excised vein grafts have been directed towards the prevention of these injuries,[6] none is perfect. At present we believe that the closest approximation to an ideal conduit (i.e. one with normal, viable, physiologically functioning endothelium and a natural taper) is a vein that has been retained in situ and is minimally damaged during its preparation for bypass.

HISTORY OF IN SITU VEIN BYPASS TECHNIQUES

In 1962, Hall[7] published a preliminary report of successful in situ vein bypasses done by the method of valve excision through transverse venotomies. This necessarily tedious procedure was practical only because most of the operations were carried out to the above-knee popliteal artery with veins of large size. By 1973, Hall[8] had developed an instrument for serial transluminal retrograde valve disruption, as had Cartier[9] and Samuels.[10] Valve excision has now been largely abandoned, as has the method of prograde blind blunt valve fracture.[11] However, a continuing experience with retrograde valve disruption using the instruments of Hall and Cartier has accumulated in Europe.[12–14]

These instruments appear to have two serious disadvantages. The first is that blunt avulsion of the valve leaflets may cause serious damage to the adjacent vein wall. The second is that both instruments must be introduced and withdrawn through the distal divided end of the vein, which invariably has the smallest diameter and is most prone to spasm. Both factors thus combine to produce the greatest potential for the most devastating injury to the vein wall, i.e. circumference endothelial avulsion. These limitations preclude the successful use of these instruments in veins less than 4 mm in diameter.

Valve incision achieves the goal of an efficient and minimally traumatic method of producing valvular incompetence by division of valve leaflets in their major axes while they are in the functionally closed position.

PREOPERATIVE SAPHENOUS VEIN ANATOMY

An invaluable aid to all saphenous vein operations and in situ techniques in particular has been the preoperative definition of the anatomy of the greater saphenous vein, previously by phlebography and, at present, by duplex Doppler ultrasound.[15–17] With the patient standing, the position of the saphenous vein should also be marked before operation by inducing a pressure wave distally. This is done by tapping or brushing the distended vein and detecting its propagation digitally or by Doppler ultrasound methods.

Surface duplex mapping of the saphenous vein has been found to be an effective and noninvasive method of determining the venous anatomy provided that the procedure is performed by an experienced technician. This method provides a detailed three-dimensional map of the course of the saphenous vein, which may be traced onto the overlying skin. This map aids in the placement of skin incisions and the location of venous access points for instrumentation (Figure 19.1).

During the past 15 years, we have utilized B-mode imaging to preoperatively assess and map the greater saphenous vein in more than 10,000 limbs.[18,19] With the patient's limb in a dependent position, the greater saphenous vein is marked on the overlying skin for its entire course from the saphenofemoral junction to the level of the medial malleolus. All branches, especially deep perforators, are noted. The internal diameter of the vein is measured at both the upper and lower thigh and calf. Diameter measurements are also made of any double systems to determine which is dominant. Valves are easily detected, but their positions are not marked unless they are stenotic or abnormal. If there is a complex system or B-mode imaging is felt to be otherwise inadequate or in question, the patients then undergo phlebography. However, our results demonstrate that in over 90% of patients, B-mode imaging is the optimal technique of venous assessment. In the patients in whom complex systems are encountered, phlebography may be utilized since it provides additional information for accurate planning of the procedure.

In spite of these considerations, many surgeons remain resistant to these preoperative assessments, preferring to determine anatomic variations at operation. However, such attempts to define anatomic variations surgically may be frustrating and ineffective and may result in inappropriate excessive dissection, increasing the potential for significant spasm, postoperative wound complications and other forms of injury to the vein that can lead to failure and abandonment of the procedure.

SURGICAL TECHNIQUE

After sterile preparation and draping of the entire extremity, warm (378°C) papaverine solution 1 mg/mL N.S. is injected percutaneously into the subcutaneous tissue adjacent to the saphenous vein along its course below the knee. The proximal saphenous vein, which lies immediately deep to the superficial fascia, is then exposed, and additional papaverine solution is infiltrated into the surrounding tissue to minimize spasm.

Although the common femoral artery has been considered the proper site for proximal anastomosis of all

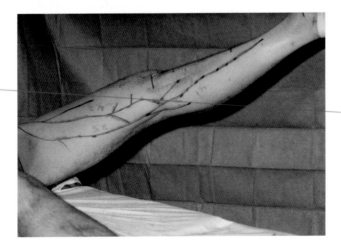

Figure 19.1 Duplex 'vein map' illustrating a double saphenous system. It is important to remember that the diameter measured by duplex is an internal dimension under relatively low venous pressure, whereas surgeons are accustomed to gauging its attributes as a conduit in terms of outside (external) diameter when under arterial pressure.

distal bypasses, there is evidence that use of the superficial femoral artery in the limb-salvage patient population is equally satisfactory. Furthermore, technical circumstances such as a previous surgical scar or exposure of the common femoral artery or its involvement with circumferential calcification may make either the deep femoral (profunda femoris) or the superficial femoral artery a better alternative inflow source.[20,21] Offsetting its less accessible anatomic location, the deep femoral artery is usually less invested with thick, calcified plaque than either the common or superficial femoral artery and, therefore, frequently provides the most satisfactory site for proximal anastomosis.

It is best approached from the medial aspect (with the surgeon on the opposite side of the table) by incision of the subcutaneous tissue immediately lateral to the saphenous vein and down to the underlying investing myofascia (Figure 19.2). Dissection laterally in this fusion plane to the superficial femoral artery is bloodless. The fascia is incised over the superficial femoral artery, and, if it is occluded, a segment of 3–5 cm can be excised, thus facilitating exposure of the deep femoral artery. If patent, a plane is developed between the femoral vein and the superficial femoral artery. The lateral circumflex femoral vein is divided, exposing the proximal deep femoral artery which lies immediately deep to it (Figure 19.3).

Having determined the most satisfactory site of proximal anastomosis, the length of the proximal saphenous vein required to reach it is apparent. If the common femoral artery is to be used as the inflow source, a complete dissection of the saphenous bulb and secure ligation of its branches is performed. If additional length is required to facilitate anastomosis to the common femoral artery, a portion of the anterior aspect of the common femoral vein is removed in continuity with the saphenous bulb.

The valve leaflets at the saphenofemoral junction are excised, removing only the transparent portion, leaving the usually prominent insertion ridge intact. The second valve invariably present 3–5 cm distal to this can be incised easily with a retrograde valvulotome through a side branch distal to the valve before the vein is divided or alternatively cut with either scissors or an antegrade valvulotome

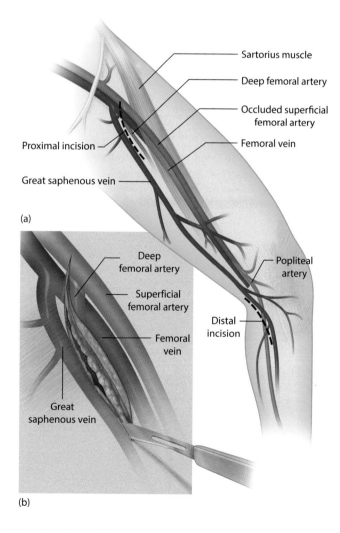

Figure 19.2   (a) Proximal and distal incisions will be used for the in situ bypass. (b) The proximal incision (inset) will start approximately at the level of the femoral artery bifurcation and will continue directly over the medial course of the great saphenous vein. The distal incision will be made later in the operation. (Illustration by B. William and M.S. Westwood, AMI, Lexington, KY.)

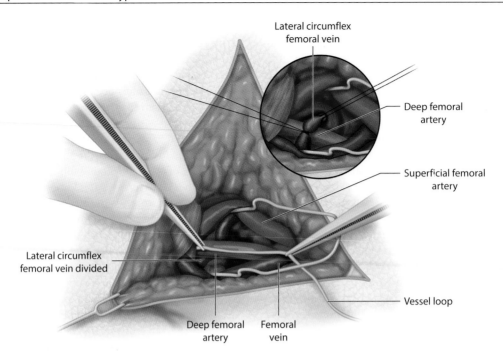

Figure 19.3 A 3–5 cm segment of the deep femoral artery has been mobilized, and a vessel loop is used to estimate the length of vein necessary for the proximal anastomosis. A portion of the great saphenous vein 2 cm longer than the 5–7 cm length required for anastomosis will be dissected free, clipped and divided at the saphenofemoral junction. (Illustration by B. William and M.S. Westwood, AMI, Lexington, KY.)

through the open end of the vein, as is the valve immediately distal to the medial accessory branch. These valves are identified by gently distending the vein through its open end with dextran or heparinized blood and are cut with scissors with the thumb and index finger around the shank of the scissors, while the valve is held in the functionally closed position by fluid trapped between the open end of the saphenous vein and the valve (Figure 19.4).

The plane of closure of the valve cusps is invariably parallel to the skin. This dictates the orientation of all instruments with relation to the valve cusps. If a valve cutter cannot be used, the location of the next valve site is determined by advancing a No. 6 Fr catheter, with the infusion solution running through it under 200 mmHg pressure, until it impacts in the valve sinus. This valve location is marked on the adjacent skin before the proximal anastomosis is carried out.

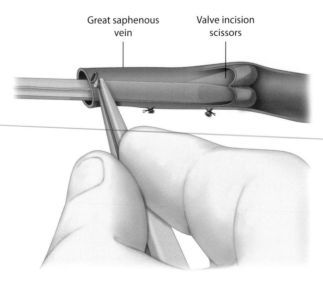

Figure 19.4 Valve incision scissors are inserted into the great saphenous vein, and the nearer valve leaflets are incised perpendicular to their plane of closure. The valves along the remaining bypass segment of the vein will be divided with the valve cutter or the retrograde valvulotome. (Illustration by B. William and M.S. Westwood, AMI, Lexington, KY.)

If the valve cutter is to be used, a 3–5 cm long incision is made 5 mm posterior to the marked position of the main saphenous vein below the knee, identifying a branch previously localized by duplex scan or venogram and using it to gain access to the lumen of the saphenous vein. A No. 3 Fogarty catheter is introduced into the saphenous vein through this side branch and passed proximally, with the leg straightened, to exit through the open end of the vein. The catheter is then divided at an acute angle at the 20 or 30 cm mark, whichever is closest to the open end of the vein. The valve cutter (2 or 3 mm) is screwed onto the catheter and a No. 6 or 8 Fr infusion catheter is then secured to the cutter with a loop of fine suture (Figure 19.3).

The leading cylinder of the valve cutter is drawn back into the open proximal end of the saphenous vein, partially obstructing venous flow while permitting visualization of the cutting blade and minimal resistance to torque. This allows precise orientation of the cutting edges at 90° to the plane of closure of the valves, that is to the plane of the overlying skin surface (Figure 19.5). The catheter–cutter assembly is then drawn slowly distally, while the dextran solution or blood is introduced through the catheter at 200–300 mmHg pressure, sealing leakage from the end of the vein by a 1 mm Silastic (polymeric silicone) 'vessel loop' secured by a small hemostat near its end (Figure 19.4). This pressurized fluid column in the proximal vein snaps each successive valve into the closed position so that the cusps can be efficiently engaged by the blades of the cutter. A slight but definite resistance is felt as the cutter encounters each valve and cuts the leaflets. Greater resistance than this should be managed by axially rotating the cutter 45° and making another attempt at advancement. If this does not produce the desired result, the cutter should be withdrawn and dismounted and the area of impaction exposed directly by a longitudinal incision.

The cutter is advanced through a safe distance, predetermined by duplex scanning or venogram generally to the knee-joint level, and is then withdrawn again to the femoral exposure. Here the cutter is dismounted and the catheter removed from the saphenous vein. Proximal anastomosis of the saphenous vein to the selected inflow artery is performed using a 'no-touch' technique (Figure 19.5), and the palpable pulsatile impulse thus provided makes the location of the next competent valve readily apparent (Figure 19.6).

The remaining valves are incised by a retrograde valvulotome introduced through a side branch or the distal end of the vein. Prior to the use of this instrument, any narrowing due to spasm should be dilated with controlled pressure of 200 mmHg. In passing the valvulotome intraluminally to and from a valve site, it is important that any pressure on the vein wall resulting from its curving path be exerted on the shaft of the instrument rather than the projecting blade tip. This lessens the likelihood of the blade becoming lodged in the side branch and lacerating the vein wall when being withdrawn. This instrument is so designed that it engages a leaflet, centres itself and cuts the leaflet in its longitudinal axis. It is then readvanced, carefully rotated through 180° and withdrawn, thus engaging the remaining leaflet (Figure 19.7). However, before the cutting force is applied to the tip of the valvulotome, it should be manoeuvred towards the centre of the vein lumen by finger depression of the vein itself, allowing division of the remaining leaflet without the risk of entering a side branch, which is invariably present on the posterior wall close to every valve sinus.

Unobstructed pulsatile arterial flow is thus brought down to the desired level adjacent to the proposed distal anastomosis. Before transection and mobilization of the distal vein, exposure of the anticipated outflow

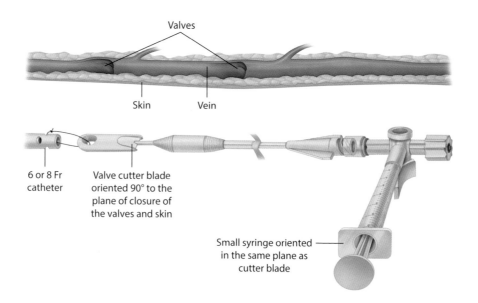

Figure 19.5 The leading cylinder of the cutter has been drawn partway into the vein to limit blood loss, and a No. 6 or 8 infusion catheter is attached with a suture loop to the opposite end. (Illustration by B. William and M.S. Westwood, AMI, Lexington, KY.)

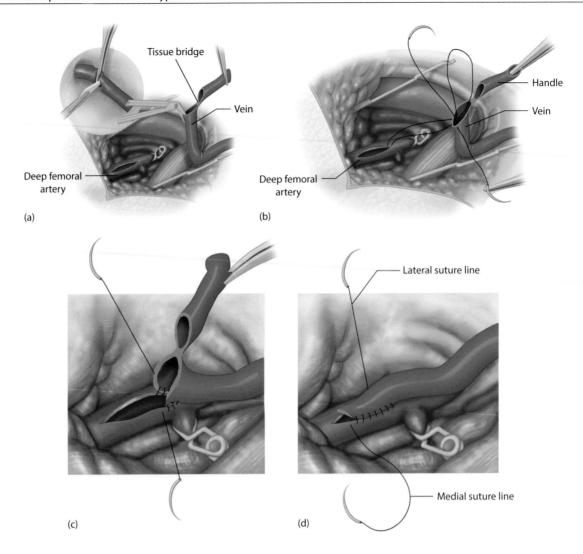

Figure 19.6 (a) The vein is partially divided with a No. 11 scalpel. A 'handle' is retained to allow traction on the vein. (b) Proximal anastomosis of the bypass vein to the deep femoral artery is carried out by the 'open parachute' technique, which allows for accurate and atraumatic placement of each individual suture in the heel portion of the anastomosis. A single, double-needle suture of 7-0 Prolene is used. (c) After placement of as many sutures as the length of suture material allows, the vein is drawn down to the artery. The *handle* will be excised. (d) Arterialization of the saphenous vein is completed by continuing the medial suture line clockwise around the end of the arteriotomy to meet the lateral suture line at the midpoint of the arteriotomy. (Illustration by B. William and M.S. Westwood, AMI, Lexington, KY.)

anastomotic site is carried out. This sequence is desirable not only to minimize the warm ischemia time of the endothelium but also to assess the appropriate length required, always allowing an additional 1–2 cm so that the manipulated (and thus traumatized) terminal segment can be excised and discarded.

After completion of the distal anastomosis, adequate flow in the bypass as well as the outflow vessel is confirmed with a quantitative appraisal made by the use of the sterile Doppler ultrasonic probe. A completion angiogram is then performed with radiopaque reference markers (19 gauge needles in their plastic containers attached to the skin by sterile adhesive strips, a radiologic strip marker or skin clips) to correlate roentgenographic position of any residual arteriovenous (A-V) fistulas with the surface anatomy.

TECHNICAL REQUIREMENTS OF IN SITU BYPASS

Efficient atraumatic functional destruction of the valves which obstruct arterial flow is both the most important and most difficult technical manoeuvre associated with the procedure. The vein may have a number of valves, ranging from 3 to 13, although the usual number for a proximal tibial bypass is between 5 and 7. Valve incision is an efficient technique for rendering the valves incompetent, and the instruments described have increased the ease and speed with which the operation can now be performed.[22] Careful follow-up has shown that the incised valve is neither a source of microemboli nor a frequent site of later pathologic degeneration.

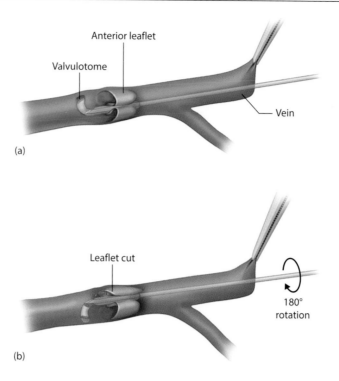

Figure 19.7 Before any intraluminal instrumentation is carried out, the mobilized segment of vein is dilated with a dextran solution at a controlled pressure of 200 mmHg. (a) A retrograde valvulotome is introduced through the distal end of the vein, and as it is withdrawn, it cuts one valve leaflet. (b) It is readvanced, rotated 180° and again withdrawn, cutting the second leaflet. (Illustration by B. William and M.S. Westwood, AMI, Lexington, KY.)

To better understand the problems encountered with valve incision, it is important to have a clear concept of venous valve function. The normal closing mechanism in a symmetrical venous valve is initiated by tension along the leading edge of the valve leaflet caused by expansion of the valve sinus as intraluminal pressures are raised. This brings the edge of the leaflet towards the centre of the lumen, where flow forces it into a closed, competent position. In any segment of vein where a valve is mechanically opened from below by passage of any instrument (e.g. a valvulotome or catheter) in the proximal direction, the potential exists for a valve leaflet to be pushed against the wall and to remain temporarily against it in an open position. This is most likely to occur in asymmetrical valves. In such valves, the normal closing mechanism may not be operative so that the valve may remain open for an indefinite period. The subsequent closure of the artificially opened valve leaflet, either spontaneous or induced by manipulation (for example palpation of the pulse in this segment), results in the partial or even complete obstruction of arterial flow. Therefore, before the distal anastomosis is performed, deliberate attempts should be made to precipitate closure of any incompletely lysed valves by the following manoeuvre. With the distal vein open and free flow observed, or high flow via a fistula distally, a sponge is rolled along the in situ conduit from top to bottom. When the valve cutter is used, the most frequent location of a missed valve is in the segment immediately distal to the point of the lowest cutter travel, at the level of exposure of the vein. This segment should be checked routinely with the valvulotome because, in the absence of flow, an undiminished pulse can be transmitted through an intact valve held in a static column of blood.

The simple expedient of assessing flow from the distal divided end of the saphenous vein before construction of the distal anastomosis is very reliable in detecting any proximal hemodynamically significant obstructive lesions. If there is steady, undiminished pulsatile flow, it is unlikely that such a lesion is present proximally.

VENOUS SPASM

Spasm of the saphenous vein is a well-known phenomenon. In excised veins, hydraulic dilatation provides a permanent solution, but the in situ vein retains its neuromuscular activity and thus its propensity for spasm. At present, there is no means of determining which patient or vein will exhibit this behaviour. All veins are prone to spasm to some degree, but in general, this is more prevalent and difficult to manage in smaller veins (i.e. below 3 mm). It is better to prevent venous spasm by minimizing surgical handling and using topical antispasmodic drugs (e.g. papaverine) and controlled intraluminal pressure than to correct it after it occurs.[23] Apart from its deleterious effect on endothelium and blood flow, spasm also makes intraluminal instrumentation dangerous because it increases endothelial abrasion.

ARTERIOVENOUS FISTULAS

Most branches of the saphenous vein drain superficial subcutaneous tissues, and their orifices are generally guarded by a competent valve, thus preventing flow away from the arterialized saphenous vein. Only valve-less branches immediately become arteriovenous fistulas. However, these branches are usually small and generally undergo spontaneous thrombosis postoperatively. This event is signalled by the development of a superficial phlebitis, the extent of which is determined by the size of this iatrogenic A-V fistula. Although occasionally a large area of induration results, it is sterile and self-limiting, and it usually resolves within a few days. Even if such superficial veins remain patent, the loss of distal arterial flow is generally small and does not threaten the continued patency of a bypass. As a rule, only branches with sufficient flow to visualize the deep venous system with radiopaque dye on the completion angiogram need be ligated.

The effects of A-V fistulas on in situ saphenous vein bypass hemodynamics and patency has been of great concern to some, even to the point of regarding these as a frequent cause of in situ bypass occlusion. For more than 10 years, following the observation that most of the residual subcutaneous iatrogenic A-V fistulas undergo spontaneous thrombosis, it has been our practice to ligate only fistulas that conduct enough dye on completion angiography to visualize the deep venous system. We have studied more than 600 such bypasses longitudinally using duplex ultrasonic scanning to assess overall hemodynamic function. The results indicate a steady reduction in fistula flow with time, with no overall effect on distal perfusion (Figure 19.1). There is a small group of patients in whom high fistula flow is poorly tolerated, usually those with limited flow due to proximal stenosis or a small vein (less than 3 mm outside diameter [OD]). However, in most (other) patients, the flow capacity of the in situ conduit far exceeds the volume demanded by a fistula and provides adequate, undiminished distal perfusion.

The allegation that fistulas are a potential cause of occlusive bypass failure is not supported by our experience.

The probable cause of failure in this setting is endothelial injury in the distal vein, the portion of the in situ conduit proximal to the fistula remaining patent because of flow down through the fistula. Therefore, we regard fistulas as, at most, an annoyance to the patient and the surgeon, but not as a potential cause of thrombosis of the bypass.

RESULTS

Among 8815 distal arterial reconstructions for limb salvage, 4079 were performed in situ in toto. In addition, 272 were completed with short segment of harvested vein (partial in situ bypass). In 1901 limbs, the vein had been harvested or previously used. In 504 limbs, the vein was spared for later use. Life-table analysis of secondary patency of bypasses for limb salvage to the popliteal level (up to the date of this writing, December 2012) is shown in Table 19.1 and to the infrapopliteal level in Table 19.2.

Early detection of stenoses and correction of defects with in situ conduits before occlusion occurs is now achieved by a comprehensive surveillance program. Our patients are seen and examined every 3–4 months up to the second year and every 6 months thereafter. Each examination includes pulse volume recordings and segmental pressures and audible Doppler assessment along the course of the bypass. Direct visualization of the conduit and estimates of volume flow by duplex ultrasonic scanning, both at rest and after reactive hyperemia induced by 3 minutes of tourniquet occlusion, have recently been used and evaluated.

Among 4079 in situ conduits constructed, 216 stenotic lesions developed in 199 patients. More than 62% of these were discovered within the first 12 months. In the distal mobilized segment, 70 occurred, and 102 were present in the proximal mobilized segment and 41 in the midportion of the bypass conduit – an even distribution. Stenotic lesions tended to occur with increased frequency in smaller veins (7% occurring in veins of 3.0 mm or less as compared with 4% in veins of 3.5 mm or larger). All of these stenoses were treated operatively, and all but 7 remained patent beyond

Table 19.1 Secondary patency popliteal in situ bypasses for salvage.

Interval	At risk	Occlusions	Int patency	Cum patency
0–1	1456	64	0.953	0.953
2–12	1222	48	0.952	0.908
13–24	742	26	0.961	0.872
25–36	566	6	0.987	0.861
37–48	386	18	0.949	0.817
49–60	300	2	0.993	0.811
61–72	232	10	0.953	0.773
73–84	186	2	0.988	0.763
85–86	152	0	1.000	0.763
97–108	122	4	0.928	0.708
109–120	92	0	1.000	0.708
121–132	56	2	0.960	0.680

Table 19.2 Secondary patency infrapopliteal in situ bypasses for salvage.

Interval	At risk	Occlusions	Int patency	Cum patency
0–1	2623	99	0.959	0.959
2–12	2168	102	0.942	0.904
13–24	1233	36	0.965	0.872
25–36	811	27	0.962	0.839
37–48	561	17	0.966	0.810
49–60	399	7	0.980	0.794
61–72	297	4	0.984	0.781
73–84	214	8	0.955	0.746
85–96	154	6	0.960	0.716
97–108	119	0	1.000	0.716
109–120	90	7	0.908	0.650
121–132	56	1	0.971	0.632

30 days. In addition, there were 198 residual A-V fistulas that required ligation under local anesthesia 3 days to 128 months after the initial procedure. Finally, there were 163 occlusions within 30 days (immediate patency rate 96%) and 159 deaths within the same period (operative mortality 3.8%).

PERSPECTIVE

Initially, the results of our prospective randomized study indicated the superiority of in situ vein bypass over reversed vein grafts.[23] With recent reports of improved patency rates using reversed vein grafts,[24] the question has again been raised as to whether the in situ vein bypass is superior to the reversed vein bypass at all levels. However, 75% of bypasses in this reported series were short bypasses. Other recent prospective randomized[25-27] and nonrandomized[28] comparison studies did not demonstrate any difference in performance between in situ and reversed vein bypasses. These studies were done using techniques that may render venous injuries, mostly for popliteal bypasses, and had patency rates much lower than those reported in recent major series of in situ bypasses.[29-31] These instruments (e.g. Hall, Cartier, LeMaitre, Bush) all use a cylindrical disruptor/cutter introduced retrogradely. Injury to the endothelial monolayer is produced by the passage of these instruments along the wall of the distal, smaller end of the saphenous vein. Thus, results with these instruments are satisfactory only in a high-flow situation (i.e. femoropopliteal) with larger ($4 OD) veins. When applied to smaller veins going to more distal tibial or pedal arteries, the importance of this degree of endothelial injury increases. In distal bypasses, with their inherently lower flow volumes and velocities, these instruments exhibit a high 30-day failure rate (20%).[32] Currently, a multicentre prospective randomized study[33] reports no difference in overall patency rates for long tibial bypasses between in situ and reversed vein bypasses. This study has a small number of cases for each centre and patency rates are also low. In addition, 15% of veins were deemed inadequate suggesting selection bias

to larger veins. In spite of these shortcomings, this study shows that in situ bypasses are superior to reversed vein bypasses for small (4.0 mm OD) veins, although this difference is not yet statistically significant.[33] Indirect evidence of in situ bypass superiority is its patency which is insensitive to length, whereas it is generally accepted that harvested vein bypass patency is clearly inversely proportioned to length (shorter is better). Our technical methodology for performing the in situ bypass has been developed with the primary goal of universal application. An in situ bypass can be performed by this technique in virtually all cases, regardless of the vagaries of venous anatomy, while minimizing the extent of exposure of the vein necessary for consistently safe and atraumatic valve incision. The high incidence of venous anomalies (up to 30% of double systems) and smaller veins distally (greater than 50%, 3.5 mm OD) makes the use of a cylindrical transluminal retrograde valve disruptor such as the Hall, Cartier or LeMaitre strippers hazardous. To date, the in situ vein arterial bypass seems to be the best conduit for long bypasses to distal arteries particularly with small diameter veins.

Use of an angioscope in performing in situ bypass has its enthusiasts and is industry driven.[34,35] This new technology demands accommodation and training with a new instrumentation that requires not only a large initial investment ($60,000–$75,000) but an ongoing disposable/replacement expense ($1,000/case). Although application of this approach produces comparable results, our experience with the method, which evolved in Albany and is essentially unchanged in over a decade, is that it is simpler, safe and reliable with all anatomic venous variations.

Clearly, problems with rendering the valves fully incompetent while at the same time not injuring the wall of the vein or its endothelium have discouraged some from using in situ techniques. So also have difficulties in locating and controlling arteriovenous fistulas. Nevertheless, we believe that the potential benefits of in situ vein bypasses outweigh the disadvantages of having to master critical new operative techniques to overcome the difficulties associated with their use.

REFERENCES

1. McGeachie J., Campbou P, Pendergast F. Vein to artery grafts: A quantitative study of revascularization of vasa vasorum and its relationship to intimal hyperplasia. *Ann Surg.* 1981;194:100.

2. Abbott W, Wieland S, Anstone WG. Structural changes during preparation of autogenous venous grafts. *Surgery.* 1974;76:1031.

3. Brody WR, Kosek JC, Angell WW. Changes in vein grafts following aorto-coronary bypass induced by pressure and ischemia. *J Thorac Cardiovasc Surg.* 1982;64:847.

4. Baumgartner HR. The role of blood flow in platelet adhesion, fibrin deposition and formation of mural thrombi. *Microvasc Res.* 1973;5:167.

5. O'Mara CS, Flinn WR, Neiman HL, Bergan JJ, Yao JST. Correlation of foot arterial anatomy with early tibial bypass patency. *Surgery.* 1981;89:743.

6. LoGerfo FW, Quist WC, Carwshaw HW, Haudens-Child C. An improved technique for preservation of endothelial morphology in vein grafts. *Surgery.* 1981;90:1015.

7. Hall KV. The great saphenous vein used in situ as an arterial shunt after extirpation of the vein. *Surgery.* 1962;51:492.

8. Skagseth E, Hall KV. In situ vein bypass. *Scand J Thorac Cardiovasc Surg.* 1973;7:53.

9. Cartier, P. Personal Communication.

10. Samuels PB, Plested WG, Haberfelde GC, Cincotti JJ, Brown CE. In situ saphenous vein arterial bypass: A study of the anatomy pertinent to its use in situ as a bypass graft with a description of a new venous valvulotome. *Am Surg.* 1968;34:122.

11. Barner HB, Judd DR, Kaiser GC et al. Late failure of arterialized in situ saphenous vein. *Arch Surg.* 1969;99:781.

12. Gruss JD, Bartels D, Vargas H et al. Arterial reconstruction for distal disease of the lower extremities by the in situ vein graft technique. *J Cardiovasc Surg.* 1982;23:231.

13. Langeron P, Puppinck P, Cordonnier D. La technique de la greffe veineuse in situ dans la chirurgie arterielle restauratrice des membres inferieurs. *J Chir.* 1978;115:171.

14. Galland RB, Young AE, Jamieson CW. In-situ vein bypass: A modified technique. *Ann R Coll Surg Engl.* 1981;63:186.

15. Veith FJ, Moss CM, Sprayregen S, Montefusco CM. Pre-operative saphenous venography in arterial reconstructive surgery of the lower extremity. *Surgery.* 1979;85:253.

16. Shah DM, Chang BB, Leopold PW et al. The anatomy of the greater saphenous venous system. *J Vasc Surg.* 1986;3:273.

17. Kupinski AM, Leather RP, Chang BB, Shah DM. Preoperative mapping of the saphenous vein. In: Bernstein EF, ed. *Vascular Diagnosis.* St. Louis, MO: Mosby; 1993, pp. 897–901.

18. Leather RP, Powers SR, Karmody AM. A reappraisal of the in situ saphenous vein arterial bypass. *Surgery.* 1979;86:453.

19. Leather RP, Shah DM, Karmody AM. Infrapopliteal arterial bypass for limb salvage: Increased patency and utilization of the saphenous vein used in situ. *Surgery.* 1981;90:1000.

20. Darling RC III, Shah DM, Chang BB, Lloyd WE, Leather RP. Can the profunda femoris artery reliably be used as an inflow source for infrainguinal reconstructions? Long term results in 563 patients. *J Vasc Surg.* 1994;20:889–895.

21. Veith FJ, Gupta SK, Samson RH et al. Superficial femoral and popliteal artery as inflow sites for distal bypass. *Surgery.* 1981;90:980.

22. Leather RP, Shah DM, Corson JD, Karmody AM. Instrumental evolution of the valve incision method of in situ saphenous vein bypass. *J Vasc Surg.* 1984;1:113.

23. Buchbinder D, Singh JK, Karmody AM et al. Comparison of patency rate and structural changes of the in situ and reversed vein arterial bypass. *J Surg Res.* 1981;30:213.

24. Taylor LM, Edwards JM, Phinney ES, Porter JM. Reversed vein bypass to infrapopliteal arteries: Modern results are superior to or equivalent to in situ bypass for patency and for vein utilization. *Ann Surg.* 1987;205:90.

25. Harris PL, How TV, Jones DR. Prospectively randomized clinical trial to compare in situ and reversed saphenous vein grafts for femoropopliteal bypass. *Br J Surg.* 1987;74:252.

26. Watelet J, Cheysson E, Poels D et al. In situ versus reversed saphenous vein for femoropopliteal bypass: A prospective randomized study of 100 cases. *Ann Vasc Surg.* 1986;1:441.

27. Moody AP, Edwards PR, Harris PL. In situ versus reversed femoropopliteal vein grafts: long term follow up of a prospective, randomized trial. *Br J Surg.* 1992;79:750–752.

28. Veterans Administration Cooperative Study Group 141. Comparative evaluation of prosthetic, reversed, and in situ vein bypass grafts in distal popliteal and tibial-peroneal revascularization. *Arch Surg.* 1988;123:434.

29. Fogel MA, Whittemore AD, Couch NP, Mannick JA. A comparison of in situ and reversed saphenous vein grafts for infra-inguinal reconstruction. *J Vasc Surg.* 1987;4:46.

30. Bandyk DF, Kaebnick HW, Steward GW, Towne JB. Durability of the in situ saphenous vein arterial bypass: A comparison of primary and secondary patency. *J Vasc Surg.* 1987;5:256.

31. Shah DM, Darling RC III, Chang BB, Fitzgerald KM, Paty PSK, Leather RP. Long term results of in situ saphenous vein bypass: Analysis of 2058 cases. *Ann Surg.* 1995;222:438–448.

32. Harris PL, Veith FJ, Shanik GD, Nott D, Wengerter KR, Moore DJ. Prospective randomized comparison of in situ and reversed infrapopliteal vein grafts. *Br J Surg.* 1993;80:173–176.

33. Wengerter KR, Veith FJ, Gupta SK et al. Prospective randomized multicentered comparison of in situ and reversed vein infrapopliteal bypass. *J Vasc Surg.* 1991;12:189.

34. Mehigan JT. Angioscopic control of in situ bypass: Technical consideration. In: Rutherford RE, ed. *Seminars in Vascular Surgery.* Philadelphia, PA: W.B. Saunders; 1993, pp. 176–179.

35. Rosenthal D, Piano G. Endovascular technique in in situ vein graft. In: Yao JST, Pearce WH, eds. *Progress in Vascular Surgery.* Stamford, CT: Appleton and Lange; 1997, pp. 271–276.

20

Adventitial cystic disease and entrapment syndromes involving the popliteal artery

JUAN CARLOS JIMENEZ and SAMUEL ERIC WILSON

CONTENTS

ADVENTITIAL CYSTIC DISEASE OF THE POPLITEAL ARTERY

Adventitial cystic disease (ACD) was first discovered by Atkins in 1947 in a case report describing its involvement with the external iliac artery.[1] Ejrup and Hiertonn, in Stockholm, Sweden, first described this clinical entity of the popliteal artery in 1954.[2] Hiertonn, with coauthors Lindberg and Rob, produced a subsequent publication, which described cystic degeneration of the popliteal artery.[3] They reviewed four known cases encountered up to 1957. A number of valuable descriptive terms were applied to the lesion including 'clear, jelly-like material similar in appearance to that seen in a ganglion', 'the specimen looked like a sausage and was 7 cm in length' and 'the lumen was compressed by an intramural cyst containing jelly under high tension'.

Due to its infrequent presentation, the majority of publications are limited to case reports and small case series. Diagnosed mostly in younger patients, this disorder results from formation of a mucinous material in the form of a cyst, which develops in the adventitial layer of arteries and veins. These cysts can contribute to luminal compression and occlusion with resultant clinical sequelae. The most commonly affected vessel is the popliteal artery, although its presence in various peripheral arteries and veins as well as the abdominal aorta has been reported.[4] The most frequent clinical presentation is intermittent claudication in young, active patients. Although the lesion has been reported between 11 and 70 years of age, it usually presents in patients in their twenties or thirties.[5,6]

Incidence and demographics

ACD of the popliteal artery is rare and the true incidence is not known. Desy and Spinner published a contemporary study following a comprehensive review of the literature on ACD.[4] The authors identified 586 studies describing ACD in 724 patients. Arteries were involved exclusively in 660 cases and 53 venous cysts were identified. Nine cases were demonstrated in the pediatric population. The most common location was the popliteal artery (81% of all cases). Evidence suggests a 4:1 male predominance with ACD for arterial lesions; however, a 1:1 male–female ratio has been demonstrated for venous cysts.[4]

Aetiology and pathogenesis

The exact cause of cystic degeneration of the adventitia in the popliteal artery remains uncertain, and there are several possible theories explaining the pathogenesis of this disorder. Repetitive trauma has been implicated; however, the lesion's occurrence in pediatric patients makes it unlikely as the sole cause. Adventitial degeneration from a systemic connective tissue disorder is another theory. A developmental mechanism for inclusion of remnant mesenchymal cells in the arterial wall has also been postulated[7] as well as an articular (synovial) theory.

Recent evidence to support a synovial source for ACD was presented by Desy and Spinner, who demonstrated joint connections between affected vessels near the hip, knee and wrist.[8] In their paper, they identified knee joint connections, which were initially unrecognized in five cases of ACD and treated at their institution. They hypothesized that adventitial cyst formation begins with a capsular defect that leads to tracking of synovial fluid through a vascular articular branch. This may be caused by trauma or degeneration of the joint and may be similar to the pathogenesis of intraneural ganglion cysts.[8] There have been suggestions that an enlargement of the knee joint capsular synovial cyst could develop along a geniculate artery to involve the adventitia of the popliteal artery or that synovial cysts can be sequestered into the arterial wall during development. This could explain why the cysts can be either entirely adventitial or involve other layers of the artery wall and why not all cysts can be enucleated.

Pathophysiology

Although there is wide variation, the sudden onset of ischemic symptoms in the leg in men in their third decade of life can be associated with cystic adventitial disease of the popliteal artery. The rapid change in the size of the cyst, which has been developing over a long period of time, causes these sudden symptoms. Some degree of stenosis may be associated with the cyst for a long period of time with preservation of luminal patency in the popliteal artery until the intracystic pressure exceeds that of the artery, causing occlusion with or without thrombosis and the resultant sudden onset of associated symptoms. Intermittent claudication without severe ischemia is a common finding because collateral circulation develops.

The nature of the content of the cyst has been the subject of numerous studies. Endo and colleagues isolated and identified proteohyaluronic acid in the cyst, and they believe that this represents cystic mucoid degeneration.[9] Leaf performed amino acid analysis of the protein present in ACD of the popliteal artery and showed similarities between ganglia and adventitial cysts by both chemical and histologic analyses.[10] Both lesions involve mucoproteins and mucopolysaccharides.

Clinical presentation

Typically, a patient in his twenties, thirties or forties presents with the sudden onset of intermittent claudication that is quite limiting. Both the pedal and popliteal pulses may be present if there is only a stenosis of the popliteal artery associated with the cyst. Depending on the degree of stenosis, there may be an associated bruit audible over the popliteal fossa. Palpable distal pulses may disappear during acute flexion of the knee. In other patients, both pedal and popliteal pulses may be absent, indicating arterial occlusion, which is less frequent than stenosis. After the initial sudden onset of cramping pain in the calf, the patient may experience some relief followed by typical intermittent

claudication as good collateral circulation develops. This results from the gradual stenosis of the popliteal artery prior to the rapid enlargement of the cyst, which produces either a more significant stenosis or occlusion. Occasionally, ischemic neuropathy may also be present.

Evaluation of the patient with adventitial cystic disease

Although physical examination as alluded to the aforementioned is the essential first step of evaluation, the noninvasive vascular laboratory can be employed to corroborate the initial physical findings. This evaluation can be performed in a manner similar to that for conventional atherosclerotic occlusive disease. Comparison with the opposite non-affected lower extremity may demonstrate significant differences, however, may not be useful in the rare patient with bilateral disease. In contrast to the normal segmental limb pressures, the affected limb below the cystic lesion will show a decrease in segmental limb pressures. Also, in contrast to the normal pulse waveforms in the unaffected limb, the affected limb will show a flattening of the pulse wave below the cystic lesion. Because of the excellent collateral circulation that usually develops in young men, total absence of pulse waves over the distal tibial arteries is rare. Duplex examination may reveal increased flow velocities at the level of the affected vessel and may reveal hypoechogenic nodules against the arterial wall.[11–13]

Advances in both magnetic resonance and computed tomography imaging have improved the diagnosis and characterization of ACD. Magnetic resonance angiography (MRA) can accurately identify the presence of the cyst within the vessel wall as well as connections with the adjacent joint, especially on T2-weighted or fluid-sensitive short tau inversion recovery sequences, where the lesions appear bright with no or only rim enhancement on gadolinium-enhanced sequences.[14–16] Evaluation of the affected limb with computed tomography angiography or venography (CTA or CTV) may also reveal the site or extent of obstruction, identify collateral vessels and aid with preoperative planning.[17,18]

Conventional angiography, once routinely performed to diagnose this disorder, is less frequently required due to advances in CTA and MRA; however, it is still the *gold standard* to outline normal arteries and the location of the lesion. Frequently, a smooth wall stenosis will be identified, usually at the midportion of the popliteal artery extending from 1 to 8 cm in length (Figure 20.1). There may be a curvilinear defect, which has been described as a 'scimitar sign', caused by displacing the contrast column within the arterial lumen (Figure 20.2). With the expansion of the cyst to encircle the arterial lumen, a concentric smooth taper of this lesion has been described as resulting in an *hourglass* appearance. It is important to have both lateral

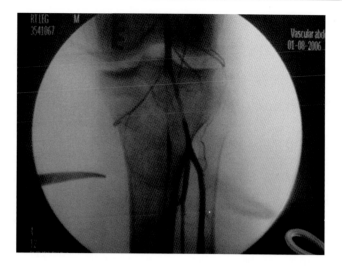

Figure 20.1 Conventional angiogram of a patient with adventitial cystic disease of the popliteal artery resulting in smooth, tapered narrowing of the vessel.

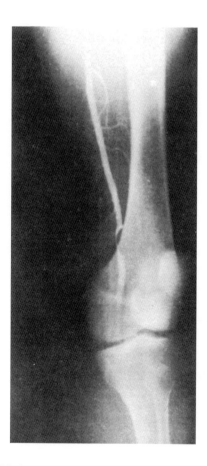

Figure 20.2 This angiogram of the popliteal artery reveals smooth tapering above and below the popliteal artery cyst that created severe stenosis of the popliteal artery. The *scimitar sign* is diagnostic for adventitial cystic disease of the popliteal artery. (Reproduced from McAllister HA, Armed Forces Institute of Pathology, Washington, DC. With permission.)

and anteroposterior angiographic views to ensure that the lesion is not missed. In contrast to typical angiographic findings with popliteal artery entrapment (PES), there will be no medial deviation of the popliteal artery with the cystic lesion. The angiographic findings combined with the clinical evaluation of the patient should allow certain diagnosis of the lesion and differentiate it from arteriosclerotic occlusive disease. There may, on occasion, be some confusion with PES if total occlusion of the middle portion of the popliteal artery has occurred. Thus, there might be a localized complete occlusion of the midpopliteal artery, with the remainder of the lower extremity arterial anatomy having a normal appearance and with excellent collateral circulation around the limited occlusion. In these instances, noninvasive imaging with MRA may be preferable to evaluate the surrounding musculotendinous structures.

Treatment

Treatment of ACD of the popliteal artery can be conservative depending on the level of severity of the patient's symptoms. However, due to the relatively young age at presentation and usually high patient activity levels, most will require treatment. Spontaneous resolution of ACD has been reported; however, it has been associated with recurrence of disease.[19] Adequate experience has documented that ultrasound-guided aspiration of the cyst can be successful in eradicating the cyst and resultant arterial stenosis or occlusion in some patients.[20,21] Because the cystic content is quite viscous and gelatinous, aspiration must be done with a relatively large bore needle. However, aspiration can be the treatment of choice if the cyst is diagnosed before the development of total occlusion of the artery. Suboptimal outcomes have been reported with endovascular treatment with angioplasty and this approach is generally not recommended.[22,23]

Surgical intervention can, and most frequently, provide effective treatment.[24,25] Surgical procedures have been divided into nonresectional techniques and resectional techniques. Nonresectional techniques are employed mainly when occlusion of the popliteal artery has not occurred. Evacuation of the cyst or enucleation is the most frequent, nonresectional form of therapy. The popliteal artery can be approached through either a posterior S-shaped incision or a medial incision; however, the posterior approach provides the best exposure of the affected vessel. The normal popliteal artery above and below the lesion can be easily mobilized. The popliteal artery involved by the cystic lesion will be enlarged and sausage shaped. There may be adhesions binding the cystic adventitial structure to the adjacent vein or to the posterior aspect of the joint capsule. Although the cyst is usually unilocular, there may be multilocular cysts with septa present. An incision into the cyst and evacuation

of its contents usually restore arterial patency (Figure 20.3a–c). The fluid extruding through the incision is usually crystal clear. However, the fluid may be light yellow or even currant jelly in colour if there has been recent or old hemorrhage into the cyst (Figure 20.4).

While evacuation or enucleation of the cyst is preferred if occlusion of the popliteal artery and resultant intimal damage have not occurred, resection and arterial reconstruction may be required if total occlusion of the artery has occurred, with or without thrombosis. Resection and replacement of the involved arterial segment with an autogenous greater saphenous vein graft are the operation of choice for this latter stage of the disease process. Results of such treatment should be excellent.

Recurrent stenosis and occlusion of the popliteal artery secondary to cystic adventitial lesions have been treated successfully by needle aspiration, recovering varying amounts of gelatinous material. Many advocate simple evacuation of the cyst by aspiration even for recurrent lesions because of the relatively high degree of success.[26]

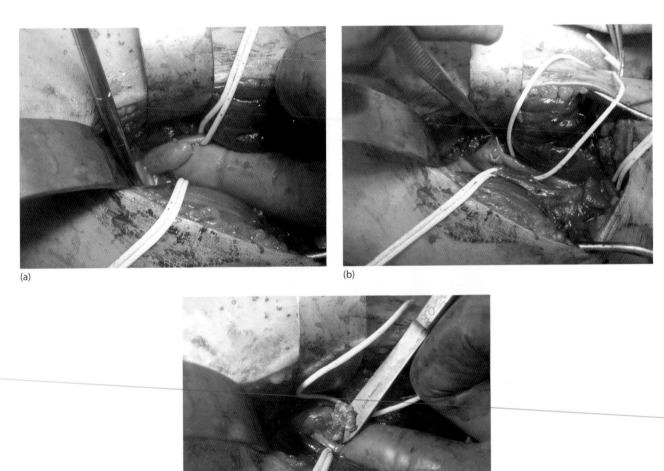

(a)

(b)

(c)

Figure 20.3 (a–c) Surgical exposure and evacuation of a popliteal cyst. Luminal patency and normal flow was restored with cyst evacuation alone.

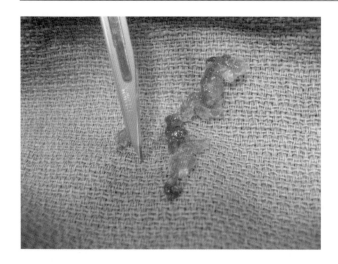

Figure 20.4 Gelatinous contents removed from a popliteal adventitial cyst.

If this is not successful, a direct surgical approach may be required with evacuation of the cyst or with replacement or bypass of the involved segment of the popliteal artery with an autogenous saphenous vein graft.

POPLITEAL VASCULAR ENTRAPMENT SYNDROMES

Popliteal entrapment syndrome (PES) refers to functional compression of the neurovascular structures located in the popliteal fossa by surrounding musculotendinous structures leading to vascular and neurogenic symptoms.[27]

The anatomic basis for PES was first described in 1879 by a medical student in Edinburgh, Scotland. T. P. Anderson Stuart was dissecting the amputated leg of a 64-year-old man, and he described the anatomic abnormality associated with the abnormal course of the popliteal artery (Figure 20.5).[28] In 1959, Hamming, at Leyden University in the Netherlands, reported a similar anomaly in a 12-year-old boy.[29] Hamming's case report is a classic reference because it represents the first successful clinical treatment of complications associated with popliteal arterial entrapment.

Classification and aetiology

The development of a definitive classification system for PES has been challenged by the infrequency of the disorder, with the majority of published data limited to case reports and small case series. Classification of this disorder has evolved as variations in the associated anatomic abnormalities were discovered.[30–33] In 1998, the Popliteal Vascular Entrapment Forum provided an updated classification system; however, it was acknowledged that the quality of available studies on which to base management guidelines was poor[27] (Figure 20.6).

Pathophysiology

The variety of anatomic variants can be associated with entrapment of either or both the popliteal artery and the popliteal vein with a variety of effects on normal lower

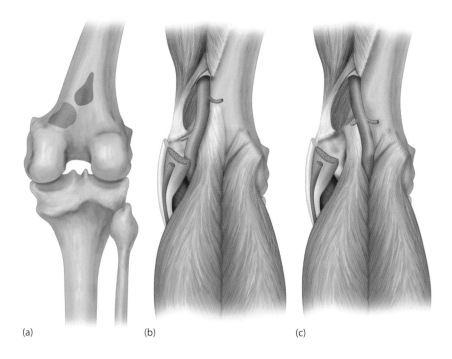

(a)   (b)   (c)

Figure 20.5 (a–c) Represent an artist's interpretation of the written description by T. P. Anderson Stuart in 1879 from the first published observation of a congenital anomaly associated with the resultant abnormal course of the popliteal artery. (b) Entrapment. (c) Usual course. (With appreciation to the artist, Gary G. Wind, MD.)

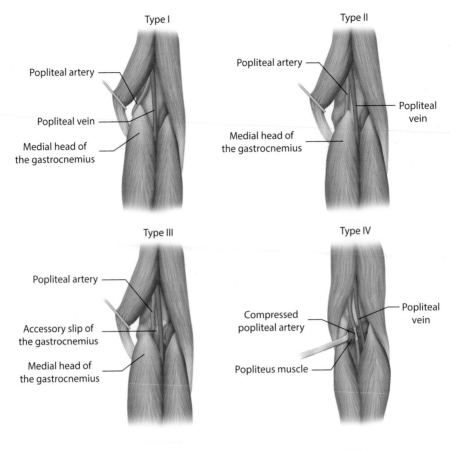

Type I	Popliteal artery running medial to the medial head of gastrocnemius
Type II	Medial head of gastrocnemius laterally attached
Type III	Accessory slip of gastrocnemius/fibrous bands arising from medial head of gastrocnemius
Type IV	Popliteal artery passing below popliteus muscle/fibrous bands arising from popliteus
Type V	Primarily venous entrapment
Type VI	Other variants
Type F	Functional entrapment

Figure 20.6 Popliteal Vascular Entrapment Forum classification for popliteal entrapment syndrome. (Adapted from Sinha S et al., *J Vasc Surg*, 55, 252, 2014.)

extremity physiology. External compression can vary from minimal in the asymptomatic patient to marked compression that causes a significant stenosis of the popliteal artery or vein. This external compression can advance to total occlusion of the popliteal vessels. This can occur either temporarily with varying positions of the patient's leg and foot or permanently with intraluminal thrombosis. The arterial pathology associated with external compression of the popliteal artery can range from poststenotic dilatation to the presence of a true aneurysm. The potential for embolization of thrombus from the aneurysm to the distal arterial run-off represents an additional threat to the patient's extremity distal to the lesion.

Midpopliteal arterial occlusion is a classic finding of PES with thrombosis. Development of extensive collateral arterial circulation can occur, and the patient may be only mildly symptomatic. Figure 20.7 demonstrates aneurysmal changes that might also develop in the entrapped popliteal vein (Figure 20.7). Thrombosis of the entrapped vein with resultant venous hypertension and/or chronic venous stasis with associated complications can develop.

An important question remains related to the segment of popliteal artery immediately distal to the area of entrapment. Even after release of the entrapment, will the recurrent trauma from the external compression cause intimal damage and subsequent thrombosis? Certainly

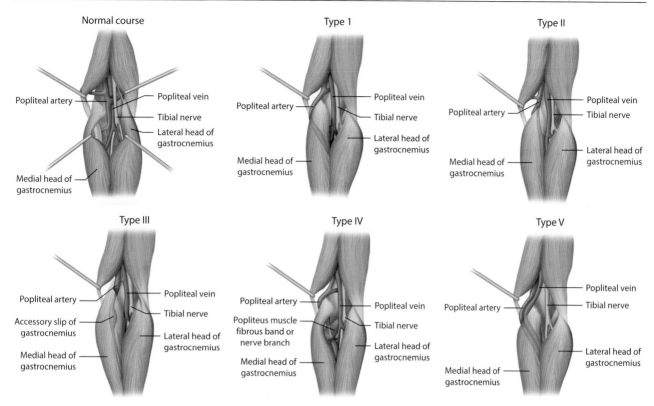

Figure 20.7 These drawings outline the normal course of the neurovascular bundle in the popliteal fossa from the posterior approach and show four generally accepted types of anomalies involving entrapment of the popliteal artery. All are usually associated with an abnormal configuration of the medial head of the gastrocnemius muscle. This classification, however, does not satisfy all anatomic variants. Empirically, type IV was expanded to include a branch of the tibial nerve as a structure compressing the popliteal artery, and type V was added to emphasize that the popliteal vein can be entrapped with the artery in all four types. (Reproduced from Rich NM et al., *Arch Surg*, 141, 726, 1979. With permission.)

the potential exists; however, no study has clarified this relationship. Similarly, it is unclear after release of the entrapment whether or not the segment of popliteal artery distal to the entrapment – minimally dilated or not – will progress to a true aneurysm and how long this process will take. Only long-term follow-up of surgically treated cases in which the compression is released and the artery is not replaced can help answer these important questions. There are so few cases of documented entrapment of the popliteal vein that answers to similar questions related to this particular structure will probably go unanswered for a long time.

Incidence and demographics

Similar to ACD of the popliteal artery, PES is rare and the true incidence is not known. In a contemporary literature review of 54 articles by Sinha and colleagues, the mean age of patients was 32 years with a median male proportion of 83%.[27] Intermittent claudication was the most common presenting symptom in 22 studies and 11 studies described a medial proportion of 11% of limbs presenting with acute ischemia.[27] Bilateral PES was estimated to be 38.25% and 17.5% of limbs were noted to be asymptomatic.[27]

Clinical presentation and diagnosis

The history of intermittent claudication in a young patient during strenuous exercise should raise the suspicion of a tentative diagnosis of popliteal vascular entrapment. Such patients might also have ACD of the popliteal artery. The absence of a history and signs of atherosclerotic disease further highlights the possibility of PES. Patients typically present with worsening symptoms associated with strenuous exercise, particularly on a graded surface. This is likely attributed to increased compression of the artery by the gastrocnemius and soleus muscles during repetitive plantar flexion.[34] Similar to patients with IC due to atherosclerotic causes, pedal pulses may or may not be present. Obliteration of pedal pulses on examination with aggressive plantar flexion has also been reported.[34]

The diagnosis of popliteal vascular entrapment may be established by noninvasive techniques in the vascular laboratory. Ankle brachial indices may be normal at rest; however, they frequently exhibit a drop in pressures with exercise treadmill testing. Duplex ultrasound examination may demonstrate abnormal deviation of the artery, an aberrant gastrocnemius and/or the presence of an accessory slip of muscle. Abnormal flow velocities also help establish the diagnosis of PES with duplex evaluation.

At our institution, we proceed with noninvasive axial imaging once PES is suspected. Computed tomography and magnetic resonance imaging may help delineate the extent of arterial disease, confirm popliteal occlusion, identify distal targets if surgical reconstruction is required and establish the presence (or absence) of collaterals. These modalities also demonstrate the position of the artery (and vein) and their relationship to the surrounding musculature and soft tissue structures.

Conventional angiography is the recognized gold standard for demonstrating the anatomic features of arterial lesions. Additionally, dynamic angiographic evaluation in conjunction with the foot in neutral positioning as well as active plantar flexion and dorsiflexion may confirm the diagnosis of PES.[35] Because PES is not generally amenable to endovascular therapy and because of the invasive nature of conventional angiography, noninvasive imaging with high resolution MRA and CTA has decreased the need for angiography prior to surgical intervention.

Treatment

When PES is identified in symptomatic patients, it is now believed that operative intervention is likely required in most patients to help protect against the development of complications from PES. If the vascular involvement extends to thrombosis and/or aneurysm formation, the operative management becomes more difficult and complicated. Operative treatment by release of the entrapping anomalous head of the gastrocnemius muscle, anomalous bands or associated structures has become widely accepted in both symptomatic and asymptomatic patients.

Although the medial approach to the popliteal artery can be utilized, exact identification of the pathology may not be obvious via medial incisions. We therefore favour a posterior S-shaped incision which provides adequate exposure of the compressive soft tissue structures and for the management of most associated complications such as popliteal artery aneurysm and thrombosis of the midpopliteal artery. The S-shaped incision also provides excellent exposure to identify the variety of anatomic anomalies that are associated with the popliteal vascular entrapment. On the other hand, some surgeons believe that the exact identification of pathology is unimportant and that the midpopliteal artery thrombosis or aneurysm can be adequately managed through the medial approach. Autogenous greater saphenous vein may also be easier to harvest in this manner. Figure 20.8 demonstrates successful surgical management of a 19-year-old male with Type II PES at our institution. He did not require arterial reconstruction after division of an aberrant accessory slip of gastrocnemius muscle. He has remained asymptomatic 5 years following his operation.

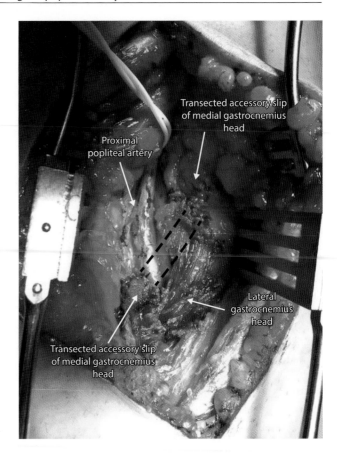

Figure 20.8 Successful management of Type II PES with surgical division of an accessory slip of gastrocnemius muscle. The underlying artery did not require surgical reconstruction. The patient remains asymptomatic 5 years following operation.

Results

Overall, the quality of available evidence for patients diagnosed with PES is poor and clear-cut clinical management guidelines cannot be made.[27] From their large contemporary review of the published literature, Sinha and colleagues determined that most papers published were noted to be at risk for bias and significant variability was found in the key outcome measures reported.[27] There is also insufficient evidence to support the superiority of individual surgical approaches. Sinha et al. also noted a significant rate of failure in a subset of studies following arterial surgical reconstruction.[27]

Optimal treatment for the asymptomatic patient is also not known. While non-surgical management of patients with popliteal stenosis and/or occlusion due to atherosclerosis yields acceptable results in clinically appropriate patients, it is unclear whether the natural history of PES is similar. Our approach to asymptomatic patients with PES involves close follow-up with noninvasive ultrasound studies (ankle brachial indices with exercise and duplex) and clinical reevaluation performed every 6 months. Patients with progression of symptoms are considered for surgical exploration.

In patients with significant lifestyle limiting claudication and/or signs of frank critical limb ischemia, restoration of arterial patency with surgical division of the compressive, extrinsic musculotendinous structures is the most common practice at our institution. The decision to reconstruct the artery with interposition reversed saphenous vein graft is made at the time of surgical exploration. Because these patients are usually young, active and have longer life expectancy than patients with atherosclerotic lesions, surgical reconstruction of diseased arterial segments is strongly considered to avoid the risk of rethrombosis.

It is likely that development of robust clinical management guidelines from retrospective single-institution studies is difficult due to the rarity of this disorder and the current heterogeneity of presentation and management. Multi-institutional cooperative databases such as the Vascular Low-Frequency Disease Consortium and the Vascular Study Group of New England may provide additional insight into the management of these and other low-frequency vascular surgical conditions.[36,37]

REFERENCES

1. Atkins HJB, Key JA. A case of myxomatous tumour arising in the adventitia of the left external iliac artery. *Br J Surg.* 1947;34:426–427.

2. Ejrup B, Hiertonn T. Intermittent claudication. Three cases treated by free vein graft. *Acta Chir Scand.* 1954;108:217.

3. Hiertonn T, Lindberg K, Rob C. Cystic degeneration of the popliteal artery. *Br J Surg.* 1957;44:348.

4. Desy NM, Spinner RJ. The etiology and management of cystic adventitial disease. *J Vasc Surg.* 2014;60:235–245.

5. Bergan JJ, Yao JST, Flinn WR. Surgical management of young claudicants: Adventitial cyst. In: Bergan JJ, Yao JST, eds. *Evaluation and Treatment of Upper and Lower Extremity Circulatory Disorders.* Orlando, FL: Grune & Stratton, 1984.

6. Flanigan DP, Burnham SJ, Goodreau JJ et al. Summary of cases of adventitial cystic disease of the popliteal artery. *Ann Surg.* 1979;189:165.

7. Tsilimparis N, Hanack U, Yousefi S et al. Cystic adventitial disease of the popliteal artery: An argument for the developmental theory. *J Vasc Surg.* 2007;45:1249–1252.

8. Spinner RJ, Desy NM, Agarwal G et al. Evidence to support that adventitial cysts, analogous to intraneural ganglion cysts, are also joint-connected. *Clin Anat.* 2013;26:267–281.

9. Endo M, Tamura S, Minakuchi S et al. Isolation and identification of proteohyaluronic acid from a cyst of cystic mucoid degeneration. *Clin Chim Acta.* 1973;47:417.

10. Leaf G. Amino-acid analysis of protein present in a popliteal artery cyst. *Br Med J.* 1967;3:415.

11. Weimar EA, Vriens PW, Heyligers JM, Moll FL. Regarding "High spatial resolution magnetic resonance imaging of cystic adventitial disease of the popliteal artery". *J Vasc Surg.* 2010;52:534–535.

12. Brodmann M, Stark G, Pabst E et al. Cystic adventitial degeneration of the popliteal artery – The diagnostic value of duplex sonography. *Eur J Radiol.* 2001;38:209–212.

13. Hai Z, Shao G. Images in vascular medicine: Cystic adventitial disease of the popliteal artery. *Vasc Med.* 2012;17:283–284.

14. Maged IM, Turba UC, Housseini AM et al. High spatial resolution magnetic resonance imaging of cystic adventitial disease of the popliteal artery. *J Vasc Surg.* 2010;51:471–474.

15. Loffroy R, Rao P, Krause D, Steinmeitz E. Use of 3.0-Tesla high spatial resolution magnetic resonance imaging for diagnosis and treatment of cystic adventitial disease of the popliteal artery. *Ann Vasc Surg.* 2011;25:385.

16. Wiwanitkit V. Cystic adventitial disease and high spatial resolution magnetic resonance imaging. *Ann Vasc Surg.* 2012;26:443.

17. Seo JY, Chung DJ, Kim JH. Adventitial cystic disease of the femoral vein: A case report with CT venography. *Korean J Radiol.* 2009;10:89–92.

18. Deutsch AL, Hyde J, Miller SM et al. Cystic adventitial degeneration of the popliteal artery: CT demonstration and directed percutaneous therapy. *Am J Roentgenol.* 1985;145:117–118.

19. Zhang L, Guzman R, Kirkpatrick I, Klein J. Spontaneous resolution of cystic adventitial disease: A word of caution. *Ann Vasc Surg.* 2012;26:422.

20. Keo HH, Baumgartner I, Schmidii J, Do DD. Sustained remission 11 years after percutaneous ultrasound-guided aspiration for cystic adventitial degeneration in the popliteal artery. *J Endovasc Ther.* 2007;14:264–265.

21. Do DD, Brauschweig M, Baumgartner I et al. Adventitial cystic disease of the popliteal artery: Percutaneous US-guided aspiration. *Radiology.* 1997;203:743–746.

22. Fox R, Kahn M, Adler J et al. Adventitial cystic disease of the popliteal artery: Failure of percutaneous transluminal angioplasty as a therapeutic modality. *J Vasc Surg.* 1985;2:464–467.

23. Khoury M. Failed angioplasty of a popliteal artery stenosis secondary to cystic adventitial disease – A case report. *Vasc Endovascular Surg.* 2004;38:277–280.

24. Sucandy I, Goldhahn R Jr, Abai B. Surgical management of cystic adventitial disease of the popliteal artery. *Am Surg.* 2012;78:E333–E334.

25. Patel SM, Patil VA, Pamoukian VN. Interposition grafting of popliteal artery cystic adventitial disease: Case report. *Vasc Endovasc Surg.* 2008;42:192–195.

26. Maged IM, Kron IL, Hagspiel KD. Recurrent cystic adventitial disease of the popliteal artery: Successful treatment with percutaneous transluminal angioplasty. *Vasc Endovascular Surg.* 2009;43:399–402.

27. Sinha S, Houghton J, Holt PJ et al. Popliteal entrapment syndrome. *J Vasc Surg.* 2012;55:252–262.

28. Stuart TPA. A note on a variation in the course of the popliteal artery. *J Anat Physiol.* 1879;13:162.

29. Hamming JJ. Intermittent claudication at an early age, due to an anomalous course of the popliteal artery. *Angiology.* 1959;10:369.

30. Insua JA, Young JR, Humphries AWS et al. Popliteal artery entrapment syndrome. *Arch Surg.* 1970;101:771.

31. Delaney TA, Gonzalez LL. Occlusion of popliteal artery due to muscular entrapment. *Surgery.* 1971;69:97.

32. Ferrero R, Baeile C, Buzzacchino A et al. La Sindrome da Costrizone dell'arteria Poplia. *Minerva Cardioangiol.* 1978;26:389.

33. Rich NM, Collins GJ Jr, McDonald PT et al. Popliteal vascular entrapment. *Arch Surg.* 1979;141:726.

34. Causey MW, Quan RW, Curry TK, Singh N. Ultrasound is a critical adjunct in the diagnosis and treatment of popliteal entrapment syndrome. *J Vasc Surg.* 2013;57:1695–1697.

35. Hai Z, Guangrui S, Yuan Z et al. CT angiography and MRI in patients with popliteal artery entrapment syndrome. *Am J Roentgenol.* 2008;191:1760–1766.

36. Lawrence PF, Harlender-Locke MP, Oderich GS et al. The current management of isolated degenerative femoral artery aneurysms is too aggressive for their natural history. *J Vasc Surg.* 2014;59:343–349.

37. Eslami MH, Rybin D, Doros G et al. Comparison of a Vascular Study Group of New England risk prediction model with established risk prediction models of in-hospital mortality after elective abdominal aortic aneurysm repair. *J Vasc Surg.* 2015;62:1125–1133.

21

Extra-anatomic bypass

EVAN C. LIPSITZ and KARAN GARG

CONTENTS

INTRODUCTION

An extra-anatomic bypass is the creation of a bypass whose pathway is normally devoid of a major arterial segment. Unlike conventional bypasses, the donor vessel is generally remote from and in line with the recipient vessel. These bypasses are commonly employed when a less physiologically stressful procedure is desirable in patients with limb ischemia with significant medical co-morbidities, or in order to avoid working in an infected, or otherwise hostile, operative field. In the peripheral circulation, the most frequently performed configurations are the axillofemoral bypass and femorofemoral bypass. These configurations are most commonly used to revascularize occlusive atherosclerotic disease affecting the aortoiliac and femoral arteries. Other configurations, performed less frequently, include the obturator bypass and thoracofemoral bypass.

The development and advancement of endovascular therapies have and will continue to impact the treatment of aortoiliac occlusive disease. In the early 1990s, reports demonstrating the efficacy and relative durability of angioplasty and stenting of focal stenoses (Trans-Atlantic Inter-Society Consensus [TASC] A and B lesions) led to widespread adoption of endovascular treatment as the preferred mode of therapy. Since the mid-1990s, advancements for crossing total occlusions (TASC C and D lesions), including the development of subintimal angioplasty, have made the treatment of an even greater number of patients with endovascular methods possible, with results comparable to open revascularization.[1,2] As a result, many of the patients who ultimately do come to require surgical repair are older, present with extensive disease, with possible failed endovascular revascularization and more significant co-morbidities. This makes them unsuitable candidates for direct aortic reconstruction, thus, necessitating an extra-anatomic bypass.

EVALUATING AORTOILIAC OCCLUSIVE DISEASE

Among the distinct patterns of arterial occlusive disease is atherosclerosis affecting the aortoiliac segment. Classic symptoms of aortoiliac occlusive disease include thigh and/or buttock claudication with absent femoral pulses on physical examination. Combined with impotence in male patients, this constellation of symptoms is known as Leriche syndrome. Aortoiliac occlusive disease can be seen in isolation or in combination with infrainguinal occlusive disease. In patients with multilevel disease, the clinical manifestation may be more severe. The diagnosis of aortoiliac occlusive disease can be made on the basis of a history and physical exam, with patients often having an extensive smoking history.

The diagnosis of aortoiliac occlusive disease can be confirmed with non-invasive diagnostic tests.

Pulse-volume recordings (PVR), a plethysmographic evaluation of lower-extremity arterial circulation, will show decreased waveforms in all segments. Arterial duplex mapping can be used to estimate the degree of stenosis or occlusion within the aortoiliac segment, as well as identify any infrainguinal disease. Computed tomography (CT) angiography is a very useful modality in this setting. CT angiography defines stenosis and occlusions in detail, delineates the extent of calcification and reveals the presence and location of previous prosthetic grafts, all of which assist in detailed operative planning. Magnetic resonance angiography (MRA) can also be useful in the evaluation of aortoiliac and lower-extremity disease; however, it may be limited in the evaluation of distal circulation and does not provide information on the extent of calcification.

Traditional angiography provides detailed anatomic information of the abdomen, pelvis and lower-extremity arterial tree. It can identify patterns of collateral flow around obstructions and provide a real-time view of blood follow patterns in the presence of aortoiliac disease. Although invasive, this modality has the advantage of allowing interventions to be performed at the time of diagnosis. In the setting of aortoiliac occlusive disease, femoral artery access may be difficult or impossible, and the use of alternative access sites, such as the brachial artery, may be required.

Disease afflicting the aorta, the bilateral iliac vessels or both generally warrants inflow from the axillary artery, with the bilateral femoral arteries as the outflow. When disease is localized to one iliac system, the contralateral unaffected femoral artery may be used as inflow and the ipsilateral femoral artery distal to the diseased iliac artery may be used as outflow.

AXILLOFEMORAL BYPASS

Axillofemoral bypass was first introduced in the early 1960s as an alternative to direct aortoiliac reconstruction with an aortoiliac or aortofemoral bypass.[3,4] The grafts are tunnelled subcutaneously, avoiding a midline laparotomy and aortic cross-clamping, which significantly reduces the operative and physiologic stresses, making this a favourable choice for reconstruction in high-risk patients.

Indications

Axillofemoral bypass is typically performed in patients with chronic arterial insufficiency and symptoms of critical limb ischemia such as disabling claudication, rest pain, ischemic ulceration or gangrene. It may be performed in the acute setting for other processes affecting the aortoiliac segment such as acute occlusion or aortic dissection that results in acute lower limb ischemia. Infectious processes affecting the aortoiliac segment, like aortoenteric fistula or infected aortic grafts, may also necessitate an axillofemoral bypass.[5] In rare circumstances, it has been used to treat aortic aneurysms in high-risk patients.[6]

Axillofemoral bypass is performed in patients with extensive aortoiliac disease who are not amenable to or who have failed endovascular therapy and who are felt to be unable to tolerate direct aortic reconstruction. Aortofemoral bypass may be deemed unfavourable on the basis of anatomic considerations such as a heavily calcified aorta, a hostile abdomen or the need for peritoneal dialysis or medical co-morbidities such as severe cardiopulmonary and renal or hepatic disease or in the presence of intra-abdominal infection. Another indication is the temporary placement of axillofemoral bypass in order to maintain visceral and renal artery perfusion during complex thoracoabdominal aortic reconstruction.

In good-risk patients in whom the abdominal aorta is unsuitable for inflow, an alternative is to use the distal thoracic aorta for inflow. This type of approach is reserved for good-risk patients with long life expectancy and who are able to tolerate the physiologic demands of the procedure.

In patients with combined aortoiliac and infrainguinal occlusive disease requiring intervention, decisions regarding the extent of reconstruction are guided by the patient's clinical status. In patients with claudication, rest pain or minor tissue loss, it is preferable to first address the proximal disease, restoring flow in the aortoiliac segment. Restoration of inflow to the femoral level alone should be sufficient to relieve symptoms in these cases with the infrainguinal component treated subsequently only if needed. In cases of severe limb-threatening ischemia, concomitant axillofemoral and infrainguinal reconstruction may be required.

Preoperative evaluation

Patients should undergo a thorough preoperative evaluation. Many patients are selected for axillofemoral bypass on the basis of their co-morbid conditions and therefore should be medically optimized to the greatest degree possible prior to surgery.

The choice of the inflow donor axillary artery is critical since unidentified stenosis may result in graft failures.[7] The axillary arteries may be evaluated by a number of invasive and non-invasive methods. Most simply, blood pressure measurements are taken in both arms and compared. If there is a significant gradient between the two sides (>20–30 mmHg), the arm with the higher pressure is chosen as the inflow artery. The presence of such a gradient in the upper extremities may itself prompt further evaluation. Upper-extremity PVR and Doppler waveforms may also be useful in guiding therapy. Direct duplex of the subclavian arteries can be used to identify proximal stenoses. In addition, the inflow arteries may be evaluated with CT angiography or MRA. Finally, digital subtraction angiography provides detailed anatomic information of the upper-extremity circulation. Full evaluation should include views of the aortic arch and great vessels. Although an invasive procedure, it does provide the opportunity to address any lesion with angioplasty and stenting, if required, prior to the bypass procedure.

In cases with no notable disease on either side, the right axillary artery is typically selected for inflow because of the somewhat higher propensity for the left subclavian artery to develop a stenosis. This choice is made despite the fact that most patients are right-handed. Some authors advocate choosing the axillary artery ipsilateral to the lower extremity with the more severe symptoms. Grafts should not be based off an upper extremity with significant distal ischemia or where dialysis access is present. Additional anatomic considerations include the presence of thoracic outlet syndrome and breast cancer or the presence of an ostomy, abdominal hernia or other previous surgery, which may complicate graft positioning. Finally, in patients undergoing axillofemoral bypass for reasons such as intra-abdominal sepsis who in the future may be a candidate for aortic reconstruction via left retroperitoneal approach, the right axillary artery should be used to avoid interference with the retroperitoneal approach by a left-sided graft.

Techniques

Although an axillofemoral bypass can be performed under local anesthesia with sedation, general anesthesia is preferred due to the large volume of local anesthetic required to cover the extensive area that includes all incisions and the subcutaneous tunnels. The room should be kept warm to prevent hypothermia, given the large body surface area that is exposed during surgery. The patient is positioned supine on a fluoroscopy-compatible table with the donor arm abducted to 90°. A rolled towel is placed between the scapulae in order to facilitate exposure of the medial-most portion of the axillary artery. This also facilitates exposure of the lateral body wall for creation of the subcutaneous tunnel. The chest, abdomen, pelvis and upper thighs are prepared and covered with impervious, sterile, plastic dressing. This permits wide exposure in the event that a thoracotomy or laparatomy is required. The donor arm is prepared and an impervious stocking is placed to the level of the mid-upper arm. This allows the operator to move the arm during the procedure in order to ensure that undue tension has not been placed on the axillary anastomosis.

A transverse, infraclavicular incision is made approximately one fingerbreadth below the lateral third of the clavicle, and the dissection is carried down through the clavipectoral fascia (Figure 21.1). The pectoralis major muscle fibres are split in the horizontal plane, exposing the deep fascia with the investing fat of the axillary artery, vein and brachial plexus below. The pectoralis minor may be retracted laterally in order to enhance exposure of the first portion of the axillary artery; however, in most cases, it is preferable to divide the pectoralis minor. This both improves exposure and reduces the risk of graft kinking. The axillary vein is first

identified, isolated and retracted caudally. Frequently, this requires ligation of venous tributaries. The axillary artery is then exposed and encircled with Silastic loops. Branches of the axillary artery are either controlled with Silastic loops under gentle tension or with removable microclips. Division of these arteries is rarely required. Because of the proximity to the brachial plexus, it is best to avoid excessive use of electrocautery in the vicinity of the vessels.

The femoral arteries are exposed through longitudinal groin incisions. This approach allows flexibility in the placement of the femoral anastomoses and facilitates the performance of any adjunctive procedures, which may be required, such as femoral endarterectomy. Oblique incisions may be used, but can limit the ability to perform adjunctive procedures in the femoral vessels. If such incisions are used, the location of the femoral bifurcation should be identified preoperatively. The anastomoses are generally placed in the distal common femoral artery over the take off of the profunda femoris artery. In cases with a concomitant superficial femoral artery occlusion, the anastomosis can still be placed onto the common femoral artery, provided there is no stenosis of the profunda femoris artery. If there is an orificial stenosis, the distal anastomosis can be used to perform a profundoplasty, with the heel of the anastomosis over the common femoral artery and the toe onto the profunda femoral artery. Direct anastomosis to the profunda femoris may also be performed. If the common, superficial and deep femoral arteries are all occluded, direct reconstruction to the popliteal artery may be required.

Once the vessels are exposed, a long, standard tunnelling device is used to create a tunnel between the axilla and the groin. The graft must initially take a lateral course under the pectoralis major and away from the axillary anastomosis before heading caudally in the subcutaneous tissue along the anterior axillary line. It then courses anteromedially over the iliac crest and inguinal ligament to the groin. The use of a counter incision below the inferior aspect of the pectoralis major on the chest wall facilitates tunnelling along the abdominal wall, thereby avoiding inadvertent injury to the abdominal contents. In the cases when a bifemoral bypass is being performed, a suprapubic tunnel for the crossover bypass is made in the subcutaneous space over the inguinal ligaments with either a tunnelling device or large aortic clamp.

An externally supported polytetrafluoroethylene (PTFE) or Dacron graft is used for conduit. An 8 mm graft is preferred; however, a 6 mm graft may be used in patients with small arteries without compromising patency. The graft is passed through the tunnels and the patient is systemically heparinized. The graft is then cut to the appropriate length. It is essential that the graft not be made too short in order to avoid undue tension on the anastomoses, as well as not too long to prevent redundancy and possible kinking of the graft. We prefer to leave external ring supports to within 1 cm of the anastomosis as a further protection against kinking.

The axillary anastomosis is fashioned so that the graft takes an acute angle relative to the artery as it travels

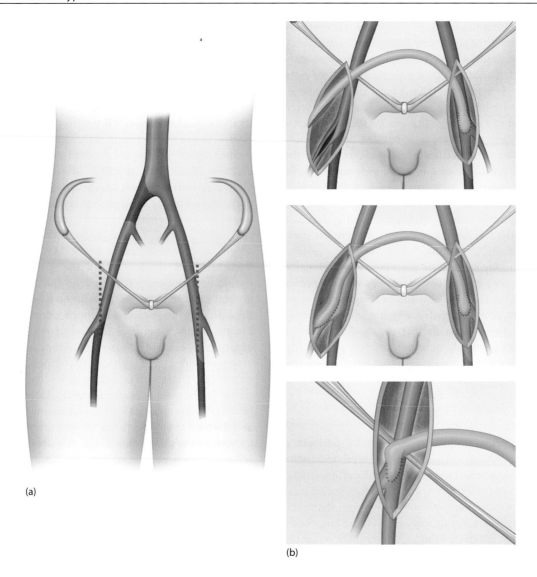

(a)

(b)

Figure 21.1 The insertion of a femorofemoral graft. Incisions are made directly over the femoral vessel (a). Arteriotomies are made (b) to ensure appropriate inflow and outflow, often involving deep femoral artery reconstruction. The graft must be carefully placed in the subcutaneous tunnel to avoid kinking (lower right).

laterally to the abdominal sidewall. This is essential to reduce tension on the anastomosis and avoid graft dehiscence. It is sewn using a 5–0 or 6–0 polypropylene suture. The axillary artery is generally soft and delicate, so it should be handled with care when dissecting or suturing to avoid tearing of the vessel. The anastomosis can be constructed either in standard fashion from heel and toe towards the centre of the arteriotomy, or the suture can be initiated at the midpoint of the posterior aspect of the anastomosis and run towards the heel and toe. In either case, it is essential to ensure that the posterior suture line is secure and without gaps because this area is difficult to repair after the suture line is completed. The femoral anastomosis is sewn in standard fashion, beginning with the heel and proximal half of the anastomosis, and then completing the distal anastomosis with the toe suture.

Confirmation of the patient's pulse status in both upper and lower extremities should be performed prior to reversal of heparin and closure. The incisions are closed in layers using absorbable polypropylene sutures. We prefer to use a subcuticular closure for all skin incisions, as staples and exposed sutures can catch clothing, requiring dressings until removed.

Graft configurations

Multiple possible graft configurations can be used when constructing the axillofemoral bypass, depending on the surgeon's preference and the patient's anatomy. There are now preformed grafts available with the femoral–femoral graft already attached to the axillary graft limb. Using such grafts reduces the total number of anastomoses from four to three, thereby reducing operative time. The order of anastomosis completion depends on the surgeon's preference as well as the number of operators.

Results

The overall 5-year patency for axillobifemoral grafts, once as low as 30%–40%, is now as high as 60%–80% since the introduction of externally supported grafts.[8–11] These external rings prevent compression of the graft when the patients lie on their sides. Although this effect has not proven by direct comparison, the use of externally supported grafts has been widely adopted on the basis of these theoretical advantages. There does not appear to be any difference in externally supported Dacron versus PTFE.[7,12]

The actual patency rates achieved vary widely according to the indication for surgery, patient selection and extent of disease. Patients undergoing axillobifemoral bypass for infected abdominal grafts originally placed for aneurismal disease, without concomitant occlusive disease, can be expected to have better patency than for patients for whom the grafts were placed for severe occlusive disease. Axillobifemoral bypass grafts are suggested to have a better 5-year patency than the axillounifemoral grafts, presumably because of the increased flow rate in the axillary limb.[13,14] Some authors, however, report no difference in patency rates.[15,16] The outflow also affects the patency. Occlusions of the superficial femoral artery may reduce the patency of the bypass.[17]

In the event of graft thrombosis, patency can frequently be re-established with thrombectomy performed under local anesthesia. We generally perform these procedures under direct fluoroscopic guidance for several reasons. First, the chance of injury to the native vessel is reduced by preventing overdistention of the balloon-thrombectomy catheters. Second, it allows the surgeon to identify and possibly treat any underlying inflow or outflow lesions with an endovascular approach. Finally, should a revision be required, an angiogram defining the patient's anatomy can be obtained.

When comparing reports in the literature regarding axillofemoral bypass grafts, it is important to note that there is considerable variability in the techniques used and the outcome measures defined, for example primary versus secondary patency. In addition, it must be noted whether graft components are considered separately in patency calculations, as some authors may consider the axillofemoral and the femorofemoral components as distinct grafts.

Complications

Potential complications of this procedure include the standard risks of bleeding and wound infection seen in all surgical procedures. The risk of graft infection is especially problematic because the majority of patients undergoing these procedures already have limited reconstructive options and significant medical co-morbidities. Another potential complication is injury to intrathoracic or intra-abdominal contents during tunnelling of the graft. As noted earlier, care must be taken to avoid injury to other neurovascular structures such as the axillary vein or brachial plexus.

Post-operative management

Patients are placed on an anti-platelet agent if not already on one preoperatively. Anticoagulation with Coumadin is reserved for patients with a known hypercoagulable state or in whom a secondary procedure was required to re-establish patency. As in all patients with peripheral artery disease, the use of a statin is recommended. Graft surveillance is performed every 3 months for the first year, every 6 months for the second year and yearly thereafter. The need for a subsequent intervention or other abnormal findings on duplex may necessitate more frequent surveillance.

FEMOROFEMORAL BYPASS

The extent of atherosclerosis in the distal aorta and iliac arteries may only have a hemodynamic affect on one of the iliac systems. In these cases, the aorta or contralateral femoral artery may serve as the donor vessel. Conditions precluding the aorta as the vessel of choice make the contralateral femoral artery a favoured candidate. Considerations to undertake a femorofemoral bypass are similar to those for an axillofemoral bypass: anatomic factors such as an unsuitable aorta as a donor vessel, patient factors such as co-morbid conditions making the patient at high risk for open abdominal surgery and indications such as chronic arterial ischemia or another disease process affecting a unilateral iliac system. Patient evaluation encompasses a thorough history and physical examination, which is further supported by non-invasive testing. It is worth noting that endovascular approaches may be worth considering, or perhaps, have failed, in the patient being evaluated for a femorofemoral bypass.

Technique

The approach to the accessing the femoral arteries has been described in the preceding section. The tunnel is placed in a suprapubic location in the subcutaneous space over the inguinal ligaments with either a tunnelling device or large aortic clamp. A Dacron or supported ringed PTFE graft, 6–8 mm in diameter, is best suited. The location makes the graft susceptible to kinking and consequently at risk for occlusion (Figure 21.2). As such, the tunnelling and potential for redundancy demand attention. A proposed modification is tacking the graft to the inguinal ligament thereby preventing kinking and creating a *ram's horn* configuration. Both ends of the graft are beveled and the anastomosis is created with the toes pointing cranially. The graft courses caudally in each groin, turns laterally, before continuing cranially to the anastomosis. The inferior curve of the graft at both anastomoses acts as a hinge, transferring pressure off the anastomosis as the pannus moves with transition from the lying to the sitting or standing position. Thus, this orientation prevents kinking of the graft and reduces the risk for anastomotic disruption.

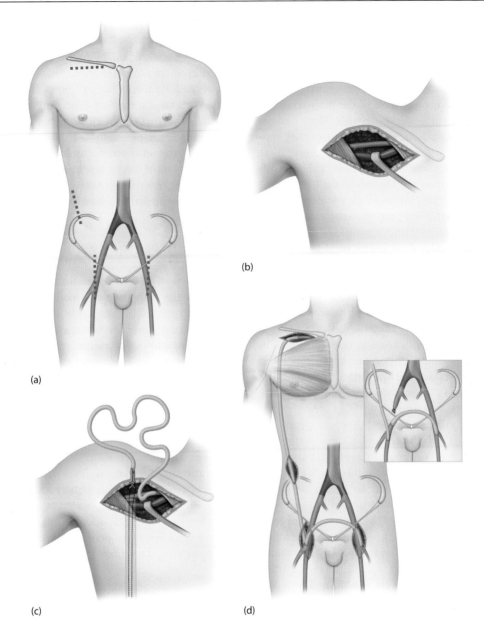

Figure 21.2 The insertion of an axillobifemoral bypass. (a) Incisions are made over the donor and recipient vessels. A separate incision for the tunnel is sometimes necessary. (b) The proximal anastomosis is aided by transection of the pectoralis minor muscle, exposing the first and second portions of the axillary artery. (c) The graft is tunnelled beneath the pectoralis major muscle. (d) The finished reconstruction is seen. An alternative anastomosis, recommended by Blaisdell[87] is noted (inset).

Patients with multilevel disease may also require distal revascularization. Reconstruction to the level of the contralateral popliteal artery may be accomplished using a single in line or crossover graft with similar patency rates.[18] The profunda femoris can also serve as a target in the setting of critical limb ischemia with promising patency and limb salvage rates.[19]

Post-operatively, patients are continued on statins and antiplatelet agents, with systemic anticoagulation reserved for those with hypercoagulable disorders or need for complex distal revascularizations with limited outflow.

Complications specific to femorofemoral bypass are wound infections given the location of the incision in the groin; as such, it is important to keep the incisions dry to prevent skin maceration and wound dehiscence, which may secondarily infect the graft. Seromas, lymph leaks and bladder injury during the tunnelling process have also been described.

Results

The reported patency rates of femorofemoral bypass grafts at 5 years have been reported between 60% and 80%.[20–22] However, they have been shown to be inferior to aortofemoral bypass. In a randomized study comparing direct versus crossover bypasses for unilateral iliac artery disease, direct reconstruction offered superior primary patency rates at 5 years, 92% versus 73%, respectively. The secondary patency rates were significantly improved, but still inferior to direct revascularization, 97% versus 90%.[23] However, the authors supported the use of crossover bypasses in high-risk patients.

Multiple factors have been shown to influence graft patency rates for crossover femorofemoral bypasses. The use of externally supported grafts improves the patency rates. Mingoli and colleagues reported superior patency rates with externally supported grafts compared to those without: 5- and 10-year rates were 80.1% and 69.9% compared to 61.1% and 21.1%, respectively.[24] Interestingly, D'Addio and colleagues reported a 76% 5-year patency rate using the femoropopliteal vein as a conduit to perform femorofemoral bypasses.[25] The indication for the bypass also influences outcomes. Lipsitz and colleagues reported a 95% 4-year primary patency rate when the bypass was performed in conjunction with aorto-uni-femoral endovascular graft placement for aneurysmal disease.[26]

THORACOFEMORAL ARTERY BYPASS

The thoracic aorta can provide arterial inflow for peripheral revascularization. This approach is reserved as an alternative for a good-risk patient, where the abdominal aorta may not be able to serve as the ideal inflow due to the anatomic factors. Stevenson and colleagues reported the use of the descending thoracic aorta to femoral artery bypass for aortic occlusive disease.[27] Schumaker et al. reported the treatment of aortic coarctation using the ascending aorta as inflow.[28]

The thoracic aorta can be accessed through a transperitoneal incision with medial visceral rotation, a retroperitoneal incision or a thoracotomy. The descending thoracic aorta may also be accessed with a minimal thoracotomy, less than 8 cm in length, along the ninth rib interspace.[29] The bypass is positioned in the extraperitoneal space, deep to the rectus muscle. When the thoracic aorta is used for inflow, the tunnel may course along the lateral abdominal wall. A PTFE prosthetic graft, 6–8 mm in diameter, serves as the ideal conduit. Five-year patencies have been reported more than 80% with minimal perioperative mortality.[30–34]

OTHER EXTRA-ANATOMIC BYPASSES

In the event that access to common femoral artery is compromised, seen most commonly in the setting of infections affected the groin, the obturator foramen can serve as an extra-anatomic route to revascularize the limb. The obturator foramen can be accessed via a retroperitoneal or transperitoneal incision (Figure 21.3).[35]

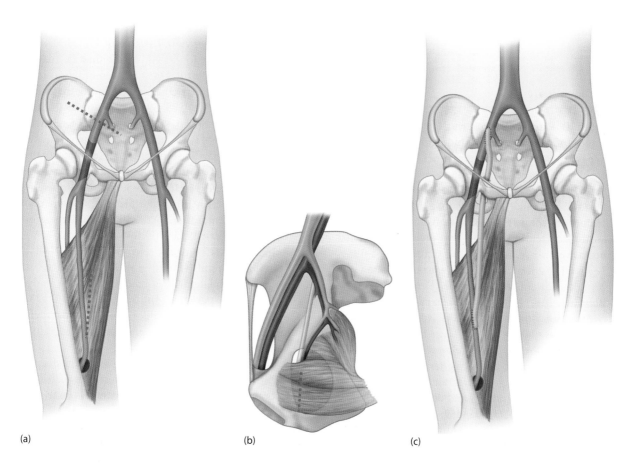

(a)   (b)   (c)

Figure 21.3 The insertion of a graft through the obturator foramen. (a) Incisions are made over the iliac artery, which is exposed retroperitoneally, and over the femoral artery proximal to the adductor canal in this illustration. (b) The obturator internus muscle and obturator fascia are incised medial to the neurovascular bundle. (c) The bypass in tunnelled superficial to the adductor muscles in this example.

The obturator neurovascular bundle penetrates the fascia laterally. The tunnel is created anterior and medial to these structures. The obturator internus muscle is divided along the direction of its fibres and the underlying fascia is divided. The outflow is the distal superficial femoral artery or popliteal artery at the level of the adductor hiatus. Next, a tunnelling instrument is used to pass the graft from the obturator foramen and adductor hiatus.

Long-term results for obturator bypasses are limited, but available series in the literature report promising results.[36–39] Among the larger studies, Nevelsteen and colleagues performed 55 bypasses over a 16-year period and reported a 37% 5-year patency.[40] As such, it remains a useful tool in the vascular surgeons armamentarium.

CONCLUSIONS

Extra-anatomic bypasses are an important and valuable treatment option for patients. For many reasons, it is the preferred or only viable option for patients with significant anatomic or medical co-morbidities, which preclude standard bypass options. Axillofemoral and femorofemoral bypasses can be performed with acceptable morbidity, mortality and long-term results, even in high-risk patients. For these reasons, surgeons should be familiar with the indications and application of this technique.

REFERENCES

1. Indes JE, Pfaff MJ, Farrokhyar F et al. Clinical outcomes of 5358 patients undergoing direct open bypass or endovascular treatment for aortoiliac occlusive disease: A systematic review and meta-analysis. *J Endovasc Ther*. 2013;20(4):443–455.
2. Burke CR, Henke PK, Hernandez R et al. A contemporary comparison of aortofemoral bypass and aortoiliac stenting in the treatment of aortoiliac occlusive disease. *Ann Vasc Surg*. 2010;24(1):4–13.
3. Lewis CD. Subclavian artery as a means of blood supply to the lower half of body. *Br J Surg*. 1961;48:574.
4. Blaisdell FW, Hall AD. Axillary-femoral artery bypass for lower extremity ischemia. *Surgery*. 1963;54:563–568.
5. Seeger JM, Pretus HA, Welborn MB, Ozaki CK, Flynn TC, Huber TS. Long-term outcome after treatment of aortic graft infection with staged extra-anatomic bypass grafting and aortic graft removal. *J Vasc Surg*. 2000;32(3):451–459; discussion 460–461.
6. Leather RP, Shah D, Goldman M, Rosenberg M, Karmody AM. Nonresective treatment of abdominal aortic aneurysms. Use of acute thrombosis and axillofemoral bypass. *Arch Surg*. 1979;114(12):1402–1408.
7. Calligaro KD, Ascer E, Veith FJ et al. Unsuspected inflow disease in candidates for axillofemoral bypass operations: A prospective study. *J Vasc Surg*. 1990;11(6):832–837.
8. Schneider JR, McDaniel MD, Walsh DB, Zwolak RM, Cronenwett JL. Axillofemoral bypass: Outcome and hemodynamic results in high-risk patients. *J Vasc Surg*. 1992;15(6):952–962; discussion 962–963.
9. Passman MA, Taylor LM, Moneta GL et al. Comparison of axillofemoral and aortofemoral bypass for aortoiliac occlusive disease. *J Vasc Surg*. 1996;23(2):263–269; discussion 269–271.
10. Martin D, Katz SG. Axillofemoral bypass for aortoiliac occlusive disease. *Am J Surg*. 2000;180(2):100–103.
11. Harris EJ Jr, Taylor LM Jr, McConnell DB, Moneta GL, Yeager RA, Porter JM. Clinical results of axillobifemoral bypass using externally supported polytetrafluoroethylene. *J Vasc Surg*. 1990;12(4):416–420; discussion 420–421.
12. Johnson WC, Lee KK. Comparative evaluation of externally supported Dacron and polytetrafluoroethylene prosthetic bypasses for femorofemoral and axillofemoral arterial reconstructions. Veterans Affairs Cooperative Study #141. *J Vasc Surg*. 1999;30(6):1077–1083.
13. Rutherford RB, Patt A, Pearce WH. Extra-anatomic bypass: A closer view. *J Vasc Surg*. 1987;6(5):437–446.
14. Taylor LM Jr, Moneta GL, McConnell D, Yeager RA, Edwards JM, Porter JM. Axillofemoral grafting with externally supported polytetrafluoroethylene. *Arch Surg*. 1994;129(6):588–594; discussion 594–595.
15. Mohan CR, Sharp WJ, Hoballah JJ, Kresowik TF, Schueppert MT, Corson JD. A comparative evaluation of externally supported polytetrafluoroethylene axillobifemoral and axillounifemoral bypass grafts. *J Vasc Surg*. 1995;21(5):801–808; discussion 808–809.
16. Ascer E, Veith FJ, Gupta SK et al. Comparison of axillounifemoral and axillobifemoral bypass operations. *Surgery*. 1985;97(2):169–175.
17. Johnson WC, Logerfo FW, Vollman RW et al. Is axillo-bilateral femoral graft an effective substitute for aortic-bilateral iliac/femoral graft?: An analysis of ten years experience. *Ann Surg*. 1977;186(2):123–129.
18. Gokalp O, Yurekli I, Yilik L et al. Crossover femoropopliteal bypass: Single graft or double grafts. *Ann Vasc Surg*. 2012;26(5):707–714.
19. Ma T, Ma J. Femorofemoral bypass to the deep femoral artery for limb salvage after prior failed percutaneous endovascular intervention. *Ann Vasc Surg*. 2014;28(6):1463–1468.
20. Rinckenbach S, Guelle N, Lillaz J, Al Sayed M, Ritucci V, Camelot G. Femorofemoral bypass as an alternative to a direct aortic approach in daily practice: Appraisal of its current indications and midterm results. *Ann Vasc Surg*. 2012;26(3):359–364.

21. Capoccia L, Riambau V, da Rocha M. Is femorofemoral crossover bypass an option in claudication? *Ann Vasc Surg*. 2010;24(6):828–832.

22. Harrington ME, Harrington EB, Haimov M, Schanzer H, Jacobson JH 2nd. Iliofemoral versus femorofemoral bypass: The case for an individualized approach. *J Vasc Surg*. 1992;16(6):841–852; discussion 852–854.

23. Ricco JB, Probst H. Long-term results of a multicenter randomized study on direct versus crossover bypass for unilateral iliac artery occlusive disease. *J Vasc Surg*. 2008;47(1):45–53; discussion 54.

24. Mingoli A, Sapienza P, Feldhaus RJ, Di Marzo L, Burchi C, Cavallaro A. Femorofemoral bypass grafts: Factors influencing long-term patency rate and outcome. *Surgery*. 2001;129(4):451–458.

25. D'Addio V, Ali A, Timaran C et al. Femorofemoral bypass with femoral popliteal vein. *J Vasc Surg*. 2005;42(1):35–39.

26. Lipsitz EC, Ohki T, Veith FJ et al. Patency rates of femorofemoral bypasses associated with endovascular aneurysm repair surpass those performed for occlusive disease. *J Endovasc Ther*. 2003;10(6):1061–1065.

27. Stevenson JK, Sauvage LR, Harkins HN. A bypass hemograft from thoracic aorta to femoral arteries for occlusive vascular disease: A case report. *Ann Surg*. 1961;27:632–637.

28. Schumaker HB, Nahrwold DL, King H, Waldhanjen JA. Coarctation of the aorta. *Curr Probl Surg*. 1968;1:64.

29. Reppert AE, Jazaeri O, Babu A et al. Minimal thoracotomy thoracic bifemoral bypass in the endovascular era. *Ann Vasc Surg*. 2014;28(6):1420–1425.

30. Passman MA, Farber MA, Criado E, Marston WA, Burnham SJ, Keagy BA. Descending thoracic aorta to iliofemoral artery bypass grafting: A role for primary revascularization for aortoiliac occlusive disease? *J Vasc Surg*. 1999;29(2):249–258.

31. McCarthy WJ, Mesh CL, McMillan WD, Flinn WR, Pearce WH, Yao JS. Descending thoracic aorta-to-femoral artery bypass: Ten years' experience with a durable procedure. *J Vasc Surg*. 1993;17(2):336–347; discussion 347–348.

32. Kalman PG, Johnston KW, Walker PM. Descending thoracic aortofemoral bypass as an alternative for aortoiliac revascularization. *J Cardiovasc Surg*. 1991;32(4):443–446.

33. Bowes DE, Youkey JR, Pharr WP, Goldstein AM, Benoit CH. Long term follow-up of descending thoracic aorto-iliac/femoral bypass. *J Cardiovasc Surg*. 1990;31(4):430–437.

34. Koksal C, Kocamaz O, Aksoy E et al. Thoracic aortobifemoral bypass in treatment of juxtarenal Leriche syndrome (midterm results). *Ann Vasc Surg*. 2012;26(8):1085–1092.

35. Guida PM, Moore SW. Obturator bypass technique. *Surg Gynecol Obstet*. 1969;128(6):1307–1316.

36. Patel A, Taylor SM, Langan EM 3rd et al. Obturator bypass: A classic approach for the treatment of contemporary groin infection. *Am Surg*. 2002;68(8):653–658; discussion 658–659.

37. van Det RJ, Brands LC. The obturator foramen bypass: An alternative procedure in iliofemoral artery revascularization. *Surgery*. 1981;89(5):543–547.

38. Pearce WH, Ricco JB, Yao JS, Flinn WR, Bergan JJ. Modified technique of obturator bypass in failed or infected grafts. *Ann Surg*. 1983;197(3):344–347.

39. Millis JM, Ahn SS. Transobturator aorto-profunda femoral artery bypass using the direct medial thigh approach. *Ann Vasc Surg*. 1993;7(4):384–390.

40. Nevelsteen A, Mees U, Deleersnijder J, Suy R. Obturator bypass: A sixteen year experience with 55 cases. *Ann Vasc Surg*. 1987;1(5):558–563.

22

Amputation in the dysvascular patient

JAMES M. MALONE and SAMUEL ERIC WILSON

CONTENTS

INDICATIONS FOR AMPUTATION

Dysvascularity accounts for approximately 75% of patients in the United Kingdom and the United States who undergo major amputation with about one third of these at the above-knee position. Diabetes mellitus is the underlying disease for amputation in more than two thirds of cases. Most patients are male and greater than 60 years of age. In general terms, the indications for amputation in the dysvascular patient are (1) complication of diabetes mellitus, (2) nondiabetic infection with ischemia, (3) osteomyelitis, (4) trauma, (5) failed limb salvage operations and (6) failed minor amputation.

INCIDENCE AND MORBIDITY OF AMPUTATION

The mortality associated with amputation depends not so much on the procedure itself as on the presence or absence of risk factors, especially cardiorespiratory insufficiency. Although above-knee amputation does carry a higher operative mortality risk than below-knee amputation,[1,2] Rush et al.[3] reported a 6% mortality for below-knee amputation and an 11% mortality for above-knee amputation. However, Bunt and Malone[4] reported an overall mortality rate of 1.5% for all major lower

extremity amputations. The higher mortality usually associated with above-knee amputation is due to more severe and widespread cardiovascular diseases in that group of patients. More than 70% of patients requiring amputation for peripheral vascular disease have other major systemic manifestations of atherosclerosis. Hospital mortality varies from 2% to 40%.[5–8] It has been reported that 50%–75% of amputee patients die within 5 years of amputation[7,8]; however, in nondiabetic patients, survival approximates the age-adjusted normal population.[6]

The amputation rate in the United States is approximately 30 per 100,000 population but is 15–20 times higher among diabetic patients, who have an incidence of amputation of 600 per 100,000.[9–11] Overall, more than 50,000–60,000 major lower-limb amputations are estimated to be performed each year in the United States. In the United Kingdom, approximately 65,000 amputees are known to the Department of Health and Social Security, with 6,000 new patients being referred to limb-fitting centres annually.[12,13]

AMPUTATIONS FOR ACUTE ISCHEMIA

Acute ischemia causing tissue necrosis presents a complex surgical management problem. If the patient has presented late, with irreversible tissue loss accompanied by systemic toxicity, with or without myonecrosis, urgent amputation is indicated. Urgent amputation is also the treatment of choice if there is extensive or invasive infection. In elderly patients with sepsis, physiologic amputation rather than urgent surgical amputation may be an important first step in lowering patient mortality.[14]

Limbs with lesser degrees of acute tissue ischemia (reversible ischemia) may often be salvageable by arterial bypass or embolectomy, usually combined with compartment fasciotomy. In some of these cases, limb salvage is not totally achieved, but the patient may at least become suitable for amputation at a more distal level.

If there are no indications for urgent operation and the associated pain is not severe, the ischemic areas may be observed for signs of improvement and heparin anticoagulation or thrombolytic therapy may be employed in selected patients to improve collateral circulation.[15]

Determination of the preferred level of amputation is difficult in the presence of acute ischemia.

Amputation in the diabetic patient

Diabetics are at special risk of developing leg ischemia and gangrene. In fact, gangrene is more than 50 times more frequent among diabetic patients over 40 years of age than among nondiabetic patients of the same age.[16]

Bacterial cultures of infected lesions in diabetic patients usually yield multiple organisms (up to 22 different organisms in one culture have been identified), with a mixture of anaerobes and aerobes.[6] The principal pathogens are usually *Staphylococcus*, *Enterococcus* and other streptococcal organisms, *Pseudomonas*, *Proteus* and *Escherichia coli*. Underlying osteomyelitis is frequently present at the time of presentation.[17] Because of the virulence and invasiveness of foot infections in the diabetic patient, delay in surgical control can lead to loss of the foot or fatal sepsis.[18] The diabetic foot should always be carefully examined for deep infection. Areas with abscess, suppuration or invasion of tendon sheaths and plantar fascia should be treated urgently by incision and drainage, wide debridement or local amputation. If the vascularity of the foot is good, then usually no further procedure will be necessary (Figure 22.1). However, with irretrievably poor vascularity, definitive amputation should be carried out only after the septic condition has been controlled and drained. In some cases, when the heel or the proximal tissues are already involved, primary below-knee amputation rather than a local foot procedure is indicated (Figure 22.2). Osteomyelitis in a diabetic foot cannot be adequately treated by antibiotics alone, and surgical excision of the infected bone is always required.

In general, surgical wounds in diabetics tend to have a higher incidence of infection[19] and delayed healing[17,20] compared to wounds in nondiabetic patients. However, the presence of diabetes does not significantly affect the rate of stump healing or wound infection after amputation.[6,21]

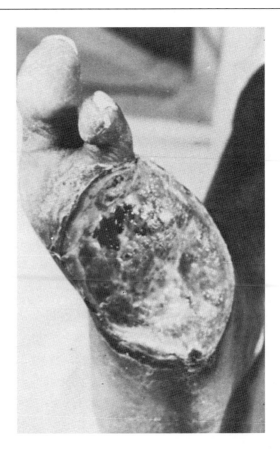

Figure 22.1 Local amputation of infected, gangrenous toes in a foot with otherwise good vascular supply resulted in successful salvage of the foot.

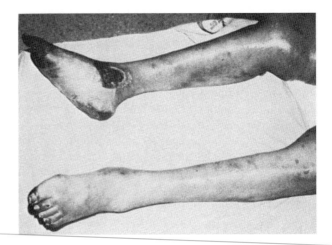

Figure 22.2 Ulceration or necrosis of the heel or ankle is a contraindication to local amputation. Below-knee amputation was necessary in this patient.

PREOPERATIVE MANAGEMENT

Preoperative care involves treatment of the affected limb and stabilization of the patient's general medical condition. The patient should not be restricted to bed. Cellulitis and lymphangitis are treated with intravenous antibiotics, while abscesses or closed-space infections require early drainage and debridement. Pain should be treated adequately with narcotic analgesics. The prevention of contractures of the knee and hip is essential in achieving eventual rehabilitation. The presence of contractures more than 15° will preclude successful ambulation on a prosthesis.

A thorough assessment of the patient's cardiac, respiratory and renal systems is made. Even if urgent amputation is required, a period of 4–8 hours for the stabilization of diabetes, cardiac failure and fluid and electrolyte imbalance can be invaluable. If longer preoperative time is available, this process of stabilizing the patient's general medical condition is a priority. In elderly patients with sepsis, physiologic amputation is a useful adjunct.[14]

For all elective major lower-limb amputations, preoperative objective amputation level selection, as described later, is an important adjunct to successful surgery and rehabilitation.

The patient is informed of the plans for a prosthesis and, if practical, should be seen by the prosthetist and physical therapist before surgery. Limb and joint mobilization exercises and strengthening procedures are commenced prior to surgery if at all possible. A team approach to rehabilitation introduced at this stage fosters a positive attitude among both staff and patient, stressing the expectation that ambulation will be restored. Amputation is a major traumatic experience for the patient and may have far-reaching effects on his or her lifestyle and employment. A multidisciplinary approach including comprehensive counselling and an optimistic, enthusiastic outlook from the entire treating team plays an integral role in achieving a successful outcome.[6]

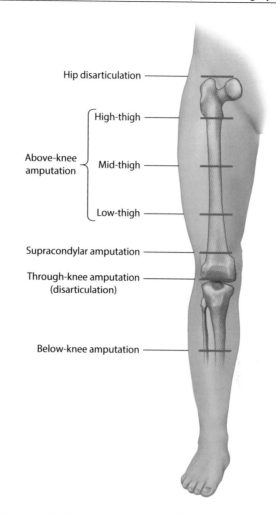

Figure 22.3 Common levels for major amputations of the lower limb.

PRINCIPLES OF AMPUTATION SURGERY

The commonly used major lower-limb amputations are shown in Figure 22.3. The main guiding philosophy is that the amputation, when necessary, should be performed at the most distal possible site to remove gangrene, infection or nonhealing lesions and where healing is likely to occur. The knee joint should be preserved in as many cases as possible. Successful ambulation is achieved after below-knee amputation in approximately 85% of patients but after above-knee amputation in only 40%. The primary objective of amputation surgery is to produce a stump that will proceed to primary, uncomplicated wound healing, allowing early limb fitting and complete rehabilitation.

In comparison to amputation below the level of the knee joint, above-knee amputation has a higher operative mortality rate,[2] with a far lower rate of patient independence and return to ambulation (with a prosthesis). The loss of mobility caused by the absence of the flexible knee joint and the loss of proprioceptive sense from the joint lining render the use of a prosthesis far more difficult and double the amount of energy that must be used for mobilization

compared to a below-knee prosthesis.[22] Even when lying in bed, the above-knee amputee is at a disadvantage, because the added length provided by a below-knee residual limb offers greater leverage for movement and rolling. A list of the principal amputations used in dysvascular patients is given in Table 22.1.

A tourniquet should never be used during amputation in the dysvascular patient because of the risk of further compromising the arterial blood supply to the area of the amputation stump. Absolute hemostasis and avoidance of stump hematomas are crucial to achieving maximum healing and rapid rehabilitation. An infected stump hematoma almost always leads to a more proximal amputation and a decrease in patient rehabilitation. Drains are not recommended, as they more often than double the risk of stump infection.[6]

Antibiotic prophylaxis is always employed because of the risk of infection in the severely ischemic limb. A first-generation cephalosporin is usually adequate, but in patients with infection or gangrene complicated by diabetes, good aerobic and anaerobic coverage is necessary. Significant distal limb infections should be drained up to and including ankle guillotine amputation at an operation

Table 22.1 Principal amputations used in the dysvascular patient.

Toe amputation
   Transphalangeal
   Transmetatarsal
Forefoot amputation
   Transmetatarsal
Amputation at the ankle
   Syme amputation
Below-knee amputation
Through-knee amputation
Above-knee amputation
   Supracondylar
   Mid-thigh
   High thigh
   Hip disarticulation

prior to definite amputation. At the definite amputation, any open or infected area(s) and necrotic tissue should be well wrapped and protected to prevent direct contamination of the amputation wound. There is evidence from several studies that, in the infected limb, guillotine amputation is the best method of elimination of the infection before definitive amputation is performed as a second-stage procedure.[23,24]

In making the skin incision, the surgeon must take care to avoid undermining and hence devascularizing the skin, especially if a flap technique is being utilized. The tissues should be handled gently at all times, and the use of traumatizing instruments such as firm clamps, retractors or sharp forceps on the skin and muscle areas should be avoided. Long plantar flaps are used in the hip, calf, foot and toes because of the superior blood supply to the plantar aspect of the lower leg.[4] A long anterior flap is used at the through-knee level for similar reasons. Bone is always transected several centimetres proximal to the other structures at a level high enough to permit the soft tissue to easily approximate over the bone, producing a good covering without skin tension. Sharp, bony spicules are smoothed from the bone edge with a file or rasp. Proximal stripping of the periosteum should be minimized. Nerves are gently pulled into the wound, ligated (especially large nerves such as the sciatic nerve) and then transected. Surrounding muscle bulk is used to cover and protect the bone end, especially for weight-bearing stumps. Coaptation of extensor muscle groups to flexor muscle groups (myoplasty) for all lower-limb amputations is important in order to create a physiologic residual limb. The author does not favour true myodesis (muscle fixation to bone) except for long above-knee amputations using a medial adductor–based flap.

Hemostasis should be meticulous so that wound drains will not be necessary. Drains probably increase the incidence of wound infection and breakdown.[2,11,21] The skin must never be sutured under tension. The author favours interrupted vertical mattress sutures and does not recommend staples or running skin closures. The latter closure

probably further compromises skin blood flow in a dysvascular patient.

Postoperatively, intensive efforts are made towards early limb and joint mobilization, and rehabilitation should commence as soon as the patient has recovered from the operation, aided by preoperative instruction, preparation and exercises.

EFFECTS OF PREVIOUS RECONSTRUCTIVE SURGERY ON AMPUTATION LEVEL

Many studies have examined the effects of previous reconstructive arterial surgery on the eventual level of amputation, some demonstrating that the resultant site was higher[25–30] and others stating that the eventual level was not affected.[31–34] There probably is no definite answer to the effect of prior arterial reconstructive surgery on eventual level of amputation, but delayed healing and local wound complication are more frequent in patients who have amputation after failed reconstruction.[35]

A patent bypass graft does not necessarily ensure limb salvage. In a review of 987 patients who had undergone infrainguinal bypass grafts, Dietzek et al.[9] identified 75 patients (7.6%) with patent grafts who failed to achieve healing of ischemic wounds and subsequently underwent a major amputation procedure. Risk factors were the presence of diabetes, extensive pedal necrosis, bypass to an isolated arterial segment and lack of improvement as measured by the ankle–brachial pressure index after bypass.

DETERMINATION OF AMPUTATION LEVEL

In the ideal situation it would be possible to determine preoperatively whether or not an amputation would heal at a chosen level, so that an inappropriately high level of amputation could be avoided and revision of an amputation to a higher level would never be necessary. In practice, when clinical observation alone is used in choosing the site of amputation, the resultant reamputation rate ranges from 15% to 40%.[6,36]

Many special investigative techniques have been advocated for the determination of amputation level (Table 22.2). Of these, the most reliable are transcutaneous P_{O_2} determination and measurement of skin clearance

Table 22.2 Preoperative determination of amputation level.

Transcutaneous P_{O_2} measurement
Skin clearance of [133]Xe
Segmental Doppler blood pressures
Laser Doppler flowmetry
Segmental skin perfusion pressures
Skin temperature measurement (thermography)
Photoplethysmography and digital plethysmography

of xenon 133, with helpful but less dependable information derived from segmental Doppler blood pressures and skin perfusion pressures. Factors that have been shown to have little predictive value include angiographic appearance of the lower limb and level of the most distal pulse.[37] In fact, the use of pulse assessment to determine amputation level has been demonstrated to result in an unacceptably high ratio of above-knee to below-knee amputations.[38]

In 1987, Malone et al.[39] published a comparative amputation series with transcutaneous oxygen, xenon (^{133}Xe) and Doppler knee and ankle blood pressures measured at the proposed level of amputation prior to surgery. The only statistically reliable measurement was transcutaneous oxygen. That publication was noteworthy because prior to that time Malone had been a co-author on many papers suggesting that ^{133}Xe skin clearance was the ideal test for preoperative amputation level selection. Since that time, the author has used transcutaneous oxygen as the single best test for preoperative prediction of healing of an amputation level.

Blood circulation in the skin is the single most important factor in determining amputation healing. Skin viability is therefore the major factor influencing selection of level in amputations for peripheral vascular disease.[40] Even in experienced hands, clinical judgement (based on factors such as skin viability, nutritional changes and physical signs of ischemia) has not been shown to be as accurate as non-invasive preamputation level testing.[6] Prediction of the healing potential of forefoot amputations may be particularly difficult even with non-invasive techniques. Accurate amputation level success prediction will also allow for correct selection of patients who will require a revascularization procedure to achieve primary healing at a lower amputation level.

Burgess and Matsen[41] have pointed out that no single technique can be expected to predict, unfailingly, the outcome of an amputation because of the effects of variables such as surgical technique (tissue handling, flap length, wound tension), alterations in blood flow caused by the procedure itself and postoperative problems such as pressure from dressings, intercurrent diseases, wound infection and malnutrition, which may compromise eventual healing. For these reasons, it is easier to predict failure due to circulatory deficiency than it is to predict success. However, Malone has reported greater than 95% success in predicting the healing of below-knee amputation with transcutaneous oxygen measurements.[6,39]

Transcutaneous P$_{O_2}$ measurement

It has been demonstrated that transcutaneous oxygen tension (Ptc$_{O_2}$) measurements, taken with a skin sensor electrode heated to 45°C, provide an accurate indication of the severity of vascular disease since blood oxygen content depends on local blood flow.[6,39,42,43] Recent studies have shown that Ptc$_{O_2}$ of the anterior and posterior skin

at the level of proposed amputation correlates well with eventual healing success or failure. Katsamouris et al.[44] found that healing was very likely if local Ptc$_{O_2}$ exceeded 40 mmHg and that failure always occurred for a Ptc$_{O_2}$ of <20 mmHg. Burgess et al.[45] also found that transcutaneous oxygen tension levels correlated well with healing outcome for below-knee amputation, but they did not identify a definite threshold value. However, all patients with a Ptc$_{O_2}$ of <26 mmHg failed to heal. Malone has reported 100% success with below-knee amputation with immediate postoperative prostheses (IPOP) with a Ptc$_{O_2}$ of ≥20 mmHg.[39]

Ameli et al.[46] used a predetermined threshold of 22 mmHg at the below-knee site in a series of 38 patients and decided on the lower level of amputation dictated by either the Ptc$_{O_2}$ or clinical judgement. They found that if Ptc$_{O_2}$ readings alone had been used as the basis for selection, 100% healing could have been achieved at the expense of three extra above-knee amputations. Wyss et al.[47] reported that Ptc$_{O_2}$ could also be used to predict which patients would require amputation after a vascular reconstruction procedure, with a postoperative Ptc$_{O_2}$ of <20 mmHg at the below-knee site predicting the occurrence of a subsequent amputation. Other research has suggested that the sensitivity of this method is greatly improved by recording the changes in Ptc$_{O_2}$ that occur on breathing 100% oxygen.[48,49]

In a prospective randomized study, Malone et al.[39] evaluated not only transcutaneous oxygen but also transcutaneous carbon dioxide. Since there are problems with oxygen diffusion through areas of edema, it was hoped that transcutaneous carbon dioxide might help improve prediction of amputation healing. However, those authors clearly showed that transcutaneous carbon dioxide was less sensitive than transcutaneous oxygen.

Clearance of ^{133}Xe

The rate of clearance of an intradermal injected dose of ^{133}Xe at the proposed site of amputation may be utilized to calculate local skin blood flow. Moore et al.[50-52] have reported that when skin blood flow was found to be >2.6 mL/100 g/min by this technique, successful primary wound healing occurred in all cases, whereas only 50% of cases healed when the skin blood flow was between 2.0 and 2.6 mL/100 g/min. Harris et al.[53] reported that no amputation healed if the skin blood flow was <1.0 mL/100 g/min. However, there was considerable overlap in the skin blood flow measurements of patients with successful and unsuccessful below-knee amputation in the Harris study.

Other studies of this technique have shown less correlation with healing rates, with some failures being seen in the presence of blood flow measured up to 7.5 mL/100 g/min.[54] For the most part, this test is no longer utilized except as a research tool, especially after the report by Malone et al.[6] on the superiority of Ptc$_{O_2}$ compared to ^{133}Xe clearance for prediction of amputation healing.

Laser Doppler flowmetry

Monochromatic light is reflected back from the skin, and the Doppler shift detected is used to evaluate skin micro-circulation. Laser Doppler flowmetry greater than 20 MV was associated with primary healing after below-knee amputation in a study reported by Kram et al.[55] However, the author has found that laser Doppler flowmetry is not as accurate as Ptc_{O_2} in predicting successful wound healing after amputation.

Segmental blood pressure

Segmental blood pressure and flow waveforms as measured by Doppler ultrasound have not in general shown good correlation with healing,[18] probably because of the high proportion of diabetics who tend to have incompressible, calcified arteries, which give false pressure measurements.[56] There is little agreement as to what pressure is necessary for primary healing; Vena et al.[57] reported failure of transmeta-tarsal amputation with ankle pressures below 35 mmHg, whereas Barnes et al.[58,59] reported that 60 mmHg was the minimal ankle pressure associated with successful healing.

When the ankle-to-brachial systolic index is considered, it seems likely that healing will occur with values above 0.35–0.45.[57,60] This technique does not give a good indication of the status of circulation in collateral vessels, and there is a significant incidence of successful healing in the presence of extremely low or undetectable segmental pressures and low ankle-to-brachial indices.[41]

Other techniques

Other techniques that have been reported include skin temperature measurement,[61,62] photoplethysmography,[63] digital plethysmography[64,65] and skin perfusion pressures.[66,67] Nuclear magnetic resonance spectroscopy may become useful as a method of non-invasive assessment of skin perfusion and muscle function,[13] but it is a research tool at the present time.

Except for Ptc_{O_2}, most of these techniques suffer from lack of widespread availability or excessive variability in results. An example of that problem is the results obtained in skin temperature thermography, which have been found to be dependent on variants other than blood flow, including ambient temperature, patient exercise and presence or absence of infection.

SURGICAL TECHNIQUES OF AMPUTATION

Amputation of the toe

TRANSPHALANGEAL LEVEL

Well-demarcated dry gangrene of the tip of a single toe or of several toes may, in many cases, be allowed to pro-ceed naturally to autoamputation (Figure 22.4). However,

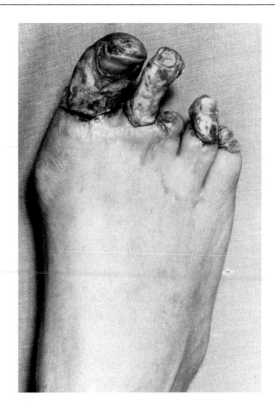

Figure 22.4 Autoamputation of necrotic toes is the pre-ferred treatment in selected patients who are free of pain or infection.

localized amputation is preferable if the involved toe is painful or if there is infection in the form of cellulitis, wet gangrene, discharging ulceration or osteomyelitis (particularly in the infected diabetic forefoot). This ampu-tation may be done at the transphalangeal level when there is no proximal spread of infection or necrosis into the forefoot and when the arterial blood supply to the rest of the foot is adequate for wound healing. It is important that all infected, ischemic or threatened tissue be removed.

The skin incision may be circular or may incorpo-rate anterior and posterior or lateral flaps (Figure 22.5a). Access to the line of incision is provided by retracting adjacent toes with a rolled gauze (rather than traumatizing the tissue with metal retractors) and gripping the toe(s) to be excised with a towel forceps. The initial incision is made to the depth of the bone, avoiding undermining the skin. The bone is then cleared of attached tendons and is usu-ally divided midway through the proximal phalanx, using bone cutters or bone rongeurs. The bone may require fur-ther shortening to allow closure of the skin without ten-sion. Under no circumstances should this amputation be completed through the proximal phalangeal meta-tarsal joint leaving exposed cartilage. In such an event, the surgeon should proceed to the next higher level (ray amputation), since exposed cartilage is prone to infection and nonhealing complications. If infection is present, it is preferable not to close the wound; otherwise the skin may be loosely approximated with interrupted sutures, usually nylon or polypropylene.

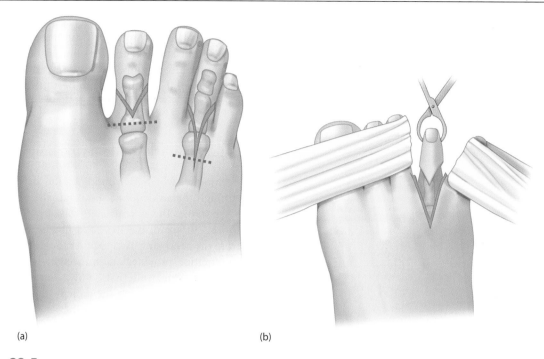

(a)   (b)

Figure 22.5 (a) Incisions for transphalangeal and transmetatarsal amputation of the toe (levels of bone division indicated). (b) Ray amputation incision onto the dorsum of the foot to expose head of metatarsal.

In most cases the patient may commence ambulation on the day following surgery. There are no prosthetic requirements after this amputation, and there is no increase in energy expenditure for ambulation compared to an age-adjusted normal population.

RAY AMPUTATION OF THE TOE

When infection or necrosis of a single toe involves all of the skin on the toe, a small part of the adjacent forefoot, goes past the plantar skin crease, then a ray (or wedge) amputation is indicated. Usually, this applies to a single toe alone; however, occasionally two adjacent toes may be amputated using this method. The initial incision should be planned so as to conserve all viable skin to allow for closure of the wound without tension. The plantar skin tends to be spared because of its better blood supply. The incision, often referred to as a racquet incision, skirts the necrotic skin of the toe and is then continued a short distance on the dorsum of the foot to allow exposure of the metatarsal head (Figure 22.5b). This incision is similarly taken directly down to the bone, dividing tendons and ligaments without undermining the skin. The metatarsal is cleared of tendons, using a periosteal elevator and taking great care to avoid injury to adjacent digital arteries. The bone is then divided through the distal part of the metatarsal, and the affected bone and soft tissues are excised free by a combination of sharp dissection with a scalpel and cutting with heavy scissors. Soft bone is indicative of osteomyelitis in the metatarsal shaft, and more proximal metatarsal shaft resection is required. Occasionally, unsuspected infection of the tendon sheaths or fascial plans may at the time of operation be found to extend into the foot. Such a finding necessitates more proximal

amputation or wide debridement and drainage in preparation for a higher level of amputation. At the conclusion of the procedure, the wound is loosely approximated with interrupted sutures, but it should be left open if there has been infection.

In most cases, the patient may commence ambulation on the day following surgery. There are no prosthetic requirements after this amputation, and there is no increase in energy expenditure for ambulation compared to an age-adjusted normal population.

Transmetatarsal amputation of the forefoot

Transmetatarsal amputation is usually employed if there is gangrene involving several toes, especially if one of these is the great toe or if the ischemic or infective process extends too far proximally up the foot to allow for the healing of a ray amputation. Once again, the ischemic process is usually more severe on the dorsal surface of the foot, so the skin incision is designed to allow for a longer plantar flap, extending to the line of the heads of the metatarsals (Figure 22.6). The line of the dorsal aspect of the skin incision is positioned slightly distal to the line of metatarsal division. This anterior or dorsal incision may be adjusted more proximally up the forefoot if resection of the metatarsal heads and part of the shafts is required. The incision is continued down to the metatarsals, and when these are cleared of tendon and ligament, the bones are divided with bone shears or an electric saw. A thick pad of subcutaneous tissue is preserved on the plantar aspect, and the other tissues are dissected away using a scalpel. Further trimming of bone and exposed tendon is performed as

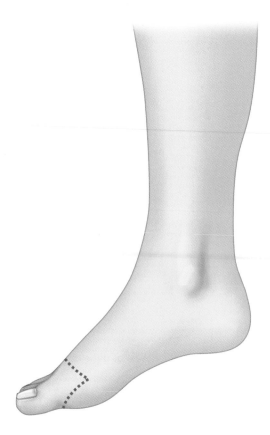

Figure 22.6 Incision for transmetatarsal amputation of the forefoot, incorporating a plantar flap.

necessary to allow for closure of the wound by plantar flap without tension.

As with all amputations for vascular disease, the skin should always be handled gently, avoiding the use of forceps wherever possible, and absolute hemostasis is mandatory. Interrupted sutures are placed loosely. The application of an IPOP is described later in this chapter. An alternative to IPOP is a non-weight-bearing short leg cast. A walking heel can be added to the cast after wound healing has occurred (10–14 days). Following healing of the transmetatarsal amputation, the patient is usually able to walk satisfactorily without significant disability.

After recovery, the patient's shoe can be modified by distal padding and a steel shank or metatarsal bar for the toe off. Compared to the age-adjusted normal population, there is a 10% increase in energy expenditure for ambulation with this level amputation.

Transmetatarsal amputation avoids the equinus and equinovalgus deformities of the more proximal midfoot amputations. However, many of these amputations, although not favoured by the author, are once again back in vogue. These amputations include (1) the Lisfranc amputation, which is a plantar flap–based metatarsal/tarsal disarticulation; (2) the Chopart amputation, which is a plantar flap–based calcaneus tarsal disarticulation; and (3) the Pirogoff amputation, a formal ankle disarticulation in which the talus is separated from the tibia and fibula, which are then transected immediately above the joint surface. In the opinion of the author, these three midfoot amputations are rarely indicated in the dysvascular patient and are best utilized in traumatic injury.

Amputation at the ankle (Syme amputation)

This technique, which is a modification of disarticulation through the ankle joint, was originally described by Syme[68] in 1982. The operation involves excision of the distal joint surface of the tibia and fibula, with a flap of skin from the heel being used to cover the transected bone. This amputation provides an end weight–bearing stump and leaves a residual limb that is only a few inches shorter than normal, thus allowing the patient to walk for short distances (at home) without a prosthesis. The addition of a prosthesis makes both legs equal in length, but the Syme prosthesis is not cosmetic in appearance and therefore may be contraindicated in women.

Because of the great potential for ischemic complication, patients should be selected carefully for this procedure. Contraindications include ischemia, ulceration or infection of the heel. This is the most technically difficult major lower extremity amputation. This amputation can be performed in one (no transection of the fibular and malleolar flares) stage or two stages (resection of the fibular and malleolar flares at a second minor operation). The main indication is well-demarcated gangrene of the forefoot that extends too far up the foot to allow for a successful transmetatarsal procedure; in addition, the vascularity of the ankle region and heel pad must be well preserved. The presence of the popliteal or posterior tibial pulse is very favourable for healing.[69,70] The author's experience suggests that this is not a good amputation level in diabetics unless sensation of the heel pad is intact, due to recurrent ulceration on the Syme residual limb requiring below-knee amputation.

The incision is shown in Figure 22.7a. The upper horizontal line begins on the lateral side of the ankle just below the lateral malleolus and is brought across the front of the ankle joint in a straight line to a point just below the medial malleolus. The lower, vertical part of the incision is carried down across the sole of the foot in front of the heel in a straight line to join the posterior aspects of the ends of the upper incision. The whole of this incision is carried down to bone, carefully avoiding undermining of the skin and preserving a maximum length of posterior tibial artery (the latter of which is crucial for healing). The ankle joint is entered through the anterior aspect, and division of the tendons and ligaments across the front of the ankle allows disarticulation of the talus. The next part of the procedure involves dissecting out the calcaneus, taking great care to avoid damage to the soft tissues and skin of the heel pad. This is performed using sharp dissection with a scalpel

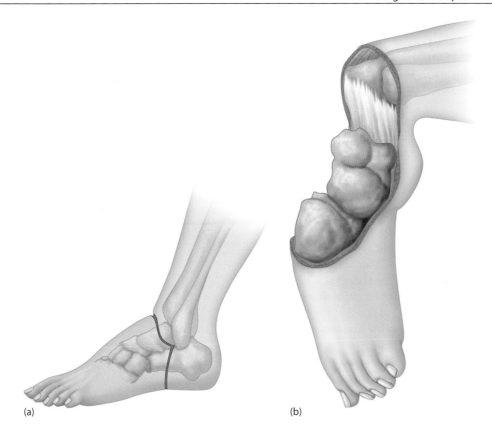

(a)   (b)

Figure 22.7 Syme's amputation: (a) skin incision; (b) the disarticulated foot is retracted downwards after the joint has been entered and the calcaneus dissected.

around the calcaneus, staying close to the bone and dissecting off surrounding fibrous tissue, ligament and fat. This is usually described as a subperiosteal removal of the calcaneus; however, because of the absence of easily identifiable planes, it is very difficult to stay within a true subperiosteal plane. Completion of excision of the calcaneus is best achieved with the partially disarticulated foot reflected down to allow better exposure. Great care must be taken to avoid perforating the skin posteriorly when transecting the insertion of the Achilles tendon. When the calcaneus has been excised, the anterior flap is gently retracted, allowing access to the distal ends of the tibia and fibula (Figure 22.7b).

The classic technique describes removal of the articular cartilage with a saw, dividing directly across the lower ends of both bones (fibula and tibia) at a level just above the joint. Hemostasis is achieved and the heel pad rotated up and secured across the cut ends of the bones. The heel pad is held in place by closure of the skin, using interrupted sutures of nylon propylene, which can be left in place for several weeks.

The wound may be dressed with layers of gauze held in place by elasticized bandaging. The dressing is applied with gentle compression so as to minimize edema. Alternatively, the stump may be placed within a well-padded plaster-of-Paris cast, which can later be fitted with a rubber stop to

allow partial weight bearing. The technique of IPOP is described later in this chapter.

In order to ambulate more than short distances in the house, a definite prosthesis is required. Due to the bulbous nature of the Syme residual limb, construction of the prosthesis requires a medial or posterior window resulting in a noncosmetic prosthesis ('fat ankle'). Compared to an age-adjusted normal population, there is a 10%–20% increase in energy expenditure for ambulation at this level of amputation.

Below-knee amputation

The general rule that amputation stumps should be as long as possible does not apply to the below-knee amputation, since fitting a prosthesis is more difficult and stump complications are increased if the below-knee stump is too long. In fact, too long a below-knee residual limb may preclude the fitting of energy absorbing/releasing prostheses such as the Flexfoot™. In addition, the problems of weight bearing and retaining adequate soft tissue to cover the stump are increased with a longer tibia, and since the more distal tissues will tend to have a less adequate blood supply, stump ulceration and pain will be more common. The ideal length for anterior skin incision is one hand's breadth (10 cm) below the tibial tubercle. After completion of the amputation, the anterior margin of the tibia must be bevelled (45°–60°) and the fibula is usually transected one quarter inch more proximally than the tibia. The posterior flap must be long enough to cover the residual limb with a good muscle myoplasty and 'plastic' skin closure of interrupted vertical mattress sutures.

Up until about 20 years ago, most amputations for vascular disease were performed at the above-knee level. Since that time, however, it has been shown that 70–85% of all vascular amputations may be performed below the knee with satisfactory healing rates.[33,71–73] The author would suggest, however, that with proper objective amputation level selection, primary healing may be expected in 95% of below-knee amputations. Clinical judgement concerning the state of the circulation and nutrition of the skin both preoperatively and intraoperatively has been shown not to be a reliable factor in predicting healing of a below-knee stump. However, if good bleeding is noted at the time of operation, the chance of wound healing has been shown to be 90%.[33] Even where there is little or no bleeding, eventual healing still occurs in 69% of patients.[33,35] It is preferable to decide on the level of amputation by objective investigations (amputation level determination) before the time of surgery rather than to commence with a below-knee incision with the idea of immediately moving to the above-knee level if necessary.

Several conditions dictate that a below-knee amputation should not be performed (Table 22.3). These are as follows:

1. Severe joint contractures of the knee or hip. Such contractions make prosthesis fitting virtually impossible. Even if fitting of a prosthesis is possible, the functional result will not be satisfactory.
2. Leg spasticity or rigidity due to previous stroke.
3. Severe arthritic changes of the knee. Painful arthritic knee joint will usually not be worth saving because of the poor functional result.
4. Skin ulceration or infection extending above the below-knee amputation level (expected anterior and/or posterior incisions). Similarly, questionable or borderline skin viability in the patient who is confined to bed should prompt selection of a higher level.
5. Deep infection or necrosis of the muscle compartments extending above the mid-calf level.

In these cases, through-knee and above-knee amputations are often acceptable alternatives.

Table 22.3 Contraindications to below-knee amputation.

Joint contracture of knee or hip
Leg spasticity or rigidity
Severe knee arthritis
Skin ulceration or infection at BKA[a] incision level
Infection or necrosis of leg muscle compartment

a BKA, below-knee amputation.

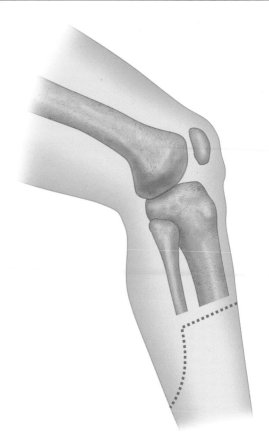

Figure 22.8 Posterior myocutaneous flap incision and level of bone section for below-knee amputation.

Several incisions are described for the below-knee amputation. These include (1) the circumferential, no-flap incision[74]; (2) short, equal anterior and posterior flaps; (3) skew flaps[75] and (4) the long posterior flap[40] ('Burgess technique', which the author favours) (Figure 22.8). As we have used the long posterior-flap technique in most cases, the following description will be of that method. The scar for end-bearing amputation residual limbs should preferably be anterior or posterior to the end of the stump; however, scar placement is not usually a concern for the below-knee amputation, where most prostheses are not of the end-bearing type. We have preferred the long posterior myoplastic flap or myocutaneous flap because of the superior blood supply of the posterior compartment, which leads to a higher rate of primary healing, and because the bulk of the gastrocnemius–soleus muscle mass gives a good cover for the end of the tibia.

The incision for this procedure is demonstrated in Figure 22.9. The operation may be performed with general, spinal or epidural anesthesia. Following skin preparation and draping, the incision is marked on the skin with a pen. The anterior or horizontal aspect of the incision continues back to a point just behind the fibula laterally and to the corresponding point on the medial side of the leg, level with posteromedial aspect of the tibia. From these (mid-shaft) points, the posterior or vertical lines of the incision are taken down the middle of the distal limb to

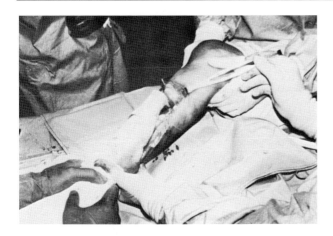

Figure 22.9 Below-knee amputation. The bone is sectioned with a saw while the skin is gently retracted.

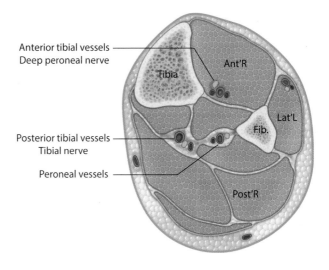

Figure 22.10 Cross-sectional anatomy of the leg at level of below-knee amputation, demonstrating position of major neuromuscular structures.

form a long, curved posterior flap of a length sufficient to cover the stump. The length of the posterior flap usually equals the diameter of the limb at the point of anterior transection plus 2–3 cm. The skin incision is deepened through the deep fascia in a single cut perpendicular to the skin so as to avoid undermining. The two saphenous veins and tributaries are ligated as they are encountered. The incision is then deepened through the fascia in all areas of the skin incision. The muscles of the anterior compartment are transected at a level several centimetres distal to the proposed line of division of the tibia, and the anterior tibial vessels are suture ligated.

Either the tibia or the fibula may be divided first, depending on the surgeon's preference. If the tibia is to be divided first, the surrounding muscles are divided in the same line as the skin incision back to the level of the posterior border of the tibia. The anterior tibial neurovascular bundle is identified and the vessels are suture ligated prior to bone section. The bone is cleared of muscle on all sides, using a scalpel and periosteal elevator. Proximal periosteal elevation should be minimized. The tibia may then be divided using a handsaw, Gigli saw or electric saw. The upper half of the anterior tibia surface is bevelled at 45°–60° after completion of removal of the distal limb. The fibula is similarly cleared of muscle and transected about one quarter of an inch proximal to the tibia. Angled bone-cutting shears aid in dividing the fibula at a higher level than the tibia. The posterior tibial neuromuscular bundle and peroneal vessels are suture ligated when exposed (Figure 22.10).

At this stage the main muscle bulk of the leg will have been divided in a line perpendicular to the skin (Figure 22.9), and the posterior myocutaneous flap may now be completed using a long amputation knife to divide the soleus and gastrocnemius muscles obliquely. Bleeding vessels and venous sinuses are suture ligated; it is important to achieve good hemostasis to avoid the formation of postoperative stump hematomas. Nerves are gently stretched down, ligated and divided and allowed to retract.

Absolute hemostasis is essential, especially if an IPOP is going to be applied.

The bone ends are smoothed with a rasp or file. Then the wound is irrigated and closed in two layers, commencing with myoplasty of the posterior flap by suturing the tendinous cut edge of the gastrocnemius–soleus forward over the ends of the bone to the thinner anterior fascia and the periosteum of the tibia. Finally, the skin is closed with interrupted sutures, avoiding tension (Figure 22.11). Skin apposition must be precise, since delay of epithelialization is likely, because of the reduced vascularity, if there are any gaps between the skin edges. The suture-line scar should be above the bevelled anterior edge of the tibia, away from regions of pressure if possible. If no attempt is made to trim the dog ears, then care must be taken with application of the postoperative dressing to not

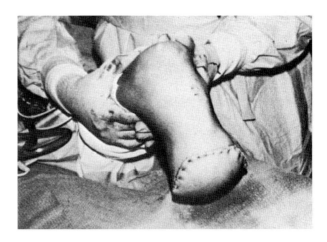

Figure 22.11 The stump is closed without tension allowing 'dog cars' to mould into the shape of the stump over several weeks.

bend or fold over the dog ears, as these will mould into the general shape of the stump after several weeks. The author favours plastic excision of the dog ears with careful closure of the surgical wound at the time of amputation. The resultant hemicylinder provides the prosthetist with a suitable shape for the manufacture of a socket. Closed suction drains may be used if needed but are generally not necessary and increase the incidence of infection.[6] A thick dressing of gauze pads and cotton–wool bandaging is then applied, and the final layer may be elastic Ace bandages or a plaster-of-Paris cast. The techniques of IPOP are described later in this chapter.

There are many variations of definite below-knee prostheses from a simple pylon with a nonmotion foot to energy-storing prostheses. Prosthetic choice depends on age and the activity level of the patient. Compared to an age-adjusted normal population, there is a 40%–60% increase in energy expenditure for ambulation at this level of amputation.

Through-knee and above-knee amputation

Many techniques of above-knee amputation have been reported; in general, these are all variations of a similar operative procedure. The distal supracondylar amputation and Gritti-Stokes techniques have lost popularity because of the realization that the through-knee amputation has the advantage of preserving proprioceptive areas of the joint and affords greater bone length, which makes manipulation of a prosthesis simpler. Otherwise, the general rule for above-knee amputation is that maximum bone length should be conserved within the bounds of the patient's vascular problem.

As with the below-knee amputation, myodesis procedures (except as described later), where the muscles are sutured or otherwise fixed to holes drilled in the bone, are generally not encouraged in the dysvascular patient. It is far simpler, just as functional, and probably allows fitting of a more cosmetic prosthesis to divide the muscles distal to the site of bone division and then to suture antagonistic groups over the end of the bone stump, anchoring them to each other and to the periosteum. This allows for the preservation of muscle activity (a 'physiologic stump') and gives a good covering for the bone.

The skin incision usually employs equal anterior and posterior flaps (fish-mouth incision), as shown in Figure 22.12; however, a circumferential skin incision is just as effective. A technique using laterally placed flaps is favoured for through-knee amputation in some centres,[76] particularly if the anterior skin-flap region is compromised by ischemia.[77]

Through-knee amputation

The through-knee level gives the amputee the advantage of a long lever with an end-bearing stump. In addition,

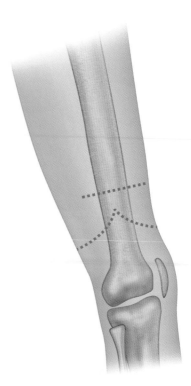

Figure 22.12 Anterior–posterior 'fish-mouth' incision for above-knee amputation.

proprioceptive information coming from the capsular structures of the knee is preserved.

The disadvantages to this level amputation are prosthetic. It is hard to get cosmetic or matching knee centres, even with new 4-bar link knees. Since the residual limb is bulbous at the distal femur flares, the prosthesis must be made with a medial or posterior window, and therefore the prosthesis is not often very cosmetic.

If a through-knee amputation is to be performed, the skin incision must be distal to the knee joint by 4–5 cm (level of the tibial tubercle), and the patella and patellar tendon are usually preserved and sutured over the exposed femoral condyles. Preferably the patient is placed prone and an anterior-based skin flap is created. The incision is deepened straight through to the depth of bone, perpendicular to the skin, and the muscles and tendons attached to the upper part of the tibia (sartorius, gracilis, semitendinosus, quadriceps expansion and gastrocnemius) are divided. The patellar tendon is separated from the tibial tubercle and the knee joint is entered anteriorly. The collateral and cruciate ligaments are divided. The resection continues below the menisci, preserving the capsular attachments to the rims of the medial and lateral meniscus. The described joint incision helps to preserve the rich proprioceptive supply of the knee joint. With the knee bent, the posterior capsule of the joint is divided, giving access to the popliteal neurovascular structures. The artery and vein are suture ligated, and the nerves are brought down, ligated and then allowed to retract up into the muscle bulk.

The patella is reflected back over the femoral condyles and may be held in place by suturing the infrapatellar tendon to the posterior capsule; however, if there is insufficient patellar tendon length, the tendon may be sutured to the stumps of the cruciate ligaments. The divided hamstring tendons are also sutured to the knee capsule. A satisfactory myoplasty is thus produced. Preservation of the patella and patellar tendon conserves the broad kneeling area of the knee.

The wound is closed in two layers. An amputation dressing is then applied, with or without a plaster cast. The techniques for application of an IPOP are described later. Compared to the normal age-adjusted population, there is a 100%–120% increase in energy expenditure for ambulation at this level of amputation.

Above-knee amputation

Because ambulation after above-knee amputation is directly related to bone length, this procedure is done with the aim of preserving the maximum possible bone length. The usual level of amputation is just above the terminal flare of the femur, allowing approximately 10 cm for the interposition of an artificial knee joint between the stump and the normal knee axis.

We have usually used anterior and posterior flaps, but a circumferential incision is also suitable. Short flaps are preferred because of the possibility of jeopardizing blood supply in long flaps. The incision passes through the skin, subcutaneous tissue and deep fascia without undermining and then is continued obliquely through the muscle layers towards the anticipated line of bone section. As the major vessels are almost certainly occluded, hemorrhage is rarely a problem. However, all large vessels should be suture ligated. The main dissection usually commences on the medial aspect of the leg to expose the femoral vessels, which are clamped and suture ligated as they are encountered (Figure 22.13). The sciatic nerve is exposed more posteriorly and ligated after being pulled down,

so that it will then retract up into the muscle bulk after it is transected and be protected from direct pressure. Ligation of this nerve is important because of the artery that accompanies it. The bone is sectioned using a hand or electric saw, and the ends are smoothed with a file. Opposing muscle groups are then sutured over the end of the bone, with special attention being given to fixation of the rectus femoris and hamstrings to each other and to the periosteum to preserve balance of contractile function. The adductor magnus and fascia lata are sutured to each other transversely over the bone. Careful approximation of muscle layers also obliterates dead space within the wound. The fasciae of the anterior and posterior flap are then approximated with interrupted, absorbable sutures. If necessary, wound drainage may be instituted with a closed suction drain or a Penrose tissue drain placed at the base of the flaps. However, absolute hemostasis is worth the effort since drains increase the possibility of infection. The skin is carefully approximated without tension. The amputation dressing is then applied, and a plaster-of-Paris cast may be added, especially if a prosthesis is to be used immediately. The techniques for application of an IPOP are described later.

One of the major prosthetic advances in the last two decades has been the move away from the quadrilateral socket (Berkeley brim) to the Catcam soft plastic socket fit for above-knee amputees. These new prostheses are lighter and more functional than their older counterparts and probably have helped to increase the percentages of ambulatory above-knee amputees. However, compared to an age-adjusted normal population, the increase in energy expenditure required to ambulate after an above-knee amputation ranges from 140% to 200%. Since the use of a wheelchair requires only a 9% increase in energy expenditure, it is easy to understand why elderly amputees, especially those with cardiovascular impairment, choose a wheelchair over walking with an above-knee prosthesis.

An important new technique for above-knee amputation has been described by F. Gottschalk (personal communication). The above-knee amputation is performed utilizing a long medial flap and shorter lateral flap in order to preserve length of the adductor magnus muscle. The adductor magnus is dissected off the distal medial femur, and after transection of the femur, the adductor magnus is wrapped over the end of the femur and then fixed to the lateral femur in a true myodesis. The medial-based skin flap allows closure of the incision on the lateral side of the leg without skin tension. The use of the adductor magnus in this fashion preserves the patient's ability to keep the residual femur in a more normal weight-bearing position relative to the pelvis and knee joint and aids with patient ambulation.

Hip disarticulation

Amputation at the hip level is rarely performed for peripheral vascular disease.[78] Usually, dysvascular

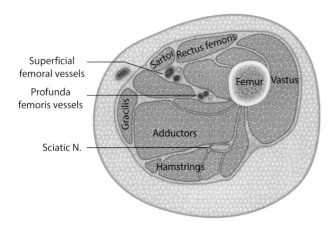

Figure 22.13 Cross-sectional anatomy of the thigh at the level of above-knee amputation.

patients requiring this level of amputation have had failed above-knee amputations. Most commonly in dysvascular patients, this amputation is performed in the face of occlusion of the common femoral, superficial femoral and profunda femoral arteries. Because of poor blood supply, healing complications and stump infection are common when this amputation is performed in dysvascular patients.

In hip disarticulation amputation, the initial step is control of the femoral artery, followed by division of the musculature of the adductor and anterolateral compartments to expose the hip joint. Anatomic considerations in this dissection have been described in detail by Boyd.[79] After disarticulation, a long posterior flap of gluteal muscle is devised and reflected anteriorly to form a broad muscle base for support of prosthesis.[77] It is important to achieve good cover of the acetabulum with muscle and soft tissue, and the suture line should be placed so as to avoid direct pressure against the prosthesis.[80]

Compared to the normal age-adjusted population, there is a 240%–500% increase in energy expenditure for ambulation at this level of amputation. Needless to say, most amputees (except children) do not ambulate at this level of amputation and use a wheelchair for mobility.

POSTOPERATIVE CARE

Adequate analgesia is important in achieving early mobility, with exercises aimed at avoidance of flexion contractures. Patients should go to physical therapy for range-of-motion and limb-strengthening exercises starting on the first postoperative day if possible. The dressing is usually not disturbed for 3 or 4 days unless there is significant pain or fever pointing to possible complication. In those instances where drainage tubes are necessary, they are removed as soon as possible, preferably within 24 hours. We prefer not to suture the drains in place, so that they may be removed gently without disturbing the dressing. The elastic stump bandage helps prevent swelling while also allowing for passive and active exercise in order to avoid contractures. If a plaster cast or IPOP has been applied, flexion contractures will not occur, but there may be some loss of joint mobility.

Conditions such as diabetes mellitus, hypertension, heart disease and chronic respiratory disorders require close monitoring and control during the postoperative period. Systemic antibiotics should be continued for several days if infection was present at the time of operation; in the absence of infection, several perioperative prophylactic doses of antibiotic are sufficient (24 hours). Early mobilization of the patient is encouraged, either by the use of temporary pneumatic air splint,[81,82] with crutches or a walking frame, or by the technique of IPOP application, as outlined later. The rehabilitation of the patient commences as soon as possible and is best achieved using a multidisciplinary approach, involving regular instruction and supervision by a physical therapist, occupational therapist, prosthetist and surgeon.[6]

Once wound healing is satisfactory, a stump dressing consisting solely of an elastic Ace bandage can be employed to prevent stump edema and to aid in moulding the residual limb shape. The patient is instructed in the proper technique of bandage application and should reapply the bandage several times a day. Correct technique is important in preventing circumferential compression, which may increase edema.

In the opinion of the author, aggressive use of temporary removable prostheses after major lower extremity amputation (even if IPOP is not used) not only improves rehabilitation results but helps control pain and swelling. In the author's personal series of over 2000 patients treated with either IPOP or early temporary prosthesis, the incidence of stump pain and phantom pain problems is <5%.[6]

After the first few days, the patient should not be allowed to lie in bed with the stump propped up on pillows, since that position tends to allow the development of contractures. Sutures should be left in place for at least 2 weeks and sometimes for longer. Narcotic analgesia will usually be required for several days; however, complaints of severe pain after 48 hours suggest a major complication and should precipitate removal of the dressing and inspection of the wound. The possible occurrence of phantom limb pain should be explained to the patient. Postoperative confusion is common because of the generally elderly population that one is dealing with and because of factors such as infection, analgesia and multiorgan disease. If the patient is confused, steps must be taken to prevent him or her from trying to get out of bed, which often precipitates injury to the amputation stump.

IMMEDIATE POSTOPERATIVE PROSTHESIS FITTING

The concept of improved stump healing and accelerated rehabilitation brought about by IPOP fitting dates back to the 1960s.[83] The main benefits claimed for this technique are faster rehabilitation of the patient with improved patient morale and motivation, coupled with early acceptance of the procedure and conditioning to accept and use the prosthesis. Other advantages have been noted with early prosthesis fitting, including better control of edema of the stump, less pain, perhaps earlier healing, protection of the wound from trauma, improved rates of rehabilitation and prevention of contractures. The earlier mobilization is thought to be associated with a lower incidence of venous thromboembolic disease, atelectasis and pneumonia. Patients have been noted to regain strength and to show earlier learning of balance control due to the increased proprioceptive input from muscles and joints of the involved limb, which occurs with early mobilization, exercise and partial weight bearing.

Obviously, this technique will not be suitable for all patients, especially those who have been severely debilitated by sepsis or long-term illness. It is possible that there is also the potential problem of compromising wound healing with IPOP use in the patient with severe vascular disease. However, with objective preoperative selection of amputation level, wound-healing problems can be reduced to a minimum. The IPOP technique also works well in diabetics. Because this technique requires the patient to wear a plaster cast over the amputation stump for 2–3 weeks, it should not be used for those patients who may be vulnerable to wound breakdown or possible infection, since the stump will then not be readily accessible for inspection.

Early involvement of the prosthetist is essential. Preferably she or he will see the patient before the operation and will assist at the time of surgery in the application of the IPOP cast. The surgical technique of amputation does not differ from that described previously except that, after the initial wound dressing is applied, an IPOP cast is built on the residual limb. The immediate fitting technique (Figure 22.14) involves application of a rigid cast socket made up of an inner layer (the stump sock), appropriate protection of bony prominences by padding (the relief pads), a polyurethane cap or pad applied over the end of the stump and application of the plaster cast.[6,84] Depending on the amputation level, a suspension strap with waist belt is incorporated into the plaster cast. An attachment plate is incorporated into the distal end of the plaster, and

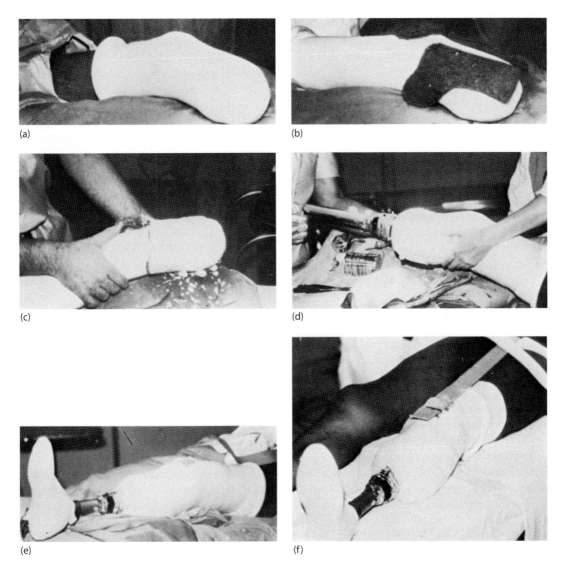

(a)

(b)

(c)

(d)

(e)

(f)

Figure 22.14 Techniques of immediate postoperative prosthesis fitting at the back knee level: (a) stump sock; (b) relief pads to protect bony prominences; (c) application of plaster cast; (d) attachment plate incorporated into the plaster, with adjustable-length pylon tube; (e) complete prosthesis with foot attached; and (f) suspension strap and waist belt attached to prosthesis.

the pylon tube with prosthetic foot will be fitted to this plate. A window is made in the cast over the patella to protect this area from pressure sores and to allow patellar movement with ambulation. Immediate postoperative prosthetic techniques work well with all levels of major limb amputation (transmetatarsal amputation, Syme, the Scottish surgeon, below knee or above knee) but work best with below-knee amputees. If the patient is well enough, mobilization may commence on the first postoperative day. On the first postoperative day, the patient stands at bedside without weight bearing. During the first week the patient progresses to standing without placing weight on the prosthesis while supported by a walking frame or crutches. By the second week the patient advances to 50% weight bearing on the amputated limb, and full weight bearing is achieved by 21–30 days after surgery. The team of prosthetist, physical therapist and surgeon supervises and encourages the patient with most of the early exercises and use of the prosthesis. The rehabilitation process is best supervised in the physical therapy department, where special equipment for ambulation, such as parallel bars, is available.

The patient progresses from standing and balancing with limited ambulation through progressive weight bearing over several weeks as previously described. The plaster cast is usually changed after 7–10 days and 14–21 days. Patients may be discharged to a rehabilitation facility (with IPOP experience) either on the second or third postoperative day or after the first cast change. After the second or third cast change, the patient makes use of temporary removable prostheses until full wound healing and moulding of the stump have occurred, at which time measurements for the permanent prosthesis may be taken and the permanent prosthesis manufactured (usually at 6 months).

COMPLICATIONS OF AMPUTATION

The complications of amputation surgery may be divided into those that are specific for the operation and those that are due to the severe cardiopulmonary disease and diabetes often seen in this patient population. Several follow-up studies have shown that approximately 50% of the diabetic amputee patients die within 2–3 years of the operation, usually because of cardiac or cerebrovascular problems, and that, of the survivors, a further 30%–50% eventually require amputation of the contralateral leg within the same time span.[6,85–88] However, survival for nondiabetic lower extremity amputees approximates the normal age-adjusted population. Until recent years, the operative mortality rate among those with amputations below the knee was approximately 10%, and among those with through-knee or above-knee amputation, the usual rates were 20%–30%.[2] With recent improvements in patient preparation for surgery, anesthetic techniques and intensive care, there should now be a mortality rate of <5% for below-knee and perhaps 10%

for above-knee operations. Bodily and Burgess[87] reported a series of 55 patients who had major amputations with an operative mortality rate of only 1.5%, and Fearon et al. reported a 3% mortality rate for below-knee amputation in 100 diabetics. There is also a relatively high incidence of postoperative cardiovascular and cerebrovascular complications such as myocardial infarction, stroke or respiratory failure.[89] The long-term survival prospects for diabetics are significantly worse than for nondiabetics, as previously stated.[90] In a series of 465 amputations, Bunt and Malone[4] reported an operative mortality rate of 1.5%. That series included amputations at all levels of the lower extremity.

If the amputation is performed for the treatment of sepsis, infective complications including septicemia and multiorgan failure may be common. A high incidence of postoperative venous thrombosis has been reported, particularly for amputation above the knee.[1] That high incidence of thromboembolic disease is most likely related to prolonged hospitalization both before and after operation and to the generally poor medical condition of patients undergoing above-knee amputation. The success rates with rehabilitation diminish dramatically in any patient who has been at bed rest for more than 30 days prior to major lower extremity amputation.[6] Malone reports that IPOP and other such aggressive rehabilitation techniques should not be utilized in patients who have been at extended bed rest prior to amputation, since the eventual successful ambulation rates are unacceptably low.

Neurological changes such as confusion, disorientation and reactive depression frequently occur and may be difficult to manage while also rendering rehabilitation difficult. Care of the skin wound is compromised in these patients, and they may require special observation to prevent accidents such as falling out of bed, which often leads to breakdown of the stump. Other common general complications include urinary tract infection and urinary retention, sacral-pressure-area bed sores, gastrointestinal bleeding and renal failure.

The main complications of the procedure itself are infections and nonhealing of the wound due to ischemia (Figure 22.15). These problems can be minimized by good objective selection of amputation level prior to surgery, preoperative treatment for infected ischemic limbs and the use of antibiotic prophylaxis. However, even with ideal management, episodes of skin-flap ischemia and suture-line infection cannot always be avoided. However, amputation level selection by objective tests (such as Ptc_{O_2}) will minimize postoperative healing failures.[6] Wound breakdown due to ischemia may be a primary problem or may occur because of excessive pressure (from the dressing, the plaster cast, a poorly fitting prosthesis or early weight bearing on a prosthesis). Small areas of wound breakdown will often heal with conservative management. Ischemic failure with or without infection usually requires revision. A failed below-knee amputation may often be revised to a

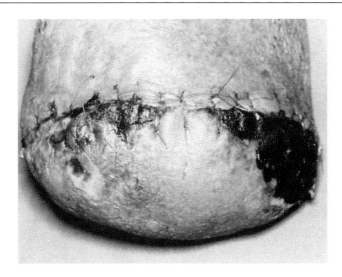

Figure 22.15 Typical wound edge necrosis of a below-knee amputation stump. This situation can often be salvaged by excision of all the necrotic tissue and primary closure, still at the below-knee level. Severe ischemia or infection usually mandates above-knee revision.

higher level while still retaining the knee joint, or it may necessitate above-knee amputation.

Phantom pain occurs frequently, and the patient should be warned of this possibility before surgery. Usually, the symptoms are not severe and no specific treatment is necessary, but occasionally narcotic or antidepressant medication may be required. In the author's experience, there is an inverse correlation between ambulation and problems with postoperative stump pain or phantom pain. Those patients who do not ambulate have a much higher incidence of pain complications, possibly as high as 30%–50%, while those patients who successfully ambulate have a pain complication rate of <5%.

Occasionally painful neuroma formation occurs at the divided nerve endings. Such neuromas require excision. Another important local complication is joint contractures. The main way to avoid contractures is to ensure that joint and leg exercises are commenced early in the postoperative period (and preoperatively too, if possible) and that rehabilitation begins immediately, with the patient being ambulated in a non-weight-bearing fashion with crutches or a walking frame. Adequate treatment of wound and stump pain in the early postoperative period aids early mobility. Failure to rehabilitate should also be regarded as a complication, since a major aim of good amputation is to achieve eventual ambulation and independent mobility. Recent experience suggests that at least 75% of amputees who have been fitted with a prosthesis will make daily use of it, although a significant proportion of these patients do not use their prosthesis outside of the home.[8] Other authors, including Malone, have reported success rates higher than 95% for periods as long as 5–10 years in those patients who were initially treated with IPOP.[6]

Physical rehabilitation, especially prosthetic training, is important for the amputee in achieving a functional state. A Cochrane database analysis showed few clinical trials to inform the choice of prosthetic rehabilitation.[91] Cumming et al. in 2015 recommended urgently trials to investigate choice of rehabilitation method and weight of prosthesis in older patients with unilateral transfemoral amputation.[91] Even if prosthetic gait training is unrealistic in older patients with co-morbidities, almost all amputees benefit from a rehabilitation programme to increase independence in transfers and wheelchair skills.[92] Outcome measures of physical function have been suggested to include a 2 minute walk distance, timed-up and go and 5 m gait speed.[93]

CONCLUSIONS

The guiding principle in amputation surgery is to obtain maximal restoration of function. Successful rehabilitation requires preservation of joint wherever such preservation is compatible with healing. Early ambulation is optimal and may best be achieved by the use of immediate prosthesis techniques in suitable patients. Amputation should thus be regarded from the rehabilitation perspective as a reconstructive procedure designed to restore function and allow the patient to return to an independent lifestyle. With the combination of low-level joint-preserving amputations and efficient, light functional prostheses (Figure 22.16), amputation is no longer regarded simply as the removal of dead tissue but as a true reconstructive procedure, which is one alternative among many in the treatment of severe limb ischemia. Attitudes towards amputation and subsequent rehabilitation should emphasize that return to ambulation is the expected outcome.

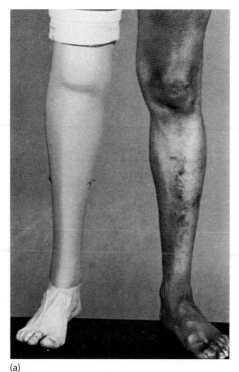 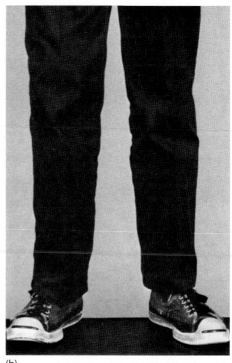

(a)　　　　　　　　　　　　　(b)

Figure 22.16 Modern lightweight, functional below-knee prosthetic limb (a) may be very difficult to differentiate from the contralateral normal limb (b).

REFERENCES

1. Little JM. *Major Amputations for Vascular Disease.* Edinburgh, UK: Churchill Livingstone; 1975.
2. Otteman MG, Stahlgren LH. Evaluation of factors which influence mortality and morbidity following major lower extremity amputation for atherosclerosis. *Surg Gynecol Obstet.* 1965;120:1217.
3. Rush DS, Huston CC, Bivins BA, Hyde GL. Operative and late mortality rates of above-knee and below-knee amputations. *Am Surg.* 1981;47:36.
4. Bunt TJ, Malone JM. Revascularization or amputation in the 70 year old. *Am Surg.* 1994;60(5):349.
5. De Frank RD, Taylor LM, Porter JM. Basic data related to amputations. *Ann Vasc Surg.* 1991;5:202.
6. Malone JM. Lower extremity amputation. In: Moore WS, ed. *Vascular Surgery, A Comprehensive Review,* 4th ed. Philadelphia, PA: W.B. Saunders; 1993.
7. Kald A, Carlsson R, Nilsson E. Major amputation in a defined population: Incidence, mortality and results of treatment. *Br J Surg.* 1989;76:308.
8. Finch DR, Macdougal M, Tibbs DJ, Morris PJ. Amputation for vascular disease: The experience of a peripheral vascular unit. *Br J Surg.* 1980;67:233.
9. Dietzek AM, Gupta SK, Kram HP et al. Limb loss with patent infrainguinal bypasses. *Eur J Vasc Surg.* 1990;4:413.
10. Bild DE, Selby JV, Sinnock P et al. Lower extremity amputation in people with diabetes: Epidemiology and prevention. *Diabetes Care.* 1989;2:24.
11. Berardi RS, Keonin Y. Amputations in peripheral vascular occlusive disease. *Am J Surg.* 1978;135:231.
12. Yao JST. Choice of amputation level. *J Vasc Surg.* 1988;8:544.
13. Sarin S, Sharmi S, Shields DA et al. Selection of amputation level: A review. *Eur J Vasc Surg.* 1991;5:611.
14. Bunt TJ. Physiologic amputation for acute pedal sepsis. *Am Surg.* 1990;56(9):520.
15. Hargrove WC, Barker FC, Berkowitz HD et al. Treatment of acute peripheral arterial and graft thromboses with low-dose streptokinase. *Surgery.* 1982; 92:981.
16. Bell ET. Atherosclerotic gangrene of the lower extremities in diabetic and non-diabetic persons. *Am J Clin Pathol.* 1957;28:27.
17. Sizer JS, Wheelock FC. Digital amputations in diabetic patients. *Surgery.* 1972;72:980.
18. Fearon J, Campbell DR, Hoar CS et al. Improved results with diabetic below-knee amputations. *Arch Surg.* 1975;120:777.
19. Cruse J, Foord RA. A five year prospective study of 23,649 surgical wounds. *Arch Surg.* 1973;107:206.
20. Kitter A. A technique for salvage of the diabetic gangrenous foot. *Orthop Clin North Am.* 1973;1:21.
21. Tripses D, Pollak FW. Risk factors in healing of below-knee amputation. *Am J Surg.* 1981;141:718.
22. Wu Y, Flanigan DP. Rehabilitation of the lower extremity amputee. In: Bergan JJ, Yao JST eds. *Gangrene and Severe Ischemia of the Lower Extremities.* New York: Grune & Stratton; 1978.

23. McIntyre KE, Bailey SA, Malone JM, Goldstone J. Guillotine amputation in the treatment of non-salvageable lower extremity infections. *Arch Surg.* 1984;119:450.

24. Fisher DF Jr., Clagett GP, Fry RE et al. One-stage vs. two-stage amputation for wet gangrene of the lower extremity: A randomized study. *J Vasc Surg.* 1988;8:428.

25. Sethia KK, Berry AR, Morrison JD et al. Changing pattern of lower limb amputation for vascular disease. *Br J Surg.* 1986;73:701.

26. Ramsburgh SR, Lindenauer SM, Weber TR et al. Femoropopliteal bypass for limb salvage operations. *Surgery.* 1977;81:453.

27. Kazmers M, Satiani B, Evans WE. Amputation level following unsuccessful distal limb salvage operations. *Surgery.* 1980;87:683.

28. Dardik H, Kahn M, Dardik I et al. Influence of failed vascular bypass procedures on conversion of below knee to above knee levels. *Surgery.* 1982;91:64.

29. Ellitsgaard N, Anderson AP, Fabrin J, Holstein P. Outcome in 282 lower extremity amputations: Knee salvage and survival. *Acta Orthop Scand.* 1990;61:140.

30. Evans WE, Hayes JP, Vermillion BD. Effect of failed distal reconstruction on the level of amputation. *Am J Surg.* 1990;160:217.

31. Bloom RJ, Stevick CA. Amputation level and distal bypass salvage of the limb. *Surg Gynecol Obstet.* 1988;166:1.

32. Murdoch G. Levels of amputation and limiting factors. *Ann R Coll Surg Engl.* 1967;40:204.

33. Kihn RB, Warren R, Beebe GW. The geriatric amputee. *Ann Surg.* 1972;176:305.

34. Larsson PA, Risberg B. Amputations due to lower limb ischaemia. *Acta Chir Scand.* 1988;154:267.

35. Rubin JR, Yao JST, Thompson RG et al. Management of infection of major amputation stumps after failed femoro distal grafts. *Surgery.* 1985;98(4):810.

36. Barber GG, McPhail NV, Scobie TK et al. A prospective study of lower limb amputations. *Can J Surg.* 1982;26:339.

37. Silbert S, Haimovici H. Results of midleg amputations for gangrene in diabetics. *J Am Med Assoc.* 1950;144:454.

38. Perry T. Below knee amputation. *Arch Surg.* 1969; 86:199.

39. Malone JM, Anderson G, Lalika S et al. A prospective randomized comparison of non-invasive techniques for amputation level selection. *Am J Surg.* 1987;154:179.

40. Burgess EM, Marsden FW. Major lower extremity amputations following arterial reconstruction. *Arch Surg.* 1974;108:655.

41. Burgess EM, Matsen FA. Determining amputation levels in peripheral vascular disease. *J Bone Joint Surg Am.* 1981;63A:1493.

42. White RA, Nolan L, Harley D et al. Noninvasive evaluation of peripheral vascular disease using transcutaneous oxygen tension. *Am J Surg.* 1982;144:68.

43. Eickhoff JH, Jacobsen F. Correlation of transcutaneous oxygen tension to blood flow in heated skin. *Scand J Clin Lab Invest.* 1980;40:761.

44. Katsamouris A, Brewster DC, Megerman J et al. Transcutaneous oxygen tension in selection of amputation level. *Am J Surg.* 1984;147:510.

45. Burgess EM, Matsen FA, Wyss CR, Simmons CW. Segmental transcutaneous measurement of P_{O_2} in patients requiring below-the-knee amputation for peripheral vascular insufficiency. *J Bone Joint Surg.* 1982;64:378.

46. Ameli FM, Byrne P, Provan JL. Selection of amputation level and prediction of healing using transcutaneous tissue oxygen tension (Ptc_{O_2}). *J Cardiovasc Surg.* 1989;30:220.

47. Wyss CR, Robertson C, Love SJ et al. Relationship between transcutaneous oxygen tension, ankle blood pressure, and clinical outcome of vascular surgery in diabetic and nondiabetic patients. *Surgery.* 1987;101:56.

48. McCollum PT, Spence VA, Walker WF. Oxygen inhalation induced changes in the skin as measured by transcutaneous oxymetry. *Br J Surg.* 1986;73:882.

49. Harward TR, Volney J, Golbranson F et al. Oxygen inhalation-induced transcutaneous P_{O_2} changes as a predictor of amputation level. *J Vasc Surg.* 1985;2:220.

50. Moore WS. Determination of amputation level. Measurement of skin blood flow with [133]xenon. *Arch Surg.* 1973;107:798.

51. Malone JM, Moore WS, Goldstone J, Malone SJ. Therapeutic and economic impact of a modern amputation program. *Ann Surg.* 1979;189:798.

52. Moore WS, Henry Re, Malone JM et al. Prospective use of [133]xenon clearance for amputation level selection. *Arch Surg.* 1981;116:86.

53. Harris JP, McLaughlin AF, Quinn RJ et al. Skin blood flow measurement with xenon-133 to predict healing of lower extremity amputations. *Aust N Z J Surg.* 1986;56:413.

54. Holloway GA, Burgess EM. Cutaneous blood flow and its relation to healing of below-knee amputation. *Surg Gynecol Obstet.* 1978;146:750.

55. Kram HB, Appel PL, Shoemaker WC. Prediction of below-knee amputation wound healing using noninvasive laser Doppler velocimetry. *Am J Surg.* 1989;158:29.

56. Gibbons GW, Wheelock FC, Siembieda C et al. Noninvasive prediction of amputation level in diabetic patients. *Arch Surg.* 1979;114:1253–1257.

57. Vena MJ, Gross WS, vanBellen B et al. Forefoot perfusion pressure and minor amputation for gangrene. *Surgery.* 1976;80:729.

58. Barnes RW, Shanik GD, Slaymaker EE. An index of healing in below-knee amputation: Leg blood pressure by Doppler ultrasound. *Surgery.* 1976;79:13.

59. Baker WH, Barnes RW. Minor forefoot amputation in patients with low ankle pressure. *Am J Surg.* 1977;133:331.

60. Wagner FW. Amputation of the foot and ankle: Current status. *Clin Orthop.* 1977;122:62.

61. Lee RY, Trainor FS, Karner D et al. Noninvasive hemodynamic evaluation in selection of amputation level. *Surg Gynecol Obstet.* 1979;149:241.

62. Henderson HP, Chir B, Hacken MEJ. The value of thermography in peripheral vascular disease. *Angiology.* 1978;29:65.

63. Abramowitz HB, Queral LA, Flinn WR et al. The use of photo-plethysmography in the assessment of chronic venous insufficiency: A comparison to venous pressure measurement. *Surgery.* 1979;86:434.

64. Standress DE, Sumner DS. Current research review: Noninvasive methods of studying peripheral arterial function. *J Surg Res.* 1972;12:419.

65. Barnes RW, Thornhill B, Nix L et al. Prediction of amputation wound healing: Roles of Doppler ultrasound and digit plethysmography. *Arch Surg.* 1981;116:80.

66. Holstein P, Sager P, Lassen NA. Wound healing in below knee amputations in relation to skin perfusion pressure. *Acta Orthop Scand.* 1979;50:49.

67. Faris I, Duncan H. Skin perfusion pressure in the prediction of healing in diabetic patients with ulcers or gangrene of the foot. *J Vasc Surg.* 1985;2:536.

68. Syme J. *Observations in Clinical Surgery.* Edinburgh, UK: Edmondson and Douglas; 1982.

69. Rosenman CD. Syme amputation for ischemic disease in the foot. *Am J Surg.* 1969;118:194.

70. McCollough NC, Shea JD, Warren WD, Sarmiento A. *The Dysvascular Amputee: Surgery and Rehabilitation. Current Problems in Surgery.* Chicago, IL: Year Book Medical Publishers; 1971.

71. Wray CH, Still JM, Moretz WH. Present management of amputations for peripheral vascular disease. *Am Surg.* 1972;38:87.

72. Sarmiento A, Warren WD. A re-evaluation of lower extremity amputations. *Surg Gynecol Obstet.* 1969;129:799.

73. Lim RC Jr., Blaisdell FW, Hall AD et al. Below knee amputation for ischemic gangrene. *Surg Gynecol Obstet.* 1967;125:493.

74. Little JM, Stewart GR, Niesche FW, Williams C. A Trial of flapless below-knee amputation for arterial insufficiency. *Med J Aust.* 1970;1:883.

75. Robinson KP. Skew-flap below-knee amputation. *Ann R Coll Surg Engl.* 1991;73:55.

76. Kjolbye J. The surgery of the through-knee amputation. In: Murdoch G, ed. *Prosthetic and Orthotic Practice.* London, UK: Edward Arnold; 1970, pp. 255.

77. Marsden FW. Amputation: Surgical technique and postoperative management. *Aust N Z J Surg.* 1977;47:384.

78. Unruh T, Fisher DF, Unruh TA et al. Hip disarticulation: An 11-year experience. *Arch Surg.* 1990;125:791.

79. Boyd HB. Anatomic disarticulation of the hip. *Surg Gynecol Obstet.* 1947;84:346.

80. Sugarbaker PH, Chretien PB. A surgical technique for hip disarticulation. *Surgery.* 1981;90:546.

81. Little JM. A Pneumatic weight-bearing temporary prosthesis for below-knee amputees. *Lancet.* 1971;1:271.

82. Kerstein MD. Utilization of an air-splint after below-knee amputation. *Am J Phys Med.* 1974;53:119.

83. Burgess EM, Romano RL. The management of lower extremity amputees using immediate postsurgical prosthesis. *Clin Orthop.* 1968;57:137.

84. Russe AS. Amputation, immediate postoperative fitting, and early ambulation. In: Haimovici H, ed. *Vascular Surgery: Principles and Techniques*, 2nd ed. Norwalk, CT: Appleton-Century-Crofts; 1984.

85. Couch NP, David JK, Tilney NL, Crane C. Natural history of the leg amputee. *Am J Surg.* 1977;133:469.

86. Mazet R. The geriatric amputee. *Artif Limbs.* 1967;11:35.

87. Bodily KC, Burgess EM. Contralateral limb and patient survival after leg amputation. *Am J Surg.* 1983;148:280.

88. Harris JP, Page S, England R, May J. Is the outlook for the vascular amputee improved by striving to preserve the knee? *J Cardiovasc Surg.* 1988;29:741.

89. Castronuovo JJ, Deane LM, Deterling RA et al. Below-knee amputation: Is the effort to preserve the knee joint justified? *Arch Surg.* 1980;115:1184.

90. Burgess EM. Pathways to diabetic limb amputation: basis for prevention. In: Kempczinski RF, ed. *The Ischemic Leg.* Chicago, IL: Year Book Medical Publishers; 1985.

91. Cumming JC, Barr S, Howe TE. Prosthetic amputation for older dysvascular people following a unilateral transfemoral amputation. *Cochrane Database Syst Rev.* 2006;18:CD005260 (Update 2015; 1:CD005260).

92. Fleury AM, Salih SA, Peel NM. Rehabilitation of the older vascular amputee: A review of the literature. *Geriatr Gerontol Int.* 2013;13:264–273.

93. Christiansen CL, Fields T, Stephenson RO et al. Functional outcomes after the prosthetic training phase of rehabilitation after dysvascular lower extremity amputation. *PM R.* 2015;15:234–238.

23

Rehabilitation of the vascular amputee

SUJIN LEE and SOPHIA CHUN

CONTENTS

Sometimes the extremities become gangrenous…you must cut off that limb as far as the disease has spread, so that the patient may escape death or greater affliction, greater than the loss of the limb.

Albucasis, c. 1001 AD

INTRODUCTION

The vast majority of amputations are performed because the arteries of the legs have become blocked due to atherosclerosis. Amputations due to vascular disease accounted for the majority (82%) of limb loss discharges and increased from 38.30 per 100,000 people in 1988 to 46.19 per 100,000 people in 1996.[1] Lower-limb amputations accounted for 97% of all dysvascular limb loss discharges, of which 25.8% were at above-knee level, 27.6% at below-knee level and 42.8% involving numerous other levels. Between 1988 and 1996, there was an average of 133,735 hospital discharges for amputation per year.[1] Dysvascular amputations accounted for 82% of limb loss discharges and increased at a rate of 27% over the period studied. About 30%–40% of amputations are performed in patients with diabetes. Approximately 7% of patients will have an active ulcer or a healed ulcer. Ulcers are recurrent in many patients and approximately 5%–15% of diabetic patients with ulcers will ultimately require an amputation.[2] Because atherosclerosis occurs most commonly in older men who smoke, the majority of amputations for vascular disease occur in this group.[2] The discussions in this chapter will primarily cover the rehabilitation and prosthetic components for lower limb amputees.

Rehabilitation aims to facilitate recovery from loss of function. Rehabilitation may involve physical and occupational therapy; psychological counselling; and social services. For some patients, the goal is complete recovery with full, unrestricted function, e.g. complete independence with ambulation in person who underwent lower-extremity amputation; for others, it is recovery of the ability to do as many activities of daily living (ADLs) as possible. Results of rehabilitation depend on the nature of the loss and the patient's motivation. Progress may be slow for elderly patients and for patients who lack muscle strength or motivation.

Rehabilitation often begins in an acute care hospital. Rehabilitation hospitals or rehabilitation units usually provide the most extensive and intensive care and should be considered for patients who have good potential for recovery and can participate in and tolerate aggressive therapy (generally, ≥3 hours/day). Many nursing homes have less intensive programmes (generally, 1–3 hours/day, up to 5 days/week) that last longer and thus are better suited to patients less able to tolerate therapy (e.g. frail or elderly patients). Less varied and less frequent rehabilitation programmes may be offered in outpatient settings or at home and are appropriate for many patients. Intensive outpatient rehabilitation programme usually consists of several hours/day up to 5 days/week.

A rehabilitation programme for vascular amputee provided by a team of interdisciplinary providers (e.g. a physiatrist, physical therapists, occupational therapists, psychologist and social worker) represents an effective model to address the complex and interwoven medical, rehabilitation and psychosocial issues that face vascular amputees undergoing rehabilitation.

STAGES OF REHABILITATION

Preoperative phase

Successful rehabilitation of vascular amputee starts with thorough preoperative rehabilitation, medical and surgical assessment. Relevant aspects of the medical and surgical assessment for rehabilitation include the level of amputation, co-morbidities, assessment of psychosocial support, vocational or leisure activities and physical accessibility issues in the home and at work.

Preoperative rehabilitation evaluation should include a detailed history and a complete physical examination.

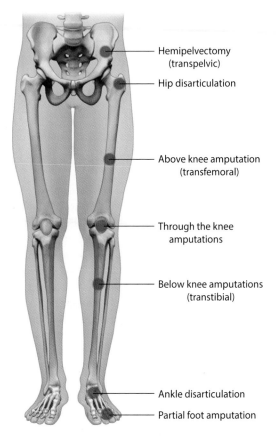

Figure 23.1 Levels of amputation. (From Levels of lower extremity amputations. http://www.cpousa.com/prosthetics/lower-extremity/, accessed August 21, 2016.)

Range of motion (ROM) and strength in the involved as well as in the noninvolved extremities, mobility, ambulation, self-care skill, social support and the patient's reaction to planned surgery should all be documented. Preoperative rehabilitation interventions include addressing issues with ROM, strengthening and cardiovascular function optimization. Treating identified contractures, assessing current ROM in joints above and on the contralateral side and education on importance of contracture prevention are essential. Assessment of preoperative strength deficits of upper extremity and lower extremity should also be performed. Preoperative home exercise programme should be determined to address identified deficits and maximize above ROM, strength, balance and cardiovascular function.

Important aspect of the preoperative medical and surgical assessment for vascular amputation is the concept of energy expenditure and preservation of limb length that is balanced with wound-healing ability and the potential for ambulation. A vascular surgery evaluation should be obtained to determine the feasibility of vascular reconstruction in the hopes of maintaining limb length. The higher the level of a lower-limb amputation, the greater the energy expenditure is required for walking.[3] See the image in the following to view the levels of amputation (Figure 23.1). As the level of the amputation moves proximally, the walking speed of the individual decreases, and the oxygen consumption increases.[4]

The velocity of the traumatic transtibial amputee is decreased by 20% with the speed of walking, and the energy expenditure was increased by 25% compared to the subjects without amputation.[5] The average measured gait velocity of dysvascular transtibial amputee however is decreased 44% with oxygen consumption increased to 33% over the distance walked. For transfemoral amputations, the energy required is 50%–65% greater than that required for those who have not undergone amputations. Additionally, those with peripheral vascular disease who have undergone transfemoral amputations may have cardiopulmonary or systemic disease and require maximal energy for walking, making independence difficult to maintain. Longer residual limbs have lower oxygen requirements than shorter residual limbs, ranging from 10% to 40% increase of oxygen consumption measured over the distance walked (Table 23.1).[6]

Table 23.1 Energy expenditure for amputation.

Amputation level	Energy above baseline (%)	Speed (m/min)	Oxygen cost (mL/kg/m)
Long transtibial	10	70	0.17
Average transtibial	25	60	0.20
Short transtibial	40	50	0.20
Bilateral transtibial	41	50	0.20
Transfemoral	65	40	0.28
Wheelchair	0–8	70	0.16

Sources: Waters RL et al., Energy expenditure of amputee gait, in *Lower Extremity Amputation*, Moore WS, Malone JM, eds., W. B. Saunders, Philadelphia, PA, 1989; pp. 250–260; Genin JJ et al., *Eur J Appl Physiol*, 103(6), 655, August 2008; Gonzales et al., *Arch Phys Med Rehabil*, 55, 111, 1974.

Assessment of wound healing is an important aspect of preoperative evaluation, especially in vascular amputation, as most amputations are performed for compromised circulation (e.g. peripheral vascular disease, damaged soft tissue involved in trauma). The integrity of the skin is an important factor in the ambulatory ability and ultimate outcome for the person who has undergone an amputation because the soft tissue end of the residual limb now becomes the proprioceptive end organ for the interface between the residual extremity and the prosthesis. For effective ambulation, the residual limb should consist of a sufficient mass of mobile nonadherent muscle and full-thickness skin and subcutaneous tissue that can accommodate axial and shear stress within the prosthetic socket. Split-thickness skin grafting is sometimes used to complete wound coverage or decrease tension on the wound closure while maintaining the limb length. However, most often these skin-grafted areas do not tolerate the axial and shear stresses within the prosthesis and may require removal at a later date, when the post-operative swelling has subsided.

Preoperative prosthetic assessment

Selecting and writing a prescription for the most appropriate prosthetic device for a dysvascular amputee has become as much of an art as a science. Revolution in prosthetic design, manufacture and fitting due to the introduction of new concepts in socket design as well as a wider array of components and new materials, including heat-mouldable plastics, lightweight metals and carbon fibre-reinforced plastics, has resulted in a multiplication of choices for prosthesis.

The first step in prosthetic prescription is prosthesis, are to enhance ambulation. Optional ambulation is accomplished by the virtue of the prosthetic providing balance, proprioceptive feedback and support for the body weight during the single limb phase of the gait cycle. In addition, the lower-limb prosthesis may allow for hands to be free for ADLs and other activities. For upper-limb amputee, motivation is a key factor to the success of fitting of the upper-limb prosthesis. While most bilateral upper-limb amputees find that prostheses enhance their function, for unilateral amputee, the prosthetic fitting is entirely optional at the discretion of the amputee especially when the amputee has become fully functional with one hand.

While no one should be excluded based on any one factor, it is important to assess the patient's cognition, motivation, goals and medical history. The patient should be assessed for their ability to learn, remember and solve problems. If a person has cognition problems to the degree that he/she might only be able to use a prosthesis with assistance from others, a prosthesis may not be a viable option if a dedicated caregiver cannot be readily identified. Level of motivation to use a prosthesis is an important factor for both determining whether to prescribe a prosthesis and in the prosthetic training phase. It is also important

to clearly define goals. Goals can be cosmetic to make a person feel like he or she looks better or goals can also be to increase function, such as for running or independence with household activities. A person with complex medical history, including chronic heart disease, lung disease, kidney disease, vascular disease and diabetes, may affect whether or not to use a prosthesis. For instance, a prosthesis may be contraindicated in persons with severe heart condition. In some cases, the fitting of bilateral dysvascular transfemoral amputees with articulated prosthese can be quite uncomfortably to sit in for prolonged periods and renders the device almost nonfunction. In addition, the device can be expensive and extremely difficult to walk with.[7] In such cases, there may be an opportunity for a focus on cosmetic restoration consisting of a lightweight cosmetic prostheses.

Some non-medical factors to consider for the choice of a prosthetic device including geographic remoteness without ready access to a prosthetist for maintenance, repair and replacement of a limb may dictate simplicity of design related to the need for self-repair of the device. Climate can also play an important role. In areas of excessive humidity, metal parts will tend to corrode and wood to rot. In areas of extreme aridity such as the desert regions of the world, fine sand particles will quickly wear out the joints of prostheses. The cost as well as limitations of benefits from the patient's insurance can be a limiting factor in determining the prescription. Fiscal limitations at the local and state levels may also mandate only a very simple prosthesis for indigent amputees, similar to those prescribed for amputees in the developing world. Local custom and knowledge are also powerful forces in determining prosthetic prescription in that they tend to limit the prescription options considered. Additional details on the prosthetic prescription and components are discussed in section on 'Special considerations for lower-limb prosthetic fitting' and 'Prosthetic components.'

Prosthetic decision should be made together with the patient and family and the interdisciplinary team that includes the amputation surgeon, the prosthetist who will be making the limb, a physiatrist, a therapist who will be providing the training in its use, a psychologist and/or social worker who will help the patient through his or her period of adjustment and the insurance nurse, especially in workmen's compensation cases. Loss of a visible part of one's body is devastating at any age. The new amputee typically experiences depression, and the response to amputation has been compared to the grieving process, to include stages of denial, anger, depression, coping and acceptance.[8] The patient's ultimate response to the psychological impact of limb loss is determined by many factors, including aetiology of amputation, patient's life experiences and ways of coping and reacting to catastrophic events, the quality of social support system available to this person and the comprehensive care provided by the prosthetic team. Amputation should be presented as a constructive option as it will end severe chronic intractable pain. The patient may also be unaware of the prosthetic options for future function and ambulation. If available, peer support or mentoring by an amputee who has successfully completed a rehabilitation programme may be an effective component that starts in the preoperative phase and continues to the end of the rehabilitation phase.

Acute post-operative phase

The main goals of acute post-operative phase are wound healing, initiation of residual limb management, pain control and emotional support. The physical examination should include evaluation of mental status, vision, peripheral vascular disease status, evaluation of the surgical incision site, skin condition, residual limb skin mobility, edema, indurations or tenderness and evaluation of any graft donor sites. ROM, joint stability, strength and sensation in all extremities should also be documented.

Wound healing is maximized by optimal nutrition, control of anemia and diabetes and appropriate antibiotic use. An open incision or wound should be covered by a Telfa pad and a sterile soft compressible dressing. The wound should be inspected regularly for odour, drainage, warmth, redness or dehiscence. For a diabetic patient, if baseline transcutaneous oxygen (T_cPO_2) is less than 40 mmHg on room air but exceeds 40 mmHg with 100% oxygen at 18TM for 20 minutes, the use of post-operative hyperbaric oxygen therapy should be considered. For non-diabetic patients, the critical value for T_cPO_2 is 30 mmHg.[9] Pinzur et al. have shown that T_cPO_2 values may be affected by the presence of infection and T_cPO_2 values increase after treating infection.[9]

Residual limb management includes the residual limb shrinkage and shaping process, which can be accomplished in one of several ways without compromising wound healing. Residual limb shrinkage and maturation permits prosthetic fit without requiring frequent changes in the size and configuration of the prosthetic socket. An ideal transtibial residual limb is cylindrical in shape, and an ideal transfemoral residual limb is conical. Residual limb management can be achieved by using different types of post-operative dressings such as soft, semi-rigid or rigid dressing. Soft dressing includes elastic bandage wraps, residual limb shrinkers and elastic stockinettes (Compressogrip; Knit Rite, Kansas City, MO). Elastic bandage is typically the least effective shrinking device because many patients do not master the wrapping technique, which requires considerable cooperation, skill and attention of the patient, family or medical staff. These wraps are done in a figure-8 configuration to avoid circumferential constriction with distal edema (Figure 23.2). These bandages are used for the transtibial limb, and double length 6 in. bandages are used for the transfemoral limb. Under this system of management, the time interval from amputation to prosthetic fit may take several months.

Elastic shrinker socks (or stump shrinkers) are easy to apply, provide uniform compression but are more expensive than elastic bandages. They should reach the

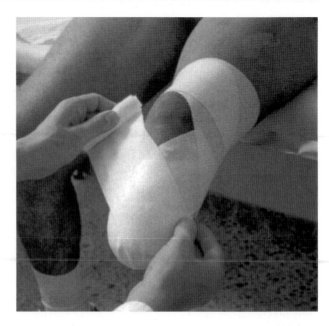

Figure 23.2 Elastic bandage wrapping. (From Blohmke F, *Otto Bock Prosthetic Compendium: Lower Extremity Prostheses*, Schiele & Schoen, Berlin, Germany, 1989.)

groin in the transfemoral amputee and should fit snugly. However, if they are not properly fitted and maintained, they can cause skin damage due to constriction. Patients who do not tolerate elastic wrap or shrinker socks may use Compressogrip socks. These elastic stockinettes are easy to apply and maintain. However, they can also cause skin damage if not properly donned or maintained.

Semi-rigid dressings are made of a fabric material impregnated with Unna paste. These are applied over the residual limb carefully to avoid proximal constriction. Studies have shown that initial immobilization and support with appropriate local pressure elevation of the injured limb will expedite healing and minimize edema.[10] These dressings should be changed every 2–3 days or less frequently, depending upon the condition of the wound.

Rigid dressing use in post-operative amputee management was revived by Berlemont[11] in France, by Weiss[12] in Poland and by Burgess in the United States.[13] The post-operative plaster or fibreglass rigid dressing prevents edema, protects from trauma and decreases post-operative pain. The goal of rigid dressing is to provide a therapeutic degree of terminal pressure and a relatively sterile dry wound surface with no restriction to tissue fluid exchanges.[13] Rigid dressings are the preferred method of residual limb care but require an experienced team. Rigid dressings consist of a plaster cast applied in the operating room immediately after surgery. The distal end is covered with soft absorbent material, and then the entire residual limb is placed in an elastic sock to prevent post-operative edema. Bony prominences are protected by using felt pads and an elastic plaster bandage, and then non-elastic plaster is applied. Suspension straps can be secured to the rigid dressing. Post-operative edema occurs within a few minutes, so immediate replacement of a dressing is mandatory.

Rigid dressing can be non-removable or removable. The non-removable rigid dressing is applied immediately after surgery in the operating room and is typically taken off and changed every 5–10 days after surgery.[14] The rigid removable dressing can be taken off and replaced whenever the wound needs to be viewed. The rigid removable dressing provides good edema control with the advantage of allowing daily inspection. Rigid dressing provides protection to the limb against trauma, in case of a fall, and it can also serve as a temporary socket to which prosthetic components can be attached to form an early post-operative prosthesis. In dysvascular amputees, early weight bearing may delay wound healing.

The amputee should wear the shrinkage device 24 hours a day, except for very short period of time for bathing or ventilating sores. A shrinkage device can be discontinued after fitting with a definitive prosthesis if the residual limb has become stabilized and the patient is wearing the prosthesis on a regular basis. However, it may still be used at night if nocturnal edema occurs.

Pain control: The initial residual limb pain is expected due to acute post-operative nerve fibre damage and ongoing stimulation of the nerve secondary to surgical incision and post-operative edema.[15] For acute post-operative pain, intravenous or intramuscular opiates are widely used and known to be effective. Acute post-operative pain usually subsides with edema control and surgical wound healing, and the need of intravenous opiate use can be discontinued within 2–3 days after the surgery. After this period, scheduled dose of oral opiates with as-needed doses can be continued for sub-acute phase of post-operative pain, with the goal of slow weaning of opiates.

Desensitization technique is an important non-pharmacological intervention that can be started within a few days after surgery to control acute/sub-acute post-operative pain and phantom sensation. The patient or a therapist can start providing sensory stimulation to the residual limb by massaging and tapping. The hypothesized mechanism of action of desensitization is that gentle stimulation can overflow the 'pain gait' to minimize the signalling of pain sensation.[16] In addition to pain control, desensitization technique can help the patient to develop a habit of taking care of his residual limb, to form a new body image and psychological adjustment to the limb loss.

Pre-prosthetic phase

Pre-prosthetic phase of rehabilitation starts with surgical wound closure and continues during and after wound healing. Many of the goals of pre-prosthetic phase overlap with those of acute post-surgical phase. While promoting wound healing, pain control, the residual limb management and providing psychological support, exercise for amputees focusing on flexibility, muscle strength, cardiovascular conditioning and balance should be initiated.

EXERCISE FOR AMPUTEE

As soon as the patient is medically and surgically stable, general endurance and strengthening exercise should be started in order to promote stabilization of muscles that will be used for ambulation with prosthesis and to prevent joint contracture. Strengthening upper extremity and improving balance are also essential for prosthetic use to accommodate transfers, wheelchair propulsion and ambulation with crutches or walker if needed. The main components of exercise for amputee include flexibility, muscle strength, cardiovascular conditioning and balance to optimize the patient's condition for prosthetic use.[17]

Flexibility: Maintaining flexibility in the residual and the intact limb is crucial to successful prosthetic use. A post-operative contracture may develop rapidly if proper care is not initiated immediately after the amputation. The residual limb needs to be placed in an extended position as much as possible when the patient is in bed and/or in a wheelchair. In order to avoid contractures, a pillow should not be placed under the knee joint, and the head of the bed should not be elevated for prolonged periods of time. Prolonged, low-load hip flexor stretch can be achieved by lying prone for extended period of time.[18] Prone lying programme should be initiated with a maximal amount of time of patient's comfort and increased gradually each day.

Along with positioning programme, the patient can be instructed to perform self-stretches by bringing one knee towards his/her chest while extending the opposite leg in supine position. Each leg is held in this position for 30 seconds with minimal five repetitions. Once the patient learns the correct technique, he/she can be instructed to repeat this stretching exercise three to five sessions a day. This provides easy and effective hip flexor and extensor stretches.[19] A stretching programme for the intact limb emphasizes the adequate ROM at the ankle, the knee and the hip. Especially patients with vascular disease can develop foot deformity in the intact limb due to limited ambulation after the amputation. This can be prevented by daily gastrocnemius soleus stretching with towel pulls while sitting or while standing with a proper foot wear and upper-extremity support for balance.[17]

Muscle strength: Muscles in residual limb need to be retrained not only as primary functional movers but also as major force distributing muscles at the socket–limb interface.[17] Electromyogram biofeedback can be used for volitional firing of specific muscle groups depending on the level of amputation.[20] Gastrocnemius soleus group, peroneal and pretibial muscles for the transtibial amputation, and residual hamstring, quadriceps, hip adductors and abductor muscle groups for the transfemoral amputation are considered to be appropriate muscles for electromyogram biofeedback.

A comprehensive total-body strengthening programme to achieve proximal stability and distal mobility can begin by the end of post-operative week 1.[17] The DeLorme protocol, a progressive resistance training programme with three sets of each ten repetitions at 50%, 75% and 100% of maximum strength, can be followed.[21] The lower-extremity exercise programme should include bilateral hip abductor (gluteus medius), hip extensors (gluteus maximus) and knee extensor (quadriceps) strengthening. Both upper-extremity shoulder depressors and wrist and elbow extensors are also strengthened for crutch or assistive device ambulation to allow improved functional gait ability in lower extremity amputees.[22]

Cardiovascular conditioning: Cardiovascular conditioning is recommended during preoperative phase and needs to be initiated as early as possible during post-operative phase. As described in the previous section, the energy expenditure during ambulation significantly increases as the level of amputation gets proximal. Low-impact aerobic activities can be initiated once the patient is medically and surgically stable, following the basic fitness principles targeting heart rate ranges 50%–65% of maximum heart rate for low-to-moderate intensity and 65%–85% of maximum heart rate for moderate-to-high intensity.[23] The cardiovascular conditioning exercise programme may start as 10 minutes of continuous activity, with the goal of 30–40 minutes of continuous aerobic exercise.[24]

Cardiovascular conditioning with ambulation may not be an optimal option for recent lower-extremity amputees with severe post-operative pain, limited functional mobility and unprotected wound. For these patients, the use of upper-body ergometer or the VersaClimber can be an alternative choice. The upper-body ergometer allows patients to perform clockwise and counterclockwise arm movement on a device similar to a bicycle wheel mechanism.[25] The VersaClimber is a vertically oriented device that allows patients to perform up-and-down climbing motion involving one or both lower and upper extremities.[17]

Balance: Adequate single-leg stance balance and stability with the intact limb in unilateral lower-extremity amputation is essential for safe and functional ambulation without the use of prosthesis and to prepare for gait training with prosthesis.[26] The balance training begins with upper-extremity supported stance with the intact limb and progresses to unilateral standing balance without upper-extremity support. Early weight-bearing activity on the residual limb prepares for prosthetic use and also is known to reduce residual and phantom limb pain.[27]

SPECIAL CONSIDERATIONS FOR LOWER-LIMB PROSTHETIC FITTING

Bilateral above-knee amputees: Stubbies are basic non-articulated (no knee joint) transfemoral sockets with rocker bottoms and appropriate suspension that can be used for new bilateral above-knee amputees. The benefit of not including a knee joint for a new bilateral above-knee amputation, is that the shorter prostheses reduce the amputee's over height, reduce impact in a tumble, and require less energy expenditure. Using stubbies can reduce heart rate and oxygen use by 7%–23% and can increase walking speed by up

to 25%.[28] They are particularly helpful in the early stages of rehabilitation, since they can help to prevent contracture and promote healing in the residual limb. Stubbies also allow the prosthetic user to master one prosthetic joint at a time: initially the ankle/foot, with the subsequent addition of the prosthetic knee unit, while building upper-body strength, which is crucial for bilateral above-knee amputees and also is used to determine if the bilateral above-knee amputee is a prosthetic candidate. Stubbies can include a variety of foot designs, ranging from standard prosthetic ankle/feet to rocker bottom platforms. If standard prosthetic feet are to be utilized, they are often set in a backward position, with the heels facing the front. This is to help prevent the amputee from falling backwards. Rocker bottoms, although not realistic, offer greater anterior and posterior horizontal support equally. This increased ground level support provides an increased level of stability for the user. For those eventually adding prosthetic knee units to the prostheses, additional gait training and therapy are highly indicated. Of note, patient with above-knee prostheses will use other assistive devices, such as crutches, walker for increased stability and wheelchairs for long-distance mobility in addition to the prosthesis.

Hip disarticulation: Hip disarticulation procedures are typically done on younger trauma or tumour patient and they often become community ambulators. In some, the slower speed of prosthetic walking compared to wheelchair results in preference of a wheelchair for longer-distance mobility. Crutches without prosthesis or prosthesis with a cane are options for shorter-distance mobility.

Age: Age should not be a factor in determining the fitting of unilateral or bilateral lower-limb prostheses. Many very elderly patients can be successfully fitted at the transtibial or Syme ankle disarticulation levels provided that they are physiologically sound and have sufficient mental capacity to comprehend the subtleties of sock adjustment for changes in residual limb volume. In borderline cases, lower-limb transtibial amputees should be fitted with inexpensive preparatory prostheses to realistically assess their potential for ambulation.

Importance of prompt and early fitting in dysvascular foot amputation: Delaying prosthetic fitting and training of the unilateral dysvascular amputee in order to prevent stress to the remaining foot will result in deconditioning. Even in patients who may need a second amputation of the other foot, early fitting is crucial because the patient may become deconditioned rendered to not be a prosthetic candidate and because patient with a unilateral prosthesis immediately fitted after each surgery has a better chance of success in learning to use a prosthesis than simultaneous fitting as a bilateral amputee.

Diabetic, blind or hemiplegic amputee: Diabetes mellitus, blindness and hemiplegia pose additional considerations for lower-limb prosthetic fitting. A blind unilateral or bilateral Syme ankle disarticulates or transtibial

Table 23.2 Patient issues to consider when prescribing a prosthesis.

Co-morbidity factors, such as cardiac, pulmonary.

Residual limb length – a longer residual limb requires less energy expenditure.

Skin and soft tissue/joint contractures, especially of the proximal joints, may preclude prosthetic fit.

Musculoskeletal problems.

Cognitive function and ability to follow directions.

Vocation/avocation.

Premorbid lifestyle, active or sedentary, as this will dictate the components that are chosen for this particular individual.

amputee should be able to walk about in familiar surroundings but may be safer with a helper for community ambulation. Additional caution should be taken for fitting of blind unilateral or bilateral above-knee amputee as there is loss of proprioceptive knee function. Patients with hemiparesis following a cerebrovascular accident can often walk with their transtibial prostheses provided that they have adequate mentation and balance and no disruptive spasticity or severe extensor or flexor patterning. Other issues to consider are noted in Table 23.2.

Prosthetic training phase

The prosthetic training phase begins when the patient starts using his or her prescribed and fabricated prosthesis. In the early prosthetic training phase, the frequent skin check is necessary to prevent skin breakdown and to correct any socket-fit problem. The daily inspection of residual limb should become a lifelong practice to prevent complication from the amputation and prosthesis use.

Tolerance of prosthetic use should increase gradually during this phase with the goal of prosthetic use during all walking hours. Along with gait training with the prosthesis, flexibility, muscle strength and endurance, and balance and coordination training should be continued. In addition, the proper care for the residual limb should be emphasized throughout the rehabilitation process.

Flexibility: The patient should continue the self-stretching programme learned during pre-prosthetic phase, since the patient can develop hip and/or knee flexion contracture even with prosthetic use. In addition, a weight-bearing stretch programme can be introduced, while incorporating the prosthesis. Hip stretching can be achieved by a long stretch, where the patient kneels on one leg and leans forward allowing the hip extension of the kneeling limb.[17] A standing hamstring stretch can be achieved by placing one limb forward of the other and then bending the trunk towards the forward placed limb. Ankle dorsiflexion of the intact limb can be accomplished by placing the intact limb in the position of knee and hip extension while the foot is kept flat on the ground.[17]

Muscle strength and endurance: The foundation of prosthetic ambulation is the ability of the residual limb with a prosthesis to sustain functional weight bearing during the single-limb stance of the gait cycle. A pre-gait programme focusing on the safety of standing with parallel bars is the first step to establish this foundation. During this pre-gait programme, the patient learns a sense of equilibrated base support and weight-shifting skills necessary for gait.[17]

Balance and coordination: Patients with new amputation feel insecure when they try to balance without upper-extremity support, mainly due to loss of the direct proprioceptive inputs and sensory feedback from the missing limb and improper hip reactions on the residual limb with a prosthesis.[29] In addition to balance training started in pre-prosthetic phase, the training continues by challenging the patients out of their base of support and then manually placing their hip into balanced position.[30]

Community integration and vocational rehabilitation phase

Once the patient makes appropriate progress during prosthetic training, he or she can make transition to community integration and vocational rehabilitation. Community integration focuses on the patient's returning to family and community, recreational activities and establishing emotional stability and developing healthy coping strategies.

Vocational rehabilitation phase often closely overlaps with community integration process and emphasizes on assessment and training for vocational activities, assessment of further education needs or job modification.[17] The safety of the patient should be always the priority, and this may impose limitations in physically demanding occupations. In general, most of amputees are advised not to walk or climb to heights exceeding 4 ft, the transtibial-level amputees are advised not to lift or transport more than 40 lb, and the transfemoral-level amputees no more than 25 lb.

Many active amputees participate in various types of recreational activities; activities of low-to-moderate intensity include gardening, walking, golfing, bicycling and swimming,[31] and activities of moderate-to-high intensity include running, aerobic dance, weightlifting, water and downhill skiing and racquet and team sports.[32] For any type of activities, the patient needs to be evaluated and medically cleared in order to participate appropriate activity based on his/her medical condition. Also, properly fitting prosthesis or special sport-specific prosthetic device (e.g. for running or skiing) and properly fitting footwear for the intact limb are critical for any amputees involving various activities.[33]

Long-term follow-up

Once the patient finishes a comprehensive rehabilitation programme, at least every 3 months' follow-up is recommended for the first 18 months by one of the team members.[17] Every 6 months' follow-up is recommended with a physician until the patient establishes stable prosthetic use. Once the patient establishes a stable prosthetic use, every 6 months to 12 months' follow-up is needed for regular lifelong prosthetic preventive maintenance. Prosthetic preventive maintenance visit includes assessment of the residual limb changes in volume as a result of muscle atrophy and weight gain or loss and check of prostheses for maintenance, repair and periodic replacement. Replacement may also be indicated as improved designs appear from time to time.

PHANTOM PAIN

Phantom limb pain is a noxious sensory phenomenon of the missing limb that can be problematic immediately after the amputation procedure and continues to be problematic in the long term. According to a recent study, 72% of amputations lead to phantom limb pain about 1 week after amputation, and 60% of amputees still have phantom pain 6 months later. Phantom limb pain was first described by Ambrose Pare (1510–1590).[34] The American neurologist Silas Mitchell (1829–1914) published his article on phantom limb anonymously in a non-scientific journal.[35] It is important to differentiate between phantom limb sensation and phantom limb pain because their management strategies are different.

Phantom limb sensation is the sensory perception of a missing limb that does not include pain. It is a common occurrence in virtually all amputees. It is usually most prominent in the early post-operative period. And the patient should be reassured that it is a normal occurrence as the cerebral pathways serving the amputated segment are still functioning. Phantom limb sensation involves sensation of willed spontaneous movement, itching, temperature and pressure. The amputee may experience all of the normal limb sensations. It occurs most common in distal limbs, which are more richly innervated. The phantom limb usually undergoes a process of telescoping, where it may shrink, and the digits of the phantom foot become attached to the end of the residual limb and may completely dissipate in 1 year.[36] Residual limb stump pain is distinct from phantom limb pain and is present in the region of amputation. It usually subsides in a few weeks after surgery.

Phantom limb pain is a noxious sensory phenomenon of the missing limb. It may be a burning or throbbing pain, or it may be an abnormal ischemic discomfort. In this situation, the phantom limb does not undergo telescoping. According to a recent study, 72% of amputations lead to phantom limb pain about 1 week after amputation, and 60% of amputees still have phantom pain 6 months later.[37]

The pathophysiology of phantom pain and sensation is not completely understood, and different mechanisms, as noted in the following, have been proposed:

1. Peripheral nerves are involved in the generation of phantom pain, e.g. neuroma from regenerating neurons might contribute to phantom limb sensation. However, this does not explain the phenomenon entirely. The sympathetic nervous system has also been implicated in phantom limb sensation. In the sympathetic efferent–somatic afferent cycle, input from the cortex excites sympathetic neurons in the spinal cord, which excite postganglionic noradrenergic cutaneous vasoconstrictor and cholinergic sudomotor fibres in the residual limb. These result in decreased blood flow to the residual limb and the perception of phantom limb sensation. Pain occurs if certain nociceptors of primary afferents are abnormally activated.[38] It is known that stress and anxiety can exacerbate phantom limb sensation and pain, while distraction, attention and diversion can reduce phantom limb sensation.

2. Loss of efferent nerves through spinal cord lesions or root avulsion causes disinhibition of dorsal root neurons, allowing transmission of phantom pian.[39]

3. Melzack has proposed a supraspinal (central) origin consisting of a neuromatrix and loops between the cortex and thalamus, as well as a cortical and limbic system.[40] The neuromatrix impact is a neurosignature on all sensory inputs or experiences. Sensory inputs modulating the neurosignature are converted to an ever-changing awareness by the sentient neural hub. Melzack states that without the inhibitory input, increased firing of spinal cells above the amputee level can trigger the neuromatrix. The overactive neuromatrix then interacts with the sentient neural hub, producing a burning, cramping pain. A corollary for the central origin of phantom limb pain states that the ensuing pain is actually a 'memory' of pain in the limb before amputation. It is well known that patients who have protracted pain in the limb before amputation develop phantom limb pain.

Treatment: Treatment of phantom pain is difficult and unsatisfactory. Some aggravating and relieving factors are noted (see Table 23.3). Sherman, in a 1980 review of phantom pain treatment, revealed 68 types of phantom pain treatment modalities in use for phantom limb treatment, but the success rate was only slightly above 30%, which is near the placebo response.[41]

Medical treatment: The use of low-dose tricyclic antidepressants (amitriptyline, imipramine, doxepin or other drugs) may achieve symptom reduction in the early postoperative period. Residual limb percussion, vibration or intense massage can help in desensitization and alleviation of pain. ROM exercises and residual limb wrapping of soft elastic or rigid dressing are helpful. Transcutaneous electrical nerve stimulation can be successful in some cases. Biofeedback and relaxation training may be beneficial.[42] Wearing a well-fitted prosthesis has been found to alleviate phantom limb pain. Other treatments that have been tried include dorsal column stimulation and various neurosurgical ablative procedures. Bach et al.[43] studied a group of dysvascular patients who were to undergo amputation under epidural anesthesia. All of them had pain for 1–6 months. These patients received continuous epidural analgesia for 3 days prior to amputation. Post amputation, none of these

Table 23.3 Factors that aggravate or relieve phantom pain.

Phantom pain aggravating factors	Relieving factors
Emotional stress	Emotional relaxation
Lack of sleep	Rest, sleep
Cold or warm weather changes	Massage, percussion, electrical stimulation
Yawning, coughing	Exercise, manipulation of residual limb
Ill-fitting prosthesis	Well-fitted prosthesis

patients had phantom limb sensation, and only 27% had phantom limb pain, which disappeared in 6 months.

PROSTHETIC COMPONENTS

General understanding of prosthetic components is an important concept to ensure that the most appropriate type of prosthesis is prescribed for the vascular amputees. A prosthetic device is a collection of component parts. Most common prosthetic devices include transtibial and transfemoral prosthetic system based on the amputation level. Both of prosthetic devices have the following components:

1. Socket: to hold the residual limb and transmit body weight to the floor.
2. Shanks: supporting systems can be exoskeletal versus endoskeletal system.
3. Suspension systems: to keep the prosthetic device on the body.
4. Joints: foot and ankle in transtibial amputation and foot, ankle and knee in transfemoral amputation (Figure 23.3).

In general, a prosthetic device can be classified as exoskeletal or endoskeletal system. The *exoskeletal system* is characterized by a hard, plastic, laminated outer shell. Its advantage is durability, but less cosmetically acceptable, and adjustments to the internal surface structure of the prosthesis are very difficult. The exoskeletal prosthesis may also weigh a little more than its endoskeletal counterpart. The *endoskeletal system* is characterized by a metal or plastic pylon covered by a soft polyurethane foam that is contoured to the shape of the sound leg. The advantage of the endoskeletal system is it is more cosmetically appealing. In addition, the internal structures can be easily accessed by removal of the polyurethane cover, and the components can be easily interchanged. The pylon allows easy length adjustments, and the assembly is quicker because of the prefabricated modules. There is also a very slight decrease in weight, especially for transfemoral and hip disarticulation amputation levels. The disadvantage of the endoskeletal system is that the cosmetic cover is much less durable than the plastic laminated of the exoskeletal construction.

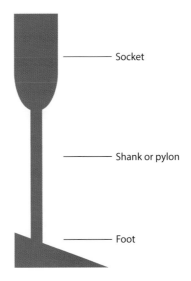

Figure 23.3 Components of a typical prosthesis.

— Socket

— Shank or pylon

— Foot

Sockets

TRANSTIBIAL PROSTHETIC SOCKETS

Prosthetic sockets support the residual limb and transmit forces from the residual limb to control the prosthesis. There are two types of transtibial sockets available. The most commonly used transtibial socket is the patellar tendon bearing (PTB) socket (Figure 23.4). It consists of a laminated or moulded plastic socket with the anterior wall extending proximal to and encapsulating the distal third of the patella. Just below the patella, at the middle of the patellar ligament, is an inner contour or bar, which is one of the major weight-bearing surfaces in the socket. However, weight is also borne on the flares of the tibia and on either side of the tibial crest. Medial and lateral walls extend proximally to above the condyles of the femur. The distal portion of the PTB socket may incorporate a soft end pad to prevent distal edema by aiding venous and lymphatic return while walking. The proper fitting should provide adequate pressure relief. However, a soft inner socket liner made of silicone gel or polyurethane foam can be used to provide comfort and skin protection. The other type of socket is total surface bearing socket, which uses suction and distributes the weight over the entire stump circumference with reduced pressure against the patellar tendon.[44]

In 1982, Kristinsson of Iceland proposed a flexible socket design for above-the-knee sockets.[45] It was developed in Sweden, and later a below-the-knee counterpart was developed in New York. In this design, an inner socket is fabricated from flexible polyethylene or a similar material, which is then inserted into a rigid plastic laminated, thermoplastic or carbon fibre-reinforced frame. The frame covers the primary weight-bearing areas, while the soft tissue and pressure-sensitive areas not requiring rigid support are enclosed in the flexible socket. The advantages of the flexible socket rigid frame

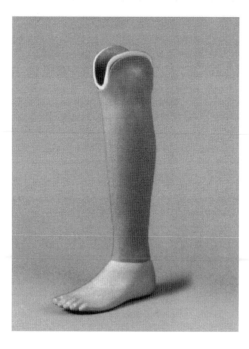

Figure 23.4 PTB socket. (From Blohmke F, *Otto Bock Prosthetic Compendium: Lower Extremity Prostheses*, Schiele & Schoen, Berlin, Germany, 1989.)

are decreased weight, increased comfort, improved heat dissipation and ease of replacement of the inner socket to accommodate minor anatomical changes. It is, however, more time consuming and difficult to fabricate, is more expensive and is considered by some to be less cosmetic.

Since the socket is the interface between the prosthesis and the residual limb, ideally, every socket should be custom-made based on the size, shape and condition of the residual limb and the degree of mobility required. Currently, computer-aided design/computer-assisted manufacturing (CAD/CAM) is used to build custom-made sockets. CAD/CAM technology can be used either as an adjunct or as an alternative to traditional methods of prosthetic fabrication. Computerized equipment can provide a positive computer model of the residual limb, which can be modified on a computer by the prosthetist. This system not only helps in designing a custom-made socket but also provides quantitative data regarding load transfer between the residual limb and the socket, which enables objective evaluation of the fit.[46]

Transfemoral prosthetic sockets

Transfemoral sockets usually provide contact of the socket over the entire residual limb including the distal end. Quadrilateral and ischial containment are the two types of transfemoral sockets. The term quadrilateral refers to the appearance of the transfemoral socket when viewed in the transverse plane because it has four distinguishable walls (Figure 23.5a). Weight bearing in the quadrilateral socket is achieved primarily through the

ischium and the gluteal musculature. The combination of skeletal and muscle anatomy rests on the top of the posterior wall of the socket, which is formed into a wide seat and is parallel to the ground. The anterior wall, especially the medial third, is carefully fitted against Scarpa's triangle and maintains the ischium and gluteals on the ischial seat. The anterior/posterior diameter of the socket walls is based on the anatomic measurements. The lateral wall is slightly higher than the medial wall, and proximal to the greater trochanter the lateral wall is contoured above the hip abductors to discourage abduction. The entire lateral wall is flattened against the shaft of the adducted femur, with the exception of the laterally projected relief for the terminal aspect of the femur. The medial wall is designed to provide even pressure on adductor muscles and contains all medial tissues to prevent an adductor roll. The quadrilateral socket is designed with initial flexion to improve the ability of the amputee to control knee stability at the heel contact and to help minimize the development of lumbar lordosis at toe-off.

The ischial containment socket narrow medial–lateral design, also known as normal shape, normal alignment,[47] is narrower mediolaterally and wider anteroposteriorly (Figure 23.5b). In this design, the ischium and/or the ischial ramus is enclosed inside the socket. The primary weight bearing in the ischial containment socket is focused primarily through the medial aspect of the ischium and the ramus. Additional weight-bearing support is provided by the gluteal muscles and the lateral aspect of the femur distal to the greater trochanter. In addition, the pressure is evenly distributed over the entire surface of the residual limb. More residual surface and volume are contained within the ischial containment socket, as compared to the quadrilateral socket, resulting in greater force distribution and lower pressures exerted within an ischial containment design.

It has been hypothesized that a quadrilateral socket is displaced laterally during mid-stance and thus results in a shearing force on the perineal tissues. Femoral abduction occurs, decreasing the effectiveness of the gluteus medius muscle.[48] In an ischial containment socket, the medial brim of the socket is extended upwards until the pressure is brought to bear against the ischial ramus, resulting in a bony lock between the ischium, trochanter and lateral aspect of the femur, providing a much more stable mechanism and resulting in increased comfort in the groin and better control of the pelvis and the trunk. It is generally believed that ischial containment sockets are desirable for short, flabby residual limbs with weak abductors. Many amputees report increased comfort and function with an ischial containment socket.

Kristinsson cited the advantages of a flexible brim for sockets, stating that a transition between the necessary rigidity of the socket structure and flexibility of the body tissue at and just proximal to the socket brim is very helpful.[45] The socket brim can be either fully or partially flexible. This type of socket design can be either quadrilateral or ischial containment and uses a flexible thermo-moulded plastic inner socket with a rigid or semi-rigid frame.

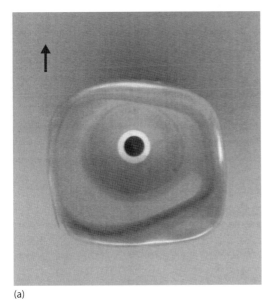
(a)

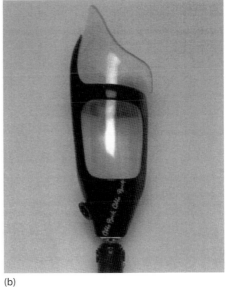
(b)

Figure 23.5 (a) Quadrilateral socket. (b) Ischial containment socket. (From Blohmke F, *Otto Bock Prosthetic Compendium: Lower Extremity Prostheses,* Schiele & Schoen, Berlin, Germany, 1989.)

Suspension systems

SUSPENSION SYSTEMS IN TRANSTIBIAL PROSTHESIS

A suspension system is required to keep the prosthesis from falling off the residual limb during the swing phase of the gait cycle. Two types of suspension systems, mechanical suspension and suction suspension systems, are used in transtibial prosthesis (Table 23.4).

Mechanical (skeletal grasp) suspension system

A mechanical suspension can be achieved using cuffs, sleeves, socket modification or thigh corset. In *cuff suspension*, a supracondylar cuff is attached to the medial and lateral socket walls and circles the thigh above the femoral condyles. The attachment point on the socket is slightly posterior to the midsagittal line in order to resist hyperextension forces to the knee and allows them to withdraw slightly from the socket during knee flexion. It does not totally eliminate relative motion between the residual limb and socket but is simple, is easily adjustable and provides adequate suspension for most amputees. The exception is a very short or painful residual limb, with a tendency towards mediolateral knee instability.

Sleeve suspension is a neoprene or a latex material sleeve that is pulled over the prosthesis and extends above the patient's knee. The suspension sleeves are very effective but do not provide enough stability for a very short residual limb or in patients with mediolateral instability. Other disadvantages include increased perspiration and heat under the sleeve and the need for good hand dexterity and strength to toll the sleeve up and down for donning and doffing.

The thigh corset is attached to the socket and the prosthetic shank by sidebars and knee joints. Sometimes a flexible waist belt and a folk strap assembly are added. Thigh corsets are not very commonly used.

Supracondylar suspension employs higher medial and lateral walls than in PTB design, which encompass the femoral condyles fully and has a proximal, smaller mediolateral diameter. Therefore, the prosthesis does not slip over the epicondyles. The most common method is to build a compressible contoured proximal medial build-up, also called a medial wedge suspension. This wedge can be either removable or non-removable, and it can be built either into the proximal socket wall or into the soft socket insert. The medial wedge supracondylar suspension eliminates the need for a cuff and provides firmer suspension with less pistoning. It also provides improved mediolateral stability and rotational control because it holds the knee above the epicondyles. This is the preferred suspension for a short residual limb, but the disadvantages are that it is more difficult to fabricate and the proximal brim protrudes above the flexed thigh in a seated position, making it less cosmetic.

In supracondylar/suprapatellar or SC/SP suspension, medial, lateral and anterior walls are high and enclose the entire patella. Any tendency for genu recurvatum is resisted because of the enclosure of the patella, and it is therefore used in a very short residual limb. The disadvantages include more difficult fabrication and the fact that the entire anterior brim of the SC/SP protrudes while sitting.

Suction (atmospheric) suspension system

Atmospheric suction suspension systems are considered to be the preferred form of suspension in lower-limb prosthetics because they provide the best suspension and virtually eliminate any motion between the residual limb and the socket. The ROM of the knee is preserved, as is the

Table 23.4 Transtibial suspension methods.

Mechanical (skeletal grasp)	Advantages	Disadvantages	General indications
Extrinsic cuff	Simple and easily adjustable. Easy to don and doff. Some control of knee. Hyperextension	Slight pistoning. No mediolateral control	Anticipated volume fluctuation
Over-the-knee sleeve	Simple and effective. Good auxiliary suspension	No mediolateral or hyperextension control. Heal and perspiration. May interfere with knee flexion. May be difficult to don	Need for auxiliary suspension during sports or other heavy activities
Thigh corset knee joint	Can unload residuum. Maximal mediolateral and hyperextension control	Pistoning. Heavy, bulky, cumbersome. Thigh atrophy	Painful, sensitive residuum. Unstable knee joint
Intrinsic supracondylar	Excellent suspension. Adds mediolateral and rotational control	Condylar fit must be precise	Shorter residua. Mild mediolateral knee instability
Supracondylar/ suprapatellar	As above, but adds recurvatum control	As above. Poor sitting cosmesis	As above. Recurvatum
Atmospheric (suction) roll-on sleeve	Secure suspension with minimal pistoning. Prosthesis feels lighter and more natural	May be difficult to don. Some discomfort with knee flexion	Preferred suspension but requires residuum of adequate length with stable volume and good skin
Hypobaric	As above. Ease of donning. Uses fabric socks which aid hygiene, comfort and ability to maintain fit	Shorter, sharply tapered residua are difficult to fit	As above

Source: Kristinsson O, *Orthot Prosthet*, 37, 25–27, 1983.

total contact throughout gait cycle. Because of the intimate fit and suspension, the prosthesis feels lighter, more natural and easier to control. However, it does require adequate length of the residual limb, stable volume and healthy skin condition. It is difficult to fabricate and fit.

The ICElandic Roll-On Silicone Socket was developed in the 1980s. The silicone sleeve is fitted very closely to the amputee's residual limb so that air is occluded and a very effective suspension is maintained throughout the gait, despite minor changes. The roll-on sleeve is a prefabricated liner that is first turned inside out and is then positioned on the end of the residual limb and rolled on proximally over the knee. It is then secured to the socket by means of a shuttle lock, in which a pin at the end of the silicone liner automatically engages with a spring-loaded plastic mechanism located at the bottom of the prosthetic socket. A release button is placed into the socket, which will permit doffing of the prosthesis. Currently, some other variations or combinations of roll-on sleeve and distal locking mechanisms are popular methods to suspend transtibial prosthesis.

The hypobaric suction system consists of a 1-inch-wide silicone band, which is impregnated into the stump sock or stump sheath. It has an automatic air release valve. The band is slightly lubricated and then is placed over the residual limb. The entrapped air is then forced out through the valve, thereby creating a vacuum. As the patient ambulates during the swing phase, the suction developed within the distal liner prevents any displacement. For the hypobaric

suspension system to work, the residual limb should be longer than 5 in. and muscular, and the patient should have a nicely contoured residual limb.

SUSPENSION SYSTEM IN TRANSFEMORAL PROSTHESIS

Suspension system in transfemoral prosthesis includes mechanical and suction (see Table 23.5). *Mechanical (skeletal grasp) suspension system* includes total elastic suspension (TES) belt, Silesian belt and hip joint and pelvic band. TES belt is a supplemental suspension system that may be used when full suction suspension system is compromised due to the residual limb contours and condition or age of the amputee. A TES is made of a neoprene type of material and can be added over the prosthetic socket. It is easy to don and comfortable. *Silesian belt* is a soft belt made of cotton webbing, leather or Dacron. It is attached to a pivot point on a socket in the area of the greater trochanter and passes around the back as a belt on the opposite iliac crest, where it achieves most of its suspension. Anteriorly, its attachment is either a singular point or, in some cases, double attachment points. *Hip joint and pelvic band* provides rotational stability and a significant mediolateral pelvic stability. However, it is not used very often.

Suction (atmospheric) suspension system includes traditional suction suspension and traditional partial or semi-suction. *Traditional suction suspension system* requires an air seal to make the prosthetic socket airtight and usually includes a distally located one-way valve through

Table 23.5 Transfemoral suspension methods.

	Advantages	Disadvantages	General indications
Mechanical (skeletal grasp)			
TES belt	Simple and effective auxiliary suspension	See 'Silesian bandage' above, plus occasional heat and perspiration problems. Limited durability	As above
Silesian bandage	Adds to retention security. Some rotational control. Easy to don and doff	No mediolateral control	Simple adjunct to suction. Provides additional physical and/or psychological security
Hip joint and pelvic belt	Very secure mechanical suspension. Maximum mediolateral and rotational control. Easy to don and doff	Increased pistoning. Restricted hip mobility. Bulky and cumbersome. Some sitting discomfort	For weak, elderly and/or obese patients. Essentially limited to non-suction wearers
Atmospheric (suction)			
Traditional 'full' suction	No restriction of hip motion by straps or belts around torso. Feels lighter and more natural	Undersized socket difficult to don requiring 'pulling in' or 'wet tit'. Some hygiene, comfort and adjustability problems	Younger, more active and agile amputees. Volumetrically stable residua of adequate length
Traditional 'partial' suction	Larger socket permits 'pushing in', hence easier donning, improved hygiene and comfort. Similar to hypobaric	Requires supplemental mechanical suspension (see below) due to transitory suction	An alternative when 'full' or hypobaric suction is not practical
Hypobaric	See 'full suction' above, plus larger, more comfortable socket simplifies donning. Uses fabric socks with air seal, improving hygiene and adjustability of fit	Shorter, sharply tapered residua are difficult to fit	Preferred for patients with donning difficulties, especially geriatric. Requires residua of adequate length, strength and musculature
Roll-on sleeve	See 'full suction' above, plus very secure retention because of considerable friction in addition to suction	Difficulties in donning especially short flabby residua. Some problems with adjustability, hygiene and comfort	For patients preferring 'roll-on' donning and more intimate feel of sleeve

Source: Kristinsson O, *Orthot Prosthet*, 37, 25–27, 1983.

which the air is expelled. A special fabric sock or elastic bandage is used to pull the residual limb into the socket, and the fabric or sock is pulled through the valve hole, thereby drawing the residual limb into the socket, past the snug proximal brim. In some cases, the patient may use a lubricant on the thigh to reduce the friction and then push or slide the limb into the socket. This is known as a 'wet-fit' socket. The air is then expelled, the valve is replaced, and full suction suspension is achieved. If the air is allowed to enter the socket, the pressure differential disappears and the prosthesis falls from the residual limb. This type of suspension allows greater freedom of movement, increased use of the remaining muscles, decreased pistoning between the residual limb and the socket and improved comfort and appearance.

Traditional partial or semi-suction can be used if the full suction socket design cannot be utilized because of difficulty in donning or significant volume fluctuation. The patient can wear socks inside the full suction socket or use a wet-fit design to push the residual limb in. However, the patient may require an additional Silesian belt of some other auxiliary suspension. Hypobaric and roll-on suction systems can also be used for transfemoral prosthesis (see Table 23.5).

PROSTHETIC KNEES

Prosthetic knees can be exoskeletal or endoskeletal. The knee units are fabricated of wood, plastic or metal. To minimize weight, aluminium, titanium and carbon fibre composites can be used. Prosthetic knees provide three functions: (1) supporting during stance phase, (2) smooth controlled swing phase and (3) unrestricted knee flexion for sitting, kneeling, stooping and related activities. Several different types of knee prostheses are currently available including single axis, polycentric, friction control, locking knees, microprocessor knee and power knee.[44]

Single axis: This consists of a simple hinge mechanism, which provides flexion and extension around the single axis with swing control. It provides stance stability dependent upon the alignment stability. This joint is simple, reliable, cheap and low maintenance, but it does not work well on irregular surface due to poor toe clearance and functions in one walking speed. Despite disadvantages, this prosthesis is best suited for patients with limited access to health care due to its simple and reliable design.[49]

Single axis with mechanical friction control: Most single axis knee units have a friction mechanism, which controls the movement of the shank during the swing phase. The friction mechanism, by applying resistance to rotation about the knee axis, helps dampen any excessive knee flexion and terminal swing impact. The resistance is adjustable with a friction adjustment screw. The single axis constant friction knee is simple, inexpensive, light in weight and quite easy to adjust and is available in both endoskeletal and exoskeletal versions. However, it does not allow change of cadence.

Polycentric axis knee: It usually consists of four-bar linkage that provides more than one point of rotation. The advantage of this knee is that it provides varied mechanical stability during the gait cycle, with enhanced stability during heel strike and decreased stability during toe-off, thus allowing for easier initiation of swing phase. The greatest advantage is the inherent shortening of the shank under the knee during sitting, thereby improving the cosmesis for very long residual limbs and for knee disarticulation amputees. The disadvantages are increased weight and bilk. However, bulk has been reduced with the carbon fibre composite and titanium materials. It is available in both child and adult sizes.

Fluid control knee: Fluid control knees contain either air (pneumatic control) or liquid (hydraulic control) to allow various walking speed. Progressive compression and transfer of air or liquid from one piston to the other during walking provide a nonlinear resistance, which controls the speed.[50] A fluid control unit can be used with either single axis or polycentric axis knee.

Pneumatic control of the prosthetic shank swing is provided by a pneumatic cylinder containing air, which is attached to the knee and is placed in the upper shank. It is more responsive to varied walking speeds and is a more advanced form of swing control than the mechanical friction. The disadvantages are increased necessity for maintenance and increased weight and expense.

Hydraulic control is similar to the pneumatic control. But oil is used instead of air and uses a cylinder and a piston rod arrangement. The oil provides resistance to motion depending on its viscosity and temperature. Silicone is the most commonly used lubricant for prosthetic hydraulic units as it avoids stiffness in cold weather and looseness in hot weather. Hydraulic units provide carried cadence and are indicated for amputees who can take advantage of the cadence response function. The disadvantages are increased weight, maintenance and expense.

Hydraulic and pneumatic controls that both swing and stance are also available. However, these units are heavier and more expensive. The weight is applied to the prosthesis while the knee is slightly flexed, thus allowing the unit a slow yielding action of the knee rather than a quick collapse, which in turn allows the young and active amputees to descend ramps and stairs in a step-over-step manner and to recover balance when stumbling. By moving a selector switch, the wearer can eliminate the slow yielding stance for control while retaining the swing phase resistance. A flexion lock can be introduced should a particular activity require it.

Microprocessor controlled or 'intelligent knee': These knees use advanced technology and allow patients to ambulate at higher speed with less energy and a precise control of the biomechanics. Microprocessor knees use either hydraulic and/or pneumatic mechanism or magneto-rheological mechanisms to control knee flexion.[44] The microprocessor knees detect the swing speed of the patient and continuously send signals to the stepper motor, which controls the resistance of the knee by adjusting the size of the valve in the pneumatic cylinder. Most of the microprocessor knees control knee flexion by calculating the average speed or by using the speed of the last few steps. Examples include the *Power Knee* by Ossur (Ossur; Figure 23.6f), *Endolite Intelligent Prosthesis Plus* by Chas Blatchford & Sons (Basingstoke, United Kingdom) and the *C-Leg* by Otto Bock (Minneapolis, MN, USA) (Figure 23.6e).

Locking mechanism (weight-activated locking knee or stance-control knee): When the weight is applied to the prosthesis, a braking mechanism mechanically prevents the knee from flexing or buckling. The amount of weight required to effectively engage the brake and prevent flexion can be adjusted depending upon the amputee's weight, activity level and stance-control needs. Locking mechanism is used very commonly for weak and debilitated individuals. Its disadvantages are increased maintenance and delayed initiation of swing phase if the stance-control brake is set for a higher degree of stance stability. *Manual locking knee*s are available for both single axis and polycentric knees in both endoskeletal and exoskeletal configurations.

Other *functional enhancement components* include torque absorber, knee shank rotation adapter and multi-axis ankle module. These elements add weight, bulk and cost to the prosthesis but may be used in some patients for specific needs. *Torque absorber* allows transverse rotation about the long axis of the prosthesis. It is useful for bilateral amputees especially when they participate in golf, tennis and other sports demanding rotational activities. The torque absorber rotator is placed between the lower end of the shank and the foot assembly, allowing rotation of the shank while the foot is placed on the ground. *Knee shank rotation adapter* is useful for sitting cross-legged on the floor by releasing a locking mechanism. The knee and shank are free to rotate and can facilitate entry and exit into cars or various sitting positions in restaurants or booths (Figure 23.7). *Multi-axis ankle module* is a modular endoskeletal component that provides multiple degree of motion within the ankle, independent of the foot. This is primarily intended for endoskeletal prosthesis but can also be used for exoskeletal prosthesis by creating a hybrid system. These modules assist in smoothing out the gait pattern and enhancing the stability in a transfemoral amputee.

FOOT–ANKLE ASSEMBLY

The foot–ankle assembly in a prosthesis substitutes for the anatomic foot and ankle. To serve its purpose, the prosthesis

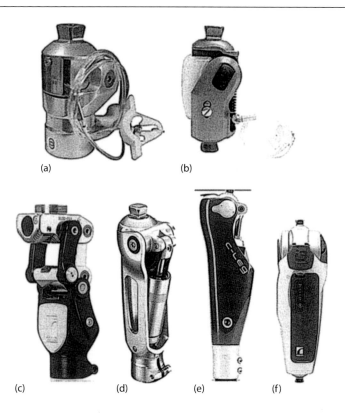

Figure 23.6 (a) Manual locking knee. (b) Single axis knee. (c) Polycentric knee. (d) Hydraulic knee. (e) C-Leg. (f) Power knee. (From Chitragari G et al., *Clin Podiatr Med Surg*, 31(1), 173, January 2014.)

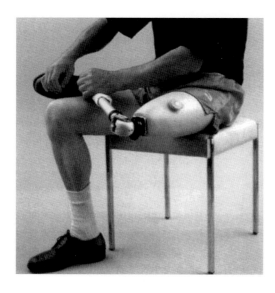

Figure 23.7 Knee shank rotation adapter. (From Blohmke F, *Otto Bock Prosthetic Compendium: Lower Extremity Prostheses*, Schiele & Schoen, Berlin, Germany, 1989.)

should provide the following functions as (1) joint simulation – plantar flexion, dorsiflexion, inversion and eversion, (2) shock absorption at heel contact and reach foot flat position rapidly after heel strike, (3) a stable weight-bearing base of support and forward propulsion and (4) cosmesis by resembling the gentle contour of the missing foot.

There are different types of foot–ankle assemblies offering additional functions such as mediolateral motion or

energy storage (Table 23.6). There are essentially two types of foot–ankle designs: non-articulated and articulated. In the non-articulated design, the basic structure is a foot-like component with a keel, which is the base supporting structure. The whole foot is made up of a resilient material, and the heel may have a lot more resilience than the rests of the foot. At heel contact, the weight compresses the heel, simulating plantar flexion and absorbing the shock, and the keel will provide a firm base of support. During the swing phase, the unloaded toe section reverts to a neutral position. Non-articulated foot ankle assemblies are generally quieter, more durable and lighter than the articulated foot–ankle assemblies.

Non-articulated foot–ankle assembly

Two types of non-articulated foot–ankle assemblies include rigid keel and flexible keel. The most commonly used rigid keel foot is the solid ankle cushion heel (SACH) foot, which is lightweight, durable, low cost and quite cosmetic. It has a solid wooden keel that extends from the toe break and has an external moulded foam with a cushioned heel wedge. It has no movable components so that joint motion is simulated by the rubber surrounding the keel. Plantar flexion is simulated by compression of the heel wedge, but no dorsiflexion is available. The cosmesis and stability are good (Figure 23.8). The disadvantages include the risk of delay in reaching foot flat in early stance, which may cause some instability. There is limited plantar flexion and dorsiflexion adjustability. However, it is a very

Table 23.6 Foot–ankle assemblies.

Foot	Advantages	Disadvantages	HCFA activity levels[a]
Rigid keel SACH	Simple, inexpensive and durable; can accommodate long residua including Syme	Rigid keel can produce 'jarring' in mid- to late-stance phase	Household ambulator (1); limited community ambulator (2)
Flexible keel Safe STEN	Smooth rollover; greater comfort with limited mediolateral motion	Increased weight and cost Limited push-off	Community ambulator (3)
Dynamic response Seattle Carbon copy Quantum Flex-Foot and derivatives	Smooth rollover: springier gait	Increased cost; some designs cannot be fitted to very long residua	Community ambulator (3); child, active adult or athlete (4)
Single axis	Provides rapid foot flat and maximum absorption of heel strike impact Readily adjustable	Weight Durability Cannot be used for Syme	Household ambulator (1)
Multiple axis	Adapts 10 uneven terrain; permits rotation	Weight; durability; cannot be used for Syme	Community ambulator (3); sports participant (e.g. golf) (4)

Source: Kristinsson O, *Orthot Prosthet*, 37, 25–27, 1983.

[a] Numbers in parentheses refer to four increasing levels of anticipated amputee function prepared by the Health Care Finance Administration (HCFA). HEW. Washington, DC, as a guide to prosthetic prescription.

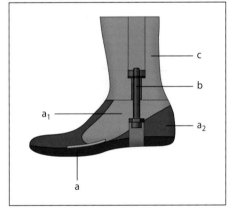

Range of applications

Suitable for all types of prostheses, especially recommended for transtibial prostheses

Description and functional properties

The foot part (a) consists of a wooden core (a_1) covered by elastic plastic material
Heel elasticity is determined by heel wedges (a_2) of different hardness
The foot part is bolted to the shaped wooden ankle block (c) thus integrating it into the prosthesis

SACH feet are available for men, women and children, offering different heel heights and different designs
The assembly bolt (b) is available in stainless steel and titanium

Figure 23.8 SACH foot with ankle block and assembly bolt. (From Blohmke F, *Otto Bock Prosthetic Compendium: Lower Extremity Prostheses*, Schiele & Schoen, Berlin, Germany, 1989.)

popular prosthetic component and is available to accommodate different heel height shoes and can also be ordered with toes for enhanced cosmesis (Figure 23.8).

Non-articular feet with flexible keel include stationary attachment flexible endoskeletal foot and the stored energy foot. Because the keel is flexible, it allows mediolateral and transverse motion. A small amount of bending of the flexible keel after heel off simulates a little dorsiflexion. However, these are heavier and more expensive than the SACH foot.

Articulated foot–ankle assembly

In these designs, an articulation is present at the anatomical ankle level and thus allows more mobility at the ankle. Different types of articulated designs are available (Table 23.6).

Single axis: Available in both exoskeletal and endoskeletal prostheses, the components include a solid wood internal keel, a moulded foam rubber shell and a single transverse metal axis joint. A rubber plantar flexion bumper allows 15° of plantar flexion, and a rubber dorsiflexion stop permits up to 5° of dorsiflexion. Push-off is simulated by the flexibility of the rubber toe section. It may be used in transfemoral prosthesis, when stability is highly desirable and very little mobility is needed. Disadvantages are increased weight, less cosmesis, tendency to squeak and higher maintenance.

Multiple axis foot/ankle: This design provides plantar flexion, dorsiflexion, inversion, eversion and a small amount of rotation and is therefore very suitable for walking on uneven terrain. It also provides excellent shock absorption in all planes due to the presence of many bumpers, thereby reducing torque on the residual limb (Figure 23.9). The disadvantages are increased bulk and weight, especially in the older Otto Bock Greissinger foot, need for more maintenance and decreased stability

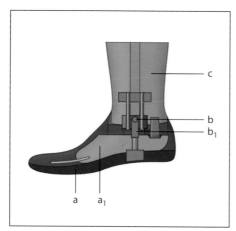

Range of applications

Suitable for all types of prostheses, except swimming prostheses

Description and functional properties

- The foamed foot part (a) with wooden core (a_1) is recessed to accept the greissinger foot joint (b) which connects the foot with the ankle block (c).
- Movement in all directions is permitted by the flexibly mounted U-joint (b_1) and the ring type rubber element.
- Rubber bumpers with different level of hardness determine the degree of plantar flexion, while an elastic bumper stop limits dorsi-flexion.
- Connection to the prosthesis is by means of the wooden ankle block.

Figure 23.9 Multi-axis ankle with ankle block. (From Blohmke F, *Otto Bock Prosthetic Compendium: Lower Extremity Prostheses*, Schiele & Schoen, Berlin, Germany, 1989.)

as compared to other feet, especially in patients with borderline coordination. Newer versions such as Endolite and Multi-Flex Ankle are made of carbon composite material and hence are much lighter.

Dynamic response or energy-storing feet

The prosthetic feet are primarily designed for walking, yet many amputees would like to be more active and require prostheses that will allow them increased activity. Dynamic response feet incorporate a shock absorption mechanism in the form of a flexible keel that will dissipate energy and provide a smoother gait. It also provides push-off that the rigid keel cannot provide. Once a patient starts to walk faster, the amount of time he/she spends on the heel decreases, while the time spent on the forefoot increases. Because more time is spent on forefoot, more forces are exerted on the forefoot, which increases dorsiflexion momentum. The new materials and new designs allow this dorsiflexion movement to allow the keel to compress, thereby absorbing energy and releasing it during push-off and aiding in propelling the patient forward. The materials currently used for the flexible keel are carbon graphite composite and flexible rubber. These feet allow more fluid motion, producing a more natural gait.

Some of the newer dynamic response feet include Seattle Foot, Carbon Copy II, Carbon Copy III and Flex-Foot. *Seattle Foot* was introduced in 1981 as the first prosthetic foot, which was able to store energy during stance phase, release it in the late stance and thereby assist in forward propulsion. This foot has a Delrin spring keel in a C shape and Kavalar-enforced toe pad in a human-looking polyurethane mould (Figure 23.10). The Seattle Foot is fitted to the patient's foot size, weight and level of activity because five degrees of keel flexibility are available. The foot is wide and heavy and has a relatively higher arch that can interfere with mediolateral stability. The Seattle Light Foot has

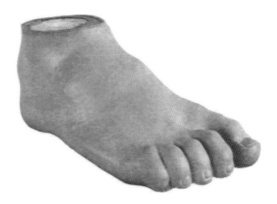

Figure 23.10 Seattle foot. (Courtesy of Seattle Limb Systems, Poulsbo, WA.)

a less pronounced medial arch, has slimmer profile and is half the weight of the original Seattle Foot. It is also available in child size (Child Play Foot). A newer version called the Voyager or Seattle Carbon Light Foot (Seattle Limb System, Poulsbo, WA) is now available and provides more springiness and reduced weight.

Carbon Copy II: This foot was introduced in 1986 and consists of a solid ankle with a rigid posterior block made of nylon in combination with two flexible anterior deflection plates made of carbon composite. These provide two levels of dynamic response. The first deflector, which ends at the level of distal interphalangeal joints, is used for day-to-day ambulation, and the second, shorter, upper deflector is used for higher-level functional activities such as running or jumping. It is encased in an elastomer shell and is available to fit adults, with different heel heights. It is lightweight, is durable and is also available for Syme's amputees.

Carbon Copy III: This is a newer model of Carbon Copy II, with a shank and ankle–foot system made from carbon fibres with a Kavalar keel. Alignment changes can be done by heating the shank and positioning it as desired. The foot provides some degree of eversion/inversion, and the shank also absorbs rotational forces. The system is

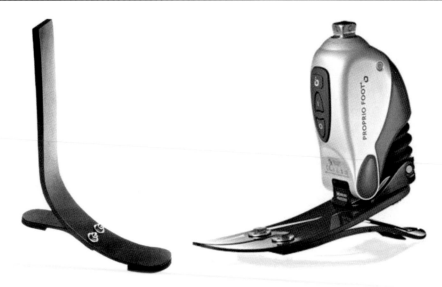

Figure 23.11 Microprocessor foot. (From Prosthetic solutions. www.ossur.in, accessed August 21, 2016.)

modular, permitting selection from two different shanks, light or heavy duty, five different heel durometers and different stiffness for each deflector plate.

Flex-Foot and derivatives (Aliso Viejo, CA) provide a unique technology in the development of a prosthetic concept where flat carbon graphite feet are extended from the metatarso-phalangeal joint lines to proximally into the prosthetic shanks. It takes advantage of the flexibility built into the pylon, storing energy during stance phase and releasing it during toe-off (Figure 23.11). Therefore, the keel forms the shank of the prosthesis, and the shank acts as a long leaf spring, bending when leading and straightening forcibly when the load is reduced. Flex-Foot feet store and return more energy than any other foot–ankle assembly, making it suitable for younger or more active amputees who pursue an active lifestyle or participate in track or field sports. The biggest improvement in this design is the achievement of body mass distribution. Also, a prosthesis incorporating the Flex-Foot design is lighter than with any other foot–ankle component. However, Flex-Foot feet require sufficient space between the floor and the end of the residual limb to take advantage of this technology. Other dynamic response feet include Springlite (Salt Lake City, UT), Endolite (Endolite N.A., Centerville, OH) and others (Figure 23.11).

Microprocessor feet

Microprocessor feet are powered prosthetic feet that provide adaptive ankle motions based on information processed through a microprocessor installed in the foot. *Proprio Foot* by Ossur and iWALK by BiOM are the main types of microprocessor feet.

The *Proprio Foot* (Ossur) is the first microprocessor foot that provides adaptive ankle motion responding to the change in speed and angle of the foot. The Proprio Foot has many accelerometers and angle sensors that send information to

the microprocessor to adjust the ankle's angle and position depending on the phase of the ambulation.[51] The Proprio Foot automatically adjusts the position of the foot including dorsiflexion or plantar flexion depending on the condition of terrain, which increases clearance of the foot. Enhanced foot clearance during swing phase minimizes gait deviation, reduces the risk of falling or tripping and improves safety and gait quality.[52] The energy expenditure of level walking with the Proprio Foot was found to be lower than with dynamic carbon fibre foot.[51] However, the energy cost of slope walking with Proprio Foot did not show significant improvement.[53] The Proprio Foot is best suited for a natural looking gait, improved symmetry and balance.[44]

iWALK by BiOM is the first powered prosthetic foot developed at the Massachusetts Institute of Technology (Boston, MA). iWALK has many sensors to detect the trajectory and motion of the prosthesis in order to adjust the position and angle of the prosthetic ankle. The device can detect the approach of a step by using pattern recognition, and the plantar flexion and dorsiflexion can occur even when the foot is loaded.[44] Increased plantar flexion during push-off and forward propel during toe-off enable amputees to walk 10% faster and decrease energy expenditure of ambulation.[54] It was also found that the use of iWALK may decrease long-term complications including socket pain and joint degeneration since it decreases the stress on the other joints.[55]

A global understanding of prosthetic components coupled with continuous efforts to learn about new developments in prosthetic components is essential in the overall success of vascular amputee's rehabilitation.

REFERENCES

1. Timothy R. Dillingham MD, Liliana E et al. Limb amputation and limb deficiency: Epidemiology and recent trends in the United States. *South Med J.* 2002; 95:875–883.

2. Moxey PW, Hofman D, Hinchliffe RJ, Jones K, Thompson MM, Holt PJE. Epidemiological study of lower limb amputation in England between 2003 and 2008. *Br J Surg.* 2010 September;97(9):1348–1353.

3. Waters RL, Perry J, Antonelli D, Hislop H. Energy cost of walking of amputees: The influence of level of amputation. *J Bone Joint Surg Am.* 1976;58:42–46.

4. Waters RL, Perry J, Chambers R. Energy expenditure of amputee gait. In: Moore WS, Malone JM, eds. *Lower Extremity Amputation.* Philadelphia, PA: W. B. Saunders; 1989, pp. 250–260.

5. Genin JJ, Bastien GJ, Franck B, Detrembleur C, Willems PA. Effect of speed on the energy cost of walking in unilateral traumatic lower limb amputees. *Eur J Appl Physiol.* 2008 August;103(6):655–663.

6. Gonzales EG, Corcoran PJ, Reyes RL. Energy expenditure in below knee amputees: Correlation with stump length. *Arch Phys Med Rehabil.* 1974;55:111–119.

7. Bowker JH. Critical choices: The art of prosthesis prescription. In: Bowker JH, Michael JW, eds. *Atlas of Limb Prosthetics,* 2nd ed. St Louis, MO: Mosby Year Book; 1992, pp. 717–720.

8. Mckechnie PS, John A. Anxiety and depression following traumatic limb amputation: A systematic review. *Injury.* 2014 December;45(12):1859–1866.

9. Pinzur MS, Sage R, Stuck R, Ketner L, Osterman H. Transcutaneous oxygen as a predictor of wound healing in amputations of the foot and ankle. *Foot Ankle.* 1992 June;13(5):271–272.

10. Burgess EM. Wound healing after amputation; effect of controlled environment treatment. *J Bone Joint Surg.* 1978;60A (2):245–246.

11. Berlemont M, Weber R. Temporary prosthetic fitting of lower limb amputees on the operating table. Technique and long term results in 34 cases. *Acta Orthop Belg.* 1966;32(5), 662–667.

12. Weiss, M. *Myoplastic Amputation, Immediate Prosthesis and Early Ambulation.* Washington, DC: Department of Health, Education and Welfare, US Government Printing Office; 1971.

13. Burgess EM, Romano RL. The management of lower extremity amputation using immediate post surgical prosthesis. *Clin Orthop.* 1968;57:137–146.

14. Wu Y, Krick H. Removable rigid dressing for below-knee amputees. *Clin Prosthet Orthot.* 1987;111:33–44.

15. Braddom RL. Rehabilitation of people with lower limb amputation. In: Braddom RL, ed. *Physical Medicine and Rehabilitation,* 4th ed. Philadelphia, PA: W. B. Saunders; 2010, p. 287.

16. Melzack R, Wall PD. Pain mechanisms: A new theory. *Science.* 1965 November 19;150(3699):971–979.

17. Esquenazi A, DiGiacomo R. Rehabilitation after amputation. *J Am Podiatr Med Assoc.* 2001 January;91(1):13–22.

18. Light KE, Nuzik S, Personius W, Barstrom A. Low-load prolonged stretch vs. high-load brief stretch in treating knee contractures. *Phys Ther.* 1984 March;64(3):330–333.

19. Beaulieu JE. Developing a stretching program. *Phys Sportsmed.* 1981;9:59–69.

20. Kegel B, Burgess EM, Starr TW, Daly WK. Effects of isometric muscle training on residual limb volume, strength, and gait of below-knee amputees. *Phys Ther.* 1981 October;61(10):1419–1426.

21. Todd JS, Shurley JP, Todd TC. Thomas L. DeLorme and the science of progressive resistance exercise. *J Strength Cond Res.* 2012 November;26(11):2913–2923.

22. Powers CM, Boyd LA, Fontaine CA, Perry J. The influence of lower extremity muscle force on gait characteristics in individuals with below-knee amputations secondary to vascular disease. *Phys Ther.* 1996 April;76:369–377.

23. Pitetti KH, Snell PG, Stray-Gundersen J, Gottschalk FA. Aerobic training exercises for individuals who had amputation of the lower limb. *J Bone Joint Surg Am.* 1987 July;69(6):914–921.

24. Wenger NK. Early ambulation after myocardial infarction. The in-patient exercise program. *Clin Sports Med.* 1984 Apr;3(2):333–348.

25. Davidoff GN, Lampman RM, Westbury L, Deron J, Finestone HM, Islam S. Exercise testing and training of persons with dysvascular amputation: Safety and efficacy of arm ergometry. *Arch Phys Med Rehabil.* 1992 April;73(4):334–338.

26. Seroussi RE, Gitter A, Czerniecki JM, Weaver K. Mechanical work adaptations of above-knee amputee ambulation. *Arch Phys Med Rehabil.* 1996 November;77(11):1209–1214.

27. Kamen LB, Chapis GJL. Phantom limb sensation and phantom pain. *Phys Med Rehabil State Art Rev.* 1994;8:73.

28. Gitter A, Paynter K, Walden G, Darm T. Influence of rotators on the kinematic adaptations in stubby prosthetic gait. *Am J Phys Med Rehabil.* 2002 April;81(4):310–314.

29. Mensch G, Ellis P. *Physical Therapy Management of Lower Extremity Amputations.* Rockville, MD: Aspen Publishers; 1986.

30. Gentile AM. Skill acquisition: Action, movement and neuromotor processes. In: *Movement Science: Foundations for Physical Therapy in Rehabilitation.* Rockville, MD: Aspen Publisher; 1987, p. 93.

31. Kegel B, Webster JC, Burgess EM. Recreational activities of lower extremity amputees: A survey. *Arch Phys Med Rehabil.* 1980 June;61(6):258–264.

32. Kegel B. *Sports for the Amputee.* Washington, DC: Medic Publishing Co.; 1986.

33. Leonard JA Jr. Lower limb prosthetic sockets. *Phys Med Rehabil State Art Rev.* 1994;8:129.

34. Postone, N. Phantom limb pain. *Psychiatry Med.* 1987;17:57–70.

35. Nathanson, M. Phantom limbs as reported by S. Weir Mitchell. *Neurology.* 1988;38:504–505.

36. Jensen T, Rasmussen P. Phantom pain and related phenomena after amputation. In: Wall PD, Melzack R, eds. *Textbook of Pain,* 2nd ed. Edinburgh, UK: Churchill Livingstone; 1989, pp. 508–521.

37. Jensen TS, Krebs B, Nielson J et al. Immediate and long term phantom limb pain in amputees: Incidence, clinical characteristics and relationship to preamputation limb pain. *Pain.* 1985;21:267–278.

38. Katz J. Psychophysiological contributions to phantom limbs. *Can J Psychiatry.* 1993;38:282–298.

39. Ribbers G, Mulder T, Rijken R. The phantom phenomenon: A critical review. *Int J Rehabil Res.* 1989;12:175–186.

40. Melzack R. Phantom limbs and the concept of neuromatrix. *Trends Neurosci.* 1990;13:88–92.

41. Sherman RA. Phantom limb pain; Mechanism-based management. *Clin Pediatr Med Surg.* 1994;11:85–106.

42. Ludenberg T. Relief of pain from a phantom limb by peripheral stimulation. *J Neurol.* 1985;232:79–82.

43. Bach S, Noreng MF, Tjellden NU. Phantom pain in amputees during the first twelve months following limb amputation, after preoperative lumbar blockade. *Pain.* 1988;33:297–301.

44. Chitragari G, Mahler DB, Sumpio BJ, Blume PA, Sumpio BE. Prosthetic options available for the diabetic lower limb amputee. *Clin Podiatr Med Surg.* 2014 January;31(1):173–185.

45. Kristinsson O. Flexible above-knee socket made from low-density polyethylene suspended by a weight-transmitting frame. *Orthot Prosthet.* 1983;37:25–27.

46. Zheng YP, Mak AF, Leung AK. State-of-the-art methods for geometric and biomechanical assessments of residual limbs: A review. *J Rehabil Res Dev.* 2001 September–October;38(5):487–504.

47. Long JA. Normal shape normal alignment (NSNA) above-knee prosthesis. *Clin Prosthet Orthot.* 1985;9:9–14.

48. Gottschalk FA, Konrosh S, Stills M. Does socket configuration influence the position of the femur in above-knee amputation? *J Prosthet Orthot.* 1989;2:96–102.

49. Michael JW. Modern prosthetic knee mechanisms. *Clin Orthop Relat Res.* 1999 April;(361):39–47.

50. Buckley JG, Spence WD, Solomonidis SE. Energy cost of walking: Comparison of "intelligent prosthesis" with conventional mechanism. *Arch Phys Med Rehabil.* 1997 March;78(3):330–333.

51. Delussu AS, Brunelli S, Paradisi F, Iosa M, Pellegrini R, Zenardi D, Traballesi M. Assessment of the effects of carbon fiber and bionic foot during overground and treadmill walking in transtibial amputees. *Gait Posture.* 2013 September;38(4):876–882.

52. Prosthetic solutions. http://www.ossur.com/prosthetic-solutions/products/feet. Accessed August 21, 2016.

53. Darter BJ, Wilken JM. Energetic consequences of using a prosthesis with adaptive ankle motion during slope walking in persons with a transtibial amputation. *Prosthet Orthot Int.* 2014 February;38(1):5–11.

54. Gates DH, Aldridge JM, Wilken JM. Kinematic comparison of walking on uneven ground using powered and unpowered prostheses. *Clin Biomech* (Bristol, Avon). 2013 April;28(4):467–472.

55. Mancinelli C, Patritti BL, Tropea P, Greenwald RM, Casler R, Herr H, Bonato P. Comparing a passive-elastic and a powered prosthesis in transtibial amputees. *Conf Proc IEEE Eng Med Biol Soc.* 2011; 2011:8255–8258.

24

Diabetes and peripheral artery disease

ROBERT S.M. DAVIES and MICHAEL L. WALL

CONTENTS

INTRODUCTION

Diabetes mellitus (DM) is a global pandemic; in 2013, there was an estimated 381 million adults living with diabetes, approximately 5% of the world population. By 2035 this figure is projected to grow by >50% such that 592 million adults, 7.5% of the world population, will be afflicted.[1] This relentless increase is secondary to the growing prevalence of obesity, urbanization, genetic susceptibility and ageing and is affecting both economically affluent countries and the developing world.

In 2013, 24.5 million adults in the United States were affected with DM causing 190,000 deaths and 38% of all deaths in people under 60 years of age.[1] However, this may only be the tip of the iceberg; an estimated further 79 million people have pre-diabetes, a condition that is independently associated with a 10%–40% increase in one's lifetime risk of cardiovascular disease compared to an individual with normal glycaemic control.[2] There has also been a steady rise in the incidence of type 2 DM amongst children with 8%–45% of new-onset paediatric DM being type 2.[3] The resulting economic burden of DM is tremendous with the total US health expenditure due to DM being $263 billion in 2013 or $800 per individual.[1]

Diabetes represents a multi-morbidity chronic condition with diabetics aged >65 years being affected by an average of six other conditions including coronary artery disease, stroke and hypertension.[4] The increasing prevalence of DM has resulted in a dramatic increase in diabetes-related complications. Vascular diseases, macro and micro, are the principal causes of morbidity and mortality in patients with diabetes. There is a fourfold increase in lifetime risk of developing macrovascular disease – coronary, cerebrovascular and peripheral artery disease (PAD) – with rates of disease severity, progression and mortality greater than in normoglycaemic patients.[5,6] Death certificates of diabetes-related deaths in the United States noted cardiovascular disease and stroke on 68% and 16%, respectively.[7]

Diabetes increases the risk and severity of lower limb symptomatic PAD proportional to the duration of affliction.[8] The Framingham Study demonstrated accelerated atherosclerotic PAD in diabetics with a threefold and eightfold increased frequency of intermittent claudication in men and women, respectively.[9] For every 1% increase in haemoglobin A1c (HbA1c), there is a 25% increase in the relative risk of PAD.[10] PAD often precedes coronary artery disease and stroke and is an independent risk factor for cardiovascular death; a 0.1 decrease in ankle brachial pressure index (ABPI) is associated with a 10% increase in the relative risk of cardiovascular events.

The single commonest cause for hospitalization in patients with DM is foot ulceration for which PAD is an independent risk factor being present in 50% of cases.[11] The lifetime risk of diabetic foot ulceration (DFU) may be as high as 25% and its occurrence increases the risk of subsequent major lower limb amputation.[12] In the United States, about 60% of non-traumatic lower limb amputations amongst people aged 20 years or older occur in people with diagnosed DM, and it is estimated that worldwide one major amputation is performed every 30 seconds due to complications from diabetes.[13] Ischaemia is reported to be a contributing factor in 90% of cases.[14,15]

PATHOPHYSIOLOGY OF MACROVASCULAR DISEASE

Cardiovascular disease is the principle cause of mortality and morbidity in patients with DM and pre-diabetes (impaired glucose tolerance and/or impaired fasting glucose). Macrovascular manifestations are sequelae of a pattern of progressive generalized arteriosclerosis, whereas retinopathy and nephropathy secondary to microvascular disease may result in blindness and end-stage renal failure. In order to optimize individual patient treatments and minimize morbidity and mortality, it is important for the vascular specialist to have a firm understanding of the underlying pathophysiological changes occurring as a result of DM in the vascular system. These can be broadly classified according to Rudolph Virchow's triad: (1) *changes in the arterial wall*, (2) *changes in the blood* and (3) *changes in blood flow*. These deleterious changes act concomitantly to increase the risk of adverse cardiovascular events through a pattern of progressive atherosclerosis, reduced blood flow and vessel thrombosis.

Changes in the arterial wall

Alterations to the structure and function of the arterial wall are central to the development of vascular disease. The initial detrimental changes pre-date the diagnosis of DM with the pre-diabetic state laying the foundations for future structural vascular wall changes. Abnormalities in endothelial and vascular smooth muscle (VSM) cell function are central to these structural changes.

The endothelium is the largest endocrine organ in the body with a surface area equivalent measuring 300–1000 m^2.[16] Strategically located between the circulating blood and the vessel wall, endothelial cells exert a central control on the maintenance of vascular homeostasis through their ability to synthesize and release autocrine and paracrine factors.

Nitric oxide (NO) is perhaps the most important molecule produced by the endothelium. Synthesized from L-arginine by endothelial NO synthase (eNOS), NO is a direct vasodilator activating guanylyl cyclase on VSM cells. NO is also important in preventing endogenous vessel wall injury through its ability to mediate platelet and leukocyte vessel wall interaction and VSM cell proliferation/migration.[17–19] Alterations in endothelial cell metabolism resulting in a reduction in NO cause the production of pro-inflammatory

chemokines and cytokines and the expression of leukocyte adhesion molecules on the cell surface. These changes promote vascular smooth cell and monocyte migration into the tunica intima with the formation of macrophage foam cells. These changes are identical to the early changes associated with atherosclerosis, and studies report reduced levels of endothelial NO production and expression in atherosclerotic lesions. Similarly, patients with type 1 and type 2 DM demonstrate aberrant endothelial-mediated vasodilatation due to impaired NO expression and production suggestive of a causal link between atherosclerosis, DM and reduced levels of NO. Indeed the metabolic derangements associated with DM – hyperglycaemia, insulin resistance and dyslipidaemia – are thought to trigger endothelial cell dysfunction through their ability to impact on the bioavailability of NO. Importantly, reduced NO bioavailability has been demonstrated to be predictive of adverse cardiovascular outcomes.[20,21]

The bioavailability of NO is a function of its synthesis versus degradation, with reactive oxygen species (ROS) being predominantly responsible for the latter. Hyperglycaemia is thought to trigger several complex cellular mechanisms that result in increased production of ROS; the process may be initiated through increased superoxide anion production via the mitochondrial electron transport chain. The generated ROS inactivates NO to form peroxynitrite, which further blunts the activity of eNOS and protective antioxidant enzymes. ROS has a positive feedback on cellular processes/pathways integral in the production of ROS, e.g. protein kinase C (PKC), causing a cascade effect of increasing ROS generation and NO inactivation.

Hyperglycaemia results in the intracellular production of advanced glycation end products (AGEs) and asymmetric dimethylarginine (ADMA). AGEs are a heterogeneous group of compounds formed through the non-enzymatic process of glycation between the amino group on proteins and the reactive glucose aldehyde moiety. AGEs have been implicated in the pathogenesis of endothelial dysfunction in DM through their ability to increase ROS production directly and indirectly through the receptor for AGE (RAGE).[22] RAGE activation causes enhanced oxidative stress, increased vascular permeability and arterial stiffness and cytokine release through its ability to up-regulate pro-inflammatory genes by increasing nuclear factor kappa-B activation.[23] These processes combined with ADMA, a NO synthetase competitive antagonist, act to reduce NO-dependent vasodilatation.[24,25]

Diabetes induces endothelial cell dysfunction through up-regulation and synthesis of endogenous vasoconstrictors, e.g. endothelin and prostanoids.[20] Hyperglycaemia induces PKC-mediated up-regulation of cyclooxygenase (COX)-2, but not COX-1, resulting in increased synthesis of thromboxane A2 (TXA$_2$) and decreased synthesis of prostacyclin (PGI$_2$). TXA$_2$ causes vasoconstriction and a prothrombotic state through its effect on platelet activation and aggregation. Endothelins are pro-inflammatory, vasoconstricting peptides produced by vascular endothelium under the influence of a variety of endogenous bio-molecules including insulin. Endothelin-dependent vasoconstrictor activity is enhanced in patients with type 2 DM, hypertension and hyperlipidaemia.[26]

Changes in the blood

Circulating levels of free fatty acids (FFA) are elevated in DM secondary to reduced skeletal muscle uptake and increased release from adipose stores.[27] Elevated levels of FFA impair endothelial function through a number of mechanisms including ROS generation and eNOS inhibition. FFA, through hepatic metabolism pathways, increase the ratio of low-density lipoproteins (LDLs) to high-density lipoproteins (HDLs) promoting an atherogenic dyslipidaemic vascular environment – the hallmark of DM.[28] Oxidized LDL (oxLDL) disrupts NO production by reducing the bioavailability of the eNOS enzymatic cofactor tetrahydrobiopterin promoting the formation of superoxide.[16] OxLDL also increases the endothelial permeability to pro-inflammatory cells.

Insulin activates and inhibits a wide spectrum of antithrombotic and pro-fibrinolytic mechanisms; insulin inhibits tissue factor preventing platelet aggregation and thrombosis and induces fibrinolysis by modulating plasminogen activator inhibitor-1 (PAI-1). Patients' with insulin resistance demonstrate a prothrombotic diathesis with a hypercoagulable and hypofibrinolytic vascular state as a result of the following: (1) First is the up-regulation of the coagulation cascade with increased plasma levels of clotting factors FI (fibrinogen), FVII (thrombin), FVIII, FXII and FXIII and decreased levels of endogenous anticoagulants, e.g. antithrombin III, protein C.[29] An elevated level of plasma fibrinogen is an independent risk factor for stroke and myocardial infarction as well as cardiovascular mortality.[30-32] An association between elevated fibrinogen and atherosclerotic peripheral vascular disease has been widely reported, and elevated levels of plasma fibrinogen are found in patients who subsequently develop peripheral artery disease. (2) Second is the hypofibrinolysis with increased PAI-1 and decreased tissue plasminogen activator (t-PA) plasma levels. t-PA is released from vascular endothelium in response to thrombin generation and becomes incorporated into the forming fibrin clot. When bound to fibrin t-PA is a potent activator of plasminogen and is therefore a marker of fibrinolysis. PAI-1 is also released from the vascular endothelium in the presence of thrombin and acts to maintain a balance between clot formation and lysis by inhibiting t-PA. (3) Third is the combination of reduced NO and PGI_2 and increased TXA_2 that enhances platelet activation and aggregation.[33-41]

Changes in blood flow

The vascular impact of DM is not limited to endothelial dysfunction. The effects of insulin resistance and hyperglycaemia on VSM cells mirror that of the endothelium; increased intracellular activity of PKC and RAGE pathways heightened ROS production. These injurious metabolic changes influence VSM regulation of vasodilatation and vasoconstriction; VSM response to both NO and endothelin demonstrates diminished vasodilatation and vasoconstriction, respectively.[42,43] Sympathetic nervous system impairment may exacerbate VSM dysfunction, and type 2 diabetics demonstrate impaired endothelial-dependent vasodilatatory responses to acetylcholine.[44,45]

Decreased VSM NO bioavailability, secondary to increased ROS, is implicated in VSM cell migration into developing atherosclerotic lesions and an increased propensity for plaque rupture. Increased VSM apoptosis, metalloproteinases and neo-intimal microvessel formation contribute to plaque destabilization, rupture and vessel thrombosis in patients with DM.[46-48]

DM-induced rheological alterations contribute to altered blood flow dynamics increasing the propensity for arterial atherothrombosis. Increased blood viscosity, secondary to increased plasma proteins, e.g. fibrinogen, reduces microcirculatory perfusion thereby increasing systemic vascular resistance and impairing local oxygen delivery. Concomitant immune system activation, increasing shear stress damage at the blood–endothelial interface and decreasing red blood cell deformability, further contributes to a pro-atherothrombotic environment.[49,50]

ANEURYSMAL DISEASE AND DIABETES

Population-based screening studies initially suggested an inverse relationship between the prevalence of abdominal aortic aneurysms (AAA) and diabetes; this has been further supported by observational studies and systematic review[51-54] (Level 3).

De Rango et al. reported that the prevalence of AAA in diabetics was lower in both male and females, odds ratio (OR) 0.9 and 0.84, respectively. This same reduction in risk was also noted in the rate of aneurysm expansion with an OR of 0.34 compared to non-diabetic controls.[55,56] However, operative intervention for AAA in diabetics is associated with a 30% higher intra- and perioperative morbidity and mortality thought to reflect the poly-morbidity nature of diabetes.[57] Long-term follow-up of AAA patients with DM who have undergone endovascular or open surgical repair demonstrate a reduced life expectancy compared to non-diabetic patients (Level 3).

The reason for this relationship is not fully understood. Aneurysm formation is in part due to a genetic predisposition coupled with bio-physiological risk factors, e.g. hypertension and dyslipidaemia.[58] An individual's genetic predisposition for AAA cannot be negated (currently), but the secondary effects of DM on the arterial wall, intraluminal thrombus (ILT) and extracellular matrix enzymatic activity could all contribute to the observed reduced prevalence.

Arterial wall thickness and stiffness are increased in DM due to increased collagen synthesis in the presence of hyperglycaemia. An elevated level of advance glycation end products forming covalent bonds between elastin and collagen promotes smooth muscle production producing a stiffened wall that is resistant to proteolysis.[51,59-63] Glycation of the extracellular matrix reduces matrix metallopeptidase (MMP)-2 and MMP-9 concentrations thereby reducing extracellular matrix breakdown. ILT has been implicated in the formation of AAA and the rate of AAA expansion. ILT reduces smooth muscle cell volume, arterial wall thickness and resistance to sheer stress. MMP's levels, a marker for increased collagenolytic activity, are also elevated in the presence of ILT. ILT in diabetics has been found to be denser than normal and maybe more resistant to fibrinolytic activity reducing the level of MMP proteolytic activation.

The discovery of DM being protective against the development of aneurysmal disease may not just reflect the disease state but also the benefits of its associated treatments. Medical management strategies for diabetics include additional pharmacological agents compared to patients with atherosclerotic disease but not diabetes. The incidence of DM in a patient cohort comparing AAA and aortoiliac disease requiring intervention was 6% versus 36%, respectively, suggesting that the protective effects of pharmacological treatments do not extend to other atherosclerotic diseases.[55] Various medications have been suggested to improve arterial wall stiffness (metformin), and the thiazolidinediones have been linked to deceased MMP activity; however, the evidence remains limited and requires further investigation.[51,63-68]

The data for the impact of DM on the natural history of popliteal artery aneurysms (PAAs) and post-operative outcomes are very limited. A series of reports have shown an incidence of DM in patients with PAA of 5%–13%, and there are currently no data to suggest that DM is an independent risk factor compared to other atherosclerotic co-morbidities.[68-70]

DIABETES AND STROKE

People with DM have more than double the risk of ischaemic stroke after correction for other risk factors, and 30% of patients requiring interventions for ischaemic stroke have concomitant diabetes.[71] Perioperative morbidity and mortality rates following carotid endarterectomy (CEA) or carotid artery stenting (CAS) in diabetic versus non-diabetic patients are variable with some reporting increased rates whilst others report equipoise.[72-75] This may reflect the heterogeneous nature of the study populations including index symptom to procedure temporal variations. At the time of selection for CEA/CAS, diabetic patients have a greater number of co-morbidities with an associated increased risk of major adverse events including short- and long-term mortality.[75] The Swedvasc group noted that the presence of DM was an independent risk

factors for adverse events in symptomatic patients intervened on in the hyper-acute time window (within 48 hours of stroke).[76] This might reflect inadequate preoperative optimization secondary to time constraints, particularly pertinent to diabetics due to the multi-morbidity nature of the disease. Life expectancy following stroke is reduced in diabetics[72] (Level 3).

Studies comparing post-CEA and post-CAS restenosis rates between diabetic and non-diabetic populations report comparable incidences, ≈6%–7% at 4 years. However, the CREST study reported DM to be an independent risk factor for the development of post-procedural restenosis with increased risk of ipsilateral stroke.[77] Female gender and dyslipidaemia were also indentified as independent risk factors for restenosis after both CEA and CAS, whilst smoking increased the rate of restenosis following CEA only. This enhanced risk was not observed in the SAPPHIRE, SPACE, CAVATAS or EVA-3S studies[76,78-80] (Level 1).

LOWER LIMB AND DIABETIC FOOT ULCERATION

The incidence of DFU in the United States and Western Europe is 2%–6% with a lifetime risk and recurrence rate of 10%–25% and 25%, respectively.[12,81,82] Ignored or inadequately treated, these ulcers are usually the first step to lower limb amputation with 5% of patients undergoing an amputation within 1 year of DFU onset and 80% of all amputations in diabetics being preceded by DFU.[83] DFU is not a dermatological disease but is the product of abnormal loading and impaired perfusion secondary to the synergistic effects of infection, ischaemia and neuropathy.[12,13] (See Figure 24.1.)

Infection

Diabetic foot infection is a common and serious problem. Traditionally believed to be a contributory factor in the initial formation of foot ulceration, infection is now recognized to occur as a consequence of ulceration or other types of foot wounds, e.g. paronychia. Polymicrobial in nature, aerobic gram-positive cocci and gram-negative bacilli are the commonest causative organisms.

Infection may be initially limited to the ulcer and local integument. However, bacteria can quickly spread into deeper tissue planes including tendon sheaths and plantar fascia. The resultant oedema elevates foot compartment pressures causing hypoperfusion and ischaemia of the intrinsic foot musculature. Without emergency treatment the ensuing muscle necrosis and infection result in a non-salvageable foot and often fulminant systemic sepsis. Prompt identification and control of infection is therefore a priority in all patients with DFU.

Local infection should be suspected if ≥2 classic findings of inflammation (calor, rubor, dolor, tumour and

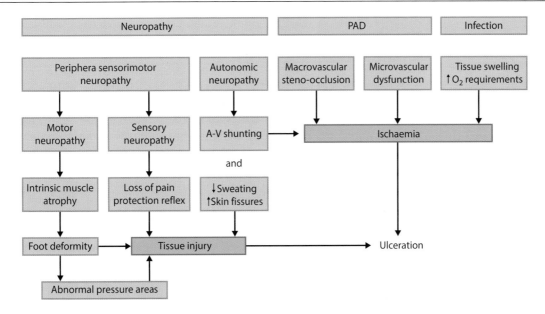

Figure 24.1 Flow chart highlighting the synergistic interactions between infection, ischaemia and neuropathy that lead to diabetic foot ulceration. (PAD, peripheral artery disease; A-V, arteriovenous.)

functio laesa), purulent secretion and malodour are present.[84] However, these clinical signs may be absent due to concomitant neuropathy, poor metabolic control, diminished leukocyte function and alterations to the foot microcirculation.[85] An increase in exudation is the commonest sign of DFU infection and an indolent ulcer present for >30 days should rouse suspicion of infection.[86] Patients with deep foot infections lack features of the systemic inflammatory response, including increased white blood cell count, C-reactive protein and fever in 50% of cases. Deterioration in glycaemic control may be the only sign of systemic upset and should raise the possibility of a deep foot infection in patients with DFU (Level 3).

Superficial necrotic tissue often hides underlying abscess formation and the extent and depth of involvement should be assessed following surgical debridement. Cultures and tissue biopsies should be obtained prior to starting empirical antibiotics. Soft tissue infection may extend down to bone. Contiguous osteomyelitis (OM) may be present in 70% of DFU cases requiring hospital admission with the first and fifth metatarsal heads and calcaneus being affected most frequently[87] (see Figures 24.2 and 24.3). The risk of OM increases with ulcers larger than 2 cm², a DFU with exposed bone or joint and an erythrocyte sedimentation rate >70 mm/h.[88,89] The presence of a continuous tract extending down to bone as evidenced by the use of a sterile probe (probe-to-bone test) is predictive of OM in up to 97% of cases[87] (Level 3).

All patients with new DFU should undergo plain radiography to look for evidence of a foreign body, deformity and soft tissue gas. The use of plain radiography for diagnosing OM may be falsely reassuring as the manifestations of OM on plain radiographs may take several weeks

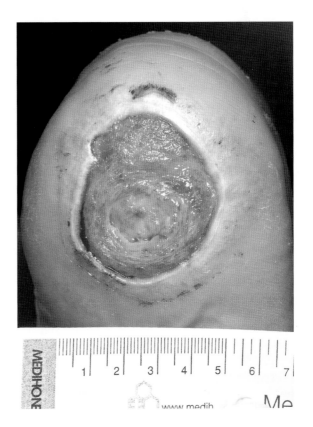

Figure 24.2 Neuroischaemic calcaneus ulceration extending to bone on bone probe test.

to develop and difficulties in differentiating OM changes from those of Charcot arthropathy.[90] Magnetic resonance imaging is the most accurate imaging investigation for OM with a sensitivity and specificity for OM of 90% and 79%, respectively[91] (Level 3).

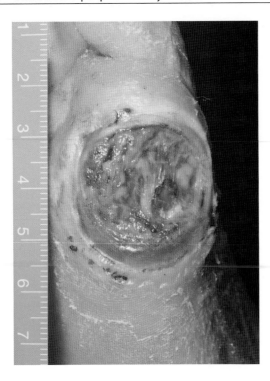

Figure 24.3 Neuroischaemic ulceration overlying first metatarsal head.

The treatment of diabetic foot infection (DFI) depends on the severity of the infection. Mild (Infectious Diseases Society of America [IDSA] infection severity classification) foot infections can be treated in the community with antibiotics, appropriate dressings, non-weight bearing and regular review by a specialist diabetic foot clinic. All patients with an IDSA severe infection and selected patients with IDSA moderate infections should be admitted to hospital for investigation and treatment. Deep foot infections require liberal surgical debridement to ensure drainage of all tissue planes and abscesses. Multiple examinations under anaesthetic and further debridement are often required. Suspected residual soft tissue infection requires a prolonged course of antibiotic therapy dictated by results from culture and tissue samples. Unfortunately a number of patients present late with fulminant foot infection, gangrene and systemic compromise and are best treated with a primary amputation as a life saving procedure (Level 2/3).

Neuropathy

Diabetic peripheral neuropathy affects both the somatic (sensorimotor) and autonomic nervous systems and is present in 80% of DFU cases. Deregulated metabolism and neural ischaemic injury are thought to be the predominant pathophysiological process underlying diabetic neuropathy. Endoneurial capillary wall thickening may result in nutrient vessel occlusion, whilst inappropriate polyol (sorbitol–aldose reductase) pathway activity may cause Schwann cell dysfunction and primary demyelination.[92,93] Polymorphisms of the Aldo-keto reductase family 1, member B1 (AKR1B1) gene, which codes for aldose reductase, may influence neuropathic decline and have been shown to influence temperature threshold discrimination in patients with type 1 DM.[94]

Peripheral sensorimotor neuropathy (PSN) is of gradual onset, initially affecting the feet and progressing proximally in a symmetrical manner – stocking distribution. The sensory component predominates in the early phase and patients may complain of numbness, altered temperature perception, paraesthesia and dysesthesia, often exacerbated at night or by touch. Impaired sensory perception renders these patients at high risk of injury as they are devoid of protective nociceptor reflexes. Early detection of diminished pinprick and vibratory sensation utilizing a Semmes-Weinstein monofilament and a tuning fork are vital to identify those at increased risk of DFU.

PSN may extend to joints with those of the foot and ankle most commonly affected. A combination of loss of proprioception and nociceptor reflexes results in a progressive cycle of chronic joint subluxation, instability and bony destruction – Charcot foot. The associated inflammatory response may be mistaken for infection and contributes to further bony degeneration and altered foot architecture (see Figure 24.4). Occasionally an acute painless foot deformity occurs. Motor neuropathy causes intrinsic foot muscle atrophy and imbalance between flexors and extensor muscle groups. Clawing of the toes and exaggeration of the longitudinal plantar arch promote abnormal pressure areas over the plantar metatarsal heads and toe pulps and dorsal aspects of the inter-phalangeal joints. These polymorphic changes act synergistically to promote the loss of normal foot biomechanics increasing the risk of ulcer formation and limb loss.

An underrecognized group of patients with DM suffer with a proximal neuropathy of the lower limbs – diabetic lumbosacral radiculoplexus neuropathy (LRN).[95] Characterized by progressive sensorimotor changes in the anterior thigh (pain, paraesthesia or numbness) and atrophy of the hip flexors, wasting of quadriceps muscles and loss of the patella are early clinical signs. Unlike distal sensorimotor neuropathy, LRN is often asymmetrical with patients making a spontaneous, if not complete, recovery over a period of months.[93] It is important to correctly identify LRN as it impacts on post revascularization/amputation rehabilitation.

Autonomic neuropathy with loss of sympathetic tone is a characteristic manifestation of diabetic peripheral neuropathy. Microvascular arteriovenous shunting reduces tissue perfusion, but may paradoxically increase overall blood flow in the absence of macrovascular disease.[96,97] A warm, pink foot may mask underlying tissue ischaemia and is a common pitfall to the unwary. Sympathetic dysfunction

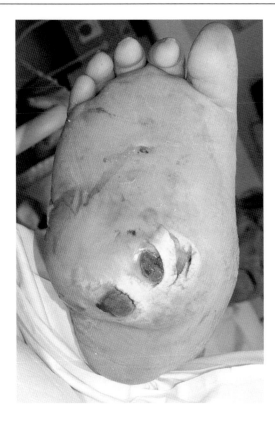

Figure 24.4 Gross mid-foot architectural deformity secondary to a combination of ischaemia, neuropathy and infection.

causes loss of sweating rendering the skin more susceptible to 'cracks' and infection. Autonomic neuropathy may alter the cardiac response to physiological stress and is strongly associated with an increased risk of silent myocardial infarction, important when assessing operative risk.[93]

Ischaemia

PAD is common in patients with diabetes. Epidemiological studies report incidence rates of 14 per 1000 patients in type 2 DM, almost three times higher than in type 1 DM.[98,99] Geographic variations exist and despite a higher incidence of DM being present in South Asian populations, there is a paradoxical reduced incidence of PAD.[100] Whereas historically neuropathy was the predominant cause for foot ulceration, PAD is increasingly implicated being present in 50% of cases. PAD rarely causes DFU in isolation, but occurs in combination with neuropathy – neuro-ischaemia. PAD is a predictor of non-healing and amputation even when only mild in severity due to increased tissue oxygen requirements.[83] Ischaemia is implicated as a contributing factor in 90% of major lower limb amputations in diabetics[14,15] (Level 3).

Historical reports of acid-Schiff positive material occluding arterioles in amputated limb specimens from

diabetics gave rise to the misconception that PAD when associated with DM represented a small vessel (arteriolar) occlusive disease.[101,102] Despite subsequent histological studies refuting these findings, a generation of surgeons falsely accepted the notion of *arteriolo*sclerosis and remained unduly pessimistic about attempting revascularization. It is now accepted that the distribution of PAD in diabetics is macrovascular, diffuse and characteristically affecting the crural vessels with relative sparing of the pedal arch[103] (Level 3).

Concomitant microvascular *functional* abnormalities potentiate the impact of macrovascular disease. Increased microcirculatory arteriolar shunting and impaired vasoreactivity cause capillary hypoperfusion.[104] Endothelial-driven collateralization of arterial steno-occlusions is impaired.[105] This synergistic macro- and microvascular dysfunction result in the circulatory requirements for healing being finely balanced. Relatively innocuous PAD disease in non-diabetics may be sufficient to prevent an ulcer healing in diabetics. This alone has considerable implications on treatment strategies and early recognition of PAD is vitally important for successful limb salvage (Level 3).

WHEN TO REVASCULARIZE

The complexity of DFU mandates a multidisciplinary approach to its treatment. DFIs require treatment tailored to their severity with moderate and severe infections undergoing surgical debridement/intervention to reduce limb amputation rates.[106] Patients with peripheral neuropathy contributing to their ulceration need suitable footwear to offload pressure areas. However, PAD is the main limiting factor in achieving healing of DFU and early recognition is vital.[11,107] Classic symptoms of severe ischaemia – claudication or rest pain – may be absent in 40% of patients with DFU, and 30%–50% of patients are 'turned down' for revascularization at the time of index vascular assessment due to the advanced extent of tissue destruction.[108,109] Thus, a high index of suspicion by the treating clinician is required to identify PAD early in patients with DFU (Level 3).

The ABPI is a sensitive and specific method of diagnosing PAD in both symptomatic and asymptomatic patients. An ABPI < 0.9 is an independent risk factor for cardiovascular morbidity and objectively identifies the presence of a haemodynamically significant major (large vessel) arterial lesion. However, patients with DM should be assessed with the knowledge that (1) up to 35% of patients with DM demonstrate mediasclerosis and calcification of the arterial wall with resultant incompressibility and a falsely elevated (>1.3) ABPI, (2) 19% of diabetic patients with critical limb ischaemia (CLI) cannot have an ABPI measured due to crural vessel occlusion and (3) there are instances in which partial incompressibility of the artery results in a normal ABPI masking underlying PAD.[110] In general, an ABPI < 0.6 indicates severe haemodynamic compromise correlating with poor ulcer healing potential.[111]

However, an ABPI ≥ 0.6 does not necessarily obviate the need for further investigation[112] (Level 3).

Digital (toe) arteries (small vessels) are rarely affected by sclerosis, and toe brachial pressure index (TBPI) measurements in combination with ABPI's are widely advocated as a more accurate and reliable diagnostic tool for the detection of significant large vessel stenosis/occlusion in patients with DM. A patient with an ABPI > 1.3 but a TBPI < 0.6 will have a haemodynamically significant lesion that may have been overlooked if ABPI was used in isolation. In addition, toe pressures (TPs) can be utilized to assess small vessel disease in the absence of large vessel disease. An absolute TP measurement of 30–40 mmHg correlates accurately with the healing potential of a diabetic toe ulcer and a TP < 30 mmHg indicates poor ulcer healing potential. There are limitations to TP with one study having reported that one in six DFU were unable to undergo TP measurement due to previous amputation or gangrene of the hallux[110] (Level 3).

Transcutaneous oxygen pressure ($TcPO_2$) measurement is theoretically the optimal indication of adequate tissue oxygenation; $TcPO_2$ < 30 mmHg is predictive of failure of ulcer healing in the absence of revascularization with $TcPO_2$ < 10 mmHg being associated with an unfavourable outcome.[113,114] A $TcPO_2$ > 50 mmHg is predictive of ulcer healing whereas a $TcPO_2$ = 30–50 mmHg particularly when the context of dynamic testing favours healing. In addition to being time consuming, there are inherent limitations in the applicability of $TcPO_2$; physiological conditions that produce peripheral oedema may lead to spurious results, whilst its usage to predict post-operative wound healing is controversial (Levels 2 and 3).

It is generally recommended that patients with an ABPI > 0.6, a TP > 40 mmHg and/or a $TcPO_2$ >50 mmHg should be treated with a 4–6-week trial period of optimal wound care consisting of infection control and treatment, pressure offloading and appropriate wound dressings.[115] Failure of a 50% reduction in DFU area following 4 weeks of conservative management predicts failure of the ulcer to heal at 12 weeks and identifies those patients requiring a more aggressive approach.[116] Irrespective of non-invasive vascular examination results, patients should undergo formal vascular imaging assessment and urgent revascularization if significant PAD is identified (Levels 2 and 3).

Patients with ABPI < 0.6 or ankle pressure <80 mmHg (whichever is lower) and a TP < 50 mmHg should undergo revascularization without a dedicated trial period of wound management (Levels 2 and 3). However, in 'real-world' experience, patients often inadvertently get a 'trial period' whilst awaiting investigations to delineate anatomy and subsequent interventions. Time to revascularization impacts on ulcer healing rates.[117] A recent Scandinavian study reported the median (IQR) time from first presentation at the diabetic foot centre to revascularization to be 8 (3–18) weeks; patients undergoing revascularization >8 weeks after index review were at an increased risk of subsequent major limb amputation (Level 3). Thus, a high index of suspicion and timely intervention are required to maximize DFU primary healing rates in patients with PAD.

DELINEATING THE ANATOMY OF DISEASE

Duplex ultrasound scanning (DUS) is a non-invasive test providing real-time imagery of arterial blood flow in the vessels. It relies on colour Doppler flow mapping of the haemodynamic parameters to delineate the severity of disease and is operator dependent. The reported sensitivity and specificity in all vessels is excellent ranging from 80% to 90% in diabetic and non-diabetic patients.[118,119] Detection rates in the infra-renal aorta and femoral segments are particularly good although overlying bowel gas may prevent adequate visualization of the iliac arteries. Heavy calcification in the vessels can be detected but limits DUS's ability to accurately quantify the degree of disease; below-the-knee diagnostics can be difficult and should not be relied on entirely when planning intervention (surgical or angiographic) (Level 3).

Digital subtraction angiography (DSA) is the gold standard imaging modality; DSA can delineate anatomy and simultaneously allow endovascular intervention as required. The ability of DSA to adequately identify patent pedal or distal crural vessels in patients with multi-level occlusive disease is a major limitation. Inadequate permeation of contrast into the distal circulation may result in patients being inappropriately labelled as unsuitable for revascularization by the inexperienced practitioner. In these patients the authors favour vessel-targeted (VT) dependent Doppler insonation to assess for patent pedal arteries and identify their dominant supply artery. Computed tomography angiography (CTA) is readily available in most institutions and may be performed as a minimally invasive alternative to DSA when contrast-enhanced magnetic resonance angiography (CE-MRA) is not available.[120] CTA enables the physician to define the degree of calcification in the vessels, which can be useful when planning intervention. With multi-slice CTA ranging from 16 to 64 detector rows, the diagnostic sensitivity in PAD has been reported at 95% (92%–97%) with correlation reported at 98% with DSA.[121] The major concern with CTA and DSA in the diabetic population is the use of iodinated contrast. A substantial proportion of the diabetic population has concomitant renal failure and this may be acutely exacerbated by iodinated contrast: contrast-induced nephropathy. One also needs to be mindful of the interactions between contrast and certain pharmacotherapies, e.g. metformin, as their inappropriate peri-procedural usage may cause dangerous metabolic injury (Level 3).

CE-MRA is becoming more widely utilized and has select advantages over DSA, CTA and DUS. It is a non-invasive test that avoids iodinated contrast and has the ability to separate outflow/contrast from the calcification in the vessel wall. Meta-analyses report an overall sensitivity and specificity of 95% and 96%, respectively, for identifying significant steno-occlusive disease.

Andreisek et al. reported a 79% sensitivity and a 90% specificity for crural vessel disease in diabetics, whilst other reports suggest CE-MRA correlates with DSA in 90% of patients.[122-125] CE-MRA images can be downgraded in the presence of metallic implants (stents) making interpretation of flow difficult. The risk of gadolinium-induced nephrogenic systemic fibrosis remains in patients with creatinine clearance of <30 mL/min with rates of 4.3 cases per thousand patient years for each scan reported in the literature (Level 3).

HOW TO REVASCULARIZE

A number of studies and meta-analyses have reported similar outcomes following successful surgical and endovascular revascularization[126-129] (see Chapters 19 and 20). However, there are no randomized trials and only limited case series reporting the outcomes of endovascular or/and surgical revascularization in a selected diabetic population (see Table 24.1).

The BASIL trial, which randomized patients with severe limb ischaemia to either bypass- or angioplasty-first treatment strategies, demonstrated survival-free-from-amputation (primary end point) was not significantly different at 12 months.[109] Surgery was associated with increased perioperative morbidity whereas patients assigned to an angioplasty-first strategy were more likely to require a secondary intervention to maintain or re-establish flow (Level 1). Of particular note for surgeons advocating a bypass-first strategy was the finding that patients undergoing a bypass procedure following failed angioplasty performed considerably worse that those undergoing a bypass procedure first.[130] At extended follow-up for those patients surviving beyond 2 years, a bypass-first strategy was associated with improved amputation-free survival over the ensuing 5 years which was not attenuated when adjusted for covariates including DM.[131] These data overall suggest that patients expected to survive beyond 2 years may benefit from a bypass-first strategy treatment. However, one should be cautious when applying the BASIL trial results to the DFU population; only 75% of the trial population had ulceration or tissue loss, <50% of the trial population had DM and no-diabetic subgroup analysis has been reported, and only 10% of distal bypass anastomoses were distal to the popliteal artery.

The PREVENT III (PIII) trial, initially designed to study the effects of a novel therapy (edifoligide) for the prevention of graft failure, is the largest prospective study reporting the outcomes of patients undergoing vein bypasses for critical limb ischaemia.[132] Of the 1404 patients randomized, 75% had tissue loss, 65% of distal anastomoses were to infra-popliteal vessels including 12% to pedal/plantar arteries and 64% were diabetic. Perioperative mortality was 2.7% and 6.1% suffered a myocardial injury or cerebrovascular event; patient survival at 12 months was 84%. Primary, primary-assisted and secondary patency rates were 61%, 77% and 80%, respectively, and 12-month limb salvage rate was 88%.

Subgroup analyses reported that DM was not a risk factor for vein graft failure, a finding corroborated by 'real-world' single-centre studies[133] (Level 3).

When choosing between surgical and endovascular revascularization, numerous patient-orientated, anatomical and technical factors should be considered by a multidisciplinary team. Bypass surgery involves a long anaesthetic, blood loss and significant surgical trauma, which for patients with limited life expectancy or physiological dysfunction may be unsuitable. Similarly, patients with extensive tissue loss overlying proposed incision sites or poor wound healing potential with low albumin or gross peripheral oedema are poor candidates for bypass surgery. Pedal bypass surgery can be performed in the presence of foot infection safely provided that deep infection is controlled before surgery.[134] The presence of a suitable bypass conduit is also paramount when considering a patient for surgery; autologous great saphenous vein is the best conduit, but cephalic or basilic veins used in continuity or spliced are suitable alternatives and preferential to prosthetic[132,135,136] (see Figure 24.5).

Perhaps the most important anatomical considerations in bypass surgery relate to the selection of the inflow and outflow vessels. The 'short-bypass principle' originally proposed by Veith in 1981 advocates the use of more distal vessels for the origin of a bypass reducing the length of the bypass.[137] The inflow vessel should ideally be free from significant disease, and in many diabetic patients, the popliteal and superficial femoral arteries can be utilized thereby avoiding dissection in the groin; this is often not the case in non-diabetics with 'true' atherosclerotic-induced CLI. The ability to perform a high percentage of bypasses utilizing the 'short-bypass principle' may explain reports that DM is not a risk factor for graft failure.

Selection of the outflow vessel is of paramount importance and in general the most proximal vessel with in-line flow to the foot is optimal. Since Attinger et al. introduced the concept of the ankle and foot consisting of six angiosomal regions supplied by specific crural vessels or their terminal branches, a great debate as to the merits of VT revascularization has ensued.[138] A number of studies have reported improved outcomes (wound healing and limb salvage) following VT treatment in patients with DFU although the quality for evidence is low.[139-141] In the authors' experience, a large proportion of patients are not suitable for direct angiosomal revascularization as often there is only one remaining patent crural vessel or the ulcer affects multiple angiosomes. Despite non-targeted revascularization, the majority of ulcers are successfully healed following revascularization adding anecdotal support to studies reporting the quality of the pedal arch rather than the angiosome revascularized, which is the primary factor influencing wound healing following successful bypass surgery.[142,143]

Risk-prediction models have been recently developed in an attempt to aid the identification of patients to whom a bypass procedure would be beneficial. The PIII risk

Table 24.1 Summary of studies reporting outcomes of endovascular or bypass revascularisation procedures in patients with diabetes.

Study	Date	Number of patients	Intervention	Percentage of lesion infra-popliteal	Technical success	Clinical success	Primary patency (months)	Secondary patency (months)	Limb salvage (months)	Survival (months)
Alexandrescu	2009	161	SIA + PTA	61%	84%	/	45 % (24), 38% (48)	69% (24), 66% (48)	83% (24), 80% (48)	/
Ferraresi et al.	2009	101	PTA	100%	94%	/	58% (12)	/	93% (36)	92% 36
Bargellini et al.	2008	60	SIA	43%	92%	98%	/	/	93% (12)	83% (36)
Faglia et al.	2005	1188	PTA	93%	84%	/	88% (60)	/	17 Major amputations and 478 minor amputations were performed peri-operatively	74% (60)
Lazaris et al.	2004	33	SIA	47%	81%	63% (24)	69% (24)	NA	82% (36)	57% (36)
Neufang	2003	79	Pedal bypass	100%	92%	92%	68% (60)	75% (60)	78% (60)	/
Faglia et al.	2002	219	Bypass + PTA	81%	87%	/	/	/	10 major and 83 minor amputations were performed peri-oepratively	/
Dorweiler et al.	2002	46	Pedal bypass	100%	98%	96%	89% (48)	/	87% (48)	45% (28)
Schneider et al.	2001	110	Bypass +/- Inflow PTA	100%	100%	100%	78% (24), 63% (60)	89% (24), 78% (60)	89 (24), 81% (60)	77% (24), 35% (60)
Wolfle et al.	2000	125	Bypass	100%	90% (30 days)	90% (30 days)	76% (12), 46% (84)	83% (12), 49% (84)	80% (12), 63% (84)	/
Wolfle et al.	2000	84	PTA	100%	93%	95% (30 days)	/	/	82% (12), 63% (72)	/
Hanna et al.	1997	29	PTA	100%	90%	79%	/	/	83% {12}	97% (12)
Rosenblum et al.	1994	39	Bypass	79%			92% (21)	92% (21)	95% (21), 83% of ulcers healed	97% (21)

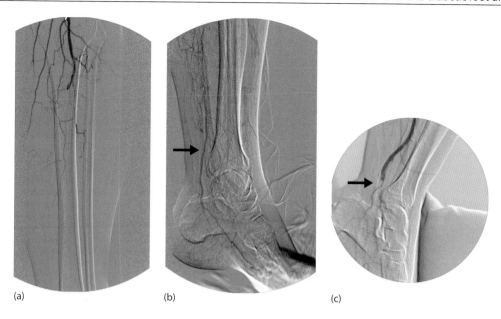

(a)   (b)   (c)

Figure 24.5   (a) Digital subtraction angiography demonstrating classic diabetic crural vessel disease with popliteal sparing. (b) Reconstitution of posterior tibial artery (black arrow) at the medial malleolus. (c) On table angiogram following popliteal to posterior tibial bypass with LSV; angiogram demonstrates good flow in graft and outflow into foot at distal anastomosis (white arrow).

score assesses for the presence of five preoperative variables and assigns the patient an overall score: dialysis (4 points), tissue loss (3 points), age ≥75 years (2 points), anaemia (2 points) and coronary artery disease (1 point). Those patients categorized as low risk (≤3 points) or moderate risk (4–7 points) preoperatively can expect survival-free-from-amputation rates following bypass surgery of 73%–86% at 1 year. However, only 45%–55% of patients classified as high risk (≥8 points) can expect to be alive without amputation at 1 year post bypass. The PIII risk-prediction score needs formal prospective validation, but can aid in decision making in a broad sense. The Finnvasc and BASIL risk-prediction scores share many features of the PIII score of which end-stage renal failure or dialysis is consistently found to have a profound negative impact on outcome[144,145] (Level 3).

Surgical revascularization achieves excellent limb salvage rates; however, patient co-morbidities, local tissue considerations and technical expertise often reduce its clinical applicability. Endovascular treatment offers an attractive alternative due to its minimally invasive nature. Diabetic lesions are often long, calcified segmental occlusions affecting more than one crural vessel. Concomitant iliac and femoral artery disease may occur, but rarely in the absence of below-the-knee disease.[146] This combination of morphological features increases the complexity of endovascular revascularization. In the authors' experience, subintimal angioplasty (SIA) offers greater scope than an intraluminal technique for the successful endovascular treatment of these complex lesions.

SIA was first introduced in 1987 as a minimally invasive percutaneous technique for the treatment of femoropopliteal occlusive disease in patients with intermittent claudication.[147] Encouraging early results extended its application to the popliteal artery and crural vessels, where it has proved to be an invaluable addition to the armamentarium for the treatment of CLI. Recent results have confirmed its applicability and durability for the treatment of CLI, and in the authors' institution, it has become the first-line treatment option for many patients with this condition[148–172] (Levels 3 and 4).

SIA has made its biggest impact in diabetic patients with CLI because it has the ability to reconstitute bifurcations and trifurcations and is very effective in recanalizing long tibial artery occlusions.[162–164,166,167,173–176] Long occlusions of the femoropopliteal and tibial arteries can be recanalized through a subintimal channel, in cases in which it would be difficult to maintain an intraluminal position of the guidewire. A popliteal occlusion that extends into the trifurcation vessels can be treated with SIA, whereby the recanalization can be extended into all three run-off vessels re-establishing three vessel run-offs. Short tibial occlusions can be easily crossed intraluminally, but a subintimal technique is more applicable for longer (>3 cm) occlusions. Technical success rates are reported in excess of 90% but vary considerably reflecting institutional experience. However, DM and crural vessel occlusion are associated with inferior technical success rates.[167,177] Perioperative complications, including perforation and distal embolization, are more frequent in diabetics and occur in 16% of cases, but the overall incidence of patients requiring surgery for a complication is ≤1%.[178] Perioperative mortality is low (0%–3%) irrespective of diabetes.[165] Primary patency rates for patients with CLI are reported as being in excess of 90% at 12 months and

60% at 5 years. The impact of DM on primary patency varies within the literature. A single-centre review of 1000 infrainguinal endovascular interventions reported a 24-month secondary patency for patients with DM as 59% compared with 76% for non-diabetics (p < 0.0001).[179] However, the heterogeneous nature of the patient group and endovascular techniques employed prevent any meaningful conclusion being reached from this study. Other studies have not found DM to be associated with patency inferiority.[177,180,181] The number of run-off vessels and quality of the plantar arch affect patency rates. Patients with two or more patent run-off vessels have three times less risk of occlusion compared to those with one patent run-off vessel.[177] Ingle et al. reported limb salvage rates of 94% at 36 months in patients who had CLI and tibial vessel disease.[167] Isolated tibial disease predicts worse limb salvage and is more prevalent in diabetics.[181] Below-the-ankle angioplasty is a useful adjunct to maximize outflow with technical success rates reported in 88% of cases[182] (Level 3).

Occlusion following successful subintimal recanalization does not necessarily cause clinical deterioration. Lower limb diabetic ischaemic ulceration is very rarely secondary to acute or acute-on-chronic arterial occlusion. The majority occurs as a result of disequilibrium between a finely balanced tissue oxygenation demand and supply. Arterial disease is often long standing, but adequate to maintain tissue integrity. Minor injuries resulting in increased tissue oxygen demand alter this equilibrium setting into motion a cascade effect. An initially successful SIA may allow minor limb amputation or ulcers to heal recreating the vascular 'entente cordial' that is not disrupted by subsequent occlusion in the absence of injury. This theory is supported by clinical studies paradoxically reporting patency rates of 70% at 12 months, but limb salvage rates between 80% and 90%.[165,171]

In the authors' view, the initial revascularization strategy is influenced by a selected number of factors; life expectancy, surgical risk, anatomy of disease, healing potential and availability of autologous vein. A patient with multi-segment occlusions and single vessel run-off with a life expectancy >24 months and is deemed physiologically fit to undergo surgery should be offered a bypass procedure if adequate vein is available. Likewise, unfit patients with limited life expectancy or no suitable vein should be considered for an endovascular first strategy. The difficulty exists in those patients between these two extremes and in the authors' experience, this represents the majority of patients. We always ask the question: is the going to live long enough for the increased short-term risks associated with bypass surgery to be offset by the improved long-term outcome? It is worth noting that as a result of a combination of better management of risk factors and co-morbidities, patients with DM and PAD have improved short-, medium- and long-term survival rates compared to as little as a decade ago.

Key points

- In 2013 24.5 million adults in the United States were affected with DM causing 190,000 deaths and 38% of all deaths in people under 60 years of age.
- The total US health expenditure for DM was $263 billion in 2013.
- Cardiovascular disease is the principle cause of mortality and morbidity in patients with diabetes.
- Endothelial cell dysfunction with reduced bioavailability of nitric oxide (NO), increased production of AGEs, ADMA and endogenous vasoconstrictors are the principle causes of macrovascular disease in diabetics.
- DM increases the risk and severity of lower limb symptomatic PAD proportional to the duration of affliction.
- The single commonest cause for hospitalization in patients with DM is DFU and PAD is implicated in 50% of cases.
- PAD in diabetics classically affects the crural vessels with relative sparing of the pedal arch.
- Patients with an ABPI > 0.6, a TP > 40 mmHg and/or a $TcPO_2$ > 50 mmHg should be treated with a 4–6 weeks trial period of optimal wound care.
- There is limited evidence supporting an endovascular- or bypass-first revascularization strategy in diabetics with critical limb ischaemia.

BEST CLINICAL PRACTICE FOR DIABETIC FOOT ULCERATION

- DFU should be treated by a multidisciplinary team (Grade D).
- Identification and control of infection are priorities in all patients with DFU (Grade B).
- An indolent ulcer present for >30 days should rouse suspicion of infection (Grade D).
- Deterioration in glycaemic control should raise the possibility of a deep foot infection in patients with DFU (Grade D).
- A continuous tract extending to bone as evidenced by the use of a sterile probe (probe-to-bone test) is predictive of OM in up to 97% of cases (Grade B).
- All patients with an IDSA severe infection and selected patients with IDSA moderate infections should be admitted to hospital for investigation and treatment (Grade B).
- All patients with DFU should be formally examined for peripheral neuropathy and PAD (Grade B).
- An ABPI < 0.6 indicates severe haemodynamic compromise correlating with poor ulcer healing potential (Grade B).
- Patients with an ABPI > 0.6, a TP > 40 mmHg and/or a $TcPO_2$ > 50 mmHg should be treated with a 4–6 weeks trial period of optimal wound care (Grade B).
- Patients with ABPI < 0.6 or ankle pressure < 80 mmHg (whichever is lower) and a TP < 50 mmHg should undergo revascularization (Grade B).

- DUS, CTA, MRA and DSA are acceptable methods of imaging the infra-popliteal vascular tree (Grade B).
- Patients requiring revascularization with a life expectancy >2 years should be considered for a bypass-first strategy (Grade B).

LEVELS OF EVIDENCE

Level 1: Systematic reviews, meta-analyses of randomized controlled trials (RCTs) and RCTs
Level 2: Non-randomized studies
Level 3: Observational or non-experimental studies
Level 4: Expert opinion

CLINICAL RECOMMENDATIONS

Grade A: Based on evidence from meta-analyses of RCTs
Grade B: Based on evidence from high quality case-controlled or cohort studies
Grade C: Based on evidence from low quality case-controlled or cohort studies
Grade D: Based on evidence from clinical series or expert opinion

DEFICIENCIES IN CURRENT KNOWLEDGE AND AREAS FOR FUTURE RESEARCH

- Impact of early revascularization on outcomes in patients with DFU
- Impact of the angiosome model of revascularization on wound healing and limb salvage in patients with DFU
- Short-, medium- and long-term outcomes of infra-popliteal open versus endovascular revascularization in patients with DFU
- Quality of life comparison for revascularization versus primary amputation in those patients with limited life expectancy

REFERENCES

1. International Diabetes Federation. *e-Atlas*, 6th ed. Brussels, Belgium, http://www.idf.org/diabetesatlas, accessed August 2013.
2. Milman S, Crandall JP. Mechanisms of vascular complications in prediabetes. *Med Clin North Am*. 2011 March;95(2):309–325.
3. Copeland KC, Becker D, Gottschalk M, Hale D. Type 2 diabetes in children and adolescents: Risk factors, diagnosis, and treatment. *Clin Diabetes*. 2005;23(4):181–185.
4. Guthrie B, Payne K, Alderson P, McMurdo ME, Mercer SW. Adapting clinical guidelines to take account of multimorbidity. *Br Med J*. 2012 October 4;345:e6341.
5. Franco OH, Steyerberg EW, Hu FB, Mackenbach J, Nusselder W. Associations of diabetes mellitus with total life expectancy and life expectancy with and without cardiovascular disease. *Arch Intern Med*. 2007;167(11):1145–1151.
6. Haffner SM, Lehto S, Rönnemaa T, Pyörälä K, Laakso M. Mortality from coronary heart disease in subjects with type 2 diabetes and in nondiabetic subjects with and without prior myocardial infarction. *N Engl J Med*. 1998;339(4):229–234.
7. Centers for Disease Control and Prevention. *National Diabetes Fact Sheet: National Estimates and General Information on Diabetes and Prediabetes in the United States*. Atlanta, GA: CDC, 2011.
8. Nilsson SE, Nilsson JE, Frostberg N, Emilsson T. The Kristianstad Survey II. *Acta Med Scand (Suppl.)* 1967;469:1–42.
9. Kannel WB, McGee DL. Update on some epidemiologic features of intermittent claudication: The Framingham Study. *J Am Geriatr Soc*. 1985;33:13–18.
10. Selvin E, Marinopoulos S, Berkenblit G et al. Meta-analysis: Glycosylated hemoglobin and CVD disease in diabetes mellitus. *Ann Intern Med*. 2004;21:421–431.
11. Prompers L, Huijberts M, Apelqvist J et al. High prevalence of ischaemia, infection and serious comorbidity in patients with diabetic foot disease in Europe. Baseline results from the Eurodiale study. *Diabetologia*. 2007;50(1):18–25.
12. Singh N, Armstrong DG, Lipsky BA. Preventing foot ulcers in patients with diabetes. *J Am Med Assoc*. 2005;293:217–228.
13. Jeffcoate W, Bakker K. World Diabetes Day: Footing the bill. *Lancet*. 2005;365:1527.
14. Eskelinen E, Lepäntalo M, Hietala EM et al. Lower limb amputations in Southern Finland in 2000 and trends up to 2001. *Eur J Vasc Endovasc Surg*. 2004;27:193–200.
15. Heald CL, Fowkes FG, Murray GD, Price JF; Ankle Brachial Index Collaboration. Risk of mortality and cardiovascular disease associated with the ankle-brachial index: Systematic review. *Atherosclerosis*. 2006 November;189(1):61–69.
16. Jingli W, Widlansky ME. Cytoskeleton, cytoskeletal interactions, and vascular endothelial function. *Cell Health Cytoskeleton*. 2012;4:119–127.
17. Sarkar R, Meinberg EG, Stanley JC et al. Nitric oxide reversibly inhibits the migration of cultured vascular smooth muscle cells. *Circ Res*. 1996;78:225–230.
18. Radomski MW, Palmer RM, Moncada S. The role of nitric oxide and cGMP in platelet adhesion to vascular endothelium. *Biochem Biophys Res Commun*. 1987;148:1482–1489.

19. Kubes P, Suzuki M, Granger DN. Nitric oxide: An endogenous modulator of leukocyte adhesion. *Proc Natl Acad Sci U S A.* 1991;88:4651–4655.

20. Hink U, Li H, Mollnau H et al. Mechanisms underlying endothelial dysfunction in diabetes mellitus. *Circ Res.* 2001;88:E14–E22.

21. Lerman A, Zeiher AM. Endothelial function: Cardiac events. *Circulation.* 2005;111:363–368.

22. Yan SF, D'Agati V, Schmidt AM, Ramasamy R. Receptor for Advanced Glycation Endproducts (RAGE): A formidable force in the pathogenesis of the cardiovascular complications of diabetes & aging. *Curr Mol Med.* 2007 December;7(8):699–710.

23. Tan KC, Chow WS, Ai VH, Metz C, Bucala R, Lam KS. Advanced glycation end products and endothelial dysfunction in type 2 diabetes. *Diabetes Care.* 2002 June;25(6):1055–1059.

24. Ahmed N. Advanced glycation end products – Role in pathology of diabetic complications. *Diabetes Res Clin Pract.* 2005 January;67(1):3–21.

25. Sydow K, Mondon CE, Cooke JP. Insulin resistance: Potential role of the endogenous nitric oxide synthase inhibitor ADMA. *Vasc Med.* 2005 July;10(Suppl. 1): S35–S43.

26. Campia U, Tesauro M, Di Daniele N, Cardillo C. The vascular endothelin system in obesity and type 2 diabetes: Pathophysiology and therapeutic implications. *Life Sci.* 2010;39(2):200–207.

27. Kelley DE, Simoneau JA. Impaired free fatty acid utilization by skeletal muscle in non-insulin-dependent diabetes mellitus. *J Clin Invest.* 1994 December;94(6):2349–2356.

28. Ginsberg HN, Zhang YL, Hernandez-Ono A. Regulation of plasma triglycerides in insulin resistance and diabetes. *Arch Med Res.* 2005 May–June;36(3):232–240.

29. Alzahrani SH, Ajjan RA. Coagulation and fibrinolysis in diabetes. *Diab Vasc Dis Res.* 2010 October;7(4):260–273.

30. Danesh J, Lewington S, Thompson SG et al. Plasma fibrinogen level and the risk of major cardiovascular diseases and nonvascular mortality: An individual participant meta-analysis. *J Am Med Assoc.* 2005 October 12;294(14):1799–1809.

31. Ernst E. Plasma fibrinogen – An independent cardiovascular risk factor. *J Intern Med.* 1990 June;227(6):365–372.

32. Smith FB, Lee AB, Fowkes FG et al. Hemostatic factors as predictors of ischemic heart disease and stroke in the Edinburgh Artery Study. *Arterioscler Thromb Vasc Biol.* 1997 November; 17(11):3321–3325.

33. Davies RS, Abdelhamid M, Wall ML, Vohra RK, Bradbury AW, Adam DJ. Coagulation, fibrinolysis, and platelet activation in patients undergoing open and endovascular repair of abdominal aortic aneurysm. *J Vasc Surg.* 2011 September;54(3):865–878.

34. Dormandy JA, Hoare E, Colley J, Arrowsmith DE, Dormandy TL. Clinical, haemodynamic, rheological, and biochemical findings in 126 patients with intermittent claudication. *Br Med J.* 1973 December 8;4(5892):576–581.

35. Meade TW, Mellows S, Brozovi M et al. Haemostatic function and ischaemic heart disease: Principal results of the Northwick Park Heart Study. *Lancet.* 1986 September 6;2(8506):533–537.

36. Kannel WB, Wolf PA, Castlli WP, D'Agostino RB. Fibrinogen and risk of cardiovascular disease. The Framingham Study. *J Am Med Assoc.* 1987 September 4;258(9):1183–1186.

37. Grant PJ. Diabetes mellitus as a prothrombotic condition. *J Intern Med.* 2007 August;262(2):157–172.

38. Carr ME. Diabetes mellitus: A hypercoagulable state. *J Diabetes Complications.* 2001 January–February; 15(1):44–54.

39. Ceriello A, Giugliano D, Quatraro A, Marchi E, Barbanti M, Lefèbvre P. Evidence for a hyperglycaemia-dependent decrease of antithrombin III-thrombin complex formation in humans. *Diabetologia.* 1990 March;33(3):163–167.

40. Ren S, Lee H, Hu L, Lu L, Shen GX. Impact of diabetes-associated lipoproteins on generation of fibrinolytic regulators from vascular endothelial cells. *J Clin Endocrinol Metab.* 2002;87(1):286–291.

41. Ceriello A, Quatraro A, Dello Russo P, Marchi E, Barbanti M, Milani MR, Giugliano D. Protein C deficiency in insulin-dependent diabetes: A hyperglycemia-related phenomenon. *Thromb Haemost.* 1990 August 13;64(1):104–107.

42. Williams SB, Cusco JA, Roddy MA, Johnstone MT, Creager MA. Impaired nitric oxide-mediated vasodilation in patients with non-insulin-dependent diabetes mellitus. *J Am Coll Cardiol.* 1996 March 1;27(3):567–574.

43. Nugent AG, McGurk C, Hayes JR, Johnston GD. Impaired vasoconstriction to endothelin 1 in patients with NIDDM. *Diabetes.* 1996 January;45(1):105–107.

44. McDaid EA, Monaghan B, Parker AI et al. Peripheral autonomic impairment in patients newly diagnosed with type II diabetes. *Diabetes Care.* 1994;17:1422–1427.

45. McVeigh GE, Brennan GM, Johnston GD, McDermott BJ, McGrath LT, Henry WR, Andrews JW, Hayes JR. Impaired endothelium-dependent and independent vasodilation in patients with type 2 (non-insulin-dependent) diabetes mellitus. *Diabetologia.* 1992 August;35(8):771–776.

46. Kim HJ, Kim MY, Jin H et al. Peroxisome proliferator-activated receptor {delta} regulates extracellular matrix and apoptosis of vascular smooth muscle cells through the activation of transforming growth factor-{beta}1/Smad3. *Circ Res.* 2009 July 2;105(1):16–24.

47. Rosenson RS, Fioretto P, Dodson PM. Does microvascular disease predict macrovascular events in type 2 diabetes? *Atherosclerosis*. 2011 September;218(1):13–18.

48. Kadoglou NP, Daskalopoulou SS, Perrea D, Liapis CD. Matrix metalloproteinases and diabetic vascular complications. *Angiology*. 2005 March–April;56(2):173–189.

49. Bhavsar J, Rosenson RS. Adenosine transport, erythrocyte deformability and microvascular dysfunction: An unrecognized potential role for dipyridamole therapy. *Clin Hemorheol Microcirc*. 2010;44(3):193–205.

50. Jaap AJ, Pym CA, Seamark C, Shore AC, Tooke JE. Microvascular function in Type 2 (non-insulin-dependent) diabetes: Improved vasodilation after one year of good glycaemic control. *Diabet Med*. 1995;12:1086–1091.

51. Shantikumar S, Ajja R, Porter KE, Scott DJA. Diabetes and the abdominal aortic aneurysm. *Eur J Vasc Endovasc Surg*. 2010;39:200–207.

52. Simoni G, Pastorino C, Perrone R et al. Screening for abdominal aortic aneurysms and associated risk factors in a general population. *Eur J Vasc Endovasc Surg*. 1995;10(2):207–210.

53. Lederle FA, Johnson GR, Wilson SE et al. Prevalence and associations of abdominal aortic aneurysm detected through screening. Aneurysm Detection and Management (ADAM) Veterans Affairs Cooperative Study Group. *Ann Intern Med*. 1997;126(6):441–449.

54. Kanagasabay R, Gajraj H, Pointon L, Scott RA. Co-morbidity in patients with abdominal aortic aneurysm. *J Med Screen*. 1996;3(4):208–210.

55. Shteinberg D, Halak M, Shapiro S et al. Abdominal aortic aneurysm and aortic occlusive disease: A comparison of risk factors and inflammatory response. *Eur J Vasc Endovasc Surg*. 2000;20(5):462–465.

56. Sweeting MJ, Thompson SG, Brown LC, Powell JT; RESCAN Collaborators. Meta-analysis of individual patient data to examine factors affecting growth and rupture of small abdominal aortic aneurysms. *Br J Surg*. 2012;99:655–665.

57. De Rango P, Farchioni L, Fiorucci B, Lenti M. Diabetes and abdominal aortic aneurysms. *Eur J Vasc Endovasc Surg*. 2014 March;47(3):243–261.

58. Saratzis A, Bown MJ. The genetic basis for aortic aneurysmal disease. *Heart*. 2014 June;100(12):916–922.

59. Norman PE, Davis TM, Le MT, Golledge J. Matrix biology of abdominal aortic aneurysms in diabetes: Mechanisms underlying the negative association. *Connect Tissue Res*. 2007;48(3):125–131.

60. Jones SC, Saunders HJ, Pollock CA. High glucose increases growth and collagen synthesis in cultured human tubulointerstitial cells. *Diabet Med*. 1999;16(11):932–938.

61. Astrand H, Ryden-Ahlgren A, Sundkvist G, Sandgren T, Lanne T. Reduced aortic wall stress in diabetes mellitus. *Eur J Vasc Endovasc Surg*. 2007;33(5):592–598.

62. Portik-Dobos V, Anstadt MP, Hutchinson J, Bannan M, Ergul A. Evidence for a matrix metalloproteinase induction/activation system in arterial vasculature and decreased synthesis and activity in diabetes. *Diabetes*. 2002;51(10):3063–3068.

63. Aronson D. Cross-linking of glycated collagen in the pathogenesis of arterial and myocardial stiffening of aging and diabetes. *J Hypertens*. 2003;21(1):3–12.

64. Torsney E, Pirianov G, Cockerill GW. Diabetes as a negative risk factor for abdominal aortic aneurysm – Does the disease aetiology or the treatment provide the mechanism of protection? *Curr Vasc Pharmacol*. 2013;11:293–298.

65. Golledge J, Cullen B, Rush C et al. Peroxisome proliferator-activated receptor ligands reduce aortic dilatation in a mouse model of aortic aneurysm. *Atherosclerosis*. 2010;210:51–56.

66. Kaya MG, Calapkorur B, Karaca Z et al. The effects of treatment with drospirenone/ethinyl oestradiol alone or in combination with metformin on elastic properties of aorta in women with polycystic ovary syndrome. *Clin Endocrinol (Oxf)*. 2012;77:885–892.

67. Jones A, Deb R, Torsney E et al. Rosiglitazone reduces the development and rupture of experimental aortic aneurysms. *Circulation*. 2009;119:3125–3132.

68. Kauffman P, Puech-Leão P. Surgical treatment of popliteal artery aneurysm: A 32-year experience. *J Vasc Br*. 2002;1(1):5–14.

69. Davies RS, Wall M, Rai S, Simms MH, Vohra RK, Bradbury AW, Adam DJ. Long-term results of surgical repair of popliteal artery aneurysm. *Eur J Vasc Endovasc Surg*. 2007 December;34(6):714–718.

70. Martelli E, Ippoliti A, Ventoruzzo G, De Vivo G, Ascoli Marchetti A, Pistolese GR. Popliteal artery aneurysms. Factors associated with thromboembolism and graft failure. *Int Angiol*. 2004 March;23(1):54–65.

71. Luitse MJ, Biessels GJ, Rutten GE, Kappelle LJ. Diabetes, hyperglycaemia, and acute ischaemic stroke. *Lancet Neurol*. 2012 March;11(3):261–271.

72. Parlani G, De Rango P, Cieri E, Verzini F, Giordano G, Simonte G, Isernia G, Cao P. Diabetes is not a predictor of outcome for carotid revascularization with stenting as it may be for carotid endarterectomy. *J Vasc Surg*. 2012 January;55(1):79–89.

73. Dorigo W, Pulli R, Pratesi G, Fargion A, Marek J, Innocenti AA, Pratesi C. Early and long-term results of carotid endarterectomy in diabetic patients. *J Vasc Surg*. 2011 January;53(1):44–52.

74. Mizuhashi S, Kataoka H, Sano N, Ideguchi M, Higashi M, Miyamoto Y, Iihara K. Acta impact of diabetes mellitus on characteristics of carotid plaques and outcomes after carotid endarterectomy. *Neurochir (Wien)*. 2014 May;156(5):927–933.

75. Protack CD, Bakken AM, Xu J, Saad WA, Lumsden AB, Davies MG. Metabolic syndrome: A predictor of adverse outcomes after carotid revascularization. *J Vasc Surg*. 2009 May;49(5):1172–1180.

76. Arquizan C, Trinquart L, Touboul PJ, Long A, Feasson S, Terriat B, Gobin-Metteil MP, Guidolin B, Cohen S, Mas JL; EVA-3S Investigators. Restenosis is more frequent after carotid stenting than after endarterectomy: The EVA-3S study. *Stroke*. 2011 April;42(4):1015–1020.

77. Lal BK, Beach KW, Roubin GS et al.; CREST Investigators. Restenosis after carotid artery stenting and endarterectomy: A secondary analysis of CREST, a randomised controlled trial. *Lancet Neurol*. 2012 September;11(9):755–763.

78. Gurm HS, Yadav JS, Fayad P et al.; SAPPHIRE Investigators. Long-term results of carotid stenting versus endarterectomy in high-risk patients. *N Engl J Med*. 2008 April 10;358(15):1572–1579.

79. Eckstein HH, Ringleb P, Allenberg JR, Berger J, Fraedrich G, Hacke W, Hennerici M, Stingele R, Fiehler J, Zeumer H, Jansen O. Results of the Stent-Protected Angioplasty versus Carotid Endarterectomy (SPACE) study to treat symptomatic stenoses at 2 years: A multinational, prospective, randomised trial. *Lancet Neurol*. 2008 October;7(10):893–902.

80. McCabe DJ, Pereira AC, Clifton A, Bland JM, Brown MM; CAVATAS Investigators. Restenosis after carotid angioplasty, stenting, or endarterectomy in the Carotid and Vertebral Artery Transluminal Angioplasty Study (CAVATAS). *Stroke*. 2005 February;36(2):281–286.

81. Muller IS, de Grauw WJ, van Gerwen WH, Bartelink ML, van Den Hoogen HJ, Rutten GE. Foot ulceration and lower limb amputation in type 2 diabetic patients in Dutch primary health care. *Diabetes Care*. 2002 March;25(3):570–574.

82. Margolis DJ, Malay DS, Hoffstad OJ et al. Incidence of diabetic foot ulcer and lower extremity amputation among Medicare beneficiaries, 2006 to 2008: Data Points #2. 2011 February 17. In: Data Points Publication Series. Rockville, MD: Agency for Healthcare Research and Quality, 2011.

83. Prompers L, Schaper N, Apelqvist J et al. Prediction of outcome in individuals with diabetic foot ulcers: Focus on the differences between individuals with and without peripheral arterial disease. The EURODIALE Study. *Diabetologia*. 2008 May;51(5):747–755.

84. Lipsky BA, Berendt AR, Cornia PB et al.; Infectious Diseases Society of America. 2012 Infectious Diseases Society of America clinical practice guideline for the diagnosis and treatment of diabetic foot infections. *Clin Infect Dis*. 2012 June;54(12):e132–e173.

85. International Working Group on the Diabetic Foot (IWGDF) Editorial Board. The diabetic foot. *Diabetes Metab Res Rev*. 2008;24(Suppl. 1):S1–S193.

86. Eneroth M, Apelqvist J. Clinical characteristics and outcome in diabetic patients with deep foot infections. *Foot Ankle*. 1997;18:716–722.

87. Aragon-Sanchez J, Lipsky BA, Lazaro-Martinez JL. Diagnosing diabetic foot osteomyelitis: Is the combination of probe-to-bone test and plain radiography sufficient for high-risk inpatients? *Diabet Med*. 2011;28:191–194.

88. Newman LG, Waller J, Palestro CJ et al. Unsuspected osteomyelitis in diabetic foot ulcers. Diagnosis and monitoring by leukocyte scanning with indium in 111 oxyquinoline. *J Am Med Assoc*. 1991;266:1246–1251.

89. Michail M, Jude E, Liaskos C et al. The performance of serum inflammatory markers for the diagnosis and follow-up of patients with osteomyelitis. *Int J Low Extrem Wounds*. 2013;12:94–99.

90. Game FL. Osteomyelitis in the diabetic foot: Diagnosis and management. *Med Clin North Am*. 2013;97:947–956.

91. Dinh MT, Abad CL, Safdar N. Diagnostic accuracy of the physical examination and imaging tests for osteomyelitis underlying diabetic foot ulcers: Meta-analysis. *Clin Infect Dis*. 2008;47:519–527.

92. Johnson PC, Doll SC, Cromey W. Pathogenesis of diabetic neuropathy. *Ann Neurol*. 1986;19:450–457.

93. Said G. Diabetic neuropathy – A review. *Nat Clin Pract Neurol*. 2007 June;3(6):331–340.

94. Thamotharampillai K, Chan AK, Bennetts B, Craig ME, Cusumano J, Silink M, Oates PJ, Donaghue KC. Decline in neurophysiological function after 7 years in an adolescent diabetic cohort and the role of aldose reductase gene polymorphisms. *Diabetes Care*. 2006 September;29(9):2053–2057.

95. Knopp M, Rajabally YA. Common and less common peripheral nerve disorders associated with diabetes. *Curr Diabetes Rev*. 2012 May;8(3):229–236.

96. Wyss CR, Matsen FA III, Simmons CW, Burgess EM. Transcutaneous oxygen tension measurements on limbs of diabetic and nondiabetic patients with peripheral vascular disease. *Surgery*. 1984;95:339–346.

97. Boulton AJ, Scarpello JH, Ward JD. Venous oxygenation in the diabetic neuropathic foot: Evidence of arteriovenous shunting? *Diabetologia*. 1982 January;22(1):6–8.

98. Norman PE, Davis WA, Bruce DG et al. Peripheral arterial disease and risk of cardiac death in type 2 diabetes: The Fremantle Diabetes Study. *Diabetes Care*. 2006;29:575–580.

99. McAlpine RR, Morris AD, Emslie-Smith A, James P, Evans JM. The annual incidence of diabetic complications in a population of patients with Type 1 and Type 2 diabetes. *Diabet Med*. 2005 March;22(3):348–352.

100. Sebastianski M, Makowsky MJ, Dorgan M, Tsuyuki RT. Paradoxically lower prevalence of peripheral arterial disease in South Asians: A systematic review and meta-analysis. *Heart*. 2014 January;100(2):100–105.

101. Goldenbeg S, Alex M, Joshi RA, Blumenthal HT. Nonatheromatous peripheral vascular disease of the lower extremity in diabetes mellitus. *Diabetes.* 1959 July–August;8(4):261–273.

102. Handelsman MB, Morrione TG, Ghitman B. Skin vascular alterations in diabetes mellitus. *Arch Intern Med.* 1962 July;110:70–77.

103. Jude EB, Oyibo SO, Chalmers N, Boulton AJ. Peripheral arterial disease in diabetic and nondiabetic patients: A comparison of severity and outcome. *Diabetes Care.* 2001 August;24(8):1433–1437.

104. Abularrage CJ, Sidawy AN, Aidinian G, Singh N, Weiswasser JM, Arora S. Evaluation of the microcirculation in vascular disease. *J Vasc Surg.* 2005 September;42(3):574–581.

105. Abaci A, Oğuzhan A, Kahraman S, Eryol NK, Unal S, Arinç H, Ergin A. Effect of diabetes mellitus on formation of coronary collateral vessels. *Circulation.* 1999 May 4;99(17):2239–2242.

106. Johannesson A, Larsson GU, Ramstrand N, Turkiewicz A, Wiréhn AB, Atroshi I. Incidence of lower-limb amputation in the diabetic and nondiabetic general population: A 10-year population-based cohort study of initial unilateral and contralateral amputations and reamputations. *Diabetes Care.* 2009;32:275–280.

107. Norgren L, Hiatt WR, Dormandy JA, Nehler MR, Harris KA, Fowkes FG. Inter-society consensus for the management of peripheral arterial disease (TASC II). *J Vasc Surg.* 2007;45(Suppl. S):S5–S67.

108. Elgzyri T, Larsson J, Thörne J, Eriksson KF, Apelqvist J. Outcome of ischemic foot ulcer in diabetic patients who had no invasive vascular intervention. *Eur J Vasc Endovasc Surg.* 2013 July;46(1):110–117.

109. Adam DJ, Beard JD, Cleveland T et al. Bypass versus angioplasty in severe ischaemia of the leg (BASIL): Multicentre, randomised controlled trial. *Lancet.* 2005;366:1925–1934.

110. Faglia E, Clerici G, Clerissi J et al. Long-term prognosis of diabetic patients with critical limb ischemia: A population-based cohort study. *Diabetes Care.* 2009;32(5):822–827.

111. Bakker K, Apelqvist J, Schaper NC. Practical guidelines on the management and prevention of the diabetic foot 2011. *Diabetes Metab Res Rev.* 2012;28(Suppl. 1):225–231.

112. WGDF-PAD Working Group 2011. Specific guidelines on diagnosis and treatment of PAD in the diabetic patient with a foot ulcer. www.idf.org, 2011.

113. Got I. Transcutaneous oxygen pressure (TcPO2): Advantages and limitations. *Diabetes Metab.* 1998 September;24(4):379–384.

114. Takolander R, Rauwerda JA. The use of noninvasive vascular assessment in diabetic patients with foot lesions. *Diabet Med.* 1995;13(Suppl. 1):S39–S42.

115. Apelqvist JA, Lepantalo MJ. The ulcerated leg: When to revascularize. *Diabetes Metab Res Rev.* 2012;28(Suppl. 1):30–35.

116. Sheehan P, Jones P, Caselli A, Giurini JM, Veves A. Percent change in wound area of diabetic foot ulcers over a 4-week period is a robust predictor of complete healing in a 12-week prospective trial. *Diabetes Care.* 2003 June;26(6):1879–1882.

117. Elgzyri T, Larsson J, Nyberg P, Thörne J, Eriksson KF, Apelqvist J. Early revascularization after admittance to a diabetic foot center affects the healing probability of ischemic foot ulcer in patients with diabetes. *Eur J Vasc Endovasc Surg.* 2014 August 5.

118. Moneta GL, Yeager RA, Lee RW, Porter JM. Noninvasive localization of arterial occlusive disease: A comparison of segmental Doppler pressures and arterial duplex mapping. *J Vasc Surg.* 1993;17:578–582.

119. Koelemay MJ, den Hartog D, Prins MH, Kromhout JG, Legemate DA, Jacobs MJ. Diagnosis of arterial disease of the lower extremities with duplex ultrasonography. *Br J Surg.* 1996;83:404–409.

120. National Institute for Health and Clinical Excellence. Lower limb peripheral arterial disease: Diagnosis and management. Clinical guideline 147, http://guidance.nice.org.uk/CG119, 2012.

121. Met R, Bipat S, Legemate DA, Reekers JA, Koelemay MJ. Diagnostic performance of computed tomography angiography in peripheral arterial disease: A systematic review and meta-analysis. *J Am Med Assoc.* 2009;301:415–424.

122. Andreisek G, Pfammatter T, Goepfert K et al. Peripheral arteries in diabetic patients: Standard bolus-chase and time-resolved MR angiography. *Radiology.* 2007;242:610–620.

123. Menke J, Larsen J. Meta-analysis: Accuracy of contrast-enhanced magnetic resonance angiography for assessing steno-occlusions in peripheral arterial disease. *Ann Intern Med.* 2010;153:325–334.

124. Dellegrottaglie S, Sanz J, Macaluso F, Einstein AJ, Raman S, Simonetti OP, Rajagopalan S. Technology Insight: Magnetic resonance angiography for the evaluation of patients with peripheral artery disease. *Nat Clin Pract Cardiovasc Med.* 2007;4:677–687.

125. Hoch JR, Tullis MJ, Kennell TW, McDermott J, Acher CW, Turnipseed WD. Use of magnetic resonance angiography for the preoperative evaluation of patients with infrainguinal arterial occlusive disease. *J Vasc Surg.* 1996;23:792–800.

126. Romiti M, Albers M, Brochado-Neto FC, Durazzo AE, Pereira CA, De Luccia N. Meta-analysis of infrapopliteal angioplasty for chronic critical limb ischemia. *J Vasc Surg.* 2008 May;47(5):975–981.

127. Pereira CE, Albers M, Romiti M, Brochado-Neto FC, Pereira CA. Meta-analysis of femoropopliteal bypass grafts for lower extremity arterial insufficiency. *J Vasc Surg.* 2006 September;44(3):510–517.

128. Bakken AM, Palchik E, Hart JP, Rhodes JM, Saad WE, Davies MG. Impact of diabetes mellitus on outcomes of superficial femoral artery endoluminal interventions. *J Vasc Surg.* 2007 November;46(5):946–958.

129. Moxey PW, Hofman D, Hinchliffe RJ, Jones K, Thompson MM, Holt PJ. Trends and outcomes after surgical lower limb revascularization in England. *Br J Surg.* 2011 October;98(10):1373–1382.

130. Bradbury AW, Adam DJ, Bell J et al. Bypass versus Angioplasty in Severe Ischaemia of the Leg (BASIL) trial: Analysis of amputation free and overall survival by treatment received. *J Vasc Surg.* 2010;51:18S–31S.

131. Bradbury AW, Adam DJ, Bell J et al. Bypass versus Angioplasty in Severe Ischaemia of the Leg (BASIL) trial: An intention-to-treat analysis of amputation-free and overall survival in patients randomized to a bypass surgery-first or a balloon angioplasty-first revascularization strategy. *J Vasc Surg.* 2010;51:5S–17S.

132. Conte MS, Bandyk DF, Clowes AW et al.; PREVENT III Investigators. Results of PREVENT III: A multicenter, randomized trial of edifoligide for the prevention of vein graft failure in lower extremity bypass surgery. *J Vasc Surg.* 2006 April;43(4):742–751.

133. Monahan TS, Owens CD. Risk factors for lower-extremity vein graft failure. *Semin Vasc Surg.* 2009;22:216–226.

134. Tannenbaum GA, Pomposelli FB, Marcaccio EJ et al. Safety of vein bypass grafting to the dorsal pedal artery in diabetic patients with foot infections. *J Vasc Surg.* 1992;15:982–988; discussion 989–990.

135. Pomposelli FB, Kansal N, Hamdan AD, Belfield A, Sheahan M, Campbell DR, Skillman JJ, Logerfo FW. A decade of experience with dorsalis pedis artery bypass: Analysis of outcome in more than 1000 cases. *J Vasc Surg.* 2003 February;37(2):307–315.

136. Alexander J, Gutierrez C, Katz S. Non-greater saphenous vein grafting for infrageniculate bypass. *Am Surg.* 2002 July;68(7):611–614.

137. Veith FJ, Gupta SK, Samson RH, Flores SW, Janko G, Scher LA. Superficial femoral and popliteal arteries as inflow sites for distal bypasses. *Surgery.* 1981 December;90(6):980–990.

138. Attinger CE, Evans KK, Bulan E, Blume P, Cooper P. Angiosomes of the 267 foot and ankle and clinical implications for limb salvage: Reconstruction, incisions, and revascularization. *Plast Reconstr Surg.* 2006;117(Suppl.):261S–293S.

139. Iida O, Takahara M, Soga Y et al. Worse limb prognosis for indirect versus direct endovascular revascularization only in patients with critical limb ischemia complicated with wound infection and diabetes mellitus. *Eur J Vasc Endovasc Surg.* 2013;46:575–582.

140. Acín F, Varela C, López de Maturana I, de Haro J, Bleda S, Rodriguez-Padilla J. Results of infrapopliteal endovascular procedures performed in diabetic patients with critical limb ischemia and tissue loss from the perspective of an angiosome-oriented revascularization strategy. *Int J Vasc Med.* 2014;2014:270539.

141. Bosanquet DC, Glasbey JC, Williams IM, Twine CP. Systematic review and meta-analysis of direct versus indirect angiosomal revascularisation of infrapopliteal arteries. *Eur J Vasc Endovasc Surg.* 2014 July;48(1):88–97.

142. Rashid H, Slim H, Zayed H, Huang DY, Wilkins CJ, Evans DR, Sidhu PS, Edmonds M. The impact of arterial pedal arch quality and angiosome revascularization on foot tissue loss healing and infrapopliteal bypass outcome. *J Vasc Surg.* 2013 May;57(5):1219–1226.

143. Azuma N, Uchida H, Kokubo T, Koya A, Akasaka N, Sasajima T. Factors influencing wound healing of critical ischaemic foot after bypass surgery: Is the angiosome important in selecting bypass target artery? *Eur J Vasc Endovasc Surg.* 2012 March;43(3):322–328.

144. Biancari F, Salenius JP, Heikkinen M et al. Risk-scoring method for prediction of 30-day post-operative outcome after infrainguinal surgical revascularization for critical lower-limb ischemia: A Finnvasc registry study. *World J Surg.* 2007;31:217–225; discussion 226–217.

145. Bradbury AW, Adam DJ, Bell J et al. Bypass Versus Angioplasty in Severe Ischaemia of The Leg (BASIL) Trial: A survival prediction model to facilitate clinical decision making. *J Vasc Surg.* 2010;51:52S–68S.

146. Graziani L, Silvestro A, Bertone V, Manara E, Andreini R, Sigala A, Mingardi R, De Giglio R. Vascular involvement in diabetic subjects with ischemic foot ulcer: A new morphologic categorization of disease severity. *Eur J Vasc Endovasc Surg.* 2007;33(4):453–460.

147. Bolia A, Brennan J, Bell PR. Recanalization of femoropopliteal occlusions: Improving success rate by subintimal recanalization. *Clin Radiol.* 1989;40:325.

148. Bolia A, Miles KA, Brennan J, Bell PRF. Percutaneous transluminal angioplasty of occlusions of the SFA by subintimal dissection. *Cardiovasc Intervent Radiol.* 1990;13:357–363.

149. Reekers JA, Kromhout JG, Jacobs MJ. Percutaneous intentional extraluminal recanalisation of the femoropopliteal artery. *Eur J Vasc Surg.* 1994;8:723–728.

150. Yilmaz S, Sindel T, Ceken K et al. Subintimal recanalisation of long SFA occlusions through the retrograde popliteal approach. *Cardiovasc Intervent Radiol.* 2001;24:154–160.

151. Laxdal E, Jenssen GL, Pederson G, Aune S. Subintimal angioplasty as a treatment for femoropopliteal occlusions. *Eur J Vasc Endovasc Surg.* 2003;25:578–582.

152. Shaw MB, De Nunzio M, Hinwood D et al. The results of subintimal angioplasty in a district general hospital. *Eur J Vasc Endovasc Surg.* 2002;24:524–527.

153. McCarthy RJ, Neary W, Roobottom C et al. Short term results of femoropopliteal subintimal angioplasty. *Br J Surg.* 2000;87:1361–1365.

154. Siablis D, Diamantopoulos A, Katsanos K, Spiliopoulos S, Kagadis GC, Papadoulas S, Karnabatidis D. Sub-intimal angioplasty of long chronic total femoropopliteal occlusions: Long-term outcomes, predictors of angiographic restenosis, and role of stenting. *Cardiovasc Intervent Radiol.* 2012 June;35(3):483–490.

155. Köcher M, Cerna M, Utikal P, Kozak J, Sisola I, Thomas RP, Bachleda P, Drac P, Sekanina Z, Langova K. Subintimal angioplasty in femoropopliteal region-mid-term results. *Eur J Radiol.* 2010 March;73(3):672–676.

156. Sidhu R, Pigott J, Pigott M, Comerota A. Subintimal angioplasty for advanced lower extremity ischemia due to TASC II C and D lesions of the superficial femoral artery. *Vasc Endovascular Surg.* 2010 November;44(8):633–637.

157. Scott EC, Biuckians A, Light RE, Burgess J, Meier GH 3rd, Panneton JM. Subintimal angioplasty: Our experience in the treatment of 506 infrainguinal arterial occlusions. *J Vasc Surg.* 2008 October;48(4):878–884.

158. Scott EC, Biuckians A, Light RE, Scibelli CD, Milner TP, Meier GH 3rd, Panneton JM. Subintimal angioplasty for the treatment of claudication and critical limb ischemia: 3-year results. *J Vasc Surg.* 2007 November;46(5):959–964.

159. Trocciola SM, Chaer R, Dayal R et al. Comparison of results in endovascular interventions for infrainguinal lesions: Claudication versus critical limb ischemia. *Am Surg.* 2005 June;71(6):474–479.

160. Desgranges P, Boufi M, Lapeyre M, Tarquini G, van Laere O, Losy F, Mellière D, Becquemin JP, Kobeiter H. Subintimal angioplasty: Feasible and durable. *Eur J Vasc Endovasc Surg.* 2004 August;28(2):138–141.

161. Laxdal E, Eide GE, Wirsching J, Jenssen GL, Jonung T, Pedersen G, Amundsen SR, Dregelid E, Aune S. Homocysteine levels, haemostatic risk factors and patency rates after endovascular treatment of the above-knee femoro-popliteal artery. *Eur J Vasc Endovasc Surg.* 2004 October;28(4):410–417.

162. Tisi PV, Mirnezami A, Baker S et al. Role of subintimal angioplasty in the treatment of chronic lower leg ischaemia. *Eur J Vasc Endovasc Surg.* 2002;24:417–422.

163. Lipsitz EC, Ohki T, Veith FJ et al. Does subintimal angioplasty have a role in the treatment of severe lower extremity ischaemia? *J Vasc Surg.* 2003;37:386–391.

164. Molloy KJ, Nasim A, London NJM et al. Percutaneous transluminal angioplasty in the treatment of critical limb ischaemia. *J Endovasc Ther.* 2003;10:298–303.

165. Lazaris AM, Tsiamis AC, Fishwick G et al. Clinical outcomes of primary infrainguinal subintimal angioplasty in diabetic patients with critical lower limb ischaemia. *J Endovasc Ther.* 2005;11:447–453.

166. Vraux H, Hammer F, Verhelst R. Subintimal angioplasty of tibial vessel occlusions in the treatment of critical limb ischaemia: Mid-term results. *Eur J Vasc Endovasc Surg.* 2000;20:441–446.

167. Ingle H, Nasim A, Bolia A et al. Subintimal angioplasty of isolated infragenicular vessels in lower limb ischaemia: Long-term results. *J Endovasc Ther.* 2002;9:414–416.

168. Spinosa DJ, Harthun NL, Bissonette EA et al. Subintimal arterial flossing with antegrade-retrograde intervention (SAFARI) for subintimal recanalisation to treat chronic critical limb ischaemia. *J Vasc Interv Radiol.* 2005;16:37–44.

169. Hynes N, Mahendran B, Manning B, Andrews E, Courtney D, Sultan S. The influence of subintimal angioplasty on level of amputation and limb salvage rates in lower limb critical ischaemia: A 15-year experience. *Eur J Vasc Endovasc Surg.* 2005 September;30(3):291–299.

170. Akesson M, Riva L, Ivancev K, Uher P, Lundell A, Malina M. Subintimal angioplasty of infrainguinal arterial occlusions for critical limb ischemia: Long-term patency and clinical efficacy. *J Endovasc Ther.* 2007 August;14(4):444–451.

171. Setacci C, Chisci E, de Donato G, Setacci F, Iacoponi F, Galzerano G. Subintimal angioplasty with the aid of a re-entry device for TASC C and D lesions of the SFA. *Eur J Vasc Endovasc Surg.* 2009 July;38(1):76–87.

172. Sultan S, Hynes N. Five-year Irish trial of CLI patients with TASC II type C/D lesions undergoing subintimal angioplasty or bypass surgery based on plaque echolucency. *J Endovasc Ther.* 2009 June;16(3):270–283.

173. Nydahl S, London NJM, Bolia A. Technical report: Recanalisation of all three infrapopliteal arteries by subintimal angioplasty. *Clin Radiol.* 1996;51:366–367.

174. Bolia A, Sayers RD, Thompson MM, Bell PR. Subintimal and intraluminal recanalisation of occluded crural arteries by percutaneous balloon angioplasty. *Eur J Vasc Surg.* 1994;8:214–219.

175. London NJM, Varty K, Sayers RD et al. Percutaneous transluminal angioplasty for lower limb critical ischaemia. *Br J Surg.* 1995;82:1232–1235.

176. Varty K, Nydahl S, Nasim A et al. Results of surgery and angioplasty for the treatment of chronic severe lower limb ischaemia. *Eur J Vasc Endovasc Surg.* 1998;16:159–163.

177. Lazaris AM, Salas C, Tsiamis AC, Vlachou PA, Bolia A, Fishwick G, Bell PR. Factors affecting patency of subintimal infrainguinal angioplasty in patients with critical lower limb ischemia. *Eur J Vasc Endovasc Surg.* 2006 December;32(6):668–674.

178. Hayes PD, Chokkalingham A, Jones R et al. Arterial perforation during infrainguinal lower limb angioplasty does not worsen outcome: Results from 1409 patients. *J Endovasc Ther.* 2002;9:422–427.

179. DeRubertis BG, Faries PL, McKinsey JF, Chaer RA, Pierce M, Karwowski J, Weinberg A, Nowygrod R, Morrissey NJ, Bush HL, Kent KC. Shifting paradigms in the treatment of lower extremity vascular disease: A report of 1000 percutaneous interventions. *Ann Surg.* 2007 September;246(3):415–422.

180. Giles KA, Pomposelli FB, Spence TL et al. Infrapopliteal angioplasty for critical limb ischemia: Relation of TransAtlantic InterSociety Consensus class to outcome in 176 limbs. *J Vasc Surg.* 2008;48:128–136.

181. Gray BH, Grant AA, Kalbaugh CA et al. The impact of isolated tibial disease on outcomes in the critical limb ischemic population. *Ann Vasc Surg.* 2010;24:349–159.

182. Abdelhamid MF, Davies RS, Rai S, Hopkins JD, Duddy MJ, Vohra RK. Below-the-ankle angioplasty is a feasible and effective intervention for critical leg ischaemia. *Eur J Vasc Endovasc Surg.* 2010 June;39(6):762–768.

25

Prevention and management of prosthetic vascular graft infection

MAX ZEGELMAN, OJAN ASSADIAN and FRANK J. VEITH

CONTENTS

INTRODUCTION

Vascular graft infection is one of the difficult challenges vascular surgeons may face. Traditional management of infected arterial grafts includes mandatory excision of the entire graft with subsequent revascularization. Due to the high morbidity and the related risk of limb loss and even death, various new strategies of prevention, but also complete or partial graft salvage that may be useful in the management of these difficult conditions, have been investigated. These include total graft excision (including implanted stent grafts), debridement of infected tissue and in situ reconstruction or revascularization through non-infected tissue planes or antimicrobial prosthetic grafts if inadequate collateral circulation exists. Veith was one of the first to suggest graft preservation as a possible special exception for high-risk patients.[1] The use of negative-pressure wound therapy (NPWT) is a promising adjunct measure not only to close dehiscent surgical sites but may also change therapeutic-operative concepts for graft infections.[2]

This chapter outlines current modalities important in preventing, diagnosing and treating these serious complications.

INCIDENCE

Vascular graft infection remains a serious limb-threatening and often life-threatening complication reported after 0.5%–6% of all arterial reconstructions. The morbidity associated with prosthetic graft infection is high. For peripheral vascular prostheses, morbidity of up to 41% has been reported, mostly resulting in amputation, with an attributable mortality of 17%. In aortic vascular grafts, a mortality rate of 24%–75% was observed, with a 5-year survival rate less than 50%.[3,4] Prosthetic graft infections, including infections of stent grafts, are more common after emergency operations.[5] Because of the placement technique, endovascular aneurysm repair (EVAR) largely eliminates the risk of intraoperative graft contamination to a certain extent. However, the reduced level of sterility in interventional suites as compared to traditional operation rooms may compensate this advantage. Infections are reported after EVAR as well.[6]

During a 5-year collection period (2005–2009), the database of the German Hospital Infection Surveillance System, KISS,[7] included pooled data on a total of 21,780 vascular surgical procedures (carotid artery reconstruction n = 4,260; surgery of aorta abdomina-lis n = 2,130; arterial reconstruction of lower extremities n = 15,390). Among these, 540 well-documented cases of infection after vascular surgical procedures, strictly based on the CDC/NHSN surveillance definitions,[8] resulted in a pooled mean soft tissue infection (SSI) rate of 2.48%. Compared to other indicator surgeries, the incidence of infection after vascular surgery is equal to nephrectomy (pooled mean infection rate, 2.48%; median, 1.66; IQR, 0.88–2.30) and is only topped by open colon surgery (9.36%), laparotomic cholecystectomy (5.33%), appendectomy (4.11%) and thoracic wound infection after coronary bypass with or without autologous removal of blood vessels from extremities (3.12% and 3.55%, respectively).

The incidence of vascular graft infection varies considerably and depends on a number of factors, such as graft location, circumstances at the time of implantation and technique of the procedure. The risk is lowest in carotid artery reconstruction (pooled mean infection rate, 0.14%; median, 0.00; IQR, 0.00–0.00), increased in surgery of the aorta abdominalis (pooled mean infection rate, 1.08; median, 0.00; IQR, 0.00–2.03) and highest in arterial reconstruction of lower extremities (pooled mean infection rate, 3.32; median, 3.33; IQR, 1.13–5.12).[6]

PATHOGENESIS AND MICROBIOLOGY

The pathogenesis of prosthetic graft infection involves complex interaction of the graft surface, microorganism, inflammatory response to the graft and host defences. Graft infection occurs when bacteria or, more rarely, fungi contaminate the vascular prosthesis. Disrespectable of the source of the causative microorganisms, vascular graft infection starts with contamination of the graft, bacterial colonization and formation of biofilms on the graft's surface. Reversible van der Waals forces and electrostatic bonds, dipole interactions, hydrogen bonds and covalent bonds support the initial microbial attachment. If the attached microorganisms are not immediately inactivated by the immune system, they will start colonizing the surface permanently, supported by cell adhesion structures and active, progressive movement. Within the formed biofilm, bacteria may communicate by the release of signal molecules ('quorum sensing') that coordinate the formation of structured and stable biofilms.[9]

Once colonization begins, the biofilm will grow by a combination of cell division and by genesis of a matrix of excreted extracellular polymeric substance. This matrix protects the microorganisms embedded within the biofilm. From the microorganism's perspective, one major benefit of this matrix is the increased protection against the immune system and considerably decreased susceptibility to antiseptics and antibiotics, which explains the difficulty to clear microorganisms by administration of systemic anti-infectives. Furthermore, prosthetic graft materials incite an immune foreign body reaction that produces a microenvironment in the peri-graft space that is conducive to bacterial adhesion and microbial colony formation within a biofilm. This foreign body reaction around prosthetic grafts is distinct from autogenous grafts. Prosthetic grafts fail to develop rich vascular connections, and, therefore, host defences and antibiotics are less likely to be effective in the face of contamination. Neutrophil chemotaxis and bactericidal function are impaired. Indolent peri-graft infection may result, and ultimately, the infection may progress and manifest as sepsis, anastomotic breakdown with pseudo-aneurysm formation or hemorrhage.[10] Additionally, in the case of aortic prostheses, graft-enteric erosions or fistulas can occur and are associated with a high mortality.

The two most common aetiologies are direct contamination at operation and hematogenous seeding. By far, the most common cause of vascular graft infection is direct contamination at implantation. This may occur with breaks in sterile technique that exposes the graft to bacteria from the surgical team, the endogenous flora of the patient or the patient's skin. Another potential source of inoculation is through infected lymph that comes into contact with the prosthesis when lymphatic vessels are disrupted during implantation. These lymph vessels that drain infected tissues such as a lower extremity infection or gangrene may predispose the graft to contamination and increase the risk of infection.[11]

In addition to direct methods of bacterial graft contamination, the prosthetic may become contaminated and hence infected due to hematogenous spread from a distant focus of infection, such as intravascular line sepsis, urinary tract infection or pneumonia. Using an experimental animal model,[12] it was demonstrated that intravenous administration of 10^7 CFU of *Staphylococcus aureus* immediately after aortic graft implantation resulted in a 100% incidence of graft infection. During the process of incorporation, the peri-graft environment becomes less vulnerable to a bacterial contamination and infection, since the development of the pseudo-intimal layer inside the graft and ingrowth of a fibrous capsule along the outer surface correlates with a gradual decrease in the rate of clinical graft infection over time.[13] Hence, transient bacteremia associated with a damaged or poorly developed pseudo-intima may result in a prosthetic graft infection, even years after implantation.

This mechanism may explain the phenomenon of late graft infection. Presentation of vascular graft infection may be distinguished as early- or late-onset infection. This clinical presentation distinguishes patients with early- or late-onset vascular graft infection significantly.

In early-onset infections (<4 months after graft implantation), the patient may be systemically septic with fever and leukocytosis. Systemic infection, local wound infection, abdominal discomfort and graft dysfunction may be present. Late-onset infections (>4 months after graft implantation) present more masked with non-specific clinical signs and symptoms.

Mostly, fever is present, and the patients are more likely to present with signs of complications of graft infection, such as gastrointestinal bleeding in the course of erosion of the graft into the gastrointestinal tract, false aneurysm or hydro-nephrosis.

Prosthetic infections with a single organism (mono-infections) seem to lose significance over the past years, whereas infections with multiple organisms constitute increasingly microbiological constellation. Also, infections with resistant bacterial strains have been increasing in number over the past years and deserve special consideration. It remains unclear, if both aspects are due to a true epidemiological change or the result of advances in molecular microbiological diagnostic methods. However, the vast majority of vascular graft infections are caused by three organisms: *S. aureus*, *S. epidermidis* and *Escherichia coli* (Table 25.1). Together with *Enterococcus spp.* and *Pseudomonas aeruginosa*, these organisms account for 90% of reported graft infections.

Yield of *S. epidermidis* and other coagulase-negative staphylococci (CoNS) is difficult to interpret, since such findings may reflect false positive microbiological results due to contamination at the time of sampling. However, also false negative results may be generated since these microorganisms, particularly *P. aeruginosa*,[14] are more difficult to isolate and as such are often associated with negative results in cultures of peri-graft fluid. Many strains of these microorganisms are able to generate biofilms with a glycocalyx that prevents their isolation using standard microbiological techniques. Prosthetic infections caused by *S. aureus* and Gram-negative bacteria such as *Pseudomonas sp.* are more virulent and usually present as an early graft infection within 4 months of implantation. Infections due to *Pseudomonas* are especially aggressive and are associated with a high rate of anastomotic dehiscence and rupture. Fungal infections are extremely rare and usually occur in immune-compromised patients.

Table 25.1 Microbial spectrum of infections in vascular surgery.

Microorganisms	Proportion (%)	Comment
S. aureus	36	Thereof MRSA: 20%
CoNS	20	Thereof CoNS as sole organism: 8%
Enterococcus spp.	16	
E. coli	12	
P. aeruginosa	8	
Enterobacter spp.	6	
Klebsiella spp.	5	
Proteus spp.	1	
C. albicans	1	

Source: Modified according to Cernohorsky P et al., *J Vasc Surg*, 54, 327, 2011.

DIAGNOSIS

Diagnosis of graft infection can be difficult and is based on clinical findings, microbiological cultures and various imaging techniques. The vascular surgeon must have a high index of suspicion to make an early diagnosis of an indolent graft infection. Timely diagnosis and management are necessary to avoid the serious consequences of sepsis, bleeding and death. Any patient with a prosthetic vascular graft that presents with signs of sepsis without an obvious source should be considered to have a graft infection until proven otherwise. Making the diagnosis is frequently challenging because the clinical manifestations may be non-specific and subtle. While graft infection can be established with positive bacterial cultures from the prostheses, this is not always possible until the graft is removed. The most accurate method of diagnosis is operative exploration and may be required to exclude infection as well.

History and physical examination

Graft infections may present as unexplained fever or sepsis. When infection involves aortic grafts confined to the abdomen, septicemia of unknown aetiology, prolonged postoperative ileus or abdominal pain or distension may be the only signs or symptoms. A history of recent illness, infection or invasive procedure that produces a transient bacteremia can prove important. Unexplained gastrointestinal bleeding in a patient with an aortic graft must be considered to have an aorto-enteric fistula or erosion until proven otherwise.[15,16] If the infection involves an extracavitary graft, local signs are usually evident and include cellulitis, draining sinus tracts, tenderness or a pulsatile mass. Extremities should be examined for evidence of septic embolization.

Laboratory studies

Routine laboratory studies including complete blood count, erythrocyte sedimentation rate, urinalysis, urine and blood cultures and cultures from any other potential sites of infection. Stool for occult blood is indicated in patients with possible aorto-enteric fistula. All laboratory tests may be normal in cases of *S. epidermidis* graft infection. Sometimes, an unexplained leukocytosis with concomitant increase of C-reactive protein and fever may be the only clinical or laboratory sign of the infection.

Imaging studies

Many modalities are available to diagnose or determine the extent of graft infection. Vascular imaging is essential for the diagnosis, treatment and pre- and postoperative management of vascular graft infection.[17,18]

Contrast-enhanced CT angiography remains the most specific and feasible examination[16,18] and is usually necessary in the planning of revascularization when the time permits. It is especially sensitive for imaging thoracic and abdominal aortic grafts. Ultrasonography is a readily available imaging technique that can be performed urgently at bedside in critically ill patients or in emergency.[19] Upper gastrointestinal endoscopy or ureteroscopy remains an important diagnostic modality for graft-enteric and graft-ureteral fistula. Contrast sinography is a method of percutaneous localization of a communication of the skin to the peri-graft space. This study relies on gentle introduction of the contrast agent into the sinus tract. Care must be exercised because forceful introduction of the contrast agent may disrupt a tenuous anastomosis. [18]FDG–PET–CT has been proposed as an additional investigation for the diagnosis of vascular graft infection, although its specificity and sensitivity have been challenged.[18,19] The accuracy of indium-111-labelled white blood cell scan approaches 80%–90% to detect a vascular graft infection. A drawback remains that all radionuclide imaging techniques still do not provide exact anatomic details and that in early postoperative course (3–6 months) the uptake is non-specific in the framework of healing and peri-graft inflammatory reaction.[18,20] Finally, ultrasonography- or CT-guided aspiration of cavitary peri-graft fluid collections may be used to differentiate uninfected seroma from bacterial abscess formation.

Microbiological study techniques

Microbiological investigations may support the diagnosis of vascular graft infection, if specimens are obtained in such manner that microorganisms potentially causative for the infection are yielded and not colonization flora with any relevance for a suspected vascular graft infection. Optimal results will be achieved with specimens obtained directly from the infection site. Such direct material may include explanted grafts, extra- or intraoperatively obtained tissue biopsies from the infected area and material aspirated from peri-graft fluid collection, but also indirect material such as blood cultures may yield important information. Blood cultures may be often negative, particularly in late-onset, less frequently in early-onset infection.[21]

Specimens may be investigated using a number of techniques such as direct streaking swabs on agar plates, broth culture, homogenization of tissue specimens with serial dilution techniques and sonication of the graft to enhance the recovery of biofilm-forming organisms from graft or infected material.[21] The report of microbiological specimens is decisive for a valuable evaluation of therapy and clinical results.[20,22] The demonstration of specimens from preoperative, intraoperative and postoperative phase is considered ideal, if feasible and possible.[23]

Relevant *preoperative samples* are blood cultures through central and peripheral venous catheters or direct vein puncture, wound specimens, drainage fluid (in cases of an early-onset postoperative vascular graft infection), nose/throat swabs in case of methicillin-resistant *S. aureus* (MRSA) colonization and urinary samples. Careful assessment is needed for microorganisms isolated from overlying wounds or sinuses, as such microorganisms may represent colonizing flora, e.g. MRSA but may be wrongly interpreted as causative agent.[24]

Relevant *intraoperative samples* are standard specimens obtained from the graft surfaces, the peri-graft fluid/pus and the explanted graft. Noteworthy, a considerable number of specimens may be negative. However, this fact does not necessarily exclude an infection. In cases of allograft (homograft) implantation, specimens from the homograft as well as from the storage medium in case of cryopreserved arterial allografts should be performed and reported in order to assess the absence of contamination of the homograft and to exclude any association to postoperative infection.

Finally, relevant *postoperative samples* are blood cultures, drainage fluid and wound specimens (e.g. in case of wound healing delay). Microbiological specimens of adjacent organs (urinary tract, gut) stay as equally relevant.

Endoscopy

Endoscopy is an essential tool used in patients with aortic grafts that present with gastrointestinal bleeding. Graft-enteric fistula or erosion should be suspected in these cases, and endoscopy of the upper gastrointestinal tract is necessary to rule out another source of hemorrhage. Special attention must be paid to the third and fourth portions of the duodenum because these are the most likely locations of aorto-enteric fistulas. If the patient has had a recent massive bleed, then endoscopy should be performed in the operating room in the event massive bleeding recurs.[25] The prosthetic may be visualized eroding into the duodenal lumen. If blood clot is visualized in the duodenum, no attempt should be made to dislodge it as this may result in massive exsanguinating hemorrhage.

PREVENTION

Graft infections are commonly associated with preoperative or intraoperative events that lead to bacterial contamination of the graft or selection of more resistant organisms. Prevention of such events is integral to the reduction of vascular graft infection. Additionally, patients tend to have a higher incidence of wound complications and infections if they have concomitant immune or nutritional compromises.[26]

An outlook of recent trends indicates that all efforts are needed to improve the current situation, as during the past years, the situation has been complicated further by the increased emergence of multiresistant microorganisms. Because of the consequences of infection in vascular surgery and the increasing resistance of causative microorganisms, the future strategy to deal with vascular graft infection needs to shift from reliance on systemic antibiotics and treatment of manifest infection to a strong focus on primary prevention of infection, particularly before surgical procedures involving prosthetic materials. Simply looking for new antibiotics will not lead to further decrease in the rate of infection in vascular surgery.

There are a number of strategies for prevention of vascular graft infection. Many of them, however, were established in the pre-antibiotic area, and therefore, the level of evidence supporting them is low. Preventive strategies used in vascular surgery, such as maximal sterile barrier precautions, routine change of surgical gloves before graft implant, performing surgical procedures in HEPA-filtered turbulence-free, laminar flow ventilated operation rooms, implementation of perioperative surgical checklists, preoperative screening for S. aureus carriers including MRSA together with eradication, the choice and concentration of preoperative skin antiseptics, or performing or not preoperative shaving and how, have not been studied in vascular surgery well enough and indicate areas for future research. Meticulous sterile technique is paramount. The graft must be handled carefully and avoid contact with the skin and wound edges. Antiseptic-impregnated incision drapes[27] should be used to cover the skin. Any lymphatic vessel should be carefully ligated during the dissection, especially in the groin. Careful handling of tissues, good hemostasis to prevent hematoma formation and closure of the wound in several layers are also important in the reduction of postoperative wound complications.

An example for the increasing interest for simple preventive infection control measure is a recently published randomized controlled trial (RCT) investigating the effect of supplemental postoperative oxygen on the prevention of surgical site infection after lower limb revascularization.[28] Patients were randomly allocated to the study group (n = 137) or a control group (n = 137). The study group received supplemental inspired oxygen for the first 2 days after surgery. The rate of surgical site infection was 23% in total, mostly superficial wound infection. Two vascular graft infections were observed. While not statistically significant, the incidence of surgical site infection was lower in the study group (18%) than in the control group with 28% (OR, 0.56; 95% CI, 0.30–1.04; p, 0.07). In isolated groin incisions, 6% of patients in the study group and 24% patients of the control group developed infection (OR, 0.20; 95% CI, 0.04–0.95; p, 0.04).

For suction groin-wound drainage, a meta-analysis investigating 4 RCTs with a total of 429 groin wounds found no significant effect on wound infection, seroma/lymphocele formation or hematoma formation and concluded that suction groin-wound drainage should

therefore not be routinely used[29]; yet with availability of modern NPWT devices, this may change.

Other infection prevention measures include simply preventing exposure to high-risk procedures. When placing a prosthetic aortic graft, other simultaneous gastrointestinal operations should generally be avoided due to the increased risk of infection.[30] One exception to this is cholecystectomy. Some vascular surgeons discourage the performance of cholecystectomy at the same time as aortic graft implantation.[31,32] Others have reported incidences of postoperative acute cholecystitis as high as 18% when gallstones were present in patients that had aortic aneurysm repair without cholecystectomy.[33] Removal of the gallbladder should be considered if the patient is stable after completion of vascular grafting and closure of the retroperitoneum.

Antibiotic prophylaxis

During the past five decades, prevention of vascular graft infection predominantly relied on the availability of effective perioperative antibiotic prophylaxis or the use of systemic antibiotics for treatment of infections after their clinical manifestation. However, evidence for the prophylactic effect of systemic antibiotics exists only for patients with vein grafts, who are at lower risk of infection compared to patients receiving prosthetic material. Furthermore, because of the changed epidemiology of bacterial susceptibility against antibiotics today, reliance of the efficacy of systemic antibiotic prophylaxis must be made with caution.

The analysis of 10 RCTs on systemic antibiotics versus placebo[34] demonstrates a consistent benefit in reduction of wound infection in 1297 patients (RR fixed, 0.25; 95% CI, 0.17–0.38; p = 0001). Although no single study demonstrated a statistically significant reduction in early vascular graft infection, the pooled results of these 10 RCTs appeared homogeneous with a reduction in early graft infection evident on meta-analysis (RR fixed, 0.31; 95% CI, 0.11–0.85; p = 02). There are, however, two aspects of these results, which need to be highlighted. First, 6 of 10 RCTs included a case mix of patients with both prosthetic and vein grafts. If the individual results are stratified by the type of graft, the RR for wound infection with prosthetic graft is non-significant at 0.51 (95% CI, 0.24–1.11). The administration of prophylactic antibiotics yielded only a significant benefit for patients with vein grafts (RR = 0.13; 95% CI, 0.04–0.41). Therefore, evidence for the prophylactic effect of systemic antibiotics exists only for patients with vein grafts, who are at lower risk of infection compared to patients receiving prosthetic material. Second, the meta-analysis is based on 10 studies comparing the effect of systemic antibiotics versus placebo conducted between 1978 and 1987, and thereof, 7 studies conducted before 1985. For S. aureus, the most frequent bacterial organism causative for vascular infection, resistance to methicillin was first noted clinically in 1961.[35] In the United States, MRSA only emerged in the period 1975–1981 onwards in tertiary care centres. The percentage of major US acute care hospital reporting greater or equal to 50 MRSA cases per year increased from 18% in 1987 to 32% in 1989.[36] Therefore, the result of meta-analyses of RCTs chiefly investigating beta-lactam antibiotics demonstrating efficacy of antibiotic prophylaxis needs to be noted with caution today, as MRSA already has become the most frequent cause of skin and SSIs presenting to the emergency departments in the United States.[37]

If the earlier considerations are followed, prophylactic administration of antibiotics should be administered intravenously prior to skin incision and at regular intervals during the procedure. The optimal time for administration of preoperative doses is within 60 minutes before surgical incision. For all patients, intraoperative re-dosing is needed to ensure adequate serum and tissue concentrations of the antimicrobial if the duration of the procedure exceeds two half-lives of the drug or there is excessive blood loss during the procedure. The recommended regimen for patients undergoing vascular procedures associated with a higher risk of infection, including implantation of prosthetic material, is cefazolin.[38] Clindamycin and vancomycin should be reserved as alternative agents. If local surveillance data indicate that Gram-negative organisms are a cause of SSIs for vascular surgical procedures, vascular surgeons may consider combining clindamycin or vancomycin with another agent (cefazolin if the patient is not β-lactam allergic; aztreonam, gentamicin or single-dose fluoroquinolone if the patient is β-lactam allergic), due to the potential for gastrointestinal flora exposure.[38]

Antimicrobial prosthetic vascular grafts

The rationale behind the idea of using antimicrobial vascular grafts is to prevent bacterial attachment to the prosthetic material and start forming biofilms. If the antimicrobial compound used in or on the graft is leaching, already approaching bacteria will be killed off, while a non-leaching antimicrobial graft will prevent formation of bacterial biofilm on its surface. Both concepts have their advantages and restrictions. The antimicrobial activity in the surrounding of leaching grafts follows, depending on the selected antimicrobial compound and the graft material, a release kinetic of the first or second order, resulting in a terminal antimicrobial efficacy, once the compound is completely released. While a non-leaching antimicrobial graft will show little protective effect in the surrounding tissue, the antimicrobial efficacy of its surface will remain intact much longer. Today, antimicrobial grafts of both concepts are available on the market. Which one of these concepts is more suitable to prevent infection will be an issue of future studies. Possibly, the indication for a leaching antimicrobial graft would be in a manifest infection, while a non-leaching graft could be preferred for

prevention of bacterial attachment and subsequent biofilm formation.[39]

> ## Key points/best clinical practice
>
> Treatment of graft infection is becoming complicated by the increased emergence of multiresistant microorganisms (Level 1/Grade A). Therefore, primary prevention is imperative. During implantation, the graft must be handled aseptically and contact with the skin and wound edges must be avoided (Level 1/Grade B). Antiseptic-impregnated incision drapes should be used to cover the skin (Level 2/Grade C). All patients shall receive preoperative antibiotic prophylaxis, preferably with a β-lactam antibiotic (Level 1/Grade A). The preoperative administration shall occur within 60 minutes before surgical incision (Level 2/Grade B).

MANAGEMENT OF GRAFT INFECTION

Traditional management of vascular graft infection includes total graft excision. If perfusion to an organ or limb is threatened, then revascularization is indicated. Many authors have described various alternative techniques for addressing these complex issues including selective complete graft preservation, partial excision and replacement of graft in situ or extra-anatomic with various autogenous, prosthetic and allograft conduits. The availability of NPWT seems to offer a promising adjunct to operative measures[2] (Table 25.2).

Aortic anastomosis: Extra-anatomic procedure

Aortic anastomosis and extra-anatomic procedures may be considered as the traditional approach to restore perfusion. Over a long period, graft infections involving aortic tube or aorto-iliac grafts were generally managed with axillo-bifemoral bypass grafting through non-infected tissue planes, closure of the incisions with placement of impermeable adhesive dressings, abdominal exploration with removal of the infected graft, ligation or closure of the aortic stump with monofilament suture, debridement

Table 25.2 Grafts to treat infections.

Autologous vein (deep or superficial)
Cryopreserved allograft (artery or vein)
Biosynthetic collagen prosthesis
Self-made pericardial tubes
Polyester graft soaked with antibiotics/antiseptics
Silver-protected polyester graft (metallic or silver acetate/ triclosan)
Silver-protected polyester graft soaked with antibiotics or antiseptics

of infected tissue and finally placement of retroperitoneal drains together with irrigation using antimicrobial or non-antimicrobial solutions. This strategy was regarded as the 'gold standard' treatment and was supported by sufficiently acceptable results derived from analysis of published case series, reporting an average amputation rate of 22.5% and an average mortality rate of 21%.[40]

However, detailed preoperative planning may be needed to achieve favourable results. Preoperative arteriography may demonstrate the location of the proximal aortic anastomosis in relation to the renal and visceral vessels. If an inadequate infrarenal cuff exists, then supra-celiac support and control is necessary. There may be insufficient non-infected tissue of the aorta below the renal arteries to allow aortic stump closure. In such cases, renal perfusion is probably best obtained by hepato-renal or spleno-renal bypass prior to graft excision.[41] If graft-enteric fistula or erosion is present, debridement of the necrotic or inflamed bowel may be required. The bowel defect then is closed with sutures or additionally a jejunal patch, or a primary anastomosis of the bowel is performed following bowel resection, if the small bowel is involved.

Aortic stump disruption is one of the most common early and late causes of death in patients with total aortic graft excision for infected vascular graft prosthesis. This catastrophic and often lethal condition typically occurs 2–6 weeks postoperatively and is caused by residual infection. Techniques to buttress or support the aortic stump include the use of autogenous vein pledgets, a patch of prevertebral fascia, or an omental flap.

Aortobifemoral grafts can be more difficult to treat with extra-anatomic grafts, since involvement of the groin complicates secondary bypasses and mandates lateral or obturatoral approaches to avoid infected groin wounds when performing secondary distal reconstructions. Through combined abdominal and groin incisions, femoral ends of the graft are excised, the femoral artery oversewed or ligated, and the wound packed open with antimicrobial-soaked dressings.[42,43] If the entire aortobifemoral graft is infected, then total excision with extra-anatomic bypass is indicated as described earlier. Revascularization may be best achieved with bilateral axillo-femoral bypasses to a non-involved section of patent superficial or deep femoral arteries or to the popliteal artery.

If graft infection is limited to a single patent femoral limb and confined to the groin with no infection of the proximal graft, an attempt can be made to save the non-infected portion of the graft by excising only the infected graft limb. The proximal limb is explored through a supra-inguinal, retroperitoneal incision. Graft incorporation is determined and Gram stains and microbiological cultures are submitted to prove no presence of bacterial colonization or early infection. Revascularization may be performed by using the proximal non-involved limb of the graft as inflow with the graft tunnelled laterally to a non-involved segment of patent superficial or deep femoral arteries. NPWT may now play an adjunct role in conditioning or saving the critical part of the infected graft and/or conditioning the wound bed after successful explantation.[2]

> ## Key points/best clinical practice
>
> The extra-anatomical approach is not the first choice, yet, it still may have its place in selected cases. All infected material shall be removed (Levels 2–3/Grade B). NPWT may be an important adjunct therapy option (Level 3/Grade C).

Aortic anastomosis: In situ repair

While the traditional management of aortic graft infection with total graft excision provides an acceptable solution to some patents, its success may be only temporary because of the concomitant risk of aortic stump blowout and the overall poor long-term patency rate with an axillo-bifemoral bypass. Although in situ replacement with rifampin-impregnated grafts has been described before,[44–46] in situ reconstruction with various antimicrobial materials has been reinvestigated as a new strategy option.[47] Recently, longitudinal results of patients with graft-enteric fistulae treated by in situ repair with rifampin-soaked grafts and omental coverage were published.[48] Over a 5-year period, the reinfection rate of such managed patients was acceptably low at 4%. Recently, daptomycin-soaked grafts have been discussed to be more effective than rifampin-soaked grafts[49] (Figure 25.1).

Following all of the earlier procedures, however, it is important to explant the infected graft material completely together with intensive debridement of adjacent tissue. Biological safeguarding with omentum is always recommended, as well as perioperative administration of antibiotics selected on the basis of preoperative microbiological antibiogram. The use of local antiseptics such as povidone–iodine, octenidine–dihydrochloride or polyhexanide either for antimicrobial washout or to soak prosthetic grafts prior to implantation may be useful; however, no systematic research exists for this measure in vascular surgery.

The availability of antimicrobial graft material based on various silver preparations or silver–triclosan combination may foster an evolution from axillo-femoral to in situ prosthetic reconstruction for the management of aortic graft infections. Silver-coated grafts have shown no healing impairment[50,51] and good clinical results with less than 8% reinfection rates after complete removal of the infected graft and in situ replacement with an antimicrobial graft based on silver.[52] However, if the infected graft material was not completely removed, incomplete removal resulted in a not acceptable infection rate of 30%.[52] In order to achieve not only an antimicrobial efficacy on the surface of the graft but also in its environment, silver-based grafts have also been soaked with rifampin.[53,54] However, it remains open if such additional measure provides added benefit (Figure 25.2).

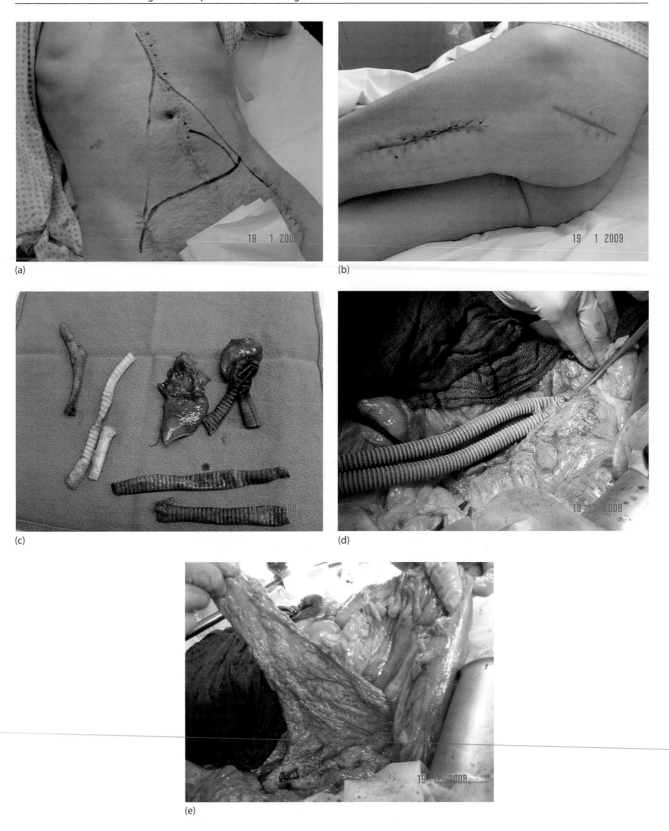

Figure 25.1 (a) Patient with an iliacofemoral bypass (left) followed by an iliacofemoral (left to right) cross-over bypass and finally an aortobifemoral bypass. The picture was taken after complete healing of the in situ reconstruction as shown in (c–e). (b) Development of gluteal and dorsal abscesses on the left thigh. (c) The causative pathology was a graft-enteric fistula. After an extensive debridement, all graft material was removed and the duodenum was reconstructed. (d) An in situ repair with a silver-protected graft soaked with rifampin (aortobifemoral) was performed. (e) Biological protection with omentum is preferred.

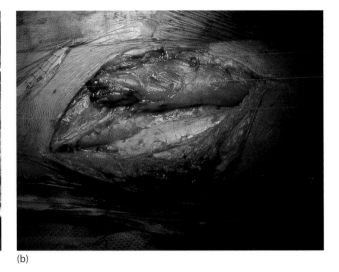

Figure 25.2 (a) Reconstruction of a destroyed common femoral artery (CFA) (intravenous drug abuser) with a silver-protected graft. (b) Biological protection with a *musculus sartorius* flap.

The use of subsidiary biological graft material has repeatedly been proposed as an alternative to reconstruct an infected aorto-iliac system. Particularly, the use of autogenous superficial femoral–popliteal veins was repeatedly demonstrated to provide a functional and durable technique for reconstruction of the infected aorto-iliofemoral axis.[55,56] Subsequent long-term follow-up suggests that this technique is durable and feasible in view of reinfection.[57] Although it is more challenging for both the patient and the surgeon, younger patients with lower surgical risk and a good life expectancy are suitable for this procedure.[56]

A modification of the earlier technique is the use of human cadaveric allografts in situ.[58] However, late deterioration of the allograft wall could be a restriction together with the limited availability of cadaveric allografts because of logistic and regulatory hurdles in some countries. Although a feasible option, the use of cryopreserved aorto-iliac allograft for infected aortic reconstruction is associated with a 24% complication rate.[59] In view of the logistic challenges coming with the use of cryopreserved allografts, management of graft infection by the use of antimicrobial prosthetic grafts seems to be an attractive alternative. Indeed, two studies comparing complete removal of infected aortic grafts and in situ repair with either silver acetate grafts or cryopreserved allografts showed comparable outcomes.[60,61]

A further strategy is to use endografts as a bridging procedure in emergency situations such as in critically ill patients with graft-enteric fistulae in order to increase chances for a definitive operation at better conditions.[62] Later, the infected endograft needs to be explanted, followed by in situ repair.[63–65] Although it was demonstrated in singe cases that high-risk patients with infected stent grafts can survive for a prolonged time if treated conservatively with antimicrobial therapy and percutaneous drainage, most authors agree that an infected endograft shall be removed, if the patient's condition allows such intervention.[66] Treatment strategies are similar to those described for graft infection after open repair.[67] Conservative treatment of an infected EVAR shows a 36% mortality, whereas surgical treatment with complete excision is associated with a 14% mortality.[68]

NPWT provides surgeons a possibility to change from a one-stage procedure, explantation and in situ repair, to a multistage repair.[2] This treatment option requires an intensive debridement with preparation of the infected graft and a complete wrap with the NPWT sponge. This procedure, however, must not be performed in cases with acute bleeding of infected stent grafts. A topical application of antiseptics may be possible, whereas systemic antibiotic administration is mandatory. The NPWT sponge then is covered with a polytetrafluoro-ethylene (PTFE) membrane to avoid adherence to the bowel. While the NPWT sponge shall be changed after 4–5 days, the PTFE membrane is only flushed with antiseptics such as povidone–iodine and is reused. If the graft remains covered by a biofilm, explantation cannot be avoided. If, however, the in situ site cleans up, any attempt to save the infected graft may be justified in certain circumstances such as a graft with a very short neck or the presence of an anastomosis of the *arteria renalis*. This multistage procedure is convenient for the surgeon and avoids excessive surgical manipulation and burden to the patient, since the in situ repair will be easier to perform if the infected graft was already liberated from surrounding connective tissue. Furthermore, the new graft will then be implanted in a microbiologically improved wound bed.

Key points/best clinical practice

In situ repair is the preferable concept. All infected material shall be removed. The use of deep veins has the lowest risk of reinfection. Infection protected grafts have shown good results comparable to allografts (Levels 2–3/Grade B). NPWT may further improve these results and the chance for graft preservation (Level 3/Grade C).

Peripheral bypass graft infections

Various graft-saving techniques to salvage patent, infected prosthetic grafts have been described. These all include aggressive wound debridement and intravenous administration of antibiotics specific to the sensitivity of the organisms cultured. However, even today graft preservation is reserved for very special cases. The use of autologous veins and complete excision of the infected graft is still recommended whenever feasible.

Extra-anatomic revascularization of ischemic limbs may be feasible, provided that adequate sites for anastomoses are available. If harvesting a patient's vein is not possible, patches of xenogene pericardium may be used to close abandoned anastomoses.[69] This material can also be used to construct a graft, e.g. in the case of bleeding from an infected CFA.[70]

Because of the higher risk of infection and occlusion of peripheral bypass, synthetic materials are not the first choice for vascular repair of infected peripheral grafts. However, if needed, antimicrobial alloplastic grafts coated or impregnated with rifampicin, silver or silver–triclosan should be used. The other option is the use of biological-synthetic grafts, yet also associated with a significant risk for reinfection.[71,72]

Cryopreserved arterial or venous allografts are not frequently used, as they frequently carry the risk of deterioration and occlusion and have the disadvantage of restricted availability at high costs.[73–76]

In most cases, additional coverage of a critical region with muscle flaps is part of the therapy. However, in some situations an amputation cannot be avoided. Yet, if the infection involves an anastomosis of an occluded graft to a peripheral artery, Calligaro and Veith demonstrated that subtotal excision of the graft can be performed, leaving an oversewn 2–3 mm graft remnant on the artery.[77] Such patch will progressively become covered by granulation tissue and may be allowed to close by secondary intention. Here, NPWT can also be helpful to improve the results and the duration of the healing procedure.

Key points/best clinical practice

Whenever possible, autologous veins should be implanted for peripheral use (Level 1/Grade A). Infection-protected grafts or xenogene pericardium is the second choice (Level 3/Grade B-C). NPWT may be used in addition (Level 3/Grade C).

DEFICIENCIES IN CURRENT KNOWLEDGE AND AREAS FOR FUTURE RESEARCH

Currently, there are only limited RCTs in the field of graft infections available. Due to the difficulties in conducting such trials, which mostly will need to be designed as multicentre trials, it is unlikely that in near future RCTs will be available to answer still open questions. One option to overcome the current challenges in generating large patient numbers may be the introduction of vascular surgical graft registries.

Even if 'infection-protected' grafts are used today, a zero percent infection rate cannot be achieved. For primary implantations, the advantage of primary infection-protected grafts is not proven. Studies in this field are further limited in different registration conditions, as, e.g. silver-coated or silver-impregnated grafts are not approved in all countries. However, further research and improvements are necessary.

The use of NPWT in vascular surgery is still in its infancy but already plays an important role in surgery of infected sites and helps to change surgical practice. It remains to be proven if NPWT may support preservation of non-infected grafts.

REFERENCES

1. Veith FJ. Surgery of the infected aortic graft. In: Bergan JJ, Yao JST, eds. *Surgery of the Aorta and Its Body Branches*. New York: Grune and Stratton, 1979, pp. 521–533.
2. Mayer D, Hasse B, Koelliker J, Enzler M, Veith FJ, Rancic Z, Lachat M. Long-term results of vascular graft and artery preserving treatment with negative pressure wound therapy in Szilagyi grade III infections justify a paradigm shift. *Ann Surg*. 2011;254:754–759.
3. Seeger JM. Management of patients with prosthetic vascular graft infections. *Am Surg*. 2000;66:166–177.
4. Oderich GS, Panneton GM. Aortic graft infections: What have we learnt during the last decades? *Acta Cir Belg*. 2002;102:7–13.
5. Cernohorsky P, Reijnen MMPJ, Tielliu IFJ, van Sterkenburg SMM, van den Dungen JJAM, Zeebregts CJ. The relevance of aortic endograft prosthetic infection. *J Vasc Surg*. 2011;54:327–333.
6. Laser A, Baker N, Rectenwald J, Criado-Pallares JLE, Upchurch GR. Graft infection after endovascular aneurysm repair. *J Vasc Surg*. 2011;54:58–63.
7. National Reference Centre for the Surveillance of Nosocomial Infections. KISS Hospital Infection Surveillance System, OP-KISS component Reference Data, Calculation period: January 2005 to December 2009, prepared on 13 March 2010: www.nrz-hygiene.de.
8. Horan TC, Andrus M, Dudeck MA. CDC/NHSN surveillance definition of health care-associated infection and criteria for specific types of infections in the acute care setting. *Am J Infect Control*. 2008;36:309–332.

9. McBain AJ, Bartolo RG, Catrenich CE et al. Exposure of sink drain microcosms to triclosan: Population dynamics and antimicrobial susceptibility. *Appl Environ Microbiol.* 2003;69:5433–5442.

10. Bandyk DF. Vascular graft infections: Epidemiology, microbiology, pathogenesis and prevention. In: Bernhard VM, Towne JB, eds. *Complications in Vascular Surgery.* St. Louis, MO: Quality Medical Publishing, 1991, pp. 223–234.

11. Calligaro KD, Veith FJ, Schwartz ML, Dougherty MJ, DeLaurentis DA. Differences in early vs. late extracavitary arterial graft infections. *J Vasc Surg.* 1995;22:680–685.

12. Malone JM, Moore WS, Campagna G, Bean B. Bacteremic infectability of vascular grafts: The influence of pseudointimal integrity and duration of graft infection. *Surgery.* 1975;78:211–216.

13. Moore WS, Swanson RJ, Campagna G, Bean B. Pseudointimal development and vascular prosthesis susceptibility to bacteremic infection. *Surg Forum.* 1974;25:250–252.

14. Bergamini TM. Vascular prostheses infection caused by bacterial biofilms. *Semin Vasc Surg.* 1990;3:101.

15. O'Hara PJ, Hertzer NR, Beven EG, Krajewski LP. Surgical management of infected abdominal aortic grafts: A review of a 25-year experience. *J Vasc Surg.* 1986;3:725–731.

16. Walker WE, Cooley DA, Duncan JM, Hallman GL Jr, Ott DA, Reul GJ. The management of aortoduodenal fistula by in situ replacement of the infected abdominal aortic graft. *Ann Surg.* 1987;205:727–732.

17. Low RN, Wall SD, Jeffrey RB Jr, Sollitto RA, Reilly LM, Tierney LM Jr. Aortoenteric fistula and perigraft infection: Evaluation with CT. *Radiology.* 1990;175:157–162.

18. Bruggink JL, Glaudemans AW, Saleem BR et al. Accuracy of FDG-PET-CT in the diagnostic work-up of vascular prosthetic graft infection. *Eur J Vasc Endovasc Surg.* 2010;40:348–354.

19. Back MR. Local complications: Graft infection. In: Cronenwett JL, Johnston KW, eds. *Rutherford's Vascular Surgery,* 7th ed. Philadelphia, PA: Saunders Elsevier, 2010, pp. 643–661.

20. Keidar Z, Nitecki S. FDG-PET in prosthetic graft infections. *Semin Nucl Med.* 2013;43:396–402.

21. Bergamini TM, Bandyk DF, Govostis D et al. Identification of *Staphylococcus epidermidis* vascular graft infections: A comparison of culture techniques. *J Vasc Surg.* 1989;9:665–670.

22. Teebken OE, Bisdas T, Assadian O, Ricco JB. Recommendations for reporting treatment of aortic graft infections. *Eur J Endovasc Surg.* 2012;43:174–181.

23. Bisdas T, Mattner F, Ella O et al. Significance of infection markers and microbiological findings during tissue processing of cryopreserved arterial homografts for the early postoperative course. *Vasa.* 2009;38:365–373.

24. FitzGerald SF, Kelly C, Humphreys H. Diagnosis and treatment of prosthetic aortic graft infections: Confusion and inconsistency in the absence of evidence or consensus. *J Antimicrob Chemother.* 2005;56:996–999.

25. Kleinmann LH, Towne JB, Bernhard VM. A diagnostic and therapeutic approach to aortoenteric fistulas: Clinical experience with twenty patients. *Surgery.* 1979;86:868.

26. Kwaan JHM, Dahl RK, Connolly J. Immunocompetence in patients with prosthetic graft infection. *J Vasc Surg.* 1984;1:45.

27. Kramer A, Assadian O, Lademann J. Prevention of postoperative wound infections by covering the surgical field with iodine-impregnated incision drape (Ioban 2). *GMS Krankenhhyg Interdiszip.* 2010;5:pii: Doc08.

28. Turtiainen J, Saimanen EI, Partio TJ, Mäkinen KT, Reinikainen MT, Virkkunen JJ, Vuorio KS, Hakala T. Supplemental postoperative oxygen in the prevention of surgical wound infection after lower limb vascular surgery: A randomized controlled trial. *World J Surg.* 2011;35:1387–1395.

29. Karthikesalingam A, Walsh SR, Sadat U, Tang TY, Koraen L, Varty K. Effect of closed suction drainage in lower limb arterial surgery: A meta-analysis of published clinical trials. *Vasc Endovasc Surg.* 2008;42:243–248.

30. Goldstone J, Moore WS. Infection in vascular prostheses: Clinical manifestations and surgical management. *Am J Surg.* 1974;128:225–230.

31. Thomas JH, McCroskey BL, Iliopoulos JI, Hardin CA, Hermreck AS, Pierce GE. Aortoiliac reconstruction combined with nonvascular operations. *Am J Surg.* 1983;146:784–787.

32. Fry RE, Fry WJ. Cholelithiasis and aortic reconstruction: The problem of simultaneous surgical therapy. Conclusions from a personal series. *J Vasc Surg.* 1986;4:345–350.

33. Ouriel K, Green RM, Ricotta JJ, DeWeese JA. Acute acalculous cholecystitis complicating abdominal aortic aneurysm resection. *J Vasc Surg.* 1984;1:646–648.

34. Stewart AH, Eyers PS, Earnshaw JJ. Prevention of infection in peripheral arterial reconstruction: A systematic review and meta-analysis. *J Vasc Surg.* 2007;46:148–155.

35. Boyce JM. Methicillin-resistant *Staphylococcus aureus* in hospitals and long-term care facilities: Microbiology, epidemiology, and preventive measures. *Infect Control Hosp Epidemiol.* 1992;13:725–737.

36. Boyce JM. Increasing prevalence of methicillin-resistant *Staphylococcus aureus* in the United States. *Infect Control Hosp Epidemiol.* 1999;11:639–642.

37. Moran GJ, Krishnadasan A, Gorwitz RJ et al. Methicillin-resistant *S. aureus* infections among patients in the emergency department. *N Engl J Med.* 2006;355:666–674.

38. Bratzler DW, Dellinger EP, Olsen KM et al. Clinical practice guidelines for antimicrobial prophylaxis in surgery. *Am J Health Syst Pharm.* 2013;70:195–283.

39. Ricco JB, Assadian O. Antimicrobial silver grafts for prevention and treatment of vascular graft infection. *Semin Vasc Surg.* 2011;24:234–241.

40. Curl GR, Ricotta JJ. Total prosthetic graft excision and extraanatomic bypass. In Calligaro KD, Veith FJ, eds. *Management of Infected Arterial Grafts.* St. Louis, MO: Quality Medical Publishing, 1994, pp. 82–94.

41. Moncure AC, Brewster DC, Darling RC, Atnip RG, Newton WD, Abbott WM. Use of the splenic and hepatic arteries for renal revascularization. *J Vasc Surg.* 1986;3:196–203.

42. Calligaro KD, Veith FJ. Diagnosis and management of infected prosthetic aortic grafts. *Surgery.* 1991;110:805–813.

43. Calligaro KD, Veith FJ, Gupta S, Ascer E, Dietzek AM, Franco CD, Wengerter KR. A modified method for management of prosthetic graft infections involving an anastomosis to the common femoral artery. *J Vasc Surg.* 1990;11:485–492.

44. Colburn MD, Moore WS, Chvapil M, Gelabert HA, Quinones-Baldrich WJ. Use of an antibiotic-bonded graft for in situ reconstruction after prosthetic graft infections. *J Vasc Surg.* 1992;16:651–658.

45. Goeau-Brissonniere O, Mercier F, Nicolas MH, Bacourt F, Coggia M, Lebrault C, Pechere JC. Treatment of vascular graft infection by in situ replacement with a rifampin-bonded gelatin-sealed dacron graft. *J Vasc Surg.* 1994;19:739–741.

46. Gupta AK, Bandyk DF, Johnson BL. In situ repair of mycotic abdominal aortic aneurysms with rifampin-bonded gelatin-impregnated Dacron grafts: A preliminary case report. *J Vasc Surg.* 1996;24:472–476.

47. Oderich GS, Bower TC, Cherry KJ Jr et al. Evolution from axillofemoral to in situ prosthetic reconstruction for the treatment of aortic graft infections at a single center. *J Vasc Surg.* 2006;43:1166–1174.

48. Oderich GS, Bower TC, Hofer J et al. In situ rifampin-soaked grafts with omental coverage and antibiotic suppression are durable with low reinfection rates in patients with aortic graft enteric erosion or fistula. *J Vasc Surg.* 2011;53:99–106.

49. Bisdas T, Beckmann E, Marsch G et al. Prevention of vascular graft infections with antibiotic graft impregnation prior to implantation: In vitro comparison between daptomycin, rifampin and nebacetin. *Eur J Vasc Endovasc Surg.* 2012;43:448–456.

50. Zegelman M, Guenther G, Florek HJ, Orend KH, Zuehlke H, Liewald F, Storck M. Results from the first in man German pilot study of the silver graft, a vascular graft impregnated with metallic silver. *Vascular.* 2009;17:190–196.

51. Zegelman M, Guenther G, Waliszewski M et al. Results from the International Silver Graft Registry for high-risk patients treated with a metallic-silver impregnated vascular graft. *Vascular.* 2013;2:137–147.

52. Zegelman M, Guenther G, Eckstein HH, Kreißler-Haag D, Langenscheidt P, Mickley V, Ritter R, Schmitz-Rixen T, Wagner R, Zühlke H. In-situ-Rekonstruktion mit alloplastischen Prothesen beim Gefäßinfekt (Evaluation mit Silberacetat beschichteter Prothesen). *Gefässchirurgie.* 2006;11:402–408.

53. Hardman S, Cope A, Swann A, Bell PR, Naylor AR, Hayes PD. An in vitro model to compare the antimicrobial activity of silver-coated versus rifampicin-soaked vascular grafts. *Ann Vasc Surg.* 2004;18:308–313.

54. Gao H, Sandermann J, Prag J, Lund L, Lindholt JS. Rifampicin-soaked silver polyester versus expanded polytetrafluoro-ethylene grafts for in situ replacement of infected grafts in a porcine randomised controlled trial. *Eur J Vasc Endovasc Surg.* 2012;43:582–587.

55. Clagett GP, Bowers BL, Lopez-Viego MA, Rossi MB, Valentine RJ, Myers SI, Chervu A. Creation of a neo-aortoiliac system from lower extremity deep and superficial veins. *Ann Surg.* 1993;218:239–249.

56. Dorweiler B, Neufang A, Chaban R, Reinstadler J, Duenschede F, Vahl CF. Use and durability of femoral vein for autologous reconstruction with infection of the aortoiliofemoral axis. *J Vasc Surg.* 2014;59:675–683.

57. Clagett GP, Valentine RJ, Hagino RT. Autogenous aortoiliac/femoral reconstruction from superficial femoral-popliteal veins: Feasibility and durability. *J Vasc Surg.* 1997;25:255–270.

58. Kieffer E, Bahnini A, Koskas F et al. In situ allograft replacement of infected infrarenal aortic prosthetic grafts: Results in 43 patients. *J Vasc Surg.* 1993;17:349–355.

59. Harlander-Locke MP, Harmon LK, Lawrence PF et al. The use of cryopreserved aortoiliac allograft for aortic reconstruction in the United States. *J Vasc Surg.* 2014;59:669–674.

60. Bisdas T, Wilhelmi M, Haverich A, Teebken OE. Cryopreserved arterial homografts vs silver-coated Dacron grafts for abdominal aortic infections with intraoperative evidence of microorganisms. *J Vasc Surg.* 2011;53:1274–1281.

61. Pupka A, Skora J, Janczak D, Plonek T, Marczak J, Szydełko T. In situ revascularisation with silver-coated polyester prostheses and arterial homografts in patients with aortic graft infection – A prospective, comparative, single-centre study. *Eur J Vasc Endovasc Surg.* 2011;41:61–67.

62. Lonn L, Dias N, Veith Schroeder T, Resch T. Is EVAR the treatment of choice for aortoenteric fistula? *J Cardiovasc Surg (Torino).* 2010;24:994–999.

63. Moulakakis KG, Mylonas SN, Antonopoulos CN, Kakisis JD, Sfyroeras GS, Mantas G, Liapis CD. Comparison of treatment strategies for thoracic endograft infection. *J Vasc Surg.* 2014;60:1061–1071.

64. Herdrich BJ, Fairman RM. How to manage infected aortic endografts. *J Cardiovasc Surg (Torino).* 2013;54:595–604.

65. Fatima J, Duncan AA, de Grandis E, Oderich GS, Kalra M, Gloviczki P, Bower TC. Treatment strategies and outcomes in patients with infected aortic endografts. *J Vasc Surg.* 2013;58:371–379.

66. Setacci C, De Donato G, Setacci F, Chisci E, Perulli A, Galzerano G, Sirignano P. Management of abdominal endograft infection. *J Cardiovasc Surg.* 2010;51:33–41.

67. Moll FL, Powell JT, Fraedrich G et al. Practice guidelines of the European society for vascular surgery. *Eur J Vasc Endovasc Surg.* 2011;41:S1–S58.

68. Veger HTC, Hederman Joosten PP, Thoma SR, Visser MJT. Infection of endovascular aortic aneurysm stent graft after urosepsis: Case report and review of the literature. *Vascular.* 2013;21:10–13.

69. McMillan WD, Leville CD, Hile CN. Bovine pericardial patch repair in infected fields. *J Vasc Surg.* 2012;55:1712–1715.

70. Czerny M, von Allmen R, Opfermann P et al. Self-made pericardial tube graft: A new surgical concept for treatment of graft infections after thoracic and abdominal aortic procedures. *Ann Thorac Surg.* 2011;92:1657–1662.

71. Fellmer PT, Wiltberger G, Tautenhahn HM, Matia I, Krenzien F, Jonas S. Early results after peripheral vascular replacement with biosynthetic collagen prosthesis in cases of graft infection. *Zentralbl Chir.* 2014;139:546–551.

72. Töpel I, Betz T, Uhl C, Wiesner M, Bröckner S, Steinbauer M. Use of biosynthetic prosthesis (Omniflow II°) to replace infected infrainguinal prosthetic grafts – First results. *Vasa.* 2012;41:215–220.

73. Boyle JR. Superficial femoral vein is superior to cryopreserved allografts for in situ aortic reconstruction. *Eur J Vasc Endovasc Surg.* 2014;48:300.

74. Castier Y, Paraskevas N, Maury JM, Karsenti A, Cerceau O, Legendre AF, Duprey A, Cerceau P, Francis F, Leseche G. Cryopreserved arterial allograft reconstruction for infected peripheral bypass. *Ann Vasc Surg.* 2010;24:994–999.

75. Hartranft CA, Noland S, Kulwicki A, Holden CR, Hartranft T. Cryopreserved saphenous vein graft in infrainguinal bypass. *J Vasc Surg.* 2014;60:1291–1296.

76. Chang CK, Scali ST, Feezor RJ, Beck AW, Waterman AL, Huber TS, Berceli SA. Defining utility and predicting outcome of cadaveric lower extremity bypass grafts in patients with critical limb ischemia. *J Vasc Surg.* 2014;60:1554–1564.

77. Calligaro KD, Veith FJ, Schwartz ML, Goldsmith J, Savarese RP, Dougherty MJ, DeLaurentis DA. Selective preservation of infected prosthetic arterial grafts—Analysis of a 20-year experience with 120 extracavitary-infected grafts. *Ann Surg.* 1994;200:461–471.

SECTION IV

Aneurysms

26

Abdominal aortic aneurysm

Pathophysiology, endovascular and surgical therapy

DENIS W. HARKIN and PAUL H. BLAIR

CONTENTS

INTRODUCTION

Abdominal aortic aneurysm (AAA), derived from the ancient Greek word *aneurysma* which describes 'a widening', is a pathological enlargement of the abdominal aorta. Whilst aneurysmal change can affect any vessel, they most commonly affect the infrarenal abdominal aorta, to cause an AAA. These AAAs are most common in men, in whom they are sixfold more prevalent than women, and most commonly above the age of 60 years. The commonest clinical definition of an AAA is based on the diameter of the abdominal aorta, which is considered aneurysmal at a diameter of 3.0 cm or more.[1,2] This widely held definition does not take account of individual variation in aortic diameter or take account for gender variation as one would expect on average a female aorta to be comparatively smaller. Therefore, some researchers have considered the alternate definition of an aneurysm as an increase of 1.5 times the expected normal diameter, and on radiological assessment, this may be assessed by comparison to the adjacent unaffected vessel. An arterial aneurysm may be *true* when it affects all layers of the arterial wall or *false* when it does not. The majority of *true* aneurysms are associated with atherosclerotic (AS)

disease in the vessel wall, but unlike typical AS which tends to stenosis or occlusion of the vessel, in these individuals with an underlying genetic predisposition, it causes the vessel to dilate. Whilst all aneurysm have some degree of chronic inflammatory change within the arterial wall, about 10% of aneurysm have pronounced inflammatory response extending beyond the wall to involve the surrounding tissues of the retroperitoneum, often described as 'inflammatory' aneurysm. Aneurysm growth can be complicated by rupture, with bleeding outside the arterial wall, and this is most often fatal unless treated by open or endovascular repair. Therefore, known small aneurysms should be placed under radiological surveillance and large aneurysms should be considered for active treatment by endovascular or open repair, to prevent fatal rupture. In this chapter, we will discuss the management principles for AAA.

EPIDEMIOLOGY

AAA is widely recognized as commoner in men than women and has increasing prevalence in those in their sixth decade of age and older. Prevalence rates vary according to age, gender, risk-factor profile and geographical location. Several population screening studies have provided evidence on the prevalence of AAA across varied geographical regions (MASS, Western Australia, Viborg and Chichester) (Lindholt, 1995).[3–8] In population screening studies, the prevalence of AAA increases with age,[9–11] occurring in 7%–8% in men over the age of 65 years.[9,11] For those aged between 65 and 80 years, the incidence of an AAA is 7.6% in men and 4.2% in women.[11] The prevalence of AAA is sixfold greater in men than women and can have increased prevalence within patient populations with multiple cardiovascular risk factors such as a smoking history, hypertension, hyperlipidaemia, family history and prior peripheral vascular disease.[10] Perhaps the most important risk factors which affect the relative risk (RR) of AAA development are male sex (4.5-fold RR) and smoking history (5.6-fold RR).[10] Incidence of AAA can be high in certain families who appear susceptible to aneurysm formation, but as yet no universal genetic anomaly has been identified to explain this at-risk phenotype. Several connective tissue disorders, such as Marfan's syndrome (MFS) and Ehlers–Danlos syndrome, are also associated with aneurysm of the aorta and other large arteries. Individuals with an AAA also have an increased risk of other peripheral artery aneurysm, with approximately 25% having an aneurysm of the popliteal or femoral artery in the leg.

PATHOPHYSIOLOGY

AAA is typically associated with advanced age and atherosclerosis, with attendant risk factors such as hypercholesterolaemia, hypertension and/or diabetes. In these patients, the aortic wall degenerates and weakens to allow a dilation or aneurysmal change. This is pathologically characterized by atheromata, invasion of inflammatory cells, destructive extracellular matrix remodelling and depletion and dysfunction of vascular smooth muscle cells. Although it is now clear that genetic determinants influence the expression of AAA, there has been no description as yet of a single major gene or locus effect that is sufficient to cause isolated abdominal aneurysm in the absence of evidence for a more systemic arteriopathy. The weight of evidence therefore indicates that AAA is a complex disorder that integrates the influence of predisposing genes with lifestyle-associated risk factors. In contrast to AAA, a subtype of thoracic aortic aneurysm (TAAA), the familial or inherited TAAA, appears to have a much stronger genetic influence, and study of these and a range of congenital connective tissue disorders (such as MFS) is now shedding new light on the pathogenesis of aneurysmal disease. Historical focus on elastic fibres in pathogenetic models of inherited aneurysms derives from the near-uniform histological observation of reduced elastin content and elastic fibre fragmentation in the aortic media (the middle aortic layer), known as cystic medial necrosis. Arteries exposed to pulsatile arterial blood pressure rely on collagen and elastin within the aortic wall to provide strength but also allow compliance of the vessel to expand and contract, and without this will expand. However, many elastin-deficiency states do not associate with aneurysm as a prominent phenotype. Aortic aneurysm is an extremely rare manifestation of cutis laxa syndromes caused by mutations in the elastin gene and is not observed in mice or humans with dominant and recessive forms of cutis laxa caused by deficiency of fibulin-5,[12] a crucial mediator of elastogenesis. By contrast, aneurysmal disease is highly penetrant in inherited cutis laxa caused by fibulin-4[13] and fibrillin-1 deficiency which leads to failed elastic fibre homeostasis and highly penetrant aortic root aneurysms in the context of an MFS.[14] Pseudoxanthoma elasticum caused by ABCC6 deficiency in humans also shows postnatally acquired elastic fibre fragmentation in the aorta, but does not typically show aneurysm. These observations raise the important question of what molecular events, besides elastin-related issues, are common to the fibrillin-1- and fibulin-4-deficiency states but not in fibulin-5 deficiency. The focus on the aortic media and elastic fibres may have been a distraction. The discovery that the genes mutated in MFS and vascular Ehlers–Danlos syndrome (FBN1 and COL3A1, respectively) encode extracellular matrix elements (fibrillin-1 and collagen α-1) led to the generation of pathogenetic models that singularly invoke inherent structural weakness of the tissues. Gene identification has allowed the creation of mouse models of inherited aortic aneurysm, and has highlighted the involvement of diverse cytokine pathways, and in particular the role of the transforming growth factor-β (TGF-β) pathway in aortic aneurysm. Perhaps the most direct evidence for a major role of TGF-β in aneurysm pathogenesis came from the finding that mutations in the TGFBR1 and TGFBR2 genes, which encode the TGF-β receptor subunits TGFR-1 (also known as ALK-5) and TGFR-2, respectively, result in aneurysm conditions with undeniable phenotypic overlap with MFS, a notable example of which is Loeys–Dietz syndrome (LDS).[15,16] Similar to MFS, patients with LDS show highly penetrant arterial tortuosity (an elongation of an artery resulting in a twisted course) and a strong predisposition for aneurysm and dissection throughout the arterial tree. Vascular disease in patients with LDS is more aggressive than in those with MFS, with rupture at a younger age (as young as 6 months) and at smaller aortic dimensions.[17] Little is known about the precise pathogenetic sequence downstream of TGF-β that is involved in aneurysm progression. Enhancement of matrix metalloproteinase (MMP) activity is frequently invoked. Evidence includes high MMP expression and activity in many natural and experimentally induced presentations of aneurysm and the ability of MMP inhibitors (such as doxycycline) to attenuate aneurysm progression, including in mouse models of MFS.[18] Whilst TGF-β has been associated with reduced expression and activity of multiple MMPs in many tissues and contexts, it has been shown to specifically induce MMP2 and MMP9 expression: the MMPs that are most closely associated with aneurysm conditions such as MFS.[18,19]

The implication of TGF-β signalling in the pathogenesis of aortic aneurysm has suggested an opportunity for targeted pharmacotherapy. Blockade of angiotensin (AT)-2 signalling through AT-1 receptor (AT1R) had previously been shown to limit TGF-β signalling and fibrosis in rodent models of chronic kidney disease (CKD). Indeed, in a mouse model of MFS, the AT1R blocker losartan prevented progressive aortic aneurysm.[20] Potential mechanisms for aneurysm treatment include the prevention of AT1R-induced expression of TGF-β ligands, receptors and activators such as thrombospondin-1 or MMPs. Prenatal initiation of losartan treatment in MFS mouse models resulted in full normalization of aortic root size, aortic root growth rate and aortic wall architecture. Importantly, postnatal initiation of therapy in the context of established aneurysmal dilatation and medial degeneration also achieved full suppression of aortic root growth and productive remodelling of the aortic wall, with decreased elastin fragmentation and matrix deposition. Several observations pointed to TGF-β antagonism as the relevant mechanism. First, the protection achieved by losartan correlated with reduced nuclear accumulation of pSMAD2 and reduced expression of TGF-β-driven gene products such as plasminogen activator inhibitor-1 and CTGF. Second, other agents with comparable blood-pressure-lowering effects that did not alter TGF-β signalling were associated with a small decline in aortic root growth rates when compared with losartan and had no effect on aortic wall architecture. Third, losartan limited the growth of the aortic root, which showed pathological dilatation and increased TGF-β signalling, but had no effect on the growth of other aortic segments, which showed neither. Losartan also limited aortic root growth in a subset of children with severe and rapidly progressive MFS.[20] However, these promising developments have not as yet given us an effective pharmacological treatment for AAA, and the search continues.

Two other distinct forms of AAA are worthy of mention, inflammatory and mycotic aneurysm (MA). Inflammatory abdominal aortic aneurysm (IAAA) represents an interesting subset of AAA where excessive inflammation within the aortic wall and peri-aortic tissues is characterized by a dense retroperitoneal fibrosis, which can involve adjacent structures such as the ureters, duodenum and small bowel. These IAAAs can be associated with abdominal and back pain and weight loss and can complicate when retroperitoneal fibrosis encases the ureter and causes obstructive uropathy and acute kidney failure. MA can arise due to infection of the aortic wall and microbial aneurysmal arteritis. Whilst rare, these infective processes can cause rapid degeneration of the arterial wall and early rupture. MA can develop when septic emboli from the heart (endocarditis) implant in the microvascular vasa vasorum of the artery wall. In these patients, the infecting agents reflect the endocardial source and as such are often Gram-positive cocci, such as *Streptococcus* spp. and *Staphylococcus aureus*. MA may also be caused by bacteraemia or septicaemia. This microbial aneurysmal arteritis develops when blood-borne bacteria seed into diseased arterial wall in an area of AS plaque, ulcerated plaque or luminal thrombus. Suppuration degeneration of the wall can be rapid with perforation and pseudo-aneurysm formation, and the septic process can affect surrounding structures such as the anterior vertebral bodies. MA may affect any age group and usually involve aortic branches rather than the main arterial trunk and often in multiple different arterial territories.

DIAGNOSIS, SCREENING AND SURVEILLANCE

The majority of AAAs are asymptomatic and detected incidentally through radiological investigation or as part of a radiological screening study. Very large AAA may produce symptoms due to pulsatile mass effect on adjacent structures causing lumbar back pain or rarely abdominal pain. Indeed, in many cases, in open surgery, the anterior spinal ligament and in some cases the anterior vertebral bodies show signs of degenerative change from the repetitive trauma of the pulsating aneurysm. However, pain is more commonly a sign of complication due to rapid expansion, impending or actual rupture. Occasionally a patient or their partner will observe or palpate signs of a pulsatile mass in the abdomen. Plain radiographs of the abdomen or lumbar spine may identify the calcified outline of an AAA, but more commonly the diagnosis is made incidentally on abdominal ultrasound scan (USS) or computed tomographic (CT) scan requested for the investigation of an unrelated condition.

Patients with large AAA should have a contrast-enhanced computed tomography angiogram (CTA) to assess the anatomical suitability of the AAA for open or endovascular repair (Figure 26.1). Contrast-induced nephropathy should be considered in those with CKD, and if contrast cannot be given safely with pre-hydration, a non-contrast scan may be sufficient and combined with either USS or magnetic resonance imaging (MRI) for additional detail. Ideally, one would scan the entire thoracoabdominal aorta, iliac systems to the femoral bifurcation to assess endovascular access, and identify thoracic aorta pathology. Image processing with modern computer packages allows accurate analysis of the anatomical suitability for endovascular device implantation (Figure 26.1).

Many aneurysms remain undetected until they become large, presenting for the first time when symptomatic or complicated. The commonest complication of AAA is rupture, which is fatal in over 80% affected. The risk of an AAA rupturing increases with aneurysm growth and

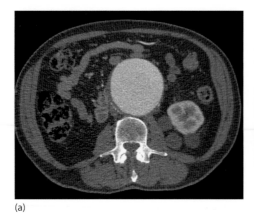
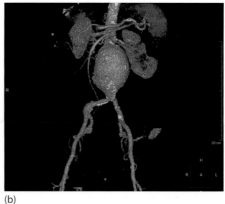

(a)   (b)

Figure 26.1 Contrast-enhanced computed tomography angiography of an abdominal aortic aneurysm on cross-sectional imaging (a) and after 3D reconstruction (b).

is related to maximum aneurysm diameter. Evidence suggests most small AAAs grow by 1–3 mm per annum and the rate of growth increases as aneurysm gets larger above 60 mm.[21,22] However, growth is not linear and some AAA will have periods of relatively little growth and some will undergo rapid growth, usually considered as >5 mm in 6 months. The natural course of an AAA is continued expansion of between 2 and 3 mm per year and a rupture risk which is exponentially related to AAA diameter.[23] Rupture is usually lethal with overall mortality rates of up to 90% common.[24] In the United Kingdom, currently around 7000 people in England and Wales die each year as a result of ruptured AAA (rAAA).[25] AAA may also complicate when laminar thrombus, which often forms a lining to the capacious aneurysmal sac, embolizes to the lower limb arteries causing painful digital micro-embolic infarcts, recurrent occlusions of the tibial arteries leading to critical limb ischaemia or occlusion of a major artery with acute limb ischaemia.

Growth rates and risk of rupture in AAA

The risk of AAA rupture is based on the maximum diameter at last scan or presentation and an estimation of growth rate. The average growth rate of small AAA, 3.0–5.5 cm, ranges from 0.2 to 0.3 cm per year, on the basis of several large screening and surveillance study populations. Large AAA (>5.5 cm) are associated with a higher rate of growth which increases with increasing AAA diameter.[23,26–36] Smoking has been implicated both as a cause of AAA and associated with AAA growth[6,7,27,28,30,36–40] and smoking cessation should be recommended. Smoking is also associated with chronic obstructive pulmonary disease (COPD) and several studies have suggested AAA growth and rupture is greater in these patients.[32,33,37,41] There is also some evidence of increased risk of AAA growth in patients with coexisting cardiovascular disease and peripheral vascular disease. The evidence is conflicting on the effect on growth of age, gender, diabetes mellitus, hyperlipidaemia, obesity

Table 26.1 Annual (every 12 months) rupture risk by abdominal aortic aneurysm diameter.

AAA diameter (mm)	Annual rupture risk
30–39	0
40–49	1
50–59	1–11
60–69	10–22
>70	30–33

Sources: Reed WW et al., *Arch Intern Med*, 157, 2064, 1997; Scott RA et al., *J Vasc Surg*, 28, 124, 1998; Conway KP et al., *J Vasc Surg*, 33, 752, 2001.
Abbreviation: AAA, abdominal aortic aneurysm.

and a variety of drug therapies (NSAIDs, beta-blockers, AT-converting enzyme inhibitors, AT II receptor blockers, antibiotics, steroids, statins and chemotherapeutic drugs).

Large AAAs are more likely to rupture, and several studies have shown a correlation between AAA diameter and rupture risk[32,33,42–50] (Table 26.1). AAAs with increased growth rate[48,49,51–53] are also more likely to rupture and indeed rapid expansion (>1.0 cm/12 months or >0.5 cm/6 months) is often an indication for active treatment. More recently, other AAA factors have been suggested such as increased intra-luminal thrombus, wall stiffness, wall tension and peak wall stress. Rupture risk is also considered greater in females, hypertension, smokers and COPD.

Screening and surveillance for small AAA

The majority of AAAs detected incidentally or by population screening are considered small AAA, 3.0–5.5 cm in diameter. The decision to offer surveillance, previously referred to as 'watchful waiting', for a small AAA is based on an assessment that the risk of death from aneurysm rupture is less than the risk of death from aneurysm repair (by open or endovascular technique). Surveillance is conducted almost exclusively using ultrasound surveillance scans by measuring the maximum AAA diameter. There is a consensus that for very small AAA, 3.0–3.9 cm, the risk of rupture is negligible. Therefore, these aneurysms should not be offered active treatment, unless in those rare cases when symptomatic, and should be kept under surveillance with USS at 12 monthly intervals. These patients should be offered cardiovascular risk-reduction measures.

The management of small AAA, 4.0–5.5 cm, has been assessed in two large multicentre RCTs comparing elective surgery to surveillance, the United Kingdom Small Aneurysm Trial (UKSAT) and in the United States, the American Aneurysm Detection and Management (ADAM) study,[48,49,54] and more recently in two smaller trials comparing endovascular repair to surveillance, the Comparison of surveillance versus Aortic Endografting for Small Aneurysm Repair (CAESAR) trial and PIVOTAL study (only AAA, 4.0–5.0 cm).[55,56] The UKSAT and ADAM trials were designed to provide evidence on the RR of elective surgical repair versus conservative management of AAA on aneurysm-related and all-cause mortality.[9,54] The UKSAT trial randomized 1090 patients with asymptomatic AAA between 4 and 5.5 cm diameter to either initial ultrasound surveillance (527 patients) or surgery (563 patients). Interestingly, in the surveillance group, 321 patients eventually underwent surgery due to rapid expansion or growth above 5.5 cm threshold. In the early surgery group, the 30-day mortality rate was 5.8%. The rupture rate for small aneurysms (<5.5 cm) was less than 2%. There was no difference in survival between the groups and the authors concluded that early surgery for small aneurysms was not indicated. The ADAM trial drew similar conclusions. Indeed, a meta-analysis combining both the UKSAT and the ADAM trials found that immediate open repair offered no significant survival benefit, even in patients with the largest AAAs and highest risk of rupture. However, when applying these results published in 1998 to contemporary practice, one must recognize that the risks of active treatment for AAA have reduced significantly in recent years with the risk from open surgery less than 2% and endovascular aneurysm repair (EVAR) less than 1% in many large volume centres.

More recently, investigators have reassessed the role of early intervention for small AAA using endovascular repair which carries a lower risk of early mortality as compared to open surgery. The European CAESAR trial failed to demonstrate any advantage of early EVAR over traditional surveillance. Whilst 30-day mortality rates for EVAR were low (0.6%) and the overall aneurysm-related mortality and rupture rates were low in both groups such that early treatment conferred no benefit.[57] Similarly, the US PIVOTAL trial showed that early all-cause mortality for both EVAR and surveillance groups were equal (4.1%).[58] Therefore, the consensus would suggest that first-line management for these patients with small AAA should be surveillance.[59] However, the early intervention policies used in the trial should also be considered for surveillance AAA which have rapid growth (>1 cm/year) and symptoms attributable to the aneurysm. There remains some uncertainty about the management of small AAA in certain subgroups (e.g. young patients, female patients, connective tissue disorders), who are perceived to be at greater risk of rupture at a smaller size. The UKSAT was the only large trial to recruit significant numbers of female patient to allow worthwhile analysis of the effect of gender in small AAA. The UKSAT found females as compared to men with small AAA were three to four times more likely to rupture whilst under surveillance, more likely to rupture at a smaller size and less likely to survive that rupture.[54] This has led many to adopt a policy in female patients of surveillance for small AAA, 3.0–5.0 cm diameter, and consider active treatment for females with an AAA of 5.0 cm or larger.

Surveillance intervals for small AAA, which are not part of a population screening programme, should take account of the increasing risk of rupture as small AAA increases in size. A consensus would recommend surveillance intervals for very small AAA, 3.0–4.5 cm, should be at 12 monthly intervals and small AAA, 4.5–5.5 cm, should be at 3 or 6 monthly intervals dependent on local policies.

Population screening for AAA

Population screening for AAA to prevent rupture and aneurysm-related death is now available in many countries where it is targeted to the at-risk population. Several large randomized population screening trials in geographically remote populations have shown benefit to screened male population in their seventh and eighth decades in respect to reduced risk of AAA-related mortality[3–7,60] (Table 26.2). These trials also demonstrate a halving of the incidence of aneurysm rupture in the screened populations. In the United Kingdom, the Multicentre Aneurysm Screening Study (MASS) trial has provided good evidence that aneurysm-related death is significantly reduced in a screened population of men aged 65–74 years, with a 53% reduction in those who attended for screening.[11] Furthermore, the cost-effectiveness ratio for screening was considered comparable with existing breast and cervical cancer screening programmes.[4,5] Screening is conducted using abdominal USS, which is non-invasive, inexpensive and portable (screening patients in community). Its sensitivity and specificity for AAA is close to 100%.[27,28,61] The majority of USS screening studies,[3–7,60,62,63] have defined an AAA as an external infrarenal aortic diameter of ≥3.0 cm, although the largest population screening study, the MASS trial, used internal aortic diameter which would provide a smaller diameter by comparison.[4,5] Measuring the anterior–posterior diameter appears more repeatable.[27,28,61,64] In some patients, iliac artery aneurysm is detected during USS screening for AAA, and if over 3.0 cm, it should be referred for consideration of active treatment. Given the prevalence of AAA is greater in men, the majority of population screening have studied men only. However, the first large-scale population screening study in Chichester (UK) did include both gender but found no reduction in AAA rupture after 10 years

Table 26.2 Tabulated results from population-based randomized screening trials.

Screening trial	Year	*n*	Age (years)	AAA prevalence	AAA mortality OR (95% CI)
Chichester, UK (16)	1995	15,775	65–80	4.0% (Men 7.6%)	0.59 (0.27–1.29)
Viborg, Denmark (17)	2002	12,628	65–73	4.0%	0.31 (0.13–0.79)
Mass, UK (19)	2002	67,800	65–74	4.9%	0.58 (0.42–.78)
Western Australia (18)	2004	41,000	65–79	7.2%	0.72 (0.39–1.32)

Notes: Year (year published), *n* (number), AAA mortality odds ratio (OR) screened versus not screened (95% confidence intervals).

follow-up.[65] There are several other subgroups of the population that may benefit from targeted screening, such as smokers, peripheral arterial disease and those with a family history of AAA. The incidence of AAA increases in older age groups, above 80 years, and as life expectancy increases and this population grow, thought must be given to extending screening to these older age groups.

The rescreening intervals should shorten as the AAA enlarges and risk of rupture increases. The majority of screening studies have recommended scanning intervals for very small AAA, <4.4 cm, to be every 12 months and for small AAA, 4.5–5.5 cm, to be every 3 months. Screening is associated with a reduction in AAA-related mortality but can increase anxiety levels in the screened population, and this in turn has a potential negative effect on quality of life.

Medical management of small AAA

Patients with AAA have increased risk of cardiovascular disease and at presentation often have several age-related co-morbid medical conditions. Therefore, all patients with a small AAA should have an assessment of cardiovascular risk and be considered for cardiovascular risk-reduction strategies (CVRRS) including lifestyle modification and pharmacotherapy. A history of current or prior smoking significantly increases the risk of AAA development. Smoking cessation appears to reduce AAA growth rate by 20%–30%.[22] COPD is exceedingly common in smokers and is associated with increased aneurysm expansion rates and higher rates of AAA rupture.[66] Therefore, there is a consensus that smoking cessation is beneficial in all patients with an AAA. Several cohort studies have suggested that statins, commonly used as lipid-lowering therapy, are associated with lower AAA growth rates.[37,67] However, a more recent study has suggested statins may have no effect on AAA growth.[67] However, their use as part of overall CVRRS is recommended and they may also reduce risk of perioperative cardiovascular complication when treating large AAA.

MANAGEMENT OF LARGE OR SYMPTOMATIC AAA

Patients with large AAA are at risk of fatal rupture, and to prevent this, they should be considered for active treatment. Many believe symptomatic AAA of any size should also be considered for active treatment. Patients with a known AAA with abdominal or mid-lumbar back pain without evidence of rupture but without alternate diagnosis for pain should be considered for active treatment especially with large AAA or any AAA which have undergone rapid growth. rAAA is a fatal event in nearly all patients who do not receive treatment, and as such all patients presenting with rAAA should be considered for active treatment when appropriate.

Comparison of open surgery and endovascular repair for AAA

The choice between open surgery and EVAR is complex and must be considered based on human factors (anatomical suitability, medical fitness and patient preference), healthcare factors (institutional experience, follow-up surveillance and cost) and the balance of risk and benefit. Several large randomized trials have compared outcomes of open surgery and EVAR. Clearly, EVAR has reduced early mortality and morbidity, at 30 days (EVAR, Dutch Randomised Endovascular Aneurysm Management [DREAM], Veteran Affairs Open Versus Endovascular Repair [OVER], ACE). However, we also now know that EVAR has increased late mortality and morbidity, beyond 2 years of follow-up. Furthermore, EVAR has been associated with an increased risk of late rupture (0.7% per 100 person-years). The early benefits of less invasive EVAR must be carefully balanced against the risks of late re-intervention (and associated morbidity and mortality), rupture, and the need for long-term radiological surveillance. So too the early risks of more invasive open surgery must be balanced against the potential late benefits of durability and freedom from late rupture.

The UK EVAR 1 trial, DREAM trial and US OVER trial provide evidence on the RR of conventional open surgery compared to EVAR for elective AAA treatment.[68,69] EVAR 1 showed a significant advantage in 30-day mortality for EVAR (1.7%) when compared to open surgery (4.7%).[70] However, after 4 years whilst aneurysm-related mortality remained better after EVAR (4% vs. 7%), complications were greater (41%), and all-cause mortality was similar for both groups (28% at 4 years).[69] Over the long term for EVAR, the early mortality benefit was offset by a higher rate of complications and late mortality and perhaps the most worrying several late fatal ruptures.[71]

Similarly, the DREAM trial group[72] showed an advantage in early 30-day mortality for EVAR (1.2%) compared to open surgery (4.6%). However, again no overall survival difference was observed during the mid and long term, and by 6 years again the EVAR group had increased complications and re-interventions.[73] Like the European trials, in the United States the OVER trial demonstrated lower 30-day mortality for EVAR (0.5%) compared to open surgery (3.0%).[74] Interestingly, a more recent French randomized trial reported no significant differences in 30-day mortality between EVAR (0.6%) and open surgery (1.3%) and with higher re-intervention rates for EVAR (24%) compared to open surgery (14%).[75] This newer trial contrasts with the findings of the three previous trials, which all showed early mortality benefit for EVAR, and this perhaps is explained by the exceptionally low 30-day mortality after open surgery in selected trial centres. One important consideration in interpreting these trials, which have been conducted over nearly two decades, is the progressive reduction in early procedure-related and all-cause mortality not only for EVAR but also for open surgery. Outside of selected trial centres, the early mortality benefit for EVAR has been reproduced, such as in the United States published Medicare analysis (45,660 patients) which showed a reduction of post-operative mortality for EVAR (1.2%) compared to open surgery (4.8%).[76] Worldwide amalgamated outcomes (31,427 patients) from national vascular registries (Australia, Denmark, Finland, Hungary, Italy, Norway, Sweden, Switzerland and the United Kingdom) have shown that the overall perioperative mortality after intact AAA repair is low at 2.8% and now stable over time. The perioperative mortality rate varied from 1.6% in Italy to 4.1% in Finland. The proportion treated by EVAR varied between countries from 14.7% (Finland) to 56.0% (Australia). Poorer outcomes were noted with increasing age, open repair and presence of co-morbidities.[77] The dilemma for the advising clinician and the consenting patient is therefore the balance between early mortality benefit for EVAR (at 30 days and up to 2 years), set against increased risk after EVAR of late complication, re-intervention, rupture and late mortality (after 4 years).

Comparison open and endovascular repair for ruptured AAA

rAAA is fatal complication in most and even those treated by emergency open surgery or emergency EVAR (eEVAR); mortality (30-day and in-hospital) remains significant (30%–50%). EVAR is less invasive and has been shown to reduce early mortality for elective AAA and as such should be considered in suitable patients presenting with rAAA. Unfortunately, patients with rAAA are often haemodynamically unstable and often have AAA which are anatomically unfavourable for standard EVAR, and this has meant that the excellent results achieved in selected

patients with rAAA using eEVAR have not resulted in a reduction in overall mortality. A Cochrane review of treatment of rAAA by eEVAR or open surgery has found no significant difference in outcomes overall.[78] The IMPROVE trial is the largest and most recent study to compare open surgery and eEVAR for rAAA but has shown no overall survival benefit for either technique. As expected haemodynamically unstable patients had a high mortality with either technique. The use of local anaesthesia may improve outcomes in some selected patients undergoing eEVAR.[79] More recently, an updated Cochrane meta-analysis of three RCTs, with a total of 761 patients with a clinical or radiological diagnosis of rAAA randomized to receive either eEVAR or open surgery, again showed no clear evidence to support a difference between the two interventions in respect to 30-day (or in-hospital) mortality.[80] Elective EVAR is associated with increased risk of late morbidity, re-intervention and late mortality (including rupture). In rAAA, aneurysm anatomy is often unfavourable for EVAR and eEVAR is more often conducted in hostile-neck anatomy which itself is associated with poor long-term outcome, and late endovascular complications in these patients are likely. Therefore, the late follow-up of the eEVAR studies is eagerly awaited. At present, most units will consider eEVAR in a haemodynamically stable patient with suitable anatomy, and when possible, this should be conducted under local anaesthetic with a suitable aorto-bi-iliac endovascular device,[81] and open surgery should be considered as an alternative when eEVAR is not possible or not appropriate.

Procedural risk assessment for open or endovascular repair

Treatment of AAA is a complex major intervention in often elderly patients with a variety of significant medical co-morbidities. To reduce the risk of major complications, careful patient selection is essential and in those more elderly patients with co-morbid disease careful consideration should be given to the risk–benefit analysis based on aneurysm size, and alternative endovascular options should be fully considered and in some cases conservative management should also be discussed. Patients should undergo pre-assessment for the identification of major vital organ dysfunction including an assessment of cardiac function and performance both at rest and under stress. The established risk factors are increasing age, ischaemic heart disease, COPD and renal impairment. Predictive scoring systems may be of value such as the physiological and operative severity score for the enumeration of mortality and morbidity[82] and Glasgow aneurysm score which predicts risk of morbidity and mortality after elective open AAA repair using an algorithm based on age, co-morbidity and operative factors.[83] It is clear from the major randomized trials (EVAR, DREAM, OVER, French) that the mortality from elective AAA repair by both endovascular and open techniques has reduced in recent years, and this is also reflected in data from large population-based registries (such as Medicare in the United States and National Vascular Registry in the United Kingdom). It is also clear that mortality is reduced in high-volume centres,[84] when teams of specialist vascular surgeons deliver care to elective and emergency AAA patients.

Coronary artery disease (CAD) is the leading cause of early and late mortality after elective AAA repair. In the presence of active CAD (unstable or severe angina, myocardial infarction within 1 month), decompensated heart failure (new onset, worsening or New York Heart Association Class IV), significant arrhythmia (atrioventricular block, poorly controlled atrial fibrillation, new-onset tachycardia) or severe valvular heart disease (symptomatic, aortic valve pressure gradient >40 mmHg), patients should have elective AAA treatment deferred until optimal management of cardiac disease can be achieved. Optimization in some cases will involve referral to a cardiologist for consideration of coronary revascularisation by coronary angioplasty and stent (CAS) placement or even to cardiac surgery for coronary artery bypass surgery (CABG). Care should be taken in determination of the requirements for anticoagulation therapy after CAS as these patients are often on dual antiplatelet therapy for 6 or 12 months and this would present a bleeding risk if open surgery were considered in that period. Two trials have assessed the role of prophylactic coronary revascularisation in vascular surgical patients (CARP and DECREASE-V).[85,86] Both studies demonstrated no benefit in respect to mortality or risk of myocardial infarction in patients who had undergone revascularisation (by CABG or CAS) prior to vascular surgery. However, high-risk patients who require major vascular surgery and are at risk of perioperative cardiac event should ideally have their treatment in a facility with access to primary CAS, if needed.

Initial trials looking at the benefit of perioperative beta-blockade (POBBLE) to reduce cardiovascular risk had been encouraging, but subsequent analysis has shown that this is only of value if indicated on clinical grounds in high-risk patients and commenced at least 1 month prior to surgery.[87,88] Several large clinical trials (POBBLE, POISE and MaVS) assessed the role for commencing beta-blockers a few days before open surgery to reduce cardiac risk and have found this provide no benefit and, in some cases, can be harmful.[89–91] Beta-blockade commenced acutely may cause more harm than good.[92] Most vascular surgery patients will already be on anti-platelet therapy (aspirin or alternative) as these have been shown to be of benefit as part of CVRRS.[93] When used as part of secondary prevention of cardiovascular risk, low-dose aspirin is associated with a reduction in major coronary events and ischaemic stroke.[93] Most vascular surgeons will prescribe perioperative low-dose aspirin and this does not appear to be associated with any increase in haemorrhagic complications. Newer anti-platelet agents such as clopidogrel have been associated with a slight increase risk of bleeding complication and some surgeons prefer to change to aspirin therapy 7 days prior to surgery. Patients on oral anticoagulant therapy should have this stopped prior to surgery (warfarin 5–7 days, thrombin inhibitors 2–3 days) and are most commonly managed by subcutaneous low-molecular-weight heparin perioperatively.

Respiratory optimization with bronchodilators or a short course of steroid therapy for patients with COPD may be necessary, and smoking cessation is worthwhile provided it can be achieved at least 2 weeks prior to surgical date. When possible, those with COPD should be considered for pulmonary optimization by a respiratory physician. Endovascular repair, which can be conducted under local anaesthetic, should also be considered where possible in these patients. CKD is common in patients presenting for treatment of AAA. All patients should have consideration given to discontinuation of nephrotoxic medications prior to surgery and during the perioperative period. Hydration in the perioperative period should also be optimized and monitored.

Enhanced recovery programmes (ERPs), also known as 'fast-track' surgery, have delivered significant benefits for patients undergoing colorectal and hepato-biliary surgery, and some recent evidence suggests it may also benefit patients undergoing open AAA repair. Several studies have reported that ERP can reduce need for intermediate or higher care (HDU or ICU) and reduce time to ambulation and discharge.[94–97] There is as yet no clear evidence that it significantly reduces major morbidity or mortality.

High-risk patients unfit for open repair

Some patients despite pre-assessment and pre-optimization remain at excessively high risk of mortality from open or endovascular repair. If the AAA is not very large (<8 cm), a conservative approach may be appropriate as the increased procedural-related mortality risk may be significantly greater than the annual aneurysm-related mortality due to rupture. In these patients, a record of the discussion should include a decision on whether or not active treatment should be considered if they represent with rupture. If the AAA is very large (>8 cm), active treatment should be considered even in high-risk patients, unless they have known terminal illness, are in decompensated major organ failure or decline treatment. Endovascular repair, which is less invasive and can be conducted under loco-regional anaesthesia, is often considered in these patients. The EVAR 2 trial looked at patients considered unfit for open surgery and randomized to active treatment by EVAR or conservative management. In EVAR group, these high-risk patients had a respectable 30-day mortality of 7.3%, and those who lived beyond 4 years had a reduced AAA-related mortality, but overall there was no benefit in all-cause mortality.[98] During the trial, there were 305 deaths, and only 78 were AAA related, and the authors concluded that due to the reduced life expectancy in this patient population, it was more expensive and unlikely that active treatment by EVAR would benefit these patients, especially when life expectancy was less than 3 years.[98]

CONVENTIONAL OPEN SURGERY AAA TREATMENT

In 1952, Dubost, a surgeon in Paris, France, reported the first successful open surgery AAA repair and thus one could comment that the era of modern vascular surgery was born.[95] On March 29, 1951, Dubost became the first surgeon to resect an AAA and replace it with a homograft. His patient was a 50-year-old man, and the operation was performed via a left thoraco-abdominal incision. A 15 cm homograft, taken from the thoracic aorta of a 20-year-old woman who died 3 weeks earlier, was anastomosed to the aorta and right common iliac artery (CIA). An endarterectomy of the occluded left CIA was performed before its anastomosis to the homograft. The patient survived for 8 years, succumbing to a myocardial infarction at his home in Brittany. The report of this operation rocked the surgical world and inspired surgeons throughout Europe and the United States. Several years later, Michael DeBakey performed a similar operation with a synthetic prosthesis and coined it 'Dubost's operation'.

Anatomical suitability for open surgery

Not all patients with AAA have favourable anatomy for standard open surgery. Pre-procedural assessment must reliably reject unsuitable patients, identify potential difficulties and allow selection of an appropriate approach and surgical repair. Common conditions which require variation in technique include hostile abdomen (previous abdominal surgery or intraperitoneal sepsis), associated aneurysm (iliac or femoral arteries), anatomical anomalies (horseshoe kidney, retro-aortic left renal vein [LRV]) and extensive aneurysmal disease (pararenal, thoraco-abdominal or dissected aneurysm). In some patients, the retroperitoneal approach[100] to an AAA is preferable. This approach may be considered in patients with prior abdominal surgery in order to avoid the lysis of adhesions which would be necessary with the trans-peritoneal approach, and especially in those with prior incisional hernia. It can also give improved proximal access for pararenal aneurysm especially if suprarenal or supra-coeliac clamp is necessary. It should also be considered for some inflammatory aneurysms and in the presence of a horseshoe kidney.

Open surgery operative technique

Informed consent for a high-risk operation such as open AAA surgery should be a process involving verbal and written information to cover the risks, benefits and alternative. The discussion should include common risks of wound complications such as incisional hernia and, in male patients, the risks of erectile dysfunction. The operative technique has been long established, but outcomes have improved dramatically in recent years due to careful patient selection, pre-optimization, expert surgery by high-volume surgeons and refinements in perioperative care (combined general and epidural anaesthesia, antibiotic prophylaxis, venous thromboembolism prophylaxis, blood product and fluid replacement and post-operative care).

For the vast majority of vascular surgeons, the conventional open surgery for the treatment of AAA involves a general anaesthetic, a midline abdominal incision and a trans-peritoneal approach to the aneurysm (Figure 26.2). This technique is a modification of the graft inclusion technique previously described by Ref. 101 and modified from Ref. 99. The patient is pre-assessed by the anaesthetic

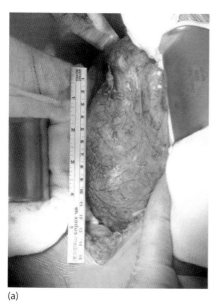
(a)

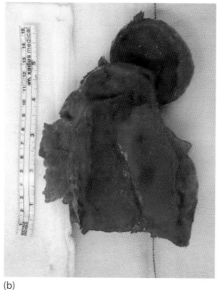
(b)

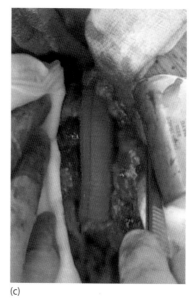
(c)

Figure 26.2 Clinical images from open surgery of abdominal aortic aneurysm (a), mural thrombus from aneurysm sac (b) and after 'in-lay' repair by aorto–aorto bypass using a straight synthetic graft (c).

team and any alterations or omissions to routine medications are agreed. The majority of patients are on antiplatelet therapy and lipid-lowering therapy, and these have been shown to have a cardioprotective effect and unless contraindicated should be continued. Some surgeons will convert clopidogrel to low-dose aspirin for 7 days preoperatively, as they believe this reduces the risk of surgical bleeding, but this is not our policy. Dual-anti-platelet therapy is common particularly in patients with prior coronary artery stenting and does increase the risk of surgical bleeding; we prefer to stop one or delay surgery until one can be safely stopped or even reconsider endovascular alternatives. Oral anticoagulant therapy in the form of coumarins (such as warfarin) or direct thrombin inhibitors should be discontinued prior to surgery and anticoagulation continued using subcutaneous therapeutic enoxaparin. Caution should be exercised in respect to all anticoagulants when epidural anaesthesia is contemplated. The patient has a peripheral venous cannula for fluid and drug administration and an arterial cannula sited (commonly the radial artery) to allow for invasive blood pressure monitoring. The patient has a low thoracic epidural cannula sited and this is locked for use in the post-operative period. The patient is inducted under general anaesthesia with endotracheal intubation, sedation and muscle relaxation. The anaesthetist inserts a central venous multi-lumen cannula (jugular vein) for volume resuscitation if necessary. The patient is paced supine on the operating table with arms abducted on arm boards to allow the anaesthetist access to peripheral lines. We use the WHO surgical checklist™ as part of our standard protocol.

The patient's abdomen and groins are exposed and aseptic skin preparation and surgical drapes are applied. The abdomen is opened and explored through a midline incision extending from the pubis to the xiphoid. A transperitoneal approach to the aneurysm is aided by lifting superiorly the transverse colon and lifting the small bowel to the right, where it is packed either outside or inside the abdominal cavity protected by large swabs or by placing it into a Lahey bag. Exposure is maintained by an assistant with a handheld retractor initially and then by the use of a fixed abdominal retraction system (such as an Omni-Tract™). The retroperitoneum is now in view with the infrarenal AAA partially covered on its right side by the duodenum and bordered on its left side by the inferior mesenteric vein (IMV). The peritoneum is incised vertically between these two structures and the duodenum is carefully displaced to the right where it should be protected. The IMV can usually be preserved and mobilized to the left and superiorly, but for pararenal AAA or when high exposure is needed, it can be divided superiorly to improve access. The incision is developed directly onto the anterior wall of the aneurysm with care and extended superiorly to reveal the infrarenal aortic neck and inferiorly to the aortic bifurcation. Superiorly, the LRV can usually be retracted to gain access to the aortic neck, but for pararenal AAA, it may need to be mobilized superiorly which can be assisted by division of the left gonadal vein at

their confluence, and in rare situations, the LRV can be divided proximally to allow access. When divided, some impairment of left kidney function may be anticipated, but venous drainage is usually maintained by collaterals, and indeed some surgeons electively repair the divided renal vein after completion of aortic repair, but we do not recommend this practice and believe it risks bleeding complication. The infrarenal aortic neck is dissected to allow adequate exposure to allow application of an aortic cross-clamp under direct vision. Some surgeons prefer to encircle the neck with a tape, but we do not recommend this practice and believe it risks bleeding complication. Inferiorly, the incision is extended onto the right CIA and sharp dissection exposes the contralateral left CIA with care to minimize dissection to the nervi erigentes damage to which can in a man contribute to post-operative sexual dysfunction. In the presence of associated CIA aneurysm, dissection needs to be extended to the iliac artery bifurcation and care should be taken to avoid damage to the ureter as it crosses the iliac vessels. Dissection of the lateral walls of the aneurysm is kept to a minimum and excessive dissection on the right can risk damage to the duodenum or inferior vena cava. On the left anterior aspect of the aneurysm sac, the origin of the inferior mesenteric artery is noted, but unless exceptionally large, specific control is unnecessary as its orifice can easily be suture ligated internally once the aneurysm sac is opened. Systemic anticoagulation is induced by administration of heparin intravenously (usually 5000 iu for an average adult); some surgeons prefer to monitor and adjust anticoagulation using a rapid bedside activated clotting time test. Some surgeons prefer to avoid anticoagulation, but we do not recommend this practice and believe it risks graft or distal arterial thrombosis. Arterial cross-clamps are applied above and below the aneurysm to the aortic neck and to the iliac arteries; some surgeons prefer to apply iliac before aortic clamps to reduce the risk of distal embolization. It is prudent to palpate the aneurysm sac to ensure the expansile pulsation has ceased prior to opening the aorta. Suction should be checked and available and we prefer to use cell salvage when possible to allow for autotransfusion of blood to reduce the need for laboratory blood products. The aneurysm is then opened longitudinally and the mural thrombus, and loose AS debris is evacuated from the aneurysm sac. The integrity of the proximal and distal clamps should be confirmed intra-luminal and any bleeding lumbar arteries oversewn with figure-of-eight polypropylene sutures. So to the origin of the IMA if still patent is sutured from within the lumen. The majority of aneurysms are repaired using a straight aorto-aortic interposition graft, but in the presence of iliac artery aneurysm, a bifurcated aorto-iliac or aorto-femoral graft may be considered. The majority of implanted graft conduits are made from woven Dacron with graft diameter selected to best suit the native aorta and allow for satisfactory anastomosis. Some surgeons prefer the use of grafts impregnated with rifampicin antibiotic or silver to reduce the risk of graft infection, but evidence for this practice is lacking.

The proximal point of anastomosis to health aortic tissue above the level of the aneurysm is selected, and the vertical sac incision may be extended laterally on both sides, to form a *T*, to facilitate exposure and anastomosis. Transection of the aorta is not normally recommended as this has the potential to weaken the posterior longitudinal support for the anastomosis and may risk bleeding. The proximal end-to-end anastomosis of the graft to the aortic neck is performed using a running polypropylene double-ended (needle) suture ensuring secure full-thickness bites of the aortic wall are taken and using an eversion technique. The suture line is completed and tied anteriorly. Some surgeons prefer to 'parachute' the posterior wall of the anastomosis and this technique is useful when access is challenging. Some surgeons prefer placement of a Teflon strip or individual Teflon pledgets to reinforce the outer aortic wall, reduce risk of stitch-hole bleeding and secure their anastomosis, and this should be considered in thin-walled aortas. A variety of topical haemostats which can be applied to the anastomotic line are also now commercially available to assist with haemostasis. The proximal anastomosis once completed is tested for leaks by clamping the tube graft and releasing the aortic clamp briefly. If any anastomotic leaks are noted, the aortic clamp is reapplied, and these are repaired with simple or horizontal mattress sutures of polypropylene and may be reinforced by the addition of a Teflon pledget. The clamp can then be reapplied to the aorta or to the graft just distal to the anastomosis to allow performance of the distal anastomosis. The graft should be cleared of blood and placed under slight tension and cut to an appropriate length for the distal anastomosis to the aortic bifurcation. The distal end-to-end anastomosis of the graft to the aortic bifurcation is performed using a running polypropylene double-ended (needle) suture ensuring secure full-thickness bites of the aortic wall are taken and using an eversion technique. All vessels are flushed before completion of this suture line. Adequate back bleeding from the iliac arteries is normally sufficient to confirm patency, but if concern exists cautious iliac artery balloon embolectomy may be required. The suture line is then completed anteriorly as for the proximal anastomosis. The iliac clamps are then released and the lower anastomosis is inspected for leaks which are repaired as for the proximal anastomosis. The anaesthetists should remain vigilant throughout the surgical procedure but special alert by the surgeon should be given prior to release of clamps, as restoration of flow to the lower body can induce acute systemic hypotension. The proximal aortic clamp is then gradually released whilst the anaesthetist maintains a satisfactory blood pressure with the use of fluid or pharmacological adjuncts as required. After release of clamps, the iliac arteries are inspected for adequate pulsations, the femoral arteries are palpated for pulsations, and a circulating team member may inspect the feet for adequate perfusion. Once blood pressure has returned to baseline (greater than 100 mmHg), a final inspection is made to ensure there is no ongoing bleeding at the proximal and distal suture line or from lumbar vessels within the aortic sac. The aneurysm sac is then wrapped over the graft and sutured anteriorly with a running suture to cover the graft and both the proximal and distal anastomosis if possible. The posterior peritoneum is then closed over the aorta and re-sutured aneurysm wall with a running suture of polyglycolate. If graft coverage cannot be achieved due to deficiencies of the aneurysm wall or peritoneum, consideration should be given to mobilizing an omental pedicle and suturing this to create a protective barrier between the graft and adjacent duodenum. A final inspection of the abdominal contents is then made to ensure the left colon is adequately perfused and to exclude iatrogenic injury to surrounding structures. The abdomen is then closed using the mass closure technique with a continuous strong polypropylene.

STANDARD ENDOVASCULAR AAA TREATMENT

In 1991, Parodi reported the first successful endovascular AAA repair and thus one could comment that the era of endovascular therapy was born.[102] Using a trans-femoral intra-luminal approach, the team implanted a device within the infrarenal aorta to exclude the aneurysm custom made by attaching balloon expandable stents to the proximal and distal end of an aortic graft, and as such, the *endograft* was born. The original straight graft was quickly replaced by a modular aorto-bi-iliac stent graft, to cope with the commonest aneurysm anatomies and to increase stability and sealing zones.[103] Endograft technology continues to develop and a variety of complex endovascular solutions now exist to treat varied anatomy. Vascular surgeons have developed their endovascular skills to cope with the demands of these novel techniques.

Anatomical suitability for EVAR

Not all patients with AAA are suitable for standard endovascular stent grafting. Pre-procedural assessment must reliably reject unsuitable patients, identify potential difficulties and allow selection of an appropriate stent graft. Tertiary referral centres report that up to 60% of patients may be suitable for standard endovascular repair of AAA (EVAR). Woodburn et al., using spiral CT angiography to determine aneurysm morphology and suitability for EVAR in an unselected population presenting with large AAA, found 55% had one or more absolute contraindication, 11% had at least one relative contraindication, and only 34% had no contraindication. The authors concluded that increased use of EVAR is only possible by deploying devices in suboptimal morphology and in treating patients who would not normally be considered for open AAA repair.[104] Suitability for EVAR is also determined by the relevant stent-graft manufacturer's eligibility criteria set down in their *instructions for use*. One of the strictest criteria surrounds the aortic neck which, for the majority of devices, must be parallel for 15 mm below the lowest renal artery, free from thrombus and excessive angulation. Off-label use of stent grafts, by treating patients who do not fulfil such anatomical inclusion criteria, is associated with poorer outcomes but is known to be common practice.[105] However, whilst clinicians and manufacturers strove to perfect stent-graft technology, some concerns were being reported of new device-related complications specific to this new endovascular repair. Whilst device failure, infection, open conversion and late rupture were all reported, it could be argued that these have also been seen with conventional open surgery AAA repair. A new phenomenon of incomplete aneurysm exclusion, with persistent blood flow or pressure within the aneurysm sac and a persistent risk of late rupture, the *endoleak*, was classified.[106] The EUROSTAR registry reported that endoleaks were common after EVAR and increased the risk of re-intervention, aneurysm growth and late rupture.[107] It was also noted that many AAAs had unfavourable anatomy for standard endovascular repair,[108] and when placing standard endografts outside of their manufacturer's indications for use (IFU) in these patients with *hostile neck anatomy* (HNA), the risks of device-related complications and failure to exclude the aneurysm or prevent rupture were high.[109] However, some of these risks can be addressed by the use of fenestrated EVAR (FEVAR) in AAA with short infrarenal necks improving the proximal sealing zone by moving this proximally to the pararenal segment and with the use of fenestrations connected by bridging bare or covered stents to the renal and/or splanchnic arteries to maintain perfusion to the kidneys and viscera.[110–112] In AAA with associated aneurysm of the CIA, improvement of the distal sealing zone may be achieved by extending the graft limb to the external iliac artery and using a branched covered iliac stent to maintain flow in the internal iliac artery.[113]

Standard endovascular technique

The majority of patients receive a modular endovascular device with standard aorto-bi-iliac endograft (Figure 26.3). Informed consent for EVAR should be a process involving verbal and written information to cover the risks, benefits and alternative. The discussion should include the risks of endoleak, secondary re-intervention and late rupture and the need for long-term radiological surveillance. The majority of patients still undergo general anaesthesia, but regional anaesthesia (epidural) and local anaesthesia are also used. Indeed, in eEVAR for rAAA, local anaesthesia is now the preferred option when possible and may reduce mortality in that setting (IMPROVE trial). Antibiotic prophylaxis should be based on local protocols, but given the endograft implant, consideration should be given to specific prophylaxis (teicoplanin or vancomycin) against methicillin-resistant *S. aureus*. The procedure will require image guidance with a high-quality fixed or mobile radiological imaging system and radiolucent mobile operating

table with appropriate radiation protection for staff. The majority of patients still have open surgical exposure of the femoral artery on both sides. Some advocate a percutaneous approach for the lower-profile devices, for the contralateral limb and even for the larger main body, and if this approach is taken arteriotomy, repair can be achieved using appropriate percutaneous suture closure devices. However, failure of the percutaneous approach is likely in obese patients and in vessels that are calcified, scarred, narrowed or tortuous. The percutaneous approach, particularly as delivery systems become smaller, may prove less invasive and more likely to facilitate an earlier ambulation and discharge. All devices are delivered over the wire after appropriate digital subtraction imaging and marking of the aortic landmarks (renal arteries, aortic infrarenal neck, aortic bifurcation, iliac bifurcation) The commonest EVAR devices used electively are aorto-bi-iliac device, although alternative aorto-uni-iliac devices allow for the management of patients with only one acceptable iliac artery access and are supplemented with a surgical femoro-femoral crossover graft to restore perfusion to the contralateral limb. The commonest endograft systems are modular and are available in a range of diameters and lengths to suit the majority of patients. These consist of a main body, with proximal aortic component bifurcating distally to form a long ipsilateral and short contralateral limb which is then combined with long contralateral limb extension and short ipsilateral limb extension pieces to allow exclusion from the infrarenal aorta to the common iliac arteries bilaterally. Once deployed, it is usually balloon moulded to ensure conformation and seal proximal and distal landing zones and at any stent overlaps. Final check DSA allows confirmation of endograft patency, exclusion of the aneurysm and assessment for endoleaks. Once all access wires and sheaths are screened out, the access arteriotomy sites in both femoral arteries are closed transversely with non-absorbable suture, and once restoration of flow is restored and haemostasis achieved, the groin wounds are closed.

Pre-operative planning and advance decisions on suitability for EVAR should exclude the most unfavourable anatomy. However, commonly standard EVAR is delivered in sub-optimal anatomy and adjustments to technique must be made. Approximately 15%–30% of all adults have accessory renal arteries. These are identified on pre-operative CTA planning and are often covered electively without significant renal compromise. Consideration should be given to preservation of certain accessory renals, especially if large (>3 mm), supplying more than one-third of the kidney, in solitary kidneys, in horseshoe kidneys and in severe CKD. Associated iliac artery aneurysms are present in up to 40% of EVAR patients and often preclude a secure distal seal in one or both iliac arteries. In the presence of unilateral CIA aneurysm, the commonest approach is to coil embolize the ipsilateral internal iliac artery (IIA) and extend the iliac graft limb to the external iliac artery (EIA). Complications can arise due to pelvic ischaemia but are less

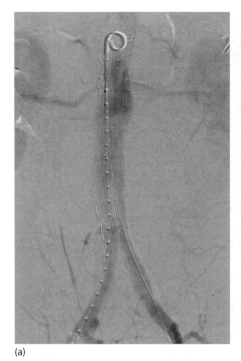
(a)

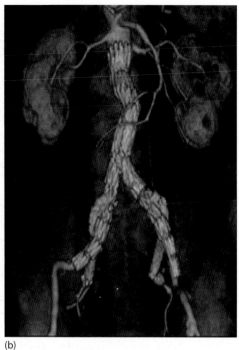
(b)

Figure 26.3 Vascular imaging of endovascular aneurysm repair showing endograft seen on (a) fluoroscopy during procedure and (b) 3D reconstruction of computed tomography angiography during post-surveillance.

common if the contralateral IIA is patent to allow for collateralization. Complications have been reported in up to one-third of patients, the commonest being buttock claudication, impotence and most worryingly colonic ischaemia. Bilateral IIA embolization is associated with higher risk of serious complication and normally is avoided, but if no other open or endovascular options are available, it should be done in a staged fashion to allow for collateralization. More recently, iliac side branched devices have been used to preserve IIA, at the expense of increased procedural time, and the long-term patency and complication rates of these devices are as yet unknown.

Radiological surveillance post-EVAR

Randomized trials have shown that whilst EVAR has reduced early mortality compared to open surgery, it is associated with increased rate of late complications and post-treatment rupture. Many of these complications are procedure-specific complications such as endoleaks and endograft failure (mechanical failure or infection). Therefore, all patients receiving EVAR should be considered for medium or long-term (>8 years) radiological surveillance. This is most commonly achieved using a combination of plain radiography and CTA. Plain radiography using a standardized protocol is an effective method for the detection of device migration.[114] Radiographs will also demonstrate junctional overlap and structural failure such as strut fracture or collapse. CTA will demonstrate patency of the endograft and visceral vessels and

allow assessment of the AAA for endoleak and diameter change. AAA diameter change is a primary parameter for determining the presence of an endoleak and assessing its impact. Whilst diameter measurement has been the most commonly used method for determining sac changes, volume measurement has now been proven superior for monitoring structural changes in the 3D sac.[115] Contrast-enhanced MRI angiogram (MRA) can be considered in non-ferrous stent grafts and may be superior to CTA for the detection of endoleaks.[116] In stable post-EVAR surveillance patients, USS is often used in preference to CTA in patients without endoleak and with significant AAA diameter reduction (<4.0 cm). Contrast-enhanced ultrasonography has been shown to have a similar sensitivity and specificity for the detection of endoleaks as CTA and MRA.[117] The standard protocol in most centres post-EVAR is for plain radiographs and CTA at 1–3 months, then 6 months and every 12 months thereafter for uncomplicated endografts.

COMPLICATIONS AFTER AAA REPAIR

The perioperative mortality for open surgery and EVAR has decreased dramatically in recent years (EVAR, DREAM, OVER, French, Medicare). The commonest early complications after either open or endovascular repair for AAA are not procedure-specific complications but the typical cardiovascular events one expects in these high-risk patients. A number of large RCTs (EVAR, DREAM, OVER) have shown that EVAR, as compared to open repair, is associated with a lower early mortality, but it is also now clear that over the medium and long term, EVAR is associated with a much higher rate of secondary re-intervention and complication documented at 20%–30% higher that open surgery. The existing published randomized trials, together with information from Medicare and Swedvasc databases, were included in a recent meta-analysis (25,078 patients undergoing EVAR and 27,142 undergoing open repair for AAA), and EVAR had a significantly lower 30-day or in-hospital mortality rate (1.3% vs. 4.7% for open repair). There was no significant difference in all-cause or aneurysm-related mortality by 2 years or longer follow-up. A significantly higher proportion of patients undergoing EVAR required re-intervention and suffered aneurysm rupture. There is no long-term survival benefit for patients who have EVAR compared with open repair for AAA. There are also significantly higher risks of re-intervention and aneurysm rupture after EVAR.[118,119]

Infective complication after either open or endovascular AAA repair may include surgical site (wound) infection, septicaemia and aortic graft infection (AGI). In a large Medicare analysis of infectious complications after elective AAA repair (open and endovascular), they found overall infective complication rates of 3%.[120] AGI is perhaps the most feared complication after synthetic graft implantation and may result in graft failure. In a large analysis (13,902 patients) in Washington State by using the Comprehensive Hospital Abstract Reporting System data, the cumulative rate of AGIs in the cohort was 0.44%, with similar rates at 2 years in open (0.19%) and EVAR (0.16%) patients and without significant difference between elective and non-elective patients. Blood stream septicaemia and surgical site infection were significantly associated with AGIs and should be treated aggressively to reduce risk of AGI.[121] The reported incidence of prosthetic graft infection varies between 0.3% and 6%.[122] Infection may occur due to implantation or later by seeding during bacteraemia from dental procedures or other septic illness. Intra-abdominal (aorto-aorto or aorto-iliac) grafts have a low risk of infection (<1%),[122-125] but the risk increases with extension of grafts to the groin (aorto-femoral) where infection rates are considerably higher (2%–4%).[125] Staphylococcal organisms are the most frequent cultured from infected grafts, with *Staphylococcus epidermis* commonest followed by *S. aureus* and *E. coli*.[125,126] One of the most feared complications seen with infected grafts is a prosthetic–enteric fistula, with the duodenum most commonly affected, occurring after open AAA surgery in less than 1%.[126] This diagnosis should be considered when gastrointestinal bleeding complicates an infected graft and may be diagnosed using CTA and endoscopy.

Procedure-related complications after open surgery for AAA

Open surgery for AAA is associated with general complications of abdominal surgery and procedure-specific complications of AAA repair. Care is taken to avoid iatrogenic injury to intra-abdominal viscera during dissection and repair and in particular to the duodenum when dissecting the aortic neck in particular with large or inflammatory AAA. Major bleeding after elective repair is fortunately uncommon. With large or inflammatory AAA, para-anastomotic aneurysm can occur after AAA repair and include false aneurysm arising from disruption of the anastomosis and true aneurysm that develop adjacent to the anastomosis. There is an increased risk of distal colon ischaemia when pelvic blood flow is significantly reduced, and it is an established surgical principle that internal iliac artery flow should be maintained on at least one side, although recently questioned by Mehta and Veith. The criteria for re-implantation of the inferior mesenteric artery are not clearly defined but certainly should be considered in the case of an unusually large inferior mesenteric artery or angiographic evidence of superior mesenteric artery stenosis or if the collateral circulation between the superior and inferior mesenteric is poorly developed. Further considerations whilst in the operating room include poor backflow from a patent inferior mesenteric artery even after completion of the distal anastomosis, concern that pelvic flow has been reduced by the reconstructive procedure and concern about the appearance of the colon. Methods such as inferior mesenteric stump pressure measurement, intraoperative Doppler, photoplethysmography or colon pH measurement provide objective assessment, but there is no evidence that these are superior to clinical assessment. In the Canadian Aneurysm Study, the inferior mesenteric artery was re-implanted in 4.8% of cases. When internal iliac flow was maintained to one or both sides, the incidence of colon ischaemia was 0.3%, whereas when it was interrupted bilaterally, the incidence increased to 2.6%. There is a significant risk of incisional hernia in the midline abdominal wound after open surgery for AAA, and this can in part be managed with meticulous attention to abdominal wall closure. If symptomatic or large, these can be revised using laparoscopic preperitoneal mesh repair at a later stage.

Procedure-related complications after EVAR

In recent years with experience and correct patient selection, the incidence of primary failure of endovascular repair requires acute conversion to open surgery has become rare. With carefully selected patients in the large RCTs (EVAR, DREAM, OVER), acute conversion was rare, and in a recent American College of Surgeons–National Safety and Quality Improvement Project (ACS–NSQIP) review, it was noted that acute surgical conversion was a rare complication affecting 1.1% of EVAR cases, with no broadly identifiable at-risk population. When conversion did occur, morbidity and mortality (3.4%) rates paralleled those observed for elective open repair.[127]

Endoleaks, re-intervention and late rupture

In the phenomenon of *incomplete aneurysm exclusion* or persistent blood flow or pressure within the aneurysm sac and a persistent risk of late rupture, the *endoleak* was defined by White in 1996.[106] Endoleaks have been classified based on the source of persistent blood flow which continues to pressurize the aneurysm sac,[128] Table 26.3. The EUROSTAR registry reported that endoleaks were common after EVAR and increased the risk of re-intervention, aneurysm growth and late rupture (EUROSTAR 2003). In general, high-pressure leaks (type I and type III) require urgent management because of the relatively high short-term risk of sac rupture. Late rupture has been reported after apparently successful EVAR and is a significant concern for late complication. By 2002, the EUROSTAR registry had enrolled 4291 patients and noted 34 patients with recorded rupture following EVAR, with the commonest endoleak associated with these being type I and III endoleaks.[129] Both type I and type III endoleaks are considered high risk and require angiographic evaluation and subsequent treatment. Low-pressure leaks (types II and V or endotension) are considered less urgent but may warrant continued endovascular evaluation if there is growth of the aneurysm sac or if the patient presents with symptoms. Once detected, endoleaks warranting correction (all type I and type III; persistent endotension and type II associated with aneurysm enlargement) are usually treated by endovascular route. A variety of techniques including extension endografts or cuff, balloon angioplasty, bare stents and a combination of transvascular and direct sac puncture embolization techniques have been used to treat endoleaks. Type II endoleak continues to be the most common but also the most controversial in terms of evaluation, the need of treatment and methods of treatment. The EUROSTAR registry also note a high and persisting rate of re-intervention after EVAR often for the

management of endoleak, with re-intervention rates at 1, 2, 3 and 4 years of 6%, 9%, 12% and 14%.[130] Gelfand et al. in their analysis of 10 EVAR trials found the incidence of the commonest type II endoleak at discharge or 30 days was 6%–17%, and whilst over one-half resolved spontaneously, persistent endoleaks were present in 1%–5% at 1 year.[131] Type II endoleaks have been shown to be associated with aneurysm sac expansion, secondary re-intervention and aneurysm rupture.[132] In a more recent large analysis of 32 non-randomized retrospective studies, totalling 21,744 patients who underwent EVAR, type II endoleak was seen in 10.2% of patients after EVAR and 35.4% resolved spontaneously. In their analysis, rupture after EVAR secondary to an isolated type II endoleak was considered rare (less than 1%), but over a third occurs in the absence of sac expansion.[133] Therefore, a conservative approach to type II endoleaks in patients with stable or reducing aneurysm sac diameter is considered safe in most patients.

Aneurysm treatment by open or endovascular repair is to prevent aneurysm-related mortality, primarily to prevent fatal aneurysm rupture. Therefore, it was a cause of considerable concern when early reports of rupture after apparently successful endovascular repair began to emerge. The EUROSTAR Registry reported the peak incidence of rupture was at 18 months (0–24) and the annual cumulative rate approximates to 1% (1.4% in the first year, 0.6% in the second year).[134] These early complications during the early evolution of endovascular practice could in part have been due to the learning-curve effect and the use of early generation endografts. However, the subsequent UK EVAR trials also reported a total of 27 post-EVAR ruptures. Eighty-two per cent of these ruptures occurred greater than 30 days following implantation, and the majority of these (63%) were in patients with previously reported complications or signs of failed EVAR. Research has identified types I and II (with sac enlargement) endoleaks, migration and graft kinking as risk factors for aortic rupture.[135] Schlösser et al. analyzed 270 patients with AAA ruptures after EVAR, and whilst many had known abnormalities such as endoleaks with aneurysm sac expansion, a significant minority had no abnormality during follow-up prior to rupture.[136] Aneurysm sac expansion in the absence of endoleak is a dilemma as there is no obvious known target for re-intervention, and some authors have suggested the risk of rupture is low, <1% over 4 years for enlargement <8 mm without detectable endoleaks.[137] Cho et al. considered whether prior endovascular AAA repair (EVAR) confers protective effects in the setting of rAAA, but found they were just as likely to be haemodynamically unstable (55.6%) and to suffer in-hospital mortality (38.9%) as primary ruptures treated in the same institution.[138] Focused surveillance for the first 2–3 years after EVAR and for those with increased risk of early rupture (relatively large initial AAA diameter or presence of endoleak or graft migration) may help identify and treat those at most risk of rupture post-EVAR.

Despite high initial technical success, the long-term durability of EVAR continues to be a concern as patients

Table 26.3 Classification of endoleaks.

Endoleak type	Subtype	Source
I	A: Proximal	Graft attachment site
	B: Distal	
	C: Iliac occluder	
II	A: Simple (single vessel)	Collateral vessel
	B: Complex (>2 vessels)	
III	A: Junctional leak	Graft failure
	B: Mid-graft hole	
	C: Other (e.g. suture hole)	
IV		Graft wall porosity
V	A: Without endoleak	Endotension
	B: With sealed endoleak	
	C: With type I or type III leak	
	D: With type II leak	

Source: Modified from Veith FJ et al., *J Vasc Surg*, 35, 1029, 2002.

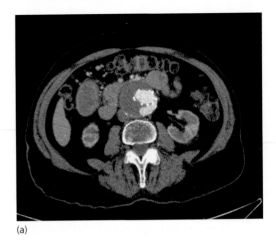
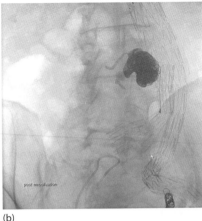

(a) (b)

Figure 26.4 Vascular imaging for surveillance after endovascular aneurysm repair, demonstrating a large endoleak with (a) cross-sectional computed tomographic angiography surveillance imaging demonstrating contrast filling the posterior aneurysm sac, and (b) on fluoroscopy during secondary endovascular re-intervention with embolization using coils and bio-glue to seal the lumbar arteries and aneurysm sac causing a type II endoleak (b).

can experience endoleaks, device migration, device fractures or aneurysm growth that may require intervention. Norden et al. looked at secondary interventions following EVAR in 32 papers (17,987 EVAR cases were reported) and found crude annual secondary intervention rates from the US population registries were 3.7%/year (range 1.7%–4.3%). Combined re-intervention-free survival estimates, from 14 series (10,365 cases), demonstrated a linear progression with 89.9%, 86.9% and 81.5% of grafts without secondary procedures at 2, 3 and 5 years, respectively.[139] The threshold for intervention with relatively common type II endoleaks is difficult to define, but many consider a conservative approach safe in the absence of significant aneurysm sac expansion.[72,140] However, persistent type II endoleaks in the presence of continued aneurysm sac expansion are more concerning and have been associated with rupture. These are often treated with coil and glue embolization of aneurysm sac and selected branch vessels (Figure 26.4), but these do not appear to yield significant benefit in many patients. Many believe a significant proportion of these treatment failures are due to an inability to diagnose and definitively treat the true cause of aneurysm expansion which is often an occult or intermittent type II or III endoleaks.[141] Evaluation should be considered in these patients to identify high-pressure endoleaks using contrast-enhanced ultrasound, dual-phase CT angiogram or catheter angiogram.

Endograft infection

Pyrexia is common after EVAR, especially in the first 48 hours, and this is often associated with raised inflammatory markers such as CRP but often due to the immune response to endograft implantation rather than true infectious complication. Microbiological investigation in the first 48 hours in these patients is unrewarding, but if persistent after this period, cultures are more likely to show growth.[142] However, with true early post-EVAR, septicaemia treatment should be aggressive with broad-spectrum intravenous antibiotics based on microbiological sensitivities and local guidelines. Endograft preservation is often possible with appropriate and extended antibiotic therapy and surveillance. Investigations to define infection may include CT scans, tagged leukocyte scan, MRI and more recently PET-CT. True endograft infection is much more serious and may require explantation with in situ (using cadaveric homograft, autologous superficial femoral vein or synthetic graft) or extra-anatomical (axillo-femoral bypass) vascular reconstruction. In high-risk patients considered unfit for explantation, they may be temporized with conservative treatment with antimicrobial therapy and percutaneous drainage.[143] Infected endografts should be explanted through a midline trans-peritoneal approach. Positive tissue cultures may help identify the infective source and direct antibiotic therapy.[144]

Delayed secondary open conversion after EVAR

Failures following EVAR occur in a small but significant number of patients. When anatomically possible, endovascular revision offers a safe means of treating these failures. A common point of failure is at the proximal sealing zone of the infrarenal aorta with development of a high-pressure proximal type I endoleak due to endograft migration or pararenal aneurysmal change. Potential endovascular solutions may include extension of the proximal sealing zone. This may be achieved with placement of a proximal cuff (covered stent) or some prefer relining of the endograft with a secondary aorto-bi-iliac or aorto-uni-iliac device.[145]

If insufficient infrarenal sealing zone exists or when pararenal aneurysmal change has occurred, the sealing zone will need to advance even more proximally, and here fenestrated endografts can be used to achieve a seal and allow bridging stents to renals and if necessary visceral arteries.[146]

Secondary open conversion (SOC) after EVAR may be required when an endograft is considered to have failed due to acute rupture or infection or for persistent malignant endoleak in the presence of an expanding aneurysm sac. The EUROSTAR Registry reported the cumulative incidence of rupture at 3 years of follow-up was 1.2%. The annual risk of secondary open conversion approximated to 2.1% (1% year 1, 3.7% year 2).[109] Occurrence of late conversion after EVAR is not negligible, affecting almost 1 in 10 patients after 6 years.[147] In a large study (14,289 patients) undergoing EVAR, 279 (1.9%) required late conversion; the mortality rate was 10%.[148] The commonest indications for SOC are endoleaks (most commonly type I or type III), material or device failure (fabric tear or strut fractures) and infections. SOC is more likely when EVAR has been carried out in challenging or unfavourable anatomy.[149] Late secondary open conversion has been reported for every major commercial endograft and the incidence of SOC does not appear to be device specific.[150,151] In the presence of an expanding aneurysm after EVAR, especially after a failed secondary endovascular re-intervention, an aggressive attitude in fit patients allows outcomes similar to those of primary open surgery.[145,152] Marone et al., in a large series of selected patients (n = 54), reported that SOC could be achieved with overall 30-day mortality of 1.9% but with significant risk of renal failure (24%).[153] SOC may involve partial explantation or complete explantation of the endograft. Infected endograft requires complete explantation, and vascular reconstruction may be achieved in situ or by oversewing of the proximal and distal aorta and extra-anatomic bypass using axillo-bi-femoral bypass. In situ reconstruction may be achieved with a variety of conduits such as arterial homograft, autologous vein (superficial femoral vein as a tube graft or 'trouser' bifurcated graft) or synthetic graft if contamination is not a concern.[154] If synthetic graft is to be used, careful debridement of the infected field and omentum patch coverage along with extended antibiotic therapy may reduce the risk of recurrent sepsis. The partial explantation technique may reduce the surgical trauma and can be achieved with a low mortality in non-infected endograft.[155] Mortality is higher in patients with rupture compared with non-ruptured SOC.[150]

PARARENAL ABDOMINAL AORTIC ANEURYSM

Whilst the majority of AAA treated are truly infrarenal in nature, in some the aneurysmal change extends proximally to impinge on the renal artery origins and is referred to as juxta- or pararenal aneurysms. In many cases, they may be considered a challenging variant of AAA with unfavourable or HNA. In extreme cases, these aneurysms should be considered part of a spectrum that includes TAAA. For true TAAA, then management options include open surgery and hybrid repair (surgical visceral artery bypass and thoracic EVAR), but increasingly these patients can also be considered for complex EVAR with branched (b-EVAR) and FEVAR endovascular repair.

Hostile neck anatomy post-EVAR

HNA is often defined as one or more of the following: neck length <15 mm, neck diameter >28 mm diameter and angulation >60°. It was also noted that many AAAs had unfavourable anatomy for standard endovascular repair,[108] and when placing standard endografts outside of their manufacturer's IFU in these patients with HNA, the risks of device-related complications and failure to exclude the aneurysm or prevent rupture were high.[109] Off-label use of stent grafts, by treating patients who do not fulfil such anatomical inclusion criteria, is associated with poorer outcomes but is known to be common practice.[105] Stather et al., in a recent large systematic review and meta-analysis of outcomes following EVAR in patients with HNA analysis of the pooled data, revealed a significant increase in 30-day mortality, intraoperative adjuncts, early and late type I endoleaks and 30-day migration. These results suggest that performing EVAR in patients with HNA increases the technical difficulty and results in poorer short-term outcomes.[118,119] In another analysis of 7 observational studies reporting on 1559 patients (hostile anatomy group, 714 patients; friendly anatomy group, 845 patients), patients with hostile anatomy had a fourfold increased risk of developing type I endoleak and a ninefold increased risk of aneurysm-related mortality within 1 year of treatment. The authors concluded that EVAR should be cautiously used in patients with anatomic neck constraints.[156] Therefore, placing standard EVAR devices into HNA is liable to result in poor outcomes and alternatives including non-standard EVAR and open surgery should be considered.

Fenestrated endovascular repair for AAA

Many patients who may benefit from an endovascular treatment option are unfavourable or unsuitable for standard endovascular repair as a result of HNA. This HNA commonly refers to infrarenal aortic necks that are short, conical and angulated but may also include pararenal extension of the aneurysm. Placing a standard endovascular device into such anatomy would risk failure with proximal type I endoleak and risk of late rupture. In these patients, consideration should be given to non-standard (complex) EVAR using FEVAR or b-EVAR devices.

Endovascular innovators have approached the challenges posed by HNA by moving the sealing zone for the endograft more proximally to the pararenal segment or distal thoracic aorta, and to maintain perfusion to the vital renal and mesenteric arteries, they created fenestrations (holes) in the graft fabric and used bridging covered stents to maintain branch vessel flow.

The first generation of fenestrated endografts was used to treat complications from existing standard endografts, with customized stents with fenestrations for the renal artery allowing extension of the proximal sealing zone to the pararenal segments to treat proximal type I endoleaks.[157] However, the potential to use fenestrated devices to electively treat AAA with unfavourable anatomy for standard EVAR, due to HNA or pararenal extension of the aneurysm, was soon recognized. Soon, fenestrations had been used for both renal arteries and also both visceral arteries (superior mesenteric and coeliac trunk) if required with comparable mortality and morbidity to the alternative of conventional open repair. Greenberg et al., in early reports of this new technique, demonstrated the feasibility of fenestrated to renal and visceral vessels and suggested the secure proximal seal provided by FEVAR which may even reduce the risk of proximal type I endoleak or endograft migration and increase the likelihood of aneurysm sac shrinkage.[110,111] Not only could FEVAR be offered in selected patients treated in experienced centres with low early mortality and morbidity, but the zenith fenestrated AAA stent graft, the first commercial fenestrated device, could provide durable results at 5 years, patient survival was 91% ± 4% and freedom from major adverse events was 79% ± 6%, primary and secondary patency of targeted renal arteries was 81% ± 5% and 97% ± 2%, freedom from renal function deterioration was 91% ± 5%, and freedom from secondary interventions was 63% ± 9%.[158] Patient selection is important, and for short-necked (<15 mm) pararenal AAA, the alternative is standard open surgery. Two recent large systematic reviews looked at open surgery or fenestrated endografts for short-necked (<15 mm) pararenal AAAs and found that there were no significant differences in early mortality, approximately 4%, and perhaps interestingly no differences were observed regarding the secondary outcomes (duration of surgery, hospital stay, post-operative renal dysfunction). They did show FEVAR was associated with a significantly higher secondary reintervention rate and may be associated with increased risk of renal insufficiency during follow-up, and perhaps, this is not unexpected given these factors are also seen after standard EVAR. However, in this high-risk patient group it remain to be seen whether endovascular or open repair can provide real benefits in respect to reduction in late aneurysm-related and all-cause mortality.[159,160]

CONCLUSIONS

This chapter provides a guide to the management of AAA based on evidence and experience. However, in clinical practice, vascular surgeons are often faced with patients who have unique combinations of clinical and anatomical factors, the management of which has not been the subject of a randomized trial, and in these cases, the surgeon must make safe decisions for the good of their patient based on available local expertise and experience. We hope this chapter will provide guidance for the practicing vascular surgeon.

REFERENCES

1. Steinberg I, Stein HL. Atherosclerotic abdominal aortic aneurysm, report of 200 consecutive cases diagnosed by intravenous aortography. *J Am Med Assoc.* 1966;195:1025.
2. McGregor JC, Pollock JG, Anton HC. The value of ultrasonography in the diagnosis of abdominal aortic aneurysm. *Scott Med J.* 1975;20:133–137.
3. Scott RA, Wilson NM, Ashton HA, Kay DN. Influence of screening on the incidence of ruptured abdominal aortic aneurysm: 5-year results of a randomised controlled study. *Br J Surg.* 1995;82:1066–1070.
4. Lindholt JS, Juul S, Fasting H, Henneberg EW. Screening for abdominal aortic aneurysms: single centre randomised controlled trial. *BMJ.* 2005;330:750.
5. Multicentre Aneurysm Screening Study Group. The Multicentre Aneurysm Screening Study (MASS) into the effect of abdominal aortic aneurysm screening on mortality in men: A randomised controlled trial. *The Lancet.* 2002;360:1531–1539.
6. Multicentre Aneurysm Screening Study Group. Multicentre aneurysm screening study MASS: Cost effectiveness analysis of screening for abdominal aortic aneurysms based on four year results from randomised controlled trial. *Br Med J.* 2002;325:1135.
7. Norman P, Spencer CA, Lawrence-Brown MM, Jamrozik K. C-reactive protein levels and the expansion of screen-detected abdominal aortic aneurysms in men. *Circulation.* 2004;110:862–866.
8. Norman PE, Jamrozik K, Lawrence-Brown MM et al. Population based randomised controlled trial on impact of screening on mortality from abdominal aortic aneurysm. *Br Med J.* 2004;329:1259–1262.
9. Lucarotti M, Shaw E, Poskitt K et al. The glouces-tershire aneurysm screening programme: The first 2 years' experience. *Eur J Vasc Surg.* 1993;7:397–401.
10. Lederle FA, Johnston GGR, Wilson SE et al. Prevalence and associations of abdominal aortic aneurysm detected through screening. Aneurysm Detection and Management (ADAM) Veterans Affairs Cooperative Study Group. *Ann Intern Med.* 1997;126:441–449.
11. Ashton HA, Buxton MJ, Day NE et al. The Multicentre Aneurysm Screening Study (MASS) into the effect of abdominal aortic aneurysm screening on mortality in men: A randomised controlled trial. *Lancet.* 2002;360(9345):1531–1539.

12. Szabo Z, Crepeau MW, Mitchell AL et al. Aortic aneurysmal disease and cutis laxa caused by defects in the elastin gene. *J Med Genet*. 2006;43:255–258.

13. Loeys B, Van Maldergem L, Mortier G et al. Homozygosity for a missense mutation in fibulin-5 (FBLN5) results in a severe form of cutis laxa. *Hum Mol Genet*. 2002;11:2113–2118.

14. Dasouki M, Markova D, Garola R et al. Compound heterozygous mutations in fibulin-4 causing neonatal lethal pulmonary artery occlusion, aortic aneurysm, arachnodactyly, and mild cutis laxa. *Am J Med Genet A*. 2007;143A:2635–2641.

15. Mizuguchi T, Collod-Beroud G, Akiyama T et al. Heterozygous TGFBR2 mutations in Marfan syndrome. *Nat Genet*. 2004;36:855–860.

16. Loeys BL, Chen J, Neptune ER et al. A syndrome of altered cardiovascular, craniofacial, neuro-cognitive and skeletal development caused by mutations in TGFBR1 or TGFBR2. *Nat Genet*. 2005;37:275–281.

17. Loeys BL, Schwarze U, Holm T et al. Aneurysm syndromes caused by mutations in the TGF-β receptor. *N Engl J Med*. 2006;355:788–798.

18. Sakalihasan N, Delvenne P, Nusgens BV, Limet R, Lapière CM. Activated forms of MMP2 and MMP9 in abdominal aortic aneurysms. *J Vasc Surg*. 1996;24:127–133.

19. Moustakas A, Heldin C-H. The regulation of TGFβ signal transduction. *Development*. 2009;136: 3699–3714.

20. Brooke BS, Habashi JP, Judge DP et al. Angiotensin II blockade and aortic-root dilation in Marfan's syndrome. *N Engl J Med*. 2008;358:2787–2795.

21. Johnston KW. Non-ruptured abdominal aortic aneurysm: Six-year follow-up results from the multicentre Canadian aneurysm study. Canadian Society for Vascular Surgery Aneurysm Study Group. *J Vasc Surg*. 1994;20:163–170.

22. Law MR, Morris J, Wald NJ. Screening for abdominal aortic aneurysms. *J Med Screen*. 1994;1:110–115.

23. Brady AR, Thompson SG, Fowkes FG, Greenhalgh RM, Powell JT. Participants UK Small Aneurysm Trial Participants. Abdominal aortic aneurysm expansion: Risk factors and time intervals for surveillance. *Circulation*. 2004;110(1):16–21.

24. Bengtsson H, Bergqvist D. Ruptured abdominal aortic aneurysm: A population-based study. *J Vasc Surg*. 1993;18(1):74–80.

25. Office for National Statistics. Leading causes of deaths in England and Wales, 2011. HMSO, London, UK, 2012.

26. Stonebridge PA, Draper T, Kelman J et al. Growth rate of infrarenal aortic aneurysms. *Eur J Vasc Endovasc Surg*. 1996;11:70–73.

27. Lindholt JS, Vammen S, Juul S, Henneberg EW, Fasting H. The validity of ultrasonographic scanning as a screening method for abdominal aortic aneurysm. *Eur J Vasc Endovasc Surg*. 1999;17:472–475.

28. Lindholt JS, Juul S, Vammen S, Lind I, Fasting H, Henneberg EW. Immunoglobulin A antibodies against Chlamydia pneumonia are associated with expansion of abdominal aortic aneurysm. *Br J Surg*. 1999;86:634–638.

29. Lindholt JS, Heickendorff L, Antonsen S, Fasting H, Henneberg EW. Natural history of abdominal aortic aneurysm with and without coexisting chronic obstructive pulmonary disease. *J Vasc Surg*. 1998;28:226–233.

30. Lindholt JS, Heegaard NH, Vammen S, Fasting H, Henneberg EW, Heickendorff L. Smoking, but not lipids, lipoprotein(a) and antibodies against oxidized LDL, is correlated to the expansion of abdominal aortic aneurysms. *Eur J Vasc Endovasc Surg*. 2001;21:51–56.

31. Santilli SM, Littooy FN, Cambria RA et al. Expansion rates and outcomes for the 3.0-cm to the 3.9-cm infrarenal abdominal aortic aneurysm. *J Vasc Surg*. 2002;35:666–671.

32. Brown PM, Sobolev B, Zelt DT. Selective management of abdominal aortic aneurysms smaller than 5.0 cm in a prospective sizing program with gender-specific analysis. *J Vasc Surg*. 2003;38:762–765.

33. Brown PM, Zelt DT, Sobolev B. The risk of rupture in untreated aneurysms: The impact of size, gender, and expansion rate. *J Vasc Surg*. 2003;37:280–284.

34. McCarthy RJ, Shaw E, Whyman MR, Earnshaw JJ, Poskitt KR, Heather BP. Recommendations for screening intervals for small aortic aneurysms. *Br J Surg*. 2003;90:821–826.

35. Schouten O, van Laanen JH, Boersma E et al. Statins are associated with a reduced infrarenal abdominal aortic aneurysm growth. *Eur J Vasc Endovasc Surg*. 2006;32:21–26.

36. Thompson AR, Cooper JA, Ashton HA, Hafez H. Growth rates of small abdominal aortic aneurysms correlate with clinical events. *Br J Surg*. 2010;97:37–44.

37. Chang JB, Stein TA, Liu JP, Dunn ME. Risk factors associated with rapid growth of small abdominal aortic aneurysms. *Surgery*. 1997;121:117–122.

38. Brady AR, Thompson SG, Greenhalgh RM, Powell JT. Cardiovascular risk factors and abdominal aortic aneurysm expansion: Only smoking counts. US small aneurysm trial participants. *Br J Surg*. 2003;90:491–492.

39. Eriksson P, Jones KG, Brown LC, Greenhalgh RM, Hamsten A, Powell JT. Genetic approach to the role of cysteine proteases in the expansion of abdominal aortic aneurysms. *Br J Surg*. 2004;91:86–89.

40. Vega de CM, Gomez R, Estallo L, Rodriguez L, Baquer M, Barba A. Growth rate and associated factors in small abdominal aortic aneurysms. *Eur J Vasc Endovasc Surg*. 2006;31:231–236.

41. Spencer C, Jamrozik K, Kelly S, Bremner P, Norman P. Is there an association between chronic lung disease and abdominal aortic aneurysm expansion? *ANZ J Surg*. 2003.

42. Cronenwett JL, Murphy TF, Zelenock GB et al. Actuarial analysis of variables associated with rupture of small abdominal aortic aneurysms. *Surgery.* 1985;98:472–483.

43. Darling RC, Messina CR, Brewster DC, Ottinger LW. Autopsy study of unoperated abdominal aortic aneurysms. The case for early resection. *Circulation.* 1997;56:II161–II164.

44. Reed WW, Hallett Jr JW, Damiano MA, Ballard DJ. Learning from the last ultrasound. A population-based study of patients with abdominal aortic aneurysm. *Arch Intern Med.* 1997;157:2064–2068.

45. Scott RA, Tisi PV, Ashton HA, Allen DR. Abdominal aortic aneurysm rupture rates: A 7-year follow-up of the entire abdominal aortic aneurysm population detected by screening. *J Vasc Surg.* 1998;28:124–128.

46. Brown LC, Powell JT. Risk factors for aneurysm rupture in patients kept under ultrasound surveillance. UK small aneurysm trial participants. *Ann Surg.* 1999;230:289–296.

47. Conway KP, Byrne J, Townsend M, Lane IF. Prognosis of patients turned down for conventional abdominal aortic aneurysm repair in the endovascular and sonographic era: Szilagyi revisited? *J Vasc Surg.* 2001;33:752–757.

48. Lederle FA, Johnson GR, Wilson SE et al. Rupture rate of large abdominal aortic aneurysms in patients refusing or unfit for elective repair. *J Am Med Assoc.* 2002;287:2968–2972.

49. Lederle FA, Wilson SE, Johnson GR et al. Aneurysm Detection and Management Veterans Affairs Cooperative Study Group. Immediate repair compared with surveillance of small abdominal aortic aneurysms. *N Engl J Med.* 2002;346:1437–1444.

50. Norman PE, Powell JT. Abdominal aortic aneurysm: The prognosis in women is worse than in men. *Circulation.* 2007;115:2865–2869.

51. Limet R, Sakalihassan N, Albert A. Determination of the expansion rate and incidence of rupture of abdominal aortic aneurysms. *J Vasc Surg.* 1991;14:540–548.

52. Hatakeyama T, Shigematsu H, Muto T. Risk factors for rupture of abdominal aortic aneurysm based on three-dimensional study. *J Vasc Surg.* 2001;33:453–461.

53. Powell JT, Brown LC, Greenhalgh RM, Thompson SG. The Rupture rate of large abdominal aortic aneurysms: Is this modified by anatomical suitability for endovascular repair? *Ann Surg.* 2008;247:173–179.

54. The UK Small Aneurysm Trial Participants. Mortality results for randomised controlled trial of early elective surgery or ultrasound surveillance for small abdominal aortic aneurysms. *Lancet.* 1998;352(9141):1649–1655.

55. Cao P. Comparison of surveillance vs aortic endografting for small aneurysm repair (CAESAR) trial: Study design and progress. *Eur J Vasc Endovasc Surg.* 2005;30:245–251.

56. Ouriel K. The pivotal study: A randomised comparison of endovascular repair versus surveillance in patients with smaller abdominal aortic aneurysms. *J Vasc Surg.* 2009;49:266–269.

57. Cao P, De Rango P, Verzini F, Parlani G, Romano L, Cieri E, CAESAR Trial Group Comparison of surveillance versus aortic endografting for small aneurysm repair (CAESAR): Results from a randomised trial. *Eur J Vasc Endovasc Surg.* 2011;41(1):13–25.

58. Ouriel K, Clair DG, Kent KC, Zarins CK. Positive Impact of Endovascular Options for treating Aneurysms Early (PIVOTAL) Investigators. Endovascular repair compared with surveillance for patients with small abdominal aortic aneurysms. *J Vasc Surg.* 2010;51(5):1081–1087.

59. Filardo G, Lederle FA, Ballard DJ, Hamilton C, da Graca B, Herrin J, Harbor J, Vanbuskirk JB, Johnson GR, Powell JT. Immediate open repair vs surveillance in patients with small abdominal aortic aneurysms: Survival differences by aneurysm size. *Mayo Clin Proc.* 2013 September;88(9):910–919.

60. Lindholt JS, Juul S, Fasting H, Henneberg EW. Screening for abdominal aortic aneurysms: Single centre randomised controlled trial. *Br Med J.* 2005;330:750–753.

61. Lederle FA, Walker JM, Reinke DB. Selective screening for abdominal aortic aneurysm with physical examination and ultrasound. *Arch Int Med.* 1988;148:1753–1756.

62. Pleumeekers HJ, Hoes AW, van der Does E, van Urk H, de Jong PT, Grobbee DE. Aneurysms of the abdominal aorta in older adults. The Rotterdam Study. *Am J Epidemiol.* 1995;142:1291–1299.

63. Singh K, Bonaa KH, Jacobsen BK, Bjork L, Solberg S. Prevalence and risk factors for abdominal aortic aneurysms in a population-based study: The Tromsø Study. *Am J Epidemiol.* 2001;154:236–244.

64. Ellis M, Powell JT, Greenhalgh RM. Limitations of ultrasonography for the surveillance of abdominal aortic aneurysms. *Br J Surg.* 1991;78:614–616.

65. Scott RA, Bridgewater SG, Ashton HA. Randomised clinical trial of screening for abdominal aortic aneurysm screening in women. *Br J Surg.* 2002;89:283–285.

66. The UK small aneurysm trial participants. Smoking, lung function and the prognosis of abdominal aortic aneurysm. *Eur J Vasc Endovasc Surg.* 2000;19:636–642.

67. Ferguson CD, Clancy P, Bourke B et al. Association of statin prescription with small abdominal aortic aneurysm progression. *Am Heart J.* 2010; 159:307–313.

68. Prinssen M, Verhoeven EL, Buth J et al. A randomised trial comparing conventional and endovascular repair of abdominal aortic aneurysms. *N Engl J Med.* 2004;351:1607–1618.

69. EVAR Trial Participants Endovascular aneurysm repair versus open repair in patients with abdominal aortic aneurysm (EVAR trial 1): Randomised controlled trial. *Lancet.* 2005;365(9478):2179–2186.

70. Greenhalgh RM, Brown LC, Kwong GP, Powell JT, Thompson SG, EVAR Trial Participants Comparison of endovascular aneurysm repair with open repair in patients with abdominal aortic aneurysm (EVAR trial 1), 30-day operative mortality results: Randomised controlled trial. *Lancet.* 2004;364(9437):843–848.

71. United Kingdom EVAR Trial Investigators. Greenhalgh RM, Brown LC, Powell JT et al. Endovascular versus open repair of abdominal aortic aneurysm. *N Engl J Med.* 2010;362(20):1863–1871.

72. Blankensteijn JD, de Jong SE, Prinssen M et al. Two-year outcomes after conventional or endovascular repair of abdominal aortic aneurysms. *N Engl J Med.* 2005;352(23):2398–2405.

73. De Bruin JL, Baas AF, Buth J et al. Long-term outcome of open or endovascular repair of abdominal aortic aneurysm. *N Engl J Med.* 2010;362(20):1881–1889.

74. Lederle FA, Freischlag JA, Kyriakides TC et al. Outcomes following endovascular vs open repair of abdominal aortic aneurysm: A randomized trial. *J Am Med Assoc.* 2009;302(14):1535–1542.

75. Becquemin JP, Pillet JC, Lescalie F et al. A randomized controlled trial of endovascular aneurysm repair versus open surgery for abdominal aortic aneurysms in low- to moderate-risk patients. *J Vasc Surg.* 2011;53(5):1167–1173–1181.

76. Schermerhorn ML, O'Malley AJ, Jhaveri A, Cotterill P, Pomposelli F, Landon BE. Endovascular vs. open repair of abdominal aortic aneurysms in the Medicare population. *N Engl J Med.* 2008;358(5):464–474.

77. Mani K, Lees T, Beiles B, Jensen LP, Venermo M, Simo G, Palombo D, Halbakken E, Troëng T, Wigger P, Björck M. Treatment of abdominal aortic aneurysm in nine countries 2005–2009: A vascunet report. *Eur J Vasc Endovasc Surg.* 2011 November;42(5):598–607.

78. Harkin DW, Dillon M, Blair PH, Ellis PK, Kee F. Endovascular ruptured abdominal aortic aneurysm repair (EVRAR): A systematic review. *Eur J Vasc Endovasc Surg.* 2007 Dec;34(6):673–681.

79. IMPROVE Trial Investigators, Powell JT, Hinchliffe RJ, Thompson MM et al. Observations from the IMPROVE trial concerning the clinical care of patients with ruptured abdominal aortic aneurysm. *Br J Surg.* 2014 February;101(3):216–224;discussion 224.

80. Badger S, Bedenis R, Blair PH, Ellis P, Kee F, Harkin DW. Endovascular treatment for ruptured abdominal aortic aneurysm. *Cochrane Database Syst Rev.* 2014 July 21;7:CD005261.

81. Dillon M, Cardwell C, Blair PH, Ellis P, Kee F, Harkin DW. Cochrane Database Syst Rev 1, 2007.

82. Neary WD, Heather BP, Earnshaw JJ. The physiological and operative severity score for the enumeration of mortality and morbidity (POSSUM). *Br J Surg.* 2003;90:157–165.

83. Samy AK, Murry G, MacBain G. Glasgow aneurysm score. *Cardiovasc Surg.* 1994;2:41–44.

84. Young EL, Holt PJ, Poloniecki JD, Loftus IM, Thompson MM. Meta-analysis and systematic review of the relationship between surgeon annual caseload and mortality for elective open abdominal aortic aneurysm repairs. *J Vasc Surg.* 2007;46:1287–1294.

85. McFalls EO, Ward HB, Moritz TE et al. Coronary-artery revascularization before elective major vascular surgery. *N Engl J Med.* 2004;351:2795–2804.

86. Schouten O, Poldermans D, Visser L et al. Fluvastatin and bisoprolol for the reduction of perioperative cardiac mortality and morbidity in high-risk patients undergoing non-cardiac surgery: Rationale and design of the decrease-iv study. *Am Heart J.* 2004;148:1047–1052.

87. Poldermans D, Boersma E, Bax JJ et al. The effect of bisoprolol on perioperative mortality and myocardial infarction in high-risk patients undergoing vascular surgery. Dutch echocardiographic cardiac risk evaluation applying stress echocardiography study group. *N Engl J Med.* 1999;341:1789–1794.

88. Poldermans D, Schouten O, Vidakovic R et al. A clinical randomised trial to evaluate the safety of a noninvasive approach in high-risk patients undergoing major vascular surgery: The decrease-v pilot study. *J Am Coll Cardiol.* 2007;49:1763–1769.

89. Brady AR, Gibbs JS, Greenhalgh RM, Powell JT, Sydes MR. Perioperative beta-blockade (POBBLE) for patients undergoing infrarenal vascular surgery: Results of a randomised double-blind controlled trial. *J Vasc Surg.* 2005;41:602–609.

90. Yang H, Raymer K, Butler R, Parlow J, Roberts R. The effects of perioperative beta-blockade: Results of the metoprolol after vascular surgery (MAVs) study, a randomised controlled trial. *Am Heart J.* 2006;152:983–990.

91. Devereaux PJ, Yang H, Yusuf S et al. Effects of extended-release metoprolol succinate in patients undergoing non-cardiac surgery (poise trial): A randomised controlled trial. *Lancet.* 2008;371:1839–1847.

92. Bangalore S, Wetterslev J, Pranesh S, Sawhney S, Gluud C, Messerli FH. Perioperative betablockers in patients having non-cardiac surgery: A meta-analysis. *Lancet* 2008;372:1962–1976.

93. Baigent C, Blackwell L, Collins R et al. Aspirin in the primary and secondary prevention of vascular disease: Collaborative meta-analysis of individual participant data from randomised trials. *Lancet.* 2009;373:1849–1860.

94. Hertzer NR, Mascha EJ, Karafa MT, O'Hara PJ, Krajewski LP, Beven EG. Open infrarenal abdominal aortic aneurysm repair: The Cleveland Clinic experience from 1989 to 1998. *J Vasc Surg.* 2002;35:1145–1154.

95. Brustia P, Renghi A, Fassiola A et al. Fast-track approach in abdominal aortic surgery: Left subcostal incision with blended anesthesia. *Interact Cardiovasc Thorac Surg*. 2007;6:60–64.

96. Muehling B, Halter G, Lang G et al. Prospective randomised controlled trial to evaluate "fast-track" elective open infrarenal aneurysm repair. *Langenbecks Arch Surg*. 2008;393(3):281–287.

97. Muehling B, Schelzig H, Steffen P, Meierhenrich R, Sunder-Plassmann L, Orend KH. A prospective randomised trial comparing traditional and fast-track patient care in elective open infrarenal aneurysm repair. *World J Surg*. 2009;33:577–585.

98. Brown LC, Powell JT, Thompson SG, Epstein DM, Sculpher MJ, Greenhalgh RM. The UK EndoVascular Aneurysm Repair (EVAR) trials: Randomised trials of EVAR versus standard therapy. *Health Technol Assess*. 2012;16(9):1–218.

99. Dubost C. Resection of an aneurysm of the abdominal aorta. *Arch Surg*. 1952;64:405–408.

100. Williams GM, Ricotta J, Zinner M, Burdick J. The extended retroperitoneal approach for treatment of extensive atherosclerosis of the aorta and renal vessels. *Surgery*. 1980;88:846.

101. Creech O Jr. Endo-aneurysmorrhaphy and treatment of aortic aneurysm. *Ann Surg*. 1966;164:935.

102. Parodi JC, Palmaz JC, Barone HD. Transfemoral intraluminal graft implantation for abdominal aortic aneurysm. *Ann Vasc Surg*. 1991;5:491–499.

103. Faries PL, Briggs VL, Rhee JY et al. Failure of endovascular aortoaortic tube grafts: A plea for preferential use of bifurcated grafts. *J Vasc Surg*. 2002;35:868–873.

104. Woodburn KR, Chant H, Davies JN, Blanshard KS, Travis SJ. Suitability for endovascular aneurysm repair in an unselected population. *Br J Surg*. 2001 January;88(1):77–81.

105. Schanzer A, Greenberg RK, Hevelone N et al. Predictors of abdominal aortic aneurysm sac enlargement after endovascular repair. *Circulation*. 2011;123(24):2848–2855.

106. White GH, Yu W, May J. Endoleak: A proposed new terminology to describe incomplete aneurysm exclusion by an endoluminal graft. *J Endovas Surg*. 1996;3:124–125.

107. Fransen GAJ, Vallabhaneni SR, van Marrewijk CJ, Laheij RJF, Harris PL, Buth J, on behalf of EUROSTAR collaborators. Rupture of Infra-renal Aortic Aneurysm after Endovascular Repair: A Series from EUROSTAR Registry. *Eur J Vasc Endovasc Surg*. 2003;26:487–493.

108. Arko FR, Filis KA, Seidel SA et al. How many patients with infrarenal aneurysms are candidates for endovascular repair? The Northern California experience. *J Endovasc Ther*. 2004;11:33–40.

109. van Marrewijk CJ, Fransen G, Laheij RJ, Harris PL, Buth J; EUROSTAR Collaborators. Is a type II endoleak after EVAR a harbinger of risk? Causes and outcome of open conversion and aneurysm rupture during follow-up. *Eur J Vasc Endovasc Surg*. 2004 February;27(2):128–137.

110. Greenberg RK, Haulon S, Lyden SP, Srivastava SD, Turc A, Eagleton MJ, Sarac TP, Ouriel K. Endovascular management of juxtarenal aneurysms with fenestrated endovascular grafting. *J Vasc Surg*. 2004 February;39(2):279–287.

111. Greenberg RK, Haulon S, O'Neill S et al. Primary endovascular repair of juxtarenal aneurysms with fenestrated endovascular grafting. *Eur J Vasc Endovasc Surg*. 2004;27:484–491.

112. Verhoeven EL, Prins TR, Tielliu IF et al. Treatment of short-necked infrarenal aortic aneurysms with fenestrated stent-grafts: Short-term results. *Eur J Vasc Endovasc Surg*. 2004;27:477–483.

113. Abraham CZ, Reilly LM, Schneider DB et al. A modular multi-branched system for endovascular repair of bilateral common iliac artery aneurysms. *J Endovasc Ther*. 2003;10:203–207.

114. Murphy M, Hodgson R, Harris PI et al. Plain radiographic surveillance of abdominal aortic stent grafts: The liverpool/perth protocol. *J Endovasc Ther*. 2003;10:911–912.

115. Lawrence-Brown MM, Sun Z, Semmens JB, Liffman K, Sutalo ID, Hartley DB. Type II endoleaks: When is intervention indicated and what is the index of suspicion for types I or III? *J Endovasc Ther*. 2009 February;16(Suppl. 1):I106–I118.

116. Wieners G, Meyer F, Halloul Z, Peters N, Rühl R, Dudeck O, Tautenhahn J, Ricke J, Pech M. Detection of type II endoleak after endovascular aortic repair: Comparison between magnetic resonance angiography and blood-pool contrast agent and dual-phase computed tomography angiography. *Cardiovasc Intervent Radiol*. 2010 December;33(6):1135–1142.

117. Cantisani V, Ricci P, Grazhdani H, Napoli A, Fanelli F, Catalano C, Galati G, D'Andrea V, Biancari F, Passariello R. Prospective comparative analysis of colour-doppler ultrasound, contrast-enhanced ultrasound, computed tomography and magnetic resonance in detecting endoleak after endovascular abdominal aortic aneurysm repair. *Eur J Vasc Endovasc Surg*. 2011 February;41(2):186–192.

118. Stather PW, Sidloff D, Dattani N, Choke E, Bown MJ, Sayers RD. Systematic review and meta-analysis of the early and late outcomes of open and endovascular repair of abdominal aortic aneurysm. *Br J Surg*. 2013 June;100(7):863–872.

119. Stather PW, Wild JB, Sayers RD, Bown MJ, Choke E. Endovascular aortic aneurysm repair in patients with hostile neck anatomy. *J Endovasc Ther*. 2013 October;20(5):623–637.

120. Vogel TR, Dombrovskiy VY, Graham AM, Lowry SF. The impact of hospital volume on the development of infectious complications after elective abdominal aortic surgery in the Medicare population. *Vasc Endovascular Surg*. 2011 May;45(4):317–324.

121. Vogel TR, Symons R, Flum DR. The incidence and factors associated with graft infection after aortic aneurysm repair. *J Vasc Surg.* 2008 February; 47(2):264–269.

122. O'Brien T, Collin J. Prosthetic vascular graft infection. *Br J Surg.* 1992;79:1262–1267.

123. Lehnert T, Gruber HE, Maeder N, Allenberg JR. Management of primary aortic graft infection by extra-anatomic bypass reconstruction. *Eur J Vasc Endovasc Surg.* 1993;7:301–307.

124. Calligaro KD, Veith FJ, Yuan JG, Gargiulo NJ, Dougherty NJ. Intraabdominal aortic graft infection: Complete or partial graft preservation in patients at very high risk. *J Vasc Surg.* 2003;38:1199–1205.

125. Ricco J-B. InterGard silver bifurcated graft: Features and results of a multicenter clinical study. *J Vasc Surg.* 2006;44:339–346.

126. Berqvist D, Bjo"rck M. Secondary arterioenteric fistulisation. A systematic literature analysis. *Eur J Vasc Endovasc Surg.* 2009;37:31–42; *Arch Surg.* 2008;393:281–287.

127. Newton WB 3rd, Shukla M, Andrews JS, Hansen KJ, Corriere MA, Goodney PP, Edwards MS. Outcomes of acute intraoperative surgical conversion during endovascular aortic aneurysm repair. *J Vasc Surg.* 2011 November;54(5):1244–1250;discussion 1250.

128. Veith FJ, Baum RA, Ohki T et al. Nature and significance of endoleaks and endotension: Summary of opinions expressed at an international conference. *J Vasc Surg.* 2002;35:1029–1035.

129. Fransen GA, Vallabhaneni SR Sr, van Marrewijk CJ et al. Rupture of infra-renal aortic aneurysm after endovascular repair: A series from EUROSTAR registry. *Eur J Vasc Endovasc Surg.* 2003;26:487–493.

130. Hobo R, Buth J, EUROSTAR collaborators. Secondary interventions following endovascular abdominal aortic aneurysm repair using current endografts. A EUROSTAR report. *J Vasc Surg.* 2006;43(5):896–902.

131. Gelfand DV, White GH, Wilson SE. Clinical significance of type II endoleak after endovascular repair of abdominal aortic aneurysm. *Ann Vasc Surg.* 2006 January;20(1):69–74.

132. Jones JE, Atkins MD, Brewster DC, Chung TK, Kwolek CJ, LaMuraglia GM, Hodgman TM, Cambria RP. Persistent type 2 endoleak after endovascular repair of abdominal aortic aneurysm is associated with adverse late outcomes. *J Vasc Surg.* 2007 July;46(1):1–8.

133. Sidloff DA, Stather PW, Choke E, Bown MJ, Sayers RD. Type II endoleak after endovascular aneurysm repair. *Br J Surg.* 2013 September;100(10):1262–1270.

134. Harris PL, Vallabhaneni R, Desgranges P, Becquemin JP, van Marrewijk C, Laheij RJF, and EUROSTAR Collaborators. Incidence and risk factor of late rupture, conversion, and death after endovascular repair of infrarenal aortic aneurysms: the EUROSTAR experience. *J Vasc Surg.* 2000;32:739–749.

135. Wyss TR, Brown LC, Powell JT, Greenhalgh RM. Rate and predictability of graft rupture after endovascular and open abdominal aortic aneurysm repair: Data from the EVAR trials. *Ann Surg.* 2010;252(5):805–812.

136. Schlösser FJ, Gusberg RJ, Dardik A et al. Aneurysm rupture after EVAR: Can the ultimate failure be predicted? *Eur J Vasc Endovasc Surg.* 2009;37(1):15–22.

137. Koole D, Moll FL, Buth J, Hobo R, Zandvoort HJ, Bots ML, Pasterkamp G, van Herwaarden JA; European Collaborators on Stent-Graft Techniques for Aortic Aneurysm Repair (EUROSTAR). Annual rupture risk of abdominal aortic aneurysm enlargement without detectable endoleak after endovascular abdominal aortic repair. *J Vasc Surg.* 2011 December;54(6):1614–1622.

138. Cho JS, Park T, Kim JY, Chaer RA, Rhee RY, Makaroun MS. Prior endovascular abdominal aortic aneurysm repair provides no survival benefits when the aneurysm ruptures. *J Vasc Surg.* 2010 November;52(5):1127–1134.

139. Nordon IM, Karthikesalingam A, Hinchliffe RI et al. Secondary interventions following endovascular aneurysm repair (EVAR) and the enduring value of graft surveillance. *Eur J Vasc Endovasc Surg.* 2010;39(5):547–554.

140. Karthikesalingam A, Thrumurthy SG, Jackson D, Phd EC, Sayers RD, Loftus IM, Thompson MM, Holt PJ. Current evidence is insufficient to define an optimal threshold for intervention in isolated type II endoleak after endovascular aneurysm repair. *J Endovasc Ther.* 2012 April;19(2):200–208.

141. Aziz A, Menias CO, Sanchez LA, Picus D, Saad N, Rubin BG, Curci JA, Geraghty PJ. Outcomes of percutaneous endovascular intervention for type II endoleak with aneurysm expansion. *J Vasc Surg.* 2012 May;55(5):1263–1267.

142. Corfield L, Chan J, Chance T, Wilson N. Early pyrexia after endovascular aneurysm repair: Are cultures needed? *Ann R Coll Surg Engl.* 2011 March; 93(2):111–113.

143. Setacci C, De Donato G, Setacci F, Chisci E, Perulli A, Galzerano G, Sirignano P. Management of abdominal endograft infection. *J Cardiovasc Surg (Torino).* 2010 Februray;51(1):33–41.

144. Laser A, Baker N, Rectenwald J, Eliason JL, Criado-Pallares E, Upchurch GR Jr. Graft infection after endovascular abdominal aortic aneurysm repair. *J Vasc Surg.* 2011 July;54(1):58–63.

145. Baril DT, Silverberg D, Ellozy SH, Carroccio A, Jacobs TS, Sachdev U, Teodorescu VJ, Lookstein RA, Marin ML. Endovascular stent-graft repair of failed endovascular abdominal aortic aneurysm repair. *Ann Vasc Surg.* 2008 January;22(1):30–36.

146. Katsargyris A, Yazar O, Oikonomou K, Bekkema F, Tielliu I, Verhoeven EL. Fenestrated stent-grafts for salvage of prior endovascular abdominal aortic aneurysm repair. *Eur J Vasc Endovasc Surg.* 2013 July;46(1):49–56.

147. Verzini F, Cao P, De Rango P, Parlani G, Xanthopoulos D, Iacono G, Panuccio G. Conversion to open repair after endografting for abdominal aortic aneurysm: Causes, incidence and results. *Eur J Vasc Endovasc Surg.* 2006 February;31(2):136–142.

148. Moulakakis KG, Dalainas I, Mylonas S, Giannakopoulos TG, Avgerinos ED, Liapis CD. Conversion to open repair after endografting for abdominal aortic aneurysm: A review of causes, incidence, results, and surgical techniques of reconstruction. *J Endovasc Ther.* 2010 December;17(6):694–702.

149. Pitoulias GA, Schulte S, Donas KP, Horsch S. Secondary endovascular and conversion procedures for failed endovascular abdominal aortic aneurysm repair: Can we still be optimistic? *Vascular.* 2009 January–February;17(1):15–22.

150. Kelso RL, Lyden SP, Butler B, Greenberg RK, Eagleton MJ, Clair DG. Late conversion of aortic stent grafts. *J Vasc Surg.* 2009 March;49(3):589–595.

151. Brinster CJ, Fairman RM, Woo EY, Wang GJ, Carpenter JP, Jackson BM. Late open conversion and explantation of abdominal aortic stent grafts. *J Vasc Surg.* 2011 July;54(1):42–46.

152. Lipsitz EC, Ohki T, Veith FJ, Suggs WD, Wain RA, Rhee SJ, Gargiulo NJ, McKay J. Delayed open conversion following endovascular aortoiliac aneurysm repair: Partial (or complete) endograft preservation as a useful adjunct. *J Vasc Surg.* 2003 December;38(6):1191–1198.

153. Marone EM, Mascia D, Coppi G, Tshomba Y, Bertoglio L, Kahlberg A, Chiesa R. Delayed open conversion after endovascular abdominal aortic aneurysm: Device-specific surgical approach. *Eur J Vasc Endovasc Surg.* 2013 May;45(5):457–464.

154. Marone EM, Mascia D, Coppi G, Tshomba Y, Bertoglio L, Kahlberg A, Chiesa R. Delayed open conversion after endovascular abdominal aortic aneurysm: Device-specific surgical approach. *Eur J Vasc Endovasc Surg.* 2013 May;45(5):457–464.

155. Gambardella I, Blair PH, McKinley A, Makar R, Collins A, Ellis PK, Harkin DW. Successful delayed secondary open conversion after endovascular repair using partial explantation technique: A single-center experience. *Ann Vasc Surg.* 2010 July;24(5):646–654.

156. Antoniou GA, Georgiadis GS, Antoniou SA, Kuhan G, Murray D. A meta-analysis of outcomes of endovascular abdominal aortic aneurysm repair in patients with hostile and friendly neck anatomy. *J Vasc Surg.* 2013 February;57(2):527–538.

157. Faruqi RM1, Chuter TA, Reilly LM, Sawhney R, Wall S, Canto C, Messina LM. Endovascular repair of abdominal aortic aneurysm using a pararenal fenestrated stent-graft. *J Endovasc Surg.* 1999 Novrmber;6(4):354–358.

158. Oderich GS, Greenberg RK, Farber M, Lyden S, Sanchez L, Fairman R, Jia F, Bharadwaj P; Zenith Fenestrated Study Investigators. Results of the United States multicenter prospective study evaluating the Zenith fenestrated endovascular graft for treatment of juxtarenal abdominal aortic aneurysms. *J Vasc Surg.* 2014.

159. Belczak SQ, Lanziotti L, Botelho Y, Aun R, da Silva ES, Puech-Leão P, de Luccia N. Open and endovascular repair of juxtarenal abdominal aortic aneurysms: A systematic review. *Clinics (Sao Paulo).* 2014 September;69(9):641–646.

160. Rao R, Lane TR, Franklin IJ, Davies AH. Open repair versus fenestrated endovascular aneurysm repair of juxtarenal aneurysms. *J Vasc Surg.* 2015 January;61(1):242–255.e5.

27

Thoracoabdominal aortic aneurysms

GERMANO MELISSANO, EFREM CIVILINI, ENRICO RINALDI and ROBERTO CHIESA

CONTENTS

INTRODUCTION

A thoracoabdominal aortic aneurysm (TAAA) involves the aorta at the diaphragmatic crura and variably extends proximally and/or distally from this point.[1] Conventional treatment of TAAA consists of graft replacement with reattachment of the main aortic branches. To improve mortality and morbidity rates, a multimodal approach has gradually evolved to maximize organ protection. Prognosis following surgical repair varies according to the extent and type of aneurysm undergoing repair, with extent I and II aneurysms carrying a higher post-operative complication rate, particularly regarding spinal cord (SC) ischaemia and renal failure.[2] Surgical indication must, therefore, take into account these severe and life-threatening complications, which must be balanced against the risk of aneurysm rupture. Careful pre-operative assessment of coexistent comorbidities, standardized surgical techniques and specific guidelines for post-operative management of these patients can have a favourable impact on the morbidity and mortality associated with this procedure, usually allowing for safe and effective repair.

AETIOLOGY AND NATURAL HISTORY

The most common cause of TAAA is medial degeneration associated with atherosclerosis, which involves loss of smooth muscle cells and fragmentation of elastin fibres. The second most common cause of TAAA is aortic dissection. Classic aortic dissection arises when a tear through the intima leads to progressive separation within the layers of the aortic media. The weakened aortic wall predisposes patients to aneurysm formation and rupture.[3]

Genetic conditions associated with TAAA development include connective tissue disorders.[4] In Marfan syndrome, mutations in the fibrillin-1 gene cause abnormal transforming growth factor-beta (TGF-β) activity, leading to degeneration of the aortic wall matrix and progressive dilatation. Loeys–Dietz syndrome is caused by mutations in genes that encode TGF-β receptors and is distinguished by the triad of arterial tortuosity and aneurysms, hypertelorism and bifid uvula or cleft palate.[5] Ehlers–Danlos syndrome (EDS) is a heterogeneous group of heritable connective tissue disorders characterized by articular hypermobility, skin hyperextensibility and tissue fragility. Eleven types of EDS have been characterized; the true prevalence of EDS is unknown. Aortic involvement is seen primarily in autosomal dominant EDS type IV. Given the extreme fragility of the aorta, affected patients are at a greater risk of adverse outcomes following surgery than are patients with other connective tissue disorders.[6]

In contrast to the previously reported syndromic variants, the familial non-syndromic thoracic aortic aneurysm occurs as a single manifestation, but follows a familial pattern of inheritance, often autosomal dominant, with decreased penetrance (especially in female family members) and variable expression. Six different genetic loci have been recognized in families with familial non-syndromic thoracic aortic aneurysm, and three genes have been identified so far: *TGF-BR2*, *ACTA2* and *MYH11*, the latter in familial aneurysms and patent ductus arteriosus.[7]

Giant cell arteritis, such as Takayasu's arteritis, trauma and infections, are aetiologies less commonly seen.[8]

Mycotic aneurysms are caused by infection of the aortic wall. These aneurysms typically have a saccular form and often occur in the region near the visceral branches. The pathogens in infected aneurysms are primarily bacterial. Common causative organisms include *Staphylococcus aureus*, *Staphylococcus epidermidis*, *Salmonella* and *Streptococcus*.[9]

Risk factors contributing to increased mortality and morbidity risk for patients with TAAA are chronic obstructive pulmonary disease (COPD), hypertension, smoking and pain.[10] Patients with COPD have a 3.6-fold greater rate of aneurysm rupture. This association suggests that patients with TAAA may suffer from innate connective tissue defects. Smoking has been associated with a significantly higher rate of thoracic and thoracoabdominal aneurysm dilation when compared to non-smokers (0.7 vs. 0.35, respectively). A history of smoking is found in the majority of patients with aortic aneurysms and is also a risk factor for rupture, but COPD has eclipsed smoking in several studies in which the two are looked at in the same multivariate analysis. The greater predictive power of COPD may be related to individual differences in response to the toxic effects of smoking; the presence of COPD may be a sensitive indicator of intolerance of connective tissue to smoking-related toxicity both in the lung and in the aorta.

A history of hypertension is present in most patients with aneurysms, and it is widely recognized that hypertension, especially diastolic hypertension, is very highly correlated with the initial development of aneurysms. On the other hand, hypertension failed to be linked with the rate of enlargement.[11]

The evaluation of pain as a risk factor for rupture is complicated to be assessed; however, the presence of pain, even uncharacteristic, is significantly associated with subsequent rupture, with an odds ratio of 2:3 in a multivariate analysis (p = 0.04) published by Juvonen.[12] Few studies in the literature are available on the natural history of TAAA. With time, most TAAAs increase in size

and rupture rates, with larger aneurysms expanding at a faster rate and rupturing more frequently. Although aneurysm rupture is seen most commonly in patients with large aneurysms, some large aneurysms can remain stable for years, making expansion rates and rupture unpredictable in any individual patient.[13] TAAAs, however, seem to have a worse prognosis when compared with abdominal aortic aneurysms. In a population-based study, Bickerstaff and colleagues reported a 2-year survival rate of 29% for untreated patients with large thoracic and TAAA.[14] Aneurysm rupture occurred in 74% of patients observed during this period, with an associated mortality rate of 94%. Rupture and death were seen more commonly in patients with dissecting aneurysms as opposed to non-dissecting aneurysms. The overall 5-year survival rate following diagnosis was only 13%, which compared poorly with the 75% survival rate for an age-matched population of patients without aneurysms.

Other reports confirmed the poor results associated with nonoperative management of TAAAs. In a study by Crawford and DeNatale, 76% of patients with TAAAs who remained untreated because of the small size of their aneurysms, advanced age, associated comorbidities or refusal of the operation died within 2 years of diagnosis. Fifty-two percent of these deaths occurred as a result of aneurysm rupture.[13]

More recently, Cambria and colleagues evaluated 57 patients with non-dissecting TAAAs who were initially managed nonoperatively.[15] Thirty-four of these 57 patients or 60% died during the follow-up period, which averaged 37 months. The most common cause of death was cardiopulmonary disease, accounting for 24% of all mortalities, followed by aneurysm rupture, responsible for 19% of deaths. The 2- and 5-year survival rates for those patients who remained untreated were 52% and 17%, respectively. On the other hand, as initially demonstrated by Crawford and colleagues, a 2-year survival rate of about 70% can be expected following operative intervention.[16] As a limitation, this operative procedure requires entering both the thoracic and abdominal cavities and is associated with significant morbidity and mortality. Such procedures can challenge even the most experienced vascular surgeons. Progress in the perioperative care of patients with TAAAs, however, has led to a decrease in the complication rate. Many authors now report an operative mortality rate of less than 10%, with an overall rate of paraplegia of approximately 4%–20%, depending upon the extent of the aneurysm, and a 2%–20% incidence of renal failure.[17] At present, aortic diameter is the most commonly used criterion for predicting the risk of aortic rupture. Aneurysms of the thoracoabdominal aorta tend to be larger than those of the ascending aorta (5.9 vs. 4.8 cm) at diagnosis.[18] Juvonen et al. found that a 1 cm increase in diameter of a descending aneurysm is correlated to a 1.9 increase in the relative risk of rupture.[12] Aortas with diameter of 6.0 cm had a fivefold increased risk of rupture, with a 14.1% yearly rate of rupture.[19] The risk of aortic rupture increases directly with increasing aortic size, with an abrupt increase at unique diameter 'hinge points'. In the presence of chronic dissection involving the TAAA, surgical treatment is recommended at smaller sizes since mortality from rupture is significantly higher in those patients than in patients with non-dissecting aneurysms.

> For patients with chronic dissection, particularly if associated with a connective tissue disorder, but without significant comorbid disease, and a descending thoracic aortic diameter exceeding 5.5 cm, open repair is recommended. (Class I; Level of Evidence: B)[19]

The hinge point for the ascending aorta is at 6.0 cm, while that for the descending aorta is 7.2 cm.[20] Using epiaortic echocardiography, Koullias et al. demonstrated in vivo that at 6 cm, the ascending aorta loses its distensibility.[21] The strong correlation among clinical and engineering data suggests that at 6 cm, the intrinsic durability of the aorta undergoes a significant breakdown. Davies and coworkers have demonstrated that the risk of aortic rupture is more precisely calculated when accounting for the patient's body surface area.[22] Risk could be grouped into three general categories: low risk (4% yearly incidence of adverse events) with an ASI < 2.75 cm/m², moderate risk (8% yearly incidence of adverse events) with an ASI between 2.75 and 4.25 cm/m² and high risk (yearly risk of adverse events of 20%) with an ASI > 4.25 cm/m². Aneurysmal growth should factor into clinical decisions regarding TAAA. In their 1997 study, the Mount Sinai group did not find a correlation between the rate of aneurysm growth and the risk of rupture. The authors of this study did comment that these data might be skewed, since patients with faster-growing aneurysms were more likely to undergo early surgical intervention. Descending aortic aneurysms tend to grow at a faster rate than ascending aortic aneurysms (0.19 cm/year vs. 0.07 cm/year).[18] Similarly, dissected aneurysms expand at a faster rate than non-dissected aneurysms (0.14 cm/year vs. 0.09 cm/year). Therefore, clinicians should recognize that there is, in effect, an acceleration of aneurysm growth as the diameter of an aneurysm enlarges – ultimately achieving size criteria that indicate surgical intervention.

> For patients with thoracoabdominal aneurysms, in whom endovascular stent graft options are limited and surgical morbidity is elevated, elective surgery is recommended if the aortic diameter exceeds 6.0 cm, or less if a connective tissue disorder such as Marfan or Loeys-Dietz syndrome is present. (Class I; Level of Evidence: C)[19]

CLASSIFICATIONS

In the Crawford classification scheme, TAAA repairs are classified according to the extent of aortic replacement. The Crawford classification scheme serves several important functions: it facilitates appropriate risk stratification, it provides a framework for planning the surgical approach and selecting specific treatment modalities according to the anticipated extent of aortic replacement, and it permits standardized reporting of post-operative outcomes (Figure 27.1).

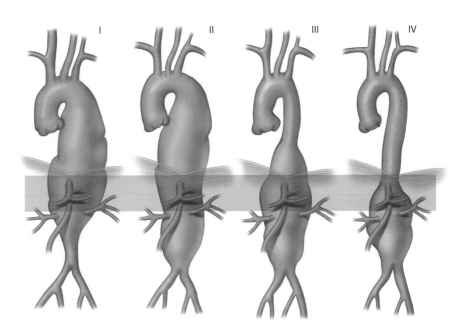

Figure 27.1 Crawford's classification: the key feature to identify a thoracoabdominal aneurysm is the involvement of the aorta at the origin of the celiac trunk (pink marker). Extent I involves the subclavian artery and extends to the level of the renal arteries. Extent II involves the subclavian artery and extends to the bifurcation of the aorta in the pelvis. This aneurysm involves the entire length of the thoracoabdominal aorta. Extent III involves the middle of the descending aorta (sixth rib) and extends to the bifurcation of the aorta in the pelvis. Extent IV involves the upper portion of the abdominal aorta and extends to the bifurcation of the aorta in the pelvis.

A modification of Crawford's classification system has been proposed by Safi and colleagues.[23] In this modified scheme, an additional extent group (i.e. extent V) comprises repairs that extend from the lower descending thoracic aorta (again, below the sixth rib) and end at or above the renal arteries, sparing the infra-renal aorta. By the original Crawford classification scheme, such repairs are categorized as either extent I (in that they spare the infra-renal aorta) or extent III (in that they spare the proximal descending thoracic aorta). Although Estrera et al.[24] have reported that extent V repairs are associated with a particularly low risk of SC complications, the modified classification scheme has not been widely adopted.

IMAGING AND OTHER DIAGNOSTIC STUDIES

Imaging is nowadays considered fundamental for diagnosis, treatment planning and follow-up of aortic diseases. In the past, imaging was based on conventional x-ray radiography, followed by invasive catheter angiography, but with the increasing number of modalities, we can now choose among a wide spectrum of different technologies and determine the most appropriate diagnostic test for each clinical situation. At present, diagnostic modalities include ultrasonography (echo-colour-Doppler, transthoracic echocardiography and transoesophageal echocardiography [TEE]), computerized tomography (CT) and magnetic resonance imaging (MRI). CT is the most important and widely used technique, thanks to its high diagnostic accuracy.

Imaging interpretation is usually done with the aid of a dedicated workstation on which individual source images are analyzed and post-processing techniques, such as multiplanar volume reformation, maximum intensity projection (MIP) reformation and volume rendering (VR) of the images, are performed. MIP images, quickly reconstructed, resemble catheter angiograms and permit a 3D appreciation of anatomy. Subvolume MIP (a thinner slab MIP reconstruction) or multiplanar reconstruction (MPR) (a single-plane reconstruction through the 3D data) should be used to evaluate cross sections of the lumen orthogonal to the long axis along the various levels. MPR and subvolume MIP are particularly helpful for evaluating the diameters of the aorta and branch vessels.

VR reconstruction has emerged as an additional method for exploiting a panoramic display of anatomy. To plan the best possible treatment strategy for each patient, our preferred modality is angio-CT. The acquisition of CT data in particular has benefited from spectacular progress, including multi-row detectors, higher rotation and translation speeds with reduced scan times (single breath-hold), cardiac cycle synchronization and better post-processing capabilities. DICOM slices of adequate thickness (≤1 mm) should be post-processed on a digital workstation using a multiplanar reformatting (MPR) tool to visualize a scan which angulation matches that of the aorta or the vessel under investigation. Nowadays, all the required post-processing may be performed on a regular desktop with dedicated software (including free and open source software) in a user-friendly and time-/resources-efficient way (Figure 27.2).

Beyond diameters and extension of the pathology, we found it particularly useful to evaluate the presence, extension and characteristics of dissection and thrombus, particularly at the clamping sites and infra-diaphragmatic

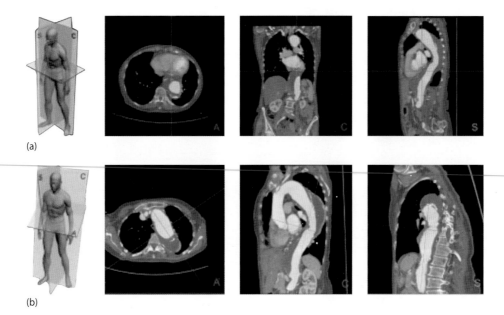

(a)

(b)

Figure 27.2 Preoperative computerized tomography (CT) scan. (a) The classic way to show a CT dataset is through the use of axial (transverse) scans and their orthogonal projections; however, the aorta has a tortuous path that curves in all directions of space. (b) An oblique multiplanar reconstruction helps us in producing a scan whose angulation matches that of the aorta or the vessel that we need to study.

aorta if cannulation of the aneurysm is chosen for distal aortic perfusion. The exact location and geometry of aortic branches are obtained to reveal possible anatomic variations or anomalies, which are particularly common at the level of the renal arteries and arch vessels. Vessel patency is also routinely evaluated; in particular, obstruction of the superior and inferior mesenteric artery and the hypogastric arteries and dominance of one vertebral artery are assessed.

Rendering tools that are 3D such as MIP, VR and surface rendering produce realistic imaging of the anatomical structures that may play a role in understanding the conformation of the patient; locating, for instance, the most appropriate intercostal space to perform thoracotomy; and studying the diseased aorta (Figure 27.3).

Perioperative SC ischaemia can cause symptoms as dramatic as paraplegia. Knowledge of the arterial supply to the SC could be extremely useful for procedure planning and risk stratification (Figure 27.4).

Recent advances in imaging techniques, especially non-invasive techniques, have increased the possibility that this knowledge will soon be available for individual patients (Figure 27.5).[25]

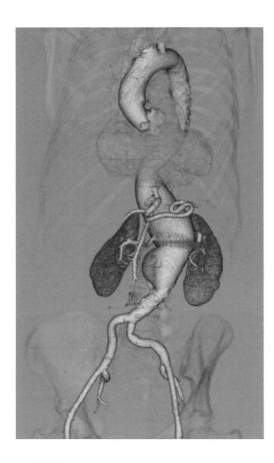

Figure 27.3 More than a merely pictorial view of the aortic pathology, 3D visualization is useful to properly identify the visceral and renal vascularization and their relationship with the aneurysm.

COMPUTERIZED TOMOGRAPHY

The development of multislice CT (MSCT) technology has revolutionized non-invasive aorta imaging, and MSCT angiography has replaced conventional angiography worldwide for the assessment of thoracoabdominal diseases. With the latest-generation CT scanners that provide high-resolution axial images with optimal contrast enhancement and advanced post-processing capabilities, CTA of the entire vascular system is available in a very short time. The volumetric data obtained with MSCT are readily processed using 2D, 3D or VR reformatting techniques to achieve angiogram-like images.

At present, CTA represents the current standard of reference for diagnosis and follow-up of TAAA or acquired aortic diseases. Because of its short time acquisition and ready availability, it is the method of choice for aortic emergency, such as dissection, intramural haematoma, aneurysm and acute traumatic injuries and other aortic diseases. It is less operator dependent than TEE and is easier and faster to perform than MR angiography (MRA); moreover, despite MR, it is possible to perform CTA in patient with stent, endograft, pacemaker and respiratory and trauma devices. The key points for aneurysm imaging are morphology, maximal aortic diameter, extension, involvement of aortic branches, relationship to adjacent structures (such as bronchi, oesophagus, duodenum and inferior vena cava), presence of mural thrombus (especially if the patient has peripheral embolization symptoms) and parietal calcifications and ulcerations. In order to estimate the aneurysmal diameters, longitudinal extent and angulation, multiplanar rendering images (MPR and curved MPR) generated orthogonal to the long axis of the aneurysm are more accurate than axial images. Mural thrombi, parietal ulcerations and atherosclerotic plaques are also better appreciated on coronal, sagittal and oblique MPRs than on standard axial images. MIPs are helpful to precisely localize visceral arteries originating from the aorta relative to the position of the aneurysmal sac, such as the Adamkiewicz artery or main and accessory renal arteries. 3D VR reconstructions, more than axial images, help to make evaluation of the spatial relationship of the aneurysm with aortic branches and surrounding structures easier for the surgeon. CTA is the modality of choice for identifying signs of impending or acute rupture in the mediastinum, pleural or pericardium, peritoneal cavity or adjacent luminal structures such as the airway, oesophagus or duodenum. CT signs of imminent rupture include a high-attenuation crescent in the wall of the aorta, discontinuous calcification in a circumferentially calcified aorta and an eccentric nipple shape to the aorta. CT findings of rupture are a high-attenuation haematoma or haemorrhage on unenhanced scans and a contrast material extravasation from the aortic lumen after contrast agent administration. In recent years, multi-detector computed tomography (MDCT) technology has developed rapidly, allowing high-resolution non-invasive imaging of the coronary

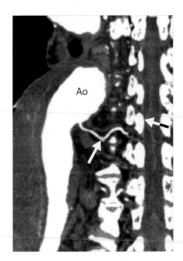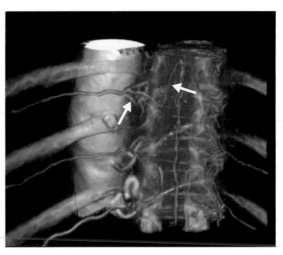

Figure 27.4 Once validation and improved understanding of the information acquired with computerized tomography–based angiography of the spinal cord (SC) vasculature are realized, pre-operative stratification of the risk of SC ischaemia and selective intercostal/lumbar artery reimplantation may be feasible.

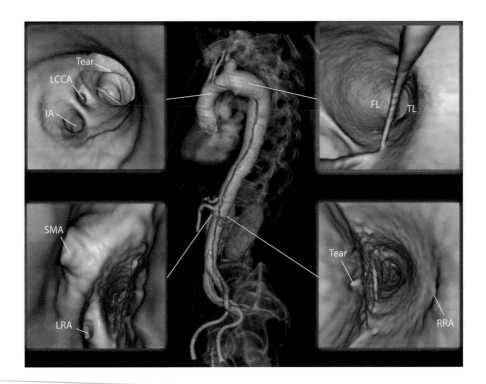

Figure 27.5 Spiral computerized tomography (CT) has dramatically improved the performance of CT by converting a 2D modality into a true 3D imaging, thus enabling the development of new applications involving volumetric imaging such as virtual angioscopy. In case of aortic dissection, for example the localization of the proximal entry tear and the relationship of the dissecting lamella with the intercostal arteries and aortic vessels may be the crucial aspect to investigate.

arteries. Thanks to faster scanning and better contrast bolus capture of multislice technology, it is now possible to study the entire aorta and the coronary tree with the same MDCT examination within a single breath-hold and with a small amount of iodinated contrast.[26] At the same time, developments in MDCT technology have focused on reduction of the radiation dose. Thus, screening of the coronary arteries of patients scheduled

for vascular surgery has become possible in a single, non-invasive examination. ECG-gated multi-detector CT may become the initial imaging modality for pre-operative cardiac risk stratification in patients with TAAA, with the potential to facilitate decision making, improve outcome and reduce the cost of surgery (Figure 27.6).

Overall, CTA allows precise classification of aortic aneurysms in all cases and correct planning of treatment.

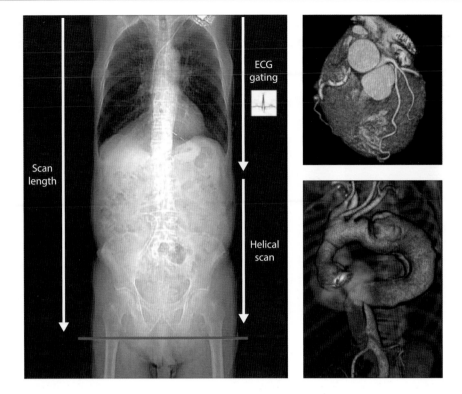

Figure 27.6 In recent years, cardiac computerized tomography (CT) angiography has emerged as a potential non-invasive technique. The availability of dose-modulation protocols and prospective electrocardiographic gating has drastically reduced patients' radiation dose, with an expanding role of this diagnostic imaging modality in clinical care. Differently from other non-invasive tests, cardiac CT allows direct visualization of the thoracoabdominal aorta and of the coronary vessels, providing valuable information on coronary atheromatous plaque components that can assist in refining patients' perioperative cardiovascular risk.

MAGNETIC RESONANCE ANGIOGRAPHY

MRA is a powerful tool for the imaging of the aorta. For optimal results, the acquisition parameters as well as imaging protocols must be tailored to the clinical request. Future technical developments providing faster image acquisition as well as specific contrast agents promise to further improve image quality.

Major advantages of MRA are the lack of ionizing radiation and iodinated contrast medium; for these reasons, the technique is usually reserved for the assessment of aortic diseases in young patients and in cases of contraindication to iodinated contrast material administration. The only main disadvantage of MRA in comparison to CT is the longer acquisition times and difficulties related to the introduction of patients requiring vital signs monitoring into the magnetic field. For these concerns, MRA is poorly suitable in the emergency setting; however, recent advances in fast imaging, such as steady-state free precession and subsecond CE-MRA (N), have enabled fast thoracic examinations with initial screening evaluations of the aorta within 4 minutes. These improvements in speed, in addition to the global improvements in clinical availability of MRI and the aforementioned advantages of MRI over CT evaluation, suggest an increasing role for MR aortography, even in the evaluation of some acute conditions.

In recent years, MRA sequences have significantly improved in terms of acquisition velocity, allowing the retrieval of 4D CE-MRA. This particular sequence allows acquisition of consecutive 3D volumes with a high temporal resolution, during the subsequent phase of contrast passage. Therefore, beyond the three dimensions in space, a temporal dimension can be also recorded. This 4D acquisition may be extremely useful for evaluation of high-flow vascular lesions, such as shunts or dissections, but also for accurate study of the arterial and venous vessels, particularly in neonatal patients who characteristically have very short circulation times.[27] The imaging volume is typically placed as a sagittal or oblique sagittal acquisition that includes the long axis of the aorta. This placement minimizes the overall imaged volume size and corresponds to a left anterior oblique radiographic projection, that is, a 'candy cane' view of the aorta. A coronal acquisition is sometimes preferred for evaluation of the arch vessels (i.e. carotid, vertebral or subclavian arteries) or for evaluation of patients with aortic dissection with suspected distal renal artery involvement (Figure 27.7).

On most 1.5 T MR scanners, a spatial resolution of roughly $1.5 \times 1 \times 1.5$ mm^3 (voxel size) can be achieved in approximately 20–30 s, for the complete study of thoracoabdominal aorta with CE-MRA.

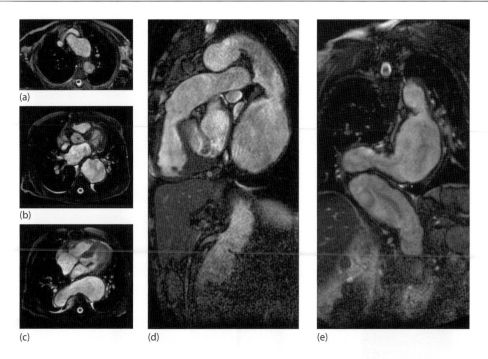

(a)

(b)

(c)

(d)

(e)

Figure 27.7 Magnetic resonance angiography (MRA). Recent advances in fast imaging have enabled fast thoracic examinations with initial screening evaluations of the aorta within 4 minutes. These improvements in speed, in addition to the global improvements in clinical availability of MR imaging, suggest an increasing role for MR aortography, even in the evaluation of some acute conditions. Also with MRA it is possible to visualize axial scan (a–c) and to perform multiplanar reconstructions (d, e).

PRE-OPERATIVE WORKUP AND PATIENT OPTIMIZATION

Patients with TAAA frequently have comorbid conditions, such as advanced age, pulmonary dysfunction, cardiovascular disease, cerebrovascular disease and renal insufficiency, which increase the morbidity and mortality associated with aneurysm repair. A thorough pre-operative evaluation, therefore, is necessary to improve the overall results associated with operative intervention. Cardiovascular and cerebrovascular diseases are also common comorbid conditions found in patients with TAAA. As demonstrated by Svensson and colleagues, over 30% of patients with TAAA will have associated significant cardiac disease, with an additional 15% having cerebrovascular disease defined by the presence of a previous transient ischaemic attack, stroke or carotid endarterectomy.[28] Echocardiography and dipyridamole thallium scan are obtained routinely in asymptomatic and in sedentary, minimally symptomatic patients, because of the high incidence of underlying silent cardiovascular disease. These studies attempt to assess cardiac risk by evaluating ventricular function, excluding valvular insufficiency and determining whether a significant segment of myocardium is at risk for ischaemia. Patients with more severe cardiac symptoms or those with poor ventricular function or evidence of significant thallium redistribution should undergo coronary angiography.[29] Cardiac revascularization before aneurysm repair is recommended in the presence of severe reconstructible coronary artery disease.

Pre-operative transthoracic echocardiography is a satisfactory non-invasive screening method that evaluates both valvular and biventricular function. Stress testing identifies patients that require cardiac catheterization with coronary arteriography. A severe coronary artery occlusive disease is treated with a percutaneous transluminal angioplasty prior to aneurysm repair, possibly avoiding use of drug-eluting stent requiring prolonged double antiplatelet therapy that increases the risk of perioperative bleeding.

The use of estimated glomerular filtration rate (GFR) is currently recommended to assess renal function in order to avoid the misclassification of patients on the basis of serum creatinine levels alone. Based on the GFR assessment, chronic kidney disease has been shown to be a strong predictor of death after thoracic aneurysm open and endovascular repair even in patients without clinical evidence of pre-operative renal disease.

A large percentage of patients undergoing TAAA repair are heavy smokers and suffer from underlying COPD. Respiratory complications have been the most common complications seen in the post-operative period and have been a major cause of morbidity and mortality. Their presence decreased the 30-day survival rate from 98% to 80%. In a study by Svensson and colleagues, only 19% of patients with TAAAs had never smoked. COPD was present in 56% of the patients, and 58% of these developed respiratory failure following surgical repair.[30] Overall, 43% of patients required ventilatory support for more than 2 days after operative intervention and 15% required a tracheostomy. Other studies have also established respiratory failure as the most common complication following TAAA repair.[31] However, certain measures, such as cessation of smoking for at least 1 week before surgical repair and the use of bronchodilators, corticosteroids and antibiotics for the treatment of bronchitis, as well as good pulmonary toilet in the post-operative period, can substantially decrease the high incidence of respiratory complications. A history of heavy smoking, productive cough, dyspnea on exertion or the diagnosis of COPD is generally considered indications for pre-operative pulmonary function tests and arterial blood gas analysis. The finding of a significant decrease in forced vital capacity or forced expiratory volume over 1 second (FEV_1) is associated with an increase in post-operative pulmonary complications. Pre-operative optimization of respiratory function in these difficult patients is of utmost importance and appears to modify the post-operative pulmonary complications. Pulmonary function evaluation with arterial blood gases and spirometry is used in all the patients undergoing open surgery of the descending aorta. In patients with a FEV_1 lower than 1.0 L and a PCO_2 higher than 45 mm/Hg, pulmonary function can be improved by smoking cessation, progressively treating bronchitis, losing weight and following a general exercise programme for a period of 1–6 months before operation. However, in patients with symptomatic aortic aneurysms, despite a poor pulmonary function, the operation may often not be delayed.

Carotid artery duplex studies are also performed routinely as part of the pre-operative assessment of patients with TAAAs, regardless of whether symptoms of cerebrovascular insufficiency are present. Carotid endarterectomy is recommended before aneurysm repair in the presence of a high-grade stenosis. This approach, which is usually well tolerated, will not significantly delay aneurysm repair yet decrease the incidence of post-operative stroke.

We use the modified European system for cardiac operative risk evaluation (EuroSCORE II) in order to perform risk stratification for patient with TAAA.[32]

The pre-operative workup is completed by a psychological intervention which is useful for establishing the kind and degree of distress being experienced by the patient. The psychological staff perform an evaluation of the defence mechanisms and support the patient during the time of hospitalization.[33]

PREPARATION FOR SURGERY

Successful repair of TAAAs requires close cooperation between the anaesthesiologist and the surgeon. Before induction of general endotracheal anaesthesia, a pulmonary artery catheter and right radial arterial catheter are placed to monitor the patient's haemodynamics and optimize cardiac function. Intraoperative TEE is also used throughout the procedure to follow the patient's volume status and detect wall-motion abnormalities suggestive of myocardial ischaemia. At least two large bore IV catheters are inserted, with one connected to a rapid infusion device (RIS, Haemonetics). Additionally, an autotransfusion device (Cell Saver, Braintree, MA) is used to minimize the need for banked blood. An indwelling urinary catheter is placed, and a dose of IV antibiotics is administered before incision.[34]

SPINAL CORD DRAINAGE

The patient is then positioned in lumbar flexion for the spinal drain insertion using a strict aseptic technique. The lower limit of SC extension should be considered when determining the level of insertion. Ideally, an intervertebral space approximately at the level of the iliac crest should be chosen. Once the dura has been punctured with the introducer needle, a drainage catheter is inserted 8–10 cm beyond the tip of the needle into the subarachnoid space. After the drain is secured to the patient, it can be connected to the pressure transducer and baseline measurements can then be made and the cerebrospinal fluid (CSF) is set to drain at a threshold of 10 cm of a preset column height. To maximize the safety of drainage, the pressure transducer can be attached to a dedicated system equipped with a roller pump that allows a volume-controlled CSF drainage (CSFD) (Figure 27.8).

> Cerebrospinal fluid drainage is recommended as a spinal cord protective strategy in open and endovascular thoracic aortic repair for patients at high risk of spinal cord ischemic injury. (Class I; Level of Evidence: B)[19]

After inserting through a 14G Tuohy needle the catheter for CSFD in the intervertebral subarachnoid space between L2 and L3 or L3 and L4, the patient is positioned

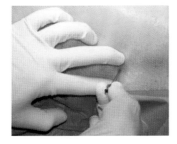
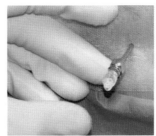
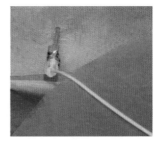

Figure 27.8 The introducer needle is entered in the dura for the spinal cord drainage.

in a right lateral decubitus with the shoulders at 60° and the hips flexed back to 30°. Prepping and draping allow for access beyond the entire left thorax, the entire abdomen and both the inguinal areas. Patient position is maintained with a moldable beanbag attached to a suction line for vacuum creation. A circulating water mattress is placed between the beanbag and the patient, in order to assist body temperature management.

Single lung ventilation by means of a double-lumen endobronchial tube is required in order to obtain adequate surgical exposure and to limit compression of the heart by retractors. Fibre-optic bronchoscopy is recommended to check correct positioning of endotracheal tube especially in large aneurysms of the descending aorta that may lead to distortion of the trachea or the left main bronchus. Correct position should be re-detached after final positioning of the patient. The insertion of a large nasogastric tube is recommended and may be helpful in identifying the oesophagus during the isolation and repair manoeuvres of the proximal thoracic aorta. A right femoral artery line is placed before draping, since the right side of the patient can be difficult to reach during surgery.

SURGICAL TECHNIQUE

Thoraco-phreno-laparotomy

The thoracic incision varies in length and level, depending on the aneurysm extent (Figure 27.9).

A gentle curve to reduce the risk of tissue necrosis is made as the incision crosses the costal margin. Usually an incision through the fifth, sixth or seventh intercostal space is employed according to the desired level of

exposure. The posterior section of the rib or, when necessary, its whole resection associated to a gently and progressive use of the retractor is useful to reduce thoracic wall trauma and fractures; anterolaterally, the incision curves gently as it crosses the costal margin, reducing the risk of tissue necrosis. The pleural space is entered after single right-lung ventilation is initiated. Monopulmonary ventilation is maintained throughout thoracic aorta replacement (Figure 27.10).

Paralysis of the left haemidiaphragm produced by its radial division to the aortic hiatus may contribute

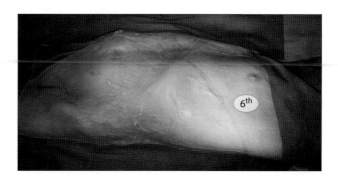

Figure 27.10 Positioning of the patient over the operation table. The left posterolateral aspect of the thorax, the abdomen and the left groin is prepped and draped. The bed is slightly bent under the right flank of the patient to improve aortic exposure after thoraco-phreno-laparotomy. A skin incision is planned from the midpoint between the spinal processes and the scapula, around the lower end of the scapula, down to the umbilicus and then to the pubis if the infra-renal aorta requires repair. Usually an incision through the sixth intercostal space is employed according to the desired level of exposure.

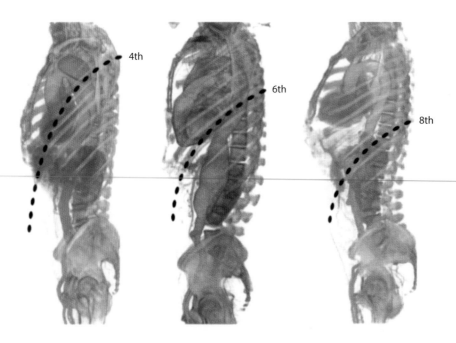

Figure 27.9 With computerized tomography scan, the volume rendering function allows us to choose the best surgical access tailored on the thoracoabdominal aortic aneurysm extension.

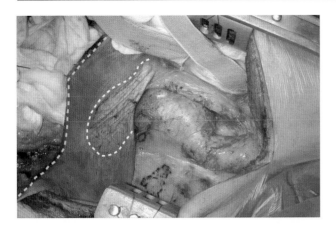

Figure 27.11 After the thoracoabdominal incision, a limited circumferential section (yellow line) of the diaphragm is performed, sparing the phrenic centre (white line).

significantly to post-operative respiratory failure; hence, after thoracoabdominal incision, a limited circumferential section of the diaphragm is routinely carried out, sparing the phrenic centre. Under favourable anatomic conditions, this has been shown to reduce respiratory weaning time (Figure 27.11).

Special care must be taken when isolating the proximal neck in the thoracic aorta, which can be supported using a vessel loop. The insertion of a large calibre oesophageal probe or of the TEE probe makes it easier to identify and preserve the oesophagus at the level of the proximal aortic neck.

The vagus nerve and the origin of the recurrent laryngeal nerve must also be identified since they can be damaged during isolation and clamping manoeuvres. Identification and clipping of some 'high' intercostal arteries can sometimes facilitate the preparation for the proximal anastomosis, thus reducing aortic bleeding. The upper abdominal aortic segment is exposed via a trans-peritoneal approach; the retroperitoneum is entered lateral to the left colon, and medial visceral rotation is performed so that the left colon, the spleen and the left kidney can be retracted anteriorly and to the right. Trans-peritoneal approach allows direct view of the abdominal organs to evaluate the efficacy of revascularization at the end of aortic repair. Extra care must be taken to avoid damage to the spleen which is particularly prone to bleed even if only small capsular lesions are produced.

Distal aortic perfusion

Cross-clamping of the descending thoracic aorta may lead to several haemodynamic disturbances, including severe afterload increase and organ ischaemia. Techniques for distal aortic perfusion with a left heart bypass (LHB) have proven to be extremely useful during aortic repair. The rationale of LHB is providing flow to the SC, viscera and kidneys during the aortic cross-clamp period together with the reduction of proximal hypertension and afterload to the heart. In preparation for LHB and aortic clamping, to reduce bleeding from the extensive tissue exposure, low dose intravenous heparin is administered. Please note that it is unsafe to stop the pump with low dose heparin (Figures 27.12 and 27.13).

> Spinal cord perfusion pressure optimization using techniques, such as proximal aortic pressure maintenance and distal aortic perfusion, is reasonable as an integral part of the surgical, anesthetic, and perfusion strategy in open and endovascular thoracic aortic repair patients at high risk of spinal cord ischemic injury. Institutional experience is an important factor in selecting these techniques. (Class IIa; Level of Evidence: B)[19]

The upper left pulmonary vein is usually cannulated for arterial blood drain that is reinfused through a centrifugal pump (Bio-Medicus) into the left femoral artery.[35] A 'Y' bifurcation is connected to the circuit and is provided with two occlusion/perfusion catheters (9 Fr.) for selective perfusion of visceral vessels (Figure 27.14).

Aortic repair

Once the proximal portion of the TAAA is isolated between clamps, the descending thoracic aorta is transected and separated from the oesophagus (Figures 27.15 and 27.16).

The proximal end of the Dacron graft is sutured to the descending thoracic aorta using a 2/0 monofilament polypropylene in a running fashion. The anastomosis is reinforced with Teflon felt pledgets or felt (Figure 27.17).

The clamp is then removed and reapplied onto the abdominal aorta above the celiac axis (sequential cross-clamping). Reimplantation of intercostal arteries to the aortic graft plays a critical role in SC protection. Critical patent segmental arteries from T7 to L2 are temporarily occluded with 4 Fr. Pruitt catheters to avoid blood steal phenomenon then selectively reattached to the graft by means of aortic patch or graft interposition (Figure 27.18).

> Moderate systemic hypothermia is reasonable for protection of the spinal cord during open repairs of the TAAA. (Class IIa; Level of Evidence: B)[20]

The distal clamp is moved below the renal arteries and the aneurysm is opened below the diaphragm. The pump maintains visceral haematic perfusion with 9 Fr. irrigation-perfusion catheters (LeMaitre Vascular) inserted selectively into the celiac trunk and the superior mesenteric artery (400 mL/min).

Previous studies have demonstrated the protective effects on renal function of hypothermia and of renal artery perfusion with cold crystalloid solutions.[36] Both perfusion with isothermic and cold blood failed to support the hypothesis that blood perfusion is more effective in renal protection than cold crystalloid.[37] In the search

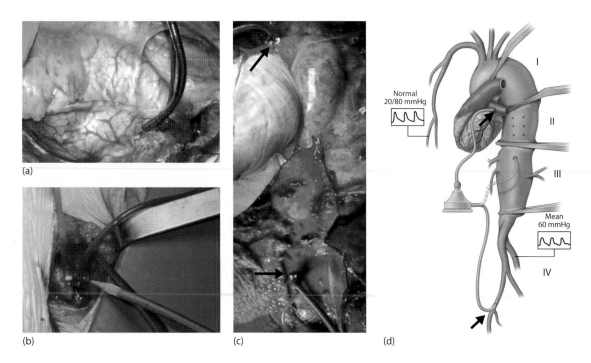

Figure 27.12 Sequential repair with distal aortic perfusion. Oxygenated blood is drained from the left pulmonary vein (a) and reinfused into the left femoral artery throughout the procedure by a centrifugal pump (b); the distal cannula is inserted over a 0.035 in. flexible guidewire in left femoral artery through a groin incision. The blood could also be drained from the descending thoracic aorta and reinfused into the subdiaphragmatic aorta (c). The aneurysm is sequentially clamped, opened and repaired in four consecutive steps (I–IV) optimizing blood flow to critical aortic branches (d).

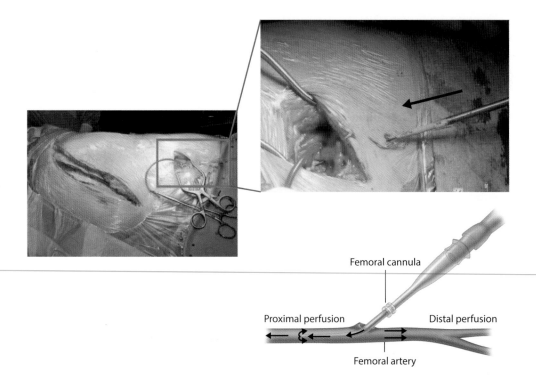

Figure 27.13 Retrograde cannulation of the common femoral artery is safely accomplished over a guidewire through a purse string. A non-occlusive cannulation prevents limb ischaemia during the intervention.

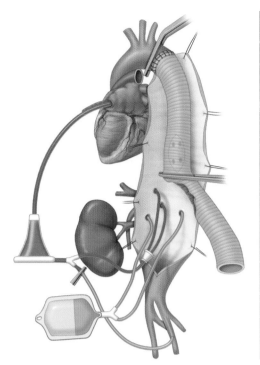

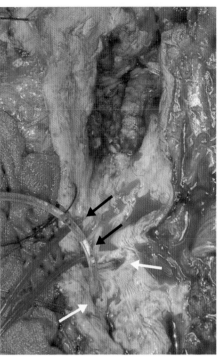

Figure 27.14 Schematic and intraoperative view of the distal aortic perfusion with left heart bypass. A 4-way infusion catheter can be used for visceral and renal blood perfusion; however, we suggest to separately protect the kidneys with cold saline perfusion (white arrows) and the visceral vessels with haematic perfusion.

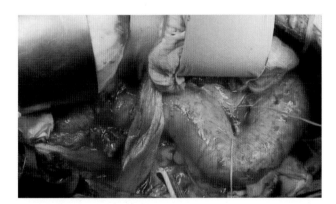

Figure 27.15 A typical Extent II thoracoabdominal aortic aneurysm exposition.

of the optimal solution for kidney protection, we recently introduced cold perfusion of both renal arteries with Custodiol (histidine–tryptophan–ketoglutarate) solution.

We reported a cohort of 104 consecutive patients treated for a thoracoabdominal aneurysm: 50 (48%) had renal perfusion with Custodiol and 54 (52%) with lactated Ringer's solution. Freedom from acute kidney injury was significantly increased in the Custodiol group (38.1% vs. 9.5%; p = 0.002) despite longer total renal ischaemic time (51.5 ± 16.4 minutes vs. 43.6 ± 16.0 minutes; p = 0.05).

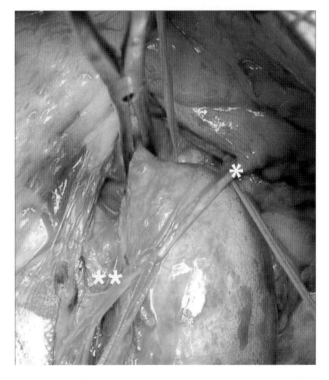

Figure 27.16 The vagus nerve (*) and the origin of the recurrent nerve (**) must be identified since they can be damaged during isolation and clamping manoeuvres.

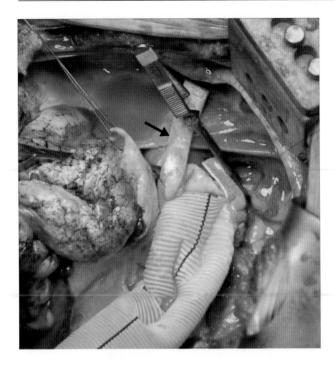

Figure 27.17 The proximal aortic anastomosis is reinforced with Teflon felt (black arrow).

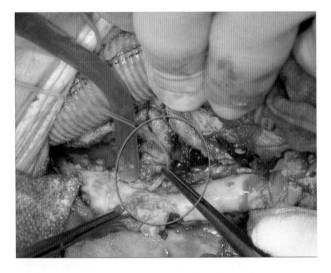

Figure 27.18 Critical patent segmental arteries from T7 to L2 are identified and temporarily occluded with Pruitt catheters to avoid blood steal phenomenon then reattached to a tailored side cut of the graft by means of island technique.

A significant upward trend of perioperative estimated GFR was observed in the Custodiol group (group × time interaction = $F_{3,66}$; $p < 0.001$), and by multivariate analysis, Custodiol perfusion was the only independent predictor of non-AKI ($p = 0.04$). The use of Custodiol in this study was safe and provided improved perioperative renal function compared with lactated Ringer's solution. Randomized trials are needed to confirm these data and to assess their clinical consequences.[38]

Pre-operative hydration and intraoperative mannitol administration may be reasonable strategies for preservation of renal function in open repairs of the descending aorta. (Class IIb; Level of Evidence: C)[19]

During thoracoabdominal repair with exposure of the renal arteries, renal protection by either cold crystalloid or blood perfusion may be considered. (Class IIb; Level of Evidence: B)[19]

Traditional methods for visceral arteries reimplantation include direct reattachment to a tailored side cut on the aortic graft (inclusion technique) as described by Crawford.[39] The inclusion in a visceral aortic patch (VAP) is relatively simple and has the advantage of decreasing the global number of anastomoses and the duration of organ ischaemia (Figure 27.19).

However, a fragile aortic wall can cause difficulties with bleeding control, the suture line may become too long in case of considerable distances between the visceral arterial ostia, and the aortic patch tissue may result in subsequent aneurysmal degeneration in time.[23]

To reduce the VAP size, separate reattachment of distant visceral vessels, namely, the left renal artery, may be employed, directly or interposing a graft. Aortorenal graft interposition allows better bleeding control, may accommodate several anatomies and presents reduced risks of late aneurysmal degeneration. Its major disadvantage is that two anastomoses are required for each vessel revascularization, and the procedure may be technically challenging.

The use of pre-shaped aortic uni- or multi-branched grafts has the advantage of reducing the number of total anastomoses to be performed. These grafts play a major role when repairing an aneurysm in the presence of a connective disease (e.g. Marfan syndrome); however, its use may be tricky and time-consuming (Figure 27.20).

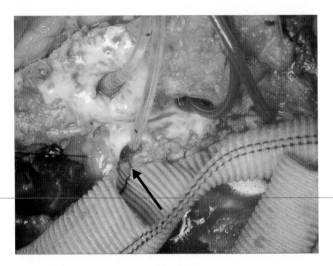

Figure 27.19 The island of reimplanted aortic tissue should be kept as small as possible to reduce risk of future aneurysm recurrences. Passing the running suture inside the vessel at its origin (black arrow) is useful to enforce the anastomosis; however, the risk of arterial dissection or fracture of an ostial plaque should be carefully evaluated.

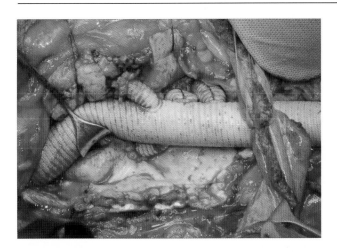

Figure 27.20 In selected cases, any aortic remnant is avoided and a multi-branched graft is used to separately reattach either the renal or the visceral arteries.

Patients with TAAAs often have occlusive disease involving the visceral branches, either related to atherosclerotic disease or caused by aortic dissection. The presence of visceral arterial occlusive disease is a significant predictor of renal complications after TAAA repair.[40] Furthermore, the presence of calcification and thrombus at the origin of the renal artery is associated with the risk of plaque disruption and dissection during vessel reattachment, leading to kidney malperfusion. Thus, renal artery endarterectomy may be required before revascularization to remove ostial plaques and to improve patency rates. This manoeuvre, however, has important limitations, including the risk of vessel thrombosis or distal dissection related to an unsatisfactory end point. Also, perforation of the friable endarterectomized wall is possible during vessel manipulation or during the insertion of balloon catheters that are used to deliver renal perfusion (Figure 27.21).[41]

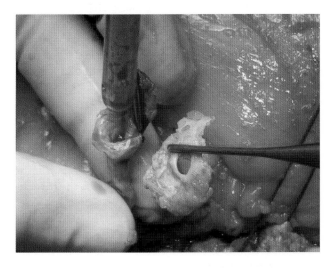

Figure 27.21 In case of ostial plaque, after exposing and controlling the renal artery, an endarterectomy can be performed.

To overcome this problem, several groups started to use bare stents during TAAA open repair, positioned and expanded within the renal artery under direct vision, both to address arterial stenosis or dissection, avoiding endarterectomy, and to tack down an unsatisfactory end point after visceral endarterectomy (Figure 27.22).[42,43]

An alternative solution to these challenging anatomies may be the use of covered self-expanding stents for sutureless anastomoses. Initially described for visceral revascularization during hybrid surgery for complex aortic repair,[44] we recently described the routine use of this technique to reattach the left renal artery with several technical advantages.[45] In our experience, short-term clinical and radiologic outcomes were satisfactory; however, larger series and longer follow-up are needed to confirm the safety and durability of the proposed technique (Figure 27.23).

After restoring antegrade flow to the visceral and renal vessels, an end-to-end anastomosis with the distal aorta is performed and the last clamp removed (Figure 27.24).

Closure

The entire aortic repair is inspected and all the pulses of the aortic branches exposed are palpated also after de-rotation of the abdominal viscera. Any bleeding or kinking of the aortic branches is carefully checked. The atrial and femoral cannulas are removed; the purse string sutures are tied and reinforced. Protamine is then given and lab tests are made to check any coagulopathy to be reversed.

The diaphragmatic pillars are approximated to reshape the aortic hiatus, and the left haemidiaphragm is loosely sutured with a running polypropylene suture. The left lung is temporarily inflated to check any air leakage.

A closed-suction abdominal drain is positioned along the repaired aorta in the left retroperitoneal space, and two chest tubes are placed in the posterior apical and basal space. Absorbable pericostal sutures are placed to approximate the intercostal space and two steel wires are used to stabilize the costal margin. The lung is inflated and the correct expansion of all the segments is carefully checked; the pericostal and diaphragmatic sutures are tightened and ligated. The steel wires are twisted and buried in the cartilaginous costal margin. The abdominal fascia is closed with a running suture. The abdominal and thoracic drains are connected to suction. The serratus and latissimus dorsi muscles are approximated with separate absorbable sutures. Subdermal layer is sutured and the skin is closed with staples.

POST-OPERATIVE CARE

Following TAAA repair, the patient is transferred to the surgical intensive care unit (SICU). Particularly, close attention is given to the patient's blood pressure, heart rate, respiratory rate and urine output. The CSFD is continued for an additional 2–3 days to minimize delayed-onset paraplegia

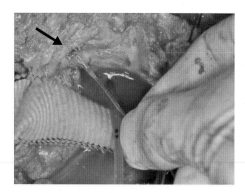
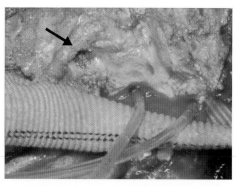

Figure 27.22 A tight ostial stenosis of the renal artery is managed by direct dilatation with a balloon-expandable stent before inserting the perfusion catheter (black arrow).

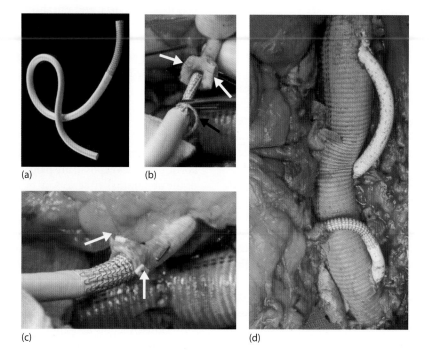

Figure 27.23 Sutureless renal reattachment with a new hybrid graft. (a) In h 'hybrid' graft the ePTFE tube graft is supported by a self expanding stent only in the distal portion. (b) The distal stent supported end of the hybrid graft in its closed configuration is inserted under direct vision in the ostium of the target vessel (the left renal artery in this case – white arrows). (c) After the distal supporting stent is released open the stented graft is secured to the artery with three pledgeted stitches in order to avoid inadvertent pull out. (d) Final appearance of a thoracoabdominal aneurysm repair in which the renal arteries were revascularized with hybrid grafts, the left in a retrograde fashion and the right in an antegrade one.

that may result from progressive SC edema. Central venous pressure, pulmonary capillary wedge pressure, cardiac output and peripheral vascular resistance are monitored frequently, and laboratory indicators such as a complete blood cell count, coagulation studies, serum electrolytes, serum creatinine and arterial blood gases are checked regularly. Blood products are often necessary in the post-operative period to optimize the patient's haemodynamics and correct any residual coagulopathy. Clinical management of acute moderate to severe bleeding is one of the major challenges for SICU team. Though substitution of erythrocytes by transfusion of red blood cells is a routine task, adequate maintenance of haemostasis may be considerably

more demanding. In fact, the underlying cause of bleeding and subsequent treatment may be completely different depending on the clinical scenario. Standard plasmatic coagulation tests such as PT/INR, aPTT and plasma fibrinogen level have several major limitations for their use in guiding perioperative management of bleeding disorders. Therapeutic options for effective haemostasis management range from the preemptive transfusion, in which blood products are transfused before laboratory abnormalities are recognized, to a targeted therapy using purified coagulation factors and/or specific procoagulant drugs. What makes this management even more complex is the fact that the underlying rationale for starting coagulation therapy might

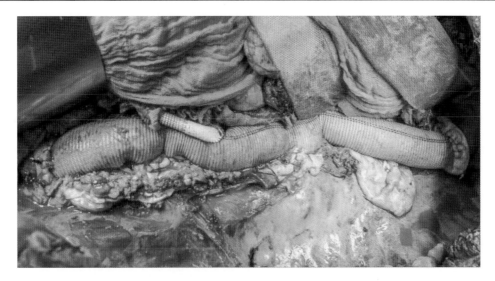

Figure 27.24 A typical type II thoracoabdominal aortic aneurysm repair. A Dacron tube graft is used to replace the aorta from the left subclavian artery to the iliacs. Intercostal and visceral arteries are reattached with the island technique. The left renal artery is reimplanted separately with a short bypass with a hybrid graft.

be either completely empiric or based on standard lab tests (which are sometimes time-consuming such that empiric therapy has already started before results are available). In addition, there is actually strong evidence that avoidance of exposure to allogeneic blood transfusion is of high importance, as it has been demonstrated to be associated with serious adverse events, such as acute lung injury, volume overload, nosocomial infections and sepsis, immunomodulation and organ dysfunction. Assessment of clot formation and strength, measured by using viscoelastic methods (thromboelastography or thromboelastometry), is useful for the diagnosis of intraoperatively acquired coagulation disturbances in a short period of time and is reflective of the specific defects in haemostasis and has resulted in the development of coagulation therapy algorithms and consequent reductions in blood transfusion and associated hospitalization costs.[46] Electrolyte disturbances, particularly hypokalemia and hypoxemia, are avoided because they may rapidly precipitate a lethal cardiac arrhythmia.

No attempts at extubation are made during the first post-operative day; rather, the patient is maintained intubated and sedated. In the presence of significant facial edema, the dual lumen endotracheal tube is not exchanged until the following day for fear of losing control of the airway. A chest x-ray and an electrocardiogram are obtained immediately post-operatively and on a daily basis until the patient is sufficiently stable to leave the SICU.

The patient's sedatives are discontinued on the second post-operative day, when weaning from the ventilator is initiated. At this time it is usually possible to more adequately assess the patient's neurologic function, which is followed closely. The spinal catheter is discontinued on the third post-operative day. If a delayed neurologic deficit occurs, reinsertion of the spinal catheter is performed rapidly, draining fluid to maintain a CSF pressure of less than 10 mmHg, while the patient's haemodynamics are optimized. In a report by Safi and colleagues, this approach

resulted in significant improvements in neurologic function in all those patients who developed a delayed deficit.[47]

Maintenance fluids initially are given at the rate of 125 mL/hour and additional IV fluids are given to match the urine output on a cc/cc basis. This is necessary. Since after the period of intraoperative renal ischaemia, there is an obligatory high output loss of fluids while the renal tubules are temporarily dysfunctional. The fluid replacement for urine losses can usually be discontinued the day after surgery and the maintenance IV fluids are usually decreased from 125 mL/hour on the first post-operative day to 100 mL/hour on the second post-operative day and 60 mL/hour on the third day, in anticipation of third-space fluid mobilization. Diuretics are frequently administered on the third post-operative day, when chest tubes, nasogastric tubes and closed-suction drains can usually be removed. An oral diet is resumed after bowel function has returned. Ambulation is encouraged after the patient has been extubated and the epidural catheter is removed. The main focus of the immediate post-operative management after thoracoabdominal aortic repair in the ICU is addressed to the early detection of any possible neurological and cardiovascular complication, to promptly deal the problem with appropriate prophylactic or therapeutic interventions.

As soon as normal pressure and body temperature are reached, the patient is allowed to wake up even if prolonged ventilation support is still required. When an SC or brain damage is suspected, CT imaging is immediately performed to exclude intracerebral bleeding or SC compression by an intradural haematoma. To detect ischaemic or embolic lesions, both of the brain and of the SC, significant results are reached usually after more than 24–48 hours after the event. In case of paraparesis or paraplegia, mean arterial pressure is forced above 80 mmHg, CSFD is drained in order to lower the CSF pressure below 10 mmHg, and methylprednisolone (1 g in bolus, then 4 g in 24 hours in continuous perfusion) and 18% mannitol (5 mg/kg 4 times/die) are administered.

If signs of lower limbs, renal or visceral malperfusion develop in the post-operative period, immediate diagnostic measures must be taken to assess organ blood supply and to appropriately plan surgical revascularization procedures. For a precise visualization of visceral organ perfusion, emergency DSA or angio-CT scanning is performed. Hypertension is common, especially in the chronically hypertensive patient, and an immediate pharmacological approach is set to reduce the risk of bleeding from suture lines, especially when a dissection is present. In uncomplicated cases, drainage tubes are removed at 36–48 hours post-operatively, while the intrathecal catheter of CSFD is usually removed only after 72 hours. A prolonged period of mechanical ventilation for several days is not unusual, especially after emergency operations, in patients with intraoperative abundant bleeding and after longer periods of circulatory arrest. In case of severe chronic kidney disease, transient temporary haemodialysis may be needed early after operation.

RESULTS

The morbidity and mortality associated with TAAA repair has decreased significantly since the procedure was first performed over 40 years ago.[48] The careful pre-operative evaluation and advancements in perioperative care and surgical technique, the introduction of the graft inclusion technique and the use of CSFD largely have been responsible for these improved results. Hollier, Safi, Acher and Brewster now report operative mortality rates of less than 10% and paraplegia rates of less than 10%. Nonetheless, despite this progress, mortality, neurologic injury and renal dysfunction rates are still greater than desirable. The incidence of these devastating complications is still noted to vary according to the extent of the aneurysm undergoing repair, cross-clamp times, age of the patient and presence of comorbid conditions. The incidence of paraplegia reported in the literature varies from 5% to 20%, with renal failure rates of 5% to 30%.

As described previously, several methods have been used successfully to decrease the incidence of these devastating complications. SC protection can be improved by CSFD, distal aortic perfusion, reimplantation of critical intercostals, mild hypothermia and IV corticosteroids.[49] Distal aortic perfusion and/or selective visceral artery perfusion can also help decrease renal failure rates and minimize haemorrhagic complications. Renal dysfunction can be minimized by adequate pre-operative hydration, administration of mannitol and furosemide prior to cross-clamping and endarterectomy or renal bypass in the presence of associated renal artery occlusive disease. Cold perfusion of the kidneys is also useful, and many authors have reported improved results using this technique. The best solution to be used is still under investigation.

CONCLUSIONS

The results of open surgical treatment of TAAA are improving with reduced post-operative mortality and morbidity. However, preventing paraplegia and other ischaemic complications remains a significant challenge. We employ a multimodal approach to spinal and visceral protection that is tailored to the specific risk factors of each patient, including the extent of aortic repair, previous aortic operations and comorbid conditions. We continue to explore and develop new protective strategies in the hope of further minimizing the risks associated with TAAA repair.

ACKNOWLEDGEMENTS

The authors gratefully acknowledge Prof. Francesco De Cobelli and Dr. Claudio Sallemi for their invaluable help with imaging of our aortic patients and for providing Figure 27.7. We also thank Dr. Pietro Spagnolo and Dr. Manuela Giglio for providing Figure 27.6.

REFERENCES

1. Johnston KW, Rutherford RB, Tilson MD et al. Suggested standards for reporting on arterial aneurysms. Subcommittee on Reporting Standards for Arterial Aneurysms, Ad Hoc Committee on Reporting Standards, Society for Vascular Surgery and North American Chapter, International Society for Cardiovascular Surgery. *J Vasc Surg.* 1991;13:452–458.
2. Wong DR, Parenti JL, Coselli JS et al. Open repair of thoracoabdominal aortic aneurysm in the modern surgical era: Contemporary outcomes in 509 patients. *J Am Coll Surg.* 2011;212(4):569–579.
3. Campa JS, Greenhalgh RM, Powell JT. Elastin degradation in abdominal aortic aneurysms. *Atherosclerosis.* 1987;65:13–21.
4. Pomianowski P, Elefteriades JA. The genetics and genomics of thoracic aortic disease. *Ann Cardiothorac Surg.* 2013;2:271–279.
5. Loeys BL, Chen J, Neptune ER et al. A syndrome of altered cardiovascular, craniofacial, neurocognitive and skeletal development caused by mutations in TGFBRß1 or TGFBR2. *Nat Genet.* 2005;37:275–281.
6. Lum YW, Brooke BS, Black JH 3rd. Lum YW, Brooke BS, Black JH 3rd. Contemporary management of vascular Ehlers-Danlos syndrome. *Curr Opin Cardiol.* 2011;26(6):494–501.
7. El-Hamamsy I, Yacoub MH. Cellular and molecular mechanisms of thoracic aortic aneurysms. *Nat Rev Cardiol.* 2009;6:771–786.

8. Borchers AT, Gershwin ME. Giant cell arteritis: A review of classification, pathophysiology, geo-epidemiology and treatment. *Autoimmun Rev.* 2012;11(6–7):A544–A554.

9. Leon LR Jr, Mills JL Sr. Diagnosis and management of aortic mycotic aneurysms. *Vasc Endovascular Surg.* 2010;44(1):5–13.

10. Griepp RB, Ergin MA, Galla JD et al. Natural history of descending thoracic and thoracoabdominal aneurysms. *Ann Thorac Surg.* 1999;67:1927–1930; discussion 1953–1958.

11. Dapunt OE, Galla JD, Sadeghi AM et al. The natural history of thoracic aortic aneurysms. *J Thorac Cardiovasc Surg.* 1994;107:1323–1332.

12. Juvonen T, Ergin MA, Galla JD et al. Prospective study of the natural history of thoracic aortic aneurysms. *Ann Thorac Surg.* 1997;63:1553–1545.

13. Crawford ES, DeNalale RW. Thoracoabdominal aortic aneurysms: Observations regarding the natural course of disease. *J Vasc Surg.* 1986;3:578–582.

14. Bickerstaff LK, Pairolero PC, Hollier LH et al. Thoracic aortic aneurysms: A population based study. *Surgery.* 1982;92:1103–1108.

15. Cambria RA, Gloviczki P, Stanson AW et al. Outcome and expansion rate of 57 thoracoabdominal aortic aneurysms managed nonoperatively. *Am J Surg.* 1995;170:213–217.

16. Crawford ES, Crawford JL, Safi HJ et al. Thoracoabdominal aortic aneurysms: Preoperative and intraoperative factors determining immediate and long term results of operations in 605 patients. *J Vasc Surg.* 1986;3:389–404.

17. Ziganshin BA, Elefteriades JA. Surgical management of thoracoabdominal aneurysms. *Heart.* 2014;100:1577–1582.

18. Davies RR, Goldstein LJ, Coady MA et al. Yearly rupture or dissection rates for thoracic aortic aneurysms: Simple prediction based on size. *Ann Thorac Surg.* 2002;73:17–27.

19. Hiratzka LF, Bakris GL, Beckman JA et al. 2010 ACCF/AHA/AATS/ACR/ASA/SCA/SCAI/SIR/STS/SVM guidelines for the diagnosis and management of patients with thoracic aortic disease. *Circulation.* 2010;121:e266–e369.

20. Coady MA, Rizzo JA, Hammond GL et al. What is the appropriate size criterion for resection of thoracic aortic aneurysms? *J Thorac Cardiovasc Surg.* 1997;113:476–491.

21. Koullias G, Modak R, Tranquilli M et al. Mechanical deterioration underlies malignant behavior of aneurysmal human ascending aorta. *J Thorac Cardiovasc Surg.* 2005;130:677–683.

22. Davies RR, Gallo A, Coady MA et al. Novel measurement of relative aortic size predicts rupture of thoracic aortic aneurysms. *Ann Thorac Surg.* 2006;81:169–177.

23. Safi HJ, Miller CC III. Spinal cord protection in descending thoracic and thoracoabdominal aortic repair. *Ann Thorac Surg.* 1999;67:1937–1939.

24. Estrera AL, Miller CC III, Huynh TT et al. Neurologic outcome after thoracic and thoracoabdominal aortic aneurysm repair. *Ann Thorac Surg.* 2001;72:1225–1231.

25. Melissano G, Civilini E, Bertoglio L. *Planning and Sizing della patologia aortica con OsiriX.* Milano, Italy: Arti Grafiche Colombo Editore, 2010.

26. Spagnolo P, Giglio M. Role of Cardiac CT in assessment of patient with thoraco-abdominal aortic aneurysm. In: Chiesa R, Melissano G, Zangrillo A, Coselli JS, eds. *Thoraco-Abdominal Aorta: Surgical and Anesthetic Management.* Cap 14(173–182). Trento, Italy: Springer-Verlag, 2011.

27. Han F, Rapacchi S, Khan S et al. Four-dimensional, multiphase, steady-state imaging with contrast enhancement (MUSIC) in the heart: A feasibility study in children. *Magn Reson Med.* 2014.

28. Svensson LG, Crawford ES, Hess KR et al. Experience with 1509 patients undergoing thoraco-abdominal aortic operations. *J Vasc Surg.* 1993;17(2):357–370.

29. Hollier LH. Cardiac evaluation in patients with vascular disease—Overview: A practical approach. *J Vasc Surg.* 1992;15:726–728.

30. Svensson LG, Hess KR, Coselli JS et al. A prospective study of respiratory failure after high risk surgery on the thoracoabdominal aorta. *J Vasc Surg.* 1991;14(3):271–282.

31. Money SR, Rice K, Crockett D et al. Risk of respiratory failure after repair of thoracoabdominal aortic aneurysms. *Am J Surg.* 1994;168:152–155.

32. Di Dedda U, Pelissero G, Ranucci M et al. Accuracy, calibration and clinical performance of the new EuroSCORE II risk stratification system. *Eur J Cardiothorac Surg.* 2013;43(1):27–32.

33. Sarno L, Di Mattei V, Motta C et al. Psychological approach to the aneurysm patient. In: Chiesa R, Melissano G, Zangrillo A, Coselli JS, eds. *Thoraco-Abdominal Aorta: Surgical and Anesthetic Management.* Cap 53(651–656). Trento, Italy: Springer-Verlag, 2011.

34. Chiesa R, Melissano G, Civilini E et al. Video-atlas of open thoracoabdominal aortic aneurysm repair. *Ann Cardiothorac Surg.* 2012 September;1(3):398–403.

35. Civilini E, Melissano G, Chiesa R. Improved cannulation: Technique for thoracoabdominal aortic aneurysm repair. *Ann Thorac Surg.* 2010;89(2):675.

36. Jacobs MJ, Mommertz G, Koeppel TA et al. Surgical repair of thoracoabdominal aortic aneurysms. *J Cardiovasc Surg.* 2007;48(1):49–58.

37. Bhamidipati CM, Coselli JS, LeMaire SA. Perfusion techniques for renal protection during thoracoabdominal aortic surgery. *J Extra Corpor Technol.* 2012;44(1):P31–P37.

38. Tshomba Y, Kahlberg A, Chiesa R et al. Comparison of renal perfusion solutions during thoracoabdominal aortic aneurysm repair. *J Vasc Surg.* 2014;59(3):623–633.

39. Crawford ES. Thoraco-abdominal and abdominal aortic aneurysms involving renal, superior mesenteric, celiac arteries. *Ann Surg.* 1974;179:763–772.

40. Kellum JA, Lameire N; for the KDIGO AKI Guideline Work Group. Diagnosis, evaluation, and management of acute kidney injury: A KDIGO summary (Part 1). *Crit Care.* 2013;4;17(1):204.

41. Clair DG, Belkin M, Whittemore AD, Mannick JA, Donaldson MC. Safety and efficacy of transaortic renal endarterectomy as an adjunct to aortic surgery. *J Vasc Surg.* 1995;21:926–934.

42. LeMaire SA, Jamison AL, Carter SA, Wen S, Alankar S, Coselli JS. Deployment of balloon expandable stents during open repair of thoracoabdominal aortic aneurysms: A new strategy for managing renal and mesenteric artery lesions. *Eur J Cardiothorac Surg.* 2004;26(3):599–607.

43. Patel R, Conrad MF, Paruchuri V, Kwolek CJ, Cambria RP. Balloon expandable stents facilitate right renal artery reconstruction during complex open aortic aneurysm repair. *J Vasc Surg.* 2010;51:310–315.

44. Lee JD, Williams JB, Winkler JL. One-stage triple hybrid arch debranching. *Innovations (Phila).* 2013;8(1):67–69.

45. Chiesa R, Kahlberg A, Mascia D et al. Use of a novel hybrid vascular graft for sutureless revascularization on the renal arteries during open thoracoabdominal aortic aneurysm repair. *J Vasc Surg.* 2014;60(3):622–630.

46. Ghavidel AA, Toutounchi Z, Shahandashti FJ et al. Rotational thromboelastometry in prediction of bleeding after cardiac surgery. *Asian Cardiovasc Thorac Ann.* 2015.

47. Safi HJ, Hess KR, Randel M et al. Cerebrospinal fluid drainage and distal aortic perfusion: Reducing neurologic complications in repair of thoracoabdominal aortic aneurysm types I and II. *J Vasc Surg.* 1996;23(2):223–228.

48. Chiesa R, Melissano G, Setacci C et al. *History of Aortic Surgery in the World.* Torino, Italy: Edizioni Minerva Medica, 2014.

49. Etz DC, Luehr M, Aspern KV et al. Spinal cord ischemia in open and endovascular thoracoabdominal aortic aneurysm repair: New concepts. *J Cardiovasc Surg.* 2014 April;55(2 Suppl. 1):159–168. Review.

28

Endovascular management of complex aortic aneurysms

GIOVANNI TINELLI, BLANDINE MAUREL, RAFAËLLE SPEAR, ADRIEN HERTAULT,
RICHARD AZZAOUI, JONATHAN SOBOCINSKI and STÉPHAN HAULON

CONTENTS

INTRODUCTION

Since the first endovascular repair of an infrarenal abdominal aortic aneurysm (AAA) published by Parodi et al.,[1] stent grafts have undergone continuous improvement.

Devices have evolved to highly complex, custom-designed devices incorporating branches and fenestrations. These developments provide an endovascular solution for complex aortic aneurysms (CAAs) incorporating the visceral branches, iliac arteries and supra-aortic trunks (SAT), expanding the indications of EVAR.

The first reported endovascular exclusion of a juxtarenal aneurysm and of an extensive thoracoabdominal aneurysm (Crawford type 3) was completed, respectively, using a fenestrated stent graft by Faruqi et al. and a branched stent graft by Chuter et al.[2,3] The first reported endovascular exclusion of an aortic arch aneurysm (AArA) using a branched stent graft was performed by Inoue et al.[4]

Following these pioneers, in the late 1990s, fenestrated–branched stent grafts (FBSGs) have been largely implanted and evaluated and are now considered a therapeutic option, especially in high-risk patients.

The management of short-neck, juxta- and para-aortic aneurysms with fenestrated endovascular aneurysm repair (f-EVAR) has been associated with favourable early and midterm results.[5–8] Most of the accumulated experience has involved the Zenith Fenestrated Graft platform (Cook have Medical Australia, Brisbane, Queensland, Australia), a custom-made stent graft (CMSG), with over 5000 implantations performed worldwide.[9]

Recently, a new fenestrated custom-made Anaconda stent graft (Vascutek, Renfrewshire, Scotland) was introduced for the treatment of juxtarenal and infrarenal AAAs with short necks.[10,11]

To reduce the manufacturing delays of CMSG, off-the-shelf fenestrated devices have been developed and currently undergoing evaluation through clinical trials: Zenith pivot branch (p-branch) device (Cook, Bloomington, Indiana)[12] and the Endologix (Irvine, California) Ventana device.[13]

Parallel grafts alongside the aortic stent graft ('chimney', 'snorkel' or 'periscope' grafts)[14,15] and surgeon-modified FBSG[16] are used in clinical practice but are used outside of device instructions for use (IFU) and thus have not been correctly evaluated. They are often used as bailout procedures in acute cases. These procedures are not described in this manuscript because they have not undergone preclinical testing and not been endorsed by any manufacturers.

DEFINITION OF COMPLEX AORTIC ANEURYSMS

CAAs are aortic aneurysms involving side branches (SAT in the arch and visceral vessels in the abdomen) that are not treatable using standard stent grafts (if IFU are respected) (Figure 28.1).

The treatment of aortic aneurysms involving visceral vessels (renal arteries, superior mesenteric artery [SMA] and celiac trunk [CT]) with an open surgical approach requires aortic cross-clamping above the visceral vessels. Suprarenal aortic clamping is associated with significantly higher morbidity and mortality rates compared to infrarenal clamping. Similarly, endovascular repair of CAAs requiring visceral stenting is associated with higher mortality and morbidity rates compared to EVAR.

CAAs include short-neck infrarenal aneurysms, juxtarenal (j-AAAs) and pararenal (p-AAAs) aneurysms, thoracoabdominal aortic aneurysms (TAAAs) and AArAs.

Short-neck infrarenal aneurysms have an unsuitable anatomy for a standard EVAR repair. They include AAA with necks that are short (<15 mm), conical, large (>32 mm) and angled (>60°) and/or with a posterior bulge (Figure 28.2).

j-AAAs are aneurysms encroaching upon but not involving the renal arteries.

p-AAAs are aneurysms involving one or both renal arteries, extending above the renal origins to the base of the SMA.

TAAAs are classified using the Crawford classification.

AArAs are located in the aorta between the origin of the innominate artery and the origin of the left subclavian artery (LSA).

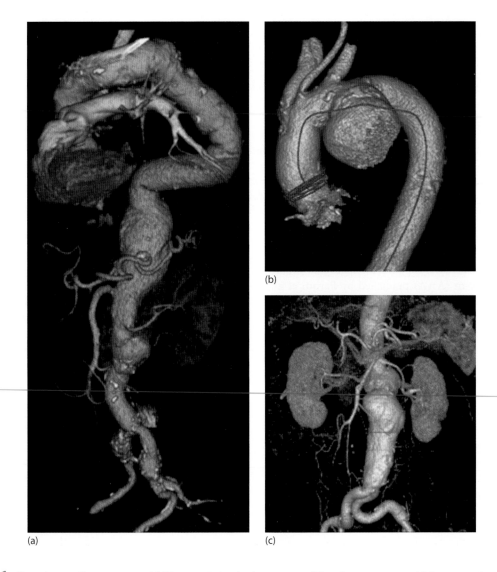

(a)　　　　(b)

(c)

Figure 28.1　Complex aortic aneurysms. (a) Thoracoabdominal aneurysm, (b) arch aneurysm and (c) pararenal aneurysm.

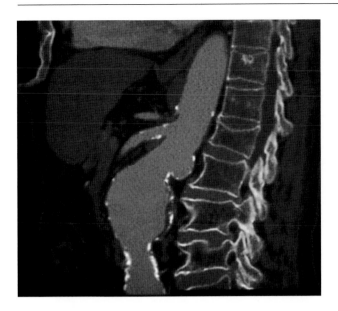

Figure 28.2 Posterior aortic bulge in a pararenal aneurysm.

The proximal sealing zone when performing endovascular procedures is a healthy aortic segment of 20 mm or more (we advocate >30 mm); thus, endovascular procedures require more extensive aortic coverage compared to open surgery. This creates a bias when analyzing outcomes of both procedures. For example, a p-AAA is often treated similarly to a type 4 thoracoabdominal with a proximal sealing stent positioned above the CT. This is why some authors classify endovascular repairs according to the post-operative amount of aortic coverage rather than according to the preoperative anatomical evaluation.[17]

TARGET POPULATION

The target patient population for FBSGs repair is primarily patients with CAAs at risk of rupture who are unsuitable for open surgery repair because of co-morbid conditions, but with a reasonable life expectancy (>2 years).

The preoperative computed tomography angiography (CTA) scan must be thoroughly analyzed on a 3D workstation to select the patients that can benefit from an endovascular approach. For example, significant atheroma or mural thrombus (shaggy aorta) within the aorta (working area) is associated with a major risk of cholesterol emboli and can be a contraindication for an endovascular repair. Vascular access requires also thorough evaluation as it can also contraindicate an endovascular repair or require adjunctive procedures.

Endovascular repair of CAAs with FBSGs generates higher radiation and contrast exposures compared to EVAR,[18] but Kirkwood et al. have reported that many patients undergoing such treatment did not know that they were exposed to radiation.[19] The risks of radiation exposure and contrast nephrotoxicity are present at the time of the procedure but also throughout the period of follow-up.

PREOPERATIVE ASSESSMENT

Medical investigation and renal optimization

The preoperative workup includes a complete physical examination, cardiac evaluation with stress cardiac echography and coronary angiography where indicated, respiratory function tests and routine blood tests. Renal function is optimized preoperatively with hydration and administration of *N*-acetyl cysteine according to our standard protocol.[20] All patients should have their serum creatinine measured and renal creatinine clearance (eGFR) estimated preoperatively. If outside the normal range, a review by a nephrologist for optimization of medications prior to aneurysm repair must be undertaken. FBSGs repairs should only be performed in hospitals where on-site haemofiltration can be performed 24/7.[21]

Computed tomography angiography

Preoperative assessment of patients includes high-resolution spiral CTA scans (0.75 mm reconstructions) that incorporate the complete thoracic aorta to the profunda femoris. High-quality contrast-enhanced computed tomography and post-processing 3D softwares used to analyze digital imaging and communications in medicine data are mandatory.

3D workstation: Planning

The preoperative planning is a foundation stone of successful EVAR in general (Figure 28.3); it is even more critical for fenestrated-branched endovascular aneurysm repair (fb-EVAR). The routine use of 3D workstations for EVAR planning significantly reduces the rate of type I endoleaks and, therefore, the rate of related secondary interventions.[22] Detailed planning requires a substantial level of experience and expertise to design devices with fenestrations aligning accurately with their respective target vessels.

The recent development of imaging workstations – Advantage Windows (GE Healthcare, CO, Unite States), OsiriX (Pixmeo, Genève, Switzerland), Aquarius iNtuition Viewer (Terarecon, San Mateo, CA, United States) and EasyVision (Philips Medical Systems, Eindhoven, Netherlands) – offers easy access to multiplanar reformatting and 3D reconstructions. Three-dimensional workstations are now intuitive and 'user friendly', which makes them accessible to vascular surgeons and radiologists alike.

There are four principle visualization techniques: multiplanar (axial, sagittal and coronal) reformation (MPR), curved planar reformation (CPR), maximum intensity projection and 3D volume rendering. The overall aortic morphology is first examined using colour volume rendering images. Multiplanar reconstructions are then generated to depict the proximal and distal sealing zones. MPR and

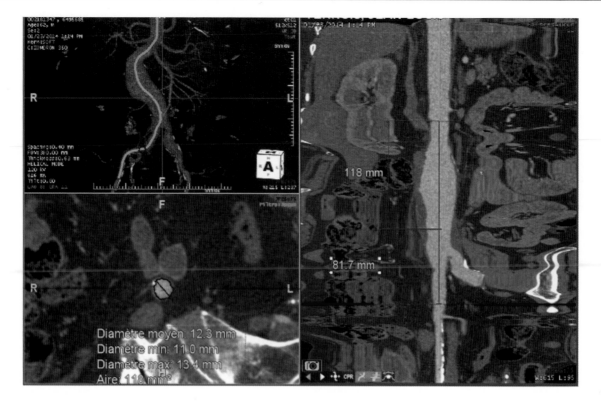

Figure 28.3 Endovascular aneurysm repair planning with a 3D workstation.

maximum intensity projection reconstructions are also performed to depict intercostal artery location and patency. CPR assesses the true cross-sectional diameters and is also obligatory in the accurate assessment of length in a curved aorta. CPR is performed following an automated vessel centre line generated between two points selected proximal and distal to the aneurysm. A variety of other layouts are then required to further estimate vessel diameters and lengths. The following measures are performed:

- True sealing zones cross-sectional diameters
- Total length of aorta to be covered by the stent graft
- The gap between the partially and fully deployed stent graft and the visceral artery-bearing aortic wall
- The longitudinal distances between target vessel origins
- Angulations of target vessels with the aorta
- Diameter and 'clock position' of the origin of each target vessel

Inexperienced clinicians may be tempted to delegate the planning phase to graft manufacturers' planning centres. This is a risky strategy because although technically accurate planning will be provided, it will be devoid of clinical judgement and compromise. Such grafts may be a 'true fit' but prove impossible to implant. Nevertheless, consultative engagement with (rather than delegation to) planning centres provides invaluable insights regarding device design limitations and should be considered mandatory for new adopters and later used as an expert resource for planning the more complex repairs. Used irresponsibly, planning centres can become a way for inexperienced physicians to gain access to a technique that they never fully control if they practice outside high-volume centres.

The following general principles apply when designing a stent graft:[23]

- The proximal and distal sealing zones of the device are positioned over healthy arterial segments (≥20 mm length). The proximal component of the device may have one or two internal sealing stents, two being preferable as it increases the length of the sealing zone in fenestrated devices. Two proximal sealing stents also provide a landing zone if a proximal extension is required during follow-up.
- Devices may incorporate scallops, small fenestrations, large fenestrations and/or branches to perfuse the target vessels.
- Usually if the gap between the deployed stent graft and the aortic wall bearing the target vessel is less than 10 mm, fenestrations are employed. If this gap is >10 mm, then the target vessels are perfused using branches. In the same stent graft, it is possible to combine fenestrations and branches. The diameter of the visceral vessel segment of the device can be modified to allow the use of either branches or fenestrations if particularly required.
- The anatomy of the target vessel also has an impact on the stent-graft design. When the angulation between the aorta and the target vessel is <60°, selective catheterization of this vessel through a fenestration, via femoral access, can be challenging. In this setting, the diameter of the aortic stent graft can be reduced to accommodate

a branch and facilitate access to the target vessel via an axillary or brachial approach. Target vessel stenosis and anatomic variations such as early branching of the target vessel may require careful selection of an appropriate bridging stent.

- The fenestrated component usually incorporates diameter-reducing ties to allow partial deployment of the graft and cannulation of the branches/fenestrations before the device is fully expanded. If the fenestration/branch is in contact with the wall of the aorta, then cannulation may be very difficult and this modification overcomes this issue, as well as allowing a degree of movement prior to final deployment.
- Large overlapping segments between the various stent-graft components and between the bridging stent grafts and fenestrations or branches are required if type III endoleaks are to be avoided.

PERIOPERATIVE ASSESSMENT

Hybrid room

Modern hybrid rooms that combine optimal open surgical environment and advanced imaging applications have been developed (Figure 28.4). These advanced applications can potentially contribute to reduce radiation dose, contrast media volume and optimize endovascular navigation.

Imaging fusion

Image fusion of aortic 3D volume rendering on live 2D fluoroscopy provides an accurate imaging guidance during endovascular procedures (Figure 28.5). As the fused aortic 3D model automatically follows table and detector movements, anatomy centring does not require fluoroscopy. Several methods are described to register the 3D volume, either from the preoperative CTA or from a contrast-enhanced cone-beam computed tomography (ceCBCT) acquired during the procedure. This latest

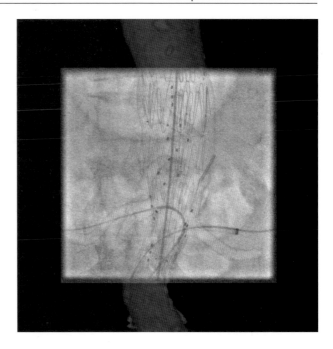

Figure 28.5 Fenestrated endograft implantation under fusion guidance. The stiff wire and sheath advanced into the left renal artery have straightened this artery. On the opposite side, the floppy wire has not modified the renal artery anatomy.

method is accurate but requires increased radiation dose and contrast media injection.

In our experience, before each procedure, a bone and an aortic 3D model are reconstructed from the preoperative CTA on a workstation (Advantage Workstation, GE Healthcare, Chalfont St Giles, United Kingdom) and then fused with live fluoroscopy (Innova Vision or Heart Vision applications, GE Healthcare). The registration of this 3D preoperative model is performed using bone landmarks visible on two fluoroscopic orthogonal shots (anterior–posterior and lateral) of the spine. During the procedure, this layout is then used to centre the region of interest and to identify the critical vessels origins. Position of the target vessels is confirmed by a 7 cc contrast-medium injection at 30 cc/s, and if necessary, registration can be refined at any time by the operator. We have reported that this

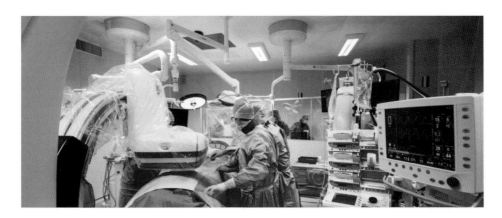

Figure 28.4 Hybrid room. (Courtesy of Discovery IGS 730, GE Healthcare.)

intraoperative guidance by preoperative CTA fusion significantly reduces radiation exposure for both patient and operator during standard and complex EVAR. Most of the other studies evaluating fusion during EVAR report a reduction in contrast media volume, but equivalent or higher radiation exposure when compared to their previous experience. Our results may partly be explained by our fusion protocol, which is contrast and almost radiation free, performed only with two fluoroscopic orthogonal shots.[24,25]

CeCBCT

ceCBCT is an advanced 3D imaging technology that is currently available on state-of-the-art flat panel–based angiography systems. Post-procedural ceCBCT has recently been proved to be adequate for assessment of incorporated vessel patency and stent-graft integrity[26] (Figure 28.6).

In our centre, ceCBCT is performed at the end of the fb-EVAR procedure in order to evaluate technical success, defined as successful deployment of the endoluminal graft, absence of a type I or type III endoleak, patent target vessels and endoluminal grafts without significant twist, kinks or obstruction.

This technique allows immediate treatment and potentially decreases the subsequent need for re-intervention. It may also potentially supplant follow-up CTA in the short-term period, minimizing the amount of radiation and contrast media delivered to the patient.[24]

Other techniques to reduce both radiation and contrast volume

New imaging systems are equipped with half-dose or low-dose modes to reduce radiation exposure with no impairment of image quality. Use of appropriate collimation allows accurate focus on the area of interest, reduces exposure of surrounding tissues for the patient and scattered radiation for the staff and increases image accuracy. Magnification induces higher exposure, with an increase of the exposure by the square of the magnification factor. To limit the need for magnification, late generation hybrid rooms are equipped with high definition large display monitors that provide large size images without magnification. The pulse mode, opposed to continuous fluoroscopy, is associated with a 90% reduction of produced images. Typical frame rate of 3.75 or 7.5 images/s is sufficient to perform aortic procedures in our daily practice.[24]

Every surgeon and endovascular therapist performing these complex procedures must undergo a dedicated radiation training programme.[18]

The use of automated contrast injector arm and contrast dilution (1:1 or 1:2 with saline) reduces the volume of contrast media injection.

DECISION MAKING IN ELECTIVE PROCEDURE FOR CAAs

Juxtarenal, pararenal and type IV thoracoabdominal aortic aneurisms

This subgroup of patients is usually referred to as 'pararenal aneurysms'. These aneurysms usually require fenestrated repair with limited coverage of the descending thoracic aorta. Their technical approach is similar and they have comparable outcomes in terms of vessels patency and (low) spinal cord ischaemia (SCI) rates.

GRAFT CONFIGURATION: f-EVAR
A custom made Zenith fenestarted stent graft (SG) by Cook Medical (Bloomington, Ind) requiring approximately

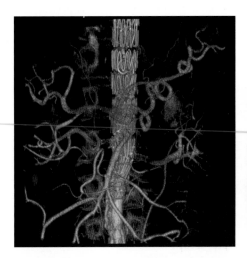
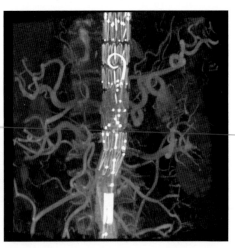

Figure 28.6 A contrast-enhanced cone-beam computed tomography is performed at the end of the procedure to check target vessel patency, stent-graft integrity and absence of endoleaks (3D volume rendering [VR] and maximum intensity projection [MIP] reconstructions of a 4-vessel fenestrated device).

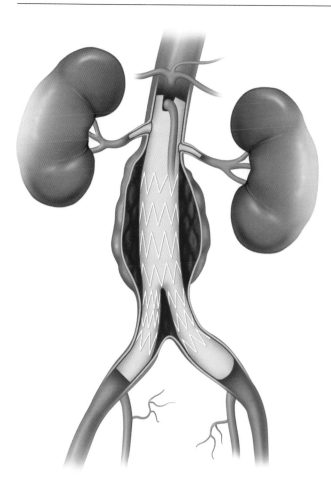

Figure 28.7 Schematic view of a fenestrated endograft designed with two small renal fenestrations and a scallop for the superior mesenteric artery.

6–8 weeks for manufacturing. These devices are modular, including a proximal tubular component with fenestrations, an uncovered proximal stent with barbs and diameter-reducing ties. It is introduced and deployed first.

There are three 'standard' configurations of fenestrations that are designed to match the ostial anatomy of the visceral arteries: small (6/8 or 6/6 mm), large (8–12 mm diameter) and scallops (6–12 mm deep, 10 mm large) (Figure 28.7). Various other fenestration designs can be manufactured (e.g. large scallops). Fenestrations are reinforced with a nitinol ring and marked with gold markers. The configuration of fenestrations and their positioning in height and on the circumference is planned according to individual patient anatomy based on preoperative CTA measurements. If the device is not properly designed, if alignment is inaccurate or if the catheterization of the visceral arteries is not possible, conversion to open surgery may become the only option.

After the visceral vessels have been mated to the fenestrated component with appropriately sized covered bridging stents, the second component, a bifurcated device similar to that used in standard infrarenal endovascular repair (without the bare-metal suprarenal

fixation stent), is introduced. It is recommended to ensure at least three stents of overlap between these two components to prevent inter-component separation and consequent type III endoleaks. The modular design serves to 'offload' the distal displacement forces of the aortic blood flow from the proximal fenestrated or branched component onto the distal bifurcated component and thus protect the visceral stents from kinking and occluding. The procedure is completed by the addition of iliac extension limb(s).

A new preloaded fenestrated delivery system is available on the zenith platform. Sheaths and wires can be advanced through the stent-graft delivery system directly to the renal fenestrations. This configuration is very useful in tortuous anatomies.

The Anaconda fenestrated stent graft is a custom-made repositionable device manufactured by Vascutek. Another fenestrated SG is the Anaconda, a custom made repositionable device manufactured by Vascutek (Inchinnan, United Kingdom).

The peaks of the proximal ring stents are placed suprarenal in a lateral position (in contrast to conventional deployment in which the peaks are positioned anteriorly and posteriorly), allowing flow to the SMA, which sits in the anteriorly oriented valley. The depth of the valley can be adjusted with the amount of oversize between the native vessel and the ring stent diameter or with an augmented anterior valley/scallop because the distance between the SMA and renal arteries is <5 mm. The fenestrations are placed in the unsupported region of the graft body. Each fenestration is supported with a nitinol ring.[10]

PROCEDURE: f-EVAR

Procedures are usually performed under general anaesthesia under invasive monitoring.

Open (or percutaneous) bilateral common femoral artery access is performed. When necessary (i.e. in the setting of severe external iliac stenosis), access to the common iliac arteries (CIAs) is an alternative (a conduit can be required). Prior to insertion, the fenestrations, branches and associated markers of the fenestrated body component (FBC) are recognized under fluoroscopy to ensure correct device orientation. After systemic heparinization with 100 international units/kg (target activated clotting time >300 seconds), the FBC is introduced on one side and a 20Fr sheath is inserted on the contralateral side, each over a stiff wire. The tip of the 20Fr sheath is positioned just proximal to the aortic bifurcation. The stiff wire is retrieved from the 20Fr sheath and 3 or 4 (depending on the number of fenestrations) and 6 or 7Fr 55 cm (depending on the diameter of the bridging stents) sheaths are introduced by direct puncture of the large sheath's valve (i.e. specifically avoiding multiple occupancy of the valve's central channel that would generate continuous bleeding). An angiography catheter is advanced over a guide wire through one sheath to an aortic position proximal to the target vessels. The FBC is advanced over its stiff guide wire to the required longitudinal position so that the fenestrations are correctly aligned with their matching target vessels. It is rotated as required to position the anterior markers in a medial position. This positioning is critical and can be repeatedly checked using small contrast volume angiography, if the procedure is performed without fusion guidance, until a satisfactory stable position is achieved. The outer sheath of the delivery system is then withdrawn to initiate device deployment. The diameter-reducing ties partially restrain the stent graft. This allows for repositioning if required. Wire access to the lumen of the stent graft is obtained via one of the contralateral sheathes. This sheath is then advanced over this wire to permit catheterization of the relevant target vessel through its corresponding fenestration. The soft guide wire is exchanged for a stiff one over a catheter advanced into the target vessel, and the access sheath is then advanced over it into the target vessel. This sequence of manoeuvres is repeated for each target vessel. Appropriately sized covered bridging stents are then advanced through the access sheaths into their target vessels. Once the bridging stents are all positioned in their target vessels, the diameter-reducing ties of the stent graft are released. If a proximal uncovered fixation stent has been included in the device design, it is

deployed at this stage. These steps fix the FBEG in position. In the final placement of each target vessel bridging stent and during catheterization of the fenestration, the C-arm tube is oriented perpendicularly to the fenestration. The bridging stent is positioned with 3–4 mm protruding into the aortic lumen and balloon expanded once the access sheath has been withdrawn. Finally, the aortic extremity of the bridging stent is the flared (rivet-like) with a 10 mm diameter and 2 cm long angioplasty balloon (Figure 28.8). To complete the procedure, the FBC is then connected to an infrarenal component as planned. Care is required in order not to dislodge or disrupt the FBC and its bridging stents when advancing the delivery system of the bifurcated component.[6]

Management of concomitant iliac aneurysms

Aneurysms of one or both CIAs, making them unsuitable for adequate distal sealing and therefore compromising the success of the endovascular repair and the feasibility of the procedure, may be present in up to 40% of EVAR patients. Coil embolization of the hypogastric artery trunk (if no concomitant hypogastric aneurysm is depicted), followed by stent-graft extension into the external iliac artery, is usually performed to prevent

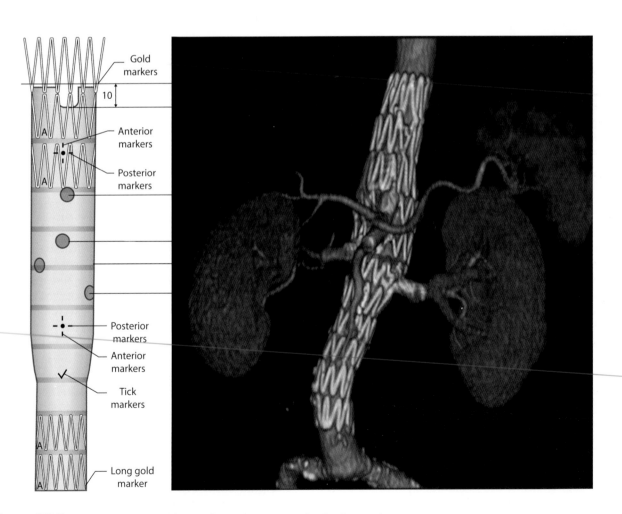

Figure 28.8 4 Vessel fenestrated device plan and post-procedural celiac trunk.

a type II endoleak. When the aneurysm involves both iliac arteries or in extensive aortic pathology, at least one hypogastric artery must be revascularized to ensure bowel and medullar perfusion. Iliac-branched stent grafts are an option to overcome this issue.

Type I, II and III thoracoabdominal aortic aneurysms

Extensive TAAAs are a major surgical challenge. Reported morbidity and mortality rates remain high (up to 20%) after open, hybrid or totally endovascular repair.[17,27]

The repair of descending thoracic and TAAAs exposes the spinal cord to ischaemic injuries and resultant paraplegia or paraparesis.[28] Over the last decade, endovascular TAAA repair has evolved from the occasional use of experimental devices by enthusiasts to become a validated routine technique for the repair of extensive aortic aneurysms. Although intuitively less invasive than open repair, thoracic and TAAA endovascular repairs are nonetheless still associated with high rates of SCI.[29] In a recent meta-analysis, SCI was described in up to 13% of patients after thoracic endovascular aortic repair (TEVAR).[30]

The mechanisms that underpin SCI are thought to be infarction secondary to absolute low perfusion (loss of intercostals covered by the fabric of the stent graft and poor collateral supply), reperfusion injury following per-procedural haemodynamic instability and micro-embolic 'trash' arising from intra-aortic manipulation. The first two are theoretically available to modification – essentially by optimization of the factors that underpin Starling's forces. The commonly described patient- and procedure-related risk factors for SCI illustrate these mechanisms.[31–34] They can be grouped into factors that directly or indirectly reduce flow/pressure in the anterior spinal artery (length of aortic coverage, poor internal iliac arteries LSA occlusion, hypotension) and those that reduce the oxygen-carrying capacity of the blood (blood loss). Other factors commonly cited as predictors of SCI are less easily explained (obesity, the use of adjunctive procedures, renal insufficiency). The question of additional SCI risk associated with previous infrarenal AAA repair is controversial. Adjunctive therapies have been reported for the prevention and treatment of SCI after TEVAR. Again, these focus on improving anterior spinal artery flow or reducing the resistance to flow after subcritical ischaemic injury and optimization of oxygen-carrying capacity and delivery. Examples include cerebrospinal fluid (CSF) drainage, LSA and hypogastric revascularization, intensification of oxygen delivery and pharmacologically induced hypertension.[35] While these strategies have substantially reduced the incidence of SCI in modern series of TEVAR, post-TEVAR paraplegia has not been eliminated. While TEVAR has been studied, to date, few reports have focused on SCI after TAAA endografting when evaluating these protocols aimed at spinal cord protection.[17,36,37]

PERI- AND POST-OPERATIVE ASSESSMENT IN THORACOABDOMINAL AORTIC ANEURYSMS

Proactive spinal cord protective protocol in our institution

CEREBROSPINAL FLUID DRAINAGE

A preoperative CSF drain was systematically established for all TAAA types I–III and V (i.e. not for type IV TAAA). A spinal drain was placed in the operating room by our dedicated cardiovascular anaesthesiology team the day before the procedure. CSF pressure was maintained <10 mmHg during and for at least 48 hours after the procedure. Continuous monitoring and recumbent positioning was performed in the ICU to avoid subdural bleeding and excessive CSF drainage. In patients without clinical evidence of SCI, CSF drains were removed 48 hours after the procedure. In the setting of documented SCI, CSF pressure was dropped to <5 mmHg and the drain was removed after neurologic recovery (or at a maximum of 5 days after the procedure).

EARLY PELVIC AND LOWER LIMB REPERFUSION

After implantation of the branch-/fenestration-bearing component and completion of any fenestrations, we immediately completed the bifurcated body and limb extensions to allow the early withdrawal of the large calibre (iliac occlusive) sheaths in order to allow early restoration of blood flow to the pelvis and lower limbs. Pelvic reperfusion enhances anterior cord perfusion via re-establishment of the internal iliac network.[38] The branches were then completed from an axillary arterial access as the final step.

PRE-EMPTIVE USE OF BLOOD PRODUCTS

At the end of the procedure, to further optimize spinal cord perfusion, blood, plasma and platelet transfusions were performed to avoid post-operative coagulopathy and blood loss. Fresh frozen plasma was transfused at 15 mL/kg and at least 1 pool of platelets was given, with therapeutic targets of haemoglobin > 10 g/dL, prothrombin time > 50%, plasma fibrinogen > 2 g/L and >100 g/L platelets.

HAEMODYNAMIC MINIMA

Volume resuscitation and vasoactive support were administered to maintain a mean arterial pressure of 85–90 mmHg (invasive haemodynamic monitoring) and a central venous oxygen saturation >75% after stent-graft deployment.

POST-OPERATIVE CARE

All patients were admitted to a dedicated cardiovascular intensive care unit for continuous haemodynamic monitoring and hourly lower limb neurological assessment for at least the first 48 post-operative hours.[39]

Staged and adjunctive procedures to preserve spinal cord flow

Following the demonstration of the potentially beneficial effects of a staged repair to encourage spinal cord preconditioning,[40] during extensive TAAA repair, we recommend implantation of the thoracic stent graft during a first procedure in all cases in which the anatomy was suitable.

Every effort to maintain the perfusion of at least one internal iliac artery is required, both whenever possible. When LSA coverage was deemed necessary for proximal seal, a carotid subclavian transposition or bypass is performed, as an initial procedure. These 'first-stage' procedures were performed 6–10 weeks before definitive TAAA repair.[39]

Branched endovascular stent graft

GRAFT CONFIGURATION

In the same stent graft, it is possible to combine fenestrations and branches.

Side arms are largely intended to be mated with self-expanding stent grafts (such as the Fluency stent, Bard Incorporated, Karlsruhe, Germany). They require a landing zone >15 mm in the target vessel for stable fixation and seal. A full overlap with the stent-graft side arm branch is mandatory. We routinely reline this bridging stent with a self-expanding nitinol stent to secure it and to provide a smooth transition between the Fluency and the target vessel (to avoid kinks). Preloaded catheters and wires can be prepositioned in the side branches to facilitate branch access, especially in the setting of challenging aortic tortuosity.[9] A larger introducer sheath for the stent-graft delivery system is then required.

PROCEDURE: b-EVAR

If the stent graft is manufactured with branches, the branch-bearing component is positioned so that the distal ends of the branches lie 10–15 mm above the ostia of the target vessels (Figures 28.9 and 28.10). If the device has only branches (i.e. no fenestrations), the distal body and iliac extensions are deployed once the branched component is in position, the large femoral sheathes are removed, and the femoral arteriotomies are closed (over small sheathes if necessary) to allow for the early restoration of blood flow to the pelvis and lower limbs. When devices are manufactured with branches and fenestrations, after implantation of the branch-/fenestration-bearing component and completion of the fenestrations, we immediately completed the bifurcated body and limb extensions to allow the early withdrawal of the large calibre sheaths.[39] The branches were then completed from an axillary arterial access as the final step. Through axillary arterial access, an 80 cm long 10Fr sheath is advanced into the stent graft, and each branch and its corresponding artery is catheterized, wired and stented with a self-expanding covered bridging stent. This sequence is completed one branch at a time, usually starting with the most distal branch first. The stents are each deployed over a stiff wire, and a bare

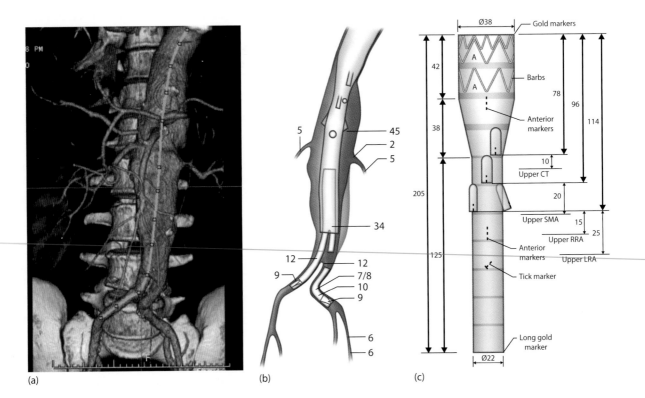

(a)   (b)   (c)

Figure 28.9 Thoracoabdominal aneurysm preoperative CTA 3D VR reconstruction (a) and anatomy sketch including the 4-branch endograft (b) and details of the device (c).

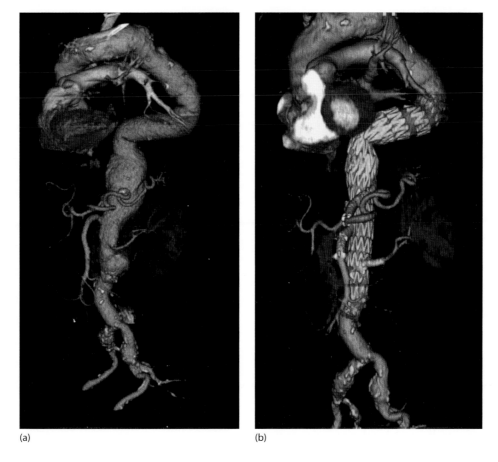

(a)   (b)

Figure 28.10 Thoracoabdominal aneurysm endovascular repair performed with a branched (celiac trunk and superior mesenteric artery) and fenestrated (renals) endograft (preoperative (a) and post-operative (b) 3D VR CTA reconstructions).

nitinol self-expandable stent is added inside each covered stent to add stability and avoid kinks.

Management of chronic aortic dissection

Total endovascular repair of chronic dissecting thoracoabdominal aneurysms including the visceral aorta with fenestrated stent graft is a challenging procedure. It is mandatory that the proximal and distal sealing zones of the stent graft are located in the true lumen. The latter is often very narrow which may hinder the ability to manipulate the main device and catheterize the target vessels located in the false lumen.

Access from the true to the false lumen and then to a target vessel via the dissection flap tear can be a challenging procedure. In our experience, access is always possible. If no flap tear is depicted, the flap can be punctured by means of different techniques, (transjugular intrahepatic portosystemic shunt needles, transseptal needle-sheath systems, simple reversed wires) using fusion or intravascular ultrasound guidance.[41] Access can be facilitated by dilating the dissection flap tear with a non-compliant balloon (8 or 10 mm diameter) during a procedure performed under local anaesthesia a few days or weeks before the fenestrated stent-graft

implantation. A new CTA is performed after this procedure to allow accurate design of the fenestrated stent graft.

A thorough analysis of the anatomical details of each individual dissection, especially the extent of the intimal flap and its fenestrations, is mandatory in planning successfully these complex endovascular repairs. This requires high-quality preoperative CTA.

Advanced imaging applications in the hybrid operating room provide important intraoperative 3D information support to facilitate the safe and effective execution of these challenging procedures.

Verhoeven et al. propose a staged approach beginning with the implantation of a proximal thoracic stent graft to expand the true lumen and thus facilitate a later fenestrated and/or branched stent-graft distal deployment.[42] The first-stage procedure (which excludes the dominant entry tear) can promote remodelling of the proximal thoracic aorta. Patients with large aortic diameters distal to the diaphragm require a second-stage fenestrated procedure 6–8 weeks after placement of the proximal thoracic stent graft. As a beneficial side effect, it is hoped that the delay between the procedures will promote the development of a collateral network at the level of the excluded intercostal arteries and thereby limit the risk of SCI associated with extensive aortic repairs.

We recommend using fenestrated devices rather than branch stent grafts to perform endovascular repairs in the narrow workspace of the true lumen. We do acknowledge that even fenestrated devices can be difficult to position and manoeuvre accurately. The use of preloaded catheters through renal fenestrations to simplify access to these target vessels and the addition of double-reducing tie wires at the posterior aspect of the device to limit its expansion during target vessel cannulation are helpful adjuncts in this setting.

We recommend sizing the various aortic components as follows:

- Thoracic stent graft: Proximal diameter is oversized by 10% according to the distal arch diameter, and distal diameter is equivalent to the maximum true lumen diameter.
- Fenestrated stent graft: Proximal diameter is oversized by 2 mm with reference to the thoracic stent-graft distal diameter. Diameter at the level of fenestrations should be equivalent to the maximum true lumen diameter at that level.[43]

The optimal strategy for the management of extensive post-dissection aortic aneurysms has not yet been determined; however, staged strategies are now recommended in the setting of extensive aortic disease.[44] If there is a satisfactory proximal sealing zone distal to the LSA, we use standard commercially available thoracic stent grafts for the first stage of these reconstructions. Where no such sealing zone exists, more complex options can be considered. The minimum length of the proximal thoracic sealing zone should be longer than 20–25 mm distal to the origin of left common carotid (LCC), and the maximal trans-aortic diameter should be no larger than 40 mm. When the sealing zone length or diameter distal to the LCC origin is inadequate for endografting, the options include open arch surgery, endovascular arch replacement and arch debranching with extra-anatomical reconstruction. We strongly advocate the first option, open surgery, as chronic dissections are associated with an increased risk of iatrogenic type A dissections when performing hybrid or total endovascular arch repairs.

Aortic arch aneurysms

The specific challenges of arch endovascular repair are related to the potential for neurologic complications, the inherent arterial angulation, the high blood flow and pulsatile movement of the aorta in this area and the proximity of the aortic valve.

In the literature, the largest experience of complete arch endovascular repair was performed using a branched device with two inner branches manufactured by Cook Medical (Bloomington, Ind)[45] (Figure 28.11). These two internal side branches have an enlarged external opening at their distal ends. The more proximal side branch is 12 mm (for the innominate trunk) in diameter and the distal one is 8 mm (for the LCC). Markers are placed on both ends

of each inner side branch to facilitate positioning under fluoroscopy. The extremities of the stent graft are wide for sealing, whereas the middle – the side branch-bearing portion – is narrow and straight to allow continuous supra-aortic perfusion and to facilitate branch cannulation. The device is loaded into a curved introducer, with a hydrophilic sheath. The curved system facilitates alignment of the branches with the greater curve of the aortic arch. The bridging component for the innominate artery is manufactured with low-profile graft fabric and loaded into a short 14F Flexor delivery system (Cook Medical). A commercially available covered stent Fluency (CR Bard, Murray Hill, NJ) or Viabahn (WL Gore, Flagstaff, Ariz) is used as the bridging component for the LCC artery.[45]

Others devices are now under study:

- Dual inner branch device (Bolton Medical, Inc., Sunrise, FL, United States) for arch aneurysms encroaching the supra-aortic trunks. This device is also manufactured with two inners branches for the innominate trunk and the left carotid artery.[46]
- Valiant Mona LSA Medtronic (Santa Rosa, California) branch stent-graft system is designed to enable the repair of thoracic aortic aneurysms encroaching on the LSA.
- Gore TAG thoracic branch endoprosthesis LSA also designed for the treatment of thoracic aortic aneurysms that require coverage of the LSA.[47]

PROCEDURE: TOTAL ENDOVASCULAR ARCH REPAIR

A LSA revascularization is performed before the arch endovascular repair in a 1-step or 2-step procedure (preferred option). To deliver the components, three arterial accesses are needed: The first access is the femoral access to insert the stent graft over a stiff wire positioned through the aortic valve into the left ventricle. The second one is the right common carotid or right axillary access to catheterize the innominate internal side branch and to insert the covered stent bridging the side branch to the innominate trunk. And finally, the third is the left axillary access to catheterize the LCC through the LSA transposition or bypass and the LCC internal side branch to deliver the covered stent bridging the side branch to the LCC. After systemic heparinization with 100 international units/kg (target activated clotting time >300 seconds), catheters and/or sheaths are placed to mark the origins of the innominate artery and LCC, a pigtail catheter is positioned into the apex of the left ventricle from the femoral access, and a stiff wire (Lunderquist; Cook Medical) is advanced through this catheter. The position of the tip of the stiff wire is constantly visualized. Under fluoroscopy, the orientation of the main body of the graft is verified outside the patient and then delivered over the stiff wire to the aortic arch. The tapered short tip is brought through the aortic valve into the left ventricle. An angiogram is performed, the branches along with their associated markers are positioned adequately, and the graft is deployed under rapid pacing (or other cardiac output suppression technique). Normal cardiac output is resumed before withdrawing

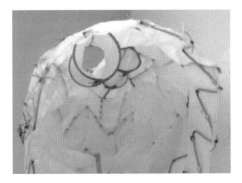
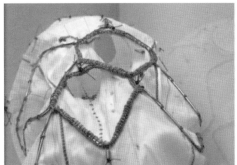
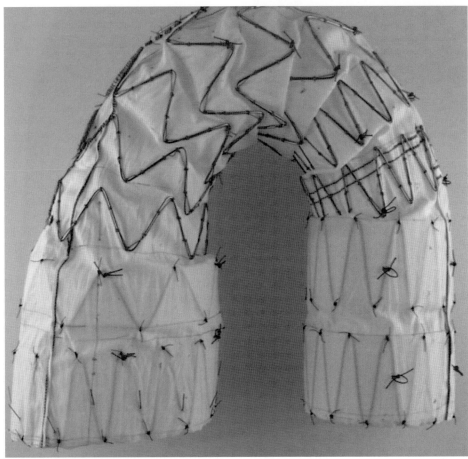

Figure 28.11 Inner branch arch device. (Courtesy of Cook Medical, Bloomington, IN.)

the tapered tip of the delivery system and the stiff wire from the left ventricle. The side branches are catheterized from the target vessels and sheaths are positioned into the inner side branches (Figure 28.12). Appropriate bridging limbs and covered stents are advanced through the access sheaths into the target vessels and deployed. On-table angiography is conducted to confirm complete exclusion of the aneurysm and patency of the branches.

LITERATURE ANALYSIS

Several studies have evaluated j-AAA and p-AAA repair with custom-made fenestrated stent grafts.[5–7,48]

In a recent literature review and meta-analysis, the outcomes of 776 patients undergoing fenestrated repair were analyzed. The pooled estimate for the 30-day mortality rate was 2.52%. The most common causes of death were bowel ischaemia and myocardial infarction. The technical success rate was 92.84% (95% CI: 87.48%–96.01%). The pooled estimate for primary target vessel patency rates was 98.26% (95% CI: 97.40%–98.84%) at 30-day and 94.52% (95% CI: 92.1%–96.2%) at 12 months. The post-operative permanent dialysis rate was 2.6%. Loss of vessel patency was caused by in-stent stenosis, stent fracture and stent-graft rotation. The re-intervention rate was 17.6%, with renal arteries thrombosis and type III and I endoleaks as leading causes.[49]

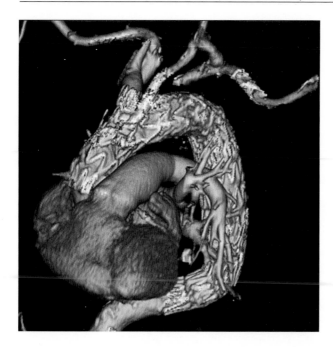

Figure 28.12 Arch and descending thoracic aorta aneurysm repair performed with a proximal arch branch endograft and a distal thoracic endograft extension.

Type IV TAAA fenestrated endografting was evaluated by combining the experience from 2 high-volume centres (231 patients from the Cleveland Clinic and Lille Aortic Centre). The 30-day mortality rate was 2.6%, the SCI rate was 1%, and the post-operative dialysis rate was 1%.[50]

Mastracci et al. show the midterm results of durability of branches in branched and fenestrated stent grafts. In 650 patients that underwent fb-EVAR, secondary procedures were performed for 0.6% of celiac, 4% of SMA, 6% of right renal artery and 5% of left renal artery stents. The mean time to re-intervention was 237 (354) days. The 30-day, 1-year and 5-year freedom from branch intervention was 98%, 94% and 84%, respectively. Death from branch stent complications occurred in three patients, two related to SMA thrombosis and one due to an unstented SMA scallop.[8]

Endovascular repair of TAAA with f-EVAR or b-EVAR has been associated with encouraging short-term results, with 30-day mortality ranging from 5% to 12% and SCI from 3% to 17%.[20,27,51,52]

However, patients undergoing fb-EVAR for TAAA remain fragile in the post-operative period and are particularly at risk of SCI and acute renal failure.

Verhoeven published outcomes in his series which included 50 patients (9 type I, 13 type II, 19 type III and 9 type IV). The primary technical success was 88% and the 30-day mortality rate 8%.[53]

The largest published series was performed at the Cleveland Clinic Foundation.[54] A total of 406 patients (16 type 1, 172 type 2 or 3 and 218 type 4) were treated. The estimated 1-year survival rates were, respectively, 70% for type 1, 74% for types 2 and 3 and 82% for type 4 TAAA.

At our institution, in December 2013, we had performed 204 TAAA endovascular repairs using custom-made devices manufactured with branches and fenestrations to maintain visceral vessel perfusion. We have compared the early post-operative results in patients treated before (group 1, 43 patients) and after (group 2, 161 patients) implementation of the modified implantation and perioperative protocols.

In this study, the early restoration of arterial flow to the pelvis and lower limbs and aggressive perioperative management significantly reduced SCI following TAAA endovascular repair. The 30-day mortality rate was 11.6% in group 1 versus 5.6% in group 2. The SCI rate was 14% versus 1.2%. If we exclude type 4 TAAA from this analysis, the SCI rate was 25% (6/24 patients) in group 1 versus 2.1% (2/95 patients) in group 2.[39]

The aforementioned data are retrospective analysis from single high-volume centres. A recent multicentre prospective study (WINDOWS trial) proposed a 'real-world' picture of endovascular repair of CAAs with FBSGs. Overall, technical success, aneurysm exclusion and target vessel's patency rates were satisfactory. Outcomes were related to aneurysm location and extent rather and also to patient's general status. In this study, mortality and morbidity rates were much higher than previously reported. The 30-day mortality rate was 6.7%, 4.3% for j-AAAs and 11.9% for p-AAAs and 11.9% for TAAAs. The in-hospital mortality rate was 10.1% (6.5% for j-AAAs, 14.3% for suprarenal and type IV TAAA and 21.4% for types III, II and I TAAA). The most frequent complications were severe renal insufficiency and SCI. The most frequent primary cause of death was multi-organ failure (26%). Of note, most centres had limited experience with f-EVAR for j-AAA and no experience at all for TAAA endografting. This study thus included the learning curve in patient selection, planning and implantation of most centres enrolling patients.[55]

The development of the total endovascular repair of arch aneurysms utilized the experience gained from the endovascular repair of TAAA using custom-designed FBSGs.[20,27] The initial results from a multicentric study confirmed that an exclusive endovascular approach to the arch may be an option in selected patients. A significant learning curve was observed in the study compared the first 10 patients (early experience group) with the subsequent 28 patients. Intraoperative complications and secondary procedures were significantly higher in the early experience group. Although not statistically significant, the early mortality was higher in the early experience group (30%) versus the remainder (7.1%).[45]

O'Callaghan et al. in the study evaluating outcomes of supra-aortic branch vessel stenting in the treatment of thoracic aortic disease reported the midterm results of fenestrated stent grafts (custom group) and compared them with results from chimney procedures (non-custom group) for proximal aortic aneurysm disease. Overall, the rate of technical success was 97%. There were 4 branch stent-related problems in the follow-up period, 1 of 15 (7%) in the custom group and 3 of 18 (17%) in the non-custom group. There were 3 proximal sealing failures in the immediate post-operative and follow-up period, 1 of 15 (7%) in the custom group and 2 of 18 (11%) in the non-custom group. Overall, 10 patients underwent secondary procedures, 4 of 15 (27%) in the custom group and 6 of 18 (33%) in the non-custom group.[56]

The technique and devices used today are evolving, and minimal long-term data are available on the durability of these repairs. For this reason, the endovascular approach to arch pathology has been reserved for patients deemed unfit for open and/or hybrid repair.

DECISION MAKING IN ACUTE CAAs

The risk of aneurysm rupture is 9.4% per year for a 5.5–5.9 cm aneurysm and up to 32.5% per year for a >7.0 cm aneurysm.[57] Considering a 6-week wait for a custom device, the rupture risk is expected to be approximately 1.1%–3.8% based on the size of the aneurysm. Standardized 'off-the-shelf' devices will solve this issue, facilitate manufacturing process and probably increase access to this technology.[41] Much effort has gone into the evolution of 'off-the-shelf' devices, and detailed analysis of the aortic anatomy of patients undergoing branched or fenestrated stent grafting has led to proposals for standard device designs that would fit the majority of patients, including emergency cases.

Off-the-shelf grafts

The p-branch (Cook Medical) device is a combination of two 'off-the-shelf' fenestrated stent-graft design (with pivot fenestrations for both renals, a large fenestration for the SMA and a scallop for the CT) to exclude juxta- and pararenal aortic aneurysms. The delivery systems incorporate preloaded renal sheaths. The diameters of both stent grafts range from 26 to 32 mm. The distance between the scallop for the CT and the SMA fenestration and the distance between both renal fenestrations differ on grafts #1 and #2.

Endologix (Irvine, California) has developed an alternative design named the Ventana device. It includes two 3 mm diameter renal fenestrations that can be dilated up to 10 mm. Its delivery system also comes with preloaded renal sheaths.[13]

A new off-the-shelf b-EVAR (t-branch; Cook Medical, Bloomington, Ind)[58] is now available for use in Europe. Its 'standard design' adapts to over 50% of TAAAs anatomies currently treated with a custom-made mbEVAR.[58–60] Early clinical evaluation of technical success and perioperative outcomes confirmed the safety and effectiveness of this device.[61,62]

Early experience with off-the-shelf devices does not demonstrate any significant renal risks.[63] However, the experience is limited and should be interpreted with caution until larger studies are published. Further studies comparing the outcomes of these techniques are required to establish the best approach to handle endovascular repair of CAA in an acute setting.

PATIENT FOLLOW-UP

CTA scan is the most widely used modality for follow-up after fb-EVAR and currently the standard method for evaluating target vessel patency and detecting endoleaks. All patients should have a CTA within 30 days of their procedure. If no endoleak is depicted on the post-operative CTA and if component overlap and visceral patency are satisfactory, follow-up can be broadly performed with ultrasound or contrast-enhanced Doppler ultrasound (ce-DU).[64] However, we currently still advocate performing a CTA 12 months after the procedure. Follow-up with ce-DU, non-contrast CT imaging and plain radiographs seems reasonable for patients with renal insufficiency.

Any increasing aneurysm diameter or new endoleak, after prior imaging studies have suggested incomplete aneurysm sac exclusion, should lead to prompt realization of a new CTA.

In our institution, an intraoperative ceCBCT is routinely performed at the end of the procedure in replacement of the completion angiogram. Immediate treatment of any technical issue can thus be performed before the patient leaves the hybrid room. A ce-DU is performed before the discharge. At 6 months, only a DU is performed and a CTA at 12 months.

All type I and III endoleaks, including visceral stent endoleaks, should be treated promptly during follow-up. Type II endoleaks without increased sac diameter can be observed.

WHERE TO PERFORM FENESTRATED–BRANCHED STENT-GRAFT PROCEDURES?

There is a learning curve in sizing, planning, implantation, intraoperative imaging and perioperative patient management. It is mandatory to be efficient with the use of 3D workstations and understand the influence of varying vessel tortuosity, calcification and calibre on device design. Various technical sequences, tips and tricks and salvage manoeuvres must be understood. It is important to develop a specialist team including surgeons, radiologists, anaesthetists, radiographers and nurses. The current centres of excellence have been involved in the development of the techniques and have acquired the range of 'soft skills' required (so often impossible to name, document and disseminate) over extended periods and many cases. We contend that fenestrated stent-graft repairs should only be performed in selected high-volume centres with appropriately dedicated teams, experience and technical infrastructure if the results currently reported for this technique are to persist. In our view, it is inappropriate for a novel high-risk solution for complex aneurysm repair in fragile patients to be generally disseminated to occasional institutions and operators.[65]

CONCLUSION

Technologies in endovascular aneurysm repair have evolved rapidly in recent years and there are now few situations where an endovascular option does not exist. Advances in imaging techniques have had a major role in the development of these complex endovascular procedures.

Several strategies are now being employed to apply endovascular solutions to complex aortic problems. The introduction of fb-EVAR in the management CAAs has improved outcome in patients at high risk for open repair.

However, mortality and complications are still important. A subset of patients is at a higher risk of death and complications. Thus, it is advisable to select patients appropriately for this technology to reduce the occurrence of intraoperative technical complications and post-operative mortality and morbidity rates.

The delay to manufacture FBSGs limits their applicability in the emergency setting. Significant effort has gone into the development of 'off-the-shelf' devices, and detailed analysis of the aortic anatomy of patients undergoing branched or fenestrated stent grafting has led to various options for 'standard' device designs that would fit the majority of patients.

There is currently industry emulation to develop new devices and improve delivery systems. These new developments will probably increase the applicability of this technique and its outcomes.

DECLARATION OF CONFLICTING INTEREST

Stéphan Haulon is a consultant for Cook Medical and GE Healthcare.

REFERENCES

1. Parodi JC, Palmaz JC, Barone HD. Transfemoral intraluminal graft implantation for abdominal aortic aneurysms. *Ann Vasc Surg.* 1991;5:491–499.
2. Faruqi RM, Chuter TA, Reilly LM et al. Endovascular repair of abdominal aortic aneurysm using a pararenal fenestrated stent-graft. *J Endovasc Surg.* 1999;6:354–358.
3. Chuter TA, Gordon RL, Reilly LM, Pak LK, Messina LM. Multi-branched stent-graft for type III thoracoabdominal aortic aneurysm. *J Vasc Interv Radiol.* 2001;12:391–392.
4. Inoue K, Hosokawa H, Iwase T et al. Aortic arch reconstruction by transluminally placed endovascular branched stent graft. *Circulation.* 1999;100:II316–II321.
5. Greenberg RK, Sternbergh WC, Makaroun M et al. Intermediate results of a United States multicenter trial of fenestrated endograft repair for juxtarenal abdominal aortic aneurysms. *J Vasc Surg.* 2009;50:730–737.e1.
6. Haulon S, Amiot S, Magnan PE et al. An analysis of the French multicentre experience of fenestrated aortic endografts: Medium-term outcomes. *Ann Surg.* 2010;251:357–362.
7. Verhoeven EL, Vourliotakis G, Bos WT et al. Fenestrated stent grafting for short-necked and juxtarenal abdominal aortic aneurysm: An 8-year single-centre experience. *Eur J Vasc Endovasc Surg.* 2010;39:529–536.
8. Mastracci TM, Greenberg RK, Eagleton MJ, Hernandez AV. Durability of branches in branched and fenestrated endografts. *J Vasc Surg.* 2013;57:926–933; discussion 933.
9. Greenberg RK, Qureshi M. Fenestrated and branched devices in the pipeline. *J Vasc Surg.* 2010;52:15S–21S.
10. Bungay PM, Burfitt N, Sritharan K et al. Initial experience with a new fenestrated stent graft. *J Vasc Surg.* 2011;54:1832–1838.
11. Dijkstra ML, Tielliu IF, Meerwaldt R et al. Dutch experience with the fenestrated Anaconda endograft for short-neck infrarenal and juxtarenal abdominal aortic aneurysm repair. *J Vasc Surg.* 2014;60(2):301–307.
12. Kitagawa A, Greenberg RK, Eagleton MJ, Mastracci TM. Zenith p-branch standard fenestrated endovascular graft for juxtarenal abdominal aortic aneurysms. *J Vasc Surg.* 2013;58:291–300.
13. Mertens R, Bergoeing M, Marine L, Valdes F, Kramer A, Vergara J. Ventana fenestrated stent-graft system for endovascular repair of juxtarenal aortic aneurysms. *J Endovasc Ther.* 2012;19:173–178.
14. Ohrlander T, Sonesson B, Ivancev K, Resch T, Dias N, Malina M. The chimney graft: A technique for preserving or rescuing aortic branch vessels in stent-graft sealing zones. *J Endovasc Ther.* 2008;15:427–432.
15. Donas KP, Torsello G, Austermann M, Schwindt A, Troisi N, Pitoulias GA. Use of abdominal chimney grafts is feasible and safe: Short-term results. *J Endovasc Ther.* 2010;17:589–593.
16. Ricotta JJ, Tsilimparis N. Surgeon-modified fenestrated-branched stent grafts to treat emergently ruptured and symptomatic complex aortic aneurysms in high-risk patients. *J Vasc Surg.* 2012;56:1535–1542.
17. Greenberg RK, Lu Q, Roselli EE et al. Contemporary analysis of descending thoracic and thoracoabdominal aneurysm repair: A comparison of endovascular and open techniques. *Circulation.* 2008;118:808–817.

18. Kirkwood ML, Arbique GM, Guild JB et al. Surgeon education decreases radiation dose in complex endovascular procedures and improves patient safety. *J Vasc Surg.* 2013;58:715–721.

19. Kirkwood ML, Arbique GM, Guild JB, Timaran C, Valentine RJ, Anderson JA. Radiation-induced skin injury after complex endovascular procedures. *J Vasc Surg.* 2014;60(3):742–748.

20. Guillou M, Bianchini A, Sobocinski J et al. Endovascular treatment of thoracoabdominal aortic aneurysms. *J Vasc Surg.* 2012;56:65–73.

21. Moll FL, Powell JT, Fraedrich G et al. Management of abdominal aortic aneurysms clinical practice guidelines of the European society for vascular surgery. *Eur J Vasc Endovasc Surg.* 2011;41(Suppl. 1):S1–S58.

22. Sobocinski J, Chenorhokian H, Maurel B et al. The benefits of EVAR planning using a 3D workstation. *Eur J Vasc Endovasc Surg.* 2013;46:418–423.

23. O'Brien N, Sobocinski J, d'Elia P et al. Fenestrated endovascular repair of type IV thoracoabdominal aneurysms: Device design and implantation technique. *Perspect Vasc Surg Endovasc Ther.* 2011;23:173–177.

24. Maurel B, Hertault A, Sobocinski J et al. Techniques to reduce radiation and contrast volume during EVAR. *J Cardiovasc Surg (Torino).* 2014;55:123–131.

25. Hertault A, Maurel B, Sobocinski J et al. Impact of hybrid rooms with image fusion on radiation exposure during endovascular aortic repair. *Eur J Vasc Endovasc Surg.* 2014.

26. Dijkstra ML, Eagleton MJ, Greenberg RK, Mastracci T, Hernandez A. Intraoperative C-arm cone-beam computed tomography in fenestrated/branched aortic endografting. *J Vasc Surg.* 2011;53:583–590.

27. Greenberg RK, Lytle B. Endovascular repair of thoracoabdominal aneurysms. *Circulation.* 2008;117:2288–2296.

28. Svensson LG, Crawford ES, Hess KR, Coselli JS, Safi HJ. Experience with 1509 patients undergoing thoracoabdominal aortic operations. *J Vasc Surg.* 1993;17:357–368; discussion 368.

29. Feezor RJ, Martin TD, Hess PJJ et al. Extent of aortic coverage and incidence of spinal cord ischemia after thoracic endovascular aneurysm repair. *Ann Thorac Surg.* 2008;86:1809–1814; discussion 1814.

30. Wong CS, Healy D, Canning C, Coffey JC, Boyle JR, Walsh SR. A systematic review of spinal cord injury and cerebrospinal fluid drainage after thoracic aortic endografting. *J Vasc Surg.* 2012;56:1438–1447.

31. Czerny M, Eggebrecht H, Sodeck G et al. Mechanisms of symptomatic spinal cord ischemia after TEVAR: Insights from the European Registry of Endovascular Aortic Repair Complications (EuREC). *J Endovasc Ther.* 2012;19:37–43.

32. Buth J, Harris PL, Hobo R et al. Neurologic complications associated with endovascular repair of thoracic aortic pathology: Incidence and risk factors. a study from the European Collaborators on Stent/Graft Techniques for Aortic Aneurysm Repair (EUROSTAR) registry. *J Vasc Surg.* 2007;46:1103–1110; discussion 1110.

33. Khoynezhad A, Donayre CE, Bui H, Kopchok GE, Walot I, White RA. Risk factors of neurologic deficit after thoracic aortic endografting. *Ann Thorac Surg.* 2007;83:S882–S889; discussion S890.

34. Ullery BW, Cheung AT, Fairman RM et al. Risk factors, outcomes, and clinical manifestations of spinal cord ischemia following thoracic endovascular aortic repair. *J Vasc Surg.* 2011;54:677–684.

35. Grabenwoger M, Alfonso F, Bachet J et al. Thoracic Endovascular Aortic Repair (TEVAR) for the treatment of aortic diseases: A position statement from the European Association for Cardio-Thoracic Surgery (EACTS) and the European Society of Cardiology (ESC), in collaboration with the European Association of Percutaneous Cardiovascular Interventions (EAPCI). *Eur J Cardiothorac Surg.* 2012;42:17–24.

36. Khan SN, Stansby G. Cerebrospinal fluid drainage for thoracic and thoracoabdominal aortic aneurysm surgery. *Cochrane Database Syst Rev.* 2012;10:CD003635.

37. Etz DC, Luehr M, Aspern KV et al. Spinal cord ischemia in open and endovascular thoracoabdominal aortic aneurysm repair: New concepts. *J Cardiovasc Surg (Torino).* 2014;55:159–168.

38. Bicknell CD, Riga CV, Wolfe JH. Prevention of paraplegia during thoracoabdominal aortic aneurysm repair. *Eur J Vasc Endovasc Surg.* 2009;37:654–660.

39. Maurel B, Delclaux N, Sobocinski J et al. The impact of early pelvic and lower limb reperfusion and attentive peri-operative management on the incidence of spinal cord ischemia during thoracoabdominal aortic aneurysm endovascular repair. *Eur J Vasc Endovasc Surg.* 2015;49:248–254.

40. Etz CD, Zoli S, Mueller CS et al. Staged repair significantly reduces paraplegia rate after extensive thoracoabdominal aortic aneurysm repair. *J Thorac Cardiovasc Surg.* 2010;139:1464–1472.

41. Sobocinski J, Resch T, Midulla M et al. Fenestrated and branched technology: What's new? *J Cardiovasc Surg (Torino).* 2012;53:73–81.

42. Verhoeven EL, Paraskevas KI, Oikonomou K et al. Fenestrated and branched stent-grafts to treat post-dissection chronic aortic aneurysms after initial treatment in the acute setting. *J Endovasc Ther.* 2012;19:343–349.

43. Sobocinski J, Spear R, Tyrrell MR et al. Chronic dissection – indications for treatment with branched and fenestrated stent-grafts. *J Cardiovasc Surg (Torino).* 2014;55:505–517.

44. Amr G, Sobocinski J, Koussa M, El Arid JM, Nicolini P, Haulon S. Staged procedure to prevent major adverse events in extensive aortic aneurysm repair. *J Vasc Surg.* 2013;57:1671–1673.

45. Haulon S, Greenberg RK, Spear R et al. Global experience with an inner branched arch endograft. *J Thorac Cardiovasc Surg.* 2014;148(4):1709–1716.

46. Kuratani T. Best surgical option for arch extension of type B dissection: The endovascular approach. *Ann Cardiothorac Surg.* 2014;3(3):292–299.

47. Monahan TS, Schneider DB. Fenestrated and branched stent grafts for repair of complex aortic aneurysms. *Semin Vasc Surg.* 2009;22:132–139.

48. Cross J, Gurusamy K, Gadhvi V et al. Fenestrated endovascular aneurysm repair. *Br J Surg.* 2012;99:152–159.

49. Di X, Ye W, Liu CW, Jiang J, Han W, Liu B. Fenestrated endovascular repair for pararenal abdominal aortic aneurysms: A systematic review and meta-analysis. *Ann Vasc Surg.* 2013;27:1190–1200.

50. Haulon S, Greenberg RK. Part Two: Treatment of type IV thoracoabdominal aneurysms – Fenestrated stent-graft repair is now the best option. *Eur J Vasc Endovasc Surg.* 2011;42:4–8.

51. Haulon S, D'Elia P, O'Brien N et al. Endovascular repair of thoracoabdominal aortic aneurysms. *Eur J Vasc Endovasc Surg.* 2010;39:171–178.

52. Chuter TA. Fenestrated and branched stent-grafts for thoracoabdominal, pararenal and juxtarenal aortic aneurysm repair. *Semin Vasc Surg.* 2007;20:90–96.

53. Verhoeven E, Tielliu IF, Zeebregts CJ et al. Results of endovascular repair of TAAA in the first 50 patients. *Zentralbl Chir.* 2011;136:451–457.

54. Greenberg R, Eagleton M, Mastracci T. Branched endografts for thoracoabdominal aneurysms. *J Thorac Cardiovasc Surg.* 2010;140:S171–S178.

55. Marzelle J, Presles E, Becquemin JP. Results and factors affecting early outcome of fenestrated and/or branched stent grafts for aortic aneurysms: A multicenter prospective study. *Ann Surg.* 2014;261(1):197–206.

56. O'Callaghan A, Mastracci TM, Greenberg RK, Eagleton MJ, Bena J, Kuramochi Y. Outcomes for supra-aortic branch vessel stenting in the treatment of thoracic aortic disease. *J Vasc Surg.* 2014;60:914–920.

57. Lederle FA, Johnson GR, Wilson SE et al. Rupture rate of large abdominal aortic aneurysms in patients refusing or unfit for elective repair. *J Am Med Assoc.* 2002;287:2968–2972.

58. Sweet MP, Hiramoto JS, Park KH, Reilly LM, Chuter TA. A standardized multi-branched thoracoabdominal stent-graft for endovascular aneurysm repair. *J Endovasc Ther.* 2009;16:359–364.

59. Bisdas T, Donas KP, Bosiers M, Torsello G, Austermann M. Anatomical suitability of the T-branch stent-graft in patients with thoracoabdominal aortic aneurysms treated using custom-made multibranched endografts. *J Endovasc Ther.* 2013;20:672–677.

60. Gasper WJ, Reilly LM, Rapp JH et al. Assessing the anatomic applicability of the multibranched endovascular repair of thoracoabdominal aortic aneurysm technique. *J Vasc Surg.* 2013;57:1553–1558; discussion 1558.

61. Bosiers MJ, Bisdas T, Donas KP, Torsello G, Austermann M. Early experience with the first commercially available off-the-shelf multibranched endograft (t-branch) in the treatment of thoracoabdominal aortic aneurysms. *J Endovasc Ther.* 2013;20:719–725.

62. Bisdas T, Donas KP, Bosiers MJ, Torsello G, Austermann M. Custom-made versus off-the-shelf multibranched endografts for endovascular repair of thoracoabdominal aortic aneurysms. *J Vasc Surg.* 2014;60:1186–1195.

63. Farber MA, Vallabhaneni R, Marston WA. "Off-the-shelf" devices for complex aortic aneurysm repair. *J Vasc Surg.* 2014;60(3):579–584.

64. Perini P, Sediri I, Midulla M, Delsart P, Gautier C, Haulon S. Contrast-enhanced ultrasound vs. CT angiography in fenestrated EVAR surveillance: A single-center comparison. *J Endovasc Ther.* 2012;19:648–655.

65. Haulon S, Barilla D, Tyrrell M, Tsilimparis N, Ricotta JJ. Debate: Whether fenestrated endografts should be limited to a small number of specialized centers. *J Vasc Surg.* 2013;57:875–882.

29

Aortic dissection

BENJAMIN O. PATTERSON and MATT M. THOMPSON

CONTENTS

INTRODUCTION

Aortic dissection is the most common of the acute aortic syndromes and occurs when the aortic intima separates from the media and adventitia.[1] Once a dissection flap is initiated via an 'entry tear', intimal disruption can propagate in either an anterograde or a retrograde direction, before re-entering the normal circulation. The resulting false lumen may compress the true aortic lumen, the ostia of aortic branches or expand rapidly due to weakening of the aortic wall. An insidious clinical presentation can delay diagnosis and this contributes to the high pre-hospital and in-hospital mortality observed in population studies.[2] The incidence of this condition appears to be increasing, with a 9/100,000 rate of dissection-related hospital admissions reported per year in the United Kingdom and 3/100,000 per year operations for dissection reported in the United States.[3,4]

Various attempts have been made to classify aortic dissections based mainly on the management options available in each situation. The most commonly used of these are the Stanford (type A/B) or DeBakey (types I, II and III) classification systems.[1,5] Both type I/II DeBakey and Stanford type A dissections originate within the ascending aorta, whereas type III DeBakey and Stanford type B begin in the descending aorta and extend into the aorta distally. DeBakey type III is subdivided into IIIa which terminates above the diaphragm and IIIb which continues

distally into the abdominal aorta and beyond. The classification of dissections that originate in the aortic arch is controversial.

Acute Stanford type A and complicated type B dissection requires immediate interventional treatment, whereas uncomplicated type B dissection has classically been managed with medical therapy alone. This is because open surgical repair of type B dissection has been associated with high mortality, morbidity and relatively poor long-term outcomes.[6] Subsequently, the first-line management of complicated acute and aneurysmal chronic type B dissections has shifted towards minimally invasive endovascular treatment, which has better short-term results (Figure 29.1).[7–9] Despite these advantages, the long-term durability of this approach is not comprehensively proven, especially with regard to chronic dissection.

CLASSIFICATION OF AORTIC DISSECTION

Anatomical classification

The anatomical classification of aortic dissection is dependent on disease configuration within the aortic arch, the distal extent and the relation of the entry tear to the origin of the great vessels (Table 29.1). As imaging techniques improve and treatment strategies become more defined, the classifications according to DeBakey and Stanford

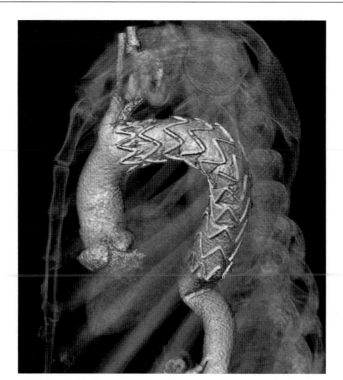

Figure 29.1 3D reconstruction of axial computed tomography images showing an endovascular stent graft in situ in a patient treated for acute complicated aortic dissection. The false lumen has completely collapsed leaving a widely patent true lumen.

based on conventional open surgical techniques may need supplementing with additional information. An attempt was made by Dake et al. to revise anatomical and clinical classification in line with advanced imaging techniques and endovascular management options based on the mnemonic DISSECT (*d*uration, *s*ize, *s*egmental *e*xtent, *c*linical complications of the dissection and *t*hrombus within the aortic false lumen).[10] This classification system includes information regarding the location of the primary entry tear and the segmental extent of aortic involvement as well as the size of the aorta based on centre-line measurements at different levels. It describes clinical presentation and

temporal manifestation as well as false lumen patency and thrombosis with regard to anatomical landmarks.

Temporal classification

Aortic dissection has classically been defined as being 'acute' during the first 2 weeks of presentation before becoming 'chronic'. This was based on the idea that most major adverse events will have occurred during this time frame. Of 384 patients with acute type B dissection in the International Registry of Acute Aortic Dissection (IRAD), the in-hospital mortality of those managed conservatively was 13%, and most of these patients died within 1 week.[11] More recently, a subacute phase has been described, between 2 and 12 weeks after presentation. This may be the optimum time to undertake interventional treatment for uncomplicated lesions, as the patient will have recovered from the acute physiological insult, but the dissection flap may still retain enough plasticity to allow remodelling.

Clinical classification

Aortic dissection can be further classified as complicated or uncomplicated, which determines the immediate management strategy in type B aortic dissection. Malperfusion (lower limb or visceral), rupture of the false lumen, the presence of rapid expansion, a large false lumen size or any other factor constituting a risk of imminent rupture defines complicated dissection and mandates

Table 29.1 Anatomical classification of aortic dissection.

DeBakey classification	
I	Originates in the ascending aorta; propagates at least to the aortic arch and often beyond it distally
II	Originates in and is confined to the ascending aorta
III	Originates in the descending aorta and extends distally down the aorta or retrograde into the arch
Stanford classification	
A	All dissections that affect the ascending aorta regardless of origin
B	All dissections that do not affect the ascending aorta

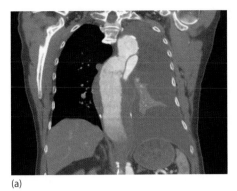 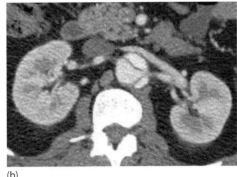

(a)   (b)

Figure 29.2 Computed tomography images showing patients with acute complicated type B aortic dissections. (a) There is a left-sided pleural effusion that is suggestive of rupture into the left hemi-thorax. (b) The true lumen is being compressed by the false lumen at the origin of the left renal artery causing malperfusion.

consideration of surgical intervention (Figure 29.2).[12] Other factors that may prompt consideration for intervention are refractory hypertension or pain during the acute phase. In the subacute or chronic phase, the main indication for treatment is ongoing expansion of the false lumen or extension of the dissection. Non-surgical treatment has historically been the standard of care for non-complicated acute type B aortic dissection as it is associated with less early morbidity than traditional surgical treatment and appears to be effective in preventing early aortic death.[13–15]

EPIDEMIOLOGY AND RISK FACTORS

The causes of aortic dissection are multifactorial, with inherited susceptibility and acquired degenerative disease contributing. Several modifiable and non-modifiable risk factors are recognized, the most important of which are discussed in the following texts.

Hypertension

Systemic hypertension is an important risk factor in the pathogenesis of aortic dissection, and many patients presenting with the condition will have high blood pressure that may have previously been undiagnosed. A relatively higher systolic blood pressure will increase the velocity of ejection from the left ventricle and increase the shear stress experienced by the outer curvature of the aortic arch. This is compounded by the fact that the aortic arch is relatively mobile in comparison with the descending thoracic aorta. As well as chronic hypertension, acute rises in blood pressure such as those occurring with physical exertion or emotional stress can lead to tears in the aortic intima and the development of a dissection flap.

Race and sex

A study of the IRAD revealed that 68% of all patients presenting with the condition were male and 79% were white.[16]

Although aortic dissection is less commonly found in black patients, the risk-factor profile is different. This group is often considerably younger (mean age 54 vs. 64 for white patients), more likely to be hypertensive (90% vs. 74%) and more than twice as likely to have left ventricular hypertrophy on echocardiogram (44% vs. 20%).[17]

Connective tissue diseases

Connective tissue diseases lead to a weakening of the aortic wall, increasing the risk of dissection. Younger patients with a dissection or aneurysm of the thoracic aorta will often suffer from some form of familial connective tissue disorder. Important conditions include Marfan's syndrome with fibrillin defects (found in 15%–50% of dissection patients under 40 years), Ehlers–Danlos type IV with abnormal synthesis of type III procollagen and other connective tissue disorders associated with cystic medial necrosis[16,18] (Figure 29.3).

Congenital cardiovascular abnormalities

There is a 5-fold to 18-fold increased risk of dissection in patients with bicuspid aortic valves due to association with a developmental defect of the proximal aorta which leads to aortic medial necrosis and dilation.[16] This is particularly found in younger patients (9% under 40 vs. 1% over 40). Coexistence of coarctation of the aorta and a bicuspid aortic valve increases the risk of acute aortic complications such as dissection by a factor of 5.[19] A group of familial aneurysmal syndromes also predispose to aortic dissection (Table 29.2).

Miscellaneous risk factors

Other risk factors include aortic vasculitic disease, cocaine misuse, pregnancy and cardiac interventions, including percutaneous revascularization and coronary artery

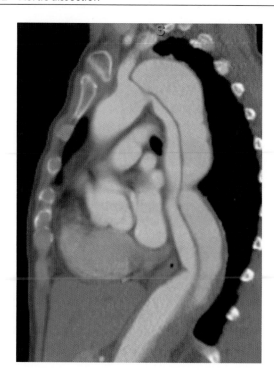

Figure 29.3 Computed tomography images showing an extensive type B dissection with acute dilatation of the false lumen in a patient with Marfan's disease who had a thoracic aortic aneurysm which was under surveillance.

bypass grafting. Patients with diabetes appear to have a lower rate of aortic dissection, although the exact mechanism of this protective effect is unclear.[20]

CLINICAL FEATURES

Acute aortic dissection often manifests clinically as the abrupt onset of sharp tearing or stabbing chest pain which radiates to the neck and back. Pain is absent in 10% of patients, and asymptomatic presentation is more common in diabetics.[21] Acute rupture or malperfusion may lead to rapid collapse and death, neurological deficits, symptomatic limb ischaemia or visceral ischaemia. Hypotension is seen in some patients with type A dissection, whereas hypertension is often present in patients with type B dissection. Chronic dissection is often asymptomatic but can be associated with ongoing back pain or compressive symptoms related to an aneurysm.

Table 29.2 Familial aortic aneurysmal syndromes associated with aortic dissection.

- Congenital contractural arachnodactyly
- Familial thoracic aortic aneurysm
- Erdheim's cystic medial necrosis
- Familial aortic dissection
- Familial ectopia lentis
- Marfan-like habitus

Table 29.3 Differential diagnosis of acute aortic dissection.

Patients with acute chest pain	
	Myocardial infarction
	Pulmonary embolism
	Spontaneous pneumothorax
Patients with acute abdominal or back pain	
	Ureteric colic
	Perforated viscus
	Mesenteric ischaemia
Patients with pulse deficit	
	Non-dissection-related embolic disease
Patients with focal neurological deficit	
	Stroke
	Cauda equina syndrome

There are many differential diagnoses (Table 29.3), but the presence of specific features may increase the likelihood of a dissection. Consensus guidelines from the American Heart Association place high-risk features into three categories.[22] *High-risk predisposing conditions* include aortic instrumentation, Marfan's syndrome or thoracic aortic aneurysmal disease. *High-risk pain features* include an abrupt onset of ripping, tearing or stabbing pain in the chest, back or abdomen. *High-risk features of the examination* include discrepancy in limb perfusion, focal neurological signs, a new murmur of aortic regurgitation and circulatory shock. Urgent imaging should be undertaken if clinical suspicion of aortic dissection is sufficient based on the presence of these features.[23]

INVESTIGATION OF SUSPECTED AORTIC DISSECTION

Axial imaging to visualize the whole aorta is mandatory if a diagnosis of aortic dissection is suspected. Serum D-dimer levels can be raised in the acute phase, and concentrations above 500 ng/mL are often detectable in patients with an acute dissection, although this test has been found to have a relatively low specificity.[24]

Computed tomography angiography

Multidetector computed tomography angiography (CTA) is the preferred investigation, as the images are acquired rapidly and immediate visual assessment of aortic morphology is possible, especially where the facility to perform 3D multiplanar reconstructions is available. The presence of complications such as contained rupture or malperfusion can be rapidly ascertained, and any intervention that may be necessary can be planned. A meta-analysis of 1139 patients with aortic dissection found that CTA had a sensitivity of 100%, specificity of 98% and diagnostic odds ratio of 6.5. The disadvantages of CTA are the need to use potentially nephrotoxic contrast media, exposure to ionizing radiation and inability to assess functional aortic insufficiency.

Echocardiography

The application of this technique is limited due to inability to reliably visualize the descending aorta, although it can diagnose aortic valve insufficiency and pericardial tamponade more effectively. Transoesophageal echocardiography can more accurately visualize the entire thoracic aorta and, despite the requirement for oesophageal intubation, can be performed at the bedside.[25] Transoesophageal echocardiography can also be an adjunct to endovascular repair due to the ability to see devices within the aortic lumen. The operator dependency of transthoracic and transoesophageal echocardiography limits their reliability.

Magnetic resonance angiography

Magnetic resonance angiography has a high sensitivity and specificity when used to diagnose aortic dissection. Gadolinium contrast agents used are less nephrotoxic than iodinated substances used for CTA, and there is no associated ionizing radiation. Disadvantages include its limited use in patients with claustrophobia or metal devices, although it can be used in those with nitinol aortic stent grafts. Long acquisition times and limited availability reduce its usefulness in the emergency setting, for which CTA is ideal. The use of newer '4D' cine MRI techniques may offer the potential for dynamic assessment of aortic dissection to determine the nature of blood flow within the true and false lumen. This information may be used to determine which patients are likely to benefit from earlier treatment due to an increased risk of subsequent aortic expansion.[26]

INITIAL MANAGEMENT OF AORTIC DISSECTION

The short-term goal of management is to resuscitate the patient and arrange definitive investigations to confirm the diagnosis. Persistent hypertension should be managed with intravenous beta-blockade using an agent such as labetalol to reduce aortic wall shear stress in the arch. A target heart rate of 60–80 beats/min and systolic blood pressure of 100–120 mmHg should be the aim, taking into account the patient's normal blood pressure. Glycerol trinitrate should be avoided as the reduction in diastolic blood pressure it causes may lead to a widened pulse pressure and a reflex tachycardia, which increases left ventricular ejection velocity. Invasive cardiovascular monitoring will be required and transfer of the patient to level II or III environment in a sufficiently experienced cardiovascular centre is mandatory. Whilst maintaining a low blood pressure is ideal, it is important to ensure adequate organ perfusion by monitoring urine output, neurological status checks and checking peripheral perfusion. Regular arterial blood gas analysis and examination for trends in markers of tissue perfusion may provide clues that malperfusion is developing.

DEFINITIVE MANAGEMENT OF ACUTE TYPE A DISSECTION

If not treated surgically, acute proximal (Stanford type A or DeBakey type I or II) dissection carries a 1-week mortality of up to 90% due to aortic rupture, stroke, visceral ischaemia, cardiac tamponade and circulatory failure. Urgent transfer to a dedicated aortic dissection centre is therefore required as soon as possible. The detailed surgical management of acute type A aortic dissection is outside the remit of this chapter. Simplistically, surgery involves replacing the section of the ascending aorta that contains the entry tear and potentially the whole arch with a prosthetic graft. If there is proximal extension of the dissection flap to the aortic valve, then this may require resuspension, and involvement of the aortic root may require the coronary arteries to be reimplanted. Adjunctive measures such as hypothermic circulatory arrest and selective perfusion of the cerebral circulation may be necessary. Surgery for proximal aortic dissection has a 5-year survival rate of up to 73%, and some of this mortality may be related to persistence of aortic dissection beyond the extent of the initial repair.[27] Some advocate complete arch replacement of the aortic arch and placement of an elephant trunk (frozen or conventional) at the time of initial surgery. This allows for subsequent endovascular treatment of any remaining dissection, to prevent subsequent expansion and rupture in the future (Figure 29.4).

The application of endovascular techniques to the management of type A dissection is often limited by the proximity of the entry tear to the coronary ostia and is presently only offered to patients who are not candidates for open surgical repair. A retrospective study of 105 patients who underwent open surgery for type A dissection showed that 35% would have been suitable for endovascular repair alone if this treatment had of been available. A further 8% would have become suitable if the distal landing zone had been extended with a carotid-to-carotid bypass.[28] Although many patients are not morphologically suitable for this form of treatment at present, it is likely that advances in device design will allow more aggressive endovascular approaches to arch in the future (Figure 29.5).[29]

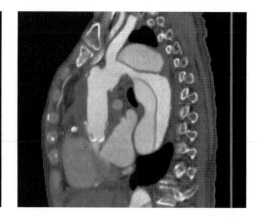

Figure 29.4 An acute type A dissection shown at time of diagnosis (above) and after surgical replacement of the ascending aorta. Note the persistence of the false lumen beyond the distal aortic arch which will almost certainly need further intervention in the future.

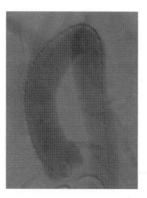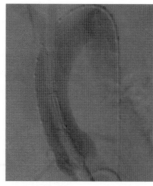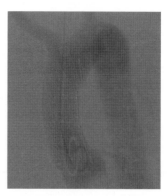

Figure 29.5 Endovascular treatment of a focal type A dissection using an endovascular stent graft. Access was achieved through the right carotid artery and the device covered an entry tear in the mid-ascending aorta.

MANAGEMENT OF TYPE B DISSECTION

If there is evidence from either imaging or physiological monitoring that the dissection is complicated by rupture, malperfusion or impending rupture, then intervention should be planned. If the patient remains stable, relatively normotensive and pain free (uncomplicated), then intravenous beta-blockade can be weaned down, whilst oral antihypertensives are introduced. If the clinical situation changes, there should be a low threshold for re-imaging. After 48–72 hours, further imaging should be arranged to reassess the aorta for expansion, extension of dissection or any clue that the rupture may be imminent, such as a left pleural effusion.

Early interventional treatment for acute complicated type B dissection

Open surgical repair was the mainstay of treatment for acute complicated dissection for many years, but this is associated with high levels of mortality and morbidity. The reason for this is the physiological insult caused by posterolateral thoracotomy, single-lung ventilation,

cross-clamping of the aorta, cardiopulmonary bypass, hypothermia and cerebrospinal fluid drainage to prevent paraplegia. With mortality rates as high as 30% reported in multinational registry data, endovascular repair is now seen as an attractive alternative.[30]

Endovascular treatment is undertaken by placement of a self-expanding endograft into the aorta via peripheral access, with the aim of covering the entry tear and promoting expansion of the true lumen and decompression of the false lumen by sealing the entry tear, preventing aortic branch vessels from being occluded or threatened. Secondary interventional procedures may be required to revascularize specific vessels, such as the common iliac artery or the visceral aortic branches. The long-term goal is to avoid subsequent aortic dilation that may later lead to rupture or other complications by promoting aortic remodelling.

Although conceptually endovascular treatment is an attractive first-line treatment for complicated acute type B dissection, there are relatively few good quality prospective studies with appropriate comparator groups. This is reflected in the lack of firm consensus in existing guidelines for practice.[22] The ongoing pathophysiological process itself and perioperative complications such as retrograde type A

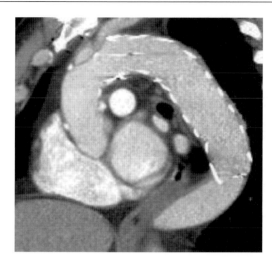

Figure 29.6 A Retrograde type A dissection following TEVAR for acute complicated type B dissection. This was managed conservatively as it was asymptomatic, relatively localized and remained stable at follow-up.

dissection means that all interventions are still associated with significant risk[31,32] (Figure 29.6). A meta-analysis of 942 patients showed an in-hospital mortality rate of 9%, with a serious morbidity rate of 8%. Re-intervention was required in 10% but subsequent aortic rupture occurred in <1%.[33] This is in agreement with more recent combined registry data which demonstrated an early mortality rate of 11%.[32] The VIRTUE registry contained 50 patients with acute type B dissections with 24 subacute dissections treated with endovascular stent grafts. The in-hospital mortality amongst the acute group was 12%, with a serious neurological complication rate of 10%. More patients in the subacute group were treated due to expansion, but there was a significant number who had developed malperfusion and some contained ruptures. No serious complications were recorded in this group during the perioperative period. In the setting of distal malperfusion, bare metal stents have been used to extend the main covered stent into the visceral aorta, with the aim of physically pinning back the false lumen whilst allowing flow into side branches, which has been termed the PETTICOAT (*p*rovisional

*ex*tension *to* induce *c*omplete *at*tachment) technique.[34] This has shown promise but required further evaluation due to relatively high levels of perioperative morbidity.

In patients that were followed up after endovascular repair of an acute complicated type B dissection, the dissection-related death rate was 0.6 per 100 patient-years for those who were followed up beyond 90 days. This suggests that early definitive treatment protects against aortic-related death in the midterm. The rate of aortic re-intervention was high in this group however, and there were 6.7 re-interventions per 100 patient-years of follow-up, three times that observed in the thoracic aortic aneurysm group.[32] This suggested that for some patients, the price for protection against aortic-related death is an increased risk of aortic re-intervention. Aortic remodelling is seen more in patients undergoing thoracic endovascular aortic repair (TEVAR) for acute aortic dissection in comparison with patients treated later, and this is usually observed during follow-up imaging as a significant reduction in false lumen diameter and an increase in true lumen diameter (Figure 29.7).[35] This has been seen to commence immediately following surgery and continue for many years in some and is associated with a lower incidence of endoleak/distal reperfusion and resultant re-intervention.[36]

Early treatment of uncomplicated aortic dissection

Studies reporting morphological changes in patients with untreated dissections of the aorta are few, but a recent study from the IRAD database has demonstrated that aortic expansion can be expected to occur in 59% of patients with acute uncomplicated dissection managed medically at 1–2 years. Paradoxically, those with a smaller aortic diameter initially exhibited the biggest expansion, whereas female gender, intramural haematoma and the use of calcium channel blockers were protective. Defining the natural history of aortic dissection and the factors that influence this in the different subgroups of patients is key to choosing the correct treatment options for individuals. Other factors that may predict aortic growth in patients with uncomplicated dissection include connective tissue

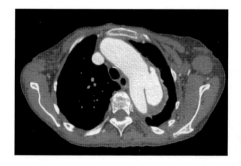
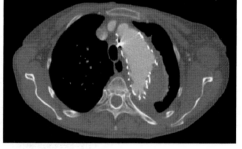

Figure 29.7 Computed tomography images of an acute type B aortic dissection with a large entry tear in the distal aortic arch before and after endovascular treatment that resulted in complete false lumen thrombosis and partial remodelling of the aorta at 6 weeks post-operatively.

disease, elliptical false lumen configuration, saccular false lumen, false lumen originating in the lesser curve of the aortic arch, large entry tear and multiple entry tears.[37] A study which described the likelihood of requiring surgical intervention based on the status of the false lumen in patients with acute uncomplicated type B dissection reported that in those with a completely thrombosed false lumen, none needed treatment as an inpatient. Conversely, 16% with a partially thrombosed false lumen and 26% with a patent false lumen required treatment. Of interest, mortality at long-term follow-up did not differ, but by 4 years follow-up almost 60% of those with a patent false lumen had undergone intervention compared with approximately 20% in the complete and partially thrombosed false lumen groups. Some preliminary work has suggested that increased metabolic activity within the aorta measured by PET scanning may also be at higher risk of adverse aortic events.[38,39]

The ADSORB study compared interventional treatment and medical management of uncomplicated aortic dissection, using aortic remodelling as the main end point. There were three crossovers from medical to the interventional group due to development of definite indications for surgery. One-year results from this study suggest that patients undergoing interventional treatment in addition to best medical therapy achieve better aortic remodelling within the first year.[40]

It would appear from recent studies that the outcome of immediate endovascular (and surgical) treatment of acute type B aortic dissection is consistently worse than for patients intervened on in the subacute phase, but in the presence of immediately life-threatening complications treatment clearly cannot be delayed. There is a subgroup of patients who do not have an absolute indication for intervention that may benefit from delayed treatment. In selected cases, those with labile blood pressure, persistent pain or a large but stable false lumen volume may be stabilized physiologically by a suitable interval of observation and maximal medical therapy. They could then undergo interval surgery performed by an experienced specialist on a semi-elective basis or continue with medical treatment if endovascular treatment is considered to be more hazardous (usually owing to adverse aortic morphological features or patient co-morbidity) than continued observation. Such measures may help to reduce the clear excess in mortality that is observed in patients undergoing intervention in the hyper-acute phase of presentation. There is evidence from large national databases that surgery for acute uncomplicated aortic dissection is safe.[41]

The investigation of stent grafts in aortic dissection (INSTEAD)-XL trial randomized 140 patients with a diagnosis of uncomplicated type B dissection to be treated either by TEVAR or best medical therapy (72 patients) or by best medical therapy alone (68 patients).[42] Although technically these patients were classified as being 'chronic', the median time to randomization was 39 days in the intervention group, which put many of these patients in a 'subacute' rather than a 'chronic' phase of aortic dissection. The primary end point of the study was all-cause death at 2 years but this was later extended to 5 years. Secondary end points were aortic-related death, aortic remodelling and a composite indicator of progressive aortic pathology that included crossover of medically management patients, additional procedures, expansion and malperfusion. In the intervention group, the peri-procedural mortality and morbidity was low, with two deaths, two serious intra-procedural technical complications and three serious neurological complications. A total of 14 patients were crossed-over from best medical therapy to the intervention group, with 5 of these performed as an emergency and 4 requiring open repair. Although the risk of midterm all-cause death was similar in both groups (11.1% vs. 19.3%), aortic specific mortality was lower (6.9% vs. 19.3%) and later disease progression was less frequent in the TEVAR group (27% vs. 46.1%). These results have prompted some to suggest that uncomplicated type B dissection should be treated with early TEVAR in the subacute phase.

Timing of treatment after acute type B dissection and effect on aortic remodelling

Recent data suggest that the outcome of immediate endovascular treatment of acute type B aortic dissection is worse than for patients intervened on in the subacute phase, but in the presence of immediately life-threatening complications, treatment clearly cannot be delayed. There is a subgroup of patients who do not have an absolute indication for intervention that may benefit from delayed treatment. In selected cases, those with labile blood pressure, persistent pain or a large but stable false lumen volume may benefit from a period of intense observation and medical therapy before undergoing surgery after a short interval, and recent evidence suggests that endovascular treatment of acute uncomplicated aortic dissection is relatively safe.[41] Alternatively, medical treatment could be continued if intervention is considered to be more hazardous due to adverse aortic morphology or patient co-morbidity than continued observation. Such measures may help to reduce the relatively high mortality observed in patients undergoing intervention in the hyper-acute phase of presentation.

Studies of the fate of false lumen in acute dissection patients have shown that there is a significant reduction in FL diameter following TEVAR with corresponding increase in the true lumen diameter.[35] The greatest changes were observed more proximally at the level of the stent graft. Total thrombosis of the false lumen was seen in 80.6%–90% of patients at this level at follow-up, which varied between 36 and 48 months on average. Unsurprisingly, the most marked change was seen in immediate post-operative period up to 1 year. Below the level of the diaphragm, total thrombosis of the false lumen was observed in fewer patients (22%–76.5%).

It has also been demonstrated that progressive growth of the true lumen and regression of the false lumen is associated with a lower incidence of endoleak/distal reperfusion and subsequent re-intervention. In chronic type B dissection, the maximum aortic diameter was observed to decrease or remain stable in the most studies, although in one study the diameter of the abdominal aorta increased. The occurrence of total false lumen thrombosis varied from 38% to 92.6%, and this occurred more commonly in less extensive dissections. In 15%–17% of patients, an increase in false lumen size was seen in at least one location. As for acute dissection, the occurrence of complete false lumen was reduced below the diaphragm in only 12.5%–45%, with some reports showing no reduction in the diameter of the false lumen at this level. One study demonstrated an increase in overall survival in those that showed signs of aortic remodelling. The VIRTUE study is one of the few studies to compare remodelling in subacute with acute and chronic dissection and found that the subacute group showed a similar degree of aortic remodelling to the acute group, especially at the level of the coeliac axis.[43]

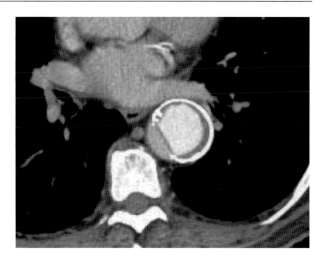

Figure 29.8 Computed tomography images of a chronic type B dissection at the level of the mid-descending thoracic aorta. Note the calcified, rigid appearance of the false lumen.

TREATMENT OF CHRONIC TYPE B DISSECTION

Uncomplicated chronic type B dissection with no indication to intervene is preferably managed conservatively, with regular surveillance scanning performed on an annual basis. Despite these, many patients develop aortic dilatation which may eventually require intervention, and following the results of the INSTEAD-XL study, this strategy could be questioned.[42,44] There is no way to predict with any certainty which patients will develop this complication. Generally, patients are considered for surgery when the aorta measures over 5.5 cm or when the false lumen measures over 4 cm. Open surgical repair has the perceived benefit of completely replacing the diseased segment of aorta, therefore reducing the need for re-intervention in the future, but even modern series from specialized centres report high levels of debilitating perioperative adverse events.[45]

Endovascular treatment can be performed with a relatively low morbidity and mortality in comparison with open surgical repair and protects against aortic-related death in the midterm[46,47] although there remain some concerns regarding long-term durability due to the relatively high rate of aortic re-intervention rates observed in studies such as the MOTHER registry.[32] The reason for the high level of aortic re-intervention after endovascular treatment of chronic type B dissection is due to the tendency of the dissection flap to become relatively fixed and immobile and therefore resistant to remodelling (Figure 29.8). The success of TEVAR for chronic dissection is dependent on maximizing the chances of aortic remodelling, and there is some evidence to suggest that certain factors relating to the repair may influence this.

A longer length of aortic coverage is intuitively preferable in chronic dissections, as a greater proportion of false lumen should be directly compressed as well as covering the main entry tear and any minor fenestrations in the descending thoracic aorta. A longer length of aortic coverage (>162 mm) has been shown to result in more false lumen thrombosis at 36 months in one study, although this did not necessarily translate into reduction in the whole aortic volume.[48] Dissection with infrarenal extension displays less tendency to remodel, potentially because treating the segment of aorta above the diaphragm will often not address the main re-entry tear.[35] This would suggested that longer coverage is necessary, as some re-interventions are linked to patent fenestrations.[49] Despite this, high rate of false lumen thrombosis was achieved in the INSTEAD trial where only a single stent graft was used in 83% of patients.[42]

A short stent graft which ends in the proximal descending thoracic aorta and does not conform correctly to the side walls may pose a risk of damage to the aortic wall due to the distal end moving with the cardiac cycle.[50] In combination with generous oversizing of the stent graft, this can traumatize the aortic wall and potentially perforate the intimal flap.[51] This may be avoided by sizing the stent graft according to the dimensions of the distal true lumen and may require the placement of tapered devices.

Retrograde aortic dissection is a particularly lethal complication of TEVAR for type B dissection and occurs in 4% of patients.[31] Most of these events occur in the immediate post-operative period and lead to mortality rate of up to 33.6%. According to the results of a systematic review, acute aortic dissection (odds ratio 10.0) and device oversizing (odds ratio 1.14 per 1% increase in oversizing above 9%) increase the risk of retrograde dissection significantly. The use of endografts with proximal bare stents was not associated with increased risk in the same study, but as it is likely that direct trauma to the aortic wall during TEVAR increases the risk of retrograde type A dissection, they should probably be avoided.

There are limited data regarding which type of endovascular device is most suited to treating aortic dissection and how to correctly plan endovascular repair. Most stent-graft systems are primarily designed to treat thoracic aortic aneurysms, and their indications for use reflect this. There is evidence to suggest that proximal and distal oversizing of endografts should be less aggressive to avoid unnecessarily excessive radial force, which has been associated with damage to the aortic wall and retrograde dissection.[31] Stents which employ active proximal fixation with bare stents and barbs should probably also be avoided for the same reason.

Timing of treatment

According to existing published current definitions, the cut-off point at which a dissection becomes 'chronic' varies, with some using 14 days from presentation and others using 90. There is no upper limit however, and some studies group patients who are 2 weeks from presentation with those who presented up to 15 years previously.[52] The INSTEAD trial intervention arm recruited patients at a median of 3.5 weeks after the diagnosis, meaning many would be categorized as subacute dissections. This partially explains why a 90.6% total false lumen thrombosis at 5 years was achieved in a group of patients with chronic dissection. Another study treated patients at a mean of 100 weeks post-diagnosis and only achieved false lumen thrombosis in 39% at 3-year follow-up.[53] This further supports the idea of a subacute group which may exist for up to a year in some cases.[43]

Branch vessel involvement and fenestrations

More aortic branches arising from the false aortic lumen and more visible fenestrations in the dissection flap may decrease the changes of false lumen thrombosis after TEVAR for chronic dissection.[49,52,54] Addressing this with uncovered bare stents may be possible, as placing a fenestrated or branched endograft is not possible if the aorta is not aneurysmal. Attempting to individually recanalize aortic branches from the true lumen is possibly not well described. If antegrade flow in the false lumen is not sufficiently sealed, then remodelling is unlikely to take place. If the entry tear is completely sealed, then flow is 'to and fro' locally through residual fenestrations as opposed to linearly in antegrade or retrograde direction, which is likely to produce lower mean pressures in the false lumen and promote remodelling or at least prevent expansion.[55]

Active false lumen thrombosis

If the aorta continues to expand and it is felt that remodelling is unlikely to occur, active management of persistent flow within the aortic false lumen can be considered. This may avoid recourse to further invasive surgery in those that may not be fit or where these is no conventional treatment option. This can be done using a covered stent, such as an iliac plug, a nitinol embolization plug or custom-made spindle-shaped devices that can be easily occluded after placement into the false lumen.[56,57] It has not yet been determined if this is a safe and durable technique although early results are promising.

SUMMARY POINTS

- Aortic dissection is diagnosed and managed according to its anatomical extent and chronicity.
- White men aged over 40 years with hypertension, or those under 40 with Marfan's syndrome or bicuspid aortic valves, are at highest risk.
- Patients often present with acute onset sharp chest pain, sometimes with loss of consciousness or poor perfusion of end organs.
- Computed tomography angiography is the first-line diagnostic investigation.
- Initial management should involve invasive cardiovascular monitoring and intravenous beta-blockade.
- Surgery is the first-line treatment for type A dissection.
- Endovascular treatment is the first-line treatment for acute complicated type B dissection, although some may benefit from a short period of observation prior to this.
- Endovascular repair uncomplicated type B dissection in the subacute phase appears safe and may prevent long-term complications.
- All patients need lifelong antihypertensive therapy and surveillance imaging.
- Chronic type B dissection should be treated if the aorta becomes aneurysmal, with endovascular treatment and open surgery offering effective prevention from aortic-related death.

REFERENCES

1. Tsai TT, Nienaber CA, Eagle KA. Acute aortic syndromes. *Circulation.* 2005 December 13;112:3802–3813.
2. Olsson C, Thelin S, Ståhle E, Ekbom A, Granath F. Thoracic aortic aneurysm and dissection: Increasing prevalence and improved outcomes reported in a nationwide population-based study of more than 14,000 cases from 1987 to 2002. *Circulation.* 2006;114(24):2611–2618.
3. Allmen von RS, Anjum A, Powell JT. Incidence of descending aortic pathology and evaluation of the impact of thoracic endovascular aortic repair: A population-based study in England and Wales from 1999 to 2010. *Eur J Vasc Endovasc Surg.* 2013 February;45:154–159.

4. Jones DW, Goodney PP, Nolan BW et al. National trends in utilization, mortality, and survival after repair of type B aortic dissection in the Medicare population. *J Vasc Surg.* 2014 July;60:11–19.e1.

5. Debakey ME, Beall AC, Cooley DA et al. Dissecting aneurysms of the aorta. *Surg Clin North Am.* 1966 August;46:1045–1055.

6. Fann JI, Smith JA, Miller DC et al. Surgical management of aortic dissection during a 30-year period. *Circulation.* 1995 November 1;92:II113–II121.

7. Dake MD, Miller DC, Semba CP, Mitchell RS, Walker PJ, Liddell RP. Transluminal placement of endovascular stent-grafts for the treatment of descending thoracic aortic aneurysms. *N Engl J Med.* 1994 December 29;331:1729–1734.

8. Nienaber CA, Fattori R, Lund G et al. Nonsurgical reconstruction of thoracic aortic dissection by stent-graft placement. *N Engl J Med.* 1999 May 20;340:1539–1545.

9. Dake MD, Kato N, Mitchell RS et al. Endovascular stent-graft placement for the treatment of acute aortic dissection. *N Engl J Med.* 1999 May 20;340:1546–1552.

10. Dake MD, Thompson M, van Sambeek M, Vermassen F, Morales JP, Investigators TD. Dissect: A new mnemonic-based approach to the categorization of aortic dissection. *Eur J Vasc Endovasc Surg.* 2013 May 27;1–16.

11. Suzuki T, Mehta RH, Ince H et al. Clinical profiles and outcomes of acute type B aortic dissection in the current era: Lessons from the International Registry of Aortic Dissection (IRAD). *Circulation.* 2003 September 9;108(Suppl. 1):II312–II317.

12. Fattori R, Cao P, De Rango P et al. Interdisciplinary expert consensus document on management of type B aortic dissection. *J Am Coll Cardiol.* 2013;1661–1678.

13. Tefera G, Acher CW, Hoch JR, Mell M, Turnipseed WD. Effectiveness of intensive medical therapy in type B aortic dissection: A single-center experience. *J Vasc Surg.* 2007 June;45:1114–1118, discussion 1118–1119.

14. Svensson LG, Kouchoukos NT, Miller DC et al. Expert consensus document on the treatment of descending thoracic aortic disease using endovascular stent-grafts. *Ann Thorac Surg.* 2008 January;85:S1–S41.

15. Estrera AL, Miller CC, Safi HJ et al. Outcomes of medical management of acute type B aortic dissection. *Circulation.* 2006 July 4;114:I384–I389.

16. Januzzi JL, Isselbacher EM, Fattori R et al. Characterizing the young patient with aortic dissection: Results from the International Registry of Aortic Dissection (IRAD). *J Am Coll Cardiol.* 2004 February 18;43:665–669.

17. Bossone E, Pyeritz RE, O'Gara P et al. Acute aortic dissection in blacks: Insights from the International Registry of Acute Aortic Dissection. *Am J Med.* 2013 October;126:909–915.

18. Albornoz G, Coady MA, Roberts M et al. Familial thoracic aortic aneurysms and dissections – Incidence, modes of inheritance, and phenotypic patterns. *Ann Thorac Surg.* 2006 October;82:1400–1405.

19. Oliver JM, Alonso-Gonzalez R, Gonzalez AE. Risk of aortic root or ascending aorta complications in patients with bicuspid aortic valve with and without coarctation of the aorta. *Am J Cardiol.* 2009;104(7):1001–1006.

20. Theivacumar NS, Stephenson MA, Mistry H, Valenti D. Diabetics are less likely to develop thoracic aortic dissection: A 10-year single-center analysis. *Ann Vasc Surg.* 2014 February;28:427–432.

21. Kodolitsch von Y, Schwartz AG, Nienaber CA. Clinical prediction of acute aortic dissection. *Arch Intern Med.* 2000 October 23;160:2977–2982.

22. Hiratzka LF, Bakris GL, Beckman JA et al. ACCF/AHA/AATS/ACR/ASA/SCA/SCAI/SIR/STS/SVM guidelines for the diagnosis and management of patients with Thoracic Aortic Disease: A report of the American College of Cardiology Foundation/American Heart Association Task Force on Practice Guidelines, American Association for Thoracic Surgery, American College of Radiology, American Stroke Association, Society of Cardiovascular Anesthesiologists, Society for Cardiovascular Angiography and Interventions, Society of Interventional Radiology, Society of Thoracic Surgeons, and Society for Vascular Medicine. *Circulation.* 2010;e266–e369.

23. Rogers AM, Hermann LK, Booher AM et al. Sensitivity of the aortic dissection detection risk score, a novel guideline-based tool for identification of acute aortic dissection at initial presentation: Results from the International Registry of Acute Aortic Dissection. *Circulation.* 2011 May 24;123:2213–2218.

24. Shimony A, Filion KB, Mottillo S, Dourian T, Eisenberg MJ. Meta-analysis of usefulness of d-dimer to diagnose acute aortic dissection. *Am J Cardiol.* 2011 April 15;107:1227–1234.

25. Shiga T, Wajima Z, Apfel CC, Inoue T, Ohe Y. Diagnostic accuracy of transesophageal echocardiography, helical computed tomography, and magnetic resonance imaging for suspected thoracic aortic dissection: Systematic review and meta-analysis. *Arch Intern Med.* 2006 July 10;166:1350–1356.

26. Clough RE, Waltham M, Giese D, Taylor PR, Schaeffter T. A new imaging method for assessment of aortic dissection using four-dimensional phase contrast magnetic resonance imaging. *J Vasc Surg.* 2012 April;55:914–923.

27. Ince H, Nienaber CA. Diagnosis and management of patients with aortic dissection. *Heart.* 2007 February;93:266–270.

28. Sobocinski J, O'Brien N, Maurel B et al. Endovascular approaches to acute aortic type A dissection: A CT-based feasibility study. *Eur J Vasc Endovasc Surg.* 2011 October;42:442–447.

29. Ronchey S, Serrao E, Alberti V et al. Endovascular stenting of the ascending aorta for type A aortic dissections in patients at high risk for open surgery. *Eur J Vasc Endovasc Surg.* 2013 May;45:475–480.

30. Tsai TT, Fattori R, Trimarchi S et al. Long-term survival in patients presenting with type B acute aortic dissection: Insights from the International Registry of Acute Aortic Dissection. *Circulation.* 2006 November 21;114:2226–2231.

31. Canaud L, Ozdemir BA, Patterson BO, Holt PJE, Loftus IM, Thompson MM. Retrograde aortic dissection after thoracic endovascular aortic repair. *Ann Surg.* 2014;260(2):389–395.

32. Patterson B, Holt P, Nienaber C, Cambria R, Fairman R, Thompson M. Aortic pathology determines midterm outcome after endovascular repair of the thoracic aorta: Report from the Medtronic Thoracic Endovascular Registry (MOTHER) database. *Circulation.* 2013 January 2;127:24–32.

33. Parker JD, Golledge J. Outcome of endovascular treatment of acute type B aortic dissection. *Ann Thorac Surg.* 2008 November;86:1707–1712.

34. Canaud L, Patterson BO, Peach G, Hinchliffe R, Loftus I, Thompson MM. Systematic review of outcomes of combined proximal stent grafting with distal bare stenting for management of aortic dissection. *J Thorac Cardiovasc Surg.* 2013 June;145:1431–1438.

35. Patterson BO, Cobb RJ, Karthikesalingam A et al. A Systematic review of aortic remodeling after endovascular repair of type B aortic dissection: Methods and outcomes. *Ann Thorac Surg.* 2014;97(2):588–595.

36. Kim KM, Donayre CE, Reynolds TS et al. Aortic remodeling, volumetric analysis, and clinical outcomes of endoluminal exclusion of acute complicated type B thoracic aortic dissections. *J Vasc Surg.* 2011 August 1;54:316–325.

37. van Bogerijen GHW, Tolenaar JL, Rampoldi V et al. Predictors of aortic growth in uncomplicated type B aortic dissection. *J Vasc Surg.* 2014 April;59:1134–1143.

38. Tanaka A, Sakakibara M, Ishii H et al. Influence of the false lumen status on short- and long-term clinical outcomes in patients with acute type B aortic dissection. *J Vasc Surg.* 2013 October 16;1–6.

39. Sakalihasan N, Nienaber CA, Hustinx R et al. (Tissue PET) Vascular metabolic imaging and peripheral plasma biomarkers in the evolution of chronic aortic dissections. *Eur Heart J Cardiovasc Imaging.* 2015;16(6):626–633.

40. Brunkwall J, Kasprzak P, Verhoeven E et al. Endovascular repair of acute uncomplicated aortic type B dissection promotes aortic remodelling: 1 year results of the ADSORB trial. *Eur J Vasc Endovasc Surg.* 2014 September;48:285–291.

41. Shah TR, Rockman CB, Adelman MA, Maldonado TS, Veith FJ, Mussa FF. Nationwide comparative impact of thoracic endovascular aortic repair of acute uncomplicated type B aortic dissections. *Vasc Endovasc Surg.* 2014 April;48:230–233.

42. Nienaber CA, Kische S, Rousseau H et al. Endovascular repair of type B aortic dissection: Long-term results of the randomized investigation of stent grafts in aortic dissection trial. *Circ Cardiovasc Interv.* 2013 August;6:407–416.

43. Virtue Registry Investigators. Mid-term outcomes and aortic remodelling after thoracic endovascular repair for acute, subacute, and chronic aortic dissection: The virtue registry. *Eur J Vasc Endovasc Surg.* 2014 October;48:363–371.

44. Winnerkvist A, Lockowandt U, Rasmussen E, Rådegran K. A prospective study of medically treated acute type B aortic dissection. *Eur J Vasc Endovasc Surg.* 2006 October;32:349–355.

45. Bashir M, Shaw M, Fok M et al. Long-term outcomes in thoracoabdominal aortic aneurysm repair for chronic type B dissection. *Ann Cardiothorac Surg.* 2014 July;3:385–392.

46. Tian DH, De Silva RP, Wang T, Yan TD. Open surgical repair for chronic type B aortic dissection: A systematic review. *Ann Cardiothorac Surg.* 2014 July;3:340–350.

47. Thrumurthy SG, Karthikesalingam A, Patterson BO et al. A systematic review of mid-term outcomes of thoracic endovascular repair (TEVAR) of chronic type B aortic dissection. *Eur J Vasc Endovasc Surg.* 2011 November;42:632–647.

48. Qing K, Yiu W, Cheng SWK. A morphologic study of chronic type B aortic dissections and aneurysms after thoracic endovascular stent grafting. *J Vasc Surg.* 2012 May 1;55:1268–1276.

49. Hughes GC, Ganapathi AM, Keenan JE et al. Thoracic endovascular aortic repair for chronic DeBakey IIIb aortic dissection. *Ann Thorac Surg.* 2014 December; 98:2092–2098.

50. Manning BJ, Dias N, Ohrlander T et al. Endovascular treatment for chronic type B dissection: Limitations of short stent-grafts revealed at midterm follow-up. *J Endovasc Ther.* 2009;16:590–597.

51. Zhang L, Zhou J, Lu Q, Zhao Z, Bao J, Jing Z. Potential risk factors of re-intervention after endovascular repair for type B aortic dissections. *Cathet Cardiovasc Intervent.* 2016;16(1):59.

52. Kitamura T, Torii S, Oka N et al. Key success factors for thoracic endovascular aortic repair for non-acute Stanford type B aortic dissection. *Eur J Cardiothorac Surg.* 2014 September;46:432–437, discussion 437.

53. Kang WC, Greenberg RK, Mastracci TM et al. Endovascular repair of complicated chronic distal aortic dissections: Intermediate outcomes and complications. *J Thorac Cardiovasc Surg.* 2011 November 1;142:1074–1083.

54. Tolenaar JL, Kern JA, Jonker FHW et al. Predictors of false lumen thrombosis in type B aortic dissection treated with TEVAR. *Ann Cardiothorac Surg.* 2014 May;3:255–263.

55. Rudenick PA, Bijnens BH, García-Dorado D, Evangelista A. An in vitro phantom study on the influence of tear size and configuration on the hemodynamics of the lumina in chronic type B aortic dissections. *J Vasc Surg.* 2013 February;57:464–474.e465.

56. Idrees J, Roselli EE, Shafii S, Reside J, Lytle BW. Outcomes after false lumen embolization with covered stent devices in chronic dissection. *J Vasc Surg.* 2014 December;60:1507–1513.

57. Kölbel T, Lohrenz C, Kieback A, Diener H, Debus ES, Larena-Avellaneda A. Distal false lumen occlusion in aortic dissection with a homemade extra-large vascular plug: The candy-plug technique. *J Endovasc Ther.* 2013 August;20:484–489.

30

Popliteal artery aneurysm

SAMUEL ERIC WILSON and JUAN CARLOS JIMENEZ

CONTENTS

Popliteal artery aneurysms are the most common peripheral aneurysms accounting for approximately 70%. Surgical treatment dates back to Antyllus, a third-century Greek physician who ligated both poles of the aneurysm and incised and packed the aneurysm sac. In 1785, John Hunter treated a coachman with a popliteal aneurysm by simply ligating the superficial femoral artery above the aneurysm (in what today is called Hunter's canal).[1] Matas performed endoaneurysmorrhaphy by ligating all branch vessels from within the aneurysm and suturing the walls of the aneurysm together. He performed this operation on 154 popliteal aneurysms between 1888 and 1920. In the 1950s, aneurysm exclusion and bypass with reversed saphenous vein interposition became the primary method of treatment. More recently endovascular repair has become common.

EPIDEMIOLOGY

Although popliteal aneurysms (Figure 30.1) are the most common form of peripheral artery aneurysms, the prevalence in the general population is low. In Detroit, at Henry Ford Hospital, popliteal aneurysm accounted for 1 in 5000 hospital admissions; there was 1 popliteal aneurysm per 15 abdominal aortic aneurysms. Popliteal aneurysm is a disease found almost exclusively in men, most often in the sixth decade of life (Table 30.1). Most popliteal aneurysms are fusiform and associated with atherosclerosis. They can also occur after trauma such as posterior knee dislocation, operative injury such as knee replacement or knee arthroscopy,[2] popliteal artery entrapment syndrome, inflammatory arteritis such as Behcet's or Kawasaki disease[3] and infected emboli and as a complication of bacteremia with organisms such as *Staphylococcus* and *Salmonella*.[4-9] Diseases associated with atherosclerosis are found in patients with popliteal aneurysm. Coronary artery disease and cerebral vascular disease occur, respectively, in 35% and 10% of patients; hypertension is present in 45% and diabetes mellitus in 13%.[3,7-13]

There is an astonishingly high rate of additional aneurysms in patients with popliteal aneurysm (Table 30.1). Bilateral popliteal aneurysms are found in about 50% of patients. Extrapopliteal aneurysms are found in 40%–75% of patients with a single popliteal aneurysm, and if bilateral popliteal aneurysms are present, there is a 68%–87% incidence of extrapopliteal aneurysm disease.[5,6,14,15] The abdominal aorta is most often affected, followed by the femoral and iliac arteries. The specific genetic defects that lead to arterial dilation are yet to be fully elucidated.[16,17]

In the patient found to have a popliteal aneurysm, a thorough examination must be made for additional aneurysms, particularly of the abdominal aorta and contralateral popliteal artery.

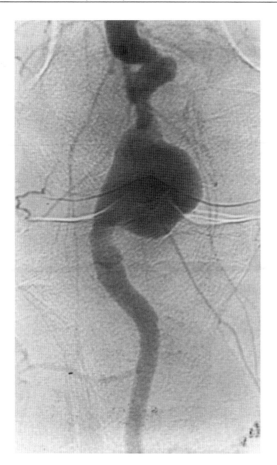

Figure 30.1 A typical angiogram of a popliteal aneurysm.

CLINICAL FEATURES

Approximately 70% of patients with popliteal aneurysms present with symptoms, often complications of thrombo-embolic disease ranging from claudication to rest pain and ischemic gangrene. Popliteal aneurysms, in contrast to aortic aneurysms, present with rupture less than 5% of the time.[13,17–19] Symptoms may also be caused by compression of neighbouring structures such as the sciatic nerve and popliteal vein in up to 10% of patients.[13,15,18,19] Compression may lead to radiculopathy, venous thrombosis and rarely arteriovenous fistula.[20]

DIAGNOSIS

Physical examination of the popliteal fossa and palpation of the popliteal pulse is usually an accurate and adequate screening test for low-risk patients; however, a very prominent popliteal pulse may signify dilation of the artery. Occasionally, a nonvascular mass such as a Baker's cyst may be mistaken on exam for an aneurysm.

Duplex ultrasound provides non-invasive confirmation of the diagnosis. A popliteal artery greater than 2 cm in diameter is usually considered aneurysmal.[14] To avoid mis-interpretation of a general dilatation, as in patients with arteriomegaly, it is appropriate to compare the diameter of the dilated vessel to the diameter of the distal superficial femoral artery. In such instances a vessel with a diameter 1.5–2.0 times the diameter of the proximal vessel is considered aneurysmal.[12,14]

Before elective intervention, it is prudent to screen for other aneurysms because of their relatively high coincidence. Depending on the findings of these screening tests, the order of treatment may need to be altered.

Ultrasound provides adequate sensitivity and specificity for most clinical decisions. Preoperative computed tomographic angiography, especially given recent advances to allow 3D reconstruction, gives high-quality images to the level of the popliteal artery and often below. Arteriography is reserved for the operating room to guide endovascular repair.

MANAGEMENT

Symptomatic aneurysms

Thromboembolic disease arising from the popliteal arterial aneurysm typically causes ischemic symptoms and physical findings. Given the relatively low rates of limb salvage once extensive embolization has occurred, any embolization should be considered a strong indication for surgery. Complete aneurysm thrombosis without embolization may also occur. The natural history of this condition is worsened by the relative paucity of collateral vessels around the bony and ligamentous knee joint.

Table 30.1 Epidemiology and percentage of additional aneurysms in patients with popliteal aneurysm.

| Series | Number of patients | Mean age | Male–female ratio | Percentage of other aneurysms | | | |
				AAA	Iliac	Femoral	Bilateral popliteal
Reilly et al.[11]	70	70	15:1	32	8	15	53
Whitehouse et al.[12]	61	67	30:1	62	36	38	44
Vermillion et al.[13]	87	60	28:1	40	25	34	68
Shortell et al.[21]	39	63	39:0	39	18	14	24
Halliday et al.[5]	40	64	19:1	30	5	22	50

Despite surgical intervention, 16%–50% of extremities that present with acute thrombosis or thromboembolism go on to minor or major amputation as either a primary or secondary procedure.[5,12–14,21]

Asymptomatic aneurysms

The management of asymptomatic popliteal aneurysms is more successful than treatment once symptoms have occurred. Accumulation of prospective natural history data on asymptomatic popliteal aneurysms is difficult as even large centres usually see fewer than 10 of these lesions per year. Retrospective analyses suggest that between 29% and 59% of popliteal aneurysms will become symptomatic over time.[6,22–24] The variables that will predispose to thromboembolism likely include size and extent of intraluminal thrombus, but this is not well defined. Dawson et al.[24] studied 42 patients over an average of 6.2 years who had asymptomatic popliteal aneurysms with an average aneurysm size of 3.1 cm. After 18 months, 59% developed symptoms, culminating in three leg amputations, one peroneal nerve palsy and eight limbs with claudication.

Delaying therapy until the onset of symptoms avoids operation in high-risk individuals, but adversely effects surgical outcome because of the pruning of outflow vessels. Varga et al.[25] followed 137 patients who were newly diagnosed with popliteal aneurysms to examine variables affecting results of repair. Grafts placed emergently had a 10% early bypass failure rate as opposed to 1.2% of those placed electively. With regard to safety and efficacy, in four series reporting operations on patients with asymptomatic aneurysms, there were no operative deaths; long-term limb loss was 0%–3%, and 89%–97% of patients remained symptom-free for years.[5,11,13,14]

In summary, the indications and timing of popliteal aneurysm repair require astute surgical judgement. In contrast to aortic aneurysms, the complications of popliteal aneurysms are limb but not life-threatening. In the high-risk patient, a case can be made for nonoperative management; however, this is less common today given the low risk of endovascular repair. For most patients, elective repair of a popliteal aneurysm (femoral–popliteal bypass or interposition with autologous vein) or exclusion by a stent graft is a definitive, safe operation that has clinical results that equal or exceed similar operations done for occlusive disease.[26] We recommend that an isolated asymptomatic popliteal aneurysm large enough to cause arterial turbulence or thrombus formation be considered for operative repair. These criteria would typically include aneurysms greater than 2.5 cm. The presence of thromboembolism discovered either clinically or radiologically should be considered a strong indication for surgery to avoid limb loss. Repair of the asymptomatic popliteal aneurysm has results much superior than intervention after ischemic symptoms develop.

Thrombolytic therapy

Thrombolytic agents, such as tissue plasminogen activator, catalyze endogenous fibrinolytic pathways. They have demonstrated efficacy in lysis of thrombus both acute and chronic, venous and arterial and in situ and embolic. Whether vascular patency will be preserved after thrombolytic recanalization depends on the nature of the primary lesion.

The use of thrombolytics in the treatment of popliteal aneurysms has a strong appeal since the most frequent cause of reconstruction failure is thromboembolic occlusion of outflow vessels.

The use of surgical thrombectomy is not necessarily easier because of frequent concomitant atheroocclusive disease and the difficulty in rescuing inframalleolar thromboembolism operatively. Thrombolysis may release additional embolism from the aneurysm sac. Catheter-based infusion directly into the distal embolus may help prevent or resolve this complication. Preoperative thrombolysis of a known thrombosed popliteal aneurysm which has not caused embolization is unnecessary and perhaps unwise.

The diagnosis of popliteal aneurysm is occasionally made incidentally after therapeutic thrombolysis for presumed atherosclerotic occlusion.

The overall effect of thrombolytics in a patient with thromboembolic outflow compromise appears to be beneficial. For example, Hoelting et al.[27] retrospectively compared 11 patients who received primary bypass surgery for acute popliteal aneurysm–related ischemia to nine similar patients who received thrombolytics prior to bypass surgery. There were five "occlusive complications" and one secondary amputation in the primary bypass group as opposed to none in the thrombolytic group. In a similar retrospective review, Carpenter et al.[26] compared 38 patients who received primary bypass surgery for acute popliteal aneurysm–related ischemia to seven similar patients who received thrombolytics prior to bypass surgery. These seven patients were described as having thrombosis of all three of their run-off vessels. The patients treated with preoperative thrombolysis had better graft patency and limb salvage than the patients that underwent emergency primary operation. Varga et al. prospectively compared 23 patients who received thrombolytics to 56 patients who had primary bypass surgery and concluded that "intra-arterial thrombolysis is of value in restoring the distal run-off before bypass in popliteal aneurysms presenting with acute limb-threatening ischemia."[25]

Surgery

The open operation of choice for popliteal aneurysm is construction by a reversed saphenous vein arterial bypass and exclusion of the aneurysm (should an autologous vein not be available, a polytetrafluoroethylene graft may be used as the arterial conduit.) A medial approach to the popliteal artery is taken, as classically described by Szilagyi et al.[15] Definitive treatment of popliteal aneurysms consists of aneurysm ligation and bypass. The typical bypass usually consists of an above-knee popliteal to below-knee popliteal bypass, although this can vary considerably in either direction, depending on the extent of aneurysmal disease. The best conduit for bypass is autologous vein.

The popliteal aneurysm can be exposed and bypassed by either the medial or posterior approach. The medial approach allows exposure of the greater saphenous vein, the above- and below-knee popliteal artery and the tibial vessels for selective tibial thrombectomy or more distal bypass. Without division of the hamstring tendons, the medial approach does not permit surgery directly on the aneurysm sac. When direct sac exposure is required, as in a patient with compressive symptoms requiring sac debridement, and when the extent of the aneurysm is clearly defined, many surgeons find the posterior approach simplest. The posterior approach allows a bloodless and superficial dissection of the entire popliteal artery. This exposure readily allows dissection and debridement of the aneurysm off neighbouring structures. For aneurysms limited to the popliteal fossa, the posterior approach may also permit a shorter interposition because of the better exposure. When necessary an additional 4–5 cm of superficial femoral artery can be exposed posteriorly by division of overlying adductor muscle fibres. Distal tibial exposure through the posterior approach, whilst possible, is more difficult than from a medial approach. One disadvantage of the posterior approach is that an additional incision will be required for harvesting of the greater saphenous vein. In general, patients with repaired asymptomatic aneurysms have higher long-term graft patency rates than do patents with symptomatic aneurysms.[18,21]

Endovascular repair

The advantages of lowered morbidity and earlier recovery are especially important in popliteal aneurysm, where many of the lesions are asymptomatic and none are life-threatening. Early reports include that of Puech-Leaao et al., who, through a posterior popliteal artery exposure, passed a Palmaz stent sewn to a saphenous vein graft superiorly into the superficial femoral artery to perform a proximal anastomosis (stent expansion) beyond the limits of surgical exposure.[28] May et al. reported successful deployment of an endovascular graft to exclude a popliteal pseudoaneurysm caused by knee replacement surgery.[29]

These early interventions were not uniformly successful. Mercadae reported six patients with popliteal aneurysms that were percutaneously treated with an endoluminal graft.[30] In this series, with follow-up less than 1 year, there was one case of thrombosis and one case of incomplete exclusion with recurrence. Mercadae concluded that 'stent grafting of popliteal aneurysms seems still to be reserved for elderly and poor condition patients'.

Contemporary outcomes are more favourable. Spesiale et al. treated 53 popliteal aneurysms using the peripheral Viabahn endograft with neither in-hospital mortality nor reintervention resulting in a primary patency of 74% after a mean follow-up of 3 years.[31] Wagenhauser et al. were cautious in their 2015 report, considering endovascular treatment 'an alternative' but pointing out that 'long-term results are pending' and stating that surgery was still the gold standard.[32] The Cochrane 2014 analysis concluded that 'endovascular repair should be considered as a viable alternative to open repair' and called for a randomized, multicentre trial.[33]

CONCLUSIONS

Popliteal aneurysms are not uncommon in the older male. The natural history consists of progression to aneurysm thrombosis or embolic occlusion of the infrapopliteal vessels. Approximately one third of untreated patients will become symptomatic within 3 years. If treatment is delayed until the onset of limb-threatening ischemia, the rate of limb loss is higher than if treated electively when asymptomatic. Popliteal aneurysms may be managed by ligation and bypass or endovascular repair. When outflow vessels are compromised, consideration should be given for preoperative thrombolytic therapy. Open repair of popliteal aneurysms can be accomplished through either the medial or posterior approaches. Endovascular exclusion is replacing open surgery but some reservations remain about long-term outcome.

REFERENCES

1. Schechter DC, Bergan JJ. Popliteal aneurysm: A celebration of the bicentennial of John Hunter's operation. *Ann Vasc Surg*. 1986;1:118.
2. Potter D, Morris-Jones W. Popliteal artery injury complicating arthroscopic meniscectomy. *Arthroscopy*. 1995;11(6):723.
3. Bradway MW, Drezner AD. Popliteal aneurysm presenting as acute thrombosis and ischemia in a middle-aged man with a history of Kawasaki disease. *J Vasc Surg*. 1997;26(5):884.
4. Wilson P, Fulford P, Abraham J, Smyth JV, Dodd PD, Walker MG. Ruptured infected popliteal artery aneurysm. *Ann Vasc Surg*. 1995;9(5):497.
5. Halliday AW, Taylor PR, Wolfe JH, Mansfield AO. The management of popliteal aneurysm: The importance of early surgical repair. *Ann R Coll Surg Engl*. 1991;73:253.
6. Farina C, Cavallaro A, Schultz RD et al. Popliteal aneurysms. *Surg Gynecol Obstet*. 1989;169:7.

7. Jimenez F, Utrilla A, Cuesta C et al. Popliteal artery and venous aneurysm as a complication of arthroscopic meniscectomy. *J Trauma*. 1988;28:1404.

8. Gillespie DL, Cantelmo NL. Traumatic popliteal artery pseudo-aneurysms: Case report and review of the literature. *J Trauma*. 1991;31:412.

9. Rosenbloom MS, Fellows BA. Chronic pseudoaneurysm of the popliteal artery after blunt trauma. *J Vasc Surg*. 1989;10:187.

10. Cole CW, Thijssen AM, Barber GG et al. Popliteal aneurysms: An index of generalized vascular disease. *Can J Surg*. 1989;32:65.

11. Reilly MK, Abbott WM, Darling RC. Aggressive surgical management of popliteal artery aneurysms. *Am J Surg*. 1983;145:498.

12. Whitehouse WM, Wakefield TW, Graham LM et al. Limb-threatening potential of arteriosclerotic popliteal artery aneurysms. *Surgery*. 1983;93:694.

13. Vermilion BD, Kimmins SA, Pace WG, Evans E. A review of one hundred forty-seven popliteal aneurysms with long-term follow-up. *Surgery*. 1981;90:1009.

14. Dawson I, Van BJ, Brand R, Terpstra JL. Popliteal artery aneurysms. Long-term follow-up of aneurysmal disease and results of surgical treatment. *J Vasc Surg*. 1991;13:398.

15. Szilagyi DE, Schwartz RL, Reddy DJ. Popliteal arterial aneurysms. *Arch Surg*. 1981;116:724.

16. Kontusaari S, Tromp G, Kuivaniemi H et al. A mutation in the gene for type III procollagen (COL 3AI) in a family with abdominal aneurysms. *J Clin Invest*. 1990;86:1465.

17. Kuivaniemi H, Tromp G, Prockop DJ. Genetic causes of aortic aneurysms: Unlearning at least part of what the textbooks say. *J Clin Invest*. 1991;88:1441.

18. Schellack J, Smith RB, Perdne GD. Nonoperative management of selected popliteal aneurysms. *Arch Surg*. 1987;122:372.

19. Hands LJ, Collin J. Infra-inguinal aneurysms: Outcome for patient and limb. *Br J Surg*. 1991;78:996.

20. Reed MK, Smith BM. Popliteal aneurysm with spontaneous arteriovenous fistula. *J Cardiovasc Surg (Torino)*. 1991;32:482.

21. Shortell CK, DeWeese JA, Ouriel K, Green RM. Popliteal artery aneurysms: A 25-year surgical experience. *J Vasc Surg*. 1991;14:771.

22. Gifford RW, Hines EA, Janes JM. An analysis and follow-up of one hundred popliteal aneurysms. *Surgery*. 1953;33:284.

23. Wychulis AR, Spittel JA, Wallace RB. Popliteal aneurysms. *Surgery*. 1970;68:942.

24. Dawson I, Sie R, van Baalen JM, van Bockel JH. Asymptomatic popliteal aneurysm: Elective operation versus conservative follow-up. *Br J Surg*. 1994;81(10):1504.

25. Varga ZA, Locke-Edmunds JC, Baird RN. A multicenter study of popliteal aneurysms. Joint Vascular Research Group. *J Vasc Surg*. 1994;20(2):171.

26. Carpenter JP, Barker CF, Roberts B, Berkowitz HD, Lusk EJ, Perloff LJ. Popliteal artery aneurysms: Current management outcomes. *J Vasc Surg*. 1994;19(1):65.

27. Hoelting T, Paetz B, Richter GM, Allenberg JR. The value of preoperative lytic therapy in limb-threatening acute ischemia from popliteal artery aneurysm. *Am J Surg*. 1994;168(3):227.

28. Puech-Leaao P, Kauffman P, Wolosker N, Anacleto AM. Endovascular grafting of a popliteal aneurysm using the saphenous vein. *J Endovasc Surg*. 1998;5(1):64.

29. May J, White GH, Yu W, Waugh R, Stephen MS, Harris JP. Endoluminal repair: A better option for the treatment of complex false aneurysms. *Aust NZ J Surg*. 1998;68(1):29.

30. Mercadae JP. Stent graft for popliteal aneurysms. Six Cases with Cragg Endo-pro System I Mintec. *J Cardiovasc Surg*. 1996;37(Suppl. 1):41.

31. Spesiale F, Siriggnano P, menna D et al. Ten years' experience in endovascular repair of popliteal aneurysm using the Viabahn prosthesis: A report from two Italian registries. *Ann Vasc Surg*. 2015;29:941–949.

32. Wagenhauser MU, Herma KB, Sagban TA et al. Long term results of open repair of popliteal artery aneurysm. *Ann Med Surg (Lond)*. 2015;4(1):58–63.

33. Joshi D, James RL, Jones L. *Cochrane Database Syst Rev*. 2014 August 31;8:CD010149.

31

Splanchnic artery aneurysms

RUSSELL A. WILLIAMS, JUAN CARLOS JIMENEZ and SAMUEL ERIC WILSON

CONTENTS

Splanchnic artery aneurysms involve the celiac, superior mesenteric and inferior mesenteric arteries and their branches. They occur relatively infrequently when compared to aneurysms of the aorta and iliac vessels, partly because there is a lower overall incidence of atherosclerosis in the splanchnic circulation. Atherosclerosis, associated with the great majority of aortic and iliac aneurysms, is present in less than half of splanchnic artery aneurysms. Whilst atherosclerosis can be found in some splanchnic artery aneurysms, it is thought to be a secondary process.[1]

Splanchnic artery aneurysms have a diverse aetiology and a correspondingly diverse natural history, but less is known about the natural history of splanchnic aneurysms than aortic aneurysms.[2]

Inflammation is an important primary cause of splanchnic artery aneurysms. It may occur from a primary vasculitis such as polyarteritis nodosa, a metastatic infection such as emboli from endocarditis or an extravascular process such as pancreatitis or a penetrating peptic ulcer. Peripancreatic pseudoaneurysms are estimated to occur in 10% of patients with chronic pancreatitis.[3] Polyarteritis nodosa is an autoimmune vasculitis which causes multiple aneurysms, typically less than 1 cm in diameter, of the small- and medium-sized muscular arteries of the abdominal viscera and kidneys. Due to their small size, intraparenchymal location and natural history, these aneurysms rupture only occasionally and do not often require surgery. In contrast, embolomycotic aneurysms have a very unpredictable natural history, which often end in fatal rupture and, unless completely resolved on follow-up angiography, are best treated with surgery. Other important causes of splanchnic artery aneurysms include haemodynamic and connective tissue alterations as well as trauma. Splanchnic artery aneurysms may be single or multiple depending on aetiology, and the wall may contain the three layers of the normal arterial wall or they may be false aneurysms.[4] Approximately 50% of splanchnic artery aneurysms occur in the splenic artery, 12% in the hepatic artery and 7% in the pancreaticoduodenal artery and to a varying degree in the celiac artery, the gastric and gastroepiploic arteries and colonic arteries.[5]

Splenic artery aneurysms (SAAs), the most common splanchnic artery aneurysms, have been variously estimated to occur in 0.8%–4% of patients undergoing angiography,[6] 10% of elderly patients at autopsy and 0.05% of autopsies of the general population.[7]

In general, a majority of splanchnic artery aneurysms are asymptomatic prior to rupture.[8] False aneurysms and peripancreatic, true aneurysms are reported to have a high but unpredictable rate of rupture.[9] When pain is present, it often signifies acute aneurysmal growth. Rupture rates and subsequent mortality rates are reported to be 2%–90% and 25%–75%, respectively, depending on location and aetiology.[6] Rupture may occur into the peritoneal cavity, causing haemorrhagic shock, or, as is common with inflammatory aneurysms, into adjacent structures such as the pancreas or the GI tract, causing related symptoms.

Angiography provides the anatomical detail necessary for the diagnosis and the planning of treatment of splanchnic artery aneurysms mainly because these aneurysms are often small, multiple and surrounded by or in direct connection with neighbouring vasculature or viscera. Other less invasive modalities, such as x-ray, ultrasound, computed tomographic angiography (CTA) and magnetic resonance imaging, are often diagnostic and useful in following aneurysmal growth over time. CTA can provide excellent images without arterial injection.

Surgical therapy, consisting of ligation or resection of an aneurysm with or without reconstruction, is the most conservative method of treatment and is effective in many instances.[10] Percutaneous embolization is often a less invasive alternative and is considered by some to be the procedure of choice for visceral aneurysms where the risk of end-organ ischemia from embolization is low or where the associated surgical morbidity is substantial, as with peripancreatic pseudoaneurysms.[11] In a limited number of situations, as with small atherosclerotic SAAs, these lesions may be safely observed.

SPLENIC ARTERY ANEURYSMS

SAAs have been recognized with certainty since 1770, when Beaussier[12] described one in a woman aged 60, at autopsy.

A majority of patients with SAA are 50–70 years of age, but 20% are 20–50 years of age, and among these younger patients, the female-to-male ratio is 20:1.[8] Overall, 87% of patients with SAA are females, and 80% are multiparous females. Ninety-five percent of patients who experience SAA rupture are pregnant.[7] Such epidemiology has led to the common speculation that changes in arterial connective tissue as well as increases in blood volume, portal congestion and splenic arteriovenous shunting related to pregnancy all contribute to splenic artery medial degeneration and aneurysm formation. One-eighth of women with SAA will also have fibromuscular dysplasia, an arteriopathy which predisposes to aneurysm formation.[1,13]

Nonpregnant patients with splenic artery hyperdynamic flow from causes such as cirrhosis, portal-systemic shunts or liver transplantation are also at increased risk of developing SAA. Splenic artery flow in cirrhotics has been found, on average, to be at least twice that in noncirrhotics. Seven percent of patients with portal hypertension undergoing angiography will have incidental SAA, and additional patients will have generalized splenic artery dilatation. Patients may also develop SAA from trauma, infected emboli and extravascular inflammatory processes, most notably pancreatic (historical note, President James A. Garfield died secondary to rupture of a traumatic SAA produced by a bullet wound during his attempted assassination).

Clinical presentation

Approximately 80% of patients with SAA are asymptomatic. In these patients the diagnosis is evident from the appearance of typical aneurysmal calcifications seen on a plain radiograph, incidental findings on angiography or symptoms of spontaneous aneurysmal rupture (Figure 31.1). Characteristic curvilinear aneurysmal calcifications can be found in 70% of patients with SAA. These findings, whilst easily identifiable, are not associated with lower incidence of rupture. Spontaneous aneurysmal rupture may cause bleeding into the peritoneal cavity or, as happens with inflammatory aneurysms, into adjoining structures such as the pancreas, the GI tract or (rarely) the splenic vein. Some 25% of the time, intraperitoneal rupture is transiently contained within the lesser sac, after which massive uncontained bleeding occurs through the foramen of Winslow or a rupture of the lesser omentum. This clinical phenomenon of 'double rupture' provides a window of opportunity for diagnosis and surgical intervention before the onset of hemorrhagic shock. The symptoms of aneurysmal rupture during pregnancy or after delivery may be mistaken for other common obstetric emergencies such as uterine rupture, abruptio placentae or amniotic fluid embolism especially since SAA rupture may occur during labour. Inflammatory aneurysms rupturing into pancreatic pseudocysts may create symptoms of abdominal pain and hypotension, as these cysts, when large, may sequester a large amount of blood. When such cysts communicate with the pancreatic duct, patients may develop acute or chronic GI bleeding. The syndrome, described as haemosuccus pancreatitis, usually requires angiography for a definitive diagnosis.[14]

Patients with noninflammatory SAA have a 2%–10% incidence of aneurysm rupture. The mortality of rupture may be as high as 70% in pregnancy and up to 25% in those who are not pregnant. The foetal mortality under these circumstances is high. Since the risk of mortality from prophylactic surgical treatment of noninflammatory SAA is low, patients should undergo surgery if they are or may become pregnant, if the aneurysm is greater than 2.0 cm or if they have referable abdominal symptoms.[9]

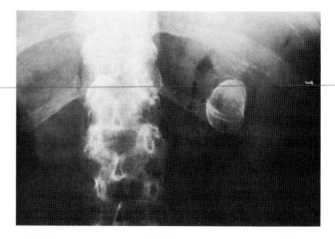

Figure 31.1 Calcified splenic artery aneurysm in a 60-year-old woman.

Operation for SAA due to pancreatitis has an associated mortality of 30% because of the persistent intra-abdominal sepsis presence of extensive inflammatory adhesions, pancreatic pseudocysts, multiple feeding vessels and enteric erosions as well as the possible need for splenectomy and partial pancreatectomy. Once rupture has ensued, the mortality increases to 50%.

Exposure for the surgical treatment of SAA provided by an upper midline incision or, alternatively, a left subcostal incision, which can be extended in a chevron fashion by adding a right subcostal incision, is also useful, especially in the obese or pregnant patient. The latter incision is more time-consuming to perform and inadvisable in an emergency, even if the diagnosis is known. The aneurysm itself is exposed by dividing the gastrocolic ligament to enter the lesser sac. Splenic preservation should be attempted, but this may not be possible if the aneurysm extends into the hilum of the spleen or if emergency surgery is being done for rupture.

SAAs secondary to pancreatitis may be densely adherent to the pancreas or may have ruptured into a pseudocyst or the pancreatic duct. They pose a more difficult technical problem because the dense inflammatory adhesions usually make operation difficult. Double ligation may even be very difficult; percutaneous arterial embolism and thrombosis of the aneurysm are often preferable and safer. Management of the patient who has rupture of a SAA into a very large pseudocyst that extends high under the left diaphragm and liver and which may be adherent to portal vein or even the inferior vena cava can be technically different and hazardous. Opening the pseudocyst to control the bleeding point usually leaves the surgeon with an obscured field that wells full of blood, at times making haemostasis impossible. In this situation the authors have introduced a balloon catheter into the abdominal aorta via the femoral artery to occlude the origins of mesenteric vessels. The gross size and situation of the cyst may preclude the use of a cross clamp of the aorta at the diaphragmatic hiatus. Once control of bleeding within the pseudocyst is achieved, a drain is placed, as many of these cysts communicate with the pancreatic duct and a pancreatic fistula or even pancreatic ascites is likely to ensue. Patients at high operative risk – such as cirrhotics – the elderly or those with extensive fibrosis from pancreatitis may benefit from nonoperative percutaneous catheter embolization of the splenic artery and aneurysm. An increasing number of reports of success using this technique are emerging. With the patient under local anaesthesia, the catheter is selectively placed within the lumen of the aneurysm.[15] The more commonly used small embolic particles of Teflon, Ivalon or Silastic are not used to cause thrombosis, as they are not retained in the aneurysm but embolize distally to the spleen. Instead, a Gianturco steel coil, which has woolly thrombogenic strands attached, is introduced. This expands after extrusion from the catheter, wedging itself within the lumen and making

embolization unlikely. Once in place, the coil acts as a baffle and the other thrombogenic materials can be injected.

HEPATIC ARTERY ANEURYSM

Hepatic artery aneurysms (HAAs) are one-third as common as SAA and affect males two to three times as often as females, which is a reversal of the sex ratio found in SAA. The reversal in gender occurrence may be because medial degeneration, responsible for most SAA, accounts for only 25% of HAP. Other important causes of HAA are trauma, atherosclerosis and inflammation. Trauma, which may be environmental or iatrogenic, accounts for 22% of HAP. Both blunt and penetrating trauma causes HAA, which may be true or false and intrahepatic or extrahepatic. Twenty percent of all HAA are intrahepatic, and a majority of these are caused by environmental trauma.[16] Iatrogenic trauma typically occurs from biliary surgery such as cholecystectomy, causing extrahepatic aneurysms of the right or common hepatic arteries. Percutaneous transhepatic procedures also can lead to HAA, usually of the intrahepatic type.

Inflammation, which accounts for 28% of HAA, occurs most frequently from embolism in a patient with infective endocarditis. Other less common causes of inflammation causing HAA include periarteritis nodosa, cholecystitis and pancreatitis.

Clinical presentation

Most patients with HAA are asymptomatic prior to rupture.[17] In these patients the diagnosis is based on vascular calcifications or detection of spontaneous aneurysmal rupture. In patients who have large aneurysms, displacement of neighbouring structures such as the biliary and GI tracts provides a diagnostic clue. Pain, when it does occur, is often associated with aneurysmal growth.

Spontaneous

HAA rupture occurs into the biliary tract as frequently as into the peritoneal cavity. One-third of patients with haemobilia will have the classic triad of haemobilia, pain and jaundice.[18] Rarely, these aneurysms will rupture into the portal vein, creating acute portal hypertension and bleeding varices. Rupture rates and subsequent mortality rates for HAA are 20%–44% and 35%, respectively.[16,19]

Investigations

On plain x-rays, atherosclerotic aneurysms will often appear as a rim of eggshell-like calcification;

ultrasonography and CTA delineate the aneurysm, showing its relation to the bile ducts or portal vein.

The definitive study for planning treatment is selective celiac or hepatic artery angiography. Angiography delineates the site and extent of the aneurysm, shows an arteriovenous fistula and demonstrates any arterial collaterals that have formed or enlarged portal venous collaterals if portal hypertension is present. It also outlines the anatomy of the liver's blood supply, which is via aberrant vessels in up to 40% of people. This is important information, as the arterial blood supply to the liver should be maintained following treatment, either through collaterals, normal aberrant arteries or a prosthetic or autologous vein graft to replace the excised, diseased segment of the artery.

Operations

Aneurysms located on the main hepatic artery proximal to the origin of the gastroduodenal artery may be excised or ligated, with the blood supply to the liver being maintained through collaterals from the superior mesenteric artery entering the gastroduodenal branch of the common hepatic artery. Excision, rather than double ligation, is desirable if the aneurysm is infected, large enough to produce obstructive symptoms of the biliary or intestinal system or if it communicates with part of the GI tract. In some cases it is safer to remove the aneurysm only partially, reducing its size by 'debridement' and leaving the sac, which may be adherent to the adjacent vital tissues. Occasionally patients may have had the gastroduodenal artery divided at a previous operation on the biliary system or the duodenum. In these patients, if collaterals are poorly developed, a saphenous vein graft can be used to restore arterial continuity after aneurysmal resection.

The 40% of patients who are found on arteriogram to have alternative origins of the hepatic arteries will have the origin of the anomalous artery from the left gastric or superior mesenteric artery. Identification of such vessels on preoperative angiography usually precludes the need to restore hepatic artery continuity. At operation, adequacy of arterial collateral blood flow to the liver is demonstrated if there is profuse back bleeding from the distal, divided end of the hepatic artery. Liver blood flow may also be restored by anastomosing the distal divided stump of the hepatic artery to an artery other than the celiac, such as the splenic, utilizing a segment of prosthetic material or a venous autograft. Invasive angiography has been used to thrombose HAAs and is the preferred method for treatment of intrahepatic aneurysms that otherwise would be treated by ligation of the right or left hepatic artery or even by hepatic lobectomy. Percutaneous embolization and thrombosis are generally not recommended for the treatment of an extrahepatic aneurysm because of the importance of maintaining the arterial blood supply to the liver. However, there are reports of extrahepatic aneurysms being successfully treated by arteriographic embolization in patients with additional illnesses, such as staphylococcal endocarditis, involving several heart valves where multiple mycotic aneurysms and liver malignancy had developed or previous surgery at which the diagnosis of leaking HAA was missed but subsequently found on an angiogram. There is one cautionary report of percutaneous hepatic aneurysm embolization proving fatal in a 73-year-old man with malignant obstruction of the bile duct who was treated by introducing an endoprosthesis for biliary drainage. A HAA complicated the initial procedure and was embolized, resulting in extensive hepatic necrosis.[20] Postoperatively, hepatic viability may be aided by inspired oxygen, bowel rest and hypertonic dextrose until liver function tests return to normal.

SUPERIOR MESENTERIC ARTERY ANEURYSMS

Unlike SAA and HAA, superior mesenteric artery aneurysms (SMAAs) are rarely caused by trauma or medial degeneration; thus, their overall incidence is proportionately lower. Most patients have subacute bacterial endocarditis or are intravenous drug abusers. Streptococcus species are commonly grown from the aneurysm, although in narcotic addicts Staphylococcus is also likely. Approximately 60% of SMAA are caused by embolism from infective endocarditis. Medial degeneration, when present, causes not only SMAA but also dissections. Embolomycotic aneurysms and dissections happen more often in the SMA than in the other splanchnic vessels. In the minority of patients, SMAA are atherosclerotic in origin, and plain radiograph may show ring-like calcification in the upper abdomen near the midline.

Clinical presentation

SMAAs are also unique in that the majority of these patients will manifest symptoms, usually of intestinal ischemia, prior to rupture.

In patients who have had bacterial endocarditis, the development of a SMAA should be considered, especially if there are complaints of abdominal symptoms, such as epigastric pain unrelated to meals. In some patients, especially those who are thin, a palpable, tender mass which is mobile from side to side may be felt. At times, a pulsation can be appreciated and the patient may have positive blood cultures.

Those patients who have a SMAA from another cause can present with similar pain but no antecedent history. The aneurysm will then be discovered during investigation (see Figure 31.2). With an atherosclerotic aneurysm, a plain radiograph of the abdomen often shows signet-ring-like

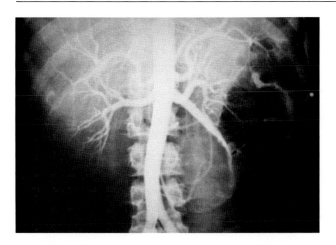

Figure 31.2 Mycotic superior mesenteric artery aneurysm in an intravenous drug abuser. (Courtesy of Dr. Albert Yellin, Haleiwa, HI. Emeritus Professor of Surgery, University of Southern California.)

calcification to the side of the midline with a posterior defect in the circumference, representing the origin of the superior mesenteric artery from the aorta. Otherwise, the aneurysm may be identified incidentally by CTA for another issue and occasionally only at laparotomy.

The natural history of mycotic aneurysms with persistence of infection in the arterial wall is of unrelenting enlargement and ultimately rupture. The history of atherosclerotic or other types of aneurysms is uncertain, though one could expect progressive enlargement and ultimate rupture.

Operations

The first SMAA to be treated successfully was a mycotic aneurysm operated upon by DeBakey and Cooley in 1949 by resection without restoring continuity of the SMAA. Following aneurysmectomy, the viability of the small bowel surprisingly may not be threatened, obviating the need for any additional procedure to restore arterial continuity. Progressive constriction of the aneurysmal lumen of the SMA and other splanchnic arteries is believed to stimulate hypertrophy of arterial collaterals. However, should aneurysmectomy result in an inadequate blood supply, the jejunal continuation of the artery may be anastomosed to the remaining SMA directly or by interposing a saphenous vein graft.

Following resection of a mycotic aneurysm, the use of a prosthetic graft or even a venous homograft, especially if it courses through the aneurysm bed, is best avoided. If flow is to be restored, an 'extra-anatomic' route from adjacent vessel such as the aorta to the jejunal or ileal segment of the superior mesenteric artery is chosen.

Other techniques for the treatment of saccular aneurysms include endoaneurysmorrhaphy. After inflow and outflow control, the aneurysm is opened and its orifice with the main artery, which may be only an ovoid slit several centimetres long, is oversewn from within the aneurysm, maintaining patency of the native vessel. This technique is particularly recommended for mycotic and traumatic false aneurysms, of which both originate from a limited area of weakness in the arterial wall.[21] As part of the management of mycotic aneurysms, the infected aneurysmal sac and contents are excised or debrided without necessarily excising the native vessel. A prolonged course of the appropriate antimicrobial agent is given, starting before operation and continuing for 6 weeks or more after operation. If this is discontinued too early, residual arterial infection may lead to reformation of an aneurysm.

A variant of aneurysmorrhaphy may be helpful to treat large saccular or fusiform aneurysms; the sac is opened after control of its inflow and outflow, and the orifices of native artery attached to the aneurysmal segment are oversewn from inside the sac. This, in fact, obliterates the involved segment of the artery, so it should be ascertained that no distal ischemia results.

Excision of many of these SMAAs may be difficult, as they can be adherent to important adjacent structures, including the superior mesenteric vein. An injury or deliberate surgical procedure that occludes the superior mesenteric vein is poorly tolerated and may produce ischemia of the small bowel along with ascites.

Operations of the main trunk of the SMA are usually done through a vertical abdominal incision. To expose the artery and its origin more proximally, the duodenojejunal flexure is mobilized and reflected medially and the pancreas elevated. The patient with a ruptured, freely bleeding SMAA often requires clamp control of the aorta at the diaphragmatic hiatus to stop bleeding and so permit operation on the aneurysm itself. Some very proximally situated aneurysms of the SMA may be operated on by exposing the origin of the artery extraperitoneally, reflecting the left colon and duodenum to the right. In some cases a thoracoabdominal incision facilitates this manoeuvre.

OTHER SPLANCHNIC ARTERY ANEURYSMS

These are very uncommon and include aneurysms of the celiac, gastric, gastroduodenal and pancreaticoduodenal arteries, the ileal and jejunal branches of the superior mesenteric trunk and – most rarely of all – the inferior mesenteric artery. The majority are atherosclerotic degenerative aneurysms, but some arise following trauma to the arterial wall or from local inflammation, particularly in the case of the pancreaticoduodenal and gastroduodenal arteries in patients with pancreatitis.

The rarity of these aneurysms makes them reportable and has led to many sporadic case reports from which recommendations have been extrapolated. It is thought

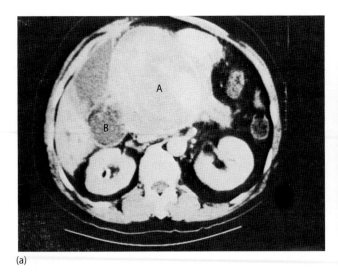
(a)

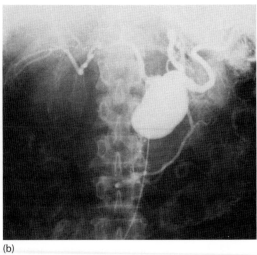
(b)

Figure 31.3 (a) CT scan with enhancement of celiac artery aneurysm (CAA) (A) compressing the extrahepatic bile ducts (B) producing biliary obstruction. (b) Angiogram of the same CAA.

that they, like aneurysms elsewhere, will all enlarge and, depending on their site, will obstruct adjacent organs, particularly the biliary system, and will ultimately thrombose or rupture (Figure 31.3a and b).

Pancreaticoduodenal and gastroduodenal artery aneurysms caused by pancreatitis usually present as bleeding following rupture into the pancreatic duct, the biliary system or adjacent bowel. These aneurysms should always be considered as possible points of origin of intestinal bleeding in patients with pancreatitis.

Celiac artery aneurysms

The celiac artery does not appear to be predisposed to a particular type of aneurysm, although it has been reported that 38% of patients with celiac artery aneurysms (CAA) have other splanchnic artery aneurysms and 18% have abdominal aortic aneurysms.[22] Atherosclerosis is associated with 27% of CAA.[22] Trauma and embolism are unusual causes of CAA.

As in the case of SMA, 60% of patients with CAA have abdominal discomfort prior to rupture and 30% have a pulsatile mass.[21] Rupture rates and subsequent mortality rates are 13% and 40%, respectively. Operation is successful in about 90% of cases. Surgical exposure, unless the aneurysm is small, will require a thoracoabdominal incision. Also, as in the case of SMAA, approximately one-third of patients with CAA will tolerate celiac ligation without reconstruction. Whether ligation is feasible should be determined from temporary intraoperative celiac artery occlusion. In 50% of cases, revascularization is performed.

Often, only the hepatic artery will require revascularization. In other instances complete revascularization, from either celiac artery reapproximation or placement of an interposition graft, is required.

Gastroduodenal and pancreaticoduodenal aneurysms

The close anatomic relationship of the gastroduodenal and pancreaticoduodenal arteries to the pancreas puts these arteries, like the splenic artery, at risk for development of inflammatory aneurysms (Figure 31.4). Sixty percent of gastroduodenal and 30% of pancreaticoduodenal aneurysms are caused by pancreatitis.[23] Patients with pancreatitis-related aneurysms may have symptoms prior to rupture, but these may be difficult to differentiate from symptoms of pancreatitis. When these aneurysms

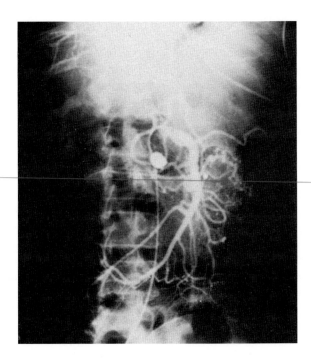

Figure 31.4 Pancreaticoduodenal artery aneurysm.

rupture, over half will do so into adjacent structures, including the GI tract, the pancreas and (rarely) the biliary tract, creating symptoms of acute or chronic GI bleeding.[24] Other aneurysms will rupture directly into the peritoneal cavity. Surgical intervention may be complicated and has an associated mortality of up to 30% leading to endovascular intervention as favoured treatment.[25]

Gastric and gastroepiploic aneurysms

Aneurysms of the gastric and gastroepiploic arteries occur through various mechanisms, the most common of which are atherosclerosis and medial degeneration. An unusual cause of gastric artery aneurysms is the so-called calibre-persistent artery of the stomach, also called cirsoid aneurysm, miliary aneurysm of the stomach or Dieulafoy's vascular malformation. These lesions are probably congenital anatomic variants in which gastric vessels penetrate the submucosa without decreasing in size or joining in the normal submucosal anastomotic plexus of vessels. In the presence of a calibre-persistent artery of the stomach, even the smallest of mucosal disruptions may lead to massive and usually lethal gastric bleeding.[26,27]

Gastric artery aneurysms most commonly develop in the gastric and not the gastroepiploic vessels. Unlike other splanchnic aneurysms, the majority of gastric artery aneurysms (70%) will rupture into the GI tract and not the peritoneal cavity. Ninety percent of patients with these lesions present with aneurysm rupture as their initial symptom. Because of the high rate of rupture, emergency surgery is the most common form of treatment. Ligation of the affected gastric vessel will not cause gastric ischemia. Arterial pathology may extend into the gastric wall, in which case local gastric resection should be performed.

INTESTINAL BRANCH ARTERY ANEURYSMS

Aneurysms of the jejunal, ileal and colic arteries are rare, usually appearing in case reports. The aetiology of solitary intestinal branch aneurysms is often difficult to ascertain; they may therefore be called 'congenital'. Multiple intestinal branch aneurysms are usually associated with a vasculitis, either autoimmune or embolomycotic. Symptoms of these lesions may include a palpable mesenteric mass or symptoms referable to intraluminal or intraperitoneal aneurysm rupture. These aneurysms tend to be small; preoperative angiography, if the patient's condition permits, is often very helpful in operative localization and in ruling out the possibility of multiple lesions. Surgical treatment can include arterial ligation, aneurysm resection and, if necessary, resection of involved bowel.

REFERENCES

1. Stanley JC, Fry WJ. Pathogenesis and clinical significance of splenic artery aneurysms. *Surgery.* 1974;76:898.
2. Pasha SF, Gloviczki P, Stanson AW, Kamath PS. Splanchnic artery aneurysms. *Mayo Clin Proc.* 2007;82:472–479.
3. Hofer BO, Ryan J Jr, Freeny PC. Surgical significance of vascular changes in chronic pancreatitis. *Surg Gynecol Obstet.* 1987;164:499.
4. Deterling RA. Aneurysms of the visceral arteries. *J Cardiovasc Surg.* 1971;12:309.
5. Pulli R, Dorigo W, Troiso N et al. Surgical treatment of visceral artery aneurysms: A 25 year experience. *J Vasc Surg.* 2008;48:334–342.
6. Owens JC, Coffey RJ. Aneurysms of the splenic artery, including a report of six additional cases. *Int Abstr Surg.* 1953;97:313.
7. Moore W, Guida PM, Schmacher HW. Splenic artery aneurysm. *Bull Soc Int Chir.* 1970;29:210.
8. Trastek VF, Bairolero PC, Joyce JW et al. Splenic artery aneurysms. *Surgery.* 1982;91:694.
9. Tetreau R, Beji H, Henry L, Valette PJ, Pilleul F. Arterial splanchnic aneurysms: Presentation, treatment and outcome in 112 patients. *Diag Interv Imaging.* 2015;15:229.
10. Marone EM, Mascia D, Kahlberg A et al. Is open repair still the gold standard in visceral artery aneurysm management? *Ann Vasc Surg.* 2011;25:936–946.
11. Cochennec F, Riga CV, Allaire E et al. Contemporary management of splanchnic and renal artery aneurysms: Results of endovascular compared with open surgery from two European vascular centers. *Eur J Endovasc Surg.* 2011;42:340–346.
12. Beaussier M. Sur un Aneurisme de l'artere Splenique Dont les Parios se Sont Ossifees. *J Med Toulouse.* 1770;31:157.
13. Bedford PD, Lodge B. Aneurysm of the splenic artery. *Gut.* 1960;1:312.
14. Lambert CJ Jr, Williamson JW. Splenic artery aneurysm: A rare cause of upper gastrointestinal bleeding. *Am Surg.* 1990;56:543.
15. Probst P, Castaneda-Zuniga WR, Gomes AS et al. Nonsurgical treatment of splenic artery aneurysms. *Diagn Radiol.* 1978;128:619.
16. Stanley JC, Thompson NW, Fry WJ. Splanchnic artery aneurysms. *Arch Surg.* 1971;101:689.
17. Salo JA, Aarnio PT, Jarvinen AA, Kivilaakso EO. Aneurysms of the hepatic arteries. *Am Surg.* 1989;5:705.
18. Countryman D, Norwood S, Register D et al. Hepatic artery aneurysm: Report of an unusual case and review of the literature. *Am Surg.* 1983;49:51.
19. Busuttil RW, Brin BJ. The diagnosis and management of visceral artery aneurysms. *Surgery.* 1980;88:619.
20. Sjovall S, Hoevels J, Sundqvist K. Fatal outcome from emergency embolization of an intrahepatic aneurysm. *Surgery.* 1980;87:347.

21. Olcott C, Ehrenfeld W K. Endoaneurysmorrhaphy for visceral artery aneurysms. *Am J Surg.* 1977;133:636.

22. Graham LM, Stanley JC, Whitehouse W Jr et al. Celiac artery aneurysms: Historic (1745–1949) versus contemporary (1950–1984) differences in etiology and clinical importance. *J Vasc Surg.* 1985;5:757.

23. Eckhauser FE, Stanley JC, Zelenock GB et al. Gastroduodenal and pancreaticoduodenal artery aneurysms: A complication of pancreatitis causing spontaneous gastrointestinal hemorrhage. *Surgery.* 1980;88:335.

24. Gangahar DM, Carveth SW, Reese HE et al. True aneurysm of the pancreaticoduodenal artery: A case report and review of the literature. *J Vasc Surg.* 1985;2:741.

25. Stabile BE, Wilson SE, Debas HT. Reduced mortality from bleeding Pseudocysts and Pseudoaneurysms caused by Pancreatitis. *Arch Surg.* 1983;18:45.

26. Eidus LB, Rasuli P, Manion D, Heringer R. Caliber-persistent artery of the stomach (Dieulafoy's vascular malformation). *Gastroenterology.* 1990;99:1507.

27. Miko TL, Thomazy VA. The Caliber persistent artery of the stomach: A unifying approach to gastric aneurysm, Dieulafoy's lesion, and submucosal arterial malformation. *Hum Pathol.* 1988;19:914.

32

Infected aneurysms

MICHOL A. COOPER, JAMES H. BLACK III, BERTRAM M. BERNHEIM,
BRUCE A. PERLER and JULIUS H. JACOBSON II

CONTENTS

Arterial infection is one of the most demanding problems encountered by the vascular surgeon. Although improvements in surgical technique and better antimicrobial prophylaxis have reduced septic complications of vascular reconstruction, the infected aneurysm continues to pose a threat to life and limb. Even in an era of rapidly expanding diagnostic and endovascular therapeutic technology, diagnosis remains difficult and is often delayed, treatment is challenging, and the results, while improving, are far from satisfactory. It is the purpose of this chapter to offer a pragmatic definition of infected aneurysms, to highlight the appropriate diagnostic approach, to provide an overview of the microbiology and anatomic distribution of these lesions and to outline therapeutic options.

HISTORY AND EVOLUTION OF TERMINOLOGY

Infected aneurysms are among the oldest arterial lesions described in the western literature. Sir William Osler,[1] in the first of his Gulstonian Lectures to the Royal College of Physicians in London in March 1885, coined the term mycotic aneurysm. Osler described several cases in which he believed valvular vegetations characteristic of endocarditis spread directly to the aortic wall and led to aneurysmal degeneration. Osler's work firmly established mycotic aneurysms as a clinical entity and stimulated other workers to make further observations.

Terminology

Confusion exists concerning the classification and nomenclature of infected aneurysms. Review and study of the pathophysiology, bacteriology and epidemiology of these lesions support a natural distinction between mycotic aneurysms associated with bacterial infective endocarditis (as defined by Osler) and other infected aneurysms that occur spontaneously, haematogenously or via direct extension.

MYCOTIC ANEURYSMS

Incidence

Mycotic aneurysms are a complication of infective endocarditis.[1,2] The introduction of antimicrobial drugs has reduced the mortality and morbidity of bacterial endocarditis, with a consequent reduction in, but not eradication of, mycotic aneurysms.

Pathogenesis

Mycotic aneurysms develop from infected heart valves either through direct extension or by embolization. Direct spread of infection from the aortic valve to the ascending aorta occurs in a substantial number of cases.[3] Embolization of the infected debris also occurs to the vasa vasorum or to small arterial branches of the main vessel. Finding intact intima in the aorta at sites of the mycotic aneurysm development suggests that these intramural abscesses were seeded from the vasa vasorum.[4] The infected emboli may cause thrombosis of the vasa vasorum and resulting vessel wall ischemia; compounded by the local sepsis, degeneration of elastic and muscular elements may ensue, resulting in aneurysm development. The lodgement of septic emboli in small peripheral arterial branches and the subsequent destructive infectious process result in infected aneurysms of peripheral vessels.

In some patients, histologic examination of mycotic aneurysms has documented intramural abscesses in the intima and inner portions of the media, areas supplied not by the vasa vasorum but by the intraluminal circulating blood. Such transmural inoculation leads to intimal and medial damage, resulting in aneurysmal dilatation. This mechanism is probably operative in the smaller, more peripheral arteries. The final common pathway is the destruction of the arterial wall, with progressive aneurysmal dilatation and eventual rupture.

Histology

The grossly normal vessel adjacent to the aneurysm may harbour microscopic signs of inflammation. Although histologic findings may be quite variable, the inflammatory reaction is less acute in mycotic than in infected aneurysms. The most characteristic findings in mycotic aneurysm are the damage and loss of intima, destruction of elastic lamellae – especially the internal elastic lamina – periarteritis or mesoarteritis. When the inflammatory reaction is less acute, plasma cells and lymphocytes may predominate. Usually, the inflammatory reaction is most prominent around the vasa vasorum, which may be thickened or obliterated in areas of the greatest inflammation. In chronic aneurysms, an infiltration of fibroblasts and calcification may be identified.[5]

INFECTED ANEURYSMS (MYCOTIC ANEURYSM WITHOUT ENDOCARDITIS)

Incidence

As our population ages and the incidence of aneurysmal disease increases, more patients are being identified with secondary infection of pre-existing arterial aneurysms, usually of the abdominal aorta.[6] In addition, microbial inoculation of a diseased but nonaneurysmal arterial wall may result in infection, mural weakening and aneurysm formation. As with mycotic aneurysms, it is difficult to determine the incidence of infected aneurysms. Most studies have evaluated aortic aneurysms. In a review of 2585 aortic aneurysm cases, the incidence of infection was 0.9%.[7] Additionally, Reddy et al. reported an overall incidence of infected aortic aneurysms of 0.65% at Henry Ford Hospital over a 30-year period.[8]

Pathogenesis

Since intact intima is known to be highly resistant to bacterial infection, a defect in the intimal surface appears necessary for microbial arteritis to develop.[9,10] Arteriosclerosis significantly diminishes resistance of the arterial wall to bacterial infection and is the underlying abnormality in the majority of patients with infected aneurysms.[11] Thrombus within arterial aneurysms and the large area of intimal disruption makes these lesions particularly susceptible to infection. Whether the infection develops in a nonaneurysmal atherosclerotic plaque or within an aneurysm, results are similar. Localized sepsis results in a disintegration of mural elastic and muscular elements, with resultant progressive dilatation of the vessel. Once a nidus of infection is established within a plaque or aneurysm thrombus, it becomes difficult or impossible for systemic antimicrobial agents to eradicate the infection.

Although atherosclerosis is the most common lesion predisposing to the development of infected aneurysms, any condition that causes irregularity of the luminal surface, such as coarctation, may predispose to secondary bacterial infection.[12] Infected aneurysms may also develop secondary to chronic arteriovenous fistulas.[13] Progressive dilatation of the proximal artery and associated degenerative changes of the arterial wall appear to increase susceptibility to bacterial infection.[14] An infected aneurysm may develop at the re-entry site of a chronic aortic dissection.[15] Spontaneous arterial infections have also developed in segments of cystic medionecrosis and areas of syphilitic aortitis.[2,16]

Some infected aneurysms have been identified with apparently intact intimal surfaces. Under these circumstances, it is presumed that haematogenous infection seeded the arterial wall via the vasa vasorum.[17] An association has been demonstrated between infected aortic aneurysms and both lumbar osteomyelitis and infected para-aortic lymph nodes. In one study,[18] 18% of the patients with infected aneurysms of the abdominal aorta also had apparent involvement of adjacent lumbar vertebrae. It is possible that infection within the vertebrae or lymph nodes reaches the aorta via the lymphatic channels or the vasa vasorum, although evidence in support of this mechanism is speculative.[17] In addition to these anatomic factors, depressed host immunity has been implicated in the genesis of infected aneurysms in at least 25% of cases reviewed.[19]

Histology

Infected aneurysms can usually be distinguished from the classic mycotic aneurysms histologically. In an infected aneurysm, the inflammatory reaction is very localized, in contrast to the diffuse inflammatory involvement in mycotic aneurysms. Whereas the intima may be absent in mycotic aneurysms, identifiable fragments of all layers of the arterial wall are usually found in the infected aneurysms. Inflammatory reaction is consistently acute in infected aneurysms, whereas subacute or even more chronic changes may be noted in mycotic aneurysm.[20]

ANATOMIC DISTRIBUTION

Mycotic and infected aneurysms have involved almost every artery (Table 32.1).[9,21–25] Excluding intracranial vessels, the most common sites are the aorta, visceral arteries and upper and lower extremity vessels.

Aorta

All segments of the aorta (Figure 32.1) have been affected, from the ascending thoracic aorta to the bifurcation. When bacterial endocarditis was prevalent, mycotic aneurysms frequently developed in the ascending aorta and arch.

As infected arteriosclerotic aneurysms have become more prevalent than true mycotic aneurysms, the infrarenal abdominal aorta, due to its predilection for arteriosclerotic degeneration, has been more commonly involved.[9] The incidence of infected aneurysms of the suprarenal abdominal and descending thoracic aorta also appears to be increasing.[26]

Carotid artery

Fortunately, since they represent special problems in management, infected aneurysms involving the extracranial carotid artery are uncommon. In a review of the literature, Pirvu et al. identified 99 cases of infected carotid artery aneurysms.[27] Prior to availability of antimicrobial drugs, many infected carotid aneurysms resulted from pharyngeal or cervical streptococcal infections. Most recently, infected carotid aneurysms have been associated with intravenous drug use and other penetrating trauma.[28,29] Nevertheless, bacterial endocarditis continues to be a cause of mycotic carotid aneurysm.[30]

Visceral arteries

Infection remains one of the most common causes of visceral artery aneurysms (Figure 32.2).[31] In the pre-antibiotic

Table 32.1 Anatomic distribution of mycotic and infected aneurysms.

	Stengel[23]	Lewis[25]	Revell[24]	Mundth[9]	Anderson[21]	Brown[22]	Total
Aorta	66 (25%)	12 (11%)	21 (75%)	13 (76%)	2 (12%)	3 (30%)	117 (27%)
Visceral	69 (26%)	31 (29%)	4 (14%)	1 (6%)	0	0	105 (24%)
Arm	23 (9%)	13 (12%)	2 (7%)	0	3 (19%)	1 (10%)	42 (10%)
Leg	31 (12%)	11 (10%)	1 (4%)	2 (12%)	7 (44%)	2 (20%)	54 (12%)
Iliac	10 (4%)	3 (3%)	0	1 (6%)	4 (25%)	1 (10%)	19 (4%)
Others	65 (34%)	37 (35%)	0	0	0	3 (30%)	105 (24%)
Total	264	107	28	17	16	10	442

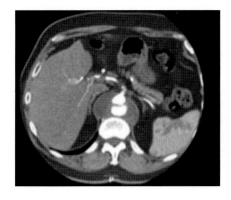 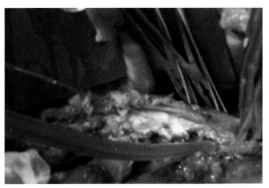

Figure 32.1 Mycotic thoracoabdominal aortic aneurysm (preoperative CT on the left and intraoperative picture of aneurysm on the right) in a 64-year-old male with a history of bladder cancer treated with multiple rounds of BCG bladder therapy complicated by mycobacterium bovis bacteremia. He underwent repair using a rifampin-soaked Dacron graft with bilateral cold renal artery and superior mesenteric artery perfusion intraoperatively in 2012. The ragged posterior edge of the aorta represents the result after surgical debridement. He did well post-operatively and remains infection-free.

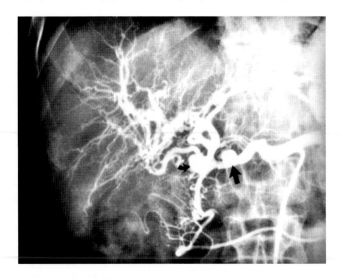

Figure 32.2 Selective celiac arteriogram of mycotic common hepatic (large arrow) and proper hepatic (small arrow) arterial aneurysms.

era, it was estimated that 20% of splenic artery aneurysms were mycotic. In a 1969 review[32] of 350 splenic artery aneurysms, only 38 mycotic or infected lesions were identified. Although superior mesenteric artery (SMA) aneurysms are not common, infection has been responsible for about 60% of these lesions and parenteral drug abuse has also contributed to their development.[33]

The hepatic artery is rarely aneurysmal (Figure 32.2). As with the SMA, however, infection is the most common aetiology with the majority resulting from endocarditis.[34] Most recently, infected hepatic artery aneurysms have been seen as a complication of orthotopic liver transplantation with an estimated incidence of 1%–3%.[35] Aneurysms have involved the main hepatic as well as the donor gastroduodenal artery.[36]

Deitch et al. reported the first case of an infected renal artery pseudoaneurysm secondary to renal artery percutaneous transluminal angioplasty (PTA) and stent placement.[37] In this case, prophylactic antibiotics had not been administered. In view of the dramatic increase in the performance of endovascular interventions, one may anticipate an increase in angioplasty and/or stent-related infections. Although experience to date is anecdotal, prophylactic antibiotic administration may be appropriate peri-procedurally in this scenario.

Extremities

Mycotic and infected aneurysms involve arm and leg arteries in about 20% of cases (Table 32.1). Infection has resulted from arteriographic catheterization procedures, indwelling arterial cannulas for hemodynamic monitoring and parenteral drug abuse.[38–40] There has also been an increase in the incidence of infected iliac artery aneurysm as a complication of kidney and pancreas transplantation.[41] Finally, sporadic cases of infected iliac artery aneurysms, secondary to PTA and stent placement, have been reported.[42]

BACTERIOLOGY

Key points

- *Salmonella* is the most commonly isolated organism in patients with mycotic and infected aneurysms.
- Patients with mycotic aneurysms may not have positive blood cultures.

Numerous organisms have been isolated from mycotic and infected aneurysms (Table 32.2). The organism isolated depends upon the aetiology of the aneurysm.

In three large reviews[42–45] of aortic infection, *Staphylococcus* (25%) and *Salmonella* (31%) species predominate.

Aneurysm cultures are not always revealing. In one study,[4] only 53% of aneurysm tissue sampled yielded growth of organisms. In another,[9] 71% of aneurysm cultures were positive. Universal failure to grow organisms from obviously infected aneurysms relates to culture techniques, fragility of the organism and intercurrent antibiotic therapy.

In addition to failure to culture organisms consistently, the source of infection has been determined in only 54%–71% of cases.[9] Osteomyelitis, gastroenteritis and endocarditis were formally common etiologies. Less commonly encountered were urinary tract sepsis, oesophageal fistula, diverticulitis, otitis media, pulmonary infection, cellulitis and perforated appendicitis.[55] Clearly, transient bacteremias from unknown foci are an important factor in the pathogenesis of infected aneurysms.

In addition to identifying appropriate antibiotic therapy, culture data may have some prognostic significance. Gram-negative infections of abdominal aortic aneurysms appear more ominous than gram-positive infections. In Jarrett's review,[18] the mortality rate was 84% among patients with gram-negative infections, contrasted to only 50% when the aneurysm contained gram-positive

Table 32.2 Microbiology of infected aneurysms (excluding colonized aneurysms).

Organisms	No. of positive cultures		
	Pre-1984	1984–1997	1997–2009
Salmonella	17	38	35
Staphylococcus	23	35	21
MRSA	–	–	6
Escherichia coli	10	8	4
Streptococcus	7	26	16
Pseudomonas	7	1	–
Enterobacter	5	3	–
Klebsiella	4	4	6
Proteus	4	1	–
Pneumococcus	2	1	–
Mycobacterium	2	1	2
Yersinia	1	–	–
Arizona hinshawii	1	–	–
Enterococcus	1	1	6
Campylobacter fetus	1	7	–
Citrobacter	–	3	2
Haemophilus	1	3	3
Edwardsiella	–	1	–
Brucella	–	2	–
Anaerobes	7	18	18
Fungal	5	3	1

Sources: Scher LA et al., *Arch Surg*, 115, 975, 1980; Reddy DJ et al., *Arch Surg*, 126, 873, 1991; discussion 878; Mundth ED et al., *Am J Surg*, 117, 460, 1969; Anderson CB et al., *Arch Surg*, 109, 712, 1974; Jebara VA et al., *Tex Heart Inst J*, 25, 136, 1998; Woods JM et al., *J Vasc Surg*, 7, 808, 1988; Uno M et al., *J Jpn Surg Assoc*, 67, 1763, 2006; Hachimaru T, *Jpn J Cardiovasc Surg*, 38, 344, 2009; Akiyama T MK, *Jpn J Cardiovasc Surg*, 37, 174, 2008; Skandalos I et al., *Surg Today*, 39, 141, 2009; Bito A et al., *Jpn J Cardiovasc Surg*, 37, 333, 2008; Maeda H et al., *Surg Today*, 41, 346, 2011; Marques da Silva M et al., *J Vasc Surg*, 38, 1384, 2003.

organisms. Rupture of the aneurysm occurred in 5 of 6 patients with gram-negative infections, compared to 1 of 10 with gram-positive organisms.

Salmonella infection

One of the more fascinating yet incompletely understood aspects of infected aneurysms is the tendency for *Salmonella* species to cause arterial infection. Three types of vascular lesions may result from *Salmonella* infection. First, a diffuse suppurative arteritis may cause arterial rupture, resulting in a saccular or false aneurysm. Second, *Salmonella* may initiate a focal arteritis that leads to the weakening of the arterial wall and formation of a true infected aneurysm. Third, *Salmonella* species may infect a pre-existing aneurysm. *Salmonella* arterial infections affect 75% of the aorta and 50% involve the abdominal aorta.[2,55,56] Recent studies continue to demonstrate that *Salmonella* is a frequent source of arterial infection.[53,54]

Inoculation of the organisms on a diseased intimal surface appears to be the initiating event in most cases,[57] although invasion of previously healthy intima can occur.[58]

Unusual bacteria

Several unusual organisms have been increasingly isolated from infected aneurysms. *Arizona hinshawii* and *Campylobacter fetus* have been isolated from infected aneurysms.[53,54,59] Bacteraemia of the genus *Arizona* are among the Enterobacteriaceae that have been noted to cause a variety of diseases in humans, including gastroenteritis, urinary tract infection, cholecystitis, septic arthritis, osteomyelitis and septicemia. Although taxonomically distinct from other Enterobacteriaceae, these organisms were at one time considered to belong to the genus *Salmonella*, since there are a number of biochemical and serologic similarities between these two groups of organisms.[60] *Campylobacter*, like *Salmonella*, lacks the enterotoxin production, cytotoxicity and invasive properties exhibited by other enteric organisms. Thus, although precise mechanisms of arterial infection are not known, *Campylobacter* and *Arizona* infections may share similar characteristics with *Salmonella*.

Clostridium septicum is a relatively uncommon anaerobic pathogen responsible for approximately 1% of all clostridial infections and often is identified in patients with underlying malignant disease. To date, 26 patients, ranging in age from 60 to 91, have been reported with infected aneurysms due to *Clostridium septicum*. At least 20 of these patients had documented malignancies.[61,62]

Fungal infection

Despite the widespread use of the word mycotic to describe infected aneurysms, such aneurysms only rarely result from fungal infection. *Histoplasma capsulatum*, *Aspergillus*, *Candida*, *Actinomyces* and *Penicillium* species are the most common reported causative agents.[63] Like systemic fungal infections, these arterial infections tend to be associated with chronic immunosuppressive states.[63] The precise mechanism of arterial infection varies but is similar to that for bacterial involvement.

Fungal infection of arterial aneurysms may occur long after recognition of the original fungal infection. Such aneurysms are usually saccular; when they involve the abdominal aorta, vertebral body erosion is frequently noted. The risk of rupture of these lesions is significant. In a review[63] of aortic aneurysms infected with *H. capsulatum*, survival was only 33%. When fungal infection of an aneurysm is suspected at operation, frozen section specimens should be examined for confirmation.

Infected anastomotic aneurysms

Anastomotic aneurysms occur following 2%–5% of bypass grafts, and a majority involve the femoral anastomosis.[64]

Traditionally, the development of anastomotic aneurysms has been attributed to a variety of factors such as structural weakness of the artery (often after endarterectomy), suture fracture, graft deterioration and mechanical stress from patient activity or hypertension. In a series of 45 anastomotic aneurysms, Seabrook et al.[65] identified 32 bacterial isolates from 27 (60%) of these lesions. Coagulase-negative staphylococci accounted for 24 (88%) of the isolates. These findings suggested that bacterial contamination and colonization may occur at implantation, resulting in a chronic, low-virulence infectious process at the arterial suture line, with late pseudoaneurysm formation.

ENDOVASCULAR STENT-GRAFT INFECTION

Arterial infection secondary to endovascular stent placement also bridges the gap between pure arterial infection and prosthetic graft sepsis. As noted earlier, it is being increasingly seen in a variety of anatomic locations. The reported incidence of endograft infection is very low. In a recent series of 945 patients from 2006 to 2011, the incidence of endograft infection was 0.6%.[66]

NATURAL HISTORY

Key points

- Without surgical intervention, infected aortic aneurysms are almost always fatal.
- Infected aneurysms often rupture at smaller size that non-infected aneurysm

Complications of infected aneurysms include progressive enlargement and rupture, thrombosis and embolization. Without surgical intervention, infected aortic aneurysms are almost always fatal. In one review, the mortality among patients with *Salmonella* aortic aneurysms was 95% when treated medically.[67] Furthermore, ruptured infected aneurysms are usually smaller than ruptured non-infected aneurysms, and progression to rupture usually occurs rapidly. Less commonly, a slow, insidious course precedes rupture of an infected aneurysm.

The outcome once an infected aneurysm has ruptured depends upon the vessel involved. Infected aortic aneurysms represent the greatest risk to life. Aortocaval and aortoenteric fistulas have been reported secondary to mycotic and infected aneurysms[59] (Figure 32.3). Limited perforation, particularly of a peripheral vessel, results in pseudoaneurysm formation with persistent sepsis.

Prior to rupture, both aortic and peripheral aneurysms may shed emboli, causing septic arthritis and purpura.[68] Although less common than rupture, thrombosis of mycotic and infected aneurysms has been noted both in the aorta and peripheral vessels.

DIAGNOSIS

Key points

- Diagnosis of infected aneurysms relies upon clinical suspicion and examination.
- Diagnosis does not require infected blood cultures.

Clinical presentation

The clinical presentation (Table 32.1) of patients with mycotic and infected aneurysms depends upon the pathogenesis, underlying aetiology and vessel involved. Earlier reports documented these lesions most commonly in the second, third and fourth decades, reflecting the association with bacterial endocarditis.[23] More recently, however, there has been a shift in incidence to the elderly. In a 2011 report

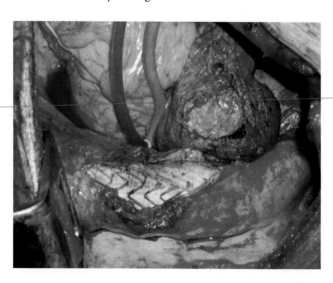

Figure 32.3 Endograft stent infection with erosion into the adjacent lung. The stent graft was excised under partial left heart bypass (cannula in inferior pulmonary vein into left atrium, with distal femoral inflow).

of patients with infected aneurysms of the thoracic, thoracoabdominal and abdominal aorta, patients ranged from 50 to 84 (mean, 67) years of age.[69] The increasing age of patients affected with aortic infection emphasizes the importance of diseased arterial intima, usually by arteriosclerosis, in the pathogenesis of microbial arteritis, as well as the rising incidence of infected arteriosclerotic aneurysms.

There is a male predominance of infected aneurysms with approximately two-thirds occurring in men.[69] Fever or history of a recent febrile illness, noted in 70%–94% of patients with infected arterial lesions, is the most common complaint of patients.[9,18,21] The fever may be steady or intermittent and is usually associated with chills and sweats.[2] Frequently, a long history of malaise, weight loss and increasing weakness is present. Pain is an almost universal complaint. In patients with infected aortic aneurysms, the discomfort may be localized to the abdomen or back. In those with peripheral aneurysms, it is usually localized to the site of the lesion, where there may be overlying erythema, induration and tenderness. Nearly 90% of infected peripheral aneurysms, but only 50%–65% of abdominal aortic aneurysms, are palpable.[9] Hepatic artery involvement may cause right-upper-quadrant or epigastric pain suggestive of cholecystitis or pancreatitis. Likewise, SMA lesions may be confused with inflammatory diseases of the small or large bowel.

Laboratory data

Leukocytosis is the most consistently abnormal laboratory finding in patients with mycotic or infected aneurysms. A leukocytosis above 10,000/mm^3 has been noted in 65%–83% of patients with proven infected aneurysms.[9,18] Antibiotic therapy, however, may blunt this elevation. Furthermore, leukocytosis may be noted following leakage from a non-infected aneurysm. Elevation of the erythrocyte sedimentation rate is a frequent but non-specific finding. With infected hepatic arterial aneurysms, liver function tests are usually unremarkable.[70]

Bacteriologic studies

Positive preoperative blood cultures provide strong confirmatory evidence for the presence of an infected aneurysm, although negative cultures do not rule out the diagnosis. In a report from Henry Ford Hospital, positive blood cultures were obtained from 69% of patients with infected aortic aneurysms, and positive cultures were noted more often in patients with ruptured in contrast to intact aneurysms.[8] As many patients with infected aneurysms may be receiving antibiotics at the time blood samples are drawn, multiple samples may be required before bacteremia is confirmed. Furthermore, the sampling of blood from an arterial site downstream from the presumed focus of infection may improve the yield of positive cultures.[71]

As with preoperative blood cultures, antibiotics may mask bacterial growth from samples obtained at operation and it is important to perform a Gram-stain examination in addition to bacterial cultures. In most patients with negative cultures, organisms will be identified on histologic examination of tissue sections. Reddy et al.[8] reported positive intraoperative Gram stains in 50% of patients with rupture but in only 1 of 8 patients with intact infected aortic aneurysms. Operative cultures were positive in all patients with ruptured and 89% of those with intact infected aortic aneurysms.

RADIOLOGIC STUDIES

Computed tomography

The contrast-enhanced computed tomography scan is extremely helpful in evaluating patients with suspected infected aortic aneurysms. Several findings are highly suggestive of the diagnosis, although none are pathognomonic (Table 32.3).[72] An irregular, saccular aneurysm noted in a febrile patient is highly suggestive, particularly if there is the disruption or absence of intimal calcification. Gas within the aortic wall is also suggestive of an infected aneurysm (Figure 32.4).[72] More often, air or fluid is identified adjacent to the aortic wall. An encasing or adjacent mass – reflecting either hematoma, abscess or inflammatory nodal tissue – has also been seen with infected aortic aneurysms. Entrapment of the ureters by a midline infectious process, particularly in the setting of prior aortic surgery should raise concern for an infected aortic aneurysm. Finally, vertebral osteomyelitis adjacent to an aortic aneurysm should raise the question of aneurysmal infection.

Radioisotope examinations

Two methods using radioisotopes are currently available for the evaluation of septic processes, particularly within the abdomen. Labelling of human leukocytes with indium-111, a gamma-emitting agent, is based upon external gamma camera detection of labelled leukocytes that have accumulated at sites of infection or inflammation. Leukocyte scintigraphy may complement CT evaluation of patients with suspected arterial infection. Ho and colleagues reported the use of leukocyte scintigraphy for early diagnosis of an infected aneurysm with a subsequent CT for further characterization.[73]

Table 32.3 CT findings of infected aneurysms.

Saccular aneurysm
Irregular aneurysm lumen
Absence of calcification
Gas within aortic wall
Perianeurysmal gas
Perianeurysmal fluid
Encasing or contiguous mass
Associated para-aortic or psoas abscess
Vertebral osteomyelitis

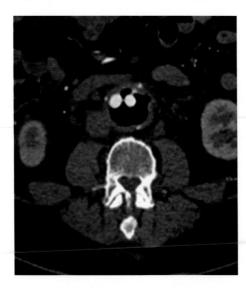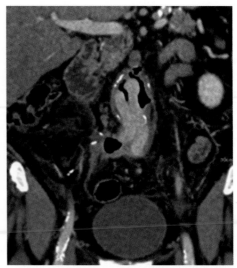

Figure 32.4 CT scan of a 72-year-old man who presented with an aortic graft infection. He had a history of failed endovascular repair of an abdominal aortic aneurysm for which he underwent an open conversion to an aortobiiliac graft at an outside hospital. Seven years later, he presented to our clinic with an aortoenteric fistula. On CT, he has a large amount of gas within the aortic wall tracking along the graft. We performed excision of the graft with in situ reconstruction with a rifampin-soaked Dacron graft.

Gallium-67 isotopic scans have been used to localize intra-abdominal abscesses. Radioactive gallium-67 collects in areas of inflammation and may be detected by external scanning cameras. Successful use of gallium-67 scanning in the diagnosis of a Dacron aortic graft infection and aortoenteric fistula has been reported.[74]

TREATMENT

Key points

- Infected aneurysms often require radical debridement and extra-anatomic versus in situ reconstruction; if the latter is applied, then muscle flap coverage is encouraged.
- The treatment of infected aortic grafts has evolved to include in situ reconstruction en par with extra-anatomic reconstruction.
- There are no strict guidelines for the duration of postoperative antibiotic therapy for infected aneurysms, but the Johns Hopkins approach is to continue IV antibiotics until serum ESR and CRP are normalized.

The aim of the therapy is to eradicate all infection while maintaining adequate circulation. Principles of successful management are independent of the specific lesion, mechanism of infection or organism responsible (Table 32.4).

Preoperative management

Establishing the correct diagnosis preoperatively is the first step in treatment. Multiple blood cultures should be obtained, including several samples from a source downstream of the presumed site of the aneurysm. Other potential sources of infection such as urine, sputum and open wounds should be cultured. High-dose intravenous organism-specific antibiotic treatment must be started to prevent continued haematogenous spread of infection and possible contamination of a vascular prosthesis that might be required for arterial reconstruction. When attempts at identifying the offending organism(s) prove futile, any combination of broad-spectrum bactericidal antibiotics for both gram-positive and gram-negative organisms (specifically *Salmonella*) is appropriate.

Operative management

Appropriate intravenous lines should be inserted. The insertion of a radial artery cannula in the non-dominant wrist or the side-opposite anticipated axillofemoral

Table 32.4 Clinical characteristics of infected aneurysms.

Epidemiology	Males, females (2:1)
	All age groups
	Bacterial endocarditis
	Atherosclerosis; illicit drug use
History	Intermittent febrile episodes
	Malaise
	Weight loss
	Pain
Exam	Fever with chill (70%–94%)
	Rapidly expanding mass (50%–90%)
Laboratory	Leukocytosis (65%–83%)
	Positive blood cultures (50%)
Operative findings	Thin-walled aneurysm
	Surrounding inflammatory reaction
	Succulent lymph nodes
	Positive Gram stain

reconstruction provides ready access for blood sampling as well as systemic blood-pressure measurements. Antibiotic prophylaxis is given within 60 minutes of starting the procedure and is re-dosed as appropriate for the half-life of the antibiotic and for blood loss of 1.5 L. Antibiotics for prophylaxis should cover MRSA as well as gram-negative bacteria. Treatment with a cephalosporin and daptomycin has been shown to decrease SSI rates by more than 60%.[75]

Once the aneurysm has been exposed, infection must be confirmed. When gross perivascular purulence is encountered, the diagnosis is obvious. In the absence of obvious signs of sepsis, Gram stains should be obtained, and frozen sections of the aneurysm wall examined for bacteria or fungi. Identification of microorganisms within the aneurysmal wall or contents in the patient with fever, leukocytosis, positive blood cultures, a particularly friable-appearing aneurysm or an aneurysm surrounded by large lymph nodes is diagnostic of aneurysm infection. Aerobic, anaerobic and fungal cultures must be obtained and plated immediately in appropriate culture media.

Principles for managing infected aneurysms are generally similar to those for dealing with an infected arterial prosthesis. Wide debridement and copious irrigation of all involved tissue is required. This includes complete resection of the aneurysm if technically possible. If rupture has occurred, a wider area will be involved in the septic process, and more aggressive debridement may be required. Ligation of arteries should be performed in a clean, healthy-appearing tissue with synthetic monofilament or wire sutures. Preoperative vascular laboratory data help document adequacy of collateral circulation around the infected lesion. If, at the initial operation, collateral circulation is adequate to support the distal bed without arterial reconstruction, arterial ligation only should be performed. If revascularization is necessary, the method of reconstruction will depend upon the location and extent of arterial involvement and the magnitude of the septic process.

Abdominal aorta

EXTRA-ANATOMIC RECONSTRUCTION

The previous standard of care was excision of all septic tissue and extra-anatomic arterial reconstruction. It has fallen out of favour due to the high mortality (up to 27%), the risk of aortic stump blowout (2%–33%), the high amputation rates (up to 24%), and the inferior patency (40%–73% at 5 years) compared to in situ reconstruction.[76] In a meta-analysis, O'Connor and colleagues calculated the combined mean event rates for amputations, graft failure, reinfection, early mortality and late mortality for extra-anatomic bypass versus in situ reconstruction with different conduits. They found event rates were 0.16 for extra-anatomic bypass, 0.07 for rifampicin-coated prostheses, 0.09 for cryopreserved allografts and 0.10 for autogenous vein grafts, pointing to EAB as the procedure with the highest combined event rates.[77] Extra-anatomic bypass is still a good option in emergency situations and in fragile or older patients where a faster procedure that can be staged is a better option.

Whether one is dealing with a ruptured or intact abdominal aortic aneurysm, secure closure of the proximal aortic stump distal to the renal arteries is mandatory for a successful result and constitutes one of the more difficult aspects of repair. Healthy tissue that will hold sutures may not be readily available. Under these circumstances, temporary suprarenal aortic occlusion, at the diaphragm through the lesser sac, permits complete mobilization of the infrarenal aorta. A two-layer aortic closure with monofilament suture has been recommended, and prevertebral fascia may be used to strengthen the closure.[78,79] A pedicle of omentum transposed through the transverse mesocolon may facilitate the resolution of periaortic infection (Figure 32.5). Copious irrigation of the retroperitoneum is performed and irrigating-drainage catheters may be placed in the aortic bed for drainage and post-operative through-and-through irrigation with

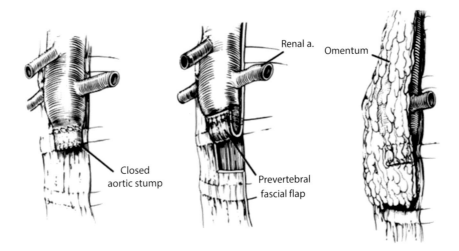

Figure 32.5 Methods of closing infrarenal aorta following aneurysm excision. A proximal row of continuous horizontal mattress sutures is followed by a distal row of continuous over-and-over sutures (left). Prevertebral fascial flap buttress sutured over an aortic stump (centre). Omental graft passed through transverse mesocolon provides additional protection (right). (From Ernst CB, Aortoenteric fistulas, in: Haimovici H, ed., *Vascular Emergencies*, Appleton-Century-Crofts, New York, 1982, pp. 365–385. Reproduced by permission.)

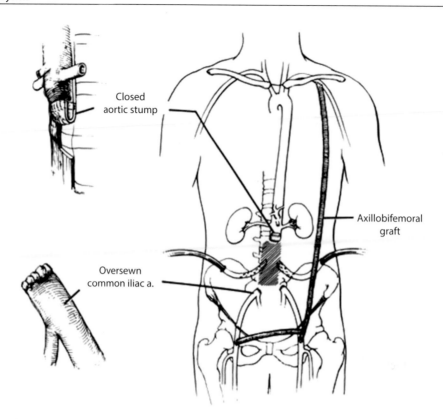

Closed
aortic stump

Axillobifemoral
graft

Oversewn
common iliac a.

Figure 32.6 Infected aneurysm has been excised. The axillobifemoral bypass maintains pelvic and leg circulation. Irrigation drainage catheters are placed in a retroperitoneal space (optional). (From Ernst CB, Aortoenteric fistulas, in: Haimovici H, ed., *Vascular Emergencies*, Appleton-Century-Crofts, New York, 1982, pp. 365–385. Reproduced by permission.)

saline or povidone–iodine solutions during the early post-operative period.[80,81]

For reconstruction, axillofemoral grafting as a means of extra-anatomic bypass has gained popularity since it was first introduced in the United States by Blaisdell and Hall[82] (Figure 32.6). When the infected aneurysm is small and limited to the aorta, following excision and distal closure of the aortic bifurcation, there is no significant iliac occlusive disease, and unilateral axillofemoral reconstruction is appropriate. Under these circumstances, the contralateral leg will be perfused retrograde around the bifurcation. If the bifurcation must be excised and the common iliac vessels are free of significant disease, they may be mobilized and anastamosed end to end to form a neobifurcation, again allowing the use of unilateral axillofemoral reconstruction (Figure 32.7).[6] If recurrent occlusion of the axillofemoral graft becomes a late problem, anatomic aortic reconstruction may be performed.[78]

IN SITU RECONSTRUCTION

In situ revascularization following resection and debridement of the infected tissues has replaced extra-anatomic bypass as the standard of care for infected aortic aneurysms due to comparatively fewer complications and better outcomes. There are a number of potential conduits that have been utilized.

In a systematic review and meta-analysis of treatments for aortic graft infection, O'Connor and colleagues report outcomes for in situ revascularization with rifampin-soaked prosthetic grafts, cryopreserved homograft and autogenous vein graft. They found the best outcomes with rifampin-soaked grafts followed by cyropreserved allografts and then autogenous vein grafts.[77] Saturating Dacron grafts in rifampin (60 mg/mL) inhibits the growth of organisms commonly involved in both primary aortic infections and aortoenteric fistulas. Standard prosthetic grafts with no antibiotic are also used, although studies have found a trend towards worse outcomes with them compared to rifampin-soaked grafts.[83] Cryopreserved allograft has mostly replaced fresh allograft due to the propensity of fresh allografts to dilate over the long term. Additionally, cryopreserved allografts are processed so that they do not require ABO matching. They can also be selected to match the normal aorta and its branches in diameter and anatomy and are thereby superior to allografts constructed on the backtable.[84] Autogenous vein grafts are more broadly available than cryopreserved grafts, and femoral vein harvest is well tolerated. Furthermore, autologous reconstruction has been shown to need only a limited course of antibiotics (4–6 weeks) and has the lowest rate of reinfection and late mortality when compared with prosthetic graft and allografts.[85]

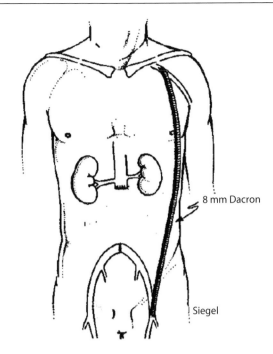

8 mm Dacron

Siegel

Figure 32.7 After resection of infected aortic aneurysm and ligation of infrarenal aortic stump, common iliac arteries have been anastamosed and unilateral axillofemoral bypass has been performed. (From Scher LA et al., *Arch Surg*, 115, 975, 1980. Reproduced by permission.)

JOHNS HOPKINS IN SITU RECONSTRUCTION OF A MYCOTIC AORTIC ANEURYSM

Prior to starting the procedures, ureteral stents are placed and large bore IV access is obtained. Preoperative antibiotics are given in the earlier discussion. The patient is placed supine and a midline laparotomy is performed. The omentum is mobilized for later flap creation. A Kocher manoeuvre is performed to expose the aorta and the aortoenteric fistula, if present. The graft is excised to native tissue. If an aortoenteric fistula is present, the duodenum is resected through the ligament of Treitz to prevent enteric flow near the new graft. In situ aortic replacement with a rifampin-soaked graft is performed. This is followed by meticulous haemostasis to prevent hematoma and decrease the risk of reinfection. The omental flap is then brought through a window in the mesentery of the transverse colon and placed over the graft. If the duodenum has been resected, a retrocolic duodenojejunostomy to the right of the middle colic artery is performed. The abdomen is then copiously irrigated and closed.

ENDOVASCULAR REPAIR

Endovascular repair for thoracic and abdominal aortic aneurysms has become widely accepted in the last two decades.[86] The main advantages of endovascular over open repair are avoidance of a large incision, aortic cross-clamping, interference with respiratory function, revascularization and significant blood loss.[87,88] Following the principles of rifampin use in open vascular repairs, a novel technique for endovascular repair is rifampin soaking of endografts. In a report of two patients, Escobar and colleagues implanted rifampin-soaked grafts. The grafts were prepared by injecting a rifampin into the sheath containing the Dacron grafts via the side port of a cook device or with minimal *pre-deployment* of the sheath for a Medtronic graft. The graft was allowed to soak for about 1 hour before being deployed. The 30-day mortality was 0. One patient ultimately required definitive repair at 1.5 years and the other remains without evidence of recurrence at 1 year.[89]

Visceral arteries

The surgical approach required for treatment depends upon the size and location of the lesion, as well as the adequacy of collateral development. Goals of operative management are to prevent rupture of the aneurysm while preserving adequate distal perfusion.

SUPERIOR MESENTERIC ARTERY

DeBakey and Cooley[90] performed the first successful resection of a mycotic aneurysm of the SMA in 1949. By 1987, a total of 19 patients with infected SMA aneurysms had been successfully treated by ligation with or without aneurysm excision.[91,92] Attempts to excise these aneurysms completely may be hazardous, since they are usually densely adherent to important adjacent structures. With adequate drainage and long-term antibiotic therapy, recurrent infection should not be a problem even with only a partial excision and endoaneurysmorrhaphy.[93]

Following ligation of the vessel, the bowel should be observed for 30 minutes to assess viability. Short segments of apparently non-viable intestine must be resected. If long segments of bowel appear compromised, mesenteric revascularization will be required, preferentially utilizing autogenous artery or vein conduits.[93]

Endoaneurysmorrhaphy, another method of treating arterial aneurysms, has proven successful in managing infected SMA aneurysms.[93] Restorative endoaneurysmorrhaphy requires obtaining proximal and distal control of the involved artery, opening the aneurysm and oversewing the aneurysm orifice, that is, performing an arteriorrhaphy, which preserves the vessel lumen. An intraluminal shunt facilitates vessel repair by maintaining bowel circulation and provides a stent around which the arteriorrhaphy is performed. The shunt is removed before placing the last few sutures. If the aneurysm is not saccular and involves both afferent and efferent vessels, obliterative endoaneurysmorrhaphy may be performed by oversewing the orifices of these vessels from within the open aneurysmal sac. By limiting dissection and working from within the aneurysm, maximum collateral circulation is preserved. Use of intraluminal balloon occlusion of the inflow and outflow vessels facilitates endoaneurysmorrhaphy because the extensive dissection required for proximal and distal clamp occlusion is not required.

HEPATIC ARTERY

Most infected hepatic arterial aneurysms can be successfully managed by ligation or ligation with aneurysm excision. When the aneurysm involves the proper hepatic artery or when preoperative angiography documents poor collateral development, an attempt at arterial reconstruction should be made to prevent liver ischemia.[70] Saphenous vein or autogenous hypogastric arterial segments are the preferred bypass materials.

Infected aneurysms of intrahepatic arteries are most often treated by hepatic lobectomy. Transcatheter arterial embolization can be used for treatment of infected visceral arterial aneurysms when surgical intervention is not advisable or technically possible. Jones et al. reported successful treatment using radiologic coil embolization of the hepatic artery followed by excision with hepatic artery ligation and antibiotic therapy.[94]

OTHER VISCERAL VESSELS

Mycotic or infected aneurysms involving the celiac, splenic or inferior mesenteric arteries (IMA) have been successfully treated by the surgical options described.[95] Most splenic arterial lesions may be ligated or excised, with or without splenectomy. Likewise, rich mesenteric collateral circulation may permit IMA ligation and aneurysm resection. Measurement of IMA stump pressure or use of a sterile Doppler helps document adequacy of colonic collateral blood flow, permitting safe IMA ligation.[96]

Carotid artery

The principals of management of infected aneurysms of the extracranial carotid arteries are the same as those for infected arterial lesions elsewhere, namely, excision, wide debridement and drainage, restoration of arterial continuity when feasible and intensive antibiotic therapy. The question of arterial reconstruction versus ligation for infected carotid artery aneurysm remains unsettled. Risks of neurologic deficit after ligation must be balanced against risks of recurrent infection, arterial disruption and potentially fatal haemorrhage following arterial reconstruction in a contaminated field.

Historically, most workers have favoured ligation.[97] However, with this approach, the incidence of a major stroke is 30%–50% and the mortality rate is 17%–40%.[98,99] Endovascular repair with covered stents is another option that has been reported, but its efficacy and safety are not well established.[100,101] Carotid ligation is now reserved for cases in which vascular reconstruction is technically impossible.

Extremity vessels

The subclavian or axillary artery between the thyrocervical and subscapular branches can usually be safely ligated because of profuse protective collateral circulation around the shoulder. Resection of lesions involving the distal axillary artery, however, may require reconstruction. When reconstruction is required, autogenous tissue should be used.[102] The brachial artery distal to the profunda branch may be safely ligated. Aneurysms of the radial and ulnar arteries can usually be excised without reconstruction. Documentation of adequacy of collateral circulation through the superficial and deep volar arches by Doppler or Allen's test assures safe ligation of these vessels.

The femoral artery is the most common site of infected peripheral aneurysms. The management of these lesions continues to generate debate. The most conservative approach, especially in the setting of gross purulence, is excision and arterial ligation. In young individuals, common or superficial femoral artery ligation usually results in a viable extremity, although these patients will often experience claudication. If these symptoms are disabling, subsequent reconstruction, after infection has resolved, is appropriate. In 1 series of 18 infected femoral pseudoaneurysms secondary to intravascular drug injections, no deaths and no complications occurred among 6 patients who underwent ligation alone. The mean ankle-brachial index after ligation in this group was 0.63.[103] There were 12 patients who underwent the revascularization procedures, and among this group, there were 13 reoperations for vascular complications and 3 (25%) major amputations. When aneurysm resection also requires sacrifice of the profunda femoris artery, arterial reconstruction will often be necessary to maintain limb viability. It is clear that ligation and extensive debridement offers the best chance of controlling the septic process and minimizing the risk of subsequent haemorrhage. Among patients in whom limb perfusion is inadequate, a number of reconstructive options exist.

An anatomic reconstruction may be performed through the bed of the resected aneurysm (Figure 32.8). The use of an autogenous conduit, usually saphenous vein, is mandatory. There is some evidence that coverage of the graft with a formal muscle flap may reduce the likelihood of recurrent infection in this setting.[104,105] Rotating a muscle from a separate bed, based upon a pedicled blood supply that is independent of the site of infection, ensures maximum vascularity of the rotated muscle. A well-vascularized muscle bundle will deliver a high level of antibiotics and immunocompetent cells to the wound and will raise the oxygen tension within the wound, which may promote eradication of residual infection through stimulation of leukocyte function and thus promote healing.[106] For these reasons and others, it has been suggested that performance of a formal rotational muscle flap procedure is a superior approach when compared to local sartorius transfer.[107,108]

Another alternative for management of mycotic extremity aneurysms is endovascular repair. Kwon and colleagues report successful endovascular repair of a common femoral artery aneurysm immediately proximal to its bifurcation with a covered stent graft. The stent was placed across the profunda femoris artery without associated

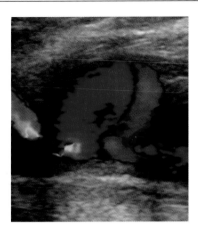
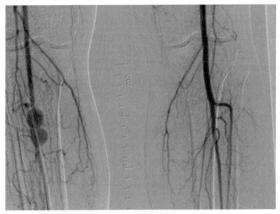

Figure 32.8 Preoperative ultrasound (left) and angiogram (right) of a 60-year-old man with a history of endocarditis complicated by a large mycotic aneurysm of the right tibioperoneal trunk treated with a vein interposition graft.

complications. The patient's symptoms resolved within 1 week and there was radiographic resolution of the aneurysm at 3 months. At 18 months, the patient remained asymptomatic and free of any radiographic evidence of aneurysm.[109] The role of endovascular management in extremity artery mycotic aneurysms is still evolving.

A novel technique for treating patients with lower extremity vascular graft infections is the use of antibiotic-based polymethymethacrylate (ab-PMMA) beads. Infection involving prosthetic material is difficult to eradicate. Complete removal of the infected prosthetic material with extensive local debridement and extra-anatomic bypass is the traditional treatment approach. However, this leads to high rates of thrombosis and reinfection.[110] The beads deliver high local and low systemic levels of antibiotics. Antibiotic beads are prepared intraoperatively on the back table with PMMA powder (40 mg), antibiotic powder (including vancomycin (1–4 g), tobramycin (1–2 g) and/or gentamicin (1–2 g)). These are then polymerized with methacrylate (20 mL). The antibiotic-impregnated PMMA cement is moulded into 5–8 mm beads and threaded through with a 0-Prolene suture. Once the cement hardens, the beads are placed in the wound (Figure 32.9), and the wound is temporarily closed with nylon sutures. The wound is then re-explored and beads are either replaced until the wound cultures clear and/or there is good granulation tissue, depending on the surgeon's approach.[111,112] In a study by Stone and colleagues, 40 patients were treated for 42 graft infra-inguinal infections using ab-PMMA beads. The antibiotic beads were replaced on average of 1.4 times. A wound-vacuum dressing was placed in 27 (64%) of the surgical sites and a sartorius flap was used in 15 (36%). The 30-day mortality was 0. Overall, long-term limb salvage was 77.5% and reinfection rate was 20%.[111] In a recent review, Poi and colleagues report 31 patients treated for 37 graft infra-inguinal graft infections using ab-PMMA beads. On average, the antibiotic beads were replaced two to three times. Formal wound closure with a muscle flap was performed for all patients when granulation tissue was seen around the graft and with negative cultures.

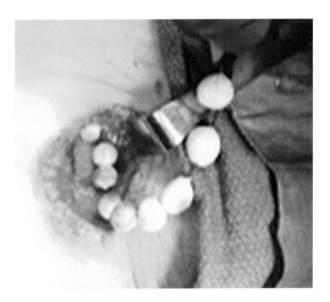

Figure 32.9 Ab-PMMA beads being placed into the wound of an infected graft. (Courtesy of Carlos Bechara MD, Baylor College of Medicine, Houston, TX.)

At 30 days, patient mortality was 0 overall, long-term limb salvage was 86.5% and reinfection rate was 12.5%.[112]

POST-OPERATIVE MANAGEMENT

Regardless of the surgical procedure performed, prolonged post-operative antibiotics are mandatory to protect arterial suture lines and vascular grafts from potential reinfection. Although the duration of antibiotic coverage required has not been firmly established, most authors[9,21] recommend at least 6 weeks of intravenous organism-specific antibiotic treatment. Our approach includes maintaining IV antibiotics until monthly ESR, CRP and white count normalize (usually 3–6 months); after which, the patient is transitioned to oral antibiotics for 1–2 years. After that time, antibiotics are discontinued if serial imaging and ESR remain normal.

RESULTS OF TREATMENT

Prior to the advent of antimicrobial drugs, mycotic or infected aneurysms were invariably fatal. With the introduction of antibiotics, better understanding of the pathophysiology of these lesions, and greater appreciation of the proper therapeutic principles, survival has improved.

Aortic aneurysms

Infected aortic aneurysms present a much greater risk to life than peripheral aneurysms. In the early experience,[80] the majority of survivors underwent extra-anatomic bypass. However, as noted earlier, it has fallen out of favour due to inferior results compared to in situ reconstruction.[76] In view of this, in the late 1990s, there was a shift towards performing in situ revascularization following resection of infected aortic aneurysms. A recent systematic review and meta-analysis found that late mortality for extra-anatomic bypass grafts was 24%, compared with 14%–16% for in situ revascularization. With all outcomes combined, including amputation rate, conduit failure, reinfection rate, early mortality and late mortality, there was a significantly lower rate of morbidity and mortality associated with in situ revascularization for all grafts (rifampin-bonded prosthetic, cryopreserved allograft and autogenous vein).[77] For this reason, in situ revascularization following resection and debridement of the infected tissues has replaced extra-anatomic bypass as the standard of care for infected aortic aneurysms.

As noted earlier, endovascular repair is also being used with increasing frequency for treatment of infected aortic aneurysms. A recent systematic review of outcomes after endovascular stent-graft treatment for mycotic aortic aneurysms by Kan and colleagues demonstrated a 30-day survival of 89.6% and a 2-year survival of 82.2%. Age over 65, rupture of the aneurysm and fever at the time of the operation were predictors of persistent infection.[87]

Peripheral aneurysms

Infected aneurysms of peripheral vessels are more easily diagnosed; consequently, mortality is less than for lesions in the aorta or the visceral circulation. Reddy et al.[113] performed selective revascularization in 54 patients with no mortality and an 11% amputation rate. Padberg et al.[114] reported 18 patients with infected femoral pseudoaneurysms secondary to illicit drug abuse, including 6 patients who underwent ligation alone, with no deaths and no amputations. Among 12 patients who underwent attempted reconstruction, there were 3 (25%) amputations and 13 reoperations for arterial complications.

A novel technique for treating patients with lower extremity vascular graft infections is the use of ab-PMMA beads. In a 2006 study by Stone and colleagues, 40 patients were treated for 42 graft infra-inguinal infections using ab-PMMA beads.[111] Overall, long-term limb salvage was 77.5% and reinfection rate was 20%. In a 2013 study by Poi and colleagues, 31 patients were treated for 37 graft infrainguinal graft infections using ab-PMMA beads. Overall, long-term limb salvage was 86.5% and reinfection rate was 12.5%.[112]

Visceral artery aneurysms

Results of treatment of infected visceral artery lesions are unclear, since individual experiences are limited and only anecdotal reports are available for study. In 1981, Howard and Mazer[92] collected 24 patients from the literature who had survived operative treatment for an infected SMA aneurysm. In 10 patients, ligation of the SMA without arterial reconstruction was performed, and 6 of these underwent aneurysm resection. Only 30% of this group required bowel resection. Of the 24 patients, 9 were successfully treated by aneurysmorrhaphy alone, and 5 underwent aneurysm resection with some form of revascularization. In two of these patients, a prosthetic graft was used, and recurrent infection developed in one, necessitating replacement with a vein graft.

Deficiencies in current knowledge

- In vivo imaging to correlate exact sites of graft infection in patients with outward clinically normal presentation would be a great advance.
- Can antibiotic bead therapy rival the results of debridement and muscle flap coverage?
- Long-term results of stent-graft therapy for aorta-enteric fistula have not been reported and would greatly aid in clinical management.

REFERENCES

1. Osler W. The Gulstonian lectures, on malignant endocarditis. *Br Med J.* 1885;1:467–470.
2. Wilson SE, Wagenen PV, Passaro Jr E. Arterial infection. *Curr Prob Surg.* 1978;15:1–89.
3. Thompson TR, Tillei J, Johnson DE et al. Umbilical artery catheterization complicated by mycotic aortic aneurysm in neonates. *Adv Pediatr.* 1979;27:275–318.
4. Bennett DE. Primary mycotic aneurysms of the aorta: Report of case and review of the literature. *Arch Surg.* 1967;94:758–765.
5. Sommerville R, Allen E, Edwards J. Bland and infected arteriosclerotic abdominal aortic aneurysms: A clinicopathologic study. *Medicine.* 1959;38:207–222.
6. Scher LA, Brener BJ, Goldenkranz RJ et al. Infected aneurysms of the abdominal aorta. *Arch Surg.* 1980;115:975–978.

7. Chan FY, Crawford ES, Coselli JS, Safi HJ, Williams TWJ. In situ prosthetic graft replacement for mycotic aneurysm of the aorta. *Ann Thorac Surg.* 1989;47:193–203.

8. Reddy DJ, Shepard AD, Evans JR, Wright DJ, Smith RF, Ernst CB. Management of infected aortoiliac aneurysms. *Arch Surg.* 1991;126:873–878; discussion 878.

9. Mundth ED, Darling RC, Alvarado RH, Buckley MJ, Linton RR, Austen WG. Surgical management of mycotic aneurysms and the complications of infection in vascular reconstructive surgery. *Am J Surg.* 1969;117:460–470.

10. Mendelowitz DS, Ramstedt R, Yao JS, Bergan JJ. Abdominal aortic salmonellosis. *Surgery.* 1979;85:514–519.

11. Davies OGJ, Thorburn JD, Powell P. Cryptic mycotic abdominal aortic aneurysms: Diagnosis and management. *Am J Surg.* 1978;136:96–101.

12. Schneider JA, Rheuban KS, Crosby IK. Rupture of postcoarctation mycotic aneurysms of the aorta. *Ann Thorac Surg.* 1979;27:185–190.

13. Perdue GDJ, Yancey AG. Mycotic aneurysmal change in the dilated artery proximal to arteriovenous fistula. *South Med J.* 1972;65:1142–1144.

14. Shumacker HBJ. Aneurysm development and degenerative changes in dilated artery proximal to arteriovenous fistula. *Surg Gynecol Obstet.* 1970;130:636–640.

15. Riester WH, Serrano A. Infrarenal mycotic pseudoaneurysm. A late complication of coronary bypass surgery with proximal aortic dissection. *J Thorac Cardiovasc Surg.* 1976;71:633–636.

16. Williams MJ. Perforating suppurative aortitis associated with idiopathic cystic medial necrosis; report of a case. *Am J Clin Pathol.* 1952;22:160–165.

17. Buxton RW, Holdefer WFJ. Primary mycotic aneurysms: Review and report of a case. *Am Surg.* 1963;29:863–867.

18. Jarrett F, Darling RC, Mundth ED, Austen WG. Experience with infected aneurysms of the abdominal aorta. *Arch Surg.* 1975;110:1281–1286.

19. Johansen K, Devin J. Mycotic aortic aneurysms. A reappraisal. *Arch Surg.* 1983;118:583–588.

20. Bennett DE, Cherry JK. Bacterial infection of aortic aneurysms. A clinicopathologic study. *Am J Surg.* 1967;113:321–326.

21. Anderson CB, Butcher HRJ, Ballinger WF. Mycotic aneurysms. *Arch Surg.* 1974;109:712–717.

22. Brown SL, Busuttil RW, Baker JD, Machleder HI, Moore WS, Barker WF. Bacteriologic and surgical determinants of survival in patients with mycotic aneurysms. *J Vasc Surg.* 1984;1:541–547.

23. Stengel A, Wolferth CC. Mycotic (bacterial) aneurysms of intravascular origin. *Arch Int Med.* 1923;31:527–554.

24. Revell S. Primary mycotic aneurysms. *Ann Int Med.* 1945;22:431–440.

25. Lewis D, Schrager VL. Embolomycotic aneurisms. *J Am Med Assoc.* 1909;53:1808–1814.

26. Moneta GL, Taylor LMJ, Yeager RA et al. Surgical treatment of infected aortic aneurysm. *Am J Surg.* 1998;175:396–399.

27. Pirvu A, Bouchet C, Garibotti FM, Haupert S, Sessa C. Mycotic aneurysm of the internal carotid artery. *Ann Vasc Surg.* 2013;27:826–830.

28. Ferguson LJ, Fell G, Buxton B, Royle JP. Mycotic cervical carotid aneurysm. *Br J Surg.* 1984;71:245.

29. Grossi RJ, Onofrey D, Tvetenstrand C, Blumenthal J. Mycotic carotid aneurysm. *J Vasc Surg.* 1987;6:81–83.

30. Hubaut JJ, Albat B, Frapier JM, Chaptal PA. Mycotic aneurysm of the extracranial carotid artery: An uncommon complication of bacterial endocarditis. *Ann Vasc Surg.* 1997;11:634–636.

31. Stanley JC, Thompson NW, Fry WJ. Splanchnic artery aneurysms. *Arch Surg.* 1970;101:689–697.

32. Vansant JH. Massive gastric hemorrhage secondary to rupture of mycotic aneurysm of the splenic artery: Resection and survival. *Am Surg.* 1969;35:497–500.

33. Sharma G, Semel ME, McGillicuddy EA, Ho KJ, Menard MT, Gates JD. Ruptured and unruptured mycotic superior mesenteric artery aneurysms. *Ann Vasc Surg.* 2014;28:1931.e5–1931.e8.

34. Lovezzola MM. Resection of mycotic aneurysm of the small-bowel mesentery. *N Engl J Med.* 1958;259:1076.

35. Houssin D, Ortega D, Richardson A et al. Mycotic aneurysm of the hepatic artery complicating human liver transplantation. *Transplantation.* 1988;46:469–472.

36. Zajko AB, Bradshaw JR, Marsh JW. Mycotic pseudoaneurysm of the gastroduodenal artery – An unusual cause of lower gastrointestinal tract hemorrhage following liver transplantation. *Transplantation.* 1988;45:990–991.

37. Deitch JS, Hansen KJ, Regan JD, Burkhart JM, Ligush JJ. Infected renal artery pseudoaneurysm and mycotic aortic aneurysm after percutaneous transluminal renal artery angioplasty and stent placement in a patient with a solitary kidney. *J Vasc Surg.* 1998;28:340–344.

38. Swanson E, Freiberg A, Salter DR. Radial artery infections and aneurysms after catheterization. *J Hand Surg Am.* 1990;15:166–171.

39. Berry MC, Van Schil PE, Vanmaele RG, De Vries DP. Infected false aneurysm after puncture of an aneurysm of the deep femoral artery. *Eur J Vasc Surg.* 1994;8:372–374.

40. Yeager RA, Hobson RW, Padberg FT, Lynch TG, Chakravarty M. Vascular complications related to drug abuse. *J Trauma.* 1987;27:305–308.

41. Tzakis AG, Carroll PB, Gordon RD, Yokoyama I, Makowka L, Starzl TE. Arterial mycotic aneurysm and rupture. A potentially fatal complication of pancreas transplantation in diabetes mellitus. *Arch Surg.* 1989;124:660–661.

42. Weinberg DJ, Cronin DW, Baker AGJ. Infected iliac pseudoaneurysm after uncomplicated percutaneous balloon angioplasty and (Palmaz) stent insertion: A case report and literature review. *J Vasc Surg*. 1996;23:162–166.

43. Chalmers N, Eadington DW, Gandanhamo D, Gillespie IN, Ruckley CV. Case report: Infected false aneurysm at the site of an iliac stent. *Br J Radiol*. 1993;66:946–948.

44. Therasse E, Soulez G, Cartier P et al. Infection with fatal outcome after endovascular metallic stent placement. *Radiology*. 1994;192:363–365.

45. Bitseff EL, Edwards WH, Mulherin JLJ, Kaiser AB. Infected abdominal aortic aneurysms. *South Med J*. 1987;80:309–312.

46. Jebara VA, Nasnas R, Achouh PE et al. Mycotic aneurysm of the popliteal artery secondary to tuberculosis. A case report and review of the literature. *Tex Heart Inst J*. 1998;25:136–139.

47. Woods JM, Schellack J, Stewart MT, Murray DR, Schwartzman SW. Mycotic abdominal aortic aneurysm induced by immunotherapy with bacille Calmette–Guerin vaccine for malignancy. *J Vasc Surg*. 1988;7:808–810.

48. Uno M, Yamada N, Yamada I, Nagano I, Kagimoto K, Kanazawa H. A case of infected abdominal aortic aneurysm. *J Jpn Surg Assoc*. 2006;67:1763–1767.

49. Hachimaru T, Watanabe M, Kawaguchi S, Nakahara H. In situ replacement with rifampin-soaked vascular prosthesis in a patient with abdominal aortic aneurysm infected by Listeria monocytogenes and presenting with symptoms of Leriche syndrome. *Jpn J Cardiovasc Surg*. 2009;38:344–348.

50. Akiyama T, Matsubara K. Tuberculous mycotic pseudoaneurysm of abdominal aorta. *Jpn J Cardiovasc Surg*. 2008;37:174–176.

51. Skandalos I, Christou K, Psilas A, Moskophidis M, Karamoschos K. Mycotic abdominal aortic aneurysm infected by *Vibrio mimicus*: Report of a case. *Surg Today*. 2009;39:141–143.

52. Bito A, Narahara Y, Murata N, Yamamoto N. A case of infected thoracoabdominal aortic aneurysm caused by Citrobacter koseri. *Jpn J Cardiovasc Surg*. 2008;37:333–336.

53. Maeda H, Umezawa H, Goshima M et al. Primary infected abdominal aortic aneurysm: Surgical procedures, early mortality rates, and a survey of the prevalence of infectious organisms over a 30-year period. *Surg Today*. 2011;41:346–351.

54. Marques da Silva M LPS, Geiran O, Tronstad L, Olsen I. Multiple bacteria in aortic aneurysms. *J Vasc Surg*. 2003;38:1384–1389.

55. Jewkes AJ, Black J. Infection of an abdominal aortic aneurysm from an appendix abscess. *J Cardiovasc Surg (Torino)*. 1989;30:870–872.

56. Katz SG, Andros G, Kohl RD. Salmonella infections of the abdominal aorta. *Surg Gynecol Obstet*. 1992;175:102–106.

57. Thompson JE, Garrett WV. Peripheral-arterial surgery. *N Engl J Med*. 1980;302:491–503.

58. Oz MC, McNicholas KW, Serra AJ, Spagna PM, Lemole GM. Review of Salmonella mycotic aneurysms of the thoracic aorta. *J Cardiovasc Surg (Torino)*. 1989;30:99–103.

59. McIntyre KEJ, Malone JM, Richards E, Axline SG. Mycotic aortic pseudoaneurysm with aortoenteric fistula caused by *Arizona hinshawii*. *Surgery*. 1982;91:173–177.

60. Edwards PR, Fife MA, Ramsey CH. Studies on the Arizona group of Enterobacteriaceae. *Bacteriol Rev*. 1959;23:155–174.

61. Takano H, Taniguchi K, Kuki S, Nakamura T, Miyagawa S, Masai T. Mycotic aneurysm of the infrarenal abdominal aorta infected by *Clostridium septicum*: A case report of surgical management and review of the literature. *J Vasc Surg*. 2003;38:847–851.

62. Seder CW, Kramer M, Long G, Uzieblo MR, Shanley CJ, Bove P. Clostridium septicum aortitis: Report of two cases and review of the literature. *J Vasc Surg*. 2009;49:1304–1309.

63. Miller BM, Waterhouse G, Alford RH, Dean RH, Hawkins SS, Smith BM. Histoplasma infection of abdominal aortic aneurysms. *Ann Surg*. 1983;197:57–62.

64. Szilagyi DE, Smith RF, Elliott JP, Hageman JH, Dall'Olmo CA. Anastomotic aneurysms after vascular reconstruction: Problems of incidence, etiology, and treatment. *Surgery*. 1975;78:800–816.

65. Seabrook GR, Schmitt DD, Bandyk DF, Edmiston CE, Krepel CJ, Towne JB. Anastomotic femoral pseudoaneurysm: An investigation of occult infection as an etiologic factor. *J Vasc Surg*. 1990;11:629–634.

66. Murphy EH, Szeto WY, Herdrich BJ et al. The management of endograft infections following endovascular thoracic and abdominal aneurysm repair. *J Vasc Surg*. 2013;58:1179–1185.

67. Oskoui R, Davis WA, Gomes MN. Salmonella aortitis. A report of a successfully treated case with a comprehensive review of the literature. *Arch Intern Med*. 1993;153:517–525.

68. Merry M, Dunn J, Weismann R, Harris EDJ. Popliteal mycotic aneurysm presenting as septic arthritis and purpura. *J Am Med Assoc*. 1972;221:58–59.

69. Weis-Muller BT, Rascanu C, Sagban A, Grabitz K, Godehardt E, Sandmann W. Single-center experience with open surgical treatment of 36 infected aneurysms of the thoracic, thoracoabdominal, and abdominal aorta. *Ann Vasc Surg*. 2011;25:1020–1025.

70. Porter III LL, Houston MC, Kadir S. Mycotic aneurysms of the hepatic artery: Treatment with arterial embolization. *Am J Med*. 1979;67:697–701.

71. Rosenthal D, Deterling RA, O'Donnell TF, Callow AD. Positive blood culture as an aid in the diagnosis of secondary aortoenteric fistula. *Arch Surg*. 1979;114:1041–1044.

72. Vogelzang RL, Sohaey R. Infected aortic aneurysms: CT appearance. *J Comput Assist Tomogr.* 1988;12:109–112.

73. Ho Y, Hennessy O. Indium-111 WBC scan to diagnose mycotic aneurysm. *Clin Nucl Med.* 1999;24:903.

74. Hsu C-C, Huang Y-F, Chuang Y-W. Detection of an infected abdominal aortic aneurysm with three-phase bone scan and gallium-67 scan. *Clin Nucl Med.* 2008;33:305–307.

75. Hodgkiss-Harlow KD, Bandyk DF. Antibiotic therapy of aortic graft infection: Treatment and prevention recommendations. *Semin Vasc Surg.* 2011;24:191–198.

76. Berger P, Moll FL. Aortic graft infections: Is there still a role for axillobifemoral reconstruction? *Semin Vasc Surg.* 2011;24:205–210.

77. O'Connor S, Andrew P, Batt M, Becquemin JP. A systematic review and meta-analysis of treatments for aortic graft infection. *J Vasc Surg.* 2006;44:38–45.

78. Cooke PA, Ehrenfeld WK. Successful management of mycotic aortic aneurysm: Report of a case. *Surgery.* 1974;75:132–136.

79. Perdue G Jr, Smith R III. Surgical treatment of mycotic aneurysms. *Southern Med J.* 1967;60:848–851.

80. Ewart JM, Burke ML, Bunt TJ. Spontaneous abdominal aortic infections. Essentials of diagnosis and management. *Am Surg.* 1983;49:37–50.

81. Ernst CB. Aortoenteric fistulas. In: Haimovici H, ed. *Vascular Emergencies.* New York: Appleton-Century-Crofts, 1982, pp. 365–385.

82. Blaisdell FW, Hall AD. Axillary-femoral artery bypass for lower extremity ischemia. *Surgery.* 1963;54:563–568.

83. Lai CH, Luo CY, Lin PY et al. Surgical consideration of in situ prosthetic replacement for primary infected abdominal aortic aneurysms. *Eur J Vasc Endovasc Surg.* 2011;42:617–624.

84. Harlander-Locke MP, Harmon LK, Lawrence PF et al. The use of cryopreserved aortoiliac allograft for aortic reconstruction in the United States. *J Vasc Surg.* 2014;59:669–674.

85. Dorweiler B, Neufang A, Chaban R, Reinstadler J, Duenschede F, Vahl CF. Use and durability of femoral vein for autologous reconstruction with infection of the aortoiliofemoral axis. *J Vasc Surg.* 2014;59:675–683.

86. Farhat F, Attia C, Boussel L et al. Endovascular repair of the descending thoracic aorta: Mid-term results and evaluation of magnetic resonance angiography. *J Cardiovasc Surg (Torino).* 2007;48:1–6.

87. Kan CD, Lee HL, Yang YJ. Outcome after endovascular stent graft treatment for mycotic aortic aneurysm: A systematic review. *J Vasc Surg.* 2007;46:906–912.

88. Semba CP, Sakai T, Slonim SM et al. Mycotic aneurysms of the thoracic aorta: Repair with use of endovascular stent-grafts. *J Vasc Interv Radiol.* 1998;9:33–40.

89. Escobar GA, Eliason JL, Hurie J, Arya S, Rectenwald JE, Coleman DM. Rifampin soaking dacron-based endografts for implantation in infected aortic aneurysms – New application of a time-tested principle. *Ann Vasc Surg.* 2014;28:744–748.

90. DeBakey ME, Cooley DA. Successful resection of mycotic aneurysm of superior mesenteric artery; case report and review of literature. *Am Surg.* 1953;19:202–212.

91. Friedman SG, Pogo GJ, Moccio CG. Mycotic aneurysm of the superior mesenteric artery. *J Vasc Surg.* 1987;6:87–90.

92. Howard TC, Mazer MJ. Case report. Mycotic aneurysm of the superior mesenteric artery: Report of a successful repair. *Am Surg.* 1981;47:89–92.

93. Olcott C, Ehrenfeld WK. Endoaneurysmorrhaphy for visceral artery aneurysms. *Am J Surg.* 1977;133:636–639.

94. Jones VS, Chennapragada MS, Lord DJ, Stormon M, Shun A. Post-liver transplant mycotic aneurysm of the hepatic artery. *J Pediatr Surg.* 2008;43:555–558.

95. Zeppa R, Petrou HD, Womack NA. Collateral circulation to the liver: A case of mycotic aneurysm of the celiac artery. *Ann Surg.* 1966;163:233–236.

96. Ernst CB, Hagihara PF, Daugherty ME, Griffen WOJ. Inferior mesenteric artery stump pressure: A reliable index for safe IMA ligation during abdominal aortic aneurysmectomy. *Ann Surg.* 1978;187:641–646.

97. Lueg EA, Awerbuck D, Forte V. Ligation of the common carotid artery for the management of a mycotic pseudoaneurysm of an extracranial internal carotid artery. A case report and review of the literature. *Int J Pediatr Otorhinolaryngol.* 1995;33:67–74.

98. Ehrnefeld WK, Stoney RJ, Wylie EJ. Relation of carotid stump pressure to safety of carotid artery ligation. *Surgery.* 1983;93:299–305.

99. Archie J. Carotid endarterectomy. In: Jack L Cronenwett, Robert B Rutherford, eds. *Decision Making in Vascular Surgery.* Philadelphia, PA: WB Saunders, 2001, pp. 38–43.

100. Lee SH, Cho YK, Park JM, Chung C, Kim HS, Woo JJ. Treatment of an acute mycotic aneurysm of the common carotid artery with a covered stent-graft. *Yonsei Med J.* 2012;53:224–227.

101. Wales L, Kruger AJ, Jenkins JS, Mitchell K, Boyne NS, Walker PJ. Mycotic carotid pseudoaneurysm: Staged endovascular and surgical repair. *Eur J Vasc Endovasc Surg.* 2010;39:23–25.

102. Pasic M, von Segesser L, Turina M. Implantation of antibiotic-releasing carriers and in situ reconstruction for treatment of mycotic aneurysm. *Arch Surg.* 1992;127:745–746.

103. Cheng SW, Fok M, Wong J. Infected femoral pseudoaneurysm in intravenous drug abusers. *Br J Surg.* 1992;79:510–512.

104. Kaufman JL, Shah DM, Corson JD, Skudder PA, Leather RP. Sartorius muscle coverage for the treatment of complicated vascular surgical wounds. *J Cardiovasc Surg (Torino).* 1989;30:479–483.

105. Meyer JP, Durham JR, Schwarcz TH, Sawchuk AP, Schuler JJ. The use of sartorius muscle rotation-transfer in the management of wound complications after infrainguinal vein bypass: A report of eight cases and description of the technique. *J Vasc Surg.* 1989;9:731–735.

106. Mixter RC, Turnipseed WD, Smith DJJ, Acher CW, Rao VK, Dibbell DG. Rotational muscle flaps: A new technique for covering infected vascular grafts. *J Vasc Surg.* 1989;9:472–478.

107. Perler BA, Vander Kolk CA, Dufresne CR, Williams GM. Can infected prosthetic grafts be salvaged with rotational muscle flaps? *Surgery.* 1991;110:30–34.

108. Perler BA, Kolk CA, Manson PM, Williams GM. Rotational muscle flaps to treat localized prosthetic graft infection: Long-term follow-up. *J Vasc Surg.* 1993;18:358–364; discussion 364.

109. Kwon K, Choi D, Choi SH et al. Percutaneous stent-graft repair of mycotic common femoral artery aneurysm. *J Endovasc Ther.* 2002;9:690–693.

110. Herscu G, Wilson SE. Prosthetic infection: Lessons from treatment of the infected vascular graft. *Surg Clin North Am.* 2009;89:391–401, viii.

111. Stone PA, Armstrong PA, Bandyk DF et al. Use of antibiotic-loaded polymethylmethacrylate beads for the treatment of extracavitary prosthetic vascular graft infections. *J Vasc Surg.* 2006;44:757–761.

112. Poi MJ, Pisimisis G, Barshes NR et al. Evaluating effectiveness of antibiotic polymethylmethacrylate beads in achieving wound sterilization and graft preservation in patients with early and late vascular graft infections. *Surgery.* 2013;153:673–682.

113. Reddy DJ, Smith RF, Elliott JPJ, Haddad GK, Wanek EA. Infected femoral artery false aneurysms in drug addicts: Evolution of selective vascular reconstruction. *J Vasc Surg.* 1986;3:718–724.

114. Padberg FJ, Hobson R, Lee B et al. Femoral pseudoaneurysm from drugs of abuse: Ligation or reconstruction? *J Vasc Surg.* 1992;15:642–648.

Cerebrovascular Disease

33

Extracranial vascular disease

Natural history and medical management

ANKUR THAPAR, IEUAN HARRI JENKINS and ALUN HUW DAVIES

CONTENTS

INTRODUCTION

Definitions

Stroke is a clinical syndrome defined by the World Health Organization as a rapidly developing focal neurological deficit lasting longer than 24 hours or leading to death from a presumed vascular cause.[1] In the special case of subarachnoid hemorrhage, this deficit may be global. Strokes may be ischemic or hemorrhagic. If the focal symptoms resolve within an arbitrary cut-off of 24 hours, this is referred to as a transient ischemic attack (TIA).[2] Amaurosis fugax is defined as transient monocular loss of vision lasting seconds to minutes attributable to ischemia or vascular insufficiency of the retina and is usually grouped with TIA.[3]

Ischemic stroke affects distinct neurovascular territories: the anterior circulation/ophthalmic artery (carotid territory) and the posterior circulation/anterior spinal artery (vertebrobasilar territory).[4] As Table 33.1 shows signs such as hemiparesis, hemisensory loss and hemianopia can be found in both territories. With the advent of diffusion-weighted MRI (dwMRI), there has been an understanding that in those clinically diagnosed with TIA, up to one-third have radiological evidence of acute cerebral infarction, despite experiencing only transient symptoms.[5] Conversely, it is also recognized that cerebral infarction can be found in patients with no clinical neurological deficit, termed a 'silent' infarct. However, radiological acute infarction identifies those at high risk of further stroke and has been incorporated into the recent ABCD2I stroke risk prediction algorithm.[6]

Carotid plaque is defined histologically as an atherosclerotic thickening of the arterial intima, commonly found close to the carotid bifurcation, and is defined using ultrasound criteria as a focal structure that encroaches into the arterial lumen of at least 0.5 mm or 50% of the surrounding intima-media thickness or demonstrates a thickness >1.5 mm as measured from the media–adventitia interface to the intima–lumen interface.[7] There is no similar ultrasound consensus for vertebral atheroma. Arterial dissection is defined as a tear in the arterial wall allowing entry of blood which separates the layers of the arterial wall.

Table 33.1 Symptoms of anterior and posterior circulation ischemia.

Anterior circulation (carotid territory)	Posterior circulation (vertebrobasilar territory)
Ipsilateral amaurosis fugax or retinal infarction (branch or central retinal artery)	Ipsilateral cranial nerve palsy, e.g. III nerve palsy
Contralateral sensory loss	Contralateral sensory loss in limbs, which may be combined with ipsilateral facial sensory loss
Contralateral homonymous hemianopia	Contralateral homonymous quadrantanopia or hemianopia or bilateral cortical visual loss
Contralateral motor weakness	Contralateral/bilateral motor weakness
Contralateral visuospatial neglect with intact visual fields (especially in right-sided cerebral infarction)	Nystagmus and diplopia
Dysphasia in left-sided cerebral infarction	Ataxic hemiparesis
	Ataxia and other cerebellar signs
	Vertigo
	Impaired conscious level
	Emesis

EPIDEMIOLOGY AND PATHOPHYSIOLOGY OF ISCHEMIC STROKE

Epidemiology of stroke

Stroke is responsible for 9% of global mortality in males and 11% in females,[8] following infectious disease (≈16%), ischemic heart disease (≈12%), cancer (≈12%) and trauma (≈10%). The age-adjusted incidence of stroke ranges from 94 per 100,000 persons in high-income countries rising to 117 per 100,000 persons in low- to middle-income countries.[9] Stroke is projected to become the second leading cause of worldwide disability in developed countries in 2020 and the fifth in developing countries[10] and is a major public health concern.

Causes of stroke

In high-income countries, the approximate breakdown of stroke subtypes are ischemic stroke (≈82%), followed by primary intracerebral hemorrhage (≈11%), subarachnoid hemorrhage (≈3%) and finally cryptogenic (≈4%).[9]

Ischemic stroke can be subclassified using the TOAST classification[11] as large artery atherosclerosis, cardioembolic, small artery occlusion, other known cause and cryptogenic. In Europe, it is estimated that 10%–15% of ischemic strokes are secondary to carotid atherosclerosis.[12,13] The mean age of patients with carotid atherosclerotic stroke in Europe is 62 (SD ± 8) years and over two-thirds of patients are male.[14] Figures for vertebral disease are less well studied.

The focus of this chapter will be large artery stroke in the extracranial vasculature, namely, the carotid and vertebral arteries. The mechanism of stroke in these vessels is commonly thromboembolic, but trauma, dissection and flow limitation (e.g. subclavian steal) are also encountered.

Mechanism of stroke

Carotid and vertebral stroke commonly occurs from two distinct processes: rupture of a vulnerable atherosclerotic plaque in the vessel intima causing local thrombosis with artery to artery embolism in the presence of inadequate distal collateral circulation from the circle of Willis or dissection through a weakened vessel media causing compression of the true vessel lumen. The resulting symptoms reflect the ischemic neurovascular territory in question (Table 33.1),[15,16] the central area of which may undergo permanent infarction and part of which may have reversible ischemia if blood flow is re-established: the penumbra. This is the area of interest targeted by new therapies such as stroke thrombolysis.

Differential diagnosis

Aside from intracerebral and subarachnoid hemorrhage, stroke mimics are important conditions to consider prior to thrombolysis. They include traumatic intracranial hematoma, seizure and postictal states such as Todd's paresis, presyncope and syncope, migraine, carotid sinus hypersensitivity, peripheral vestibular disturbance, cerebral space occupying lesion, peripheral nerve palsy and functional weakness.

Similarly, stroke chameleons are atypical presentations of stroke including vertigo, coma, amnesia and ophthalmoplegia. These are more common in the posterior circulation. These require a high index of suspicion and dwMRI to detect.

Transient ischemic attacks

Approximately a quarter of ischemic stroke patients will have experienced a preceding TIA.[17] TIAs are considered a neurovascular emergency for two reasons. First, there are time-dependent interventions available to prevent stroke, including thrombolysis and antiplatelet agents, anticoagulants and carotid intervention, as discussed in the next chapter. Second, a new appreciation that when a subsequent stroke occurs, it does so in the 7 days following the most recent TIA in 43% of patients.[17] Therefore, in the words of Rothwell and Warlow 'the window for prevention is very short'. The EXPRESS study demonstrated that a rapid access TIA clinic and early initiation of antiplatelet therapy reduced the 90-day risk of stroke from 10% to 2%[18] (level of evidence 2b, grade of recommendation B).

Patients are recommended to be risk stratified after a TIA using the ABCD2 risk score, with points for risk derived from multivariate analysis, age ≥60 years (1 point), blood pressure 140/90 mmHg (2 points), and clinical features, unilateral weakness (2 points) or speech impairment without weakness (1 point), duration of symptoms ≥60 minutes (2 points) or 10–59 minutes (1 point) and the presence of diabetes (1 point).[6] Those who are at high risk (ABCD2 score 6–7) have an 8% risk of stroke over the following 2 days, allowing triage of patients to an acute stroke centre.[19] Evidence of brain infarction on computed tomography or dwMRI improves accuracy of subsequent stroke prediction from a c-statistic of 0.66 for ABCD2 to 0.78 for ABCD2I.[6] The presence of brain infarction increases the risk of stroke sixfold[6] (level of evidence 2). Unfortunately, the ABCD2 score does not predict the presence of carotid stenosis or the benefit of revascularization.[20]

A SHORT HISTORY OF CAROTID ATHEROSCLEROSIS

Initial thoughts on the mechanism of carotid atherosclerotic stroke focused on flow limitation. Ambroise Paré, the Napoleonic surgeon commented that the carotid arteries were essential for cerebral perfusion: 'there are two branches which they call carotids or *soporales* [the sleep arteries] because they being obstructed or any way stopt we presently fall asleep'.[21] Ramsay Hunt in 1914 recommended the carotid pulse be examined in patients with neurological symptoms: 'While inequality of pulsation on the two sides might be accidental, its occurrence in four cases all presenting with symptoms of extensive brain softening [stroke] is rather significant and the thought naturally arises that some obstructive lesion of the vessel…has interfered with the free flow of blood to the brain'.[22]

However, there were problems with this hypothesis in that carotid ligation was historically practiced to limit the growth of intracranial aneurysms,[23] made possible due to collateral circulation from the circle of Willis, complete in around 90% of healthy persons.[24]

Chiari in a post-mortem study in 1905 detected carotid atheroma surface thrombus in patients who had died of stroke, the first evidence for carotid atheroma rupture causing thromboembolism.[25] In the 1970s, post-mortem studies revealed embolic showers in the anterior and middle cerebral artery distribution in patients with a ruptured carotid plaque.[26] In 1992, transcranial Doppler was used to insonate the middle cerebral artery of patients with carotid atherosclerosis in the immediate period post stroke, allowing identification of microembolic particles which were postulated to originate from ruptured carotid plaques.[27] These findings were not found in healthy controls. Today, dwMRI can visualize the sequelae of an embolic shower in the hours after a TIA.[28]

NATURAL HISTORY OF CAROTID ATHEROSCLEROSIS

Carotid atherosclerosis is a common problem, with >2% of the general European population over 60 estimated to have unilateral >50% carotid stenosis.[29] Historically, the ipsilateral stroke risk in patients with no recent stroke symptoms treated with early medical therapy was just over 2% per annum in the 1995 ACAS trial.[30] More recently, this fell below 1% in the 2010 asymptomatic carotid surgery trial-1 (ACST-1).[31] This is mirrored by the results of non-randomized studies.[32]

Recent cohort studies such as OXVASC and SMART have reported lower stroke risks (≈0.3% per year) for patients treated medically than in ACST-1[33,34] and demonstrate that the majority of individuals with carotid atherosclerosis can be treated safely with medical treatment (level of evidence 2, grade of recommendation B). One criticism of non-randomized studies is selection bias towards low-risk patients who might never require surgical intervention.

The reasons for this temporal improvement are hypothesized to include increased awareness of cardiovascular risk factors, improvements in primary prevention of stroke through public health programmers for cardiovascular disease and smoking cessation and the introduction of statins and multimodal antihypertensive therapy into primary prevention guidelines.

Two further questions are of interest. First, what is the rate of progression of carotid disease? Progression through one stenosis category (50%–69%, 70%–89%, 90%–99% and occlusion) was noted in the medical arm of ACST-1, at a rate of approximately 5% per year; however, one must take this with caution as 5% of patients also regressed, due to either imaging discrepancy or true regression of disease.[35] In a single-centre retrospective US cohort study of 900 patients with 50%–69% NASCET equivalent stenosis, the 5-year incidence of plaque progression was 39%, equivalent to an 8% annual rate of progression.[36] These two studies found opposite effects of plaque progression on risk of future stroke.

The second question is what is the effect of carotid artery occlusion on stroke risk? The ACST-1 investigators looked at this in detail and found that in their deferral of surgery arm, the risk of new carotid occlusion in patients with 50%–99% carotid stenosis was about 1% per annum.[37] In these patients, only 17/30 (57%) developed a contemporaneous stroke, suggesting their circle of Willis was intact. In multivariate analysis, occlusion was an independent prognostic risk factor for stroke (adjusted HR 1.73 [95% CI 1.15–2.61]). These data demonstrate plaque progression towards occlusion to be quite slow and confer only a small added stroke risk (level of evidence 2, grade of recommendation B). With modern medical therapy, this situation may become less common.

PREVENTION OF CAROTID ATHEROSCLEROTIC STROKE

Risk factors for carotid atherosclerosis

The Framingham cohort study examined the risk factors for development of carotid atherosclerosis.[38] Independent predictors of the degree of stenosis were age (OR 1.6–1.7/ decade), cigarette smoking (1.3–1.5/10 cigarettes smoked per day), systolic blood pressure (1.2/10 mmHg increase) and total cholesterol (1.1–1.2/0.5 mmol/L increase). These were confirmed in an independent cohort study.[39] Three key risk factors are modifiable: hypertension, smoking and dyslipidemia (level of evidence 2). In recent European guidelines,[40] the presence of asymptomatic carotid disease is considered to be a very high risk marker for future cardiovascular events, obviating the need for risk scoring and mandating aggressive anti-atherosclerotic therapy. We consider here the key risk factors, evidence for primary prevention of ischemic stroke and recommendations from UK, US and European guidelines.

Hypertension

Hypertension is defined by consensus as a systolic blood pressure ≥140 mmHg and a diastolic blood pressure of ≥90 mmHg.[41] Hypertension can be primary or secondary to other vascular pathology such as coarctation of the aorta or renal artery stenosis. Stroke risk is directly related to blood pressure as demonstrated in a meta-analysis of nine prospective studies. In this analysis, a 10 mmHg decrease in diastolic BP was independently associated with a 56% reduction in stroke incidence over a mean of 10 years, with no evidence of a threshold below which risk reduction stopped.[42] Similarly, a seminal meta-analysis of 61 cohort studies in 2002[43] demonstrated a constant relationship between blood pressure and stroke mortality across genders and age groups, with a 20 mmHg fall in systolic blood pressure equating to a risk reduction of around 60% for the next decade for a man aged 60 (HR 0.41 [95% CI 0.39–0.44] (level of evidence I) (Figure 33.1).

Recently, it has been established that episodic hypertension is at least as strong a predictor of future stroke as mean systolic blood pressure, leading to ambulatory monitoring to identify episodic hypertension and minimize white coat hypertension.[44]

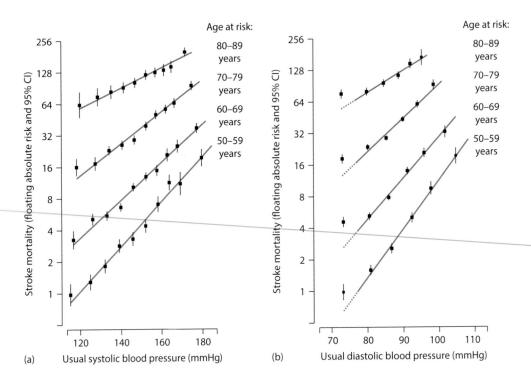

Figure 33.1 Stroke mortality rate in each decade of age versus usual blood pressure at the start of that decade. (a) Systolic blood pressure. (b) Diastolic blood pressure. (Reprinted from Lewington S et al., *Lancet*, 360(9349), 1903, 2002. With permission.)

Current international recommendations are summarized in a recent article in the *Journal of the American Medical Association*.[45] The 2014 US guidelines set a target of <150/90 mmHg for the general population ≥60 years and 140/90 mmHg for those younger or with diabetes or renal impairment.[45] The 2013 European Society of Cardiology (ESC) guidelines set a target of <150/90 mmHg for those ≥80 years and 140/90 mmHg for those younger or with diabetes or renal impairment but lower at 130/90 mmHg for those with proteinuria.[40] The 2011 NICE guidelines recommend 150/90 mmHg for those ≥80 years and 140/90 mmHg for others.[46]

These do not address the important questions of the degree of risk reduction with treatment and whether there is a threshold effect below a certain level of blood pressure. However, these were explored in a recent meta-analysis of 147 randomized controlled trials in patients both with and without cardiovascular disease.[47] It found first that in both subgroups, lowering blood pressure by 10 mmHg systolic or 5 mmHg diastolic consistently reduced future strokes by at least one-third during follow-up. For patients who had experienced a previous stroke, the relative risk of stroke during follow-up was 0.66 (95% CI 0.56–0.76). For patients with no clinical cardiovascular disease, the relative risk of stroke during follow-up was 0.54 (95% CI 0.45–0.65). This effect was consistent across randomized and non-randomized studies (level of evidence 1) (Figure 33.2) and relates to both ischemic and hemorrhagic strokes.

The same study found further risk reduction in stroke when patients who were normotensive were treated with antihypertensives. This was corroborated to an extent by the 2002 meta-analysis by Lewington.[43] This is a controversial area, as the evidence is sparse, the population in whom this is applicable is enormous and the risk–benefit is altered. It does suggest that no true threshold blood pressure exists and that blood pressure targets necessarily reflect an acceptable level of risk versus an acceptable level of side effects in the population being considered. The authors provided a model as to the risk reduction an individual could expect based on age, pre-treatment blood pressure and blood pressure reduction (Figure 33.3).

Larger blood pressure reductions were achieved with low-dose multimodal therapy than with high-dose single agents alone, which one would expect reduce the severity of side effects as a secondary benefit. In comparison to placebo or to another agent, beta-blockers had the least effect on recurrent stroke (rate ratio [RR] 1.18, 95% CI 1.03–1.36) versus other antihypertensive agents. Coupled with their diabetogenic properties, beta-blockers cannot be recommended as a first-line antihypertensive therapy for stroke (level of Evidence 1, grade of recommendation A).

Blood pressure treatment algorithms vary internationally, with the 2011 UK NICE algorithm recommending a calcium channel blocker in those over 55[46] and the US 2014 algorithm starting with either a thiazide, angiotensin-converting enzyme inhibitor or calcium channel blocker in non-blacks over 60 years of age.[45] Treatment targets reflect the age of the patient and the overall cardiovascular risk. As a caveat, a small group of patients with severe bilateral carotid or vertebral stenosis or occlusion may develop watershed ischemia, if their blood pressure is reduced below their elevated autoregulatory threshold.[48] These patients should have their blood pressure controlled more gently, with expert opinion that this could be up to 150 mmHg systolic[49] (level of evidence 4, grade of recommendation D).

For patients who have already experienced a TIA or stroke, secondary prevention recommendations are available from the United Kingdom, ESC and American Stroke Association (ASA). The 2012 UK Royal College of Physicians recommendations are that blood pressure be controlled to 130/80 mmHg, starting treatment before discharge or at 2 weeks, whichever is sooner.[49] The ESC recommend a target of <140/90 mmHg, except in the elderly where this has not been directly tested.[41] The 2014 ASA guideline recommendations are that a target of <140/90 mmHg is achieved, stating that there is uncertain benefit in reduction below this level.[50] In acute stroke patients who were previously on antihypertensives, they state that these can be resumed in patients without fluctuating neurology after 24 hours.

One special scenario is post-endarterectomy hypertension which has been linked to coma, seizures and hemorrhagic stroke, often preceded by headache, termed

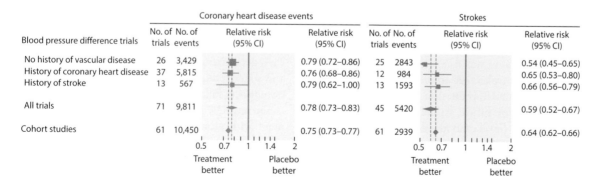

Figure 33.2 Relative risk reduction for coronary heart disease and stroke for a 10 mmHg systolic or 5 mmHg diastolic in blood pressure across randomized and non-randomized studies. (Reprinted from Law MR et al., *Br Med J*, 338, b1665, 2009. With permission.)

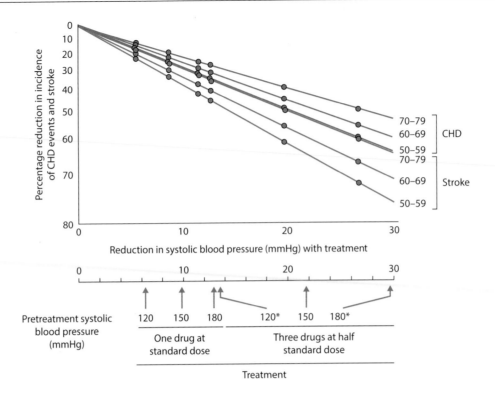

Figure 33.3 Multivariate model of reduction in incidence of coronary heart disease and stroke events in relation to reduction in sytolic blood pressure, combination of antihypertensive drugs, pretreatment blood pressure and age. *Note:* * indicates that these values are more uncertain and also the incidence of events. (Reprinted from Law MR et al., *Br Med J*, 338, b1665, 2009. With permission.)

'cerebral hyperperfusion syndrome'. Recognition and prompt treatment of patients post-endarterectomy with hypertension and headache can prevent this devastating complication of endarterectomy. Several guidelines are available with one presented here (Figure 33.4), which uses oral nifedipine retard or intravenous labetalol depending on whether headache or new neurological symptoms are present.[51,52] Urgent cerebral imaging is recommended for those with symptoms more than transient headache to determine if there is a new cerebral infarct or hemorrhage.

Dyslipidemia

The Cholesterol Treatment Trialists' Collaborative 2010 meta-analysis of 26 randomized controlled trials examined the benefits of intensive lowering of cholesterol in high risk patients using statins.[53] They found consistent reductions in total stroke risk amongst all categories of trial. For each 1 mmol/L reduction in LDL cholesterol, the risk reduction for future stroke was 16% (OR 0.84 [95% CI 0.79–0.89]) (level of evidence 1, grade of recommendation A). A significant decrease in ischemic stroke (OR 0.79 [95% CI 0.74–0.85]) was seen in comparison with a non-significant increase in hemorrhagic stroke (OR 1.12 [95% CI 0.93–1.35]). There were no significant increases in non-cardiovascular mortality or cancer through the use of intensive statin therapy. The excess

rate of rhabdomyolysis with 80 mg of simvastatin in comparison with 20 mg was estimated to be 4 per 10,000 patients. It is unknown how much publication bias there is when considering the beneficial effects of statins and this should be borne in mind.

It is clear therefore that patients with carotid and vertebral atherosclerosis benefit from intensive LDL reduction. Current UK guidelines recommend a >40% reduction in LDL, ESC guidelines recommend a ≥50% decrease in LDL aiming for <1.8 mmol/L and US guidelines recommend moderate- or high-intensity statins (e.g. atorvastatin 10–80 mg) for those with a 10-year cardiovascular risk ≥7.5% aiming for as low an LDL as possible.[40,54]

For patients who have already experienced a carotid TIA or stroke, the effect of secondary prevention through intensive lowering of cholesterol was suggested in a post hoc subgroup analysis of the SPARCL trial of atorvastatin 80 mg versus placebo in patients with ischemic stroke or TIA, demonstrating a 33% reduction in all stroke subtypes and a 56% reduction in the need for carotid revascularization during follow-up.[55]

Current UK NICE guidelines recommend initial treatment with atorvastatin 80 mg daily. The ESC guidance is identical to that in primary prevention. The 2014 ASA secondary prevention recommendation is that there is strong benefit in reducing LDL cholesterol to 2.6 mmol/L and slightly weaker evidence for reducing it below 2.6 mmol/L,[50] differing from the recommendation from the ACC, who recommend the lower the better. This is due

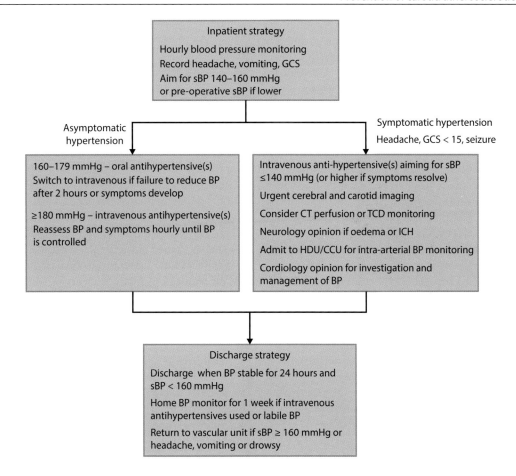

Figure 33.4 An algorithm for management of post carotid endarterectomy cerebral hyperperfusion syndrome. (Reprinted from Bouri S et al., *Eur J Vasc Endovasc Surg*, 41(2), 229, 2011. With permission.)

to the non-significant increase in hemorrhagic stroke that has been found with statin therapy.[53]

Smoking

Smoking is now banned in public areas in over 60 countries worldwide, demonstrating the strength of evidence between smoking and stroke risk which rises in an exposure-dependent fashion[56] (level of evidence 1) and can be either first hand or passively acquired. Furthermore, the effect of quitting is a return to baseline stroke risk after 5 years as demonstrated in the Framingham study[57] (level of evidence 2, grade of recommendation B).

The effects of smoking bans are difficult to tease out, but in the year after the smoking in public places ban in 2007 in England and Wales, admissions for acute myocardial infarction dropped by 2% and an extra 300,000 persons made an attempt to quit[58] (level of evidence 3).

Current UK NICE guidelines suggest validating success by carbon monoxide breath levels of <10 parts per million at follow-up visits. Both individual and group behavioural therapy are recommended in combination with either nicotine replacement therapy or varenicline or bupropion for 2–4 weeks after their target quit date, based on data from the 2012 Cochrane review. This pooled data from 40 randomized

controlled trials of combined therapy versus usual care and found that at 6 months, there was a relative risk of 1.82 (95% CI 1.66–2.00, $I^2 = 40\%$) for quitting with combined therapy[59] (level of evidence 1, grade of recommendation A).

A more controversial topic is that of e-cigarettes as an adjunct to quitting. These were introduced in 2003 and contain nicotine but a negligible concentration of carcinogens. Their long-term safety is unknown but is likely to be better than cigarettes as they lack tobacco. Two randomized trials are conflicting as to the efficacy of e-cigarettes versus conventional pharmacotherapy.[60,61] From a public health point of view, it is unknown whether they encourage more people to give up tobacco than they encourage current smokers to quit. More research is needed in this area.

In secondary prevention, there is evidence from the Cardiovascular Health cohort study that smoking is an independent risk factor for second stroke (HR 2.06, 95% CI 1.19–3.56, p = 0.010).[62] Hence, even after ischemic stroke, smoking cessation may be of benefit (level of evidence 2, grade of recommendation B).

Antiplatelet therapy

Stroke may be caused through thromboembolism or intracranial hemorrhage which may be potentiated by antiplatelet therapy. The effect of low-dose aspirin, the most commonly used primary prevention antiplatelet agent, was analyzed in 2009 by the Antiplatelet Trialists' Collaborative.[63] This was an individual patient data meta-analysis of six primary prevention trials using aspirin 75–500 mg daily versus placebo (4 trials) or no placebo (2 trials). The principal results (Figure 33.5) showed no benefit in terms of stroke overall and a trend towards more fatal stroke in those treated with aspirin. This is explained by the finding that whilst aspirin prevents as many ischemic strokes as it causes hemorrhagic strokes, the latter are more likely to be fatal. Therefore, in primary prevention, aspirin is beneficial for the prevention of non-fatal myocardial infarction rather than stroke (level of evidence 1, grade of recommendation A).

In contrast, in patients who have already had a cardiovascular event, the risk of future ischemic stroke is higher. Hence, data from the same analysis regarding secondary prevention demonstrated a small but significant benefit of aspirin in reducing future stroke in patients with a previous myocardial infarction or ischemic stroke (RR 0.78, 95% CI 0.61–0.99, p = 0.04). Therefore, low-dose aspirin is recommended in secondary prevention of stroke (level of evidence 1, grade of recommendation A).

In recent years, clopidogrel has emerged as an alternative to aspirin. The CAPRIE trial demonstrated that in secondary prevention of ischemic stroke, 75 mg of clopidogrel versus 325 mg of aspirin prevented only 23 more strokes (315 vs. 338) in the 12,033 stroke patients randomized, i.e. equivalent (level of evidence 1).[64] The intracranial hemorrhage rate was additionally lower with clopidogrel (0.35% vs. 0.49%), as was the gastrointestinal hemorrhage rate (1.99% vs. 2.66%).

Preliminary evidence from meta-analysis of small randomized controlled trials points to the combination of dual antiplatelet regimes with complementary modes of action (aspirin, dipyridamole and clopidogrel) being superior to aspirin alone in the prevention of recurrent stroke (RR 0.67, 95% CI 0.49–0.93).[65] This was at the expense of a non-significant increase in major bleeding. This strategy is being tested in the larger Platelet-Oriented Inhibition in New TIA trial. Triple combination antiplatelet therapy is also being trialled in the Triple Antiplatelets for Reducing Dependency after Ischemic Stroke trial, designed to assess the efficacy, safety and tolerability of combining clopidogrel with aspirin and dipyridamole in patients with recent ischemic stroke or TIA.

Blood sugar control

In a similar fashion to cholesterol, the effect of more intensive lowering of glycosylated hemoglobin on cardiovascular outcomes was examined through meta-analysis in 2009.[66]

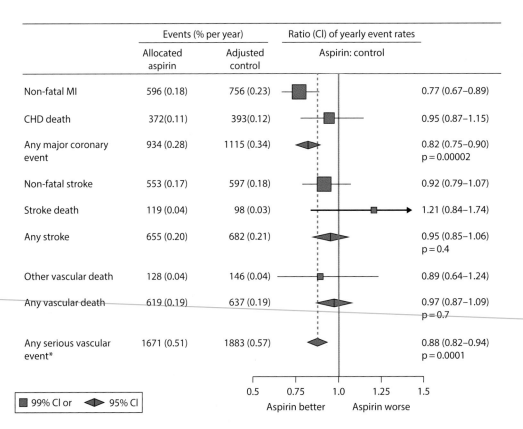

Figure 33.5 Major vascular events in primary prevention randomized trials. Rate ratios for all trials are indicated by squares and their 99% CIs by horizontal lines. MI, myocardial infarction; CHD, coronary heart disease. *Myocardial infarction, stroke or vascular death. Vascular death is coronary heart disease death, stroke death or other vascular death (which includes sudden death, death from pulmonary embolism and death from any hemorrhage, but in the primary prevention trials excludes death from an unknown cause). (Reprinted from Baigent C et al., *Lancet*, 373(9678), 1849, 2009. With permission.)

In five randomized controlled trials comparing intensive versus less standard HBA1C control (approximately a difference of 1%), with different agents, no significant difference in future stroke events was found with intensive HBA1C control (OR 0.93, 95% CI 0.81–1.06). Therefore standard care is advised (level of evidence 1, grade of recommendation A).

Effectiveness of treat to target medical therapy

The European Action on Secondary and Primary Prevention by Intervention to Reduce Events (EUROASPIRE) surveys looked at compliance with secondary prevention measure in patients with symptomatic ischemic heart disease across eight European countries.[67] EUROASPIRE I was performed in 1995–1996, EUROASPIRE II in 1999–2000 and EUROASPIRE III in 2006–2007. Across this decade, the proportion with hypercholesterolaemia decreased significantly from 95% to 46%. The proportion of smokers (≈20%) and those who suffered hypertension remained similar (≈60%). The prevalence of diabetes rose from 17% to 28%, as did the prevalence of obesity (25% to 38%).

In a contemporary US cohort study on patients with 50%–69% asymptomatic carotid stenosis,[36] 87% took statins; however, only 52% achieved an LDL < 2.6 mmol/L and only 14% achieved an LDL < 1.8 mmol/L.

These studies demonstrate that despite advances in pharmacological therapy for atherosclerosis, there are important barriers that still remain to smoking cessation and treatment of hypertension and dyslipidemia that need to be overcome. This means importantly that there is still a large population of patients with asymptomatic carotid stenosis who fail to receive best medial therapy (level of evidence 3).

HYPERACUTE TREATMENT FOR ISCHEMIC STROKE

In 1996, intravenous thrombolysis with recombinant tissue plasminogen activator (rt-PA) was licensed in the United States. This followed the results of the landmark National Institute of Neurological Disorders and Stroke trial,[68] which demonstrated a significant improvement at 3 months in disability in those treated with the fibrinolytic agent rt-PA within 3 hours of symptom onset.

Subsequent trials have supported this initial finding with a meta-analysis of 12 randomized controlled trials of rt-PA versus standard care comprising 7012 patients worldwide published in 2012.[69] This demonstrated an increased risk of death from intracranial hemorrhage within the first week (3.6% vs. 0.6%). However, at final follow-up no significant mortality difference was observed (OR for rt-PA vs. placebo 1.06, 95% CI 1.06–1.29). The benefit of thrombolysis was a small increase overall in the proportion of patients alive and independent, defined as a modified Rankin score of 0–2 (46.3% thrombolysis vs. 42.1% for placebo, OR 1.17, 95% CI 1.06–1.29) (Figure 33.6) (level of evidence 1, grade of recommendation A).

Of the subgroups analyzed, the most important finding was that those thrombolyzed within 3 hours of symptom onset had a better chance of being alive and independent than those treated between 3 and 6 hours (OR 1.53 [95% CI 1.26–1.86] vs. 1.07 [95% CI 0.96–1.20]). Age was no barrier to the benefit of thrombolysis, with >80 years thrombolyzed within 3 hours benefitting as much as those ≤80 years in their chances of being alive and independent at the end of follow-up (age ≤ 80 OR 1.51 [95% CI 1.18–1.93] vs. age >80 OR 1.68 [95% CI 1.20–2.34]).

The benefits of early intervention for acute ischemic stroke were a driver towards better organized hyperacute stroke units and public health campaigns, including the 2009 UK Face Arms Speech Time campaign, aimed at increasing public understanding of stroke symptoms and of the need to act quickly and seek urgent medical attention when such symptoms occur. In the UK, 2010 figures show that 14% of all patients with stroke were eligible for thrombolysis; however, only 5% received it. Currently, the proportion of patients receiving thrombolysis is limited by the time from symptoms to presentation of patients (ideally <2 hours) and the proportion of those of aged ≥80 receiving thrombolysis.[70]

Intra-arterial thrombolysis

Four randomized trials comprising 478 patients have so far provided no firm evidence of any benefit of intra-arterial thrombolysis with rt-PA or urokinase over conventional intravenous thrombolysis. A Cochrane meta-analysis in 2013 demonstrated an odds ratio of 1.08, 95% CI 0.75–1.55 for intravenous versus intra-arterial thrombolysis in terms of death or dependency at follow-up (level of evidence 1).[71] More research is needed as to in which setting intra-arterial thrombolysis has a benefit. Currently, intra-arterial thrombolysis is not recommended as first-line therapy over intravenous thrombolysis (grade of recommendation A).

Primary embolus retrieval

The standard of care in hyperacute ischemic stroke is now intravenous thrombolysis, analogous to the treatment of myocardial infarction 20 years ago, which subsequently evolved to primary endovascular therapy. Will ischemic stroke follow suit? A number of centres now offer mechanical clot retrieval for distal internal carotid or middle cerebral artery occlusive thrombus in selected patients; however, randomized trial data have been lacking until recently. Interestingly carotid angioplasty or stenting may need to be performed simultaneously for access to the anterior circulation.

Three recent randomized controlled trials have examined the benefits of additional intracranial thrombectomy to conventional thrombolysis alone.[72–74]

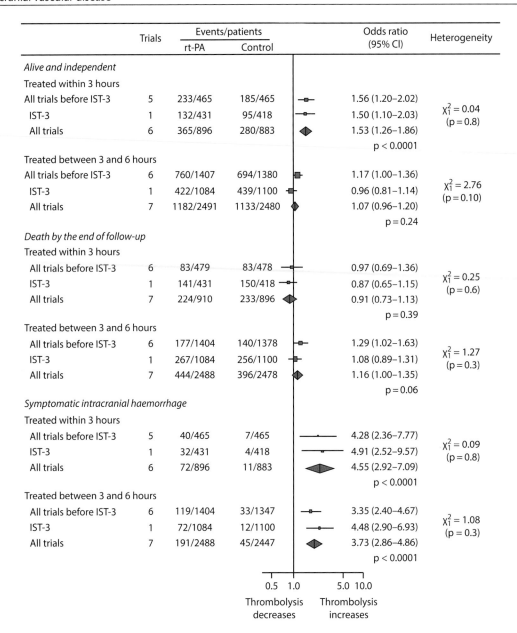

	Trials	Events/patients		Odds ratio (95% CI)	Heterogeneity
		rt-PA	Control		
Alive and independent					
Treated within 3 hours					
All trials before IST-3	5	233/465	185/465	1.56 (1.20–2.02)	
IST-3	1	132/431	95/418	1.50 (1.10–2.03)	$\chi^2_1 = 0.04$ (p = 0.8)
All trials	6	365/896	280/883	1.53 (1.26–1.86)	
				p < 0.0001	
Treated between 3 and 6 hours					
All trials before IST-3	6	760/1407	694/1380	1.17 (1.00–1.36)	
IST-3	1	422/1084	439/1100	0.96 (0.81–1.14)	$\chi^2_1 = 2.76$ (p = 0.10)
All trials	7	1182/2491	1133/2480	1.07 (0.96–1.20)	
				p = 0.24	
Death by the end of follow-up					
Treated within 3 hours					
All trials before IST-3	6	83/479	83/478	0.97 (0.69–1.36)	
IST-3	1	141/431	150/418	0.87 (0.65–1.15)	$\chi^2_1 = 0.25$ (p = 0.6)
All trials	7	224/910	233/896	0.91 (0.73–1.13)	
				p = 0.39	
Treated between 3 and 6 hours					
All trials before IST-3	6	177/1404	140/1378	1.29 (1.02–1.63)	
IST-3	1	267/1084	256/1100	1.08 (0.89–1.31)	$\chi^2_1 = 1.27$ (p = 0.3)
All trials	7	444/2488	396/2478	1.16 (1.00–1.35)	
				p = 0.06	
Symptomatic intracranial haemorrhage					
Treated within 3 hours					
All trials before IST-3	5	40/465	7/465	4.28 (2.36–7.77)	
IST-3	1	32/431	4/418	4.91 (2.52–9.57)	$\chi^2_1 = 0.09$ (p = 0.8)
All trials	6	72/896	11/883	4.55 (2.92–7.09)	
				p < 0.0001	
Treated between 3 and 6 hours					
All trials before IST-3	6	119/1404	33/1347	3.35 (2.40–4.67)	
IST-3	1	72/1084	12/1100	4.48 (2.90–6.93)	$\chi^2_1 = 1.08$ (p = 0.3)
All trials	7	191/2488	45/2447	3.73 (2.86–4.86)	
				p < 0.0001	

0.5 1.0   5.0 10.0

Thrombolysis decreases   Thrombolysis increases

Figure 33.6 Effects of recombinant tissue plasminogen activator (rt-Pa) on being alive and independent (modified Rankin score 0–2) by time to treatment at the end of follow-up of randomized trials, including the International Stroke Trial 3. Below this is the effect of rt-Pa on symptomatic intracranial hemorrhage in the first 7 days following presentation in the same trials. (Reprinted from Wardlaw JM et al., *Lancet*, 379(9834), 2364, 2012. With permission.)

All three trials were stopped early due to efficacy of additional thrombectomy in preventing medium term disability in patients with a confirmed small infarct core and internal carotid or middle cerebral artery occlusion on CT imaging. For example in the ESCAPE trial functional independence (modified Rankin score 0–2) was 53% versus 29%; in the MRCLEAN trial this was 33% versus 19% and in the SWIFT PRIME trial this was 60% versus 35%. Times from stroke onset to reperfusion were a median of 241 minutes in ESCAPE, highlighting that even 4 hours after an event, there is potential for reversal of deficit with intervention.

It is likely that these trials will result in a major restructuring of stroke services, in a fashion analogous to acute myocardial infarction. It also means that in the future there will need to be a pool of trained interventionalists to deal with the out of hours workload that will come with this paradigm shift in care.

Carotid and vertebral dissection

Carotid and vertebral dissection was first reported by Fisher[75] and is a rarer cause of ischemic stroke than thromboembolism, with an incidence of approximately 2 per 100,000 person-years.[76] Incidence peaks in the fifth decade and therefore impacts on a younger, working population. Dissections arise from an intimal tear in the media of the artery, which allow an intramural hematoma or 'false lumen' to develop. Intimal tears can be traumatic (e.g. from the impact of the carotid against an adjacent vertebral transverse process) or atraumatic (commonly associated with connective tissue disorders). These compress the true lumen causing ischemia. Occasionally, a subadventitial dissection can cause aneurysmal dilation of the artery, termed a 'pseudoaneurysm'.

The cause of spontaneous dissection is thought to be a connective tissue disorder. Those that are currently recognized are cystic medial necrosis, fibromuscular dysplasia, Ehlers–Danlos type IV, Marfan's syndrome and osteogenesis imperfecta type I.

The classic presentation of carotid dissection is unilateral neck pain, headache (typically around the ipsilateral orbit) with partial Horner's syndrome only (ptosis and miosis only, due to the sweat fibres which are responsible for anhidrosis running along the external carotid artery) and carotid territory neurology or cranial nerve palsies, particularly the hypoglossal,[75] due to compression from the expanded vessel. The presentation may mimic migraine; however, a bruit, neurological signs or lack of previous migraines may suggest otherwise. The pain of vertebral dissection is referred to the posterior neck and may mimic musculoskeletal pain and is associated with vertigo, diplopia, ataxia and dysarthria.

Investigation is as aforementioned with duplex ultrasound which may show a mobile intimal flap, a double-barrelled lumen with thrombus in the false lumen and dyssynchronous flow in the false lumen in comparison to the true lumen (video). Cross-sectional MR or CT angiography provides superior anatomical detail up to the circle of Willis and allows for simultaneous imaging of cerebral infarction (Figure 33.7).

Dissection syndromes cause stroke through thromboembolism, luminal compression but only rarely through intracranial extension of the dissection. Intracranial extension can rarely cause subarachnoid hemorrhage and compression of vital structures.

Historically, the risk of preventable thromboembolism from the damaged endothelial surface has led either anticoagulation or antiplatelet therapy to be used at diagnosis. A current meta-analysis of antiplatelet versus anticoagulant therapy in 39 non-randomized studies of carotid or vertebral dissection showed no significant difference for recurrent stroke or death between the two strategies[77] (level of evidence 2, grade of evidence B). The CADISS pilot randomized controlled trial of antiplatelet versus anticoagulant treatment for carotid and vertebral dissection showed no difference in ipsilateral stroke or death at 3 months (OR 0.35, 95% CI 0.01–4.39), with recurrent stroke occurring rarely in only 4% of those with confirmed dissection.[78]

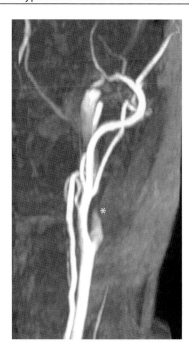

Figure 33.7 Acute carotid dissection imaged with magnetic resonance angiography using a T1 FAT–SAT sequence demonstrating acute intramural thrombus (*).

Long-term complications such as recurrent TIA or enlarging pseudoaneurysms have been treated with stenting in small case series with resolution of the pseudoaneurysm due to covering of the intimal tear.[79]

> ## Key points
>
> - Carotid and vertebral ischemia can result from thromboembolism, dissection or rarely hypoperfusion.
> - Carotid territory ischemia is well characterized; however, vertebral territory symptoms are less specific.
> - The ABCD2I score is the latest validated risk prediction tool for future stroke in patients with TIA but does not reflect the presence of carotid atherosclerosis.
> - Early initiation of antiplatelet therapy post TIA reduces subsequent stroke incidence fivefold.
> - Stroke risk is directly linked to smoking habit, LDL cholesterol levels and blood pressure in a dose-dependent fashion. EUROASPIRE demonstrated that whereas control of cholesterol was improving, smoking cessation and control of hypertension were not.
> - Ipsilateral stroke rates for asymptomatic patients with 50%–99% carotid atherosclerosis on modern medical therapy have been reported as ≤0.5% per annum.
> - Antiplatelet therapy prevents non-fatal myocardial infarction in primary prevention therapy for asymptomatic carotid atherosclerosis. In secondary prevention, it prevents both stroke and myocardial infarction; however, the main effect remains on myocardial infarction.
> - Current data suggest that intravenous thrombolysis is simpler and as effective as intra-arterial thrombolysis or embolus retrieval for hyperacute ischemic stroke and is therefore the first-line therapy.

BEST CLINICAL PRACTICE

Patients with asymptomatic carotid or vertebral atherosclerosis are very high risk for cardiovascular death and should receive the following interventions:

- Multimodal antihypertensive therapy to lower blood pressure to ≤140/80 mmHg
- Intensive statin therapy to lower LDL cholesterol to <1.8 mmol/L
- Aspirin or clopidogrel therapy to prevent non-fatal myocardial infarction
- A combined behavioural and pharmacological approach to smoking cessation
- Standard control of HBA1C in diabetes
- Follow-up to ensure treatment targets are met

AREAS FOR FUTURE RESEARCH

- Can the results of modern medical therapy be replicated internationally in asymptomatic patients with 70%–99% stenosis?
- What is the role of carotid endarterectomy for asymptomatic patients on modern medical therapy?
- Is there a benefit for intensive lowering of blood pressure in patients with carotid atherosclerosis?
- Is there a role for primary endovascular therapy for stroke in the future?

KEY REFERENCES

1. Rothwell PM, Giles MF, Chandratheva A et al. Effect of urgent treatment of transient ischaemic attack and minor stroke on early recurrent stroke (EXPRESS study): A prospective population-based sequential comparison. *Lancet*. 2007;370(9596):1432–1442.

   The EXPRESS study changed the pace at which TIA was investigated and treated.
2. den Hartog AG, Achterberg S, Moll FL et al. Asymptomatic carotid artery stenosis and the risk of ischemic stroke according to subtype in patients with clinical manifest arterial disease. *Stroke*. 2013;44(4):1002–1007.

   The SMART study demonstrated the results of modern medical therapy in asymptomatic carotid disease.
3. Baigent C, Blackwell L, Emberson J et al. Efficacy and safety of more intensive lowering of LDL cholesterol: A meta-analysis of data from 170,000 participants in 26 randomised trials. *Lancet*. 2010;376(9753):1670–1681.

   The Cholesterol Treatment Trialists' Collaboration identified the benefits of intensive statin treatment.
4. Baigent C, Blackwell L, Collins R et al. Aspirin in the primary and secondary prevention of vascular disease: Collaborative meta-analysis of individual participant data from randomised trials. *Lancet*. 2009;373(9678):1849–1860.

   The Antiplatelet Trialists' Collaborative identified the benefits of aspirin in secondary prevention of ischemic stroke.
5. Wardlaw JM, Murray V, Berge E et al. Recombinant tissue plasminogen activator for acute ischaemic stroke: An updated systematic review and meta-analysis. *Lancet*. 2012;379(9834):2364–2372.

   The Cochrane meta-analysis examined the benefits of intravenous thrombolysis in hyperacute ischemic stroke.

REFERENCES

1. World Health Organisation. *Cerebrovascular Disorders: A Clinical and Research Classification*. Geneva, Switzerland: World Health Organisation, 1978.
2. Tyrrell P, Swain S, Rudd A. Diagnosis and initial management of transient ischaemic attack. *Clin Med*. 2010;10(2):164–167.
3. The Amaurosis Fugax Study Group. Current management of amaurosis fugax. *Stroke*. 1990;21(2):201–208.
4. Bamford J, Sandercock P, Dennis M, Burn J, Warlow C. Classification and natural history of clinically identifiable subtypes of cerebral infarction. *Lancet*. 1991;337(8756):1521–1526.
5. Easton JD, Saver JL, Albers GW et al. Definition and evaluation of transient ischemic attack: A scientific statement for healthcare professionals from the American Heart Association/American Stroke Association Stroke Council; Council on Cardiovascular Surgery and Anesthesia; Council on Cardiovascular Radiology and Intervention; Council on Cardiovascular Nursing; and the Interdisciplinary Council on Peripheral Vascular Disease. The American Academy of Neurology affirms the value of this statement as an educational tool for neurologists. *Stroke*. 2009;40(6):2276–2293.
6. Giles MF, Albers GW, Amarenco P et al. Addition of brain infarction to the ABCD2 Score (ABCD2I): A collaborative analysis of unpublished data on 4574 patients. *Stroke*. 2010;41(9):1907–1913.
7. Touboul PJ, Hennerici MG, Meairs S et al. Mannheim carotid intima-media thickness consensus (2004–2006). An update on behalf of the Advisory Board of the 3rd and 4th Watching the Risk Symposium, 13th and 15th European Stroke Conferences, Mannheim, Germany, 2004, and Brussels, Belgium, 2006. *Cerebrovasc Dis*. 2007;23(1):75–80.
8. WHO. WHO Global Infobase. https://apps.who.int/infobase/Mortality.aspx. 2004, accessed 23 April, 2016.
9. Feigin VL, Lawes CM, Bennett DA, Barker-Collo SL, Parag V. Worldwide stroke incidence and early case fatality reported in 56 population-based studies: A systematic review. *Lancet Neurol*. 2009;8(4):355–369.

10. Murray CJ, Lopez AD. Alternative projections of mortality and disability by cause 1990–2020: Global Burden of Disease Study. *Lancet.* 1997;349(9064):1498–1504.

11. Adams HP Jr, Bendixen BH, Kappelle LJ et al. Classification of subtype of acute ischemic stroke. Definitions for use in a multicenter clinical trial. TOAST. Trial of Org 10172 in Acute Stroke Treatment. *Stroke.* 1993;24(1):35–41.

12. Hajat C, Heuschmann PU, Coshall C et al. Incidence of aetiological subtypes of stroke in a multi-ethnic population based study: The South London Stroke Register. *J Neurol Neurosurg Psychiatry.* 2011;82(5):527–533.

13. Kolominsky-Rabas PL, Weber M, Gefeller O, Neundoerfer B, Heuschmann PU. Epidemiology of ischemic stroke subtypes according to TOAST criteria: Incidence, recurrence, and long-term survival in ischemic stroke subtypes: A population-based study. *Stroke.* 2001;32(12):2735–2740.

14. European Carotid Surgery Trialists' (ECST) Collaborative. Randomised trial of endarterectomy for recently symptomatic carotid stenosis: Final results of the MRC ECST. *Lancet.* 1998;351(9113):1379–1387.

15. Thapar A, Jenkins IH, Mehta A, Davies AH. Diagnosis and management of carotid atherosclerosis. *Br Med J.* 2013;346:f1485.

16. Savitz SI, Caplan LR. Vertebrobasilar disease. *N Engl J Med.* 2005;352(25):2618–2626.

17. Rothwell PM, Warlow CP. Timing of TIAs preceding stroke: Time window for prevention is very short. *Neurology.* 2005;64(5):817–820.

18. Rothwell PM, Giles MF, Chandratheva A et al. Effect of urgent treatment of transient ischaemic attack and minor stroke on early recurrent stroke (EXPRESS study): A prospective population-based sequential comparison. *Lancet.* 2007;370(9596):1432–1442.

19. Johnston SC, Rothwell PM, Nguyen-Huynh MN et al. Validation and refinement of scores to predict very early stroke risk after transient ischaemic attack. *Lancet.* 2007;369(9558):283–292.

20. Walker J, Isherwood J, Eveson D, Naylor AR. Triaging TIA/minor stroke patients using the ABCD2 score does not predict those with significant carotid disease. *Eur J Vasc Endovasc Surg.* 2012;43(5):495–498.

21. Friedman SG. *A History of Vascular Surgery,* 2nd ed. Oxford, UK: Blackwell, 2005, 226pp.

22. Hunt JR. The role of the carotid arteries in the causation of vascular lesions of the brain with remarks on certain special features of the symptomatology. *Am J Med Sci.* 1914;147(5):704–712.

23. Tindall GT, Goree JA, Lee JF, Odom GL. Effect of common carotid ligation on size of internal carotid aneurysms and distal intracarotid and retinal artery pressures. *J Neurosurg.* 1966;25(5):503–511.

24. Gunnal SA, Farooqui MS, Wabale RN. Anatomical variations of the circulus arteriosus in cadaveric human brains. *Neurol Res Int.* 2014;2014:687281.

25. Chiari H. Uber das Verhalten des Teilungswinkels der Carotis communis bei der Endarteritis chronica deformans. *Verh Dtsch Ges Pathol.* 1905;9:326–330.

26. Castaigne P, Lhermitte F, Gautier JC, Escourolle R, Derouesne C. Internal carotid artery occlusion. A study of 61 instances in 50 patients with postmortem data. *Brain.* 1970;93(2):231–258.

27. Siebler M, Sitzer M, Steinmetz H. Detection of intracranial emboli in patients with symptomatic extracranial carotid artery disease. *Stroke.* 1992;23(11):1652–1654.

28. Allen LM, Hasso AN, Handwerker J, Farid H. Sequence-specific MR imaging findings that are useful in dating ischemic stroke. *Radiographics.* 2012;32(5):1285–1297; discussion 1297–1299.

29. de Weerd M, Greving JP, Hedblad B et al. Prevalence of asymptomatic carotid artery stenosis in the general population: An individual participant data meta-analysis. *Stroke.* 2010;41(6):1294–1297.

30. Endarterectomy for asymptomatic carotid artery stenosis. Executive Committee for the Asymptomatic Carotid Atherosclerosis Study. *J Am Med Assoc.* 1995;273(18):1421–1428.

31. Halliday A, Harrison M, Hayter E et al. 10-year stroke prevention after successful carotid endarterectomy for asymptomatic stenosis (ACST-1): A multicentre randomised trial. *Lancet.* 2010;376(9746):1074–1084.

32. Abbott AL. Medical (nonsurgical) intervention alone is now best for prevention of stroke associated with asymptomatic severe carotid stenosis: Results of a systematic review and analysis. *Stroke.* 2009;40(10):e573–e583.

33. Marquardt L, Geraghty OC, Mehta Z, Rothwell PM. Low risk of ipsilateral stroke in patients with asymptomatic carotid stenosis on best medical treatment: A prospective, population-based study. *Stroke.* 2010;41(1):e11–e17.

34. den Hartog AG, Achterberg S, Moll FL et al. Asymptomatic carotid artery stenosis and the risk of ischemic stroke according to subtype in patients with clinical manifest arterial disease. *Stroke.* 2013;44(4):1002–1027.

35. Hirt LS. Progression rate and ipsilateral neurological events in asymptomatic carotid stenosis. *Stroke.* 2014;45:702–706.

36. Conrad MF, Boulom V, Mukhopadhyay S, Garg A, Patel VI, Cambria RP. Progression of asymptomatic carotid stenosis despite optimal medical therapy. *J Vasc Surg.* 2013;58(1):128–135 e1.

37. den Hartog AG, Halliday AW, Hayter E et al. Risk of stroke from new carotid artery occlusion in the asymptomatic carotid surgery trial-1. *Stroke.* 2013;44(6):1652–1659.

38. Fine-Edelstein JS, Wolf PA, O'Leary DH et al. Precursors of extracranial carotid atherosclerosis in the Framingham Study. *Neurology.* 1994;44(6):1046–1050.

39. Mathiesen EB, Joakimsen O, Bonaa KH. Prevalence of and risk factors associated with carotid artery stenosis: The Tromso Study. *Cerebrovasc Dis.* 2001;12(1):44–51.

40. European Guidelines on cardiovascular disease prevention in clinical practice (version 2012): The Fifth Joint Task Force of the European Society of Cardiology and Other Societies on Cardiovascular Disease Prevention in Clinical Practice (constituted by representatives of nine societies and by invited experts). *Eur J Prev Cardiol.* 2012;19(4):585–667.

41. Perk J, De Backer G, Gohlke H et al. European Guidelines on cardiovascular disease prevention in clinical practice (version 2012): The fifth joint task force of the European society of cardiology and other societies on cardiovascular disease prevention in clinical practice (constituted by representatives of nine societies and by invited experts). *Atherosclerosis.* 2012;223(1):1–68.

42. MacMahon S, Peto R, Cutler J et al. Blood pressure, stroke, and coronary heart disease. Part 1, Prolonged differences in blood pressure: Prospective observational studies corrected for the regression dilution bias. *Lancet.* 1990;335(8692):765–774.

43. Lewington S, Clarke R, Qizilbash N, Peto R, Collins R. Age-specific relevance of usual blood pressure to vascular mortality: A meta-analysis of individual data for one million adults in 61 prospective studies. *Lancet.* 2002;360(9349):1903–1913.

44. Rothwell PM, Howard SC, Dolan E et al. Prognostic significance of visit-to-visit variability, maximum systolic blood pressure, and episodic hypertension. *Lancet.* 2010;375(9718):895–905.

45. James PA, Oparil S, Carter BL et al. 2014 evidence-based guideline for the management of high blood pressure in adults: Report from the panel members appointed to the Eighth Joint National Committee (JNC 8). *J Am Med Assoc.* 2014;311(5):507–520.

46. NICE. Guideline 127: Clinical management of primary hypertension in adults, 2011.

47. Law MR, Morris JK, Wald NJ. Use of blood pressure lowering drugs in the prevention of cardiovascular disease: Meta-analysis of 147 randomised trials in the context of expectations from prospective epidemiological studies. *Br Med J.* 2009;338:b1665.

48. Bladin CF, Chambers BR. Clinical features, pathogenesis, and computed tomographic characteristics of internal watershed infarction. *Stroke.* 1993;24(12):1925–1932.

49. Physicians RCo. Fourth National Clinical Guideline for Stroke. http://www.rcplondon.ac.uk/resources/stroke-guidelines. Accessed 16 October 2012.

50. Kernan WN, Ovbiagele B, Black HR et al. Guidelines for the prevention of stroke in patients with stroke and transient ischemic attack: A guideline for healthcare professionals from the American Heart Association/American Stroke Association. *Stroke.* 2014;45:2160–2236.

51. Bouri S, Thapar A, Shalhoub J et al. Hypertension and the post-carotid endarterectomy cerebral hyperperfusion syndrome. *Eur J Vasc Endovasc Surg.* 2011;41(2):229–237.

52. Newman JE, Ali M, Sharpe R, Bown MJ, Sayers RD, Naylor AR. Changes in middle cerebral artery velocity after carotid endarterectomy do not identify patients at high-risk of suffering intracranial haemorrhage or stroke due to hyperperfusion syndrome. *Eur J Vasc Endovasc Surg.* 2013;45(6):562–571.

53. Baigent C, Blackwell L, Emberson J et al. Efficacy and safety of more intensive lowering of LDL cholesterol: A meta-analysis of data from 170,000 participants in 26 randomised trials. *Lancet.* 2010;376(9753):1670–1681.

54. Stone NJ, Robinson J, Lichtenstein AH et al. 2013 ACC/AHA guideline on the treatment of blood cholesterol to reduce atherosclerotic cardiovascular risk in adults: A report of the American College of Cardiology/American Heart Association task force on practice guidelines. *J Am Coll Cardiol.* 2013.

55. Sillesen H, Amarenco P, Hennerici MG et al. Atorvastatin reduces the risk of cardiovascular events in patients with carotid atherosclerosis: A secondary analysis of the Stroke Prevention by Aggressive Reduction in Cholesterol Levels (SPARCL) trial. *Stroke.* 2008;39(12):3297–3302.

56. Shinton R, Beevers G. Meta-analysis of relation between cigarette smoking and stroke. *Br Med J.* 1989;298(6676):789–794.

57. Wolf PA, D'Agostino RB, Kannel WB, Bonita R, Belanger AJ. Cigarette smoking as a risk factor for stroke. The Framingham Study. *J Am Med Assoc.* 1988;259(7):1025–1029.

58. Bauld L. The impact of smokefree legislation in England: Evidence review. University of Bath, Bath, UK, 2011.

59. Stead LF, Lancaster T. Combined pharmacotherapy and behavioural interventions for smoking cessation. *Cochrane Database Syst Rev.* 2012;10:CD008286.

60. Bullen C, Howe C, Laugesen M et al. Electronic cigarettes for smoking cessation: A randomised controlled trial. *Lancet.* 2013;382(9905):1629–1637.

61. Caponnetto P, Campagna D, Cibella F et al. EffiCiency and Safety of an eLectronic cigAreTte (ECLAT) as tobacco cigarettes substitute: A prospective 12-month randomized control design study. *PLOS ONE.* 2013;8(6):e66317.

62. Kaplan RC, Tirschwell DL, Longstreth WT Jr et al. Vascular events, mortality, and preventive therapy following ischemic stroke in the elderly. *Neurology.* 2005;65(6):835–842.

63. Baigent C, Blackwell L, Collins R et al. Aspirin in the primary and secondary prevention of vascular disease: Collaborative meta-analysis of individual participant data from randomised trials. *Lancet.* 2009;373(9678):1849–1860.

64. CAPRIE Steering Committee. A randomised, blinded, trial of clopidogrel versus aspirin in patients at risk of ischaemic events (CAPRIE). *Lancet.* 1996;348(9038):1329–1339.

65. Geeganage CM, Diener HC, Algra A et al. Dual or mono antiplatelet therapy for patients with acute ischemic stroke or transient ischemic attack: Systematic review and meta-analysis of randomized controlled trials. *Stroke.* 2012;43(4):1058–1066.

66. Ray KK, Seshasai SR, Wijesuriya S et al. Effect of intensive control of glucose on cardiovascular outcomes and death in patients with diabetes mellitus: A meta-analysis of randomised controlled trials. *Lancet.* 2009;373(9677):1765–1772.

67. Kotseva K, Wood D, De Backer G, De Bacquer D, Pyorala K, Keil U. Cardiovascular prevention guidelines in daily practice: A comparison of EUROASPIRE I, II, and III surveys in eight European countries. *Lancet.* 2009;373(9667):929–940.

68. The National Institute of Neurological Disorders and Stroke rt-PA Stroke Study Group. Tissue plasminogen activator for acute ischemic stroke. *N Engl J Med.* 1995;333(24):1581–1587.

69. Wardlaw JM, Murray V, Berge E et al. Recombinant tissue plasminogen activator for acute ischaemic stroke: An updated systematic review and meta-analysis. *Lancet.* 2012;379(9834):2364–2372.

70. Rudd AG, Hoffman A, Grant R, Campbell JT, Lowe D. Stroke thrombolysis in England, Wales and Northern Ireland: How much do we do and how much do we need? *J Neurol Neurosurg Psychiatry.* 2011;82(1):14–19.

71. Wardlaw JM, Koumellis P, Liu M. Thrombolysis (different doses, routes of administration and agents) for acute ischaemic stroke. *Cochrane Database Syst Rev.* 2013;5:CD000514.

72. Randomized assessment of rapid endovascular treatment of ischemic stroke ESCAPE Trial Investigators. *N Engl J Med.* 2015;372:1019–1030.

73. A randomized trial of intraarterial treatment for acute ischemic stroke MR CLEAN Investigators. *N Engl J Med.* 2015;372:11–20.

74. Stent-retriever thrombectomy after intravenous t-PA vs. t-PA alone in stroke SWIFT PRIME Investigators. *N Engl J Med.* 2015;372:2285–2295.

75. Fisher CM, Ojemann RG, Roberson GH. Spontaneous dissection of cervico-cerebral arteries. *Can J Neurol Sci.* 1978;5(1):9–19.

76. Schievink WI, Mokri B, Whisnant JP. Internal carotid artery dissection in a community. Rochester, Minnesota, 1987–1992. *Stroke.* 1993;24(11):1678–1680.

77. Kennedy F, Lanfranconi S, Hicks C et al. Antiplatelets vs anticoagulation for dissection: CADISS nonrandomized arm and meta-analysis. *Neurology.* 2012;79(7):686–689.

78. Antiplatelet treatment compared with anticoagulation treatment for cervical artery dissection (CADISS): A randomised trial. The CADISS trial investigators. *Lancet Neurol.* April 2015;14(4):361–367.

79. Pham MH, Rahme RJ, Arnaout O et al. Endovascular stenting of extracranial carotid and vertebral artery dissections: A systematic review of the literature. *Neurosurgery.* 2011;68(4):856–866; discussion 866.

34

Extracranial carotid artery occlusive disease
Surgical management

A. ROSS NAYLOR

CONTENTS

EVIDENCE SUPPORTING INTERVENTION

Symptomatic patients

2011 AHA GUIDELINES RECOMMENDATIONS

Table 34.1 summarises the American Heart Association (AHA) recommendations for patients with recently symptomatic carotid disease.[1]

EVIDENCE UNDERPINNING THE AHA RECOMMENDATIONS
CEA versus BMT

Table 34.2 summarises a meta-analysis of 6000+ patients who were randomised between carotid endarterectomy (CEA) and best medical therapy (BMT) in the European Carotid Surgery Trial (ECST), the North American Symptomatic Carotid Endarterectomy Trial (NASCET) and the Veterans Affairs (VA) Trial.[2] CEA conferred no benefit in patients with <50% stenoses (NASCET measurement method). Maximum benefit was observed with increasing internal carotid artery (ICA) stenosis severity, but not subocclusion.

Because >6000 patients were randomised, it was possible to perform subgroup analyses to identify patients at greater (or lesser) risk of suffering a stroke. Clinical features associated with an increased risk of late stroke include (1) increasing age (especially >75 years), (2) recent symptoms (especially <2 weeks), (3) males, (4) hemispheric (vs. retinal) symptoms, (5) cortical (vs. lacunar) stroke and (6) increasing co-morbidity.[3] Imaging features associated with an increased risk of late stroke include (1) increasing stenosis severity (excluding subocclusion), (2) irregular (vs. smooth) plaques, (3) contralateral occlusion, (4) tandem intracranial disease and (5) failure to recruit intracranial collaterals.[3]

In clinical practice, the most important recent change in practice is the drive towards performing CEA as soon as possible after onset of symptoms. This is because CEA confers maximum benefit if performed <2 weeks (185 ipsilateral strokes prevented at 5 years per 1000 CEAs compared with only 8 if >12 weeks elapse)[4] and because of evidence that the risk of stroke in the first few days after symptom onset is higher than previously thought. An overview of seven contemporary natural history studies suggests that the risk of recurrent stroke in patients with 50%–99% stenoses and a recent transient ischemic attack (TIA)/minor stroke may be 5%–8% at 48 hours, 17% at 72 hours, 8%–22% at 7 days and 11%–25% at 14 days.[3]

CEA versus CAS

The 2011 AHA guidelines (Table 34.1) acknowledged carotid artery stenting (CAS) as an alternative to CEA, based upon the North American CREST trial, to the virtual exclusion of three European trials (EVA-3S, SPACE and ICSS). An overview of all of the randomised trials suggests that (1) CAS is associated with a twofold excess risk of procedural stroke; (2) using a clinical definition of myocardial infarction (MI), there is no difference between CEA and CAS; (3) when 'chemical MI' is included (biomarker elevation in the absence of chest pain or ECG changes), CEA is associated with a twofold excess risk of MI; (4) if 'chemical MI' is included within a composite endpoint of a 30-day death/stroke/MI, outcomes are similar between CEA and CAS; (5) 30-day rates of death/stroke after CAS in patients aged <70 years are similar to those after CEA

Table 34.1 Summary of American Heart Association recommendations for managing patients with recently symptomatic carotid artery disease.

Recommendation	Grade and level of evidence
CEA is recommended for patients with recent TIA/ischaemic stroke (<6 months) and an ipsilateral severe (70%–99%) ICA stenosis, provided the perioperative risk of death/stroke is <6%.	I/A
CEA is recommended (depending upon age, sex and co-morbidities) in patients with recent TIA/ischaemic stroke (<6 months) and an ipsilateral moderate (50%–69%) carotid stenosis, provided the perioperative risk of death/stroke is <6%.	I/B
If the ICA stenosis is <50%, there is no indication for carotid revascularisation by either CEA or CAS.	III/A
When CEA is indicated for patients with TIA/stroke, surgery <2 weeks is reasonable (rather than delaying surgery) provided there are no contraindications to early revascularisation.	IIa/B
CAS is an alternative to CEA for symptomatic patients at average risk of complications, when the diameter of the lumen of the ICA is reduced by >70% (non-invasive imaging) or >50% (angiography).	I/B
When performed by operators with established periprocedural morbidity and mortality rates of 4%–6%, i.e. similar to those observed in trials of CEA and CAS.	IIa/B

Source: Data derived from Furie KL et al., *Stroke*, 42, 227, 2011.

Table 34.2 Meta-analysis of outcomes in patients randomised within the ESCT, NASCET and VA Trials: 5-year risk of any stroke (including perioperative events).

Stenosis severity	n =	5-year risk of any stroke (including perioperative risk)		ARR (%)	RRR	NNT	Strokes prevented per 1000 CEAs at 5 years
		Surgery (%)	Medical (%)				
<30%	1746	18.4	15.7	−2.7	n/b	n/b	None
30%–49%	1429	22.8	25.5	+2.7	10%	38	27
50%–69%	1549	20.0	27.8	+7.8	28%	13	78
70%–99%	1095	17.1	32.7	+15.6	48%	6	156
Subocclusion	262	22.4	22.3	−0.1	n/b	n/b	None

Source: Data derived from Rothwell PM et al. for the Carotid Endarterectomy Trialists Collaboration, *Lancet*, 361, 107, 2003.
Abbreviations: n/b, no benefit conferred by CEA; ARR, absolute risk reduction; RRR, relative risk reduction.

(however, death/stroke was significantly higher after CAS in patients aged >70 years); (6) randomised trials reporting mid-to-late term outcomes following successful CAS consistently report that long-term stroke risks are similar to CEA, i.e. CAS appears durable; (7) restenosis rates were significantly higher following CAS, but this did not translate into an increased risk of late ipsilateral stroke; (8) CEA is associated with higher rates of cranial nerve injury (CNI), while (9) CAS is associated with a fivefold excess risk of new and persisting MRI lesions compared with CEA.[5]

Given that the AHA has advised that CAS is an alternative to CEA in selected patients,[1] it is important that regular audits ensure that procedural risks remain <6% (Table 34.1). Recent evidence suggests that CAS carries a threefold excess risk of stroke (compared to CEA) when performed <14 days after onset of symptoms.[6] This should be borne in mind when determining whether CEA or CAS is the preferred intervention in the hyperacute period. It would not be appropriate to delay interventions (in order to secure lower procedural risks), as the highest-risk patients will have suffered their stroke before any opportunity for treatment.

Asymptomatic patients

2012 AHA GUIDELINES RECOMMENDATIONS

Table 34.3 summarises AHA recommendations for treating patients with asymptomatic carotid disease.[7]

EVIDENCE UNDERPINNING AHA RECOMMENDATIONS
CEA versus BMT

Table 34.4 summarises outcomes from the Asymptomatic Carotid Atherosclerosis Study (ACAS) and the Asymptomatic Carotid Surgery Trial (ACST).[8,9] Note the '11%' stroke risk at 5 years in medically treated patients within ACAS refers to ipsilateral stroke, while the '11.8%' stroke risk in medically treated patients in ACST refers to

Table 34.3 Summary of American Heart Association recommendations for managing patients with asymptomatic carotid artery disease.

Recommendation	Grade and level of evidence
Selection for carotid revascularisation should be guided by assessment of co-morbid conditions and life expectancy, as well as other individual factors. It should include a thorough discussion of the risks and benefits of the procedure, with an understanding of patient preferences.	I/C
Prophylactic CEA (<3% morbidity/mortality) can be useful in highly selected patients with an asymptomatic carotid stenosis (60% by angiography, 70% by validated Doppler ultrasound). It should be noted that the benefit of surgery may now be lower than anticipated based on randomised trial results, and the cited 3% threshold for complication rates may be high because of interim advances in medical therapy.	IIa/A
Prophylactic carotid artery stenting might be considered in highly selected patients with an asymptomatic carotid stenosis (>60% on angiography, >70% on validated Doppler ultrasonography or >80% on computed tomographic angiography or MRA if the stenosis on ultrasonography was 50%–69%). The advantage of revascularisation over current medical therapy alone is not well established.	IIb/B
The usefulness of CAS as an alternative to CEA in asymptomatic patients at high risk for the surgical procedure is uncertain.	IIb/C

Source: Data derived from Goldstein LB et al., *Stroke*, 42, 517, 2011.

Table 34.4 Asymptomatic Carotid Atherosclerosis Study and Asymptomatic Carotid Surgery Trial outcomes for 5 and 10 years for the treatment of asymptomatic patients with 60%–99% ICA stenoses.

Trial	n =	5-year 'stroke' risk*		ARR	RRR	NNT	Strokes prevented per 1000 CEAs at 5 years
		CEA	BMT				
ACAS	1662	5.1%	11.0%	5.9%	54%	17	59
ACST	3120	6.4%	11.8%	5.4%	46%	19	54
Trial	n =	10-year 'stroke' risk*		ARR	RRR	NNT	Strokes prevented per 1000 CEAs at 5 years
		CEA	BMT				
ACST	3120	13.4%	17.9%	4.6%	26%	22	46

Sources: Data derived from Executive Committee for the Asymptomatic Carotid Atherosclerosis Study, *J Am Med Assoc*, 273, 1421, 1995; Asymptomatic Carotid Surgery Trial Collaborators, *Lancet*, 363, 1491, 2004.

* ACAS is reporting 'ipsilateral' stroke, while ACST is reporting 'any' stroke when describing five or ten year stroke risks.

any stroke. These data are now quite historical and there is uncertainty as to whether they should still determine modern practice. Contrary to that found in the symptomatic trials, subgroup analyses failed to identify 'high risk for stroke' asymptomatic patients, other than the fact that patients aged >75 years gained no benefit from CEA.[9]

CEA versus CAS

The only published randomised trial comparing CEA with CAS, which included asymptomatic patients, was CREST,[10] despite it having started as a symptomatic trial. When recruitment declined, approval was granted to include asymptomatic patients. CREST was not, however, powered to determine whether CEA or CAS was safer in asymptomatic patients. Overall, 1181 asymptomatic patients were randomised.

The 30-day death/stroke rate was 2.5% after CAS versus 1.4% after CEA (hazard ratio [HR] 1.9 [95% CI, 0.8–4.4]; p = 0.15).[10] Although the 2011 AHA guidelines advised that CAS might be considered in highly selected patients, the Committee on Medicare and Medicaid continues to refuse to reimburse stenting costs in average risk, asymptomatic individuals.

CAROTID ENDARTERECTOMY

Choice of anaesthesia

WHAT IS THE DEBATE?

Are procedural risks influenced by choice of anaesthesia?

RATIONALE

Performing CEA under locoregional anaesthesia (LRA) enables the surgeon to determine who needs a shunt during clamping (to prevent haemodynamic stroke). It was also suggested that LRA might reduce cardiac/pulmonary morbidity and mortality.

WHAT IS THE NON-RANDOMISED TRIAL EVIDENCE?

A meta-analysis of 41 non-randomised studies (25,000 CEAs) observed that LRA was associated with a 40% relative reduction in perioperative stroke/death,[11] as well as significant reductions in MI and pulmonary complications.

WHAT IS THE RANDOMISED TRIAL EVIDENCE?

The 2013 Cochrane Review identified 14 randomised trials (4596 patients).[12] A meta-analysis showed no evidence that type of anaesthesia influenced perioperative outcomes.

CONCLUSION

Surgeons/anaesthetists can perform CEA using whichever anaesthetic method they prefer.

Choice of incision

WHAT IS THE DEBATE?

Do transverse or longitudinal incisions influence outcomes?

RATIONALE

CEA can be performed via a smaller transverse incision with better cosmetic results and fewer CNIs.

WHAT IS THE NON-RANDOMISED TRIAL EVIDENCE?

Bastounis observed that transverse incisions were feasible and gave better cosmetic results with fewer CNIs, compared to a longitudinal incision.[13] Conversely, Marcucci reported no difference in the prevalence of CNIs and observed that it was more difficult to use a shunt if a transverse incision was used.[14] Ascher used a modified approach wherein ultrasound localised the bifurcation and a smaller longitudinal incision was made which could be extended as required. This strategy significantly reduced incision lengths and offered better cosmetic results, with no excess CNI risk.[15]

WHAT IS THE RANDOMISED TRIAL EVIDENCE?

No randomised trial has been undertaken.

CONCLUSION

Surgeons can use whichever incision they prefer. If ultrasound suggests that the bifurcation is not high and there is a focal lesion, a transverse incision will probably give the best cosmetic result. If there is any question about the bifurcation being high, or if the lesion is extensive, a longitudinal incision remains preferable.

Antegrade or retrojugular exposure?

WHAT IS THE DEBATE?

Is retrojugular exposure of the bifurcation associated with reduced CNI rates, shorter operation times and reduced procedural risks compared with the ante-jugular approach?

RATIONALE

The antegrade approach to the bifurcation involves ligation of the common facial vein (CFV) and mobilisation of the hypoglossal nerve. The retrojugular approach involves lateral retraction of sternomastoid and medial retraction of the internal jugular vein. The bifurcation is exposed with no need to mobilise the hypoglossal nerve. Advocates argue that retrograde exposure involves shorter operation times, it is easier to expose the upper ICA (without having to mobilise the hypoglossal nerve) and there is no need to mobilise the cervical fat pad containing lymph nodes and lymphatics.[16]

WHAT IS THE EVIDENCE?

A meta-analysis of four non-randomised and two randomised trials (740 CEAs) found no evidence that retrograde exposure was associated with a greater/lesser risk of perioperative death (0.6% vs. 0.5%), stroke (0.9% vs. 0.7%) or TIA (1.8% vs. 2.1%).[16] However, there were important differences regarding CNI. Five studies reported the prevalence of recurrent laryngeal nerve injury. Two used laryngoscopy, while three were based upon clinical review. The retrojugular approach was associated with significantly higher rates of recurrent laryngeal nerve injury (8.1%), versus 2.2% after antegrade exposure (odds ratio [OR] 3.2 [95% CI 1.5–7.1]; p = 0.004). This finding persisted when randomised trials and those with direct laryngoscopy were analysed separately.[16]

There was no difference between retrograde and antegrade approaches regarding hypoglossal nerve injury (1.3% vs. 1.3%) or accessory nerve injury (1.2% vs. 0%). Six patients undergoing CEA via the retrograde approach (2.1%) had a persisting CNI (all recurrent laryngeal), while only one patient (0.3%) suffered a persisting CNI using antegrade exposure (p = ns).

CONCLUSION

There is no evidence that the retrojugular approach confers significant benefit or reduces the prevalence of hypoglossal nerve injury. Proponents of the retrograde approach should carefully audit rates of recurrent laryngeal nerve palsy, especially when supervising trainees. This incision should be avoided in any patient with evidence of a contralateral recurrent laryngeal nerve palsy.

Carotid sinus blockade

WHAT IS THE DEBATE?

Does carotid sinus nerve blockade (prior to carotid clamping) reduce perioperative haemodynamic instability?

RATIONALE

Haemodynamic instability (hypotension/hypertension/arrhythmias) is relatively common during and after CEA and may predispose to cardiac/cerebral complications.

WHAT IS THE RANDOMISED TRIAL EVIDENCE?

Tang undertook a systematic review and meta-analysis and identified four randomised trials (432 patients).[17] There was no evidence that carotid sinus nerve blockade reduced the prevalence of perioperative hypotension/hypertension and arrhythmias.

CONCLUSION

There is no evidence that carotid sinus nerve blockade confers any benefit regarding perioperative haemodynamic instability. However, the quality of the trials was poor, with most being too small to have any realistic chance of being powered to reach a reliable conclusion.

Heparin and its reversal with protamine

WHAT IS THE DEBATE?

Does heparin reversal (with protamine) reduce post-operative neck haematomas without increasing the risk of thrombotic stroke?

RATIONALE

A small number of CEA patients will develop neck haematomas in the early post-operative period that can compromise the airway. In addition, evidence suggests that re-exploration for neck haematoma increases the risk of CNI, MI, stroke and death.[18] Protamine reverses intravenous unfractionated heparin, but this is at the expense of a higher risk of early post-operative thrombotic stroke.

WHAT IS THE RANDOMISED TRIAL EVIDENCE?

Only one small, randomised trial has been performed, and this was abandoned after only 64 patients had been recruited because two patients who received protamine thrombosed their ICA in the early post-operative period.[19]

WHAT IS THE NON-RANDOMISED TRIAL EVIDENCE?

Practices vary considerably. In 1994, an audit revealed that 26% of European surgeons and 54% of North American surgeons routinely reversed heparin with protamine.[20] The Vascular Study Group of New England (VSGNE) reported that 46% of surgeons used protamine between 2003 and 2007. Protamine was not associated with increased rates of perioperative stroke but was associated with significantly lower rates of re-exploration for bleeding (0.6% vs. 1.7%; p = 0.001). Perhaps more importantly, patients undergoing re-exploration for bleeding were significantly more likely to die or suffer a perioperative stroke/MI in the post-operative period.[18]

The VSGNE published a second review of practice in 2013.[21] By 2008, 52% of surgeons used protamine, increasing to 62% by 2010. Patients receiving protamine were significantly less likely to undergo re-exploration for bleeding, and there was no evidence of any increase in perioperative MI, stroke or death. The GALA Trial published a *post hoc* analysis in 2107 patients randomised to CEA.[22] There was a significant increase in neck haematomas in patients not receiving protamine (10.4% vs. 7.4%), but this did not translate into increased rates of re-exploration. Paradoxically, there was a non-significant trend towards an increased rate of perioperative stroke in patients who did not receive protamine.

Protamine, however, is not without complications. In a review of practice across Europe and North America, Wakefield observed that 5% suffered an adverse event following protamine administration.[20] The commonest was systemic hypotension (4.5%), possibly mediated via nitric oxide release. Pulmonary artery hypertension (possibly mediated via thromboxane release) affected 0.2% of patients, while anaphylaxis occurred in 0.16% and 0.02% of patients died.

CONCLUSION

Registry data suggest that protamine administration is not associated with an excess risk of perioperative thrombotic stroke, but it does appear to reduce bleeding complications. When deciding whether to use protamine, surgeons should remain aware that protamine cannot prevent bleeding problems secondary to low-molecular-weight heparin nor antiplatelet therapy, especially when aspirin and clopidogrel are combined.

Shunt policy

WHAT IS THE DEBATE?

Does a policy of routine, selective or never shunting influence stroke rates after CEA?

RATIONALE

Two-thirds of the population do not have a functioning circle of Willis, making them vulnerable to cerebral ischaemia during carotid clamping. In order to prevent haemodynamic stroke, surgeons are mostly 'routine' or 'selective' shunters, while a small minority are 'never' shunters. The argument against routine shunting is that it is unnecessary in the majority of patients, while some believe that shunts cause as many strokes as they prevent through 'ploughing' debris from the stenosis into the distal ICA, or by causing intimal injuries. Advocates of 'selective' or 'never' shunting also argue that shunts interfere with visualising the distal intimal step, possibly compromising the quality of any reconstruction. Not surprisingly, routine shunters disagree, arguing that familiarity with shunt use makes it easier to operate around them and that when a shunt really is necessary (especially during high dissections), it is much easier to complete the procedure.

WHAT IS THE NON-RANDOMISED TRIAL EVIDENCE?

In NASCET, shunt policy did not influence procedural risk.[23] Malone and Ballard reviewed outcomes from 17 published series (8323 CEAs),[24] concluding that there was no difference in perioperative stroke between routine shunters (2.5%), selective shunters (3.4%) and never shunters (3.9%). The only consensus was that patients with a stump pressure <50 mmHg in the presence of a contralateral occlusion should always be shunted.

WHAT IS THE RANDOMISED TRIAL EVIDENCE?

The 2014 Cochrane Review identified six randomised trials.[25] Three compared 'routine' with 'never' shunting, while one compared 'routine' with 'selective' shunting. The remaining trials evaluated selective shunting based upon a variety of combinations of EEG, stump pressure and near infrared spectroscopy (NIRS).

Unfortunately, most studies were underpowered and subject to bias. Three randomised trials comparing routine with never shunting (686 patients) observed non-significant trends towards reduced stroke and reduced death/stroke favouring routine shunting. In the trial comparing routine with selective shunting, the latter only received a shunt if the stump pressure was <40 mmHg. There was no difference in outcomes. Finally, EEG, stump pressure and NIRS were unable to identify subgroups with a greater or lesser risk of procedural stroke.[25]

CONCLUSION

It is not surprising that randomised trials have failed to answer this question. Many surgeons find it difficult to randomise patients to 'never' shunt, while no monitoring method (other than LRA) is reliable enough to predict who really needs a shunt. Accordingly, surgeons will have to accept the limitations/benefits of each shunting strategy and adopt a policy that they are comfortable with. For the most part, the final choice almost always reflects what they were taught by their mentor!

Patch or primary closure?

WHAT IS THE DEBATE?

Does the method of arteriotomy closure influence outcomes?

RATIONALE

There are three ways to close the arteriotomy following traditional (not eversion) CEA: routine primary closure, routine patching and selective patching. The rationale underlying patching is that primary closure causes some degree of stenosis (especially distally), predisposing towards higher rates of early thrombosis and late restenosis, and thus (by inference) a greater risk of stroke. By contrast, patching may be associated with prolonged clamp times, prosthetic patch infection and venous blow out.

WHAT IS THE NON-RANDOMISED TRIAL EVIDENCE?

There is a vast literature with totally conflicting findings and little consensus.

WHAT IS THE RANDOMISED TRIAL EVIDENCE?

Two recent meta-analyses[26,27] have reported on (1) routine patching versus routine primary closure and (2) prosthetic versus autologous vein patch closure. No randomised trials have compared selective patching with routine patching. Ten randomised trials (2157 patients) compared routine primary closure versus routine patching.[26] Seven randomised trials observed a significant reduction in perioperative ipsilateral stroke (patch 1.5% vs. 4.5% primary), giving an OR of 0.2 (95% CI 0.1–0.6; p = 0.001) favouring routine patching. There was also a significant reduction in 30-day thrombosis rates (0.5% patch vs. 3.1% primary), representing a fivefold excess risk of early thrombosis following routine primary closure (OR 5.6 [95% CI 2.4–12.5]; p = 0.0011).[26] Patients randomised to routine primary closure were three times more likely to return to theatre within <30 days (3.1% vs. 1.1%; OR 2.9 [95% CI 1.3–6.3]; p = 0.01). There was no significant difference between routine patching and routine primary closure regarding perioperative death, fatal stroke, death/stroke and CNI.[26]

When perioperative and late outcomes were combined, routine patching was associated with significant reductions in (1) late ipsilateral stroke (1.6% vs. 4.8%; OR 0.3 [95% CI 0.2–0.6]; p = 0.001), (2) any stroke (2.4% vs. 4.6%; OR 0.49 [95% CI 0.3–0.9]; p = 0.002), (3) stroke/death (13% vs. 20.6%; OR 0.6 [95% CI 0.4–0.8]; p = 0.004) and (4) restenosis (4.3% vs. 13.8%; OR 0.2 [95% CI 0.2–0.3]; p < 0.01). There were no statistically significant differences regarding fatal stroke or death.[26]

Regarding patch type, there were no differences regarding restenosis/occlusion rates, stroke, operation times or mortality. Haemostasis times were significantly longer for PTFE compared with both vein and polyester patches. One trial comparing bovine pericardial patches with polyester patches observed a significant reduction in suture line bleeding with bovine patches.[27]

CONCLUSION

A policy of routine primary closure is associated with significantly higher rates of early and late adverse events and cannot be supported. Intuitively, the optimal solution should be selective patching, but no randomised trial has ever been performed.

Eversion or traditional endarterectomy?

WHAT IS THE DEBATE?

Does eversion CEA confer any benefit over traditional endarterectomy, regarding procedural risks and late restenosis?

RATIONALE

'Traditional' endarterectomy involves a longitudinal arteriotomy from the distal common carotid artery (CCA) into the proximal ICA. A transverse plane (somewhere within the media/adventitia) is developed proximal to the stenosis, and this is then mobilised caudally so that the plaque is removed. The distal ICA 'feathers' back to normal intima or is transected and tacked down. The arteriotomy is then closed primarily or with a patch. During eversion endarterectomy, the ICA is transected obliquely at its origin and the tube of atheroma 'expelled' as the media and adventitia are everted. The distal intimal step is carefully feathered and the distal CCA endarterectomised. The ICA is then shortened (as required) and reanastomosed to the CCA.

Theoretical advantages of eversion CEA include avoidance of prosthetic patch material (avoiding patch infection), it is quicker, it preserves bifurcation geometry, and it may be associated with reduced restenosis rates. Disadvantages include not being able to insert a shunt until the plaque is removed and problems with access should the plaque extend unexpectedly high into the neck.

WHAT IS THE NON-RANDOMISED TRIAL EVIDENCE?

The literature contains a large number of single centre studies confirming that eversion CEA can be performed safely and with results at least comparable to (or better than) traditional endarterectomy.

WHAT IS THE RANDOMISED TRIAL EVIDENCE?

Five randomised trials (2465 patients, 2590 CEAs) were the subject of a systematic review by Cao.[28] When eversion CEA was compared with 'traditional' CEA, there was no statistically significant difference regarding (1) 30-day death/stroke, (2) perioperative thrombosis, (3) perioperative cardiovascular or wound complications and (4) late stroke. However, patients randomised to eversion CEA had a twofold reduction in restenosis >50% (2.5%), compared to patients undergoing 'traditional' CEA (5.2%) (OR 0.3 [95% CI 0.1–0.8]).[28] However, when the meta-analysis compared eversion with patched endarterectomy, there was no difference in late restenosis rates (2.5% vs. 3.9%; HR 0.52 (0.2–1.7).[28]

CONCLUSION

Provided the endarterectomy is patched, there is no difference in outcomes between eversion and traditional CEA. Eversion CEA is associated with significantly fewer restenoses compared with primary closure.

Monitoring and quality control

WHAT IS THE DEBATE?

Does monitoring and quality control (QC) prevent perioperative stroke during CEA?

RATIONALE

Two-thirds of perioperative strokes follow inadvertent technical error. Advocates of monitoring and QC argue that targeted strategies can reduce perioperative risks.[29] Opponents claim there is no evidence that monitoring and QC reduces procedural risk.[30]

WHAT IS THE RANDOMISED TRIAL EVIDENCE?

No randomised trials have been performed.

WHAT IS THE NON-RANDOMISED TRIAL EVIDENCE?

The New York Carotid Artery Study (9278 CEAs) reported that a minority of surgeons used intraoperative imaging and that these surgeons did not report lower procedural risks.[30] However, this type of study is flawed because (1) most 'monitoring' strategies are used to identify patients at risk of haemodynamic stroke during carotid clamping, despite the fact that <20% of intraoperative strokes follow haemodynamic failure and (2) the flawed assumption that one single monitoring/QC modality can prevent all perioperative strokes. Because there are multiple causes of perioperative stroke, this assumption was always doomed to failure, and (3) the main reason why many believe that monitoring and QC cannot prevent stroke is a simple failure to ask the right questions.

The causes of intraoperative stroke include (1) embolism during carotid mobilisation, (2) haemodynamic failure during carotid clamping, (3) embolisation of retained luminal thrombus following flow restoration and (4) on-table thrombosis. The main causes of post-operative stroke are (1) thrombosis/embolisation from the endarterectomy zone (usually first 6 hours after flow restoration), (2) intracranial haemorrhage (ICH; usually >24 hours) and (3) stroke secondary to the hyperperfusion syndrome (HS; usually >24 hours).

In order to prevent one or more of these stroke aetiologies, monitoring and QC strategies need to be targeted. Figure 34.1 details the roles for monitoring, as opposed to QC (they are not the same). Only transcranial Doppler ultrasound (TCD) warns of embolisation during carotid mobilisation. Reduced perfusion following clamping can be evaluated by ICA stump pressure or backflow, near-infrared spectroscopy, cerebral blood flow measurement, jugular venous oxygen saturation and TCD, but none are infallible. If the surgeon really does want to know who needs a shunt, CEA should be performed under LRA. Similarly, EEG and sensory evoked potential abnormalities will warn that the cellular threshold for loss of electrical activity has been crossed, but this does not mean that a neurological deficit is inevitable. This is because the perfusion threshold for cellular death is lower.

Figure 34.1 also summarises the various QC roles. TCD is the only modality for diagnosing embolisation and shunt malfunction (3% of shunts malfunction because of impingement on the arterial wall). Retained luminal thrombus and intimal flaps can be diagnosed using angioscopy, angiography or duplex ultrasound, but only

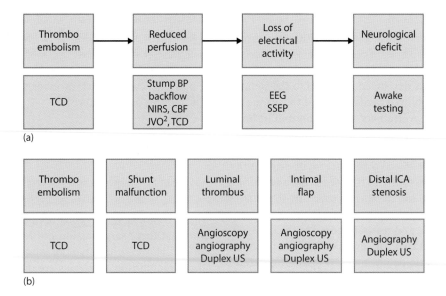

(a)

(b)

Figure 34.1 The rationales and techniques for intraoperative (a) monitoring and (b) quality control (QC). No single monitoring/QC modality can prevent all causes of perioperative stroke. They must be targeted. (Reproduced from Naylor AR, Completion angioscopy after carotid endarterectomy, in: Dieter RS, Dieter RA, eds., *Endovascular Interventions: A Case Based Approach*, Springer, New York, 2013, pp. 1253–1256. With permission.)

angioscopy can diagnose the presence of thrombus prior to flow restoration. Duplex ultrasound and angiography are useful methods for identifying residual/iatrogenic distal ICA stenoses.

In Leicester, a 21-year research/audit programme sequentially evaluated each major cause of perioperative stroke and implemented preventive strategies using targeted monitoring and QC. Intraoperative TCD and completion angioscopy virtually abolished intraoperative stroke (4% prior to 1991, 0.3% during the last 2300 CEAs).[29] There are four roles for TCD: (1) to identify embolisation during carotid mobilisation which warns the surgeon of an unstable carotid plaque, (2) to warn of shunt malfunction, (3) to ensure mean middle cerebral artery (MCA) velocity is >15 cm/s. If so, haemodynamic stroke is unlikely and (4) TCD warns of the very rare patient who is thrombosing their carotid artery during neck closure. This is because the evolving thrombus sheds increasing numbers of emboli, which can be detected using TCD.

Angioscopy (performed immediately after flushing with heparinised saline and prior to flow restoration) has three roles: (1) to confirm a normal endarterectomy zone, (2) to diagnose luminal thrombus (derived from bleeding from transected vasa vasorum [Figure 34.2]) and (3) to identify large intimal flaps requiring correction.[29] In our experience, the majority of intraoperative strokes probably followed embolisation of retained luminal thrombus following flow restoration.

In the first 6 hours after CEA, the commonest cause of perioperative stroke is thromboembolism from an evolving thrombus adherent to the endarterectomised surface. Postoperative carotid thrombosis (POCT) can be predicted and prevented using post-operative TCD monitoring. Those with increasing rates of embolisation are at high risk of

POCT and were (previously) administered incremental dose, intravenous dextran. This abolished stroke due to POCT and worked well for a decade until dextran was withdrawn.[29] However, research has shown that patients with higher rate embolisation after CEA had platelets that were more sensitive to ADP.[29] A randomised trial subsequently

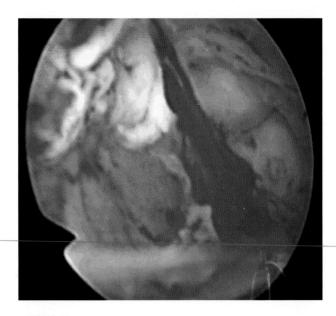

Figure 34.2 Completion angioscopy after carotid endarterectomy completed with a patch angioplasty. The carotid vessels have been clamped and the shunt removed. The endarterectomy zone has been irrigated with heparinised saline and a flexible hysteroscope inserted. There is a large residual thrombus adherent to the proximal common carotid artery intimal step. These thrombi are generally derived from bleeding from transected vasa vasorum.

showed that regular aspirin plus a single 75 mg dose of clopidogrel the night before surgery virtually abolished embolisation after surgery.[31] For the last 8 years, dual antiplatelet therapy is administered to every CEA patient undergoing CEA in Leicester. Post-operative TCD has been abandoned and no one has suffered a stroke due to POCT.[29]

However, while TCD/angioscopy prevented intraoperative stroke and selective dextran therapy (superseded by dual antiplatelet therapy) prevented stroke due to POCT, neither strategy prevented stroke due to ICH or the HS. Following a review of practice, almost every case of stroke due to ICH or HS was preceded by worsening hypertension, which was usually inadequately treated. In 2008, consensus guidance for the management of post-CEA hypertension was published (Tables 34.5 and 34.6) and a copy placed in every patient's case notes. As a consequence, post-CEA hypertension is treated much more quickly and ICH and/or stroke due to HS have all but disappeared. Interestingly, the combination of dual antiplatelet therapy and aggressive post-CEA hypertension management has also significantly reduced major perioperative cardiac events as well.[29]

Table 34.5 Guidance for the management of (i) severe hypertension in the recovery area of theatre (>170 mmHg) or (ii) back on ward (>160 mmHg) in association with severe headache and/or seizures.

First-line labetalol	100 mg labetalol in 20 mL of 0.9% saline (i.e. 5 mg/mL).
	Give 10 mg (2 mL) boluses slowly every 2 minutes up to 100 mg (i.e. 20 mL given over 20 minutes).
	If BP remains elevated after 20 minutes, move to second-line agent.
	If BP reduces and does not rebound, continue regular BP observations.
	If BP reduces but increases again, start infusion at 50–100 mg/hour, titrating dose to BP.
Second-line hydralazine	10 mg hydralazine in 10 mL of 0.9% sodium chloride (i.e. 1 mg/mL).
	Give 2 mg (2 mL) boluses slowly every 5 minutes up to 10 mg (i.e. 10 mL given over 25 minutes).
	If BP remains elevated after 25 minutes, move to third-line agent.
	If BP reduces and does not rebound, continue regular BP observations.
	If BP reduces but increases again, move to third-line agent.
Third-line glyceryl trinitrate (GTN)	50 mg GTN in 50 mL 0.9% sodium chloride (i.e. 1 mg/mL).
	Start infusion at 5 mL/hour (5 mg/hour), increasing rate to 12 mL/hour (12 mg/hour), titrated to BP.

Source: Reproduced from Naylor AR et al., *Eur J Vasc Endovasc Surg*, 46, 161, 2013. With permission.

Table 34.6 Management of the patient who becomes hypertensive on the ward (systolic blood pressure >170 mmHg) but with *no* headache, seizure or focal neurological deficit.

Patient *is not* normally taking antihypertensive therapy	
First line	Nifedipine retard (10 mg), repeated after 1 hour if no change in BP. *Do not* use crushed nifedipine capsules.
Second line	Bisoprolol 5.0 mg. If contraindicated, move to third-line agent.
Third line	Ramipril 5 mg, repeated at 3 hours if necessary.
Patient *is* normally on antihypertensive therapy	
First line	Check if the patient has received normal antihypertensive medication. If not, administer this.
Second line	A, ACE inhibitor; B, b-blocker; C, calcium channel blocker; D, diuretic.
	If patient is on A, add in C (nifedipine LA, 10 mg).
	If patient is on C, add in A (ramipril, 5 mg).
	If patient is on D, add in A (ramipril, 5 mg).
	If patient is on A + C, add in D (bendrofluazide, 2.5 mg).
	If patient is on A + D, add in C (nifedipine LA, 10 mg).
	If patient is on A + C + D, add in B (bisoprolol, 5 mg).
Patient cannot swallow tablets	Pass nasogastric tube and administer appropriate medicines in liquid form as prescribed earlier. In this situation, amlodipine should replace nifedipine.

Source: Reproduced from Naylor AR et al., *Eur J Vasc Endovasc Surg*, 46, 161, 2013. With permission.

CONCLUSION

Targeted monitoring and QC strategies can reduce procedural risks after CEA. Uncritical monitoring/QC strategies will not. No single monitoring or QC strategy can prevent procedural stroke.

PRACTICAL TIPS FOR PERFORMING CEA

Operating in the hyperacute period

The move towards operating in the first few days after symptom onset has brought new challenges to the surgeon. Most patients have unstable carotid plaques with friable, overlying thrombus (Figure 34.3), and surgical techniques must be modified accordingly.

Contrary to what was stated earlier (regarding subocclusion), no diagnosis of 'subocclusion' should be made on the basis of ultrasound in the hyperacute period after symptom onset. It is not unusual for ultrasonographers to report a very narrow lumen extending into the upper neck, with no apparent exit into a normal calibre lumen. This feature would previously have been labelled as being a 'subocclusion', but the critical difference is that there are still high peak systolic and end-diastolic velocities across the stenosis. In chronic subocclusions, there are very low peak systolic velocities (<20 cm/s) with no diastolic flow. In the acute situation, corroborative CTA/MRA imaging will usually confirm that the stenosis opens out into a normal lumen (i.e. revascularisation is appropriate). In short, no one should be 'labelled' as having subocclusion in the hyperacute period after onset of symptoms without corroborative imaging.

In the perioperative period, the anaesthetist must be vigilant when applying the oxygen mask to the patient's face prior to induction. If fingers inadvertently press on the

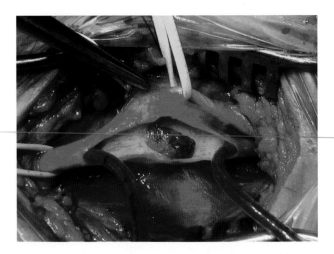

Figure 34.3 Operative image from a 39-year-old female with crescendo TIAs. Duplex ultrasound suggested there was a hypoechoic 90% stenosis in the proximal ICA. At operation, there was a large fresh thrombus overlying an ulcerated plaque, almost completely obliterating the lumen.

bifurcation, this can precipitate embolisation. Similarly, aseptic skin prep must be applied meticulously as this too can precipitate embolisation. Patients who have suffered a recent stroke with partial recovery will almost always exhibit worsening of their pre-existing neurological deficit as they recover from anaesthesia. The clue that nothing untoward has happened (intraoperatively) is that the patient awakens rapidly. The neurological deficit will usually recover to preoperative levels within an hour. This means that there is no need to immediately re-explore this type of patient.

About 25% of patients undergoing CEA within the hyperacute period after onset of symptoms will develop severe post-CEA hypertension in the first 4–6 hours after surgery, while 25% will develop hypertension on the ward. About 12% will suffer post-CEA hypertension in both locations.[32] It is essential that post-CEA hypertension is managed aggressively to prevent progression on to stroke due to ICH or HS (Tables 34.5 and 34.6).

Mobilising the cervical 'fat pad'

The surgeon will occasionally encounter a large cervical fat pad overlying the carotid bifurcation, especially in short, fat-necked male patients. Conventional teaching advises that dissection continues deep to the anterior sternomastoid border. However, this merely delays having to deal with the fat pad. The situation can become further complicated when arterial branches (usually the superior thyroid artery) emerge from the fat. The mantra 'mobilise lymph nodes towards you and branches away' will guide the surgeon. There is usually a relatively avascular crescent on the supero-medial boundary of the fat pad. This is entered by opening a pair of dissecting scissors (superiorly) and then mobilising the crescent of fat and lymph nodes towards the surgeon. Superiorly, lies digastric muscle. Deep to the mobilised fat pad lies the CFV, which is then mobilised and divided as usual.

Eversion plication

Occasionally, there is redundancy of the endarterectomy zone following CEA, or where coiling/kinking of the distal ICA has been incorporated within the arteriotomy in order to remove the plaque safely. Uncorrected, the bifurcation rotates following flow restoration (especially if patched), causing a functional distal stenosis. This is prevented by either (1) transecting the redundant arterial wall, with primary reanastomosis, or (2) performing an eversion plication. Here, the redundant segment of ICA is mobilised and two stay sutures placed on either side of the ICA to incorporate the length of ICA that needs shortening. It is the author's preference to include the distal intimal step within the eversion zone. When the two sutures are tied, the redundant segment of ICA is everted posteriorly. One of the sutures is then used to complete the anastomosis to approximate the two layers of adjacent arterial wall in order to restore arterial continuity. The shortened arteriotomy is then closed primarily or with a patch.

Carotid bypass

There are several situations when it may be necessary to perform a bypass: (1) excessive (dangerous) thinning of the arterial wall after endarterectomy, (2) excessive ICA coiling or kinking that cannot be treated by transection and primary anastomosis or eversion plication, (3) when treating prosthetic patch infection and (4) where the ICA has been removed *en bloc* with a tumour.

The first step is to harvest a segment of long saphenous vein from the thigh and place the reversed vein segment over the distal limb of a Pruitt-Inahara shunt. Once the shunt limb is reinserted into the distal ICA, the vein graft and ICA lie closely opposed, facilitating a relatively easy spatulated anastomosis. Once the distal anastomosis is completed, it is useful to deflate the distal Pruitt balloon and gently withdraw the shunt to test the distal anastomosis. This is because once the bypass is completed, it can be occasionally difficult to correct bleeding from the posterior aspect of the distal anastomosis. The distal Pruitt shunt is soft and can easily be relocated within the distal ICA while the proximal anastomosis is completed. A methylene blue line drawn down the vein (while on the Pruitt) minimises chances of the vein graft twisting (Figure 34.4). The bifurcation is reconstituted by opening up the back wall of the vein graft so that the heel of the vein graft hood lies adjacent to the orifice of the external carotid artery (ECA).

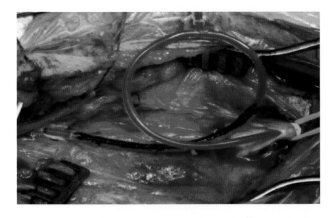

Figure 34.4 Operative image from a 46-year-old male who has undergone en bloc resection of a very large carotid body tumour. A carotid bypass is underway. The saphenous vein has been harvested from the groin, reversed and placed over the distal limb of a Pruitt shunt. Methylene blue has been used to mark the correct alignment of the graft so as to avoid twisting of the vein following flow restoration. The shunt neatly aligns the distal vein to the distal ICA which makes the distal anastomosis easier to complete.

High carotid disease

HIGH DISEASE ANTICIPATED PREOPERATIVELY

If high disease is anticipated preoperatively, consider postponing the operation. The patient's symptom status will dictate the need (urgency) to continue. If the patient is symptomatic, consider asking a more experienced colleague to either take on the case, or assist you. Alternatively, consider CAS. Practical measures to optimise exposure include (1) nasolaryngeal intubation (this opens the angle between mandible and cervical vertebrae) and (2) not using a transverse incision or eversion endarterectomy. If the patient is asymptomatic, it may be prudent to cancel the procedure as the risks of proceeding may now outweigh any potential benefits. Remember that the management of patients with asymptomatic carotid disease is highly controversial and many now believe that CEA/CAS rarely benefits the asymptomatic patient.

If a surgical approach remains the optimal treatment, consider whether you need to speak to maxillofacial colleagues to consider temporo-submandibular subluxation. This has to be planned in advance, as it cannot be performed once the procedure has started. Alternatively, a combined exposure with a parotid surgeon offers a simpler alternative (see later). Two operative scenarios now face the surgeon.

The operation has started, but the vessels have not been opened

It is still not too late to abandon the procedure and (as mentioned earlier) the decision to proceed will depend upon the patient's symptom status. The risks will now almost certainly be higher than what were quoted to the patient. If the risk/benefit favours continuing, consider once again whether you are the best person to complete the procedure, or whether you should seek assistance from a more experienced colleague.

The carotid artery has been opened

Now there are almost no alternatives to completing the operation or ligating the carotid artery. Simple manoeuvres to optimise distal access include ligating the sternomastoid branch of the ECA, followed by its occipital branch. Digastric can be divided. Distally, the hypoglossal nerve becomes closely related to the vagus and needs to be carefully dissected free. Traction to the hypoglossal nerve can be minimised by dividing the ansa cervicalis and putting a tie on the end attached to the hypoglossal nerve. This can then be used to lift the hypoglossal nerve without direct traction.

Many surgeons assume that the majority of postoperative swallowing problems follow glossopharyngeal nerve trauma. In fact, the majority probably follow injury to the small motor fibres from the vagus nerve. These traverse the distal ICA in a membrane superior to the hypoglossal nerve. Great care should be taken to avoid injuring these nerve fibres.

The next option is to fracture the styloid process (not always easy). If this fails to optimise exposure, seek the assistance of a colleague with experience in parotid surgery. The carotid incision is extended anterior to the ear and a standard mobilisation of the parotid gland is performed. Division of the parotid fascia greatly increases direct exposure of the upper ICA. The main advantage is that this can still be performed once the procedure is underway.[33]

If all strategies fail, the only alternative is ICA ligation. This can be a difficult decision, unless the procedure was started under LRA and there was no deficit with clamping. If, however, TCD monitoring is available, it should be safe to ligate the ICA if the mean MCA velocity is >15 cm/s.

Tandem inflow disease (retrograde stenting)

It is not uncommon to encounter isolated or tandem stenoses of the innominate or proximal CCA. Previously, these could only be treated by direct exposure of the arch vessels, but most can now be treated by open retrograde angioplasty ± stenting (Figure 34.5).

In practice, it is preferable to have an arch catheter placed via the common femoral artery to provide optimal road mapping. Images can be obtained via retrograde angiography via a catheter in the CCA, but image quality is never as good. In order to minimise embolisation during angioplasty or following flow restoration, the distal CCA should be clamped above the sheath. The sheath can then be removed and the puncture site opened to permit

flushing of debris. A couple of sutures will close the defect. Alternatively (if the patient requires CEA), the retrograde angioplasty is completed and an arteriotomy made across the ICA stenosis. Proximal debris is then flushed before a shunt is inserted between the CCA and distal ICA. Not only does this maintain cerebral perfusion but it also maintains flow across the recently stented innominate/CCA, thereby reducing the risk of overlying thrombus formation.[34]

When should I abandon the procedure?

A procedure should be abandoned when the risks of continuing exceed any potential benefit to the patient. This might include unanticipated proximal and/or distal disease extension that cannot be overcome or a major intraoperative medical event (myocardial infarction, anaphylactic reaction) or where the surgeon encounters a hypoplastic distal ICA.

POST-OPERATIVE COMPLICATIONS

Post-CEA hypertension and its management

With the move towards treating patients in the hyperacute period after onset of symptoms, a greater proportion will develop post-CEA hypertension, which

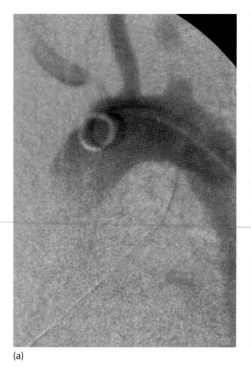 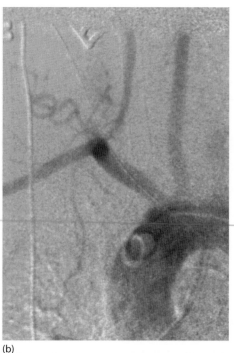

(a)   (b)

Figure 34.5 Intraoperative images from a 54-year-old female who presented with a right carotid territory stroke secondary to a severe stenosis of the innominate artery (a). This was treated by open retrograde insertion of a covered stent (b) via the right common carotid artery which was exposed using a traditional anterior sternomastoid neck incision.

increases the risk of ICH and stroke due to HS. In a prospective study involving 100 patients undergoing CEA (80% underwent CEA <14 days of the index event), 25% required treatment for hypertension in theatre recovery, 26% on the ward, while 12% required treatment in both areas. The only parameters predictive of an increased likelihood of developing post-CEA hypertension were undiagnosed or poorly controlled hypertension and impaired baroreceptor function.[33] No other demographic feature predicted post-CEA hypertension, including impaired cerebral autoregulation. The Leicester protocol for managing post-CEA hypertension is detailed in Tables 34.5 and 34.6.

Perioperative stroke

There are two types of perioperative stroke: intraoperative and post-operative. The former includes any patient who recovers from anaesthesia with a new neurological deficit. The latter includes any patient who suffers a new neurological deficit having made an otherwise uneventful recovery from the procedure. It is easier to prevent (rather than to treat) a perioperative stroke. The following sections will, therefore, offer practical advice to those who have no access to the preventive monitoring and/or QC strategies described earlier.

INTRAOPERATIVE STROKE

It is conventional to re-explore any patient who suffers an intraoperative stroke. If the patient has a hemiplegia and evidence of higher cortical dysfunction (aphasia, visuospatial neglect), it is highly likely that either the ICA has thrombosed or the MCA mainstem is occluded with an embolus. Minor neurological deficits suggest MCA branch occlusion. The Leicester experience has been that most intraoperative strokes follow embolisation of retained intra-luminal thrombus (derived from transected vasa vasorum) following restoration of flow.[29] Unfortunately, re-exploring these patients will not yield much. However (in the absence of TCD), the surgeon has no way of knowing whether thrombus has been accumulating within the endarterectomy zone while the neck wound was being closed and now requires removal.

Great care should be taken to minimise movements of the carotid bifurcation as this will precipitate embolisation. The CCA and ECA should be clamped and the anastomosis reopened. There is no need to clamp the distal ICA at this stage. Retrograde flow down the ICA will prevent embolisation while the endarterectomy zone is inspected. If no abnormality is found, an on-table angiogram may identify abnormalities in the distal ICA (dissection, embolus) or embolic occlusion of the MCA. As a rule, patients with minor deficits secondary to MCA branch occlusion will make a good recovery. Those with MCA mainstem occlusion have a poorer prognosis so that low-dose thrombolysis or clot/embolus extraction may be appropriate. The latter strategy can only be carried out by practitioners experienced in intracranial interventional procedures.

POST-OPERATIVE STROKE

Any stroke occurring after recovery from the procedure but within 24 hours of flow restoration (especially the first 6 hours) should be assumed to be embolic until proven otherwise. A CT angiogram may be helpful (provided it can be performed immediately), but it should not delay returning the patient to theatre. Any delay beyond 1 hour significantly reduces the prospect of neurological recovery. Although the stroke may be due to MCA branch embolism (as opposed to carotid thrombosis), the surgeon has no way of knowing whether there was an underlying technical error or mural thrombus with the potential for further embolisation.

An emergency CT scan should, however, be performed in any patient who suffers a neurological deficit after 24 hours has elapsed to exclude ICH. Patients suffering ICH require careful blood pressure (BP) control to avoid the extremes of rising intracranial pressure and hypoperfusion. Patients reporting severe headache and/or seizure in the early post-operative period require urgent treatment and hospitalisation. Almost all will have a grossly elevated BP and they are at high risk of suffering ICH or stroke due to HS. If the patient has been readmitted to an Acute Medical Unit, there is a general reluctance to treat post-CEA hypertension appropriately, thereby increasing the risk of ICH and stroke due to HS. The mainstay of treatment is rapid control of seizures (titrated intravenous diazepam), followed by reduction in BP (Tables 34.5 and 34.6).

Cranial nerve injuries

Surgeons have tended to 'underplay' CNIs after CEA and have rejected claims by CAS practitioners that they are equivalent to a non-disabling stroke. Pooled data from ECST, NASCET and the VA Trials reported a prevalence of 7.1%.[2] This compares with 5.6% following 6878 CEAs reported by the VSGNE[35] and 5.5% in 821 patients randomised to CEA in the International Carotid Stenting Study (ICSS).[36] Up to 0.7% of patients will have more than one CNI.[35,36] In ICSS, the mandibular branch of the facial nerve was the most commonly reported CNI (2.8%), followed by hypoglossal (1.6%), vagus (0.7%), accessory (0.12%), glossopharyngeal (0.5%) and trigeminal (0.12%).[36] In VSGNE, the commonest CNIs were hypoglossal (2.7%), mandibular branch of facial (1.9%), vagus (0.7%) and glossopharyngeal (0.5%).[35] In both ICSS and VSGNE, re-exploration for neck haematoma was associated with a significant increase in CNI.[35,36]

ICSS reported that the median time for a CNI to resolve was 30 days.[36] Overall, the vast majority of CNIs are non-disabling; ICSS reported that 1% had not resolved by 30 days, while only 0.12% were disabling at 30 days.[36] VSGNE observed that only 0.7% of CEA patients had a persisting CNI at 10 months follow-up.[35]

Prosthetic patch infection

Prosthetic patch infection complicates <1% of CEAs where the arteriotomy was closed with a PTFE/polyester patch.[37] A recent systematic review identified 123 patients who were treated for patch infection; 29% presented <2 months (original operation had been complicated by a post-operative haematoma in 19% and wound infection in 53%), while 63% presented >6 months after CEA. The latter patients rarely reported early post-operative wound complications (4%).[37]

The commonest presentations in patients presenting <2 months were wound infection/abscess (55%), patch rupture (17%), sinus discharge (17%) and false aneurysm formation (8%). The commonest clinical presentations in patients presenting >6 months were sinus discharge (36%), false aneurysm (28%), discharging sinus plus false aneurysm (8%) and wound infection/abscess (15%). Late patch rupture was rare (8%). Stroke/TIA was also an extremely rare presentation (1.6%). Staphylococci and streptococci were the infecting organism in 90% of cases.[37]

Management depends upon presentation, co-morbidity and infection severity. The literature includes highly selected cohorts who were treated by debridement/abscess drainage ± antibiotics or muscle flap closure. Reinfection rates were low, but this probably represents the preferential reporting of 'good outcomes' rather than real-world practice. The majority required debridement, patch excision and revascularisation. The systematic review observed that autologous vein repair (patch/bypass) conferred the lowest rates of late reinfection (7% at 10 years). Prosthetic reconstruction was associated with the poorest outcomes with seven of nine patients either dying in the perioperative period or suffering reinfection. The insertion of a covered stent has been described in five patients, with none suffering reinfection.[37] This may become an important treatment option in the future, but the limited data may again simply reflect selective reporting of good outcomes and there are no long-term data. For now, the 'gold standard' remains debridement, patch excision and autologous venous reconstruction.

Still to be resolved controversies

IDENTIFYING 'HIGH RISK FOR STROKE' ASYMPTOMATIC PATIENTS

In ACAS, operating upon 1000 patients with asymptomatic 60%–99% stenoses prevented 59 strokes at 5 years (Table 34.4). This means that 941 (94%) underwent an ultimately unnecessary procedure, costing US health providers $2 billion/year.[38] Even if the procedural risk could be reduced to zero, the number of strokes prevented per 1000 CEAs at 5 years would increase to 82, but this would still mean that 918 (92%) still underwent an unnecessary procedure.[38] In addition, there is compelling evidence that the annual risk of stroke in medically treated patients is diminishing, potentially further reducing any benefit from CEA.[38]

The AHA recommends that only 'highly selected' patients should undergo CEA/CAS,[7] but they never defined what this caveat meant. In reality, most surgeons and interventionists ignore this advice, if only to avoid medico-legal censure. There is, however, an urgent need to validate imaging strategies for identifying a smaller cohort of 'high risk for stroke' patients in whom to target CEA/CAS. A number of potential imaging strategies have been proposed, but these require independent validation before they can be translated into clinical practice. These include stenosis progression, a history of contralateral TIA/stroke, silent infarction on CT, TCD-detected spontaneous embolisation, plaque ulceration, MRI-diagnosed intraplaque haemorrhage, computerised plaque analysis and the presence of tandem intracranial artery disease.[39]

To date, only two randomised trials comparing CEA with CAS in asymptomatic patients includes a third limb for modern medical therapy (CREST-2, SPACE-2). Unfortunately, neither is funded to evaluate imaging strategies for identifying 'high risk for stroke' cohorts.

Concurrent carotid and cardiac disease

CURRENT GUIDELINES

The 1998 AHA guidelines considered staged/synchronous CEA and coronary artery bypass grafting (CABG) to be 'acceptable' in patients with unilateral asymptomatic stenoses >60%, provided the procedural risk was <3% and life expectancy >5 years.[40] This recommendation was downgraded to 'uncertain' should the surgical risk increase from 3% to 5% (irrespective of unilateral/bilateral disease), and it retained this 'uncertain' classification should the operative risk increase from 5% to 10%.

In 2004, the American College of Cardiology and the AHA concluded that 'CEA was probably recommended before CABG or concomitant with CABG in patients with a symptomatic carotid stenosis or in asymptomatic patients with a unilateral or bilateral internal carotid stenosis of 80%', giving it a Grade C level of evidence.[41] Subsequently, the American Society of Interventional and Therapeutic Neuroradiology, the American Society of Neuroradiology and the Society of Interventional Radiology advised that CAS was now acceptable in CABG patients with an asymptomatic or symptomatic severe stenosis associated with contralateral carotid artery occlusion requiring treatment before undergoing cardiac surgery and also in asymptomatic patients with 'pre-occlusive' lesions (defined as 90%–99% or near occlusion).[42]

By contrast, the American Association of Neurologists provided no recommendation regarding which patients should be considered for prophylactic CEA (prior to CABG), observing that *at this time the available data are insufficient to declare either CEA before or simultaneous with CABG as being superior in patients with concomitant carotid and coronary artery occlusive disease.*[43] The Society for Vascular Surgery has made no formal recommendation, while the European Society for Vascular Surgery recommends that (in the absence of randomised trials) *treatment should be individualised and based on the specific risk profile of each patient.*[44]

In short, there is no consensus as to how to best manage patients with concurrent carotid and cardiac disease.

WHY THE DEBATE?

This debate primarily relates to the management of patients with asymptomatic carotid disease undergoing CABG and whether prophylactic CEA/CAS can reduce the risk of perioperative stroke. Most surgeons and physicians agree that the small proportion of CABG patients with a prior history of TIA/stroke should undergo either staged or synchronous carotid revascularisation.

Uncritical meta-analyses suggest that the presence of a '>70%' stenosis is associated with a 7% risk of post-CABG stroke (if performed without CEA), increasing to 9% in patients with '>80%' stenoses.[45] The key issue, however, is that uncritical meta-analyses combine symptomatic with asymptomatic patients, occlusions with stenoses and unilateral with bilateral carotid disease. If symptomatic patients and carotid occlusions are excluded, the risk of stroke after isolated CABG in the presence of an asymptomatic 70%–99% stenosis falls to 2% (95% CI 1.0–5.7).[45] If one now focuses (solely) on unilateral, asymptomatic carotid disease (the majority of patients in this debate), 6 studies looked at the risk of stroke in 231 patients undergoing isolated CABG in the presence of a unilateral, asymptomatic 70%–99% stenosis, and none suffered a stroke.[45] Similarly, 143 patients with a unilateral, asymptomatic 80%–99% stenosis underwent isolated CABG with a perioperative stroke rate of 0.7%.[45] These are hardly compelling statistics supporting prophylactic intervention.

Moreover, if carotid disease really was such an important cause of post-CABG stroke, one would expect that patients with bilateral severe carotid disease undergoing a unilateral staged/synchronous CEA+CABG would have higher rates of perioperative stroke in the hemisphere ipsilateral to the non-operated severe carotid stenosis after CABG. In fact, <4% of this type of patient suffered a stroke ipsilateral to the non-operated ICA, once again casting doubt on the relevance of carotid disease in post-CABG stroke.[46]

Four natural history studies have looked at the likely causes of stroke after CABG, with particular reference to the role of carotid disease. Naylor pooled CT scan/autopsy data from 4674 patients undergoing isolated CABG and reported that 85% of post-CABG strokes could not be attributed to underlying carotid disease.[47] Stamou (16,528 CABG patients), Schoof (2797 CABG patients) and Li (4232 CABG patients) concluded that 94%–95% of post-CABG strokes could not be ascribed to carotid artery disease.[48–50]

CONCLUSION

The evidence supporting a role for prophylactic CEA/CAS in CABG patients with asymptomatic carotid disease is tenuous. Meta-analyses suggest that synchronous CEA+CABG is associated with an 8.7% risk of death/stroke <30 days, compared to 6.1% for staged CEA+CABG, 7.3% for staged CABG+CEA and 9.1% for staged CAS+CABG.[51] For the most part, these risks exceed the risk of stroke after isolated CABG. This is clearly an area where a properly powered randomised trial could determine optimal practice, rather than relying upon intuitive reasoning and misinterpretation of the data.

REFERENCES

1. Furie KL, Kasner SE, Adams RJ et al. Guidelines for prevention of stroke in patients with stroke/TIA; A guideline for healthcare professionals from the AHA/ASA. *Stroke.* 2011;42:227–276.

2. Rothwell PM, Eliasziw M, Gutnikov SA. For the Carotid Endarterectomy Trialists Collaboration. Analysis of pooled data from the randomised controlled trials of endarterectomy for symptomatic carotid stenosis. *Lancet.* 2003;361:107–116.

3. Naylor AR, Sillesen H, Schroeder TV. Clinical and imaging features associated with an increased risk of late stroke in patients with symptomatic carotid disease. *Eur J Vasc Endovasc Surg.* 2015;49:513–523.

4. Rothwell PM, Eliasziw M, Gutnikov SA, Warlow CP, Barnett HJM for the Carotid Endarterectomy Trialists Collaboration. Endarterectomy for symptomatic carotid stenosis in relation to clinical subgroups and timing of surgery. *Lancet.* 2004;363:915–924.

5. Naylor AR, MacDonald S. Extracranial carotid artery disease. In: Beard JD, Gaines PA, Series eds., Carter DC, Garden OJ, Paterson-Brown S, eds. *A Companion to Specialist Surgical Practice. Volume VI – Vascular and Endovascular Surgery*, 5th ed. New York: Elsevier, 2013, pp. 160–189.

6. Rantner B, Goebel G, Bonati LH, Ringleb PA, Mas J-L, Fraedrich G for the Carotid Stenting Trialists Collaboration. The risk of carotid artery stenting compared with carotid endarterectomy is greatest in patients treated within 7 days of symptoms. *J Vasc Surg.* 2013;57:619–626.

7. Goldstein LB, Bushnell CD, Adams RJ et al. Guidelines for primary prevention of stroke. guideline for healthcare professionals from AHA/ASA. *Stroke.* 2011;42:517–584.

8. Executive Committee for the Asymptomatic Carotid Atherosclerosis Study. Endarterectomy for asymptomatic carotid artery stenosis. *J Am Med Assoc.* 1995;273:1421–1428.

9. Asymptomatic Carotid Surgery Trial Collaborators. The MRC Asymptomatic Carotid Surgery Trial (ACST): Carotid endarterectomy prevents disabling and fatal carotid territory strokes. *Lancet.* 2004;363:1491–1502.

10. Silver FL, Mackey A, Clark WM et al. Safety of stenting and endarterectomy by symptomatic status in the carotid revascularization endarterectomy versus stenting trial (CREST). *Stroke.* 2011;42:675–680.

11. Rerkasem K, Bond R, Rothwell PM. Local versus general anaesthesia for carotid endarterectomy. *Cochrane Database Syst Rev.* 2004;(2):CD000126.

12. Vaniyapong T, Chongruksut W, Rerkasem K. Local versus general anaesthesia for carotid endarterectomy. *Cochrane Database Syst Rev.* 2013; Issue 12; CD000126.

13. Bastounis E, Bakoyiannis C, Cagiannos C, Klonaris C, Filis C, Bastouni EE, Georgopoulos S. A short incision for carotid endarterectomy results in decreased morbidity. *Eur J Vasc Endovasc Surg.* 2007;33:652–656.

14. Marcucci G, Antonelli R, Gabrielli R, Accrocca F, Giordano AG, Siani A. Short longitudinal versus transverse skin incision for carotid endarterectomy: Impact on cranial and cervical nerve injuries and esthetic outcome. *J Cardiovasc Surg.* 2011;52:145–152.

15. Ascher E, Hingorani A, Marks N, Schutzer RW, Mutyala M, Nahata S, Yorkovich W, Jacob T. Mini skin incision for carotid endarterectomy (CEA): A new and safe alternative to the standard approach. *J Vasc Surg.* 2005;2:1089–1093.

16. Antoniou GA, Murray D, Antoniou SA, Kuhan G, Serracino-Inglott F. Meta-analysis of retrojugular versus antejugular approach for carotid endarterectomy. *Ann R Coll Surg Engl.* 2014;96:184–189.

17. Tang TY, Walsh SR, Gillard JH, Varty K, Boyle JR, Gaunt ME. Carotid sinus nerve blockade to reduce blood pressure instability following carotid endarterectomy: A systematic review and meta-analysis. *Eur J Vasc Endovasc Surg.* 2007;34:304–311.

18. Stone DH, Nolan BW, Schanzer A, Goodney PP, Cambria RA, Likosky DS, Walsh DB, Cronenwett JL; Vascular Study Group of Northern New England. Protamine reduces bleeding complications associated with carotid endarterectomy without increasing the risk of stroke. *J Vasc Surg.* 2010;51:559–564.

19. Fearn SJ, Mortimer AJ, Faragher EB, McCollum CN. Carotid sinus nerve blockade during carotid surgery: A randomised controlled trial. *Eur J Vasc Endovasc Surg.* 2002;24:480–484.

20. Wakefield TW, Lindblad B, Stanley TJ, Nichol BJ, Stanley JC, Bergqvist D, Greenfield LJ, Bergentz SE. Heparin and protamine use in peripheral vascular surgery: A comparison between surgeons of the Society for Vascular Surgery and the European Society for Vascular Surgery. *Eur J Vasc Surg.* 1994;8:193–198.

21. Patel RB, Beaulieu P, Homa K, Goodney PP, Stanley AC, Cronenwett JL, Stone DH, Bertges DJ; Vascular Study Group of New England. Shared quality data are associated with increased protamine use and reduced bleeding complications after carotid endarterectomy in the Vascular Study Group of New England. *J Vasc Surg.* 2013;58:1518–1524.

22. Dellagrammaticus D, Lewis SC, Gough MJ; GALA Trial Collaborators. Is heparin reversal with protamine after carotid endarterectomy dangerous? *Eur J Vasc Endovasc Surg.* 2008;36:41–44.

23. Ferguson GG, Eliasziw M, Barr HWK et al. The North American symptomatic carotid endarterectomy trial: Surgical results of 1415 patients. *Stroke.* 1999;30:1751–1758.

24. Malone JM, Ballard JL. Carotid artery shunt: Argument for its routine use. In: Moore WS, ed. *Surgery for Cerebrovascular Disease*, 2nd ed. Philadelphia, PA: WB Saunders, 1996, pp. 347–354.

25. Chongruksut W, Vaniyapong T, Rerkasem K. Routine or selective carotid artery shunting for carotid endarterectomy (and different methods of monitoring in selective shunting). *Cochrane Database Syst Rev.* 2014;Issue 6:Art No CD000190.

26. Rerkasem K, Rothwell PM. Systematic review of randomized controlled trials of patch angioplasty versus primary closure and different types of patch materials during carotid endarterectomy. *Asian J Surg.* 2011;34:32–40.

27. Ren S, Li X, Wen J, Zhang W, Liu P. Systematic review of randomized controlled trials of different types of patch materials during carotid endarterectomy. *PLOS ONE.* 2013;8:e55050.

28. Cao P, de Rango P, Zannetti S. Eversion vs conventional carotid endarterectomy: A systematic Review. *Eur J Vasc Endovasc Surg.* 2002;23:195–201.

29. Naylor AR, Sayers RD, McCarthy MJ, Bown MJ, Nasim A, Dennis M, London NJM, Bell PRF. Closing the Loop: A 21-year audit of strategies for preventing stroke and death following carotid endarterectomy. *Eur J Vasc Endovasc Surg.* 2013;46:161–170.

30. Rockman CB, Halm EA. Intraoperative imaging: does it really improve perioperative outcomes of carotid endarterectomy? *Semin Vasc Surg.* 2007;20:236–243.

31. Payne DA, Jones CI, Hayes PD, Thompson MM, London NJM, Bell PRF, Goodall AH, Naylor AR. Beneficial effects of Clopidogrel combined with Aspirin in reducing cerebral emboli in patients undergoing carotid endarterectomy. *Circulation.* 2004;109:1476–1481.

32. Newman JE, Bown MJ, Sayers RD, Thompson JP, Robinson TG, Williams B, Panerai RB, Lacy PS, Naylor AR. Poorly controlled BP and impaired baroreceptor function (but not impaired autoregulation) are associated with a significantly higher prevalence of post-carotid endarterectomy hypertension. Paper presented at the *Vascular Society of Great Britain and Ireland*, Manchester, UK, November 2012.

33. Naylor AR, Moir A. An aid to accessing the distal internal carotid artery. *J Vasc Surg.* 2009;49:1345–1347.

34. Payne DA, Hayes PD, Bolia A, Fishwick G, Bell PRF, Naylor AR. On-table angioplasty for common carotid and innominate artery stenoses: A method for cerebral protection from embolisation. *Br J Surg.* 2006;93:187–190.

35. Fokkema M, de Borst GJ, Nolan BW et al. Clinical relevance of cranial nerve injury following carotid endarterectomy. *Eur J Vasc Endovasc Surg.* 2014;47:2–7.

36. Doig D, Turner EL, Dobson J et al. Incidence, impact and prediction of cranial nerve palsy and haematoma following carotid endarterectomy in the International Carotid Stenting Study. *Eur J Vasc Endovasc Surg.* 2014;48:498–504.

37. Mann CD, McCarthy M, Nasim A, Bown M, Dennis M, Sayers RD, London NJM, Naylor AR. Management and outcome of prosthetic patch infection after carotid endarterectomy: A single centre series and systematic review of the literature. *Eur J Vasc Endovasc Surg.* 2012;44:20–26.

38. Naylor AR. Time to rethink management strategies in asymptomatic carotid disease. *Nat Rev Cardiol.* 2011;9:116–124.

39. Naylor AR, Sillesen H, Schroeder TV. Clinical and imaging features associated with an increased risk of late stroke in patients with asymptomatic carotid disease. *Eur J Vasc Endovasc Surg.* 2014;48:633–640.

40. Biller J, Feinberg WM, Castaldo JE et al. Guidelines for carotid endarterectomy: A statement for healthcare professionals from a special writing group of the Stroke Council, American Heart Association. *Stroke.* 1998;29:554–562.

41. Eagle KA, Guyton RA, Davidoff R et al. ACC/AHA 2004 Guideline Update for coronary artery bypass graft surgery: Summary article: A report of the American College of Cardiology/American Heart Association Taskforce on Practice Guidelines (Committee to update the 1999 Guidelines for Coronary Artery Bypass Graft Surgery). *J Am Coll Cardiol.* 2004;44:1146–1154.

42. Barr JD, MD, Connors JJ, Sack Ds et al. Quality improvement guidelines for the performance of cervical carotid angioplasty and stent placemen. Developed by a Collaborative Panel of the American Society of Interventional and Therapeutic Neuroradiology, the American Society of Neuroradiology, and the Society of Interventional Radiology *Am J Neuroradiol.* 2003;24:2020–2034.

43. Clinicians Assessment: Carotid Endarterectomy – An Evidence Based Review. www.aan.com/professionals/practice/guideline/pdf/Clinician_guideline.pdf, accessed 28 October, 2014.

44. Liapis CD, Bell PRF, Mikhailidis D, Sivenius J, Nicolaides A, Fernandes e Fernandes J, Biasi G, Norgren L. ESVS Guidelines. Invasive treatment for carotid stenosis: indications, techniques. *Eur J Vasc Endovasc Surg.* 2009;37:S1–S19.

45. Naylor AR, Bown MJ. Stroke after cardiac surgery and its association with asymptomatic carotid disease: An updated systematic review and meta-analysis. *Eur J Vasc Endovasc Surg.* 2011;41:607–624.

46. Naylor AR. Synchronous cardiac and carotid revascularisation: The devil is in the detail. *Eur J Vasc Endovasc Surg.* 2010;40:303–308.

47. Naylor AR, Mehta Z, Rothwell PM, Bell PRF. Stroke during coronary artery bypass surgery: A critical review of the role of carotid artery disease. *Eur J Vasc Endovasc Surg.* 2002;23:283–294.

48. Stamou SC, Hill PC, Dangas G et al. Stroke after coronary artery bypass: Incidence, predictors, and clinical outcome. *Stroke.* 2001;32:1508–1513.

49. Schoof J, Lubahn W, Baemer M et al. Impaired cerebral autoregulation distal to carotid stenosis/occlusion is associated with an increased risk of stroke with cardiopulmonary bypass. *J Thorac Cardiovasc Surg.* 2007;134:690–696.

50. Li Y, Walicki D, Mathieson C et al. Strokes after cardiac surgery and relationship to carotid stenosis. *Arch Neurol.* 2009;66:1091–1096.

51. Naylor AR, Mehta Z, Rothwell PM. A systematic review and meta-analysis of 30-day outcomes following staged carotid angioplasty with stenting and coronary bypass. *Eur J Vasc Endovasc Surg.* 2009;37:379–387.

52. Naylor AR, Completion angioscopy after carotid endarterectomy. In: Dieter RS, Dieter RA, eds. *Endovascular Interventions: A Case Based Approach.* New York: Springer, 2013, pp. 1253–1256.

35

Occlusive disease of the branches of the aortic arch and vertebral artery

GERT J. DE BORST

CONTENTS

GENERAL INTRODUCTION

Clinically relevant occlusive disease of the aortic arch branch vessels occurs relatively infrequently. However, when associated with symptoms, occlusive disease in this area may have a serious clinical impact on the health status of the patient. Furthermore, every vascular surgeon or interventionist will be confronted with a clinical dilemma in managing patients with aortic arch branch vessel disease several times each year and, therefore, needs to understand the main features of atherosclerotic disease in this area. This chapter reviews the clinical presentation, diagnosis, imaging and treatment of occlusive lesions of the branches of the aortic arch and vertebral artery (VA).

ANATOMICAL VARIATIONS

Variations and anomalies in the anatomy of the branches of the aortic arch are important and relevant to understanding the presentation and treatment of atherosclerotic occlusive disease in these vessels. The standard anatomic arrangement is a left-sided aortic arch from which the innominate (brachiocephalic), left common carotid and left subclavian arteries take off in succession. In 16% of patients, the origins of the left common carotid and the innominate arteries are close enough that they share some part of the circumference of their ostia. In 8% of patients, a common trunk exists for the innominate and left common carotid artery (CCA) (termed as 'bovine arch'). In 0.5% of patients, the right subclavian arises as the last branch of the arch and reaches the right upper extremity via a retro-oesophageal route (arteria lusoria).

The VA takes its origin from the subclavian arteries, opposite from the origin of the internal mammary artery. In 6% of patients, the left vertebral arises directly from the aortic arch, usually between the origins of the left common carotid and the left subclavian arteries. In the majority of patients, blood supply via the posterior cerebral artery (PCA) to the occipital cortex is via the vertebrobasilar circulation. However, in a small proportion of patients, the PCA is supplied via the carotid arteries instead of the vertebrobasilar arteries.

OCCLUSIVE DISEASE OF THE MAIN ARCH VESSELS

In the general population, the incidence of significant stenosis or occlusion at the origin of an aortic arch branch vessel ranges from 0.5% to 6.4%, with a relatively higher frequency in the innominate or left subclavian artery, as opposed to the left CCA.[1] The total CCA occlusion (CCAO) is a relatively rare finding and is present in 2%–4% of patients undergoing angiography for symptomatic cerebrovascular disease.[2]

Patients with a symptomatic origin stenosis of an aortic arch artery have a relatively high risk for developing a further stenosis in another aortic arch branch vessel. Based on a total follow-up of 162 months, the risk of developing a new symptomatic lesion in another arch branch vessel was 2.3% per year.[1] Concomitant (symptomatic) coronary artery disease requiring coronary artery bypass grafting (CABG) may exist in up to 20% of patients with arch branch origin stenoses. Because proximal subclavian artery disease may affect the flow in the internal mammary artery (frequently used as a bypass conduit during cardiac surgery), the proximal subclavian artery should be screened in patients undergoing evaluation of their coronary arteries. Occlusive disease at the carotid bifurcation requiring concomitant carotid endarterectomy may be present in up to 17% of patients.[3]

OCCLUSIVE DISEASE OF THE MAIN ARCH BRANCHES: CLINICAL PRESENTATION

Occlusive disease of the branches of the aortic arch may result in either distal embolization or blood flow restriction to the brain or upper limbs. Lesions of the left CCA may give rise to left hemispheric or left retinal symptoms. Left subclavian artery lesions can give rise to both vertebrobasilar and left upper extremity symptoms, while innominate artery lesions can involve any one of three territories (right carotid, vertebrobasilar and right upper extremity). Occlusive lesions that involve the branches of

the aortic arch are generally atherosclerotic. Less commonly arteritis (Takayasu's, radiation) and dissection can be a cause of symptoms (see Chapters XX). In nearly all patients with concomitant brachiocephalic and carotid bifurcation disease, symptoms specific to brachiocephalic disease will appear distinct from symptoms related to the carotid bifurcation disease.[3]

Before duplex ultrasound (DUS) was introduced into routine clinical practice, screening and follow-up examinations relied solely upon hemodynamic and clinical evaluation. The key clue suggesting a diagnosis of occlusive disease of the branches of the aortic arch is an absent ipsilateral, radial pulse, abnormal pulse waveforms or unequal blood pressures in the upper extremities, combined with effort fatigue of the arm. Bruits at the base of the neck are common in these patients, but do not add to the diagnosis.

The diagnosis is generally considered positive if any of the following clinical or imaging features apply: new or recurrent vertebrobasilar, hemispheric or coronary (related to coronary steal syndrome) symptoms or signs; a decrease of ≥0.15 in the blood pressure index of the ipsilateral arm compared with the contralateral arm; reversal of flow in the ipsilateral vertebral or carotid artery on DUS; or vessel evaluation indicating a marked serial increase in velocity (>130 cm/s) in the CCA. The diagnosis of subclavian steal syndrome (SSS) is based on the combination of ipsilateral effort–related arm fatigue, a blood pressure gradient between both upper extremities and retrograde flow in the ipsilateral VA on DUS.

> ### Key points
>
> 1. Symptoms specific to brachiocephalic disease will appear distinct from symptoms related to carotid bifurcation disease.
> 2. Screening and follow-up examinations rely upon hemodynamic and clinical evaluation.

OCCLUSIVE DISEASE OF THE VERTEBRAL ARTERY

An atherosclerotic stenosis >50% in the vertebral or basilar artery is found in approximately 25% of patients with vertebrobasilar territory, transient ischemic attack (TIA) or stroke. This stenosis is most frequently located in the proximal VA. The consequences of finding a VA stenosis are uncertain, especially when the patient is asymptomatic. The natural course and thus the risk of ischemic stroke in patients with an asymptomatic VA stenosis are poorly understood.

In a series of 282 patients with asymptomatic VA stenosis >50% on DUS, the annual stroke rate was 0.4% during a mean follow-up of 4.6 years, versus an annual stroke rate <0.1% in patients without VA stenosis.[4] The risk of posterior circulation ischemic stroke was higher in patients with a VA stenosis than in patients without a VA stenosis (hazard ratio [HR], 4.2; 95% CI, 1.4–13.1) and was further increased in patients with combined VA and carotid artery stenosis (HR, 10.5; 95% CI, 3.0–37.3). Patients with symptomatic VA stenoses have an increased risk of stroke, but the risk of recurrent vascular events in patients with VA stenosis is uncertain. The best available data come from a systematic review, in which the risk of subsequent stroke or death in patients with vertebrobasilar events was similar to the risk in patients with carotid territory events.[5,6]

> ### Key point
>
> Patients with atherosclerotic arterial disease and asymptomatic VA stenosis have a higher risk of posterior circulation ischemic stroke than patients without such a stenosis, but the absolute risk remains low.

OCCLUSIVE DISEASE OF THE VERTEBRAL ARTERY: CLINICAL PRESENTATION

Twenty to thirty percent of all TIAs and ischemic strokes involve territories supplied by the vertebrobasilar circulation. Common causes of vertebrobasilar ischemia include embolism from the heart, aorta or small-vessel disease. Up to 32% of ischemic events are presumed to be caused by a hemodynamic mechanism. In patients with symptomatic VA stenoses, more than half of the TIAs or nondisabling ischemic strokes may be associated with nonfocal neurological symptoms. Nonfocal symptoms occur more frequently in patients with a symptomatic VA stenosis than carotid artery stenosis.[7]

IMAGING

Determination of severity and length of stenosis is of critical importance when deciding whether the patient warrants revascularization. Physicians rely most commonly on DUS when screening for atherosclerotic stenosis of the brachiocephalic and vertebral vessels using the method described by Grosveld.[8] DUS may visualize lesions in all three branches of the arch, but the standard examination may not satisfactorily image the retrosternal segments of the branches of the arch. Moreover, DUS is very much user dependent and can be limited in cases of severe calcification.

Magnetic resonance angiography (MRA) can be a valuable corroborative/diagnostic modality for imaging the arch branches, but this may require special coils and sequencing. A routine brain and neck MRA is unlikely to provide adequate visualization of the branches of the arch, mainly due to pulse artefacts. In MRA, a loss of signal can occur due to complex flow patterns in areas of severe stenosis resulting in non-perpendicular flow. In addition, slow-moving flow may appear as an occlusion. As a consequence, compared to a DUS, MRA tends to overestimate the degree of stenosis.

Computed tomographic angiography (CTA) is easy to undertake and is less prone to overestimating stenosis severity due to turbulence or tortuosity. Multidetector helical CT enables rapid scanning with lower radiation doses and less contrast administration. Correlation between CTA and MRA is associated with a sensitivity, specificity and accuracy of 93%, 100% and 98% for 70%–99% stenoses,[9] respectively. As with DUS, the degree of stenosis may be difficult to obtain in heavily calcified lesions. Furthermore, as in MRA, CTA may not provide a clear picture of hemodynamics around the origins of the arch branches due to motion defects.

Accordingly, some still consider intra-arterial angiography to be the true reference standard for providing optimal visualization. In cases of multiple arch branch lesions, it offers information on cerebral perfusion, as well as patterns of intracranial collateralization. In cases of total CCAO, neither CTA nor MRA can document the dynamic pattern of collateral flow involved in reconstituting a patent carotid bifurcation. Angiographic findings can be categorized into four types according to Riles et al.: Type 1A involves a patent internal carotid artery (ICA) and external carotid artery (ECA); type 1B, a patent ECA and occluded ICA; and type 1C, a patent ICA and an occluded ECA. Type 2 lesions include total occlusions of the CCA, ICA and ECA.[10]

Conventional angiography is particularly useful in imaging arch type and vertebral tortuosity, as well as stenosis. While superior for determining stenosis severity, angiography is limited in assessing plaque morphology and plaque ulceration. Furthermore, as an invasive procedure, angiography is associated with the risk of access site injuries, contrast-induced nephrotoxicity and an overall neurologic complication rate of 2.6%.[10] Accordingly, when planning a carotid bifurcation intervention, the severity of tortuosity, proximal disease and arch type rarely affects surgical decision-making.[11] However, this type of information is invaluable when considering patients for endovascular procedures in the arch branch vessels.

Non-invasive surveillance imaging for stented patients mostly involves DUS. However, duplex velocity criteria for assessing recurrent stenosis in a non-stented artery may not be valid in patients with a stented carotid artery, and these thresholds may require modification to reliably detect in-stent restenosis. MRA traditionally has been of limited value in assessing vessels following stent implantation, largely due to stent artefact causing artificial lumen narrowing. CTA is superior to MRA and should be the second-line imaging strategy for confirming DUS diagnosed in-stent restenosis.

For the VA, contrast-enhanced MRA is considered the most sensitive method for detecting origin stenoses, with a high specificity. CTA also has a good sensitivity and high specificity. By contrast, DUS has a low sensitivity and will miss many vertebral stenoses.[12] Conventional angiography remains the gold standard for the diagnosis of VA stenosis. No studies have compared the varying imaging modalities against intra-arterial angiography in the same cohort of patients.[13]

> ### Key points
>
> 1. DUS should be used for screening for stenoses of the brachiocephalic and vertebral vessels.
> 2. Contrast-enhanced MRA is the most sensitive non-invasive technique for detecting origin stenoses.
> 3. Conventional angiography is the true reference imaging standard.
> 4. DUS thresholds may require modification in order to reliably detect in-stent restenosis.

INDICATIONS FOR REVASCULARIZATION

Indications for revascularizing aortic branch origin lesions of the innominate or CCAs are similar to the indications intervening in the carotid bifurcation territory. A significant stenosis in the brachiocephalic artery is generally defined as being a narrowing of ≥70%. Although a conservative approach may be justifiable in patients without symptoms, in patients with neurological sequelae or upper extremity ischemia, the indication for revascularization is relatively straightforward. In symptomatic patients, the etiology may be embolic or hemodynamic secondary to low cerebral perfusion. There is not, and probably will never be, a prospective series with sufficient numbers to advise on the natural history of isolated common carotid or innominate lesions. Critical lesions of the innominate and CCA arteries may progress towards occlusion, and CCAO can be associated with a variety of neurologic symptoms and an increased risk of stroke.

Guidelines recommend 'revascularization for patients with symptomatic ischemia involving the anterior cerebral circulation caused by common carotid or brachiocephalic artery occlusive disease', without, however, referring to CCAO specifically or discussing CCAO independently.[14] Therefore, the necessity to intervene in a patient with CCAO remains controversial.[2] Occlusion of a subclavian artery rarely causes a stroke and most patients are neurologically asymptomatic. Once a decision to proceed with surgical reconstruction has been made, the next step is to decide whether it will be done by means of an endovascular approach or via an open cervical or thoracic procedure.

It is advisable that patients are discussed in a multidisciplinary panel consisting of interventional radiologists, vascular surgeons and neurologists. Although graft or intervention failures occur with either strategy, other factors (such as predicted operative risk, anatomic distribution of disease, concomitant multisystem disease, initial and late costs and patient preference) may affect decision-making in individual patients.

> ### Key points
>
> 1. The natural history of isolated common carotid or innominate stenosis is unknown.
> 2. Patients with neurological symptoms or life-limiting upper limb ischemia benefit from revascularization.

RECONSTRUCTION: ENDOVASCULAR VERSUS OPEN SURGICAL RECONSTRUCTION

There is considerable controversy regarding the optimal intervention in patients with brachiocephalic disease, as there is usually evidence of concurrent multivessel involvement. Until 30 years ago, supra-aortic trunk occlusive disease could only be treated with open surgery.[15,16] Despite the reports of good long-term patency rates, open surgery was associated with high morbidity and mortality rates. In the 1980s, percutaneous transluminal angioplasty (PTA) was introduced followed by PTA with stent placement. Nowadays, PTA with or without stenting is feasible and safe in the short term and is accepted by most interventionists as being the first-line treatment for aortic arch branch origin lesions.

OPEN SURGICAL RECONSTRUCTION: CERVICAL VERSUS TRANSTHORACIC

Operative techniques for reconstruction of the arch vessels[17-19] include bypass procedures via a transthoracic or via an extrathoracic (cervical) approach. The transthoracic approach involves either a median sternotomy or a less invasive (trapdoor) technique. The choice of operative approach should be guided by the extent and distribution of atherosclerotic disease, as determined by preoperative imaging, presence of (aortic) calcification, clinical assessment of overall operative risk and patient/surgeon preferences.

Cervical reconstructions are less invasive than transthoracic reconstructions and are associated with lower procedural risks. Conversely, in complex cases with two- or three-vessel involvement, the long-term prognosis of a cervical reconstruction may be inferior to a transthoracic approach. Lesions in the innominate artery which may be a source of distal embolization deserve special consideration because the proximal innominate artery needs to be mobilized and excluded from the circulation, and this will be challenging via a purely cervical approach.

There is clearly a need for both transthoracic and cervical approaches. Patients with a single subclavian or common carotid lesion with a fully patent ipsilateral carotid or subclavian artery should undergo a cervical transposition or bypass (Figure 35.1a and b). This approach is associated

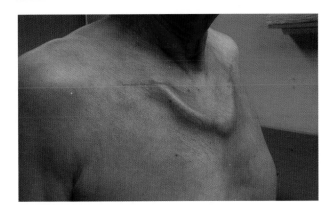

Figure 35.1 Open surgical approach aortic arch branch origins and vertebral artery. (From Valentine & Wind Lippincott Williams @ Wilkins 2nd edition.)

with durable patency rates and low morbidity.[20] At the other end of the spectrum, however, is the patient with involvement of all three branches of the aortic arch, where graft outflow needs to arise from the aorta, mandating a transthoracic reconstruction involving a median sternotomy.

CERVICAL RECONSTRUCTION

The most frequently performed surgical reconstruction for occlusive disease of the supra-aortic branches is a carotid–subclavian or subclavian–carotid bypass. The technique of carotid–subclavian bypass usually involves a single supraclavicular incision. If, because of concomitant disease or the presence of total ipsilateral CCAO, the operation has to extend towards the carotid bifurcation, two incisions may be required (a supraclavicular and a short anterior sternomastoid incision at the level of the bifurcation).

The standard approach to the subclavian artery is via an incision above the clavicle, followed by mobilization of the prescalene fat pad. The phrenic nerve should be identified and the underlying scalenus anterior muscle divided. The segment of subclavian artery chosen for anastomosis is usually lateral to the thyrocervical trunk. The CCA is exposed in the medial aspect of the wound, by retracting the jugular vein and vagus nerve. If the operation is being done for embolic disease, the proximal end of the recipient vessel must be divided (see earlier discussion). In subclavian–carotid bypasses, the proximal end of the CCA should be divided even when the operation is being done for the treatment of a hemodynamic lesion, in order to prevent thrombosis of the proximal CCA and/or distal embolization.

Originally, a vein graft was considered the first choice conduit for this type of bypass, but this has changed. Vein grafts are often too small, and they are prone to kinking and angulation more frequently than prosthetic bypass material.[21]

In most patients where revascularization of the distal carotid artery is being considered, the ipsilateral subclavian artery is usually the most suitable and convenient donor vessel. Alternatively, the ipsilateral axillary artery can be used with excellent long-term patency rates.[20]

CROSSOVER BYPASSES

Some patients do not have an adequate ipsilateral donor vessel and it may be necessary to use a contralateral inflow vessel. In this situation, the bypass crosses the midline in front of the trachea, sometimes partially hidden behind the clavicular heads of sternomastoid. This may result in a less than satisfactory cosmetic appearance. The retro-oesophageal route is more direct than the pretracheal approach, but does include a small risk of oesophageal injury. A less invasive alternative is to use the axillary artery for inflow. The exposure of the donor and recipient arteries for a crossover bypass is exactly the same, irrespective of whether a presternal, pretracheal or retro-oesophageal bypass is performed.

TRANSTHORACIC RECONSTRUCTIONS

The transthoracic approach involves a midline sternotomy. Alternatively, a limited right or left anterior thoracotomy over the third intercostal space can be used. The pectoralis muscle is divided medially, and the underlying pectoralis minor is exposed and divided to facilitate exposure of the aorta. The proximal anastomosis of any graft should be placed either at the most proximal portion of the ascending aorta or a more distal part of the descending aorta in order to minimize the potential for kinking and on the right side of the ascending or descending aorta to avoid compromise when closing the sternum. The subclavian or carotid arteries can be exposed by separate supraclavicular/sternomastoid incisions as described earlier. Following the creation of one or more tunnels deep to the clavicle and chest wall, the graft or graft limbs can be tunnelled and anastomosed to the recipient vessels in an end-to-side fashion, without excessive tension on the graft because head and neck movement might be restricted with a risk for early anastomotic complications.

Outcome

Transthoracic arch reconstructions for complex brachiocephalic disease may be done with acceptably low morbidity/mortality rates which can be similar to those involving a less invasive extrathoracic approach. Moreover, the transthoracic approach is associated with significantly better long-term patency rates. In one of the largest comparative series, 157 consecutive patients (mean age, 54 years; 48% male) with innominate artery or multivessel disease underwent open operative reconstruction using either a transthoracic approach (group A, n = 113) or a less invasive, extrathoracic approach (group B, n = 44) over a 34-year time frame.[3] Reconstruction required concomitant CEA in 26 patients (17%). No significant differences were found between group A and group B patients regarding operative mortality (2.7% vs. 2.3%) or stroke rates (2.7% vs. 6.8%). However, 10 years after surgery, freedom from graft failure was significantly better in group A (94% ± 4%) than in group B (60% ± 13%) (p = 0.002). Freedom from graft failure was adversely influenced by having a non-aortic inflow (p = 0.002) and the use of axillo-axillary cervical grafts.

Operative mortality in all patients was just under 3%. There was a trend for higher stroke rates in patients who underwent reconstruction via a cervical approach, and this may have been related to the need for manipulation and serial clamping of both CCAs.

Most authors discourage concomitant brachiocephalic reconstruction and CABG for patients with both brachiocephalic disease and CAD.[22,23] Other studies suggest that either bypass or endarterectomy techniques, when used during transthoracic reconstruction, may provide a safe and durable treatment for multivessel disease.[24-27] Each transthoracic technique maintains proximal inflow from the aorta, which may account for the excellent long-term freedom from graft failure that has been reported in recent series using either technique.[27,28] Extrathoracic bypass is associated with inferior long-term freedom from graft failure when used to treat the innominate artery or multivessel brachiocephalic disease. Although a non-aortic inflow contributes to these poorer results, the superior long-term freedom from graft failure achieved by extrathoracic bypass for single-vessel branch vessel disease suggests that other factors may be involved.[29,30]

As the long-term results of endovascular intervention are awaited, the differences in outcome between surgical and endovascular management of brachiocephalic disease will be defined. It is not yet known whether either type of management has specific advantages with regard to long-term freedom from graft or intervention failure, safety, initial and late cost, patient satisfaction, efficacy for single-vessel versus multivessel disease or efficacy for treatment of concomitant carotid bifurcation disease. Among patients with single-vessel brachiocephalic disease, midterm freedom from graft or intervention failure has been reportedly lower after endovascular intervention than after operative bypass.[31-33]

ENDOVASCULAR TREATMENT

PTA and stenting are being employed with increasing frequency for lesions involving the brachiocephalic artery. While many now consider an endovascular approach as the first line of treatment, contemporary studies do report higher rates of significant residual stenosis, restenosis, dissection and stent fracture, ultimately requiring a higher rate of secondary reintervention. In the literature, reports on endovascular treatment of atherosclerotic stenosis or occlusion of the supra-aortic arteries are relatively scarce

and most involve a limited number of cases. There are only four reports involving more than 50 procedures.[34-36] Furthermore, these studies are mostly limited to reporting procedural and/or short-term outcomes only.

Long-term results for treating lesions of the subclavian or innominate arteries have shown a significant restenosis rate. Accordingly, carotid–subclavian bypass remains an important option. Alternative methods may still be required, particularly after failure of open revascularization and percutaneous techniques. Carotid–axillary artery bypass is an underused technique that enables upper extremity revascularization following prior attempts at endovascular and/or standard open techniques.[37] Endovascular recanalization of a chronic CCAO is a therapeutic field with limited knowledge and has not been widely adopted.[2]

Endovascular procedure

Procedures can be performed in the angiosuite or in a hybrid operating theatre under local and/or general anesthesia. In all cases, initial arterial access is usually gained via the common femoral or brachial arteries. Stenting of the origin of the CCA can also be performed by retrograde stenting from the carotid bifurcation, for example in symptomatic patients with a tandem lesion in both the CCA and proximal ICA. A retrograde transbrachial approach has been preferentially used in patients who underwent PTA for the treatment of subclavian artery disease. In the remaining patients in this study who underwent PTA, a transfemoral approach was used.

Angle-tip guide wires can be used to cross lesions in the supra-aortic arteries. In patients with occlusion, recanalization from a femoral approach should be attempted first. If the lesion cannot be crossed (despite the use of selective catheters), a combined brachial and femoral approach can be used. In 10% of interventions, access may be gained through the brachial artery after initial femoral attempts.

Intra-procedural angiography–based measurements enable the calculation of balloon size and/or stent size with a length appropriate to the lesion and a diameter equal to or with a maximum of 10% oversizing, compared to the normal diameter of the target artery. When the lesion is passed, balloon angioplasty is performed either as primary angioplasty or as pre-dilatation before stent placement. The decision to use PTA alone or to use an additional stent depends on the type of lesion (e.g., extent of lesion, residual stenosis, trans-lesional pressure). Technical success is usually defined as a residual diameter stenosis less than 30% on intra-procedural control angiography.[1]

Outcome

In the largest series of primary stenting for aortic side branch origin lesions published, 145 lesions were treated in 114 symptomatic patients (mean age 66; 39 male): PTA (n = 21; brachiocephalic artery [BCA] 9; left subclavian artery [LSA] n = 12) or PTA with stenting (n = 124; BCA 58; LCCA 7; LSA 59). The initial technical success rate was 97%. Thirty-day outcomes revealed no deaths or strokes. During a mean follow-up of 52 months (range 2–163), restenosis-free survival rates were 96% and 83% at 12 and 60 months, respectively.

Analyses showed no significant difference between PTA only versus PTA with stent placement. In total, 27 patients (24%) became symptomatic during follow-up and all 27 symptomatic lesions underwent successful (repeat) endovascular procedures. Of interest, 19 patients became symptomatic following the development of a restenosis within the target vessel (mean 57 months), while 8 patients had symptoms related to a new significant stenosis in another supra-aortic artery (mean 41 months). Symptom-free survival rates were 95% and 78% at 12 and 60 months, respectively.

Initial technical and clinical success rates >90% have been reported and are in line with previous reports, both following standardized PTA with stenting[35] as for standardized PTA alone.[36] However, large series evaluating mid- and/or long-term outcomes after PTA treatment of occlusive lesions of the supra-aortic arteries are scarce (Tables 35.1 and 35.2). Due to the low incidence of occlusive disease in this area of anatomy, a randomized trial is beyond expectation. When compared to bypass surgery, midterm freedom from graft or intervention failure showed significantly better results after bypass than after endovascular intervention for the treatment of single-vessel disease.

Although the surgical management of brachiocephalic disease is well established, evolving endovascular techniques present innovative and new options for treatment. From 1966 to 2004, 391 consecutive patients (44% male; mean age, 62 years) with single-vessel brachiocephalic disease were treated by either operative bypass (group A; n = 229) or PTA and stenting (group B; n = 162).[28]

Carotid–subclavian bypass was the sole operative reconstruction technique used in this study. Group A and group B had similar operative mortality rates (0.9% vs. 0.6%) and stroke rates (1.3% vs. 0%). However, 5 years after the procedure, patients undergoing operative bypass

had significantly better freedom from graft or intervention failure (93% ± 2%) than did the group undergoing stenting (84% ± 4%; p = 0.03, Kaplan–Meier analysis; p = 0.001, Cox regression analysis).

Endovascular intervention has a potential advantage when used to treat subclavian artery disease. Endovascular treatment of SCA disease does not involve manipulation of the CCA, whereas an open procedure requires manipulation of the carotid vessel during the construction of the subclavian–carotid bypass.[29] Several other potential advantages of endovascular over surgical management include shorter hospital stay, being less invasive and the avoidance of general anesthesia. Endovascular intervention may also offer other benefits regarding cost and subjective patient satisfaction.

> ## Key points
>
> 1. Endovascular treatment of supra-aortic origin obstruction is safe and efficacious in most patients and can be considered as the preferred treatment.
> 2. Recurrent symptomatic lesions can be safely treated by endovascular interventions.
> 3. Extrathoracic bypass and endovascular intervention for single-vessel brachiocephalic disease are associated with acceptably low operative morbidity and mortality.
> 4. Operative bypass produces significantly better midterm freedom from graft or intervention failure than endovascular intervention.

Rarer techniques

Transposition of the CCA on to the subclavian artery provides a direct autogenous revascularization. However, this type of bypass is not always applicable, as it often requires additional thromboendarterectomy of the occluded CCA as well as the absence of significant disease in the ipsilateral subclavian artery. Common carotid endarterectomy can also be performed either via an open or retrograde semi-closed endarterectomy. In these cases, securing a 'sound' proximal CCA end is essential.

Treatment of vertebral artery stenoses

The benefit of revascularizing vertebral stenoses remains uncertain and many surgeons have limited experience of mobilizing this vessel beyond its origin. In the last decade, treatment of VA stenoses by PTA, usually with stent placement, has been introduced as an attractive alternative to surgery.

Endovascular access to the VA is relatively easy and the procedure can be performed without general anesthesia, thereby enabling continuous neurological monitoring of the patient. Disadvantages include the theoretical risk of distal embolization of plaque and thrombotic debris, which may lead to a stroke.

Table 35.1 Endovascular treatment of arch branch origin stenosis or occlusion.

Follow-up examination	13.5 years
Mean follow-up	52.0 months
Range follow-up	2–163 months
Total patients	114 patients
Death during follow-up	12 patients
Refused follow-up	1 patient
Total initial interventions	114 interventions
Total repeat interventions	27 interventions
Total repeat–repeat interventions	3 interventions
Total interventions	144 interventions
Symptomatic during follow-up	27 patients
Recurrent stenosis	19 stenosis
Alternative stenosis	8 stenosis

Note: Follow-up > 30 days.

Table 35.2 Literature of endovascular treatment of origostenoses of supra-aortic arteries.

Author	Year	Total Int.	% stents	Interventions	% symptomatic patients	PSR	SR	FU (months)
Vd Weijer et al.	2014	145	85.7	Brachio n = 69 Subclavian n = 69 CCA n = 7	100	96.6%	95.2% at 12 months 93.0% at 24 months 82.5 at 60 months	Mean 43.7
Muller-Hulsbeck et al.	2007	55	40.0	Brachio n = 8 Subclavian n = 36 CCA n = 6	100	100	90.6% at 20 months	Mean 22.00
Zaytsev et al.	2006	21	100	Brachio n = 2 Subclavian n = 17	100	96	100% at 6 months	Mean 21.3
Peterson et al.	2006	20	100	Brachio n = 8 Subclavian n = 3 CCA n = 9	80	100	100% at 1 month	1
Przewlocki et al.	2005	76	86.8	Brachio n = 2 Subclavian n = 72	85.3	93.40%	88.5% at 12 months 83.6% at 24 months 77.2% at 60 months	Mean 24.40
Modarai et al.	2004	Unknown	Unknown	Brachio n = 1 Subclavian n = 34	97.5	85.37%	82% at 48 months	Mean 48
Gonzales et al.	2002	9	88.9	Brachio n = 2 Subclavian n = 7	100	100%	77.8% at 40 months	Mean 37.4
Korner et al.	1999	43	0	Brachio n = 4 Subclavian n = 38	100	84%	72% at 100 months	Mean 15
Sullivan et al.	1998	87	100	Brachio n = 7 Subclavian n = 66 CCA n = 14	90.3	94.30%	85% at 35 months	Mean 14.3
Motarjeme et al.	1993	131	0	Brachio n = 9 Subclavian n = 66 CCA n = 6		93%	96.3 at 60 months	Mean 60
Selby et al.	1992	32	0	Brachio n = 2 Subclavian N = 26	81.2	100%	96.9 at 90 months	Mean 36

Abbreviations: PSR, primary success rate; SR, survival rate; FU, follow-up.

Case reports suggest that VA stenting is relatively safe with a periprocedural risk of stroke or death ranging from 2% to 14%. In a review of endovascular treatment of VA stenoses, the 30-day risk of TIA, stroke or death was 6.4%. In another review, stenting of the extracranial VA in 313 patients resulted in technical success in 98%–100% of procedures, with a 0.3% risk of death and 5.5% risk of neurological complications.[38] Stenting of the distal (intracranial) VA in 283 patients was associated with technical success in 97%–98% of patients, but with higher complication rates, including a mortality rate of 3% and a 17% risk of neurologic complications. The differences in complication rates of stenting between the proximal and distal VAs may be explained by the fact that stenting of the distal VA was more frequently performed in the acute phase of vertebral or basilar artery occlusion and was considered technically more difficult. Other neurological complications, such as VA and basilar artery dissection, occurred in 3% and 6% of cases, respectively, along with non-neurological complications, such as inguinal hematoma, in 1.3% and 2.8%.

Stenting of the proximal VA might be associated with a relatively high rate of restenosis at follow-up. After a mean follow-up of 1 year, restenosis had occurred in one quarter of patients undergoing proximal VA stenting.[38] Restenosis in the distal VA was detected in about one-fifth of cases after a mean follow-up of 7.5 months. The use of drug-eluting stents for VA stenting may reduce both the rate of restenosis and recurrence of symptoms as compared to bare metal stents.[39] Most of the patients with restenosis remained asymptomatic.

At the present moment, stenting of VA stenoses appears to be a promising technique for the prevention of recurrent vascular events in the VB territory, but is still without proven benefit. The natural course of a symptomatic VA stenosis in patients on best medical treatment alone is unknown, and the exact indications for vertebral stenting are unclear. Also, the procedure may be complicated by disabling stroke and early restenosis. Before widespread application, the procedure should be assessed in a large randomized trial. The safety and benefit of stenting of symptomatic >50% VA stenoses as compared with best medical therapy alone are currently being tested in a randomized clinical trial (the Vertebral Artery Stenting Trial).[40]

Key points

1. The natural history of symptomatic VA stenoses is unknown.
2. Surgical revascularization is rarely performed and few surgeons have experience in exposing the VA beyond its origin.
3. Primary stenting of VA stenoses looks promising, but may be hampered by procedural stroke and high rates of restenosis.

Level of evidence

Most studies in the field of aortic branch occlusive disease are non-randomized and retrospective. Despite the several studies having relatively large populations of innominate, multivessel and multisystem brachiocephalic disease, their statistical power is limited, which reflects the potential for a type II error. It is unlikely that a randomized, prospective trial of treatments for complex brachiocephalic disease will ever be performed, given the relative infrequency of this severe pattern of disease.[41]

CONCLUSIONS

Transthoracic and extrathoracic arch reconstructions can be performed with acceptably low morbidity and mortality. Transthoracic arch reconstructions may have better long-term freedom from graft failure, but this is at the expense of a more major intervention with higher morbidity and mortality rates. Extrathoracic bypass and endovascular interventions for single-vessel disease are associated with acceptably low procedural risks. Extrathoracic bypass may have better midterm freedom from graft failure than endovascular intervention. Endovascular interventions offer tangible benefits regarding cost, level of invasiveness and subjective patient satisfaction. Although the precise indications for endovascular intervention versus operative reconstruction need to be defined, an endovascular first approach is commonly accepted.

Best clinical practice

- Dual imaging in the workup: duplex for screening and CTA or MRA for planning of revascularization strategy.

- Asymptomatic patients should not undergo any revascularization procedure.
- In symptomatic patients, an endovascular first approach is safe but durability may be limited. This accounts for all aortic arch branch vessels including the VA.
- Of all optional extrathoracic bypass procedures, the carotid–subclavian bypass may offer longest benefit.
- Intra-thoracic (bypass) procedures are the most extensive procedures, but long-term patency and durability may counterbalance the invasiveness of the procedure.

Deficiencies in current knowledge

- Natural long-term neurological risk of proximal aortic arch branch origin stenosis
- Natural long-term neurological risk of significant VA stenosis
- Long-term patency of endovascular intervention for aortic arch branch origin stenosis or VA origin lesions
- Benefit of relatively new techniques such as drug-eluting balloons for PTA and drug-eluting stenting in the aortic arch branch origin level.
- Influence of dual antiplatelet therapy on patency rates after bypass surgery

Wish list

- Further development of endovascular techniques
- Multicentre collaboration in effectiveness evaluation of aortic arch atherosclerotic disease treatment
- Maximum knowledge on materials and medication including antiplatelet therapy in maintaining long-term patency

REFERENCES

1. Maarten AJ van de Weijer, Evert Jan PA Vonken, Jean-Paul PM de Vries, Frans L Moll, Jan-Albert Vos, G.J. de Borst. Durability of endovascular therapy for proximal stenosis of the supra-aortic arteries. *Eur J Vasc Endovasc Surg.* 2015;50(1):13–20.
2. Klonaris C, Kouvelos GN, Kafezza M, Koutsoumpelis A, Katsargyris A, Tsigris C. Common carotid artery occlusion treatment: Revealing a gap in the current guidelines. *Eur J Vasc Endovasc Surg.* 2013;46(3):291–298.
3. Thomas J Takach, George J Reul, Denton A Cooley, J Michael Duncan, James J Livesay, Igor D Gregoric. Brachiocephalic reconstruction I: Operative and long-term results for complex disease. *J Vasc Surg.* 2005;42:47–54.

4. Compter A, van der Worp HB, Algra A, Jaap Kappelle L, on behalf of the Second Manifestations of ARTerial disease (SMART) Study Group. Prevalence and prognosis of asymptomatic vertebral artery origin stenosis in patients with clinically manifest arterial disease. *Stroke.* 2011;42(10):2795–2800.

5. Flossmann E, Rothwell PM. Prognosis of vertebrobasilar transient ischaemic attack and minor stroke. *Brain.* 2003;126(Pt 9):1940–1954.

6. Compter A, Kappelle LJ, Algra A, van der Worp HB. Nonfocal symptoms are more frequent in patients with vertebral artery than carotid artery stenosis. *Cerebrovasc Dis.* 2013;35:378–384.

7. Grosveld WJ, Lawson JA, Eikelboom BC, Windt JM, Ackerstaff RG. Clinical and hemodynamic significance of innominate artery lesions evaluated by ultrasonography and digital angiography. *Stroke.* 1988;19:958–962.

8. Sameshima T, Futami S, Morita Y et al. Clinical usefulness of and problems with three-dimensional CT angiography for the evaluation of atherosclerotic stenosis of the carotid artery: Comparison with conventional angiography, MRA, and ultrasound sonography. *Surg Neurol.* 1999;51:301–308, discussion 308–309.

9. Riles TS, Imparato AM, Posner MP, Eikelboom BC. Common carotid occlusion. Assessment of the distal vessels. *Ann Surg.* 1984;199:363–366.

10. Akers DL, Markowitz AI, Kerstein MD. The value of aortic arch study in the evaluation of cerebrovascular insufficiency. *Am J Surg.* 1987;154:230–232.

11. Khan S, Rich P, Clifton A, Markus HS. Noninvasive detection of vertebral artery stenosis A comparison of contrast-enhanced MR angiography, CT angiography and ultrasound. *Stroke.* 2009;40:3499–3503.

12. Khan S, Cloud G, Kerry S, Markus HS. Imaging of vertebral artery stenosis: A systematic review. *J Neurol Neurosurg Psychiatry.* 2007;78(11):1218–1225.

13. Brott TG, Halperin JL, Abbara S et al. ASA/ACCF/AHA/AANN/AANS/ACR/ASN guideline on the management of patients with extracranial carotid and vertebral artery disease: Executive summary. *Circulation.* 2011;124:e54–e130.

14. Linni K, Aspalter M, Ugurluoglu A, Holzenbein T. Proximal common carotid artery lesions: Endovascular and open repair. *Eur J Vasc Endovasc Surg.* 2011;41:728–734.

15. Paukovits TM, Lukacs L, Berczi V, Hirschberg K, Nemes B, Huttl K. Percutaneous endovascular treatment of innominate artery lesions: A single-centre experience on 77 lesions. *Eur J Vasc Endovasc Surg.* 2010;40:35–43.

16. Takach TJ, Reul GJ. Total aortic arch reconstruction for multiple great vessel occlusive disease. *Semin Vasc Surg.* 1996;9:118–124.

17. Reul GJ, Jacobs MJ, Gregoric ID et al. Innominate artery occlusive disease: Surgical approach and long-term results. *J Vasc Surg.* 1991;14:405–412.

18. Takach TJ, Reul GJ, Cooley DA. Transthoracic reconstruction of the great vessels using minimally invasive technique. *Tex Heart Inst J.* 1996;23:284–288.

19. Ziomek S, Quinines-Baldrich WJ, Busuttil RW, Baker JD, Machleder HI, Moore WS. The superiority of synthetic arterial grafts over autologous veins in carotid subclavian bypass. *J Vasc Surg.* 1986;3:140–145.

20. Fry WR, Marin JD, Clagett GP, Fry WJ. Extrathoracic carotid reconstruction: The subclavian-carotid artery bypass. *J Vasc Surg.* 1992;15:83–88.

21. Berguer R, Morasch MD, Kline RA. Transthoracic repair of innominate and common carotid artery disease: Immediate and long-term outcome for 100 consecutive surgical reconstructions. *J Vasc Surg.* 1998;27:34–41.

22. Berguer R, Morasch MD, Kline RA, Kazmers A, Friedland MS. Cervical reconstruction of the supraaortic trunks: A 16-year experience (discussion). *J Vasc Surg.* 1999;29:239–248.

23. Kieffer E, Sabatier J, Koskas F, Bahnini A. Atherosclerotic innominate artery occlusive disease: Early and long-term results of surgical reconstruction. *J Vasc Surg.* 1995;21:326–337 (discussion).

24. Rhodes JM, Cherry KJ Jr, Clark RC et al. Aortic-origin reconstruction of the great vessels: Risk factors of early and late complications. *J Vasc Surg.* 2000;31:260–269.

25. Cherry KJ Jr. Direct reconstruction of the innominate artery. *Cardiovasc Surg.* 2002;10:383–388.

26. Cherry KJ Jr, McCullough JL, Hallett JW Jr, Pairolero PC, Gloviczki P. Technical principles of direct innominate artery revascularization: A comparison of endarterectomy and bypass grafts. *J Vasc Surg.* 1989;9:718–723.

27. Brewster DC, Moncure AC, Darling RC, Ambrosino JJ, Abbott WM. Innominate artery lesions: Problems encountered and lessons learned. *J Vasc Surg.* 1985;2:99–112.

28. Perler BA, Williams GM. Carotid-subclavian bypass – A decade of experience. *J Vasc Surg.* 1990;12:716–722.

29. Uurto IT, Lautamatti V, Zeitlin R, Salenius JP. Long-term outcome of surgical revascularization of supraaortic vessels. *World J Surg.* 2002;26:1503–1506.

30. Bates MC, Broce M, Lavigne PS, Stone P. Subclavian artery stenting: Factors influencing long-term outcome. *Catheter Cardiovasc Interv.* 2004;61:5–11.

31. Sullivan TM, Gray BH, Bacharach JM et al. Angioplasty and primary stenting of the subclavian, innominate, and common carotid arteries in 83 patients. *J Vasc Surg.* 1998;28:1059–1065.

32. Martinez R, Rodriguez-Lopez J, Torruella L, Ray L, Lopez-Galarza L, Diethrich EB. Stenting for occlusion of the subclavian arteries: Technical aspects and follow-up results *Tex Heart Inst J.* 1997;24:23–27.

33. Przewlocki T, Kablak-Ziembicka A, Pieniazek P et al. Determinants of immediate and long-term results of subclavian and innominate artery angioplasty. *Catheter Cardiovasc Interv.* 2006;67:519–526.

34. Muller-Hulsbeck S, Both M, Charalambous N, Schafer P, Heller M, Jahnke T. Endovascular treatment of atherosclerotic arterial stenoses and occlusions of the supra-aortic arteries: Mid-term results from a single center analysis. *Rontgenpraxis.* 2007;56:119–128.

35. Motarjeme A, Gordon G. Percutaneous transluminal angioplasty of the brachiocephalic vessels: Guidelines for therapy. *Int Angiol.* 1993;12:260–269.

36. Orozco V, Impellizzeri PP, Naftalovich R, Dardik H. Carotid axillary artery bypass: An option following failed open and percutaneous procedures. *Vascular.* 2013;22(3):198–201.

37. Takach TJ, Michael Duncan J, James J Livesay, Zvonimir Krajcer, Roberto D Cervera, Igor D Gregoric, David A Ott. Brachiocephalic reconstruction II: Operative and endovascular management of single-vessel disease. *J Vasc Surg.* 2005;42:55–62.

38. Eberhardt O, Naegele T, Raygrotzki S, Weller M, Ernemann U. Stenting of vertebrobasilar arteries in symptomatic atherosclerotic disease and acute occlusion: Case series and review of the literature. *J Vasc Surg.* 2006;43:1145–1154.

39. Langwieser N, Buyer D, Schuster T, Haller B, Laugwitz KL, Ibrahim T. Bare metal vs drug eluting stents for extracranial vertebral artery disease. A meta-analysis of nonrandomized comparative studies. *J Endovasc Ther.* 2014;21:683–692.

40. Compter* A, van der Worp HB, Schonewille WJ, Vos JA, Algra A, Lo TH, Mali WPThM, Moll FL, Kappelle LJ. VAST: Vertebral Artery Stenting Trial. Protocol for a randomised safety and feasibility trial. *Trials.* 2008;9:65.

41. Burnand KG. Distinguished guest lecture. Surgery of head and neck vessels: Is stenting going to put us out of business? Paper presented at the *29th Annual Meeting of the Southern Association for Vascular Surgery*, Marco Island, FL; January 20, 2005.

36

Carotid arterial tortuosity, kinks and spontaneous dissection

J. TIMOTHY FULENWIDER, ROBERT B. SMITH III, SAMUEL ERIC WILSON and DENNIS MALKASIAN

CONTENTS

The overwhelming majority of carotid-related ischemic brain and retinal syndromes referred to the vascular surgeon are secondary to atherosclerosis. Initiated either by intraplaque hemorrhage or by accretion of platelets and fibrin on a 'rough' plaque or in an ulcer niche, carotid emboli are presumed responsible for most target-organ ischemic events. However, carotid stenoses reducing the lumen's cross-sectional area to 25% of normal may also precipitate distal ischemic events, especially during periods of systemic hypotension or reduced cardiac output.

A heterogeneous group of extracranial carotid arteriopathies, both congenital and acquired, occur relatively infrequently and may produce ischemic central nervous syndromes virtually indistinguishable from those of atherosclerotic origin. The symptomatic loop or coil, carotid kink and spontaneous carotid dissection are among these unusual entities potentially responsible for carotid flow impairment or embolization. This chapter examines the carotid loop or coil, carotid kink and spontaneous dissection, emphasizing anatomic and pathophysiologic details, diagnostic dilemmas and contemporary medical or surgical management controversies.

CAROTID LOOP

Extracranial internal carotid tortuosity is a relatively common angiographic finding.[1-3] The carotid loop, defined as a 360° coil or spiral configuration or as an elongation and redundancy resulting in a sigmoid curvature, may be congenital in origin (Figure 36.1).[4-8] Development of this anomaly is best explained by defective embryogenesis of the carotid artery.[9] Normally, extensions of the endocardial heart tubes form the embryonic dorsal aortas, which assume an arched configuration in the fetal pharyngeal region due to rotation of the cardiogenic plate and fusion of the endocardial heart tubes. Central to an understanding of the development of the arterial tree is an appreciation of the development and regression of the dorsal aortas, appearing initially as symmetrical and parallel conduits destined to transform into the adult vascular form by as early as the 14 mm embryo stage. The dorsal aortas run parallel to the primitive foregut and fuse with the truncus arteriosus, forming the aortic sac, which contributes branch arteries to each developing pharyngeal arch. The third aortic arch ultimately forms the common carotid artery and the proximal internal carotid artery; the distal internal carotid system is formed by the cranial portion of the dorsal aorta. The external carotid artery sprouts from the third aortic arch, which joins with remaining portions of the first and second arches.

Early in development, the communication between the third and fourth aortic arches – the carotid duct – becomes obliterated, and the extracranial carotid system assumes its adult configuration. These primordial vascular changes and cardiogenesis occur in the cephalad region of the embryonic pharynx. Developmental elongation of the fetal neck subsequently leads to descent of the heart into the mediastinum, with elongation of the innominate and carotid arteries. Maldescent of the heart or persistence of embryonic anatomy is thought responsible for subsequent looping and redundancy of the internal carotid artery.[3] Evidence for the congenital origin of the carotid loop is based upon its identification in fetal post-mortem examinations.

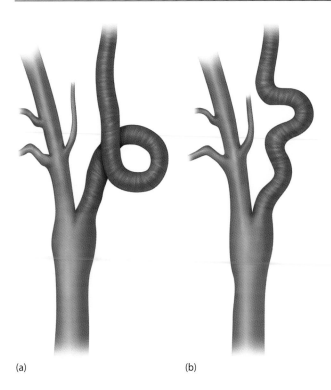

(a)   (b)

Figure 36.1 Artist's rendition of a 360° loop of the internal carotid artery and of marked tortuosity without coiling: (a) elongation (loop) and (b) tortuosity.

The anomaly is found in approximately 15% of children studied, with the prevalence rising to 25% of adults.[10]

Degenerative changes of the arterial wall with secondary elongation, along with long standing hypertension, are probably responsible for the higher prevalence in ageing populations. Others have identified elastic tissue dysplasia of the tunica media of the carotid artery, a finding supportive of the congenital origin of carotid loops and tortuosities.[11,12] The etiologic significance of degenerative changes secondary to arteriosclerosis – with accentuation by chronic arterial hypertension and other hyperdynamic circulatory states – remains speculative.

Although anatomists of the mid–eighteenth century accurately described elongation of the carotid arteries in autopsy examinations, Kelly, in the Glasgow Medical Journal in 1889, was among the first to observe the condition and to forewarn unwary surgeons of the significance of the bulging pharyngeal wall behind the posterior tonsillar pillar.[13] Edington, in an autopsy of a 34-year-old man who had died from chronic Bright's disease, identified bilateral, tortuous internal carotid arteries abutting each ipsilateral posterior pharyngeal wall. He speculated that the condition was secondary to the arteritis of chronic nephritis; however, he noted that abnormal persistence of portions of the embryonic arches could not be excluded etiologically.[13] In 1925, Kelly reported 150 consecutive cases of tortuous or redundant internal carotid arteries and ascribed the condition in young individuals to developmental abnormalities.[5] He stressed the infrequency of progressive enlargement and alleviated fears of

spontaneous rupture. On a number of occasions, tortuous internal carotid arteries have been misdiagnosed as peritonsillar abscesses, with fatal exsanguination following surgical drainage.

Since the first successful surgical correction of a tortuous extracranial artery by Riser in 1951, controversy has persisted concerning the potential association of tortuous or coiled internal carotid arteries and the risk of cerebral ischemia and infarction.[14,15] While precise figures are unavailable, the relatively high prevalence of tortuosity, looping and coiling of the cervical internal carotid artery is noteworthy. In patients with cerebral symptoms undergoing carotid arteriography, 4%–31% of adults and 15%–43% of children have demonstrated extracranial internal carotid tortuosity, coiling or looping.[1,10,16,17] The tortuosity frequently occurs in association with atheromatous plaques in adults. It is probable that tortuosity or carotid looping alone is rarely a primary cause of neurologic symptoms in adults; nevertheless, Sarkari et al.[8] described several children with seizures, transient hemiparesis, hemianopsia and dysphasia in association with an ipsilateral internal carotid loop. Unfortunately, Sarkari, who theorized that the carotid anomaly was responsible for the severe neurologic deficits, provided no pathologic studies of the vessels involved. Additionally, most other series affirming the association of carotid tortuosity and coiling with cerebral ischemia have not provided convincing evidence of such a cause-and-effect relationship. The available data suggest that carotid coiling, whether unilateral or bilateral, rarely accounts for cerebral ischemic symptoms in the absence of atherosclerotic occlusive disease in the carotid, vertebral or basilar arteries.[1,18] Thus far, proof is lacking that the risk of stroke in unselected patients with carotid tortuosity and coiling exceeds the risk of neurologic injury or death associated with operative intervention.[1] Most patients presenting with cerebral ischemic symptoms who are found to have redundancy or looping of the extracranial carotid artery are middle-aged, with peak incidence at approximately 60 years. Approximately one-fourth of adults have bilateral lesions, whereas up to 50% of children with tortuous vessels have bilateral coiling or elongation, which may be associated with other arterial anomalies such as aortic coarctation. For unknown reasons, women with elongation of the common carotid artery are four times more likely than age-matched men to have this vascular anomaly.[19]

Presenting symptoms mimic those from extracranial carotid atherosclerotic lesions and include both focal and global transient ischemic events, fluctuating deficits and fixed neurologic damage of variable severity.[20,21] Not infrequently, symptoms are most intense when the patient is supine in bed or has just woken up. Symptoms are usually considered to be secondary to hemodynamic consequences; most frequently, they are provoked by ipsilateral cervical rotation. However, contralateral cervical rotation, flexion and extension may also lead to impairment of carotid flow. As demonstrated by arteriogram, cervical rotation manoeuvres may reduce or stop carotid flow by causing critical angulation or compression of the vessel by parapharyngeal soft tissue or osseous structures.[22] While extrinsic compression by the atlas, mandible, vertebral bodies or fibrous bands is thought to limit carotid flow with cervical motion, the possibility of distal embolization has not been excluded in these cases. Albanese et al.[11] recently reported finding elastic tissue dysplasia of a coiled internal carotid artery in a 48-year-old man who suffered two episodes of transient left cerebral hemispheric ischemia prior to the development of a left hemispheric infarction. The extracranial carotid coil demonstrated a paucity of elastic fibres in the tunica media; however, in addition to focal areas of intimal hyperplasia, a small area of endothelium was covered by recent thrombus – a possible source of cerebral embolus. Theoretically, flow disturbances in looped arteries may occur, creating areas of high and low luminal surface shear stress potentially sufficient to promote deposition of platelet–fibrin aggregates with cerebral embolic potential.

Although there are no pathognomonic neurologic changes attributable to carotid tortuosity and coiling, symptoms of either hemispheric or global neurologic deficits and vertebrobasilar insufficiency provoked by cervical rotation, extension or flexion are important clues. Moreover, transient or permanent cerebral hemispheric signs in children should always arouse suspicion of the presence of internal carotid coiling. There are also no pathognomonic signs of internal carotid tortuosity. A prominent cervical pulsation below the mandibular angle that becomes more pronounced with head turning may rarely be found and is best appreciated using bidigital, peritonsillar palpation. Rarely, a bruit or thrill may be appreciated during cervical rotation manoeuvres. Carotid compression tests, as recommended by Derrick,[23] add little diagnostically and are potentially hazardous, since four of his patients developed acute neurologic deficits with these compression manoeuvres. Perhaps the simplest, most sensitive non-invasive test to identify the presence of the tortuous, looped or coiled internal carotid artery is the Doppler colour flow mapping technique. The experienced technologist may be able to delineate these carotid anatomic variants with real-time, B-mode ultrasonography of the duplex scanner. Both of these ultrasound imaging techniques may also provide important adjunctive information (e.g. atherosclerotic plaque formation). Nonetheless, these imaging techniques alone, as with arteriography, provide insufficient physiologic data and will not clarify the hemodynamic significance of the loop or coil. Additionally, the interpretation of flow data based upon Doppler spectral analysis may be difficult because of severe flow disturbances related to the geometry of the loop or coil. Most authorities agree that complete four-vessel cerebral angiography is essential and should include multiple views taken with cervical flexion, extension and bidirectional rotation.[1,18,23,24] Examples of typical internal carotid tortuosity and looping are presented in Figures 36.2 and 36.3. Prior to assignment of the carotid loop as causal in producing cerebral symptoms, other possibilities must be excluded. The most common of these include carotid atherosclerotic disease, cerebral neoplasm, intracranial

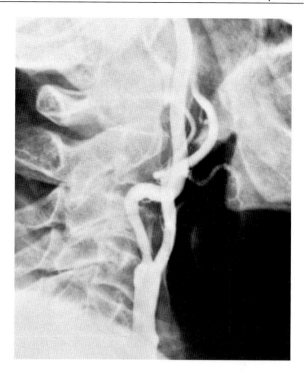

Figure 36.2 Lateral view angiogram of the extracranial carotid system, demonstrating a smooth atheromatous plaque of the proximal internal carotid artery and sigmoid curve in the vessel at the level of the angle of the mandible.

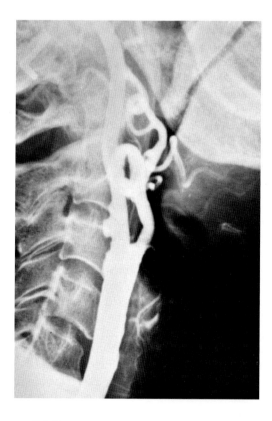

Figure 36.3 Lateral angiogram showing an ulcerated atheroma in the proximal internal carotid artery and a 360° loop just cephalad to the plaque.

vascular disease, cardiogenic emboli and arrhythmias, subdural hematoma and orthostatic hypotension. The natural history of the tortuous, or coiled, extracranial internal carotid artery is unknown; yet it is generally agreed that these anomalies, if asymptomatic and discovered coincidentally, may be safely observed without significant threat of cerebral ischemia.

Once the decision is made that the tortuous carotid is responsible for cerebral symptoms, operative correction should be considered, since the roles of systemic anticoagulation and antiplatelet compounds have not been determined in symptomatic patients. The goal of operative therapy should be to eliminate the tortuosity or loop of the carotid artery and also to remove any intrinsic obstruction from coexisting atherosclerotic plaque. Restoration of unimpeded carotid arterial flow is essential. Originally described by Riser et al.,[15] carotid arterioplexy to the sternocleidomastoid muscle to straighten the elongated artery has been abandoned. Presently, resection of the elongated artery is the operation of choice and demands proper assessment of the redundant arterial length. This determination is facilitated by complete mobilization of the distal internal carotid artery, with lysis of all fibrous bands that tether the artery near the base of the skull. Gentle manipulation of the thin-walled, friable internal carotid artery is mandatory to prevent possible dislodgment of atherothrombotic material and to minimize endothelial injury.

Endarterectomy of associated bifurcation atheromas is as essential as complete mobilization and precise geometric planning to eliminate possible kinking.

In order to minimize the dangers of suture line disruption of the friable internal carotid artery, some authors have advocated resection of a sleeve of common carotid artery, thus placing the anastomosis in this vessel of larger calibre and greater structural integrity. However, this technique frequently necessitates sacrifice of the external carotid artery – potentially an important route of cerebral collateral blood flow. To preserve the external carotid artery, others have recommended ligation at the origin of the internal carotid artery, with translocation of the orifice of the internal carotid artery more proximally onto the anterolateral common carotid artery.[25] The authors prefer instead to excise a segment of proximal internal carotid artery, to apply caudad traction and detorsion in order to eliminate the redundancy and then to construct a new anastomosis over an indwelling shunt, as previously recommended by Najafi et al.[26] Caution is essential during insertion of the internal carotid shunt; the redundant length of internal carotid artery must be straightened prior to shunt insertion to minimize the risk of creating an endothelial flap. The internal and common carotid arteries are spatulated to create an elliptical anastomosis that is twice the length of the diameter of the internal carotid artery. The anastomosis is constructed with continuous 5–0 or 6–0 monofilament suture, and the shunt is removed immediately prior to completion of the anastomosis.

Because of the extensive dissection necessary, general anaesthesia is frequently employed, but local or regional block anaesthesia is also suitable for some patients. In properly selected subjects, the results of carotid arterioplasty for congenital loops and coils are quite acceptable, with approximately 80% of patients completely relieved of symptoms. Perioperative combined neurologic morbidity and mortality rates should be under 5%.[21]

CAROTID KINK

Kinking of the extracranial internal carotid artery is defined as an acute bending or angulation of the artery, often described as 'buckling'. Acute angulation of the internal carotid artery is almost invariably associated with atherosclerosis, with the distal tip of the rigid atheroma corresponding to the vertex of the carotid angle.[17] Kinking of the carotid is most frequently an acquired condition, which appears later in life and occasionally coexists with tortuous changes of the internal carotid.[10] The relative fixation of the proximal common carotid artery by the aortic arch and the distal internal carotid artery at the base of the skull predisposes the more flexible internal carotid to angulation, particularly when elongation of the artery occurs as a result of congenital lengthening or acquired degeneration secondary to chronic hypertension. The exact incidence of acute angulation of the carotid artery is unknown; however, in selected patients with cerebral symptoms, the incidence varies from 4% to 20%.[1,2,16,17] Even more confusing is the matter of stroke risk from carotid kink alone, since the overwhelming majority of patients with carotid kinks also demonstrate significant extracranial carotid atherosclerotic disease. Nevertheless, most authorities agree that a demonstrated carotid kink represents a greater threat of ischemic stroke than does elongation or coiling of the internal carotid artery.

The first direct operation for correction of an internal carotid artery kink was performed by Hsu and Kistin[27] in 1956 but was unsuccessful. In 1959, Quattlebaum et al.[28] successfully resected the common carotid artery in three symptomatic patients with kinked internal carotid arteries. In 1962, Derrick and Smith[29] postulated that carotid kinking was more frequently causal of cerebral infarction than previously recognized and endorsed a more aggressive attitude towards the investigation and operative correction of carotid kinks. Vannix et al.[3] re-emphasized the potential lethality of cerebral complications associated with the internal carotid artery kink and urged operative correction of this potentially disabling condition. On the other hand, some have de-emphasized the importance of carotid kink alone in the production of neurologic symptoms and have correctly pointed out the high prevalence of concomitant atherosclerosis and other coexisting nonvascular pathology as potentially responsible for the apparent cerebral ischemia.[1] The role of the non-invasive vascular laboratory in screening for significant carotid kinks remains controversial. Approaching the problem directly, Stanton et al.[30] used the electromagnetic flowmeter intraoperatively to record flow during bidirectional rotation, hyperextension and flexion. He confirmed the hemodynamic significance of the carotid kink with reductions of arterial flow from 30% to 80% during testing. Interestingly, each of the 16 patients undergoing operation had atherosclerotic stenoses and presumably underwent concomitant endarterectomy of an associated carotid atheroma.

As elaborated by Metz et al.,[16] however, it is difficult to be certain of the relevance of any given factor in the production of cerebrovascular symptoms. These investigators have stated that the cessation of symptoms after the removal of a suspected cause does not necessarily establish a direct relationship between the two. In fact, some believe that removal of carotid plaque by endarterectomy alone is sufficient to relieve cerebral symptoms and that correction of redundant length is rarely necessary.

Symptoms produced by the kinked internal carotid artery are virtually indistinguishable from the transient and permanent neurologic deficits that are of atherosclerotic origin. It is generally accepted that the hemodynamic theory of cerebral hypoperfusion is operative in the majority of symptomatic cases; however, microembolic events cannot be excluded with certainty. Kinking of the vertebral or innominate arteries also may coexist. Historical clues suggestive of the presence of a carotid kink typically include the precipitation of cerebral symptoms with extremes of cervical motion. Development of an audible bruit with cervical rotation may be observed, but physical examination of the cervical region is most often entirely normal.[28] The definitive diagnostic test is the four-vessel carotid and vertebral angiographic examination with complete intracranial views (Figure 36.4). Positional angiography may confirm the anatomic significance of carotid kinks. Reduction in

carotid flow is unlikely if the carotid angulation is less than 60° or if there is the functional equivalent of less than 25% residual lumen area. The authors endorse the more conservative approach to the isolated asymptomatic kink, for it appears that the natural history of this lesion is less morbid than operative correction.

Generally accepted indications for the correction of internal carotid artery kinks are the following: (1) evidence that the kink may be responsible for cerebral ischemia by reproduction of symptoms on head rotation, flexion or extension and (2) exclusion of other craniocerebral vascular, neoplastic or developmental abnormalities which might account for similar symptoms. In actual practice, most patients with extracranial carotid kinks undergo operation primarily for correction of ulcerostenosing atheromas of the carotid with coincidental angulation of the artery noted at the apex of the rigid atheroma. Following endarterectomy and primary or patch closure of the arteriotomy, the acute angulation is frequently relieved. On other occasions, acute angulation of 90° or less is observed after performance of the endarterectomy. If such a kinked vessel creates a harsh thrill or produces significant intraoperative pressure reduction in the distal internal carotid artery, the angulation should be corrected. A variety of shortening techniques have been advocated, but direct arteriopexy is rarely indicated. The authors' preferred technique of arterioplasty for correction of acute angulation is similar to that described earlier for the correction of the internal carotid artery loop (Figures 36.5 through 36.10).

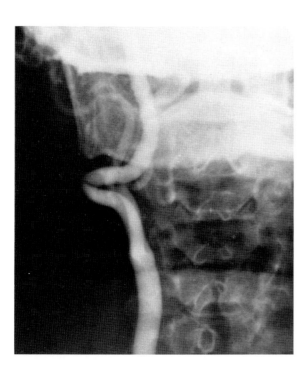

Figure 36.4 Anteroposterior carotid arteriogram showing an incidental kink or lateral angulation of the internal carotid artery.

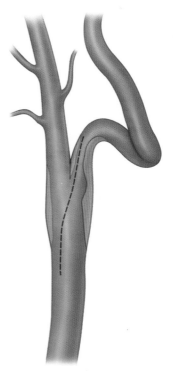

Figure 36.5 Operative repair of a carotid bifurcation atheroma with associated redundancy and kinking: location of the arteriotomy.

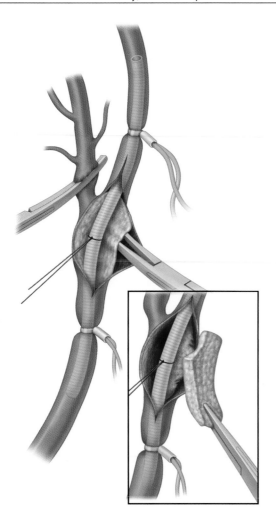

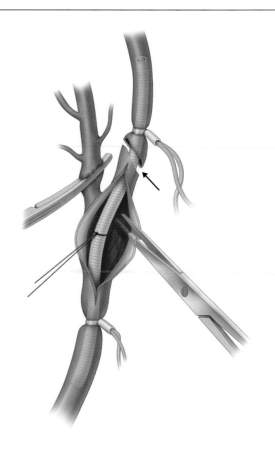

Figure 36.7 An appropriate length of redundant internal carotid is excised, taking care to prepare the ends for an oblique reanastomosis.

Figure 36.6 Following mobilization of the internal carotid artery and cautious shunt insertion, a standard bifurcation endarterectomy is performed.

Following endarterectomy, if required, resection of a cuff of proximal internal carotid is performed over an indwelling shunt, which serves additionally as a reconstruction stent. In the absence of intraluminal shunt utilization, careful internal carotid detorsion and spatial orientation are required to minimize anastomotic flow disturbances. An elliptical end-to-end anastomosis (length-to-diameter ratio of 2:1) is then constructed with running monofilament vascular sutures. Despite the infrequent need for correction of a carotid kink, operative morbidity and mortality rates are acceptably low and should parallel those of simple carotid endarterectomy in experienced hands.

SPONTANEOUS DISSECTING HEMATOMA OF THE INTERNAL CAROTID ARTERY

Dissecting hematomas of the extracranial internal carotid artery are rare yet potentially devastating causes of cerebral ischemia. The term spontaneous implies the occurrence of internal carotid dissection without recognizable

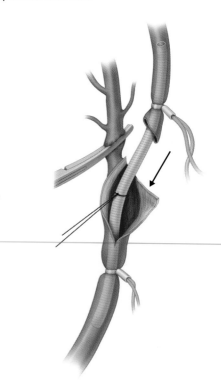

Figure 36.8 With gentle traction while the indwelling shunt is being advanced, the internal carotid stump is positioned at the cut edge of the common carotid artery.

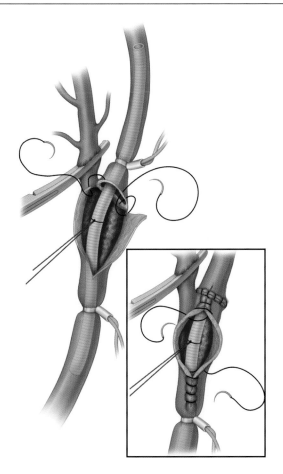

Figure 36.9 Reanastomosis is performed by use of a continuous monofilament vascular suture, producing a 'T-shaped' closure.

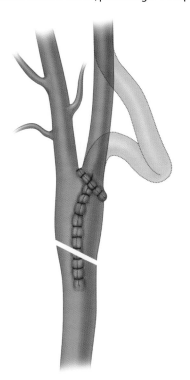

Figure 36.10 Completed endarterectomy and internal carotid shortening procedure. Note that the continuity of the external carotid is preserved by this technique.

traumatic antecedent, although – not infrequently – spontaneous dissections are observed in association with fibromuscular dysplasia, Erdheim's cystic medial necrosis, arteriosclerosis, arterial tortuosity, Marfan's syndrome and Ehlers–Danlos syndrome.[31–35] Since the original description by Anderson and Schechter in 1959,[36] over 200 cases have been reported, with the largest series from Ehrenfeld and Wylie,[37] Fisher et al.[38] and Bogousslavsky et al.[39] Blunt and penetrating cervical trauma and acceleration–deceleration cervical injuries are well recognized causes of arterial dissection. We have excluded from this discussion dissecting aneurysms of the ascending and transverse aorta, which may extend into the proximal carotid system and, rarely, into the internal carotid artery. Whether dissection of the extracranial internal carotid artery is ever clearly spontaneous remains controversial. As emphasized by Trosch et al.,[40] antecedent trauma may be trivial and either not recalled or too embarrassing to disclose. Such trauma as coughing, vigorous nose blowing, shaving, brushing teeth, head turning while leading a parade, neck flexion while scolding a child and 'head banging' during punk rock dancing have been recorded prior to 'spontaneous' carotid dissections.[40,41] Even vigorous exercise, such as running up and down 'bleachers', has been noted to cause dissection. Carotid dissection has also been described after tonsillectomy and adenoidectomy in a 12-year-old boy.[42] In many patients, however, the aetiology remains unknown.

Males and females appear to be afflicted at similar rates, with the mean age at diagnosis being 46 years (range, 11–74 years). Both internal carotids appear to be affected with similar frequency.[34,35,39] Presenting clinical manifestations of internal carotid dissection include focal cerebral neurologic deficits – whether transient or permanent – in over 80% of cases, but it appears that the regional extent of neurologic complaints in this condition is often greater than that attributable to atherosclerotic embolization.[38] Thus, many patients present with signs of both retinal ischemia and contralateral hemiparesis or hemihypesthesia, in addition to multiple cranial nerve palsies.

Noteworthy physical symptoms and signs of carotid dissection may include the rapid onset of severe hemicrania; Horner syndrome; Raeder trigeminal syndrome; scalp hyperalgesia; dysgeusia; central sixth, seventh and eighth cranial nerve palsy; and contralateral focal sensory and motor deficits. These neurologic features may occur singly or in variable combinations or may be preceded by transient cerebral ischemia in about 20% of patients.[39] Dysgeusia is felt to result from involvement of the chorda tympani branch of the seventh cranial nerve. Importantly, the evolution of a complete Horner oculosympathetic palsy may occur asynchronously or may be incomplete.

The acute onset of ipsilateral head and facial pain in the frontal, parietal or periorbital area may be followed in 24–72 hours by the development of one or more features of Horner syndrome, with anhidrosis most frequently absent.

The headaches are typically non-throbbing and fluctuating in intensity; they frequently require 2–6 months to resolve completely. During this interval, rarely is there complete relief of the cephalalgia. Other complaints include pulsatile or machinery vascular tinnitus.[37,38,43,44]

The reconciliation of symptoms to an embolic source may be difficult. For example, although fibromuscular dysplasia is usually associated with embolization to the anterior cerebral distribution, the posterior circulation may also be affected. In the event of a large, persistent fetal posterior communicating artery, emboli may pass into the posterior cerebral arteries. Such an embolus can cause permanent or transient ischemia to the visual cortex, possibly resulting in hemianopsia.[45,46] Physical findings of carotid dissection vary enormously. The multiplicity of neurologic findings mentioned earlier – in addition to tenderness over the carotid bulb, carotidynia and an evolving cervical bruit – is strongly suggestive of the diagnosis. The origin of the internal carotid dissecting hematoma is usually 2–3 cm distal to the carotid bulb. Through the usually vertically oriented intimal rent, the hematoma pulsates deep into the tunica media, creating a subadventitial cleavage plane.[37,38] The entire arterial circumference is rarely involved; however, thrombosis of the false channel severely compromises the true lumen, leading either to markedly reduced flow or to secondary complete thrombosis. The dissection seldom extends beyond the base of the skull, but cavernous sinus extension has been reported. On rare occasions, re-entry of the hematoma into the true lumen may occur acutely, restoring arterial flow. The experience of Ehrenfeld and Wylie[37] in 10 patients with dissecting aneurysms has provided the best description of the typical gross pathology. Consistent in their experience was a sharp transition between the normal colour and size of the internal carotid artery and the dark-blue discolouration and moderate cylindrical dilatation produced by the dissection. Only four patients of their series experienced termination of the dissection at a level easily visualized from the cervical incision, whereas the other six experienced dissections beyond the limits of surgical accessibility. Three patients had an arteriotomy performed, and each demonstrated the short vertical intimal rent marking the origin of the dissection. Microscopically, the typical features included organizing hematoma in the deeper layers of the tunica media with reduction of elastic tissue and fragmentation of internal elastic laminae. Smooth-muscle cells were widely separated and diminished in number. Mucopolysaccharide stains demonstrated the deposition of mucoid material indicative of degenerative changes. Atherosclerosis was consistently absent.[37]

In 1972, Ojemann et al.[45] suggested that the long stenotic segment of extracranial internal carotid artery visualized angiographically ('string sign') might be a reliable indicator of carotid dissection (Figures 36.11 and 36.12). Adopting this radiographic feature, radiologists became convinced that spontaneous carotid dissection was clearly not as rare as previously suspected. Typically, the

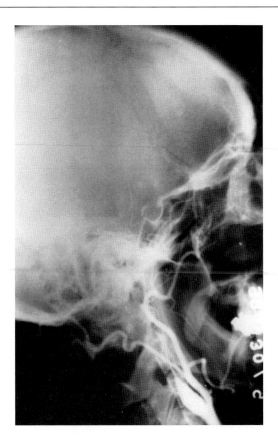

Figure 36.11 Lateral carotid arteriogram of a young patient with carotid dissection, showing severe tapering of the internal carotid lumen and a 'string sign' extending cephalad. Note the absence of atherosclerotic changes.

angiogram of the carotid dissection reveals an irregular, extremely narrow column of contrast beginning slightly above the carotid bulb, with a gradual taper ending at the base of the skull. Usually there is little or no evidence of atherosclerotic plaque. These radiographic features are highly suggestive of carotid dissection, but the 'string sign' may also occur with other types of vascular disease such as atherosclerosis, fibromuscular dysplasia, arteritis, moyamoya and vasospasm.[38] Although the degree of stenosis is usually high grade, the length of the angiographic stenotic segment can be variable. Occasionally a small cul-de-sac projecting cephalad and posteriorly is identified and is thought to represent the residual lumen at the origin of the intimal tear. If spontaneous organization of the false channel hematoma develops, retraction of the intima occurs at variable rates, producing scalloped or undulating angiographic margins of the recanalizing carotid artery walls. Traditionally, contrast arteriography remains the diagnostic standard of carotid dissection; however, confidence in magnetic resonance angiography in establishing the diagnosis is increasing. The role of helical computerized tomography in the detection and surveillance of carotid dissections is presently unclear. Carotid duplex imaging with colour flow mapping will be useful in the screening of patients with possible carotid dissections. B-mode ultrasound

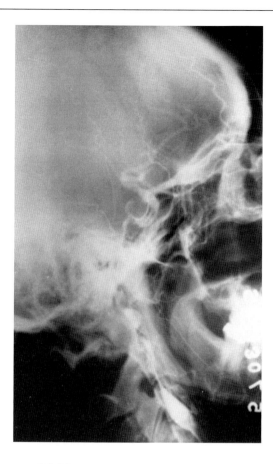

Figure 36.12 Later film from the same angiographic sequence demonstrating eventual filling of the carotid siphon and suggesting patency of the severely narrowed lumen.

findings of a double internal carotid lumen with intimal flap, intramural thrombus with overlying intact intima and minimal atherosclerotic changes are typical of carotid dissection. Spectral analysis data may show a high resistance wave form with short systolic flow signal or temporal fluctuations of systolic signals. Colour flow mapping may suggest severe arterial luminal encroachment or occlusion. The accuracy of carotid duplex scanning in the diagnosis of carotid dissection is technologist dependent; therefore, the most reliable technique for the diagnosis of carotid dissection remains contrast arteriography either conventional or CTA. Bilateral and recurrent carotid dissections are unusual.[35,38,39]

Early experience with this condition resulted in a variety of urgent attempts to restore cerebral arterial flow. These included resection of the involved segment with saphenous vein interposition grafting, dilation, balloon catheter thrombectomy, or endovascular occlusion, or ligation of the internal carotid artery.[37] The majority of these operations were unsuccessful due to technical difficulties with exposure of the distal point of dissection, the presence of residual thrombus with cerebral embolic potential or progression of frank stroke as a result of acute revascularization of a bland cerebral infarct. In 1976, taking a new approach, Ehrenfeld and Wylie[37] described experience with seven patients in whom the carotid artery was not disturbed surgically. Of these patients, three underwent cervical exploration only and four were managed non-operatively. Surprisingly, none of the patients had further progression of neurologic symptoms with up to 3 years follow-up. Repeat arteriography was obtained in six of these patients from 2 to 16 months following the original arteriogram. One carotid had progressed to total occlusion, whereas the remaining five had increased to essentially normal calibre. Others have since reported favourable results with non-operative therapy.[47] One of the larger, clinical series of 30 spontaneous carotid dissection and stroke patients was reported by Bogousslavsky et al.[39] This group represented 2.5% of stroke patients admitted to their unit. Bogousslavsky emphasizes that acute carotid dissection is frequently followed by severe, permanent neurologic impairment or even death: 7 (23%) expired within 7 days of the neurologic event and 11 of 23 survivors (48%) had severe physical limitations or required total custodial care. Maximal functional recovery was achieved within 6 months by the survivors. Of the 23 survivors, 13 (57%) demonstrated recanalization of the carotid artery, which usually occurred within 30 days of the acute dissection. The authors conclude that carotid thrombosis and distal cerebral embolization account for the larger hemispheric infarctions and that early heparin anticoagulation may favourably influence clinical outcome by maintaining carotid patency and preventing luminal thrombosis until natural clot retraction can occur. They also caution against heparin therapy whenever the dissection extends intracranially, because of commonly associated subarachnoid hemorrhage. Although the exact role of heparin, warfarin and antiplatelet drugs is uncertain, it is reasonable that the initial approach should be non-surgical.[39]

In the absence of major cerebral infarction or intracranial hemorrhage, systemic heparinization should be initiated to minimize the threat of distal cerebral embolization. It has been suggested that a minimum of systemic anticoagulation heparin therapy and subsequent warfarin (Coumadin) or dual antiplatelet therapy until remodelling or recanalization – as determined by duplex carotid scanning or computed tomographic arteriography at 6 months – is a logical approach.[47,48] Operative or endovascular intervention is reserved for continuing symptoms. Persistence of transient ischemic neurologic events with failure of recanalization may necessitate graft replacement of the diseased carotid artery or stenting placement. Technical feasibility of immediate endovascular stent recanalization of a carotid dissection has been demonstrated.[49] Precise estimates of risks and outcome of endovascular stent procedures for carotid dissections await analysis of larger numbers of patients. Very rarely, the spontaneous dissection originates in the common carotid artery, permitting reconstruction by subclavian–carotid bypass to preserve ipsilateral cerebral perfusion.[50]

REFERENCES

1. Perdue GD, Barreca JP, Smith RB. The significance of elongation and angulation of the carotid artery: A negative view. *Surgery.* 1975;77:45.

2. Brosig H-J, Vollmar J. Chirurgische Korrektur der Knickstenosen der A Carotis Interna. *Munch Med Wochenschr.* 1974;116:969.

3. Vannix RS, Joergenson FJ, Carter R. Kinking of the internal carotid artery: Clinical significance and surgical management. *Am J Surg.* 1977;134:82.

4. Desai B, Toole JF. Kinks coils and carotids: A review. *Stroke.* 1975;6:649.

5. Kelly AN. Tortuosity of the internal carotid in relation to the pharynx. *J Laryngol Otol.* 1925;40:15.

6. Gass HH. Kinks and coils of the cervical carotid artery. *Surg Forum.* 1958;9:721.

7. Ohara I, Iwarbrehi T, Yaegashi S. Abnormally twisted cervical internal carotid artery, probably congenital. *Vasc Surg.* 1969;3:1.

8. Sarkari NBS, Holmes JM, Bickerstaff ER. Neurological manifestations associated with internal carotid loops and kinks in children. *J Neurol Neurosurg Psychiatry.* 1970;33:194.

9. Gray SW, Skandalakis JE (eds.). The thoracic aorta. In: *Embryology for Surgeons, the Embryological Basis for the Treatment of Congenital Defects.* Philadelphia, PA: Saunders, 1972, pp. 809–857.

10. Weibel J, Fields WS. Tortuosity, coiling, and kinking of the internal carotid artery: I. Etiology and radiographic anatomy. *Neurology.* 1965;15:7.

11. Albanese V, Spadaro A, Iannotti F. Elastic tissue dysplasia of coiled internal carotid artery in an adult. *J Neurosurg.* 1983;58:781.

12. Ochsner JL, Hughes JP, Leonard GL. Elastic tissue dysplasia of the internal carotid artery. *Ann Surg.* 1977;185:684.

13. Edington GH. Tortuosity of both internal carotid arteries. *Br Med J.* 1901;2:1526.

14. Robicsek F, Daugherty HK. Redundancy of the carotid artery combined with intrinsic occlusion. *Vasc Surg.* 1970;4:101.

15. Riser MM, Geraud J, Ducoudray J. Dolicho-carotide interne avec syndrome vertigineux. *Rev Neurol (Paris).* 1951;85:145.

16. Metz H, Murray-Leslie RM, Bannister RG. Kinking of the internal carotid artery in relation to cerebrovascular disease. *Lancet.* 1961;1:424.

17. Bauer R, Sheehan S, Meyer JS. Arteriographic study of cerebrovascular disease: II. Cerebral symptoms due to kinking, tortuosity and compression of carotid and vertebral arteries in the back. *Arch Neurol.* 1961;4:119.

18. Weibel J, Fields WS. Tortuosity, coiling, and kinking of the internal carotid artery: II. Relationship of morphological variation to cerebrovascular insufficiency. *Neurology.* 1965;15:462.

19. Schecter DC. Dolichocarotid syndrome: Cerebral ischemia related to cervical carotid artery redundancy with kinking: Parts I and II. *NY State J Med.* 1979;79:1391–1542.

20. Harrison JH, Davalos PA. Cerebral ischemia: Surgical procedures in cases due to tortuosity and buckling of the cervical vessels. *Arch Surg.* 1962;84:85.

21. Quattlebaum JK Jr, Wade JS, Whiddon CM. Stroke associated with elongation and kinking of the carotid artery: Long-term follow-up. *Arch Surg.* 1973;177:572.

22. Freeman TR, Lippitt WH. Carotid artery syndrome due to kinking: Surgical treatment in forty-four cases. *Am Surg.* 1962;28:745.

23. Derrick JR. Carotid kinking and cerebral insufficiency. *Geriatrics.* 1963;17:272.

24. Robicsek F, Daugherty HK, Sanger PW. Intermittent cerebrovascular insufficiency: A frequent and curable cause of stroke. *Geriatrics.* 1967;22:96.

25. Rundles WR, Kimbrell FD. The kinked carotid syndrome. *Angiology.* 1969;20:177.

26. Najafi H, Javid H, Dye WS. Kinked internal carotid artery. *Arch Surg.* 1964;89:134.

27. Hsu I, Kistin AD. Buckling of the great vessels. *Arch Intern Med.* 1956;98:712.

28. Quattlebaum JK Jr, Upson ET, Neville RL. Stroke associated with elongation and kinking of the internal carotid artery. *Ann Surg.* 1959;150:824.

29. Derrick JR, Smith T. Carotid kinking as a cause of cerebral insufficiency. *Circulation.* 1962;25:849.

30. Stanton PE, McClusky DA, Lamis PA. Hemodynamic assessment and surgical correction of kinking of the internal carotid artery. *Surgery.* 1978;84:793.

31. Mettinger KL, Ericson K. Fibromuscular dysplasia and the brain. Observations on angiographic, clinical and genetic characteristics. *Stroke.* 1982;13:46.

32. Bostro"m K, Liliequist B. Primary dissecting aneurysm of the extracranial part of the internal carotid and vertebral arteries: Report of three cases. *Neurology.* 1967;17:179.

33. Luken MG, Ascherl GF, Carrell JW. Spontaneous dissecting aneurysms of extracranial internal carotid artery. *Clin Neurosurg.* 1979;26:353.

34. Treiman GS, Treiman RL, Foran RF. Spontaneous dissection of the internal carotid artery: A nineteen-year clinical experience. *J Vasc Surg.* 1996;24:597.

35. Bassetti C, Caruzzo A, Sturzeneggel M. Recurrence of cervical artery dissection: A prospective study of 81 patients. *Stroke.* 1996;27:1804.

36. Anderson R, Schechter M. A case of spontaneous dissecting aneurysms of the internal carotid artery. *J Neurol Neurosurg Psychiatry.* 1959;22:195.

37. Ehrenfeld WK, Wylie EJ. Spontaneous dissection of the internal carotid artery. *Arch Surg.* 1976;111:1294.

38. Fisher CM, Ojemann RF, Roberson GH. Spontaneous dissection of cervicocerebral arteries. *Can J Neurol Sci.* 1978;5:9.

39. Bogousslavsky J, Despland P, Regli F. Spontaneous carotid dissection with acute stroke. *Arch Neurol.* 1987;44:137.

40. Trosch R, Hasbani M, Brass L. "Bottoms up" dissection (letter). *N Engl J Med.* 1989;320:1564.

41. Jackson MA. "Headbanging" and carotid dissection. *Br Med J.* 1983;287:1262.

42. Carvalho KS, Edwards-Brown M, Golomb MR. carotid and stroke after tonsillectomy and adenoidectomy. *Pediatr Neurol.* 2007;37:127–129.

43. Waespe W, Niesper J, Imhof H-G. Lower cranial nerve palsies due to internal carotid dissection. *Stroke.* 1988;19:1561.

44. Maitland CG, Black JL, Smith WA. Abducens nerve palsy due to spontaneous dissection of the internal carotid artery. *Arch Neurol.* 1983;40:448.

45. Ojemann RD, Fisher CM, Rich JC. Spontaneous dissecting aneurysm of the internal carotid artery. *Stroke.* 1972;3:434.

46. Poppe AY, Minuk J, Glikstein RG, Leventhal M. Fibromuscular dysplasia with carotid dissection presenting as an isolated hemianopsia. *J Stroke Cerebrovas Dis.* 2006;17:330–338.

47. McNeill DH, Dreisbach J, Marsden RJ. Spontaneous dissection of the internal carotid artery: Its conservative management with heparin sodium. *Arch Neurol.* 1980;37:54.

48. Firas A-Ali, Perry BC. Spontaneous carotid artery dissection: The Borgess classification. *Front Neurol.* 2013;4:133–141.

49. Hong MK, Satler LF, Gallino R. Intravascular stenting as a definitive treatment of spontaneous carotid artery dissection. *Am J Cardiol.* 1997;79:538.

50. Graham JM, Miller T, Stinnett DM. Spontaneous dissection of the common carotid artery. Case report and review of the literature. *J Vasc Surg.* 1988;7:811.

37

Extracranial carotid artery aneurysms

JAMES A. GILLESPIE, SAMUEL ERIC WILSON and JUAN CARLOS JIMENEZ

CONTENTS

Carotid artery aneurysms are uncommon, but their clinical significance has long been recognized. Indeed, surgical treatment was first employed successfully in 1808 by Sir Astley Cooper,[1] a London surgeon, using the technique of proximal ligation, even then widely practiced in dealing with peripheral aneurysms. His patient lived for another 13 years. Since that time, reports of carotid aneurysms have appeared regularly in the literature, Winslow[2] collecting some 106 cases up to 1925. However, it was not until 1952 that a reconstructive surgical technique was used to deal with a carotid aneurysm.[3] Reconstructions, by maintaining carotid blood flow, reduce the risk of a cerebrovascular accident, often the sequel of simple ligation, and the various surgical techniques are now fairly well standardized. Approximately 1% of carotid extracranial operations are for aneurysms.[4]

INCIDENCE OF CAROTID ARTERY ANEURYSMS

The total incidence of extracranial carotid artery aneurysms is relatively small, and this is perhaps best indicated by Schechter's[5] detailed survey. He found reports of a total of only 853 carotid aneurysms in the literature up to 1977. The low incidence of carotid artery aneurysms compared to that of other extracranial aneurysms is also well demonstrated, for example in figures from DeBakey's[6] unit in Houston, where there were only 37 carotid aneurysms out of a total of 8500 aneurysms which they treated surgically in the 20 years up to 1977. Another group in Ohio reported 41 carotid aneurysms from a total of 1118 peripheral aneurysms which they evaluated over a 30-year period.[7]

Yet another report states that while 500 patients with occlusive carotid disease had been treated over a 24-year period, only 19 carotid aneurysms were managed in the same period.[8] Most reports of carotid aneurysm in the literature have been concerned with only one or two new examples, however, and although a relatively rare condition, it carries importance because of the threat of haemorrhage, stroke or death.

PATHOLOGY OF CAROTID ARTERY ANEURYSMS

Many causes of carotid aneurysms have been described, but the two most important are undoubtedly atherosclerosis and trauma. Before considering these in more detail, some of the other less common etiologies may be noted. Syphilis was an important cause in the last century and the first part of this one but rarely is today. Loss of elastic tissue in the arterial wall in Marfan's syndrome has been the cause of some reported carotid aneurysms, as has cystic medial necrosis, where carotid aneurysms are frequently associated with other peripheral aneurysms. Similarly, carotid aneurysms may occur with renal artery aneurysms in fibromuscular hyperplasia.

Extracranial carotid aneurysms, some of which can expand rapidly, have been associated with Behcet's disease, a chronic, systemic inflammatory disease causing recurrent oral and genital ulcers and uveitis.

Congenital carotid aneurysms, sometimes bilateral, have been reported and so also have primary or spontaneous dissecting aneurysms, as opposed to traumatic dissecting ones, though their etiology is somewhat obscure.[9] Carotid aneurysm has also been associated with polyarteritis nodosa. Mycotic carotid aneurysms are occasionally caused by infected emboli in bacterial endocarditis but more usually result from spread of infection from a nearby area of cellulitis or from a peritonsillar or mastoid abscess. Mycotic aneurysms may also follow a septic penetrating injury, perhaps from a heroin injection in an addict.[10] In one series of 10 post-operative aneurysms, 5 were caused by infection.[11] Diabetes seems to have been only rarely mentioned in patients with carotid aneurysms. Finally, carotid aneurysms have been described after irradiation for cervical malignancy.[12]

Atherosclerotic carotid aneurysms

These aneurysms usually occur in elderly patients and are frequently associated with atherosclerotic aneurysmal or occlusive arterial disease elsewhere. Many of these patients are hypertensive, and the aneurysm wall is frequently calcified. These aneurysms may be bilateral, are usually fusiform rather than saccular and tend to occur in the region of the carotid bifurcation.

Traumatic carotid artery aneurysms

These aneurysms are the second most common type after atherosclerotic aneurysms. They may result from blunt trauma, penetrating injuries and sudden neck hyperextension and rotation, or they may follow previous carotid artery surgery for stenotic or occlusive disease. Penetrating injuries may lead occasionally to carotid aneurysms and, if infection enters, mycotic aneurysms. Traumatic aneurysms are often of saccular type, but dissecting ones occasionally may result. Blunt trauma may cause intimal tears and medial disruption with consequent weakening of the arterial wall. Traumatic carotid aneurysms can also result from damage to the arterial wall from bone splinters, and examples in association with mandibular fractures are reported. While traumatic aneurysms involve mostly the common carotid artery, some occur in the high internal carotid artery, often extending up to the base of the skull. It is likely that fixation of the internal carotid artery as it passes into the bony carotid canal in the base of the skull base is an important factor when the more distal part of the artery is deformed and twisted by blunt trauma. Many post-traumatic aneurysms are actually false aneurysms, especially those occurring as a result of penetrating injuries and after surgery for carotid stenosis. The latter most commonly occurs when the original arteriotomy was closed with a patch graft and seldom when it was closed directly. In these patients who have prosthetic patches and pseudoaneurysms, infection of the patch is always a worry.[13]

False aneurysms have also, very rarely, been reported after needling the carotid vessels in arteriography. Aneurysms of any type involving the external carotid artery are rare.[14]

EFFECTS OF CAROTID ARTERY

Aneurysms

Like other peripheral aneurysms, carotid aneurysms may occlude spontaneously, may liberate emboli distally or, less commonly, may rupture. Their special danger lies in the effect of emboli or sudden ischemia on the brain, while rupture and haemorrhage may occur into the oropharynx with desperate airway consequences. Carotid aneurysms pose a very real threat to life, and Winslow,[2] in his extensive early survey of these lesions, made the point that four out of every five patients treated conservatively eventually died from a complication of their aneurysm, though few authorities would put the figure so high today.

Clinical presentation

The most common presentation of a carotid aneurysm is a swelling in the neck, usually pulsatile. Pain in the area is also a frequent complaint, especially when the aneurysm is expanding or dissecting, and here the mass is likely to be tender to palpation. Reports on brain damage vary greatly, some suggesting that perhaps up to half of all patients present with some neurological feature, such as a stroke, transient cerebral ischemic attacks (Figure 37.1) or a visual defect due to embolization.[15] The patient sometimes complains of a buzzing in the ear, and auscultation over the neck may reveal a loud systolic bruit. Hoarseness can result from vagal or recurrent laryngeal nerve compression, and Horner's syndrome from similar compression of the cervical sympathetic nerves. The hypoglossal nerve may also be involved.[16]

Some internal carotid aneurysms project into the oropharynx (Figure 37.2), occasionally giving dysphagia or dyspnea. It has long been recognized that here a carotid aneurysm may resemble a peritonsillar abscess and disaster attends attempted lancing. Fatal spontaneous rupture into the oropharynx has occurred. Small, high internal carotid aneurysms may not be palpable in the neck and can be a rare cause of unexplained facial pain. Occasionally they may rupture to give rise to profuse epistaxis or to bleeding from the ear. For these reasons otolaryngologists especially recognize the importance of carotid aneurysms.[17]

Differential diagnosis

In most cases the diagnosis can be made clinically without much difficulty. However, enlarged cervical lymph

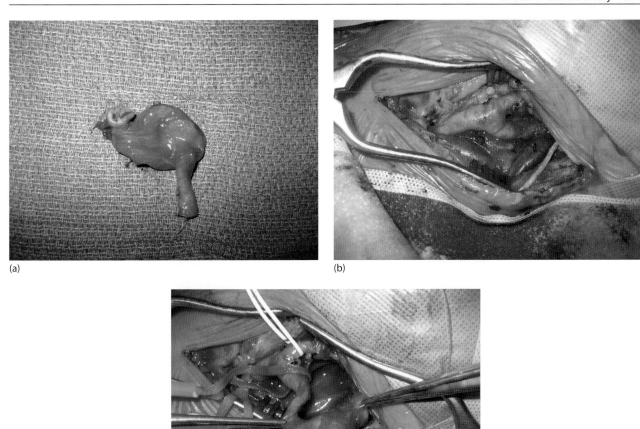

(a)

(b)

(c)

Figure 37.1 (a–c) Excision of an internal carotid artery aneurysm with primary end-to-end anastomosis. (Photo courtesy of Wesley Moore MD and Juan Carlos Jimenez MD, UCLA Division of Vascular Surgery, Los Angeles, CA.)

nodes, branchial cysts and carotid body tumours may occasionally be confused, and if the aneurysm bulges into the oropharynx, it may be misdiagnosed as a peritonsillar abscess. Perhaps the greatest difficulty in differential diagnosis arises where the carotid artery in an elderly and often hypertensive patient is elongated and kinked outward, pulsation and swelling being both visible and easily palpable. Here it may only be possible to prove or refute the diagnosis of aneurysm with ultrasound scanning or computed tomographic arteriogram (CTA).

Investigation of carotid aneurysms

While diagnosis often is certain on clinical examination, it can sometimes be difficult, for example, with high, small internal carotid aneurysms. Investigations include plain x-rays of the neck to show a soft tissue mass and perhaps calcification in the aneurysm wall. Ultrasound scanning demonstrates aneurysms well and is the best non-invasive investigative method. Examination of the fundi may reveal retinal artery emboli in patients with aneurysms complicated by transient visual field defects or transient cerebral ischemia.

CTA often provides the anatomical information necessary for operative repair. Arteriography may also be done when operation or stenting is planned. The proximal and distal carotid artery, as well as the aneurysm, must be visualized. Arteriography can be performed by selective carotid catheterization via the common femoral artery. The aneurysm itself should not be needled. Arteriography shows dissecting aneurysms well (Figure 37.3), a common appearance being a tapering narrowing with a line string of contrast extending distally. Duplex ultrasound can be used for post-operative follow-up.

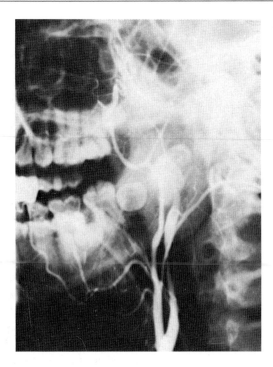

Figure 37.2 Three weeks after an apparently trivial injury to the left side of his neck, this 15-year-old male patient presented in the ear, nose and throat unit with a mass in the left tonsillar region. Arteriography showed a large, false internal carotid artery aneurysm. This ruptured into the esophagus immediately before surgery was to be undertaken, but he was resuscitated and the common carotid artery ligated. He made a complete recovery.

TREATMENT OF CAROTID

Aneurysms

Treatment is essentially surgical, there being little to offer of a non-surgical nature that is likely to be helpful. Patients who are for other reasons unfit for operation, those who have small and symptomless aneurysms discovered by chance and those whose aneurysms extend right to the base of the skull may merely be observed. However, a conservative approach to carotid aneurysms in general is likely to result in a considerable morbidity, mainly because of neurological complications, but occasionally from rupture. For example, Winslow[2] found that of 106 patients treated conservatively, 71% died as a result of a complication of their aneurysms. Even though the only active treatment then was proximal ligation, he concluded that carotid aneurysm was 'strictly a surgical problem'. Perhaps an occasional exception to this rule of active treatment arises in dealing with the rather rare dissecting aneurysms without cerebral embolic complications. Here reports suggest that the calibre of the arterial lumen may return spontaneously to normal in time, as has been shown arteriographically.[11] Long-term anticoagulation or aspirin therapy with the aim of preventing cerebral embolic symptoms in conservatively

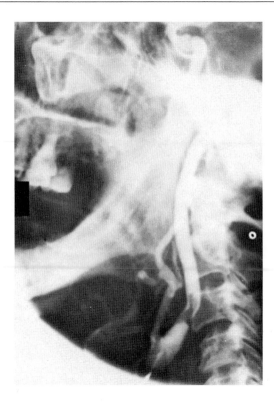

Figure 37.3 Right carotid angiogram showing a partial occlusion due to dissection of the proximal part of the right internal carotid artery in a patient who developed hemiplegia following a traffic accident. He sustained multiple facial fractures including a fracture of the right mandibular ramus.

treated patients does not appear to have been employed, and it seems unlikely that it would be effective. Mycotic aneurysms require intensive antibiotic therapy but also need urgent surgical treatment because of the high risk of rupture, and the same applies to false aneurysms, which in general are liable to continue to expand and possibly to rupture.

Techniques of surgical treatment

The techniques for surgical treatment fall into two main types, namely, simple ligation and reconstructive surgery.

Simple ligation

As has been noted, treatment of a carotid aneurysm by ligation was carried out successfully more than 175 years ago, and ligation remained virtually the only surgical option available until the advent of reconstructive arterial techniques. Ligation may be done just proximal to the aneurysm or both proximal and distal to it, or the common carotid may be ligated. Wherever the ligature is placed, however, it has long been recognized that there is a high risk of cerebral infarction post-operatively. In the early literature, for example, death rates of more than 50% were reported as a sequel to common carotid ligation. However, more recent reports put the incidence of serious neurological damage at a lower figure. McIvor reported that ligation of the internal carotid artery in 16 patients after negative balloon test occlusion led to five strokes, two of which were fatal.[18]

Simple proximal ligation is of course a good technique for dealing with the uncommon external carotid aneurysms, where there is no risk of producing cerebral ischemia.

Reconstructive approach to carotid aneurysm surgery

Reconstruction was first employed successfully in 1952. Several procedures have now been described, the most preferable being excision of the aneurysm with primary end-to-end reconstruction of the artery (Figure 37.1a through c). This is quite often feasible, but it does require the availability of a sufficient redundant length of artery. If there is not a sufficient length, interposition of a vein or prosthetic tube graft is necessary. Sise et al.[19] reported a favourable experience with PTFE interposition grafts in six patients with extracranial carotid aneurysm changes. An occasionally applicable technique for avoiding the use of an interposition graft in dealing with low internal carotid aneurysms is to divide the external carotid artery at such a level that its proximal end can be anastomosed to the distal end of the internal carotid after excision of the aneurysm (Figures 37.4 and 37.5).

Saccular aneurysms often have a relatively narrow neck, especially those saccular false aneurysms arising after previous carotid endarterectomy. Here the small defect in the arterial wall left after excision of the aneurysm may be closed with a vein or prosthetic patch graft. Mycotic aneurysms require special additional measures including antibiotic cover, vein rather than prosthetic graft material and complete excision of all the infected

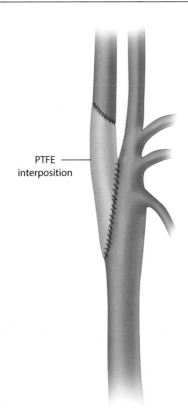

PTFE interposition

Figure 37.5 Method for reconstruction of an aneurysm of the internal carotid artery by interposition of a PTFE graft. (Reprinted from Sise MJ et al., *J Vasc Surg*, 16, 601, 1992. With permission.)

aneurysm wall. A vein bypass rather than an interposition graft may occasionally be feasible when removing mycotic aneurysms to avoid having suture lines in the infected area.[20]

Matas' endoaneurysmorrhaphy may still be employed unusually in dealing with high internal carotid aneurysms where a distal anastomosis at the base of the skull is not technically possible. In these patients, a Matas repair is done over a temporary internal shunt. This shunt may be a tapered one to allow better wedging of it into the distal internal carotid artery as it passes through the bony carotid canal in the base of the skull.[21] Much ingenuity has also been displayed in planning the distal anastomosis of grafts even in this very difficult situation.[22] Endovascular placement of a covered stent graft has been attempted at first cautiously.[23] In a subsequent, large 2015 review of 1239 patients, endovascular repair was used in only 5%.[24] In carefully selected patients, procedural success may be high (93%), but endoleaks were present in 8% and in-hospital mortality was 4% in Li's 2011 report.[25]

Carotid pseudoaneurysms are often suitable for endovascular repair. In a contemporary report (2015) of 116 pseudoaneurysms, 33 (29%) had open operation and 18 (15%) had endovascular repair.[26]

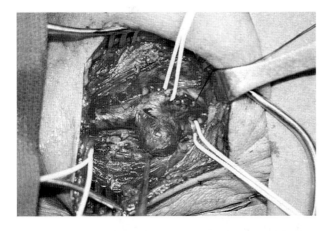

Figure 37.4 Operative exposure of a 4 cm aneurysm of the internal carotid artery. The common carotid artery is to the left in the photograph and the hypoglossal nerve to the right. This aneurysm was replaced by interposition of a PTFE graft. (See also colour plate.)

Measures to minimize the risk of cerebral embolization and ischemic damage during surgery

Cerebral embolization may occur during surgery as a result of handling an aneurysm which contains laminated and loose thrombus. It is therefore essential to disturb aneurysms as little as possible during their dissection. When an internal shunt is to be used, a clamp is first applied distal to the aneurysm, which is then incised so that the thrombotic material inside can be removed quickly before the shunt is inserted. Intravascular clotting during surgery can be minimized by the use of heparin, 100 units/kg intravenously, just before arterial occlusion. When cerebral collateral flow is inadequate, brain ischemia may be lessened by insertion of an internal shunt during the reconstructive procedure, if anatomically feasible. The interposition vein or prosthetic graft is passed over the shunt before the shunt is inserted. The distal (craniad) anastomosis is then completed first, and the shunt is removed just before the last sutures are placed in the proximal anastomosis. Occasionally an external shunt is more applicable. However used, a shunt means that internal carotid blood flow is only arrested for 3–5 minutes.

Surgical anatomy of the carotid arteries

The left common carotid artery is intrathoracic in its lower part on the left side, and in the neck, each common carotid artery is covered by the sternomastoid muscle. Surgical exposure is achieved by an incision through the skin and platysma in line with the anterior border of the sternomastoid or by an oblique, transverse incision which is a more cosmetic choice. The vagus nerve and cervical sympathetic chain lie behind the common carotid, as does the jugular vein. The internal carotid artery is closely related to the ninth to twelfth cranial nerves, as well as to the internal jugular vein and the carotid body. The uppermost third of this artery is deeply placed below the base of the skull, the temporomandibular joint and the parotid gland. It is crossed superficially by the stylohyoid ligament, the posterior belly of the digastric muscle and the styloglossus and stylopharyngeus muscles. The mastoid and styloid processes lie behind it, as do the longus capitis muscle and the prevertebral fascia. The external carotid artery lies behind the stylohyoid muscle and the posterior belly of the digastric muscle and passes up towards the parotid gland. It is closely related to the superior laryngeal, facial, hypoglossal and glossopharyngeal nerves and to the pharyngeal branch of the vagus.

Care must be taken to avoid injury to all these nerves during exposure of aneurysms. To lessen the risk of nerve damage when dealing with large non-mycotic aneurysms, portions of the aneurysm wall with adherent nerves can safely be left in situ when the bulk of the aneurysm is removed.

Results of surgery for carotid aneurysms

Apart from damage to adjacent nerves and the risk of local infection, the only serious complication of surgery is cerebral damage from ischemia or embolization. If this does not occur, the operation can be judged successful. However, the risk of neurological damage in association with surgery remains significant, though just exactly how significant it is difficult to say because widely varying figures appear in the literature. Simple ligation appears to be followed by cerebral damage in about 30% of patients in collected series,[27] while its reported incidence after reconstructive operations is less. Moreau et al. reported the outcome of 38 patients who had primary closure of the defect, reanastomosis or grafting with only 2 transient neurologic events and 8 cranial nerve injuries.[28] The severity of this neurological damage ranges from the massive fatal stroke to lesser defects with later partial or complete recovery. Occasionally, evidence of neurological damage does not appear immediately after operation but becomes manifest after several days, presumably because of late distal thrombosis of the internal carotid or its intracranial branches, occlusion of the reconstruction or late embolization.

CONCLUSIONS

Aneurysms of the extracranial carotid arteries are uncommon, but they have a special significance because of the threat they pose of cerebral embolic phenomena and, less commonly, of rupture. They appear to have been increasingly recognized, and to have generated much interest, over the last 10 or 15 years, judging by the number of case reports and reviews which have appeared in the surgical literature. The present tendency is to treat them actively, preferably by reconstructive vascular techniques, with open repair still the most common method. In suitable patients, usually carotid pseudoaneurysms, stent grafts have been used effectively.

REFERENCES

1. Cooper A. Account of the first successful operation performed on the common carotid artery for aneurysm in the year of 1808 with post mortem examination in the year 1821. *Guy's Hosp. Rep.* 1836;1:53.
2. Winslow N. Extracranial aneurysm of the internal carotid artery. *Arch Surg.* 1926;13:689.
3. Dimtza A. Aneurysms of the carotid arteries. Report of two cases. *Angiology.* 1956;7:218.
4. Pulli R, Gatti M, Credi G, Narcetti S, Capaccioli L, Pratesi C. Extracranial carotid artery aneurysms. *J Cardiovasc Surg.* 1997;38(4):339–346.
5. Schechter DC. Cervical carotid aneurysms. *NY State J Med.* 1979;79:892.
6. McCollum CH, Wheeler WG, Noon GP, DeBakey ME. Aneurysms of the extracranial carotid artery. *Am J Surg.* 1979;137:196.
7. Welling RE, Taha A, Goel T et al. Extracranial carotid artery aneurysms. *Surgery.* 1983;93:319.

8. Busuttil RW, Davidson RK, Foley KT et al. Selective management of extracranial carotid arterial aneurysms. *Am J Surg.* 1980;140:85.

9. Campbell FC, Robbs JV. Spontaneous dissecting aneurysm of the internal carotid artery. *J R Coll Surg Edinb.* 1981;26:286.

10. Ledgerwood AM, Lucas CE. Mycotic aneurysm of the carotid artery. *Arch Surg.* 1971;109:496.

11. Krupski WC, Effeney DJ, Ehrenfeld WK et al. Aneurysms of the carotid arteries. *Aust NZ J Surg.* 1983;53:521–525.

12. McCready RA, Hyde GI, Bivins BA et al. Radiation-induced arterial injuries. *Surgery.* 1983;93;306.

13. Borazjani BH, Wilson SE, Fujitani RM et al. Postoperative complications of carotid patching: Pseudoaneurysm and infection. *Ann Vasc Surg.* 2003;17:156–161.

14. Kaupp HA, Haid SP, Jurayj MN et al. Aneurysms of the extracranial carotid artery. *Surgery.* 1972;72:946.

15. Boddie HG. Transient ischaemic attacks and stroke due to extracranial aneurysm of internal carotid artery. *Br Med J.* 1972;3:802.

16. Morki B, Sundt TM Jr, Houser OW et al. Spontaneous dissection of the cervical internal carotid artery. *Ann Neurol.* 1986;19:126–138.

17. Lane JR, Weisman RA. Carotid artery aneurysms: An otolaryngologic perspective. *Laryngoscope.* 1980;90:897.

18. McIvor NP, Willinsky RA, TerBrugge KG, Rutka JA, Freeman JL. Validity of test occlusion studies prior to internal carotid artery sacrifice. *Head Neck.* 1994;16(1):11–16.

19. Sise MJ, Ivy ME, Malanche R, Ranbarger KR. Polytetrafluoroethylene interposition grafts for carotid reconstruction. *J Vasc Surg.* 1992;16:601.

20. Monson RC, Alexander RH. Vein reconstruction of a mycotic internal carotid aneurysm. *Ann Surg.* 1980;191:47.

21. Rhodes EL, Stanley JC, Hoffman GL et al. Aneurysms of extracranial carotid arteries. *Arch Surg.* 1976;111:339.

22. Pellegrini RV, Manzetti GW, DiMarco RF et al. The direct surgical management of lesions of the high internal carotid artery. *J Cardiovasc Surg.* 1984;25:29.

23. May J, White GH, Waugh R, Brennan J. Endoluminal repair of internal carotid artery aneurysms: A feasible but hazardous procedure. *J Vasc Surg.* 1997;26(6):1055–1060.

24. Welleweerd JC, den Ruijter HM, Nelissen BG et al. Management of Extracranial carotid artery aneurysm. *Eur J Endovasc Surg.* 2015;15:313–315.

25. Li Z, Chang G, Yao C et al. Endovascular stenting of extracranial carotid artery aneurysm: A systematic review. *Eur J Vasc Endovasc Surg.* 2011;42:419–426.

26. Fankhauser GT, Stone WM, Fowl RJ et al. Surgical and medical management of extracranial carotid artery aneurysms. *J Vasc Surg.* 2015;61:389–393.

27. Rittenhouse EA, Radke HM, Summer DS. Carotid artery aneurysm. *Arch Surg.* 1972;105:786.

28. Moreau P, Albat B, Thaevenet A. Surgical treatment of extracranial internal carotid aneurysm. *Ann Vasc Surg.* 1994;8(5):409–416.

38

Carotid body tumours

J.R. DE SIQUEIRA and MICHAEL J. GOUGH

CONTENTS

INTRODUCTION

Carotid body tumour (CBT), carotid paraganglioma and carotid chemodectoma are interchangeable names for an uncommon neuroendocrine tumour, which is occasionally hormonally active. Around 5% of CBTs are bilateral. Historically, surgical management was associated with significant complications, but due to its potential to metastasize (5%–10% are malignant), aggressive operative treatment is advocated.

Although the first CBT resection was recorded in 1880, it was another 6 years before a patient survived surgery without a major neurological event.[1] The technique of sub-adventitial dissection had not been developed at this time, and ligation of the carotid artery was an integral part of the procedure. In 1938, Enderlen[2] described a patient in whom successful carotid resection and reconstruction had been performed. Interestingly, it was a further 16 years before Eastcott[3] described the same technique in a patient with carotid atherosclerosis.

Following the description of sub-adventitial dissection by Gordon-Taylor[4] in 1940, complication rates fell dramatically. The risk of stroke fell from around 25% to less than 3%. Similarly, mortality was reduced from approximately 5% to 1% or less. By the late 1980s, long-term follow-up of patients undergoing CBT surgery had shown a 20-year survival equal to that of age-matched controls.[5] Despite these advances, cranial nerve injury (IX, X, XII) remained a common complication affecting up to 30% of patients.[6]

CBTs are generally highly vascular, and preoperative embolization has been suggested as a technique to facilitate their removal. Its use remains relatively controversial with some reporting significant complications with this strategy.[7]

Although advances in genetics[8] and imaging[9] have led to new strategies in diagnosis and follow-up, little has changed in respect of the operative technique in recent years.

PATHOPHYSIOLOGY OF CAROTID BODY TUMOURS

The carotid body is a small, highly vascular structure lying close to the carotid bifurcation and deriving its blood supply from the external carotid artery, usually via the ascending pharyngeal artery. It contains glomus type I (also referred to as chief cells) and type II cells (derived from neuroectoderm) and responds to variation in temperature, pH and the partial pressures of oxygen and carbon dioxide in the blood; its signals are carried by the afferent branches of the glossopharyngeal nerve to the cardiorespiratory loci of the medulla oblongata, the relay of which regulates ventilation. The mechanism by which chief cells detect physiological changes is not fully understood but is broadly linked to changes to mitochondrial function in the presence of hypoxia. Thus, it is not surprising that CBTs have been associated with chronic hypoxic states including living at altitude, chronic obstructive pulmonary disease and cyanotic heart disease. Nonetheless, the majority of CBTs arise in patients with no history of chronic hypoxia.

There is increasing evidence to suggest an underlying genetic basis for many, but not all, CBTs. In one series, over 40% of patients who underwent genetic testing had mutations in the SDH gene.[8] In familial cases, this abnormality is present in up to 70% of patients.[10] This gene, which also has links to phaeochromocytoma and other paragangliomas, codes for succinate dehydrogenase, a mitochondrial enzyme involved in Krebs cycle. It is a tumour suppressor, the dysfunction of which leads to uncontrolled cell replication. The underlying mechanism behind point mutations in SDH and the development of CBT remains unknown. Another series assessing oncogene expression by immunohistochemistry also found that c-myc expression was present in 13 of 13 cases and bcl-2 in 11 of 13 cases.[11]

Macroscopically, CBTs are well circumscribed and vary in size. The diagnosis of malignancy is predicated upon the development of metastases, there being no histological criteria for differentiating benign from malignant lesions. They are mainly composed of glomus type I cells demonstrating a prominent granular cytoplasm arranged in a nesting or cluster arrangement, referred to as a 'Zellballen' appearance from the German cell balls.

Among larger case series, malignancy is reported in 3%–13% of cases,[12] although the true incidence of this is difficult to determine due to the rarity of CBTs. Typically, metastases spread to local lymph nodes, the liver and lungs. Finally, local invasion of CBTs can involve the vagus and hypoglossal nerves thus increasing the risk of complications at resection.

The most commonly employed classification of CBTs was introduced in 1971 by Shamblin[13] and describes three morphological tumour types (Table 38.1).

Table 38.1 Shamblin classification of carotid body tumours.

Classification	Description
Shamblin I	Relatively small tumours minimally attached to carotid vessels
Shamblin II	Larger tumours with moderate attachment
Shamblin III	Large tumours usually encasing the carotid arteries

CLINICAL PRESENTATION

CBTs affect a wide age range with a peak incidence between 40 and 55 years of age.[14,15] Further, the female: male ratio varies significantly in different series but is generally higher in high altitude areas.[12] Bilateral tumours occur in around 30% of familial cases.[16]

Although the majority of patients present with a painless neck swelling,[15] there are reports of CBTs being found after investigation of syncope, Horner's syndrome or as a result of familial screening. If symptoms are present, these may include neck pain, dysphonia, hoarseness, stridor, dysphagia, odynophagia, jaw stiffness and a sore throat. Finally, around one in five patients present with a cranial nerve deficit.

CBTs are slow growing, and patients often describe symptoms that have been present for a few years. Unlike other neuroendocrine tumours, reports of hormonally active CBTs are rare, although Zeng[17] described an incidence of 12.5% in one small series. In these, the symptoms (hypertension, flushing, arrhythmias, headaches) are the same as for other functional paragangliomas (e.g. phaeochromocytoma). When symptomatic, the possibility of a glomus vagale tumour, multicentric paraganglioma or multiple endocrine neoplasia should be considered.

On examination, CBTs feel similar to a lymph node: they have a rubbery consistency and are less mobile in a cephalocaudal plane due to their attachment to the carotid bifurcation. They often appear pulsatile (but not expansile) and there may be a carotid bruit. Transverse movement of the mass should displace the carotid pulse in the same direction (Fontaine's sign). Cranial nerve deficits may also be detected.

The contralateral side of the neck should also be examined to assess the possibility of CBTs, particularly in familial cases.

The differential diagnosis includes the causes of any lateral cervical swelling:

1. Malignancy
   a. Lymphoma
   b. Other paragangliomas (jugular, sympathetic, vagal)
   c. Other primary cervical neoplasms (salivary gland, neurofibroma, schwannoma, laryngeal carcinoma)
   d. Metastatic cervical lymphadenopathy
2. Benign cervical lymphadenopathy
3. Carotid artery aneurysm

Naturally, a detailed history exploring the presence of coexisting symptoms and a thorough examination will help to distinguish between these pathologies. However, appropriate imaging is required to make the correct diagnosis.

Clinical recommendation

Suspect CBT in patients with a lateral-neck mass (Grade D).

INVESTIGATIONS

When CBT is considered a potential diagnosis, particularly in patients with a slow-growing lateral-neck mass, imaging is central to confirming the diagnosis. Fine-needle aspiration cytology (FNAC) and hormonal assays have a lesser role but warrant brief discussion.

FNAC of CBTs is considered inappropriate by most authors because of the risks of haemorrhage, stroke and vascular injury.[18] This view is based on *common sense* and dogma rather than evidence. Whilst the authors of this chapter would not go so far as to advocate the use of this technique, there is no doubt that the quality of currently available imaging modalities to guide FNAC and the appropriate technical skills have improved considerably over the last decade. Nevertheless, the diagnosis can be established without this, and it is difficult to justify the additional cost and risk for this ultimately unnecessary investigation.

Similarly, blood tests add little to establishing the diagnosis of CBT although they may be helpful in excluding some of the differential diagnoses (C-reactive protein, erythrocyte sedimentation rate and full blood count). If a hormone-secreting tumour is suspected, then 24-hour urine catecholamines and fractioned metanephrines should be assayed.

Except in possible familial cases, genetic testing is normally performed post-operatively once the diagnosis has been confirmed.

Imaging plays the largest part in establishing of the diagnosis of CBT, and traditionally catheter arteriography was considered the gold standard. Alternative modalities and the small (<0.5%) but definite risk of stroke have rendered this technique obsolete in recent years. A number of studies have demonstrated that colour flow Doppler ultrasound, computed tomography (CTA) and magnetic resonance angiography (MRA) are suitable alternatives.[19]

The two cardinal radiographic features of CBTs are their hypervascularity and splaying of the carotid bifurcation (Lyre Sign). Proponents of digital subtraction angiography (DSA) suggest that an intense tumour blush and early venous drainage are better shown by this technique and that it is superior to 3-D imaging for assessing internal carotid artery involvement (implied by an irregular stenosis).

A vascular mass splaying the internal (ICA) and external (ECA) carotid arteries is easily detectable by colour flow Doppler ultrasound, and following a 30-year retrospective, multicentre review, Sajid et al. considered it the investigation of choice.[15]

CTA also demonstrates Lyre's sign and rapid tumour enhancement. Further, it will detect concurrent contralateral tumours and better delineate local invasion.[20] MRA shares many of the advantages of CTA, and 3-D time of flight imaging was reported as being the most effective protocol in one study but with only 90% sensitivity and 92% specificity compared to DSA.[19] On T2- and T1-weighted images the typical findings are of a hyper-intense mass with flow voids (salt and pepper sign).[9] Figure 38.1 demonstrates the characteristic MRA findings of a patient with a CBT.

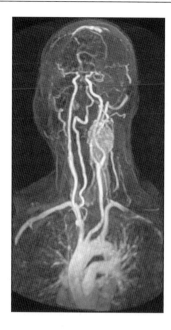

Figure 38.1 Left-sided CBT with splaying of carotid vessels and a hypervascular tumour mass.

Since reliable comparison of the efficacy of these imaging techniques is compromised by the rarity of the tumour, it seems reasonable to suggest that DSA should be reserved for a small minority of patients in whom the diagnosis is in doubt following non-invasive imaging.

Lastly, octreotide scintigraphy[21,22] and positron emission tomography (PET scanning)[22,23] have both been used for the detection of metastases in CBT patients. Previously undetected paragangliomas or metastases were identified in 36% (9 of 25) and 60% (3 of 5) of patients undergoing scintigraphy or PET, respectively.[21,23] Conversely, no additional tumours or metastases were identified in 12 patients investigated by Martinelli[22] (scintigraphy and PET). The findings of the first two studies would suggest that either the traditional view on the malignant potential of CBTs is incorrect or that these techniques have a significant false-positive rate. Alternatively, patients in these two groups may have been at higher risk of metastases than normal as 30% of Kwekkeboom's[21] series had familial CBT, and 80% of the other series had bilateral masses, many of which are likely to have been familial.

The ultimate decision on which imaging modality to employ in patients suspected of having a CBT will be based on availability and the skill set of an institution's radiologists.

Duplex ultrasound (US) is an excellent, non-invasive, screening investigation with a reported diagnostic accuracy of 100% compared to DSA which appears superior to that of CTA and MRA. However, these investigations have other advantages that have been outlined earlier.

If a CBT is still suspected after a negative ultrasound, and renal function permits, CTA (or MRA) is the next investigation of choice since it also provides valuable information to guide subsequent surgery (tumour size, the

Shamblin classification). It can also assess patency of the circle of Willis, in the event that carotid reconstruction is required. If these investigations fail to provide the necessary information then DSA may occasionally be required.

Lastly, scintigraphy or PET scans may be the optimum method of demonstrating distant metastasis or concurrent paragangliomas although the sensitivity and specificity of these investigations require confirmation. However, given the slow growth rate of CBTs, this information is unlikely to alter the decision to treat the lesion surgically.

Clinical recommendations

1. FNA should not be performed on suspected lesions (Grade D).
2. Duplex ultrasound should be the primary diagnostic modality (Grade D).
3. When Duplex ultrasound confirms the diagnosis, CTA or MRA should be performed for preoperative planning (Grade D).
4. DSA may be performed if CTA/MRA does not provide the necessary information (Grade D).
5. Patients with CBT should be offered genetic testing for SDH mutations (Grade D).

THERAPEUTIC OPTIONS

Historically, surgery for CBT has fallen in and out of favour. Two factors favour aggressive management: the inability to predict which tumours are, or will become, malignant and the significant reduction in complication rates with modern surgery. Thus, resection remains the mainstay of treatment. Preoperative tumour embolization and radiotherapy are employed in some centres and are worthy of discussion. However, the evidence base to support their routine use is weak.

It is possible that reports describing the efficacy of radiotherapy are subject to either selection (i.e. patients who are unsuitable for surgery) or publication bias. Nonetheless, results from several small series are broadly comparable to those of surgery: One series of 10 cases (1 post-operative) demonstrated no tumour growth or metastasis after a mean follow-up of 8 years.[24] This correlates well with another series that reported a 90%–100% cause-specific survival.[25] However, Mitchell[26] et al. reported a 10% risk of metastases, whilst other complications and side effects are not uncommon. These include weight loss, mucositis and radiation-related meningioma. It is unsurprising that these have led others to conclude that radiation therapy is best reserved for inoperable or recurrent tumours.[27]

Progress in endovascular intervention has led to the increased use of devascularization techniques prior to surgical resection. These include embolization with a variety of materials (Onyx, coils) or deployment of a covered stent in the external carotid artery to occlude the ascending pharyngeal artery. This is limited to cases where its origin is not too close to the carotid bifurcation. Devascularization rates of up to 90% have been reported[28] and two non-randomized studies have reported a significant reduction in intraoperative blood loss.[29,30] However, there was no reduction in the frequency of cranial nerve injury.

In a large series of CBT patients (2117) derived from the US Nationwide Inpatient Sample database (2002–2006), embolization was associated with a non-significant reduction in mortality (0% vs. 0.59%) and stroke (0% vs. 3.5%).[31]

Clinical recommendations

1. Patients in whom a CBT is technically resectable should be offered surgery (Grade D).
2. There is no definitive evidence to support routine preoperative embolization of CBTs (Grade D).
3. Radiotherapy should be reserved for patients who are not suitable for surgery (Grade D).

PREOPERATIVE PLANNING AND OPERATIVE TECHNIQUE

The following are recommended before embarking upon resection:

1. Cross-sectional imaging to assess tumour size and encroachment on surrounding structures (Shamblin classification) (CT/MR)
2. Assessment of the collateral cerebral circulation (circle of Willis) if internal carotid reconstruction or ligation is envisaged (CTA/MRA/Transcranial Doppler)
3. Assessment of hormonal activity *and* alpha- and beta-adrenergic blockade if appropriate
4. Preoperative devascularization (surgeon preference)
5. Marking of the great saphenous vein if carotid resection may be necessary (surgeon preference)

Consent should include the risk of haemorrhage and blood transfusion, cranial nerve injury (20%–30%), stroke (1%–3%) and death (0.5%). Given the risk of recurrent laryngeal nerve injury and baroreceptor reflex failure, bilateral tumours should be treated by staged procedures.

General anaesthesia is usually employed although cervical plexus block, as for carotid endarterectomy, has been described.[32] The latter may be less acceptable if significant bleeding occurs or surgery is prolonged.

As a precaution, a carotid shunt should be available within the operating room.

Surgical exposure is the same as for carotid endarterectomy with an incision over the anterior border of sternocleidomastoid (SCM) that is angled posteriorly below the mastoid to avoid injury to the parotid gland, mandibular branch of the facial nerve and the greater auricular nerve. After division of platysma, the internal jugular vein (IJV) is dissected beneath the anterior border of the SCM and the common facial vein divided to allow lateral retraction of the IJV thus exposing the carotid

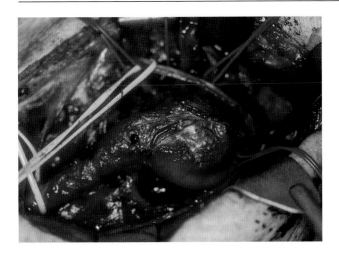

Figure 38.2 Dissection and control of the carotid vessels and hypoglossal nerve prior to CBT removal.

bifurcation. The common carotid artery (CCA), ICA and ECA and branches of the EIA are then *controlled* with atraumatic slings (Figure 38.2). Any non-essential vessels feeding the CBT are ligated.

The majority of CBTs are removed using sub-adventitial dissection starting at a point where the ECA, ICA or CCA are not involved in the tumour. Resection is facilitated by using bipolar dissecting scissors to enhance haemostasis. Meticulous attention is paid to identifying and preserving the hypoglossal, glossopharyngeal and recurrent laryngeal nerves.

An alternative technique has been described by Van der Bogt[19] in which identification and control of the distal ICA and ECA followed by craniocaudal, rather than caudal–cranial, dissection is employed. This technique allows the tumour to be pulled forward, allowing ligation of posterior feeding vessels. The tumour is then separated from the carotid bifurcation in the sub-adventitial plane. The author reported a significant reduction in blood loss and cranial nerve injury in a non-randomized trial. Further, the technique may be helpful in cases where the tumour involves part or all of the carotid bifurcation making identification of a dissection plane difficult.

In a small proportion of patients, when the bifurcation is encased by tumour, en bloc resection may be required. On these occasions, an appropriate length of great saphenous vein (circa 10 cm) should be harvested for vascular reconstruction before the resection commences. A suitable carotid shunt is passed through the lumen of the vein, which is then inserted into the proximal CCA and distal ICA (transected above the tumour mass). Tumour resection then proceeds. Balloon catheters may also be employed to control bleeding if it proves difficult to control with clamps (particularly the ECA). Although the authors' preference is to use a vein graft, satisfactory patency rates have also been reported for synthetic grafts.

Routine lymph node sampling has been suggested by some authors and in one case led to the diagnosis of a local metastasis. However, if identification of lymph node spread is required, octreotide scintigraphy is likely to be more accurate and avoids lymphadenectomy.

COMPLICATIONS

Cranial nerve injury occurs in up to 30% of patients and is directly linked to tumour size and invasion. The nerves most at risk are the glossopharyngeal, vagus and hypoglossal nerves. Also at risk are the facial and accessory nerves and the cervical sympathetic trunk. Most injuries are temporary and 80% resolve within a year.[29] Given the peak age at presentation (40–55), the implications of a cranial nerve injury should be carefully discussed preoperatively.

The second most common complication is stroke affecting around 3% of patients.

Baroreflex failure after excision of the carotid body or vagus nerve can be a serious complication, precipitating hyper- or hypotension and/or orthostatic tachycardia.[33] It is particularly prevalent following bilateral tumour excision, affecting approximately a quarter of such cases.[34] Initially, patients may need to be managed in a high dependency unit. Clonidine can be used to manage such cases, however, this only reduces the frequency of attacks, and many patients have lifelong problems.

FOLLOW-UP

Although the risk of malignancy in CBTs is low (3%–13% of cases), both local recurrence and metastases have been reported many years after resection.[7] This makes it difficult to decide if discharge or interval imaging of patients is required post-operatively.

Further, since histological examination of the tumour offers little insight as to whether it is malignant, routine post-operative radiotherapy is not recommended.

Octreotide scintigraphy and PET scans have been advocated as appropriate modalities for identifying local recurrence or metastases, but evidence for their routine use during follow-up is sparse. Further, the slow-growing nature of the tumour suggests that the interval between post-operative assessments is unlikely to be critical.

Finally, when genetic profiling of a resected tumour is positive, first-degree relatives of affected individuals should be offered counselling and screening.

OTHER CERVICAL PARAGANGLIOMAS

A vascular opinion may be sought in patients with other paragangliomas of the neck. On occasions, they may form part of the differential at the diagnosis of a CBT, depending upon their location. Glomus jugulare tumours arise from the jugular foramen of the temporal bone and glomus tympanicum from the middle ear. Both typically present with tinnitus or hearing loss and usually present to otorhinolaryngologists. However, invasion of the jugular vein or internal carotid artery may prompt vascular referral.

Glomus vagale are the least common cervical paraganglioma and are tumours of the vagal nerve. Again, involvement of vascular structures will necessitate a multidisciplinary approach to treatment. The various diagnostic and therapeutic considerations for other neck paragangliomas are the same as for CBTs.

> ## Key points
>
> - CBTs are rare but should be considered in patients presenting with a lateral cervical mass.
> - Only a minority (<10%) are malignant.
> - Historically, DSA is the gold standard for diagnosis but ultrasound, MR and CT appear equally effective.
> - Surgical resection is the mainstay of treatment; preoperative embolization may have a role in large tumours.
> - Metastases and local recurrence can occur many years later (>5 years).

DEFICIENCIES IN KNOWLEDGE AND FUTURE AREAS FOR RESEARCH

These are rare tumours, and at best, only level 3 evidence exists for their management. Thus, deficiencies in knowledge exist about most aspects of CBT management.

A number of areas would seem to be targets for further research:

- The influence of preoperative embolization on perioperative haemorrhage and stroke
- The role and frequency of whole body scintigraphy or PET scans for detecting metastatic disease
- The benefit or otherwise of screening first-degree relatives

Multicentre, international randomized trials would be required to answer these questions.

BEST CLINICAL PRACTICE

- Diagnosis should be confirmed by Duplex US or CT scan. DSA should be reserved for cases where the diagnosis remains uncertain.
- CBTs should always be resected if feasible due to the risk of malignancy.
- Genetic testing should be offered to relatives of patients who have positive tests.
- Patients should be followed up for at least 5 years and this should include an annual ultrasound scan. If recurrence is suspected, PET, CT or octreotide scintigraphy should be performed.

KEY REFERENCES

1. van der Bogt KE, Vrancken Peeters MP, van Baalen JM, Hamming JF. Resection of carotid body tumors: Results of an evolving surgical technique. *Ann Surg.* 2008;247(5):877–884.

   A detailed description of the surgical technique for CBT resection.
2. Vogel TR, Mousa AY, Dombrovskiy VY, Haser PB, Graham AM. Carotid body tumor surgery: Management and outcomes in the nation. *Vasc Endovasc Surg.* 2009;43(5):457–461.

   The largest available US series regarding the investigation and management of CBT.
3. Sajid MS, Hamilton G, Baker DM. Joint Vascular Research Group. A multicenter review of carotid body tumour management. *Eur J Vasc Endovasc Surg.* 2007 August;34(2):127–130.

   The largest available European series regarding the investigation and management of CBT.

REFERENCES

1. Gratiot JH. Carotid body tumors: Collective review. *Surg Gynecol Obstet.* 1943;77:177.
2. Enderlen E. Originalmitteilungen, Operation der Carotisdrusengeschwulste. *Zentralbl Chir.* 1938;46:2530.
3. Eastcott HHG. Reconstruction of internal carotid artery in a patient with intermittent attacks of hemiplegia. *Lancet.* 1954;2:994–996.
4. Gordon-Taylor G, On carotid tumors. *Br J Surg.* 1940;28:163.
5. Nora JD. Surgical resection of carotid body tumours: Long term survival, recurrence and metastasis. *Mayo Clinic Proc.* 1988;63(4):348–352.
6. Sen I, Stephen E, Malepathi K, Agarwal S, Shyamkumar NK, Mammen S. Neurological complications in carotid body tumors: A 6-year single-center experience. *J Vasc Surg.* 2013;57(2 Suppl.):64S–68S.
7. O'Neill S, O'Donnell M, Harkin D, Loughrey M, Lee B, Blair P. A 22-year Northern Irish experience of carotid body tumours. *Ulster Med J.* 2011;80(3):133–140.
8. Fruhmann J, Geigl JB, Konstantiniuk P, Cohnert TU. Paraganglioma of the carotid body: Treatment strategy and SDH-gene mutations. *Eur J Vasc Endovasc Surg.* 2013;45(5):431–436.
9. Arya S, Rao V, Juvenakar S, DCruz AK. Carotid body tumours: Objective criteria to predict the shambling group on MR imaging. *Am J Neuroradiol.* 2008;29:1349–1354.
10. Baysal BE, Willet-Brozick JE, Lawrence EC et al. Prevalence of SDHB, SDHC and SDHD gremlin mutations in clinic patients with head and neck paragangliomas. *J Med Genet Mar.* 2002;39(3):178–183.

11. Wang DG, Barros D'Sa AA, Johnston CF, Buchanan KD. Oncogene expression in carotid body tumors. *Cancer*. 1996;77(12):2581–2587.

12. Rodriguez-Cuevas J, Lopez-Garza J, Labastida-Almendaro S. Carotid body tumors in inhabitants of altitudes higher than 2000 meters above sea level. *Head Neck*. 1998;20(5):374–378.

13. Shamblin WR, ReMine WH, Sheps SG, Harrison EG Jr. Carotid body tumour (chemodectoma): Clinicopathological analysis of ninety cases. *Am J Surg*. 1971;122(6):732–739.

14. van der Bogt KE, Vrancken Peeters MP, van Baalen JM, Hamming JF. Resection of carotid body tumors: Results of an evolving surgical technique. *Ann Surg*. 2008;247(5):877–884.

15. Sajid MS, Hamilton G, Baker DM. Joint Vascular Research Group. A multicenter review of carotid body tumour management. *Eur J Vasc Endovasc Surg*. 2007;34(2):127–130.

16. Ridge BA, Brewster DC, Darling RC, Cambria RP, La Muraglia GM, Abbot WM. Familial carotid body tumours: Incidence and implications. *Ann Vasc Surg*. 1993;7(2):190–194.

17. Zeng G, Zhao J, Ma Y, Huang B, Yang Y, Feng H. A comparison between the treatments of functional and nonfunctional carotid body tumors. *Ann Vasc Surg*. 2012;26(4):506–510.

18. Rosa M, Sahoo S. Bilateral carotid body tumour: The role of fine needle aspiration biopsy in the preoperative diagnosis. *Diagn Cytopathol*. 2008;36(3):178–180.

19. van den Berg R, Schepers A, de Bruine FT, Liauw L, Mertens BJ, van der Mey AG, Van Buchem MA. The value of MR angiography techniques in the detection of head and neck paragangliomas. *Eur J Radiol*. 2004;52(3):240–245.

20. Muhm M, Polterauer P, Gstottner W, Temmel A, Richling B, Undt G, Niederle B, Staudacher M, Ehringer H. Diagnostic and therapeutic approaches to carotid body tumors. Review of 24 patients. *Arch Surg*. 1997;132(3):279–284.

21. Kwekkeboom DJ, van Urk H, Pauw BK, Lamberts SW, Kooij PP, Hoogma RP, Krenning EP. Octreotide scintigraphy for the detection of paragangliomas. *J Nucl Med*. 1993;34(6):873–878.

22. Martinelli O, Irace L, Massa R, Savelli S, Giannoni F, Gattuso R, Gossetti B, Benedetti-Valentini F, Izzo L. Carotid body tumors: Radioguided surgical approach. *J Exp Clin Cancer Res*. 2009;28:148.

23. Naswa N, Kumar A, Sharma P, Bal C, Malhotra A, Kumar R. Imaging carotid body chemodectomas with 68Ga-DOTA-NOC PET-CT. *Br J Radiol*. 2012;85(1016):1140–1145.

24. Dupin C, Lang P, Dessard-Diana B, Simon JM, Cuenca X, Mazeron JJ, Feuvret L. Treatment of head and neck paragangliomas with external beam radiation therapy. *Int J Radiat Oncol Biol Phys*. 2014;89(2):353–359.

25. Evenson IJ, Mendenhall WM, Parsons JT, Cassisi NJ. Radiotherapy in the management of chemodectomas of the carotid body and glomus vagale. *Head Neck*. 1998;20):609–613.

26. Mitchell DC, Clyne CAO. Chemodectomas of the neck: The response to radiotherapy. *Br J Surg*. 1985;72(11):903–905.

27. Rao AB, Koeller KK, Adair CF. Paragangliomas of the head and neck: Radiologic-pathologic correlation. *Radiographics*. 1999;19:1605–1632.

28. Kalani MY, Ducruet AF, Crowley RW, Spetzler RF, McDougall CG, Albuquerque FC. Transfemoral transarterial onyx embolization of carotid body paragangliomas: Technical considerations, results, and strategies for complication avoidance. *Neurosurgery*. 2013;72(1):9–15.

29. Power AH, Bower TC, Kasperbauer J, Link MJ, Oderich G, Cloft H, Young WF Jr, Gloviczki P. Impact of preoperative embolization on outcomes of carotid body tumor resections. *J Vasc Surg*. 2012;56(4):979–989.

30. Zhang TH, Jiang WL, Li YL, Li B, Yamakawal T. Perioperative approach in the surgical management of carotid body tumors. *Ann Vasc Surg*. 2012;26(6):775–782.

31. Vogel TR, Mousa AY, Dombrovskiy VY, Haser PB, Graham AM. Carotid body tumor surgery: Management and outcomes in the nation. *Vasc Endovasc Surg*. 2009;43(5):457–461.

32. Jones HG, Stoneham MD. Continuous cervical plexus block for carotid body tumour excision in a patient with Eisenmenger's syndrome. *Anaesthesia*. 2006;61(12):1214–1218.

33. Ketch T, Italo B, Robertson R, Robertson D. Four faces of baroreflex failure hypertensive crisis, volatile hypertension, orthostatic tachycardia, and malignant vagotonia. *Circulation*. 2002;105:2518–2523.

34. Netterville JL, Reilly KM, Robertson D, Reiber ME, Armstrong WB, Childs P. Carotid body tumors: A review of 30 patients with 46 tumors. *Laryngoscope*. 1995;105(2):115–126.

39

Carotid angioplasty and stenting

JOS C. VAN DEN BERG

CONTENTS

INTRODUCTION

Since the introduction of endovascular treatment of carotid artery stenosis (initially with balloon angioplasty, later with additional stenting using devices that were not specifically designed for the carotid artery), significant changes in technique and development of dedicated devices and optimization of pharmacotherapy around the procedure have increased the overall safety of the carotid artery stenting (CAS) procedure. This chapter will deal with the timing and technical aspects of the procedure, including the use of embolic protection devices (EPDs), and will also discuss the pharmacotherapeutic management around CAS. Finally, an overview of the major randomized controlled trials (RCTs) and current guidelines will be given.

TIMING OF CAROTID INTERVENTION

The goal of treatment of internal carotid artery (ICA) disease is the prevention of (further) neurological injury and achievement of timely cerebral reperfusion following transient ischemic attack (TIA), recurrent TIA or minor stroke. Treatment should lead to a reduction of patient disability and overall health costs. Recent studies have demonstrated that the risk of recurrent stroke is actually highest in the period immediately after the ischemic event in patients with a significant ipsilateral carotid stenosis. It has been established in various studies that the majority of patients with symptomatic carotid artery stenosis will benefit from early intervention with carotid endarterectomy (urgent treatment

has been estimated to prevent up to 80% of early recurrent strokes).[1-7] This is true even when knowing that patients with unstable neurological symptoms (stroke-in-evolution or crescendo TIA) have a significantly increased perioperative risk,[8] most probably due to high carotid plaque instability, repeated brain injury (in crescendo TIAs) and thus increased brain vulnerability.[9] Crescendo transient ischemic attacks are believed largely to result from repeated artery-to-artery carotid embolism, since such patients' carotid plaques commonly show surface irregularity and ulceration at pathologic examination,[10] and are to be considered a different entity from progressive stroke. It remains however a problem that most surgeons, interventionalists and neurologists involved in stroke management are reluctant to undertake carotid revascularization immediately after the neurological event for fear of hemorrhagic transition of the cerebral infarct. The current guidelines of the ESVS, NICE and AHA recommend instituting treatment (without mentioning the preferred treatment modality) within 2 weeks after onset of symptoms in patients with TIA or non-disabling stroke (*level 1 evidence*). The UK Department of Health recommends that carotid intervention should be regarded as an emergency procedure in stable symptomatic patients and should ideally be performed within 48 hours of a TIA or minor stroke.[7]

It has to be kept in mind that the concept of endovascular treatment in the acute phase is different[10]: a combination of artery-to-artery embolism, hemodynamic insufficiency and acute circulatory failure that has been triggered by plaque rupture or bleeding into a plaque is responsible for progression in carotid-related stroke.

The main therapeutic aim of emergency carotid stent placement is not removal of an ongoing embolic source but restoration of blood flow to rescue the ischemic penumbra in the affected hemisphere by improving cerebral perfusion thereof and secondly to reinstate sufficient distal perfusion pressure to reduce the risk of worsening of the ongoing ischemia. Additionally, the treatment should eliminate the release of new emboli from unstable plaque in the ICA.[11]

CAS in the acute phase is controversial, as outcomes, patient selection and optimal timing are still to be defined in the literature, and therefore, it is not clear whether this urgent treatment approach can also be applied to stenting. In one study[12] that evaluated patients from three large randomized trials (EVA-3S, SPACE and ICSS), it was found that patients undergoing carotid endarterectomy (CEA) within the first 7 days of the qualifying event had the lowest periprocedural stroke or death rate (2.8%); nota bene this finding is in contradiction with the findings of the studies mentioned earlier. Patients treated with CAS within the first 7 days had a 9.4% risk of periprocedural stroke or death (risk ratio CAS vs. CEA: 3.4). Those patients treated between 8 and 14 days after becoming symptomatic showed a periprocedural stroke or death rate of 3.4% for CEA and 8.1% for CAS. The patients treated more than 14 days after the onset of symptoms had 4% complications in the CEA group and 7.3% in the CAS group.

One of the disadvantages of CEA is the risk it carries of decreasing cerebral blood flow in the cerebral hemisphere during the operation and has the potential to render the affected hemisphere more vulnerable to ischemia.[10] From a theoretical point of view, CAS has the advantage of rarely reducing cerebral blood flow in the affected hemisphere during the procedure (at least when proximal flow occlusion is not used during the procedure). On the other hand, early CAS (as CEA) can provoke a further deterioration of neurological status by converting a non-hemorrhagic infarction into a hemorrhagic one and extending the infarct area. Reperfusion injury may result in hyperperfusion or hemorrhagic complications with possible impairment of autoregulation from chronic ischemia. Further, there is a risk of new emboli from plaque prolapse, anticoagulation-related hemorrhage, and postprocedural hypotension. Many aspects of patient selection regarding either urgent or delayed treatment or the selection of treatment type are yet to be defined.[7]

Preoperative considerations

With the advent of CAS as an alternative to surgical treatment of stenotic ICA disease, additional preoperative imaging has become more important and is not solely required to determine the degree of stenosis and to decide whether the patient needs invasive treatment. CT angiography and MR angiography are considered mandatory in order to judicate the feasibility of carotid stenting through the femoral route and in order to estimate the complexity of the procedure. Imaging should include the aortic arch and cervical and intracranial segments of the carotid artery, allowing evaluation of the anatomy of the access vessels and the configuration of the aortic arch and the tortuosity and length of the common carotid artery (CCA) and ICA and demonstrating the presence of disease of the external carotid artery (ECA). Additional imaging should also allow for evaluation of the intracranial circulation, since concomitant disease of the intracranial vessels can influence the efficacy of treatment.

Evaluation of patency of access vessels (common femoral artery and iliac axis) is not routinely performed, but occasionally access problems may arise. Duplex ultrasound can be used as an alternative to screen for disease of the access vessels.

In the acute stage, the role of imaging has become of paramount importance in order to properly select patients. The necessity of additional sophisticated imaging also underlines the importance of collaboration in a multidisciplinary team. From recent publications, it appears that a proper preoperative workup is crucial to improve outcome of urgent CEA in patients with unstable neurological symptoms.[9] This is probably also true for CAS.[7,13] Since reversibility of the brain tissue ischemia is strongly associated with collateral flow through leptomeningeal branches, the time window for recanalization by emergency carotid stent placement is variable in patients with carotid-related stroke and can be estimated by using second-level imaging.[10] The assessment should include evaluation of presence and extension of brain lesions by either CT or MRI, characteristics of the carotid plaque by duplex ultrasound and patency of the middle cerebral artery by CT or MR angiography. Knowledge of the degree of viability in the affected hemisphere by diffusion weighted imaging (DWI) is essential prior to attempt emergency carotid stent placement. In order to evaluate the extension of areas of brain ischemia, MRI with DWI is preferred over CT.[7] DWI is used to exclude high-risk patients (who have radiologic evidence of large irreversible ischemic stroke) from undergoing emergency stent placement. In this way one can minimize the chance that the patient will have massive hemorrhagic transformation of the infarct after recanalization.[10] Secondary imaging also allows better differentiation of TIA from minor stroke. By definition the diagnosis of TIA can only be made in a retrospective fashion, i.e. at the moment when the symptoms have completely regressed. Patient subgroups in which early intervention should be avoided are those with evidence of a zone of ischemic infarct >2.5 cm, intracranial hemorrhage, recent carotid occlusion that has lasted more than 6 hours, Rankin score >3, patients with a fluctuating level of consciousness and absence of neurological plateau (*level 2 evidence*).[14]

Arch configuration is of importance in deciding upon the suitability of an endovascular procedure, and additional imaging is needed for classification of aortic arch morphology and for visualization of anatomical variants. Knowledge of the length and degree of tortuosity of the CCA is of importance to evaluate the possibility of safe placement of the guiding catheter or long introduction sheath. Evaluation of plaque calcification and ulceration and intimal thickening is of importance in determining the optimal (endovascular) approach (including the choice of the type of protection device; see following text). Plaques that are more prone to disruption, fracture or fissuring may be associated with a higher risk of embolization, occlusion and consequent ischemic neurological events.[15] The absence of (occlusive) disease of the ECA is essential to allow for placement of a long guide wire in the ECA to perform an exchange of the diagnostic catheter for a long introduction sheath or guiding catheter.

Suitability for carotid stenting may be as low as 36% as judged by anatomical criteria (mainly carotid tortuosity and proximal arch disease).[16] Anatomical factors that increase the difficulty during CAS may be related to the access to the ICA (low carotid bifurcation/short CCA, tortuous CCA, diseased CCA and disease or occlusion of the ECA), arch (presence of severe arch atheroma, severe arch origin disease, type III arch and bovine arch) and target vessel (pinhole stenosis, angulated origin of the ICA, angulated distal ICA and circumferential calcification of the ICA).[17] It has been shown that severe angulation of the ICA–CCA junction and long segment stenosis of the ICA (>10 mm), calcified stenosis and left-sided carotid artery stenosis are related to a significant increase in stroke and/or death rate, while complications in patients with type III arch, aortic arch calcification and ulceration of the stenosis tend to be higher (*level 1 evidence*).[18]

CAS procedure

CAS is a procedure that involves a number of well-defined steps that should be performed sequentially, paying attention to every detail, and always following this sequence without skipping one of the steps.

CHOICE OF ACCESS

The most commonly used access vessel is the common femoral artery. Advantages are the size of the artery that makes it easy to puncture and allows for placement of large-bore indwelling sheaths. In addition, the artery is easily compressible and apt for the use of closure devices. Disadvantages include the distance to the target vessel. Furthermore, it requires arch navigation that may be especially cumbersome in extreme tortuous anatomy that is typically seen in the older age group.

Alternatively, a brachial or radial approach can be used.[19] Especially the carotid access route takes out the oftentimes difficult manipulation in the aortic arch. In the early years of carotid stenting, direct carotid access (either by direct puncture or surgical cut-down) has been advocated,[20] but has not been adopted widely. This approach is gaining renewed interest, with the advent of new devices. Initial results with the ENROUTE system using a direct cervical (surgical) access with flow reversal have demonstrated high technical success rate with a low occurrence of new white matter lesions on DWI post-procedure.[21]

ARCH NAVIGATION AND CANNULATION OF CCA

After placement of a femoral sheath, access to the ipsilateral CCA should be obtained. Cannulation of the CCA can be performed using a variety of 4F–5F diagnostic catheters and a standard 0.035 in. hydrophilic angled-tip guide wire. The choice of the diagnostic catheter depends on the amount of tortuosity and angulation of the aortic arch and supra-aortic vessels, respectively (in the absence of significant tortuosity, a simple curve such as vertebral, Berenstein, Judkins and Headhunter can be used, while in more difficult anatomy, more complex curves such as sidewinder, Newton and VTK are required). Subsequently, a diagnostic angiography of the carotid bifurcation is performed. This is followed by a cerebral angiography in an AP and lateral projection. In order to be able to advance a larger-diameter sheath or guiding catheter, it is necessary to have a sufficiently stiff guide wire from the aortic arch into the ipsilateral CCA. In the presence of a (high-grade) stenosis of the ICA, it is recommended to avoid crossing of the ICA stenosis with the stiff guide wire, and therefore, the tip of the guide wire should be positioned into the ECA (Figure 39.1a). After the diagnostic angiogram, a roadmap image of the carotid bifurcation is obtained, with a field of view that includes both the aortic arch and the skull base, and an angulation of the C-arm that allows maximum separation of the ECA and ICA. This projection not necessarily corresponds to the one that displays the stenosis with maximum severity. A large field of view will allow for a direct visual control of the diagnostic catheter while advancing the guide wire into the ECA and subsequently monitor the advancement of the catheter from the aortic arch into the CCA and ECA while monitoring the tip of the guide wire. In doing so optimal control over the equipment can be held. With the tip of the diagnostic catheter into one of the branches of the ECA, the standard 0.035 in. guide wire can be exchanged for a long (>260 cm) stiff (0.035 in. or 0.038 in.) guide wire that is left with its tip in a secure position in the ECA branch. Cannulation of the lingual branch of the ECA should be avoided, since perforation of this vessel may lead to (life-threatening) hematoma formation. Subsequently, the diagnostic catheter is removed, and at this point, either a (6F) long sheath with dilator (this technique is called the exchange technique) or an (8F) guiding catheter can be inserted (the so-called telescoping technique; Figure 39.1b). In order to avoid scraping of the (large-bore) guiding catheter (snow plough effect related to the presence of only a guide wire) against the

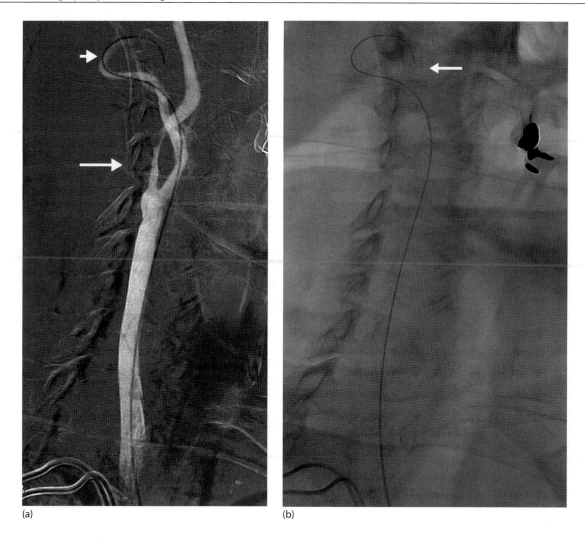

(a)   (b)

Figure 39.1 Roadmap image (a) demonstrating stenosis of internal carotid artery (arrow) and presence of exchange guide wire (arrowhead) in external carotid artery branch; fluoroscopic image with large field of view (b) allowing for monitoring of advancement of the long sheath/guiding catheter, without loss of visual control of guide wire tip (arrowhead).

vessel wall (distal aorta and aortic arch) and to facilitate entering of the guiding catheter into the origin of the CCA, the guiding catheter should be 'filled up' with a 5F 125 cm long diagnostic multipurpose catheter.[22] In extremely challenging cases (type III aortic arch), direct probing of the CCA using a specially shaped guiding catheter may be used, keeping however in mind that this carries a higher risk of dislodging atheroma from the aortic arch. Additional support during this procedure can be obtained by positioning an additional 0.014 in. guide wire ('buddy wire') into the ECA until the stent delivery system is in place. In cases where the ECA is highly stenotic or occluded, the telescoping technique is the preferred approach, taking care that the 0.035 in. guide wire is not crossing the ICA stenosis. The diagnostic catheter can be used for additional support, by letting it running well ahead of the tip of the guiding catheter. As an alternative on the right side, the subclavian artery can be used to position the stiff guide wire, and subsequently the guiding catheter or sheath can be advanced into the brachiocephalic trunk. After withdrawal of the

dilator or diagnostic catheter, a second guide wire can then be used to cannulate the CCA; the stiff wire is then withdrawn to the level of the bifurcation of the brachiocephalic trunk and advanced into the CCA. After withdrawal of the second guide wire, the dilator of long diagnostic catheter is reinserted and the whole system is advanced into the CCA.[23]

Continuous flushing with heparinized saline (using a pressure bag) of the sheath/guiding catheter should be initiated. In order to avoid/reduce blood loss through the lumen of the guiding catheter, a Y connector is connected to the guiding catheter. After securing proper flushing of either long sheath or guiding catheter, the system should be positioned in the distal CCA, with the tip 2–3 cm proximal to the carotid bifurcation. The dilator/diagnostic catheter is then removed together with the guide wire, taking care not to dislocate the position of the tip of the sheath/guiding catheter. Subsequently stenting of the ICA can be performed. The way to proceed at this point differs depending on whether a protection device is used and the type of EPD used.

CANNULATION OF THE ICA

Although most procedures are currently performed using EPDs, this section will initially describe the basic technique, using a guide wire only.

Procedure performed without EPD

After proper positioning of the 'working channel' in the distal segment of the CCA, a roadmap image is performed using a field of view that allows for visualization of the tip of the sheath/guiding catheter and the petrous part of the ICA (using the projection mentioned before displaying the origin of the ICA and stenosis). A steerable 0.014 in. guide wire with shapeable tip (a slight curve in the tip is made manually) is then inserted into the sheath/guiding catheter using a valve opener or short dilator (in order not to damage the tip). Selection of the wire depends on the tightness, location, length, angulation and eccentricity of the stenosis and on the anatomy of the carotid bifurcation. The tip of the guide wire is navigated through the stenosis under fluoroscopic control, taking care to 'steer away' the tip of the guide wire from the vessel wall/plaque. The flexible tip of the guide wire should be well advanced into the petrous part of the ICA (close to the skull base), and thus, the more rigid part of the guide wire will be beyond the stenosis, allowing for proper advancement of balloon catheters and stent. In complex stenoses, the use of a microcatheter can be of help in crossing the lesion by providing additional support to the guide wire.[24,25] After crossing of the lesion with the guide wire, predilation is performed using a small-diameter (2.5–3 mm) rapid-exchange angioplasty balloon, with a single, brief (<30 seconds) balloon inflation. Main goal of the predilation is to achieve a less traumatic crossing of the lesion with the stent delivery system, by creating a small channel. After removal of the angioplasty balloon, the stent delivery system is inserted and advanced under fluoroscopic guidance, using the previously made roadmap (no control angiography is performed after the predilation). The stent is then deployed according to the instructions for use of the manufacturer. Stent length should be chosen such that it allows for covering of the carotid artery at least 5 mm proximal and beyond the stenosis. Extreme elongation or kinks situated closely to the stenosis should also be taken into account when choosing the stent length in order to avoid relocation of arterial redundancy and increasing the amount of kinking. One must avoid placing the distal end of the stent into kinks and tortuosities of the ICA, because these kinks cannot be eliminated, are displaced distally and oftentimes will be aggravated.[26,27] The stent diameter should be oversized at least 1 mm to the reference vessel diameter (RVD). In case the stent needs to extend from the CCA into the ICA (covering the origin of the ECA), preferably tapered stents are used. At this point 0.5 mg of atropine is administered and subsequently postdilation is performed, using a rapid-exchange angioplasty balloon with a diameter equal to or slightly smaller than the RVD. Aggressive postdilation should be avoided, since this might lead to an increase in emboli (cheese grater effect). Some authors even advocate to not use postdilation at all.[28,29] Control angiography of the stented segment and intracranial series (to exclude any embolic branch occlusion) is performed using the guiding catheter/sheath. A residual stenosis of up to 30% can still be accepted. Likewise residual ulceration external to the stent is of no clinical importance.[30] The sheath is then removed, and hemostasis is typically obtained using an arterial closure device.

Procedure performed with distal EPD

Distal EPDs that are currently used are mainly filter-type devices, and these can be divided in mesh-like filters and filters that make use of a porous membrane and can be eccentric or concentric. Only in a minority of cases a distal balloon protection device is used. All filter-type EPDs allow for continuous antegrade flow throughout the procedure and are able to entrap medium- to large-sized particles (>100 μm in diameter). The devices are either premounted on a wire that comes with the delivery system (wire-mounted filters) or are inserted over a previously positioned guide wire (bare wire filters). The filter is placed in a way similar to the placement of a bare guide wire as described earlier. Predilation before passage of the filter is typically not performed. Care should be taken to deploy the filter in a segment of the ICA that is straight, in order to allow for proper wall appositioning of the filter (Figure 39.2).[25] Furthermore, the filter should be placed at a distance from the stenosis that allows the tip of the stent delivery system and distal part of the stent to cross the lesion (Figure 39.3). In case of severe tortuosity where the filter cannot be advanced, also here the use of an adjunctive wire ('buddy wire') will help in straightening out the ICA, thus facilitating passage of the protection device.[25] After deployment of the distal EPD, stent placement can be performed as described earlier. After stent placement, the EPD is retrieved using a specific retrieval catheter that allows for closing and withdrawal of the filter. Care should be taken when traversing the stent that the retrieval device does not get entangled in the stent struts. This risk is higher in stents with an open-cell design.

Procedure performed with proximal EPD

The working principle of proximal protection devices is by either completely interrupting or reversing the blood flow in the ICA, and in this way 'endovascular clamping' can be obtained. They rely on the vascular anastomoses of the circle of Willis. These devices cannot be used in all cases because complete flow occlusion/reversal is not tolerated by 6%–10% of patients. Embolic particles of all sizes can be captured, and the systems offer the advantage that the stenosis of the ICA is only crossed once the protection device is in place, and thus, all manipulation needed to cross the lesion is performed during protection. The currently available devices all create an occlusion of the ECA and ICA with two separate balloons.

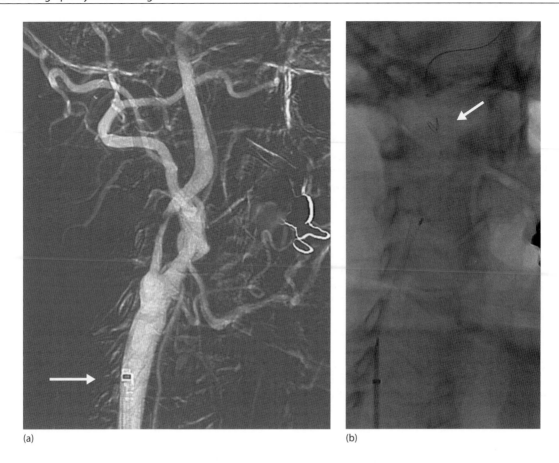

(a)

(b)

Figure 39.2 Roadmap image (a) of same patient as in Figure 39.1, after advancement of sheath (arrow) into distal common carotid artery; fluoroscopic image (b) after placement of filter-type embolic protection device (arrow).

The first system (Mo.Ma; Medtronic-Invatec) consists of an 8F or 9F sheath that provides an effective working channel of 5F or 6F, respectively, and two balloons that can be inflated independently. The distal balloon is located close to the sheath tip and aims to occlude the external carotid artery. The proximal balloon is located on the body of the sheath and is to be inflated at the level of the common carotid artery. When inflated, both balloons prevent antegrade flow from the CCA and retrograde flow from the ECA leading to complete flow blockage (Figure 39.4). The device is advanced into the ECA. The distal ECA balloon should be placed proximal to the origin of the superior thyroid artery in order to provide an adequate flow interruption/reversal. Once the device is in place, the stenting procedure can be performed along the aforementioned guidelines. After the lesion is treated, three 20 mL syringes of carotid blood are aspirated and checked for debris before deflating the distal and then the proximal balloons, re-establishing cerebral blood flow. Moratto et al. have described a modification of this standard technique.[7] Their approach (which can only be used in the absence of signs of clamping intolerance) features a second low-pressure (4 ATM) inflation of the postdilation balloon to mobilize any unstable protruding plaque. While the cerebral flow is blocked by the postdilation balloon, the occluding balloons in the ECA

and CCA are deflated for 5–10 seconds, allowing blood to flow into the ECA. Any plaque freed by the second balloon inflation would be flushed through the ECA and aspirated. The occluding balloons are then reinflated and the postdilation balloon is deflated and removed. A second aspiration is performed, checking for the absence of debris prior to reconstituting blood flow and removing the protection device.

The second commercially available system is the NeuroProtection System (WL Gore and Associates). The system is composed of a 9F sheath with an effective working lumen of 6F and an inflatable balloon at its tip and a separate balloon wire. After positioning of the sheath in the common carotid artery, the balloon wire is inserted and placed in the proximal segment of the ECA (as with the Mo.Ma device). Both balloons are subsequently inflated, leading to flow blockage. After this the proximal part of the sheath is connected to the contralateral femoral vein. This allows for blood flow reversal of blood from the cerebral circulation (i.e. the circle of Willis) down the ICA and the sheath into the venous system. The blood flows through a filter with a pore size of 180 μm. Contrary to the Mo.Ma system (where complete blockage of flow is obtained), the procedure is performed in reverse flow mode. As with the Mo.Ma device at the end of the procedure, 10–20 mL of carotid blood is aspirated before balloon deflation.

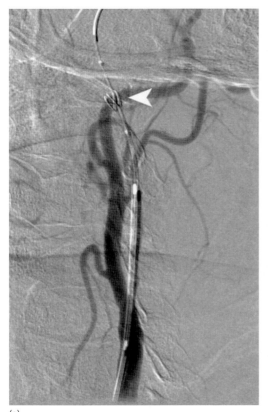
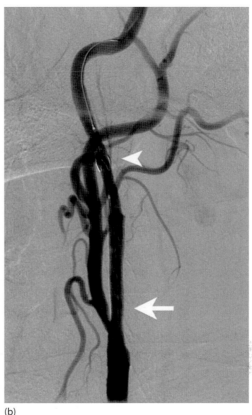

(a)   (b)

Figure 39.3 Digital subtraction angiography image after placement of filter-type protection device (arrowhead) and insertion of stent delivery system (a); note occlusion of the internal carotid artery due to the presence of the stent delivery system; control angiography after stent deployment and postdilation; embolic protection device (arrowhead) still in place, minimal residual stenosis (arrow) that does not require further angioplasty (b).

One of the theoretical advantages is that use of proximal protection devices would allow the use of (more flexible) open-cell stents (with a potentially higher embolic risk; see 'Choice of EPD' section) in elderly patients who frequently present with tortuous anatomy (which precludes the use of closed-cell stents that typically are more rigid and cannot be navigated as easily through tortuous anatomy). Furthermore, it can reduce the risk of arterial spasm, dissection or intimal damage. A disadvantage of this technique includes the larger sheath size required, which may be problematic in patients with advanced peripheral arterial disease and may be associated with an increased rate of vascular access complications.[19] Proximal protection is also contraindicated in patients with severe external or CCA disease.

A theoretical disadvantage is the possibility of retinal embolization at the point where the ECA balloon of the protection device is deflated, especially since collateral pathways from the ECA across the ophthalmic artery are widely open.

Choice of EPD

Each type of protection device has its advantages and disadvantages, with specific recommendations for their use.[31] Advantages of filter-type devices are that they allow antegrade flow preservation, permit real-time debris capture and allow for angiography during the procedure. Disadvantages are the higher crossing profile and a higher stiffness (which may not allow use in tortuous vessel), the risk of getting occluded with debris during the procedure and the risk of entanglement in the stent upon retrieval of the filter. Proximal protection devices on the other hand can avoid embolization during the stent deployment and balloon angioplasty, allow for the use of a guide wire of choice and protect also during crossing of the lesion. Downsides of these devices are the larger sheath size, risk of intimal damage to the CCA, potential intolerance of the patient to occlusion or flow reversal and the inability to perform angiography throughout the procedure.

It is still not clear whether CAS should be performed with embolic protection or not and, if protection devices are being used, which type of protection is the best. Randomized data are lacking.[32] A systematic review that evaluated a total of 71 papers published between 2006 and 2011 concluded that the intraprocedural use of EPDs did not demonstrate a consistent relationship with 1 month stroke and/or death.[33] In a substudy of the ICSS trial, it was found that protection devices do not seem to be effective in preventing cerebral ischemia

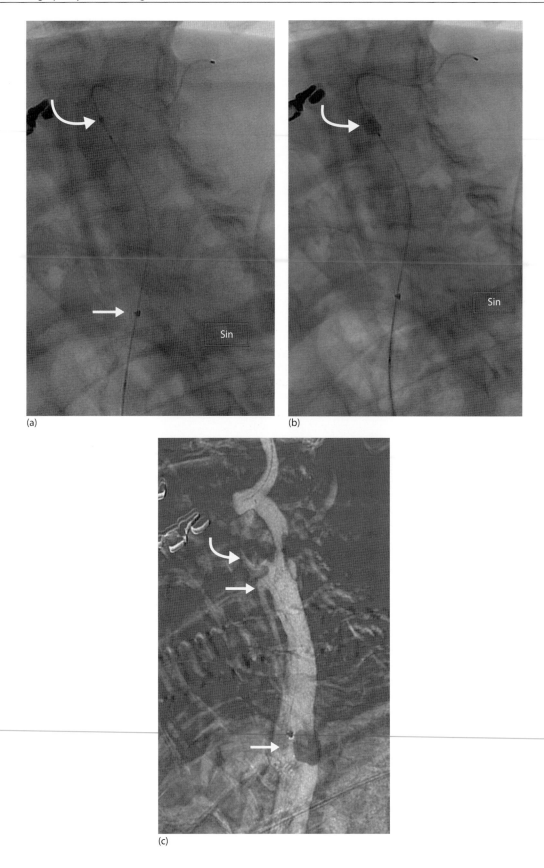

Figure 39.4 Fluoroscopic image after positioning of proximal protection device Mo.Ma (a), distal balloon marker (curved arrow) positioned in the proximal part of the external carotid artery, distal part of sheath in common carotid artery (arrow); fluoroscopic image (b) after inflation of distal balloon (curved arrow); roadmap image (c) obtained after inflation of distal balloon (curved arrow), showing low origin of superior thyroid artery, not completely occluded (arrowhead) and proximal balloon inflated (arrow)..

during stenting.[34] Similarly data from a large registry showed there was no significant difference in rates of MAE between the group where no (filter-type) embolic protection was used and those where filter-type embolic protection was used, although the patients in the unprotected group had a worse baseline neurological risk.[35] Finally, the Cochrane Review on stenting for symptomatic carotid artery stenosis (based on the outcomes of EVA-3S, SPACE and ICSS)[36] concluded that for the outcome of death or any stroke within 30 days after treatment, there are no indications that the use of embolic protection (with filter-type devices) is beneficial (*level 1 evidence*). In this review it was mentioned that only in the EVA-3S trial a positive effect was seen on outcome. As EVA-3S, also other studies indicate a beneficial effect.[31,32] Most operators currently use protection devices during carotid stent procedures, and choice of the type of device is mainly based on personal preference and the experience with a specific device. The use of proximal protection devices is typically perceived as more cumbersome. However, recent data, including a meta-analysis, indicate that with the use of proximal protection devices, the number of embolic events, micro-embolic signal on transcranial Doppler or new lesions on DW-MRI per patient can be significantly reduced.[37–41]

Given the diversity of reported outcomes with various devices (oftentimes not relating outcome to preprocedural neurological status), no definite answer to the question of which type of protection device to use can be given. There are indications that the choice of the protection device can be made by using plaque and anatomical characteristics (*level 2 evidence*).[42] The anatomic features that influence the choice of proximal protection are patency/presence of stenosis of the external and common carotid arteries as well as features of unstable plaque (irregular or ulcerated appearance of the plaque, heterogeneous plaque, intraplaque hemorrhage, presence of intraluminal thrombus). The feature that influences the choice of filter-type protection is tortuosity of the ICA beyond the lesion. Implementing these selection criteria, both approaches can be equally safe and effective.[42]

Choice of stent

Given the high probability of the presence of an unstable plaque (especially in recently symptomatic patients), the choice of stent is important, and in general a stent that provides better scaffolding is preferred by most operators. This preference is supported by data coming from an evaluation of filter content in procedures performed with either open- or closed-cell design stents: a larger mean particle size was seen with the use of open-cell design stents.[43] In this study, no difference in procedural outcome was seen. Similarly, in a small randomized trial of open-versus closed-cell design stents for CAS (with filter-type embolic protection), no difference in findings at TCD or DW-MRI could be demonstrated.[44] Data on

clinical outcome in the literature, however, remain non-equivocal. One study included 1684 consecutive patients (1010 asymptomatic, 674 symptomatic) from 10 centres.[45] CAS was performed with either closed-cell (51%) or open-cell (49%) design stents. Combined transient ischemic attack, stroke or death rates and stroke or death rates within 30 days of treatment were 6.1% and 3.1% for the closed-cell design versus 4.1% and 2.4% for the open-cell design stents (not statistically significant), respectively. No significant differences in asymptomatic and symptomatic patients were seen. Both by separate analysis and by propensity score–adjusted multivariable analysis, the open-cell carotid stent design was not associated with a differential risk for combined acute and subacute neurological complications compared with closed-cell stents. However, another study evaluated retrospectively 3179 consecutive CAS patients for the distribution of neurological complications as related to different stent types and designs. The postprocedural event rate analyzed for different stents varied from 1.2% using a closed-cell-type stent to 5.9% using an open-cell-type stent. The late event rates were significantly lower for free cell areas <2.5 mm (1.2%) as compared to free cell areas >7.5 mm (3.4%). The postprocedural event rate was 1.3% for closed cells and 3.4% for open cells. These differences were more pronounced in symptomatic patients.[46]

The evidence from some registries and randomized trials indicates that neurological events are less frequently occurring in cases where closed-cell design stents are used (*level 2 evidence*).[47]

PHARMACOTHERAPY AROUND CAS

Anticoagulation and antiplatelet therapy

During the procedure, anticoagulation should be administered in order to reduce the risk of thromboembolism that is related to the presence of intra-arterial sheaths, catheters and guide wires. Usually a bolus of heparin is given. The required dose of heparin ranges from 75 to 100 units/kg. In a standard patient a single dose of 5000–7500 units will be sufficient to provide adequate coverage throughout the entire CAS procedure (that should not take more than 45 minutes), and therefore, ACT measurement is not routinely performed. The effect of heparin is generally allowed to subside in a physiological way, and protamine sulphate reversal is not performed.

As in other vascular territories, arterial stenting causes endothelial and intimal damage and platelet adhesion, activation and aggregation and thus predisposes to thrombus formation and increases the risk of embolization.[48,49] This risk, in addition to the potential risk of (late) embolization to the brain, provides a rationale for early antiplatelet therapy with CAS.[50] Combination therapy of clopidogrel with aspirin has been demonstrated to be effective in decreasing the incidence of adverse neurological events after CEA and CAS as compared to monotherapy using aspirin without increasing the incidence of hemorrhagic complications (*level 1 evidence*).[51–54] Dual antiplatelet therapy should be commenced at least 3 days prior to the procedure. Aspirin dosage should be in the range of 75–150 mg daily, while clopidogrel should be dosed at 75 mg/day. In cases where treatment is planned in a more expedite manner (<3 days), typically a loading dose of clopidogrel (>300 mg) at least 6 hours prior to the procedure is given. Dose and regimen of other agents used for CAS are not established.[55]

In addition to this, one randomized trial involving TIA patients (also those not operated on) found that the combination of aspirin and clopidogrel significantly reduces the early risk of recurrent stroke,[56] so this should be considered in all patients.

Hypotension and asystole

During CAS procedures, hemodynamic changes are very common, with an incidence of bradycardia of 20%, hypotension of 30% and asystole as high as 17%. Adverse cerebral outcome is associated with angioplasty-induced hypotension and/or asystole,[57–59] and prolonged hemodynamic depression is associated with an increased risk of major adverse neurological events.[60] Prevention of hemodynamic instability consists of sufficient volume expansion (administration of 1 L of fluid intravenously prior to the procedure) and pharmacological support using either atropine or isoprenaline during pre-dilatation and stent tailoring. Atropine is a muscarinic antagonist and abolishes the effect of acetylcholine. It does not have an effect on the sympathetic system and causes only a modest tachycardia (80–90 beats/minutes). Isoprenaline is a β-adrenergic agonist and therefore has an advantage over atropine, since it stimulates both the heart rate and contractility of the heart by stimulating β1-receptors in the heart. In cases where hemodynamic instability persists despite the aforementioned measures, placement of a temporary transvenous pacemaker should be considered. Other causes of hypotension (e.g. retroperitoneal bleeding related to the arterial access) should be ruled out.

Hyperperfusion and hypertension

Hyperperfusion syndrome is a rare and potentially devastating entity and is a recognized complication of carotid endarterectomy. The syndrome is thought to be a failure of normal cerebral autoregulation of blood flow as a result of long-standing low perfusion pressure. Risk factors identified for the development of a hyperperfusion syndrome include severe ipsilateral stenosis, absence of collateral flow, periprocedural hypertension and the use of anticoagulative agents. Case reports of cerebral hyperperfusion injury following ICA angioplasty and stenting are few, thus suggesting a low incidence. However, two reports describe a higher incidence after stenting of up to 5% as compared to endarterectomy. Intracranial flow velocities are typically more than double. Patients most commonly complain of headache, although stroke-like signs due to edema may also occur. Major risk is the development of intracerebral hemorrhage with or without seizures. Therapy consists of lowering of blood pressure. The impairment of cerebrovascular autoregulation is more severe in the acute stroke stage. As clinical findings in cerebral hyperperfusion may be difficult to differentiate from those in cerebral ischemia, strict monitoring for evidence of hyperperfusion is necessary for at least the first 7 days after the procedure. Signs suggestive of hyperperfusion are an indication for aggressive blood pressure control even in the acute ischemic stage. Also hypertension associated with carotid baroreceptor or microvascular failure at the level of the blood–brain barrier reflecting perfusion breakthrough into a recent infarct or spontaneous hemorrhagic conversion caused by showers of microemboli may occur after stent placement.

Spasm

Spasm can occur during any procedure in the carotid artery. It has been seen in procedures using balloon-expandable stents as well as in patients where self-expanding stents are used.[61,62] Spasm seems to occur more frequently in cases where EPDs are used.[63] Transcranial Doppler monitoring is useful in the early detection of flow reduction caused by spasm[64,65] and may be used in the evaluation of whether or not flow impairment is severe enough to warrant therapy.[65] The majority of cases of spasm of the ICA is self-limiting.[66] Treatment is only necessary in cases of flow-limiting spasm and consists of the administration of vasodilating drugs intra-arterially, either nitroglycerin (100–200 μg) or nimodipine (200 μg diluted in a 10 mL solution injected slowly as a 2–3 mL bolus, or even dosage as high as 0.5–1 mg).[26,61,63,67–69] In cases where the EPD seems to be the culprit of the spasm, advancing the device or moving the device more proximally in order to eliminate the focal trigger for spasm may be useful.[63]

MONITORING AROUND CAS

During the procedure, neurological status, electrocardiogram, heart rate and blood pressure should be monitored. Blood pressure is measured preferably intra-arterially, by connecting a pressure sensing system to one of the side ports of the flush system that is connected to the long introducer sheath or guiding catheter. Neurological status is monitored by asking on a regular basis to the patient (i.e. after each step of the procedure) to squeeze a squeezing toy.[70] To adequately monitor neurological status, it is of importance to perform the procedure without sedation.[25] After the procedure, it is advised to monitor the patient in an intensive care unit or stroke unit for at least 6 hours. Special attention should be given to maintaining the blood pressure at a level 10%–20% below the baseline pressure, in order to prevent cerebral reperfusion injury.[30] A regular check of the neurological status should be made, and the presence of headache should be asked for. The latter may be an indication of the development of a hyperperfusion syndrome.

MANAGEMENT OF COMPLICATIONS

Although relatively rare, basic knowledge of neuro-rescue techniques should be acquired to be able to deal with complications. It is beyond the scope of this chapter to describe in detail the treatment of embolic complications, thrombosis and dissection. The reader is referred to an article from the Carotid Masterclass series in the EJVES (Open Access) on this subject.[71]

Overview of results of RCTs and current guidelines

Between 1995 and 2010, a total of 13 trials have been performed, randomizing more than 7000 patients to CAS versus CEA. These trials have been subject of a systematic review and meta-analysis recently.[72,73]

The first meta-analysis[72] evaluated 13 trials containing 7501 patients. The risk of stroke or death within 30 days was higher after CAS than CEA especially in previously symptomatic patients. It was found that at 1 year, the risk of stroke or death of both techniques was comparable. In a subgroup analysis, the risk of death and disabling stroke at 30 days did not differ significantly between CEA and CAS, whereas the rate of non-disabling stroke within 30 days was much higher in the CAS. The risks of myocardial infarction within 30 days and 1 year were significantly less for CAS.

The second meta-analysis[73] analyzed a slightly lower number of patients (3723 carotid endarterectomy and 3754 CAS patients, for a total of 7477). Regarding short-term outcomes, CAS was associated with a higher risk for stroke and 'death or stroke'. CAS also showed a marginal trend towards higher death and 'death or disabling stroke' rates. Carotid endarterectomy presented with higher rates of myocardial infarction and cranial nerve injury. Concerning long-term outcomes, the authors concluded that CAS was associated with higher rates of stroke and 'death or stroke'. Unlike the first study mentioned, no differentiation between disabling and non-disabling stroke was made. The difference in long-term stroke rates was more evident in patients over 68 years of age, while little difference was seen in patients younger than <68 years.

In all trials the efficacy of CAS and CEA with regard to ipsilateral stroke prevention, restenosis rates and need for repeat revascularization was similar.

More than half (7/13) of these trials are mainly of historic interest and/or have included small numbers of patients. The remaining six (more recent) trials have randomized a total of 6780 patients to CAS versus CEA and will be discussed here in more detail. The SAPPHIRE trial included both symptomatic and asymptomatic patients at high surgical risk.[74] Four trials included symptomatic patients with standard surgical risk (CAVATAS, SPACE, EVA-3S and ICSS).[75–78] The last trial (CREST) enrolled both symptomatic and asymptomatic patients at standard surgical risk.[79]

CAVATAS TRIAL[75,80]

This study was performed at the end of the twentieth century and randomized a total of 504 symptomatic patients.

Being one of the earliest studies, no dedicated stents and balloons/protection devices were available. In the endovascular arm, only 26% of patients were treated with stenting, using a balloon-expandable stent. The incidence of death or stroke at 30 days was 10.0% in the endovascular group and 9.9% in the surgical group. At 8 years, no difference in ipsilateral stroke, ipsilateral stroke or transient ischemic attack or any stroke between the two arms was seen. Although this trial demonstrated equivalence of both techniques, the results cannot be extrapolated to the current status of stenting and endarterectomy. Furthermore, the complication rate in both treatment arms is considered too high for current standards.

SAPPHIRE STUDY[74,81]

This study randomized 334 patients with a high surgical risk for surgery to CAS with the use of EPD or CEA. The majority of patients were asymptomatic (71%). In this study, a composite primary endpoint was chosen (death, stroke or myocardial infarction within 30 days after the intervention or death or ipsilateral stroke between 31 days and 1 year). There was a trend to better outcome in the CAS group (primary endpoint 12.2% vs. 20.1%, p = 0.053) and a significantly lower occurrence at 30 days of myocardial infarction (1.9% vs. 6.6%, p = 0.04). At 3-year follow-up, CAS and CEA had the same efficacy in terms of stroke prevention.

SPACE TRIAL[76,82]

This study was designed as a non-inferiority study of CAS (with or without EPD) versus CEA in patients with recent symptomatic carotid artery stenosis (treatment up to 180 days after onset of symptoms). The primary endpoint was ipsilateral ischemic stroke or death from time of randomization to 30 days after the procedure. A total of 1200 patients were included with 1183 patients available for analysis (in the 2-year follow-up, a total of 1214 patients were evaluated). The difference between rate of death and ipsilateral ischemic stroke from randomization to 30 days after the procedure was 6.84% with CAS and 6.34% with carotid endarterectomy (absolute difference 0.51%, 90% CI −1.89% to 2.91%), and thus, this trial failed to prove non-inferiority of CAS compared with carotid endarterectomy for the complication rate in the periprocedural period. At 2 years follow-up, an intention-to-treat and per-protocol analysis of the Kaplan–Meier estimates of ipsilateral ischemic strokes was performed. No difference between any periprocedural stroke or death was found between the two groups. In both analyses recurrent stenosis of 70% or more was found to be significantly more frequent in the CAS group compared with the carotid endarterectomy group.

EVA-3S TRIAL[77,83,84]

This study included 527 patients with a symptomatic carotid stenosis of at least 60%, with as primary endpoint the incidence of any stroke or death within 30 days after treatment. EPDs were not used in all cases. The trial was stopped prematurely because of safety issues. At 30 days and 6 months, the incidence of any stroke or death was 3.9% and 6.1% after CEA and 9.6% and 11.7% after CAS, respectively. The 30-day incidence of disabling stroke or death was 1.5% after endarterectomy and 3.4% after stenting. At 4 years the cumulative probability of periprocedural stroke or death and non-procedural ipsilateral stroke was higher with stenting than with endarterectomy, but this difference could be accounted for almost completely by the higher periprocedural (within 30 days of the procedure) risk of stenting compared with endarterectomy. Beyond this period, the risk of ipsilateral stroke was low and similar in both treatment groups. A late follow-up (median 7.1 years) showed that there was still no difference between the treatment groups in the rates of ipsilateral stroke beyond the procedural period. In addition to this, it was also found that severe carotid restenosis (≥70%) or occlusion, death, myocardial infarction and revascularization procedures occurred at equal rates in both groups.

ICSS TRIAL[78,85]

The ICSS trial enrolled 1713 patients, with the 3-year rate of fatal or disabling stroke in any territory as primary outcome. The first report presented the 120-day rate of stroke, death and/or myocardial infarction as part of an interim safety analysis by intention to treat. The incidence of stroke, death or procedural myocardial infarction was 8.5% in the stenting group (with or without EPD) compared with 5.2% in the endarterectomy group. The incidence of disabling stroke or death at 120 days did not show a significant difference (4.0% in the CAS group and 3.2% events in the CEA), but the risk of any stroke was higher in the stenting group than in the endarterectomy group. At long-term follow-up (median 4.2 years), the number of fatal or disabling strokes did not show a statistically significant difference between CAS and CEA (6.4% vs. 6.5%). It was found however that the excess of strokes in the CAS arm persisted, with a 5-year cumulative risk of 15.2% versus 9.4% in the CEA group. This difference did not translate into differences in functional disability and quality of life.

CREST TRIAL[79]

The CREST trial is the largest of the trials described here and randomized 2502 symptomatic and asymptomatic patients to CAS (all performed with EPDs) or CEA. This study also had a primary composite endpoint (stroke, MI or death from any cause during the periprocedural period or ipsilateral stroke within 4 years after randomization).

After a median follow-up period of 2.5 years, there was no significant difference in the estimated 4-year rates of the primary endpoint between CAS (7.2%) and CEA (6.8%), a difference that was not statistically significant. There was no differential treatment effect with regard to the primary endpoint according to symptomatic status or sex. The 4-year rate of stroke or death

was 6.4% with CAS and 4.7% with CEA. These rates were higher for symptomatic patients (8.0% and 6.4%, respectively) and lower for asymptomatic patients (4.5% and 2.7%, respectively; all differences were not statistically significant). Periprocedural rates of single components of the endpoints showed a difference between the CAS group and the CEA group: for death (0.7% vs. 0.3%, p = 0.18), for stroke (4.1% vs. 2.3%, p = 0.01) and for myocardial infarction (1.1% vs. 2.3%, p = 0.03). Beyond the periprocedural period, the incidence of ipsilateral stroke with stenting and with endarterectomy was similar (2.0% and 2.4%, respectively). A secondary analysis[86] showed that in the second half of the study, the rate of stroke in the CAS arm, but not in the CEA arm, showed a significant reduction. This finding might be explained by the presence of a learning curve effect in the endovascular arm (despite stringent selection criteria for the centres and operators that were allowed to enrol patients for treatment with CAS). The incidence of restenosis was low, and no difference between CAS and CEA was reported.[87]

None of the most recent and large trials was able to demonstrate non-inferiority or superiority of CAS in symptomatic patients. Strong advocates of CAS have argued that there were major flaws in trial design and operator experience (amongst others), and this is subject of an ongoing debate.[88] It has become clear though that CAS most probably needs technical improvements in order to make the procedure safer than it currently is (see aforementioned: stent design and optimization of embolic protection). It has also become clear that patient selection is of utmost importance, and the following categories have been identified as those benefitting most from an endovascular procedure.

A pre-planned evaluation of three large European trials (EVA-3S, SPACE and ICSS),[89] which by themselves were underpowered for investigation of specific patient subgroups, identified the following. Of all subgroup variables assessed, only age significantly modified the effect of treatment: in patients younger than 70 years, the estimated 120-day risk of stroke or death was of the same order in the carotid stenting group as in the carotid endarterectomy group. However, in patients older than 70 years, the estimated risk with carotid stenting was double the risk of that with carotid endarterectomy. This was the case for both the per-protocol and intention-to-treat analysis.

Another evaluation of these three trials revealed that operator lifetime CAS experience and general stenting experience did not influence the 30-day risk of stroke or death.[90] It showed however that annual volume plays a more important role (low annual volume doubles the risk as compared to higher annual volume), and therefore, it was concluded that carotid stenting should only be performed by operators with an annual procedure volume of more than six cases per year.

The last study that emerged from this pooled analysis investigated the effects of sex, contralateral occlusion, age and restenosis on the procedural risk of stroke or death.[91] It was found that patients with contralateral occlusion or restenosis and women younger than 75 years are at a relatively low risk of perioperative stroke or death when using CAS (similar to the risk in this group of patients with CEA [*level 1 evidence*]).

CONCLUSION

The initial enthusiasm for CAS has subsided after the publication of the results of various randomized controlled trials. It has become clear from these trials that meticulous technique and proper patient selection is of utmost importance. By taking this into account, CAS can be performed as safely as CEA. Data on new devices like mesh-covered stents and cervical access are eagerly awaited.

Key points

- CAS should only be performed by operators with an annual volume of >6 cases per year.
- It remains unclear which is the best endovascular technique to be used in CAS.
- CAS can be performed as safely as CEA in patients with contralateral occlusion or restenosis and women younger than 75 years.

DEFICIENCIES IN CURRENT KNOWLEDGE AND DIRECTIONS FOR FUTURE RESEARCH

- No large, multicentre randomized trials are available that compare various stent designs and the use of EPDs (none, distal or proximal).
- Future research should focus on ways to make CAS safer and more widely applicable.

KEY REFERENCES

1. Macdonald S, Lee R, Williams R, Stansby G. Towards safer carotid artery stenting: A scoring system for anatomic suitability. *Stroke.* 2009 May;40(5):1698–1703.
2. Bonati LH, Lyrer P, Ederle J, Featherstone R, Brown MM. Percutaneous transluminal balloon angioplasty and stenting for carotid artery stenosis. *Cochrane Database Syst Rev.* 2012;9:CD000515.
3. Stabile E, Sannino A, Schiattarella GG et al. Cerebral embolic lesions detected with diffusion-weighted magnetic resonance imaging following carotid artery stenting: A meta-analysis of 8 studies comparing filter cerebral protection and proximal balloon occlusion. *JACC Cardiovasc Interv.* 2014 October;7(10):1177–1183.
4. Schillinger M, Gschwendtner M, Reimers B et al. Does carotid stent cell design matter? *Stroke.* 2008 March;39(3):905–909.
5. van den Berg JC. Neuro-rescue during carotid stenting. *Eur J Vasc Endovasc Surg.* 2008 December; 36(6):627–636.

REFERENCES

1. Rothwell PM, Eliasziw M, Gutnikov SA, Warlow CP, Barnett HJ. Endarterectomy for symptomatic carotid stenosis in relation to clinical subgroups and timing of surgery. *Lancet.* 2004 March 20;363(9413):915–924.
2. Ois A, Cuadrado-Godia E, Rodriguez-Campello A, Jimenez-Conde J, Roquer J. High risk of early neurological recurrence in symptomatic carotid stenosis. *Stroke.* 2009 August;40(8):2727–2731.
3. Fairhead JF, Mehta Z, Rothwell PM. Population-based study of delays in carotid imaging and surgery and the risk of recurrent stroke. *Neurology.* 2005 August 9;65(3):371–375.
4. Stromberg S, Gelin J, Osterberg T, Bergstrom GM, Karlstrom L, Osterberg K. Very urgent carotid endarterectomy confers increased procedural risk. *Stroke.* 2012 May;43(5):1331–1335.
5. Naylor AR. Time is brain! *Surgeon.* 2007 February;5(1):23–30.
6. Sharpe R, Sayers RD, London NJ et al. Procedural risk following carotid endarterectomy in the hyperacute period after onset of symptoms. *Eur J Vasc Endovasc Surg.* 2013 November;46(5):519–524.
7. Moratto R, Veronesi J, Silingardi R et al. Urgent carotid artery stenting with technical modifications for patients with transient ischemic attacks and minor stroke. *J Endovasc Ther.* 2012 October;19(5):627–635.
8. Rerkasem K, Rothwell PM. Systematic review of the operative risks of carotid endarterectomy for recently symptomatic stenosis in relation to the timing of surgery. *Stroke.* 2009 October;40(10):e564–e572.
9. Capoccia L, Sbarigia E, Speziale F et al. The need for emergency surgical treatment in carotid-related stroke in evolution and crescendo transient ischemic attack. *J Vasc Surg.* 2012 June;55(6):1611–1617.
10. Imai K, Mori T, Izumoto H, Watanabe M, Majima K. Emergency carotid artery stent placement in patients with acute ischemic stroke. *Am J Neuroradiol.* 2005 May;26(5):1249–1258.
11. Avgerinos ED, Brountzos EN, Ptohis N, Giannakopoulos T, Papapetrou A, Liapis CD. Urgent CAS for patients in high neurologic risk. *J Cardiovasc Surg (Torino).* 2009 December;50(6):761–766.
12. Rantner B, Goebel G, Bonati LH, Ringleb PA, Mas JL, Fraedrich G. The risk of carotid artery stenting compared with carotid endarterectomy is greatest in patients treated within 7 days of symptoms. *J Vasc Surg.* 2013 March;57(3):619–626.
13. Setacci C, de DG, Chisci E, Setacci F. Carotid artery stenting in recently symptomatic patients: A single center experience. *Ann Vasc Surg.* 2010 May;24(4):474–479.
14. Setacci C, de DG, Setacci F et al. Carotid artery stenting in recently symptomatic patients. *J Cardiovasc Surg (Torino).* 2013 February;54(1):61–66.

15. Randoux B, Marro B, Koskas F et al. Carotid artery stenosis: Prospective comparison of CT, three-dimensional gadolinium-enhanced MR, and conventional angiography. *Radiology*. 2001 July;220(1):179–185.

16. Chong PL, Salhiyyah K, Dodd PD. The role of carotid endarterectomy in the endovascular era. *Eur J Vasc Endovasc Surg*. 2005 June;29(6):597–600.

17. Macdonald S, Lee R, Williams R, Stansby G. Towards safer carotid artery stenting: A scoring system for anatomic suitability. *Stroke*. 2009 May;40(5):1698–1703.

18. Naggara O, Touze E, Beyssen B et al. Anatomical and technical factors associated with stroke or death during carotid angioplasty and stenting: Results from the endarterectomy versus angioplasty in patients with symptomatic severe carotid stenosis (EVA-3S) trial and systematic review. *Stroke*. 2011 February;42(2):380–388.

19. Cremonesi A, Castriota F, Secco GG, Macdonald S, Roffi M. Carotid artery stenting: An update. *Eur Heart J*. 2015 January 1;36(1):13–21.

20. Mathieu X, Piret V, Bergeron P, Petrosyan A, Abdulamit T, Trastour JC. Choice of access for percutaneous carotid angioplasty and stenting: A comparative study on cervical and femoral access. *J Cardiovasc Surg (Torino)*. 2009 October;50(5):677–681.

21. Pinter L, Ribo M, Loh C et al. Safety and feasibility of a novel transcervical access neuroprotection system for carotid artery stenting in the PROOF Study. *J Vasc Surg*. 2011 November;54(5):1317–1323.

22. Kim HJ, Lee HJ, Yang JH et al. The influence of carotid artery catheterization technique on the incidence of thromboembolism during carotid artery stenting. *Am J Neuroradiol*. 2010 October;31(9):1732–1736.

23. Gupta K, Biria M, Mortazavi A. A modified technique for carotid cannulation via the transfemoral approach, during angioplasty and stent placement. *Tex Heart Inst J*. 2008;35(3):286–288.

24. van den Berg JC, Moll FL. Microcatheter technique assists stenting of complex carotid stenoses. *J Endovasc Ther*. 2002 June;9(3):381–383.

25. Maleux G, Heye S. Carotid intervention 2: Technical considerations. *Semin Intervent Radiol*. 2007 June;24(2):226–233.

26. Vitek JJ, Roubin GS, Al-Mubarek N, New G, Iyer SS. Carotid artery stenting: Technical considerations. *Am J Neuroradiol*. 2000 October;21(9):1736–1743.

27. Vos JA, Vos AW, Linsen MA et al. Impact of head movements on morphology and flow in the internal carotid artery after carotid angioplasty and stenting versus endarterectomy. *J Vasc Surg*. 2005 March;41(3):469–475.

28. Baldi S, Zander T, Rabellino M, Gonzalez G, Maynar M. Carotid artery stenting without angioplasty and cerebral protection: A single-center experience with up to 7 years' follow-up. *Am J Neuroradiol*. 2011 April;32(4):759–763.

29. Maynar M, Baldi S, Rostagno R et al. Carotid stenting without use of balloon angioplasty and distal protection devices: Preliminary experience in 100 cases. *Am J Neuroradiol*. 2007 August;28(7):1378–1383.

30. Phatouros CC, Higashida RT, Malek AM et al. Carotid artery stent placement for atherosclerotic disease: Rationale, technique, and current status. *Radiology*. 2000 October;217(1):26–41.

31. Mousa AY, Campbell JE, AbuRahma AF, Bates MC. Current update of cerebral embolic protection devices. *J Vasc Surg*. 2012 November;56(5):1429–1437.

32. Knur R. Technique and clinical evidence of neuroprotection in carotid artery stenting. *Vasa*. 2014 March;43(2):100–112.

33. Khan M, Qureshi AI. Factors associated with increased rates of post-procedural stroke or death following carotid artery stent placement: A systematic review. *J Vasc Interv Neurol*. 2014 May;7(1):11–20.

34. Bonati LH, Jongen LM, Haller S et al. New ischaemic brain lesions on MRI after stenting or endarterectomy for symptomatic carotid stenosis: A substudy of the International Carotid Stenting Study (ICSS). *Lancet Neurol*. 2010 April;9(4):353–362.

35. Giri J, Yeh RW, Kennedy KF et al. Unprotected carotid artery stenting in modern practice. *Catheter Cardiovasc Interv*. 2014 March 1;83(4):595–602.

36. Bonati LH, Lyrer P, Ederle J, Featherstone R, Brown MM. Percutaneous transluminal balloon angioplasty and stenting for carotid artery stenosis. *Cochrane Database Syst Rev*. 2012;9:CD000515.

37. Stabile E, Sannino A, Schiattarella GG et al. Cerebral embolic lesions detected with diffusion-weighted magnetic resonance imaging following carotid artery stenting: A meta-analysis of 8 studies comparing filter cerebral protection and proximal balloon occlusion. *JACC Cardiovasc Interv*. 2014 October;7(10):1177–1183.

38. Bijuklic K, Wandler A, Hazizi F, Schofer J. The PROFI study (Prevention of Cerebral Embolization by Proximal Balloon Occlusion Compared to Filter Protection During Carotid Artery Stenting): A prospective randomized trial. *J Am Coll Cardiol*. 2012 April 10;59(15):1383–1389.

39. Cano MN, Kambara AM, de Cano SJ et al. Randomized comparison of distal and proximal cerebral protection during carotid artery stenting. *JACC Cardiovasc Interv*. 2013 November;6(11):1203–1209.

40. Gupta N, Corriere MA, Dodson TF et al. The incidence of microemboli to the brain is less with endarterectomy than with percutaneous revascularization with distal filters or flow reversal. *J Vasc Surg*. 2011 February;53(2):316–322.

41. Akkaya E, Vuruskan E, Gul ZB et al. Cerebral microemboli and neurocognitive change after carotid artery stenting with different embolic protection devices. *Int J Cardiol*. 2014 September 20;176(2):478–483.

42. Mokin M, Dumont TM, Chi JM et al. Proximal versus distal protection during carotid artery stenting: Analysis of the two treatment approaches and associated clinical outcomes. *World Neurosurg.* 2014 March;81(3–4):543–548.

43. Tadros RO, Spyris CT, Vouyouka AG et al. Comparing the embolic potential of open and closed cell stents during carotid angioplasty and stenting. *J Vasc Surg.* 2012 July;56(1):89–95.

44. Timaran CH, Rosero EB, Higuera A, Ilarraza A, Modrall JG, Clagett GP. Randomized clinical trial of open-cell vs closed-cell stents for carotid stenting and effects of stent design on cerebral embolization. *J Vasc Surg.* 2011 November;54(5):1310–1316.

45. Schillinger M, Gschwendtner M, Reimers B et al. Does carotid stent cell design matter? *Stroke.* 2008 March;39(3):905–909.

46. Bosiers M, de DG, Deloose K et al. Does free cell area influence the outcome in carotid artery stenting? *Eur J Vasc Endovasc Surg.* 2007 February;33(2):135–141.

47. Macdonald S. Strategies for reducing microemboli during carotid artery stenting. *J Cardiovasc Surg (Torino).* 2012 February;53(1 Suppl. 1):23–26.

48. Jordan WD Jr, Voellinger DC, Doblar DD, Plyushcheva NP, Fisher WS, McDowell HA. Microemboli detected by transcranial Doppler monitoring in patients during carotid angioplasty versus carotid endarterectomy. *Cardiovasc Surg.* 1999 January;7(1):33–38.

49. Grewe PH, Deneke T, Machraoui A, Barmeyer J, Muller KM. Acute and chronic tissue response to coronary stent implantation: Pathologic findings in human specimen. *J Am Coll Cardiol.* 2000 January;35(1):157–163.

50. Chaturvedi S, Yadav JS. The role of antiplatelet therapy in carotid stenting for ischemic stroke prevention. *Stroke.* 2006 June;37(6):1572–1577.

51. Cunningham EJ, Fiorella D, Masaryk TJ. Neurovascular rescue. *Semin Vasc Surg.* 2005 June;18(2):101–109.

52. McKevitt FM, Randall MS, Cleveland TJ, Gaines PA, Tan KT, Venables GS. The benefits of combined antiplatelet treatment in carotid artery stenting. *Eur J Vasc Endovasc Surg.* 2005 May;29(5):522–527.

53. Bhatt DL, Kapadia SR, Bajzer CT et al. Dual antiplatelet therapy with clopidogrel and aspirin after carotid artery stenting. *J Invasive Cardiol.* 2001 December;13(12):767–771.

54. Payne DA, Jones CI, Hayes PD et al. Beneficial effects of clopidogrel combined with aspirin in reducing cerebral emboli in patients undergoing carotid endarterectomy. *Circulation.* 2004 March 30;109(12):1476–1481.

55. Gortler D, Schlosser FJ, Muhs BE, Nelson MA, Dardik A. Periprocedural drug therapy in carotid artery stenting: The need for more evidence. *Vascular.* 2008 November;16(6):303–309.

56. Wang Y, Wang Y, Zhao X et al. Clopidogrel with aspirin in acute minor stroke or transient ischemic attack. *N Engl J Med.* 2013 July 4;369(1):11–19.

57. Ackerstaff RG, Suttorp MJ, van den Berg JC et al. Prediction of early cerebral outcome by transcranial Doppler monitoring in carotid bifurcation angioplasty and stenting. *J Vasc Surg.* 2005 April;41(4):618–624.

58. Eckert B, Thie A, Valdueza J, Zanella F, Zeumer H. Transcranial Doppler sonographic monitoring during percutaneous transluminal angioplasty of the internal carotid artery. *Neuroradiology.* 1997 March;39(3):229–234.

59. Qureshi AI, Luft AR, Sharma M et al. Frequency and determinants of postprocedural hemodynamic instability after carotid angioplasty and stenting. *Stroke.* 1999 October;30(10):2086–2093.

60. Gupta R, Abou-Chebl A, Bajzer CT, Schumacher HC, Yadav JS. Rate, predictors, and consequences of hemodynamic depression after carotid artery stenting. *J Am Coll Cardiol.* 2006 April 18;47(8):1538–1543.

61. Diethrich EB, Ndiaye M, Reid DB. Stenting in the carotid artery: Initial experience in 110 patients. *J Endovasc Surg.* 1996 February;3(1):42–62.

62. Bergeron P, Becquemin JP, Jausseran JM et al. Percutaneous stenting of the internal carotid artery: The European CAST I Study. Carotid Artery Stent Trial. *J Endovasc Surg.* 1999 May;6(2):155–159.

63. Macdonald S, Venables GS, Cleveland TJ, Gaines PA. Protected carotid stenting: Safety and efficacy of the MedNova NeuroShield filter. *J Vasc Surg.* 2002 May;35(5):966–972.

64. Benichou H, Bergeron P. Carotid angioplasty and stenting: Will periprocedural transcranial Doppler monitoring be important? *J Endovasc Surg.* 1996 May;3(2):217–223.

65. Antonius Carotid Endarterectomy AaSSG. Transcranial Doppler monitoring in angioplasty and stenting of the carotid bifurcation. *J Endovasc Ther.* 2003 July;10(4):702–710.

66. Kwon BJ, Han MH, Kang HS, Jung C. Protection filter-related events in extracranial carotid artery stenting: A single-center experience. *J Endovasc Ther.* 2006 December;13(6):711–722.

67. Cremonesi A, Manetti R, Setacci F, Setacci C, Castriota F. Protected carotid stenting: Clinical advantages and complications of embolic protection devices in 442 consecutive patients. *Stroke.* 2003 August;34(8):1936–1941.

68. Theron J, Guimaraens L, Coskun O, Sola T, Martin JB, Rufenacht DA. Complications of carotid angioplasty and stenting. *Neurosurg Focus.* 1998 December 15;5(6):e4.

69. Biondi A, Ricciardi GK, Puybasset L et al. Intra-arterial nimodipine for the treatment of symptomatic cerebral vasospasm after aneurysmal subarachnoid hemorrhage: Preliminary results. *Am J Neuroradiol.* 2004 June;25(6):1067–1076.

70. Gomez CR, Roubin GS, Dean LS et al. Neurological monitoring during carotid artery stenting: The duck squeezing test. *J Endovasc Surg.* 1999 November;6(4):332–336.

71. van den Berg JC. Neuro-rescue during carotid stenting. *Eur J Vasc Endovasc Surg.* 2008 December;36(6):627–636.

72. Liu ZJ, Fu WG, Guo ZY, Shen LG, Shi ZY, Li JH. Updated systematic review and meta-analysis of randomized clinical trials comparing carotid artery stenting and carotid endarterectomy in the treatment of carotid stenosis. *Ann Vasc Surg.* 2012 May;26(4):576–590.

73. Economopoulos KP, Sergentanis TN, Tsivgoulis G, Mariolis AD, Stefanadis C. Carotid artery stenting versus carotid endarterectomy: A comprehensive meta-analysis of short-term and long-term outcomes. *Stroke.* 2011 March;42(3):687–692.

74. Yadav JS, Wholey MH, Kuntz RE et al. Protected carotid-artery stenting versus endarterectomy in high-risk patients. *N Engl J Med.* 2004 October 7;351(15):1493–1501.

75. Ederle J, Bonati LH, Dobson J et al. Endovascular treatment with angioplasty or stenting versus endarterectomy in patients with carotid artery stenosis in the Carotid and Vertebral Artery Transluminal Angioplasty Study (CAVATAS): Long-term follow-up of a randomised trial. *Lancet Neurol.* 2009 October;8(10):898–907.

76. Ringleb PA, Allenberg J, Bruckmann H et al. 30 day results from the SPACE trial of stent-protected angioplasty versus carotid endarterectomy in symptomatic patients: A randomised non-inferiority trial. *Lancet.* 2006 October 7;368(9543):1239–1247.

77. Mas JL, Chatellier G, Beyssen B et al. Endarterectomy versus stenting in patients with symptomatic severe carotid stenosis. *N Engl J Med.* 2006 October 19;355(16):1660–1671.

78. Ederle J, Dobson J, Featherstone RL et al. Carotid artery stenting compared with endarterectomy in patients with symptomatic carotid stenosis (International Carotid Stenting Study): An interim analysis of a randomised controlled trial. *Lancet.* 2010 March 20;375(9719):985–997.

79. Brott TG, Hobson RW, Howard G et al. Stenting versus endarterectomy for treatment of carotid-artery stenosis. *N Engl J Med.* 2010 July 1;363(1):11–23.

80. Endovascular versus surgical treatment in patients with carotid stenosis in the Carotid and Vertebral Artery Transluminal Angioplasty Study (CAVATAS): A randomised trial. *Lancet.* 2001 June 2;357(9270):1729–1737.

81. Gurm HS, Yadav JS, Fayad P et al. Long-term results of carotid stenting versus endarterectomy in high-risk patients. *N Engl J Med.* 2008 April 10;358(15):1572–1579.

82. Eckstein HH, Ringleb P, Allenberg JR et al. Results of the Stent-Protected Angioplasty versus Carotid Endarterectomy (SPACE) study to treat symptomatic stenoses at 2 years: A multinational, prospective, randomised trial. *Lancet Neurol.* 2008 October;7(10):893–902.

83. Mas JL, Trinquart L, Leys D et al. Endarterectomy Versus Angioplasty in Patients with Symptomatic Severe Carotid Stenosis (EVA-3S) trial: Results up to 4 years from a randomised, multicentre trial. *Lancet Neurol.* 2008 October;7(10):885–892.

84. Mas JL, Arquizan C, Calvet D et al. Long-term follow-up study of endarterectomy versus angioplasty in patients with symptomatic severe carotid stenosis trial. *Stroke.* 2014 September;45(9):2750–2756.

85. Bonati LH, Dobson J, Featherstone RL et al. Long-term outcomes after stenting versus endarterectomy for treatment of symptomatic carotid stenosis: The International Carotid Stenting Study (ICSS) randomised trial. *Lancet.* 2014 October 14.

86. Gray WA, Simonton CA, Verta P. Overview of the 2011 food and drug administration circulatory system devices panel meeting on the ACCULINK and ACCUNET Carotid Artery Stent System. *Circulation.* 2012 May 8;125(18):2256–2264.

87. Lal BK, Beach KW, Roubin GS et al. Restenosis after carotid artery stenting and endarterectomy: A secondary analysis of CREST, a randomised controlled trial. *Lancet Neurol.* 2012 September;11(9):755–763.

88. Roffi M, Sievert H, Gray WA et al. Carotid artery stenting versus surgery: Adequate comparisons? *Lancet Neurol.* 2010 April;9(4):339–341.

89. Bonati LH, Dobson J, Algra A et al. Short-term outcome after stenting versus endarterectomy for symptomatic carotid stenosis: A preplanned meta-analysis of individual patient data. *Lancet.* 2010 September 25;376(9746):1062–1073.

90. Calvet D, Mas JL, Algra A et al. Carotid stenting: Is there an operator effect? A pooled analysis from the carotid stenting trialists' collaboration. *Stroke.* 2014 February;45(2):527–532.

91. Touze E, Trinquart L, Felgueiras R et al. A clinical rule (sex, contralateral occlusion, age, and restenosis) to select patients for stenting versus carotid endarterectomy: Systematic review of observational studies with validation in randomized trials. *Stroke.* 2013 December;44(12):3394–3400.

SECTION VI

Visceral Arterial Disease

40

Renovascular disease

GEORGE HAMILTON

CONTENTS

INTRODUCTION

Few areas of vascular disease have received such intense clinical research focus with paradigm shifts in management opinions as renovascular disease. The pathologies giving rise to renovascular disease are varied ranging from fibromuscular dysplasia (FMD) to arteriosclerosis. Atherosclerotic renovascular disease is by far the most common cause for this condition. Vascular surgeons have been aware of renovascular disease and involved in its treatment since the 1970s when this disease was considered to be relatively rare and within the clinical remit of major vascular centres. With the advent of CT and MR scanning, and increased clinical awareness, atherosclerotic renal artery stenosis presents regularly to all vascular surgeons. In the days of relatively ineffective agents to control

hypertension and arteriosclerosis, there was an undoubted clinical benefit from surgical renal artery reconstruction. With the advent of the endovascular era and in particular renal stent angioplasty, there was an explosion of intervention, but during the same time period, optimal medical management of hypertension and arteriosclerosis made major advances. Recent experimental studies have given insights into the complexity of ischaemic nephropathy and renal arteriosclerosis which begins to explain the clinical realization that revascularization of renal artery stenosis in the majority of patients with atherosclerotic renal artery disease has no benefit over optimal medical therapy. This chapter will discuss the pathophysiology, diagnosis and management of renal artery disease in addition to the techniques and current indications for renal arterial revascularization.

PATHOLOGY

Several pathologies involving the renal artery give rise to hypertension and renal failure (Table 40.1).

Atherosclerotic renal artery disease is the most common cause accounting for approximately 90% with FMD as the second most common.[1]

FIBROMUSCULAR DYSPLASIA

Better understanding of this condition has resulted from the US registry for FMD.[2] This review has shown that FMD is not a disease primarily and exclusively involving the renal arteries but commonly affects other vessels. Female predominance is confirmed with 91% being of women. The mean age at diagnosis for all of the patients was 51.9 years (SD 13.4; median 52; range 5–83 years), with no difference in presentation of age between men and women. This is in contradistinction to original reports suggesting that this disease most commonly presented earlier in the third or fourth decade. This registry now confirms that FMD is really a disease of middle age but can present throughout all age groups.

Of importance, the registry showed that extra-cranial carotid and vertebral arteries were involved as commonly as renal arteries. Probably because of improved imaging, the prevalence of multi-vessel FMD was higher than previously reported and 65% of patients with renal FMD had also involvement of the cerebrovascular circulation. However, those presenting primarily with hypertension had an earlier age of onset at 43 years. The striking finding is of the multi-vessel character of FMD and the very strong association with extra-cranial arterial disease, both stenotic and aneurysmal. This is a reciprocal association and strongly supports the concept that patients with renal FMD should have their extra-cranial arterial circulation studied as part of the management process. The findings of this important registry are summarized in Table 40.2.

FMD is typically associated with a better long-term prognosis compared to atherosclerotic renal artery stenosis with a lower rate of progression to complete renal artery occlusion.

Renal artery aneurysm frequently presents with hypertension most commonly thought to be secondary to the

Table 40.1 Causes of renal artery disease.

Fibromuscular dysplasia

Renal artery aneurysm

Mid-aortic syndrome

Vasculitides including Takayasu

Neurofibromatosis type I

Arteriovenous fistula (iatrogenic, traumatic, congenital)

Aortic dissection

Atherosclerotic renal artery disease

Table 40.2 Clinical data from the US registry for fibromuscular dysplasia.

FMD involves multiple vessels most commonly the renal and cerebral vascular arteries.

Most commonly patients with FMD present with, in addition to hypertension, other symptoms such as headaches, pulsatile tinnitus, dizziness, neck pain, chest pain, abdominal pain, aneurysms or dissections.

Patients with known renal artery FMD will have cerebral vascular FMD and vice versa in up to 65%.

Generally 1 in 5 patients with FMD will have dissections and 1 in 5 patients will have aneurysms.

Although less common in men, FMD behaves more aggressively and is associated with a higher incidence of dissections and aneurysms.

Angioplasty or stent angioplasty for renal FMD is more likely to have success in either reducing or curing hypertension in comparison to atherosclerotic renal artery stenosis. Angioplasty is more effective in younger patients, with recent onset hypertension and those with focal FMD.

FMD may have a genetic association and could be an inherited vasculopathy.

Source: Adapted from Sharma AM and Kline B, *Tech Vasc Intervent Radiol*, 17, 258, 2014. With permission.

haemodynamic upset of the aneurysm on blood flow. The strong association with FMD however indicates that there may be undetected stenotic disease present in addition.

ATHEROSCLEROTIC RENAL ARTERY DISEASE

Atherosclerotic renal artery disease is by far the most common presentation of renovascular disease. In the majority of these patients, the most proximal component of the renal artery is primarily involved and indeed may be considered as an extension of severe aortic atherosclerosis. The presentation is in a much older group compared to FMD. Obviously, these patients carry a significant burden of arteriosclerotic disease elsewhere, most commonly coronary and cerebrovascular. There is also a long recognized association between increasing severity of renal artery stenosis and symptomatic arterial disease elsewhere, with more than half of patients with greater than 50% stenosis having significant coronary and cerebrovascular disease.[3] The prevalence of renovascular hypertension in patients with atherosclerotic renal artery stenosis is about 2% in unselected hypertensive patients but as high as 40% in older, arteriopathic patients with resistant hypertension. The natural history of atherosclerotic renovascular disease has changed since the first reports four decades ago. At that time higher grade renal artery stenosis had a high rate of progression of up to 44% within 2 years to severe stenosis or occlusion and up to 40% requiring renal replacement. The most recent trials now document progressive renal impairment in around 20% with less than 8% needing renal replacement therapy.

PATHOPHYSIOLOGY

Eight decades ago, Goldblatt showed that reduction of renal blood flow by clipping one artery resulted in hypertension. This observation, particularly in the days of inefficient and poorly tolerated antihypertensive agents, led to the concept that overcoming reduced renal blood flow by revascularization would cure hypertension. This simple association however has been shown to be present in only a small percentage of such patients with the realization that the pathophysiology is much more complex. Early studies implicated changes within the contralateral normal kidney in successfully revascularized patients but with persistent hypertension. Clinical presentation occurs after many years and perhaps decades of progressive arteriosclerosis and poorly controlled hypertension. This significantly increases the likelihood of chronic change taking place within the parenchyma not only of the affected but also the contralateral kidney.

Arterial blood flow is compromised only when a stenosis is >70% or if there is a significant trans-lesional gradient of 10–20 mmHg, and renal vein renin studies confirm elevated renin production only in these scenarios.[4] If the renin–angiotensin hypothesis was solely at work, then the syndrome of atherosclerotic renal artery stenosis would present only in high-grade renal artery stenoses. Textor and colleagues suggest however that even in the presence of low-grade stenosis, renal hypo-perfusion will develop because frequently there are fluctuating arterial pressures and impaired cardiac output. This recent hypothesis proposes that repeated intermittent episodes of acute kidney injury are frequent but from which the kidney can recover, however, inducing a state of chronic inflammation within the renal parenchyma. Support for this hypothesis is found in the chronically elevated bio-markers for injury such as neutrophil gelatinase–associated lipocalin, measured in renal vein sampling.[5] Further evidence is found in experimental studies of repeated acute kidney injury resulting in interstitial fibrosis and inflammation. This hypothesis provides a likely explanation for the chronic parenchymal changes associated with atherosclerotic renovascular disease even in the presence of moderate stenosis or well controlled hypertension.[6] This more global renal pathology in atherosclerotic renal artery disease is more accurately known as ischaemic nephropathy.

Further insights into the pathophysiology of ischaemic nephropathy have been provided recently from the Mayo Clinic. These focused on understanding tissue deoxygenation and microvascular injury in atherosclerotic renovascular disease. In 2010, they reported reduction of corticomedullary blood flow of 30%–40% measured by contrast transit times using multidetector CT in human studies. This was sufficient to reduce GFR and activate the renin–angiotensin system but did not produce measureable tissue deoxygenation.[7] Further important human studies by this group measured tissue oxygenation in essential hypertension and renovascular disease by corticomedullary deoxyhemoglobin measurements

using blood oxygen level–dependent magnetic resonance (BOLD MRI). All patients had standardized antihypertensive drug therapy and sodium balance correction. BOLD MRI was shown to reliably measure tissue oxygenation by assessment of deoxyhemoglobin throughout the renal cortex and medulla. These studies showed large tissue oxygenation gradients, with low levels of deoxyhemoglobin in the cortex with areas of higher deoxygenation in the deeper medulla. These studies indicate that even in the presence of severe inflow stenosis, the kidney is able to preserve normal tissue oxygenation, most probably because blood flow to the kidney has a dual purpose, not only to meet parenchymal metabolic requirements but also as a filtering organ. This finding may explain in part the stability of renal function seen in patients on effective antihypertensive therapy documented in both the ASTRAL and CORAL trails.[6] These same BOLD MRI studies have shown that in higher grade (>70%–80%) renal artery stenosis, significant hypoxia of the cortex and throughout the renal parenchyma is present. Tissue biopsies performed in these patients revealed structural damage involving the glomeruli and tubules but also marked interstitial inflammatory cell infiltration particularly from T cells and macrophages. Thus, once the degree of stenosis has become severe enough to induce cortical hypoxia, severe inflammatory injury develops which appears to become chronic.[6] Thus, the dual findings that in moderate stenosis the kidney is able to maintain good oxygenation despite reduced blood flow but that in high-grade stenosis tissue hypoxia results in a chronic inflammatory state give further insight into the lack of benefit found in the majority of patients undergoing revascularization.

Thus, ischaemic nephropathy results from complex interactions only beginning to be understood involving oxidative stress injury, a chronic inflammatory reaction and parenchymal arteriosclerotic damage, leading to fibrosis of the glomerulus and tubular structures.

DIAGNOSIS, INVESTIGATION AND ASSESSMENT

The clinical features which should raise suspicion of renovascular disease are listed in Table 40.3. In general, non-atherosclerotic causes of renovascular disease should be considered in younger patients presenting with hypertension but in the over 50s being much more likely to be secondary to arteriosclerotic renovascular disease.

Careful consideration must be given to a further diagnostic and investigation of a patient presenting with hypertension. In a patient under the age of 30 years presenting with hypertension, the probability of an underlying renovascular lesion is higher, and the threshold for further investigation should be set lower. In a patient over the age of 50 years, however, the prevalence of an underlying renovascular condition is much lower. Careful selection for further diagnostic evaluation should be based on the clinical features, particularly those indicating the presence of arteriosclerosis.

Table 40.3 Clinical features of renovascular disease.

Onset of hypertension or associated complications (fitting) in children – FMD, neurofibromatosis type 1, mid-aortic syndrome

Onset of hypertension in young adults – FMD, vasculitis, mid-aortic syndrome

Onset of hypertension after 50 years – atherosclerotic renovascular disease, renal artery aneurysm/FMD

Resistant hypertension/malignant hypertension

Renal failure complicating angiotensin-converting enzyme inhibitors or angiotensin-receptor blocker

Asymmetrical kidneys (more than 1.5 cm difference in size)

Recent onset renal failure in the absence of any other diagnosis

Sudden onset refractory pulmonary oedema (flash pulmonary oedema)

With the clinical evidence which has now become available together with the much more effective and well tolerated range of hypertensives, this diagnostic decision-making has become more complex. If a patient has hypertension that is easily and successfully controlled and where renal function remains stable, the need for extensive diagnosis evaluation is increasingly considered to be of academic interest. Diagnostic evaluation for a possible atherosclerotic renal lesion should be limited to patients who have a clinical picture including resistant hypertension, progressive renal failure, angiotensin-converting enzyme (ACE) inhibitor–induced renal failure or the possibility of a cardio-renal syndrome as evidenced by refractory or recurrent pulmonary oedema. General functional assessment of patients with hypertension and certainly patients with renal failure will obviously include the careful history and physical examination. Particular attention should be paid to the possibility of concomitant arterial disease particularly involving the carotid, cerebral vascular and peripheral circulations.

In addition to standard haematological investigations, urinalysis is important; a 24-hour urine collection for a creatinine clearance is standard. If clinically indicated where there is suspicion of phaeochromocytoma or an adrenal cortical tumour, urinary estimation for catecholamines, VMA and steroids can be undertaken.

Commonly, these patients require sequential follow-up with eGFR as a method of estimating renal function. However, there has been considerable concern expressed regarding the accuracy of this measurement in sequential analysis. The recent randomized control trial data indicate that in patients with atherosclerotic renovascular disease, the eGFR losses are small being in the range of 1–2 mL/minutes/1.73 m^2/year.[8,9] This is a rate of loss of function which is similar to that in patients of the same age group with general chronic kidney disease. This has led to an increasing realization that eGFR estimation has little accuracy and that isotopic GFR(i) performs more accurately.[10]

There has been a great deal of work identifying potential bio-markers in the circulation for atherosclerotic renovascular disease. Unfortunately no marker that performs satisfactorily has been identified thus far. In particular there has been analysis of highly sensitive C-reactive protein. This value is a good marker for systemic burden of arteriosclerosis but has not proved to be of prognostic value in renovascular disease. Further studies have considered serial BNP measurements, but the results of studies in atherosclerotic renovascular disease with regard to diagnosis and prognosis have yielded conflicting results.

DUPLEX RENAL ULTRASONOGRAPHY

This imaging method has the advantage of being inexpensive and non-invasive. In the majority of centres, it is the primary screening tool in the assessment of renovascular disease providing both functional and structural information. It has disadvantages relating to operator experience, but also to obesity and the presence of bowel gas. Nonetheless, it remains a valuable screening tool but also of value in sequential follow-up of patients following a revascularization.

Renal duplex assessment should be performed by fully trained vascular scientists or technologists in accredited vascular laboratory with full imaging of the aorta and renal artery using a flank approach. Doppler signals should be obtained from the renal parenchyma to measure peak systolic velocity (PSV) and end diastolic velocity (EDV) along the renal arteries. A PSV >285 cm/seconds gives an overall diagnostic accuracy for a >60% stenosis, with sensitivity, specificity and overall accuracy of 67%, 90% and 81%, respectively. The renal aortic ratio (RAR) cut-off value of 3.7 gives the best overall accuracy for a >60% stenosis with a sensitivity, specificity and overall accuracy of 69%, 91% and 82%, respectively.[11] A further frequently used measure is the resistive index (RI) obtained from segmental arterial flow giving an assessment of flow in the renal micro circulation beyond the main renal arteries. It is derived as the height of the PSV minus the height of the EDV divided by the PSV (RI = [PSV – EDV] over PSV).

An RI > 0.8 before angioplasty has been documented as predicting worse renal outcomes compared to an RI of <0.8 in one study, but in a second study, similar renal outcomes were reported for both groups.[12,13] This measurement is therefore rather controversial, but the general acceptance is that a lower RI results from a better preserved parenchymal renal blood flow and probable better kidney function. Our institutional practice is to request full imaging of the renal artery and kidney, measurement of longitudinal and renal length, PSV and EDV measurement with calculation of RAR and RI.

COMPUTED TOMOGRAPHIC ANGIOGRAPHY

Computed tomographic angiography (CTA) using modern multidetector technology which facilitated volumetric data acquisition with rapid scan speeds provides excellent angiographic imaging in investigation of renal artery stenosis. In addition to providing a 3D image, the cross-sectional imaging gives a full assessment of the kidney itself. CTA has sensitivity and specificity with regard to accuracy of assessing renal artery stenosis of 94% and 93%, respectively. Similar sensitivities are reported in diagnosing FMD. Furthermore, CTA is able to accurately assess renal artery stents with 100% sensitivity and 99% specificity for detecting in-stent stenosis.[14]

CTA is rapid, accurate and readily available but has certain disadvantages. The first is that it does not provide functional assessment of renal artery stenosis. The other problems and associated risks are related to radiation and to contrast-induced nephropathy particularly in repeated CT assessments.

MAGNETIC RESONANCE ANGIOGRAPHY

Magnetic resonance angiography (MRA) delivers similarly non-invasive imaging as CTA but without ionising radiation. It has been shown to be highly accurate with sensitivity and specificity of non-enhanced MRA for renal artery stenosis of 94% and 85%, respectively. For gadolinium-enhanced MRA, sensitivity is increased to 97% and specificity to 93%, and there is improved positive predicted value when compared to non-enhanced MRA.[15] A major problem even with contrast-enhanced MRA has been a tendency to overestimation of the degree of stenosis by about 25%–30% but with more modern algorithms, this has been significantly reduced.

Further major advantages of MRA are that functional data and assessment can be obtained, in particular renal parenchymal blood flow, glomerular filtration rate and measurement of renal artery and vein blood flow. The disadvantages are significant artefact in the presence of metal, particularly stents, and the absolute contraindication of pacemakers, implantable defibrillators, brain aneurysm clips or metal fragments in the eyes. There is no contraindication for vascular stents, coils or filters. A further major problem is of the association between the use of gadolinium-enhanced MR imaging in chronic kidney disease and the development of nephrogenic systemic fibrosis. The incidence of this syndrome is reported at between 1% and 6% for patients on dialysis and those with a GFR of <30. Congestive heart failure, which can be present in patients with severe renal artery stenosis, is also a relative contraindication. However, with appropriate pre-investigation protocols of hydration, the use of peri-investigation dialysis in patients in end stage renal failure and the use of the more recent preparations of gadolinium, these risks have been significantly reduced.

BOLD MRI is a well-established methodology in functional brain imaging. This methodology is based on the presence in deoxyhemoglobin of four free iron electrons making this molecule paramagnetic. This allows mapping across the kidney with the ability to distinguish between different regions and detect alterations in oxygen consumption.

Thus, renal tissue which has impaired oxygen supply but is metabolically active will produce more deoxyhemoglobin. A recent study combining BOLD MRI with i-GFR suggests that this could be a useful predictor of response to renal revascularization in an ischaemic kidney. The detection of intra-renal hypoxia relative to renal function has the potential to identify 'hibernating' renal parenchyma which could improve with revascularization. Further evaluation of this technique is underway and may provide a valuable methodology to select those patient subgroups that would benefit from renal revascularization.[16]

DIGITAL SUBTRACTION ANGIOGRAPHY

This technique is obviously invasive but offers the major advantage of the highest-resolution imaging and also truly objective assessment of the degree of stenosis by measuring pressure gradients. A gradient of >10% of the mean arterial pressure is considered as significant. There are several disadvantages related to digital subtraction angiography (DSA) mostly of complications due to its invasive nature with the most important being arterial embolization into the renal parenchyma. Furthermore, there are the risk of aortic and renal artery dissection and the significant nephrotoxic risks of contrast agents in renal injury or failure. DSA has little use as the primary investigation of renovascular disease but still has a major role to play when the results of CTA or MRA are equivocal and obviously in patients suitable and eligible for renal stent angioplasty.

FUNCTIONAL TESTS FOR RENOVASCULAR DISEASE

Radionuclide renography is commonly used to evaluate renal function. Captopril renography is no longer used as a diagnostic test because of poor sensitivity and specificity ranging from 58% to 95% and 17% to 100%, respectively. Furthermore, this test does not distinguish between unilateral and bilateral renal artery stenosis. Mercaptoacetyltriglycine renography continues to have a role however in defining the relative function of each kidney before revascularization or even nephrectomy.[17]

PLASMA RENIN ACTIVITY

Plasma renin activity (PRA) has been extensively used over the years both in diagnosis of renovascular hypertension and prediction of response to revascularization. Peripheral PRA measurement however has had disappointing results on both of these scores. Segmental renal vein renin measurements have performed better with regard to predicting response to revascularization. Calculation of a ratio of renal vein renin to IVC renin where the ratio is >1.5 is a predictive positive value for improvement of hypertension from revascularization of up to 92%.[18] In our paediatric practice, this measurement has proved to be very useful in terms of its positive predictive value in children with renal artery stenosis secondary to FMD and mid-aortic syndrome particularly in assessment of segmental renal arterial involvement. The test however is invasive and production of renin will vary according to the patients' medications, volume status and arterial pressure levels. However, given the need for more selective selection for renal revascularization in the modern era, this measurement may merit further prospective study.

MANAGEMENT OF RENOVASCULAR DISEASE

In all of aetiologies of renovascular disease, the initial management focuses on control of hypertension. With the current range of well tolerated and safe antihypertensive agents, nowadays this rarely presents a therapeutic problem. In most non-atherosclerotic causes of renovascular disease, revascularization, either endovascular or vascular, is a secondary but curative treatment. In atherosclerotic renovascular disease, however, it is now clear that most patients will not benefit from revascularization. Atherosclerotic renovascular disease requires treatment not solely on maintaining blood pressure below the guideline recommended 130/90 mmHg and maintaining of renal function, but most importantly with a focus on reduction of cardiovascular events by treatment of generalized atherosclerosis. Patients with atherosclerotic renovascular disease (ARVD) are several times more likely to die from a cardiovascular cause than from end stage renal failure.

Inhibition of ACE and angiotensin-receptor blockade (ARB).

Inhibition of the renin–angiotensin cascade is now recognized to be highly effective, not only in the control of hypertension but also in the optimization of cardiac function and endothelial cell function. ARVD patients treated with these agents have significantly lowered risk of cardiac or cardiovascular events and congestive heart failure, reduced need for renal replacement therapy and reduced mortality.[19] The current recommendation is that these agents be prescribed for both unilateral and bilateral renal artery stenosis in patients with ARVD. A minority of patients, particularly with bilateral renal artery stenosis, will suffer a decline in renal function resulting in an increase in serum creatinine of more than 30% – this possibility mandates careful review of patients after starting on renin–angiotensin inhibitors or blockers.[20]

MEDICAL THERAPY DIRECTED AT CONTROL OF ATHEROSCLEROSIS

Atherosclerotic risk factor modulation is extremely important in ARVD patients since they are a group at particularly high cardiovascular risk. Lifestyle modifications most importantly with regard to smoking, exercise and obesity reduction, in addition to control of metabolic syndrome and effective treatment for diabetes, are all of importance.

Treatment of hyperlipidaemia is a further extremely important feature in the management of these patients. Statins have been confirmed to reduce not only total and LDL cholesterol levels but also cardiovascular mortality in atherosclerotic renovascular disease.[21] The pleiotropic effects of statins and in particular their anti-inflammatory effects may also be beneficial in the modulation of the chronic inflammation of ischaemic nephropathy. The cardiovascular protective effects of antiplatelet treatment outweigh the small risk of bleeding complications, particularly in patients with chronic kidney disease. The success and safety of optimized or best medical therapy has been abundantly confirmed by both the ASTRAL and CORAL trials.

REVASCULARIZATION

There is now considerable objective evidence confirming that the role of renal artery revascularization in addition to best medical therapy in patients with ARVD is limited. Revascularization however remains important in the treatment of non-atherosclerotic renovascular disease where long-term improvement or even cure in control of hypertension and preservation of renal function can be expected.

Open renal revascularization

The primary consideration is the selection and assessment of surgical risk of patients suitable for open repair. In non-atherosclerotic renovascular disease, the patients are typically younger and fitter; thus, in this group of patients, open surgical repair remains the gold standard (Table 40.4).

Patients with ARVD have a very high prevalence of coronary, cerebrovascular and peripheral arterial disease. Furthermore, these patients may have a cardio-renal syndrome with pulmonary oedema. Meticulous preoperative assessment with input from cardiology, nephrology and vascular anaesthesia is of vital importance in selecting surgical candidates. Specialist units, in the main

Table 40.4 Indications for open surgical repair in non-atherosclerotic renovascular disease.

Failed interventional treatment for renal artery stenosis in FMD, mid-aortic syndrome, vasculitis

Mid-aortic syndrome in older children, adolescents and adults

Hostile aorta with extensive arteriosclerosis

Complex renal anatomy (segmental disease multiple renal arteries)

Renal artery aneurysm

Table 40.5 Indications for open surgical repair in patients with ARVD.

Complex renal anatomy: segmental stenotic disease, multiple renal arteries

Failed angioplasty/stent angioplasty: failed deployment, dissection, stent restenosis

Severely diseased aorta

Hybrid repair of thoraco-abdominal aneurysm

high-volume centres, have reported lower operative mortality rates between 3% and 6%. However, operative mortality in the United States using data from the National Inpatient Sample was reported in 2008 as being closer to 10% – this represents mortality across a range of centres and is quoted by many experts as being a more realistic assessment of surgical risk. These data further reinforce the importance of surgical intervention being undertaken in high-volume specialist centres (Table 40.5).

There are a range of operative approaches which can be tailored to the individual diagnosis, vascular anatomy and patient-specific risk. Aorto-renal bypass grafting is the preferred procedure because of its relative simplicity and partial cross clamping of the aorta (Figure 40.1). Careful assessment of the patency of the coeliac trunk must take place preoperatively since up to 50% of patients with ARVD will have significant coeliac artery stenosis, particularly important if extra-anatomic revascularization by hepato-renal or spleno-renal bypass is being considered. In patients with segmental renal arterial disease, bench reconstruction with auto-transplantation is a reliable procedure with acceptably low morbidity and mortality. Combined aortic reconstruction and renal revascularization should, if at all possible, be avoided because of the increased associated mortality.[22]

Some centres have reported good results for either end-arterectomy of the renal artery origin with patch repair or aortic endarterectomy in its reno-visceral component, also usually with patch repair (Figures 40.2 and 40.3). In the hands of most surgeons, this is regarded as a more complex approach with a particular disadvantage of the need for complete aortic cross clamping and increased left ventricular strain.

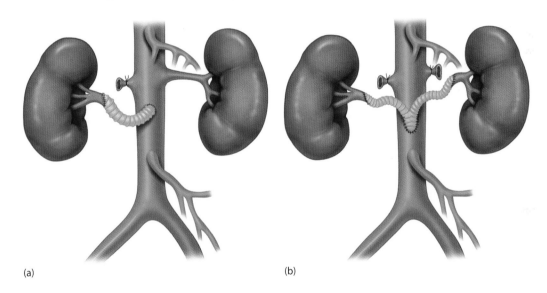

(a)   (b)

Figure 40.1 (a) Direct aorto-renal bypass graft using a prosthetic 6 or 8 mm conduit; (b) direct bilateral infrarenal aorto-renal bypass graft using 12 × 8 mm conduit NB 'normal' aorta essential and end-to-end renal anastomoses.

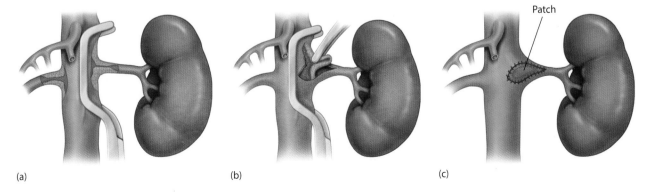

(a)   (b)   (c)

Figure 40.2 Renal endarterectomy with prosthetic patch repair: (a) partial cross clamping of the aorta after heparinisation; (b) endarterectomy of the aortic and renal ostium; (c) patch repair of completed enadarterectomy.

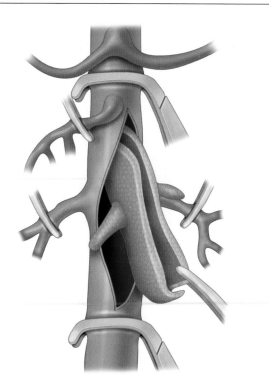

Figure 40.3 Aortic endarterectomy of the renal and visceral component of the aorta; a durable procedure in experienced hands but requires a patient able to withstand total aortic clamping.

Finally, nephrectomy of a small kidney (<8 cm in length) in a patient with refractory hypertension will infrequently be indicated. Laparoscopic nephrectomy is now established as of equivalent safety to open, with markedly reduced morbidity. However, with the advent of modern antihypertensives and in particular ACE inhibitors and ARBs, the need for nephrectomy has reduced significantly.

Percutaneous renal artery angioplasty and stenting

Percutaneous transluminal balloon angioplasty of the renal artery (PTRA) was first developed and reported by Gruntzig in 1978[23]. Simple PTRA was increasingly employed over the following decade. A small prospective randomized trial comparing PTRA versus surgical reconstruction for atherosclerotic renal artery stenosis was reported in 1993 indicating equivalent outcomes in terms of improvement of control of hypertension and renal function. The primary patency rate however was inferior for PTRA at 75% in comparison to 96% in the operative group. The secondary patency rate however was 90% for the PTRA group in comparison to 97% for the surgical group.[24] The conclusion of this first level 1 study was that there was equivalence for intervention and open surgery but that PTRA should be recommended as a first choice therapy with intensive follow-up and aggressive re-intervention. As interventional experience gathered, it was realized that

mortality rates were lower than open surgery but at the price of a higher technical failure rate of around 50% from both elastic recoil and in-stent restenosis. This elastic recoil was recognized to be secondary to the preponderance of ostial stenoses – essentially extensive calcified aortic wall disease involving the renal artery origins.

Balloon expandable stents were introduced shortly after, and throughout the 1990s the technique of PTRA with stenting (PTRAS) was widely used, with improved technical success rates. These were confirmed and summarized in a randomized study comparing PTRAS with PTRA reported in 1999 which documented a much reduced restenosis rate of 14% at 6 months compared to 48% for PTRA alone.[25] These results led to the widespread application of PTRAS in treatment of atherosclerotic renal artery stenosis. Unfortunately, in many hands, selection for PTRAS was based on poor selection culminating in the notorious practice of 'fly by' PTRAS for asymptomatic, >50% stenosis by some interventional cardiologists. The technical supremacy of PTRAS in comparison to simple PTRA however was now established.

As previously discussed, during this same period, pharmacotherapy for treatment of arteriosclerosis and hypertension had progressed significantly. This advance led to several small prospective randomized comparisons of Best Medical Therapy versus PTRAS. The results of these trials indicated a benefit in terms of reduced antihypertensive medication but with a probable higher risk of complications for intervention. The numbers involved were small with systematic analysis yielding largely inconclusive results.

The scene was therefore set for the first of two large prospective randomized comparisons between intervention by PTRAS and Best Medical Therapy and with Best Medical Therapy alone. The first of these was the ASTRAL trial performed mostly in the United Kingdom and reported in 2009.[8] This trial randomized 806 patients with the inclusion criteria of unilateral or bilateral significant atherosclerotic renal artery stenosis. Only patients where there was uncertainty or equipoise regarding a benefit from revascularization were included. The primary end points were change in renal function and control of hypertension. No difference in blood pressure control either systolic or diastolic was found, there was no difference in preservation of renal function, and there was no difference in cardiovascular events or mortality. This pragmatic trial was designed to maximize recruitment within the UK National Health Service, but without the services of a core lab. Randomization was on the basis of initial diagnosis of significant renal artery stenosis (>50%), using duplex scanning or MRA and/or DSA. At on-table angiography, overestimation of stenosis was found in 20% of patients previously randomized to intervention at time of diagnosis when the stenosis was found to be <50%, and therefore, these patients did not undergo revascularization. This significant failure of randomization together with the specific exclusion from randomization of patients in whom the clinician felt that intervention was positively indicated were major flaws in this otherwise large prospective randomized study.

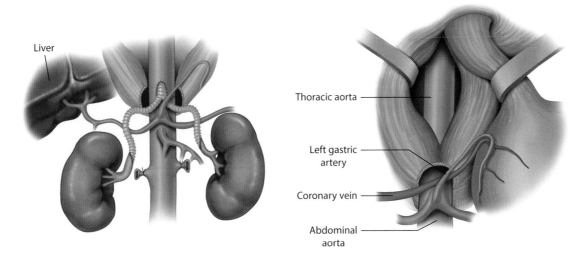

Figure 40.4 Bilateral aorto-renal bypass using supra-coeliac aortic inflow with bifurcated 12 × 8 mm prosthetic graft. The diaphragmatic crura are divided exposing 5 cm of usually 'healthy' distal thoracic aorta. The graft limbs are tunnelled retro-peritoneally and anastomosed end to end.

Subsequently, the CORAL trial similarly randomized between PTRAS with Best Medical Therapy and Best Medical Therapy alone but with a radiology core lab to strictly define estimation of renal artery stenosis. The results of the CORAL trial were reported in 2014 with a total number of randomized patients of 947.[26] The primary end point was one of a composite nature, namely death from cardiovascular and renal causes (myocardial infarction, stroke, congestive cardiac failure, progressive renal impairment or need for renal replacement therapy). On all of these outcomes, no significant difference between intervention and non-intervention could be found – results strikingly similar to those of the ASTRAL trial.

Improved blood pressure control was found in four recent trials, however, with the improvement being noted in both the interventional and non-interventional limbs.[8,27,28] Irrespective of intervention, all of these most recent prospective randomized studies confirm that modern Best Medical Therapy is highly effective in controlling hypertension and preserving renal function. The inevitable initial conclusion reached is that PTRAS confers no additional benefit over Best Medical Therapy for the majority of patients with atherosclerotic renal artery disease (Figure 40.4).

Technique of percutaneous transluminal renal artery angioplasty and stenting

As standard for arterial interventions, informed consent is taken; the patient is conscious with local anaesthesia and intravenous sedation. Non-invasive monitoring by either an experienced endovascular surgeon and his team, or a vascular anaesthetist, is mandatory usually with oxygen administration as required. Access is typically by the right common femoral artery with percutaneous puncture followed by placement of a 4F sheath, flush angiography with a 4F pigtail catheter, with selective angiography using a 4F Cobra C1 catheter. For stent insertion, a long 6F sheath is used to catheterize the renal arteries with a 4F C1 catheter and hydrophilic 035 hydrophilic guidewire, then exchange for a stiffer wire such as a 035 Rosen or 035 Terumo Advantage. Some use pre-dilation with a simple angioplasty balloon before placement of a stent, but our usual practice is a primary stent deployment using a balloon expandable uncovered stent thus minimising the risk of embolization. Where there is doubt about the severity of renal artery stenosis a trans-stenotic pressure gradient can be measured with a pressure wire. Finally, check angiography is performed to confirm technical success which is usually defined as a residual stenosis of <50% by visual assessment. The procedure is covered with intravenous administration of standard heparin, in our practice 5000 IU, without reversal of heparinization at the end of the intervention; peri-procedure intravenous hydration with optional addition of sodium bicarbonate and *N*-acetyl cysteine is important to protect and preserve renal function. The patient is then carefully monitored post procedure with blood pressure, pulse and oxygen saturation measurements for a minimum period of 4 hours. In modern practice the majority of patients are already on antiplatelet therapy, but in rare cases where this is not already instigated, a minimum period of antiplatelet therapy with either aspirin or clopidogrel of 6 weeks is recommended.

PTRA/PTRAS: Fibromuscular dysplasia and transplant renal artery stenosis

Patients with renal FMD with refractory hypertension or more rarely deteriorating renal function can be successfully treated with simple angioplasty. Technical success rates are almost 100% with significant improvement in blood pressure control. A meta-analysis of angioplasty for renal FMD revealed a 30% cure and overall clinical benefit rate of 88.3%.[29] The recommendation is that stent placement is only used as a bailout for complications of simple angioplasty such as dissection or renal artery aneurysm.[30]

Renal artery complications following transplant can be anatomical, i.e. from kinking or bending, post anastomotic or anastomotic. These latter two are mediated by immunological responses and cardiovascular risk factors. The literature clearly supports better outcomes in terms of morbidity, mortality and renal graft survival using endovascular rather than open treatment confirming significant improvement in graft function and control of blood pressure. This improvement was found with both bare metal and drug-eluting stents. A recent single-centre retrospective review of a small number of patients reported significantly higher patency rates with drug-eluting stent in comparison to bare metal stents.[31]

In-stent restenosis following PTRAS

Significant in-stent restenosis with increasing incidence over longer follow-up is a major complication, with almost 60% of patients over a 30-month period of follow-up in one series having developed duplex ultrasound criteria for recurrent stenosis.[32] In-stent restenosis can be treated in several ways including simple repeated angioplasty, cutting balloon angioplasty, stent-in-stent angioplasty, drug-eluting stents, covered stents and brachytherapy. Of these interventions, simple balloon angioplasty seems to have the highest recurrence rate with no significant difference between outcomes comparing simple balloon angioplasty versus cutting balloon angioplasty. There are little data to clearly define the best treatment, but drug-eluting stents and also covered stents may have the advantage in terms of reduced restenosis rate. There is some limited evidence that endovascular brachytherapy has promising results in the treatment of in-stent restenosis.[33]

INTERPRETATION OF CLINICAL EVIDENCE FOR PTRA/PTRAS

There are several analyses, meta-analyses and summative assessments of the many studies assessing the role of intervention. However, the majority of these studies are heterogeneous, and with the exception of the ASTRAL and CORAL trials, the prospective randomized comparisons were mostly underpowered; indeed, none were adequately powered to undertake meaningful subgroup analysis. A recent invited review updating intervention versus medical therapy from the Charleston Group attempted an analysis of all of these studies.[34]

Improvement in clinical outcome of blood pressure after intervention was reported in 79% during the follow-up period with a probable poorer outcome for blood pressure control in diabetics. For clinical outcome of renal function after intervention, most studies did not show a significant change in renal function in the majority, with deterioration in some but with improved renal function reported in 21% of 47 study treatment groups. An interesting and clinically relevant finding was that improvement or stabilization of renal function was not found in the more recent larger prospective randomized studies. A further relevant finding on the comparison of medical therapy with stent-only cohorts (these were in earlier studies) is that the stent-only group reported stable and improved renal function more commonly with a trend towards better blood pressure control, but neither difference reaching significance. The likely explanation for these findings is the marked improvement in Best Medical Therapy which has become established over these last 10–15 years.

With regard to subgroup analysis, most trials are insufficiently powered to reveal significant outcomes. With regard to increasing severity of renal artery stenosis, both the ASTRAL and CORAL trials failed to show any correlation between improved outcome in either arm in the presence of higher grade >80% renal artery stenosis. The RAS-CAD trial focused particularly on the effect of medical therapy alone versus medical therapy with PTRAS and on the progression of left ventricular hypertrophy in patients with both coronary artery disease and renal artery stenosis. In this study, there was a statistically significant improvement in systolic and diastolic blood pressure control in the medical therapy arm with a non-statistically significant drop in both measures in the stenting plus medical therapy arm. There was no difference in renal function at 1 year, and of interest both arms reported a statistically significant reduction in left ventricular mass index but with no difference between either groups for cardiovascular events. An important limitation of this study was its focus on cardiac and coronary end points but with the exclusion of patients with >80% renal artery stenosis. The question as to whether intervention in addition to Best Medical Therapy will improve left ventricular function remains unanswered.

There is consensus rather than objective evidence to support the value of intervention for treatment of patients with a cardio-renal syndrome or flash pulmonary oedema. In a recent retrospective single-centre study reported by Kalra's Group, PTRAS in 237 patients with underlying atherosclerotic renovascular disease presenting with flash pulmonary oedema, refractory hypertension or rapidly declining kidney function, survival was found to be improved after intervention. This was in patients presenting with flash pulmonary oedema and also in those presenting with a combination of rapid decline of renal function and refractory hypertension, but not when these conditions presented in isolation.[35]

MODERN MANAGEMENT OF RENOVASCULAR DISEASE

With regard to treatment of congenital renal arterial disease, renal FMD and renal transplant arterial stenosis, the endovascular approach of balloon angioplasty with or without stenting is the preferred treatment option. This is with good long-term clinical outcomes with regard to blood pressure control and preservation of renal function and with low rates of morbidity and mortality.

Endovascular treatment by simple balloon angioplasty and/or balloon stent angioplasty has an important role to play now in the management of renovascular hypertension

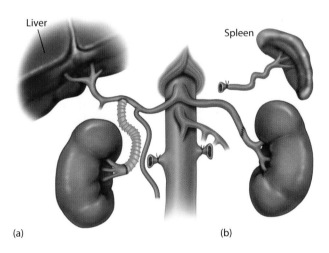

(a)   (b)

Figure 40.5 Extra-anatomic bypass grafts with end-to-end renal anastomoses. (a) Hepato-renal on the right using gastro-duodenal artery if of suitable calibre or 6 or 8 mm prosthetic bypass. (b) Splenorenal on the left using the splenic artery. NB careful preoperative inflow assessment of the coeliac artery essential as up to 50% will have a significant stenosis.

in children. Angioplasty provided clinical benefit in 63% of children in a recent series with renovascular hypertension.[36] PTRA/PTRAS will be curative in some and, in most, play an important bridging role in improved hypertension treatment and preserved renal function until a child has grown to an age and size allowing a single-stage definitive open vascular reconstruction. Open vascular reconstruction of the aorta and renal arteries will continue to play a major and definitive role in the management of renovascular hypertension in children with middle aortic syndrome and FMD. The roles of endovascular and vascular intervention are now complementary in the management of children with renovascular disease. Management of these children must be in multidisciplinary groups within specialist paediatric hospitals (Figures 40.5 and 40.6).

The picture is not so clear in the management of atherosclerotic renovascular disease, even with the current plethora of clinical evidence. All of this evidence however clearly points to the central importance of Best Medical Therapy in the baseline treatment of patients with atherosclerotic renovascular disease. The combination of meticulous and aggressive hypertension control in particular with the use of ACE inhibitors and ARBs, control of hyperlipidaemia with statins, antiplatelet therapy and lifestyle modification will reliably achieve clinical improvement in blood pressure control and preservation of renal function. The recent prospective randomized comparisons of Best Medical Therapy with or without intervention confirm that in the majority of patients with the exception of some subgroups, intervention offers little benefit and possibly increased complication rates (Figure 40.7). A major caveat is that ACE inhibitors and ARBs must be used with careful monitoring in particular to detect the deterioration of renal function that can result in a minority.

There are important subgroups of patients with atherosclerotic renal artery disease however in whom intervention should continue to be considered (Table 40.6).

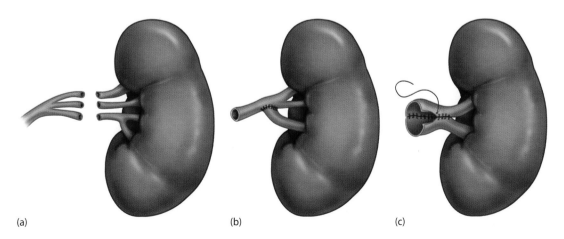

(a)   (b)   (c)

Figure 40.6 Bench reconstruction of the renal artery with auto-transplantation. (a) Using the internal iliac artery for multiple segmental arterial repair – useful in severe fibromuscular dysplasia. (b and c) Bench renal artery reconstruction after resection of truncal or proximal segmental aneurysmal or stenotic disease.

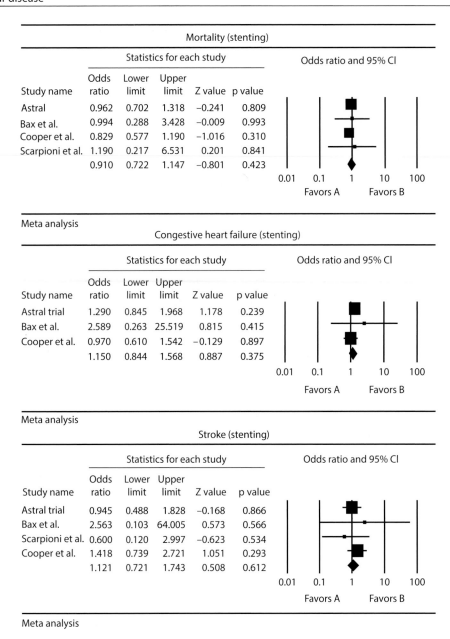

Figure 40.7 Forest plot of a meta-analysis of the major trials comparing outcomes of best medical therapy and PTRA. (From Riaz IB et al., *Am J Cardiol*, 114, 1116, 2014.)

Table 40.6 Indications for revascularization in atherosclerotic renovascular disease.

Severe or dialysis dependent, acute renal failure[a]

Intolerance of renin–angiotensin blockade[a]

Recurrent acute heart failure or flash pulmonary oedema[a]

Rapid onset of severe hypertension

Rapid onset of deteriorating renal function

Chronic heart failure

'Hibernating' renal parenchyma – as identified on BOLD MRI and isotopic single kidney GFR ratio

[a] Strongly recommended.

These indications are important to consider in individual patients in the absence of level 1 data – prospective randomized comparison in adequately powered trials for these subgroup analyses is highly unlikely ever to be performed. In the majority of these patients, because of co-morbidities, the intervention of choice will be PTRAS. Although the evidence base is heterogeneous, open revascularization is associated with better long-term outcomes in terms of control of blood pressure and preservation of renal function.[22] Selection for open repair must obviously be on the basis of multidisciplinary assessment by anaesthesiologist, nephrologist and vascular surgeon, and of necessity because of the low volume in these largely high-risk groups, open interventions should take place in specialist vascular centres.

REFERENCES

1. Safian RD, Textor SC. Renal artery stenosis. *N Engl J Med.* 2001;344:431–442.

2. Olin JW, Froehlich J, Xiaokui GU et al. The United States registry for fibromuscular dysplasia results in the first 447 patients. *Circulation.* 2012;125:3182–3190.

3. Wollenweber J, Sheps S, Davis G. Clinical course of atherosclerotic renovascular disease. *Am J Cardiol.* 1968;21:60–71.

4. Drieghe B, Madaric J, Samo G, Manoharan G, Bartunek J, Haryndrickx GR, Pijls NH, DeBruyne B. Assessment of renal artery stenosis: Side-by-side comparison of angiography and duplex ultrasound with pressure gradient measurements. *Eur Heart J.* 2008;29:517–524.

5. Eirin A, Gloviczki ML, Tang H, Rule AD, Woollard JR, Lerman A, Textor SC, Lerman LO. Chronic renovascular hypertension is associated with elevated levels of neutrophil gelatinase – associated lipocalin. *Nephrol Dial Transplant.* 2013;27:4153–4161.

6. Textor SC, Lerman LO. Paradigm shifts in atherosclerotic renovascular disease: Where are we now? *J Am Soc Nephrol.* 2015;26:1–7.

7. Gloviczki ML, Glockner JF, Lerman LO, McKusick MA, Misra S, Grande JP, Textor SC. Preserved oxygenation despite reduced blood flow in post stenotic kidneys in human atherosclerotic renal artery stenosis. *Hypertension.* 2010;55:961–966.

8. Wheatley K, Ives M, Gray R et al. Revascularisation verses medical therapy for renal artery stenosis. *N Engl J Med.* 2009;361:1953–1962.

9. Ritchie J, Green D, Chrysochou C et al. High risk clinical presentations in atherosclerotic renovascular disease: Prognosis and response to renal artery revascularisation. *Am J Kidney Dis.* 2014;63:186–197.

10. Crimmins JM, Madder RD, Marinescu V, Safian RD. Validity of estimated glomerular filtration rates for assessment of renal function after renal artery stenting in patients with atherosclerotic renal artery stenosis. *JACC Cardiovasc Interv.* 2014;7:543–549.

11. Abu Rahama AF, Srivastava M, Mousa AY et al. Critical analysis of renal duplex ultrasound parameters in detecting significant renal artery stenosis. *J Vasc Surg.* 2012;56:1052–1060.

12. Redermacher J, Chavan A, Bleck J et al. Use of Doppler ultrasonography to predict the outcome of therapy for renal artery stenosis. *N Engl J Med.* 2001;344:410–417.

13. Garcia-Criado A, Gilabert R, Nicolau C et al. Value of Doppler sonography for predicting clinical outcome after renal artery revascularisation in atherosclerotic renal artery stenosis. *J Ultrasound Med.* 2005;24:1641–1647.

14. Abu Rahama AF, Yacoub M. Renal imaging: Duplex ultrasound, computed tomography angiography, magnetic resonance angiography, and angiography. *Sem Vasc Surg.* 2013;26:134–143.

15. Tan KT, Van Beek EG, Brown PWG, Van Delden OM, Tijssen J, Ramsay LE. Magnetic resonance angiography for the diagnosis of renal artery stenosis: A meta-analysis. *Clin Radiol.* 2002;57:617–624.

16. Chrysochou C, Mendichovszky IA, Buckley DL, Cheung CM, Jackson A, Kalra PA. BOLD Imaging: A potential predictive bi-marker of renal functional outcome following revascularisation in atheromatous renovascular disease. *Nephrol Dial Transplant.* 2012;27:1013–1019.

17. Vasbinder GB, Nelemens PJ, Kessels AG et al. Diagnostic tests for renal artery stenosis in patients suspected of having renovascular hypertension: A meta-analysis. *An Intern Med.* 2001;135:401–411.

18. Maxwell MH, Rodnick MR, Waks AU. New approaches to the diagnosis of renovascular hypertension. *ADV Nephrol Necker Hosp.* 1985;14:285–304.

19. Chrysochu C, Foley RN, Young JF et al. Dispelling the myth: The use of renin – angiotensin blockade in atheromatous renovascular disease. *Nephrol Dial Transplant.* 2012;27:140–149.

20. Ahmed A. Use of angiotensin convertor enzyme inhibitors in patients with heart failure and renal insufficiency: How concerned should we be by the rise in serum creatinine? *J Am Geriatr Soc.* 2002 July;50(7):1297–1300.

21. Kalaitzidis RG, Elisaf MS. The role of statins in chronic kidney disease. *Am J Nephrol.* 2011;34:195–202.

22. Abela R, Ivanova S, Lidder S, Morris R, Hamilton G. An analysis comparing open surgical and endovascular treatment of atherosclerotic renal artery stenosis. *Eur J Vasc Endovasc Surg.* 2009;38:666–675.

23. Gruntzig A, Kuhlmann U, Vetter W et al. Treatment of renovascular hypertension with percutaneous transluminal dilatation of renal artery stenosis. *Lancet.* 1978;311:801–802.

24. Weibull H, Bergqvist D, Bergentz, SE, Jonsson K, Hulthen L, Manhem P. Percutaneous transluminal renal angioplasty versus surgical reconstruction of atherosclerotic renal artery stenosis: A prospective randomised study. *J Vasc Surg.* 1993;18:841–850.

25. Van de Ven PJG, Kaatee R, Beutler J et al. Arterial stenting and balloon angioplasty in ostial atherosclerotic renovascular disease: A randomised trial. *Lancet.* 1999;353:282–286.

26. Cooper CJ, Murphy TP, Cutlip DE et al. for the CORAL Investigators. Stenting and medical therapy for atherosclerotic renal artery stenosis. *N Engl J Med.* 2014;370:13–22.

27. Bax L, Wittiez AJ, Kouwenberg HJ, Mali WP, Buskens E, Beek FJ et al. Stent placement in patients with atherosclerotic renal artery stenosis and impaired renal function: A randomised trial. *Ann Intern Med.* 2009;150:840–848.

28. Marcantoni C, Zanoli L, Rastelli S, Tripepi G, Matalone M, Di Landro D et al. Stenting of renal artery stenosis in coronary artery disease (RAS-CAD) study: A prospective, randomized trial. *J Nephrol.* 2009 January–February;22(1):13–16.

29. Trinquart L, Mounier-Vehier C, Sapoval N, Gagnon N, Plourin PF. Efficacy of revascularization for renal artery stenosis caused by fibromuscular dysplasia: A systematic review and meta-analysis. *Hypertension.* 2010;56:525–532.

30. Anderson JL, Halperin JL, Albert NM et al. Management of patients with peripheral artery disease, [compilation of 2005 & 2011 ACCF/AHA guideline recommendations]: A report to the American College of Cardiology Foundation/American Heart Association Task Force on practice guidelines. *Circulation.* 2013;127:1425–1443.

31. Biederman DM, Fischman AM, Titiano JJ, Kim E, Patel RS, Nowakowski FS, Florman S, Lookstein RA. Tailoring the endovascular management of transplant renal artery stenosis. *Am J Transplant.* 2015;15:1039–1049.

32. Simone TAI, Brooke BS, Goodney PP, Walsh DB, Stone DH, Powell RJ, Cronenwett JL, Nolan BW. Clinical effectiveness of secondary interventions for restenosis after renal artery stenting. *J Vasc Surg.* 2013 September;58(3):687–694.

33. Silverman SH, Exline JB, Silverman LN, Samson RH. Endovascular brachytherapy for renal artery in-stent restenosis. *J Vasc Surg.* 2014 December;60:1599–604.

34. Mousa AY, Abu Rahma AF, Bozzay J, Broce M, Bates M. Update on intervention versus medical therapy for atherosclerotic renal artery stenosis. *J Vasc Surg.* 2015;61:1613–1623.

35. Ritchie J, Green D, Chrycochou C et al. High risk clinical presentations in atherosclerotic renal artery disease: Prognosis and response to renal artery revascularization. *Am J Kidney Dis.* 2014;163:186–197.

36. Kari JA, Roebuck DJ, McLaren CA, Davis M, Dillon MJ, Hamilton G, Shroff R, Marks SD, Tullus K. Angioplasty for renovascular hypertension in 78 children. *Arch Dis Child.* 2015 May;100(5):474–478.

37. Sharma AM, Kline B. The United States registry for fibromuscular dysplasia: new findings and breaking myths. *Tech Vasc Intervent Radiol.* 2014;17:258.

38. Riaz IB, Husnain M, Riaz H, Asawaeer M, Bilal J, Pandit A, Shetty R, Lee KS. Meta-analysis of revascularization versus medical therapy for atherosclerotic renal artery stenosis. *Am J Cardiol* 2014;114:1116–1123.

41

Acute and chronic mesenteric vascular disease

STEFAN ACOSTA and MARTIN BJÖRCK

CONTENTS

CLASSIFICATION

The classification of mesenteric vascular disease is shown in Figure 41.1. Hypoperfusion syndromes such as colonic ischaemia after aortoiliac surgery and abdominal compartment syndrome (ACS) belong to the same category as non-occlusive mesenteric ischaemia (NOMI).

EPIDEMIOLOGY

Unfortunately, contemporary population-based studies on the epidemiology of acute mesenteric ischaemia (AMI) are lacking owing to low autopsy rates and reporting of only patients who have surgery. The overall incidence of AMI between 1970 and 1982 in the city of Malmö, Sweden, diagnosed at either autopsy or operation, was 12.9 per 100,000 person-years. The autopsy rate in this population was 87%. Among 402 patients, 270 (67.2%) had thromboembolic SMA occlusion, 63 (15.7%) mesenteric venous thrombosis (MVT), 62 (15.4%) NOMI and 7 (1.7%) had indeterminate aetiology.[1] The embolus to thrombus ratio was 1.4:1 among the 213 patients with acute SMA occlusion diagnosed at autopsy.[2] Acute SMA occlusion was more common than ruptured abdominal aortic aneurysm

(AAA).[1] The incidence of chronic mesenteric ischaemia (CMI) is unknown and dependent on diagnostic activity.

The frequency of AMI among patients with acute abdomen varies from 2.1% in suspected peritonitis,[3] 17.7% in emergency laparotomies[4] to 31.0% in damage-control laparotomies in non-trauma patients[5] (Table 41.1).

HISTORY

Recovery following resection of infarcted intestine secondary to mesenteric vessel occlusion was first described in 1895. The first successful emergency SMA embolectomy was undertaken in 1951, SMA thromboendarterectomy (TEA) in 1958 and aortomesenteric bypass in 1973. Intra-arterial thrombolysis for SMA embolus, using a combination of streptokinase and heparin, was reported to be successful in 1979.

PATHOPHYSIOLOGY

In AMI, whatever the cause, the infarction starts from the mucosa outwards. Acute SMA occlusion, in contrast to low-flow states and left-sided colonic ischaemia, causes a more significant reduction in blood flow with rapid development of extensive intestinal infarction.[9]

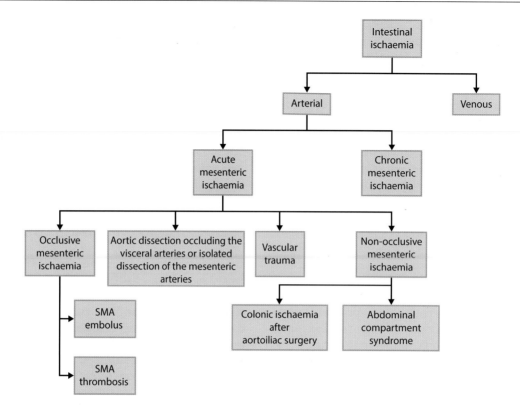

Figure 41.1 Classification of mesenteric ischaemia.

Table 41.1 Frequency of acute mesenteric ischaemia among patients with acute abdomen.

First author	Publication year	Patient selection criteria	Population	Study period	Frequency of acute mesenteric ischaemia (%)
Rozycki[4]	2002	Emergency laparotomy	Atlanta, USA	1996–2001	17.7 (53/300)
Sanna[3]	2003	Suspected peritonitis	Ferrara, Italy	1995–2001	2.1 (2/94)
Arenal[6]	2003	Emergency abdominal surgery and age ≥ 70 years	Valladolid, Spain	1986–1995	3.8 (27/710)
Weir-McCall[7]	2012	Emergency laparotomy	Eastbourne, United Kingdom	2008–2010	3.1 (3/97)
Green[8]	2013	Emergency laparotomy and age ≥ 80 years	Gillingham, United Kingdom	2005–2010	5.0 (5/100)
Khan[5]	2013	Damage-control laparotomy and non-trauma patients	Auckland, New Zealand	2008–2010	31.0 (13/42)

PATHOGENESIS

There are three main components, endothelial injury or dysfunction such as atherosclerosis, haemodynamic changes and hypercoagulability, contributing to the occurrence of thrombosis termed 'Virchow's triad'. This triad has most been related to occurrence of venous thrombosis, but is also applicable to arterial thrombosis. Patients with impaired cardiac function and lower cardiac output are at higher risk of impaired visceral blood flow than patients with a normal cardiac function. Thrombophilia plays an important role in venous mesenteric thrombosis, but the influence of hypercoagulable factors such as thrombocytosis have been less studied in the development of arterial thrombosis.

ARTERIAL MESENTERIC ISCHAEMIA

SMA atherosclerosis

Patients with advanced atherosclerosis in the SMA is often a manifestation of generalized atherosclerosis. The incidence of SMA atherosclerosis increases with age and is prevalent in 20% of the population at 65 years of age. Patients who undergo bypass operation for symptomatic iliac artery occlusive disease have simultaneous SMA atherosclerosis in 70% of the cases.[10] A collateral arterial network between the celiac trunk, SMA, inferior mesenteric artery and internal iliac arteries exists, which may become increasingly important and enlarged to compensate for the decreased visceral perfusion after gradual development of atherosclerotic occlusion or stenosis of the celiac trunk and/or SMA. Narrowing of the SMA has the greatest impact on the development of mesenteric ischaemia.

Acute thrombotic occlusion of the SMA

Thrombosis occurs at areas of severe atherosclerotic narrowing, most often at the origin of the SMA from the aorta, which also is named osteal stenosis.[2] History of other atherosclerotic manifestations such as coronary, cerebrovascular or peripheral arterial occlusive disease is common. In a substantial proportion of these patients, progressive atherosclerosis at the SMA origin may have developed over many years, resulting in collateral circulation to the SMA, mainly from the celiac trunk and inferior mesenteric artery. Dehydration, low cardiac output and hypercoagulable states are major contributing factors to thrombosis. In case of a thrombotic occlusion at the origin of the SMA, ischaemia usually develops from the proximal jejunum to the mid-transverse colon.

Embolic occlusion of the SMA

Mesenteric emboli usually originate from the heart. Aortoarterial embolism has also been described infrequently. Cardiac thrombi may be associated with atrial fibrillation, valvular disease, dilated left atrium, recent myocardial infarction and ventricular dilatation with mural thrombus. Iatrogenic embolization has been reported after cardiac catheterization, coronary arteriography and aortography.[11] Patients with emboli seldom have a history of previous intestinal ischaemia. A number of these patients have a history of prior arterial embolism and may, in addition to SMA embolus, suffer from synchronous embolism to other arterial segments. In an autopsy series of patients with lethal occlusion of the SMA, 19% had an acute myocardial infarction, 48% had remnant cardiac thrombus and 68% had synchronous embolus.[2] The embolus may occlude the arterial lumen completely or partially. Emboli tend to lodge at points of normal anatomical narrowing, usually immediately distal to the origin of a major branch. Typically, the embolus lodges a few centimetres distal to the origin of the SMA, sparing the proximal jejunal branches and allowing preservation of the proximal jejunum.

Diagnosis

CLINICAL PRESENTATION

A high index of suspicion and awareness among physicians who see patients who may have AMI is important, but not enough to improve outcomes. The typical clinical triad for an acute embolic SMA occlusion is severe abdominal pain but minimal findings at examination (pain out of proportion), bowel emptying and a source of embolus, most often atrial fibrillation. The often sudden onset of abdominal pain (*phase 1*) may decrease in intensity (*phase 2*), followed by an increase in abdominal pain associated with clinical deterioration and progression towards peritonitis (*phase 3*) (Box 41.1). This clinical triad is, however, not a consistent finding. Acute thrombotic SMA occlusion is difficult to diagnose at first evaluation. In retrospect, a high proportion of the often misunderstood patients with acute thrombotic SMA occlusion may have had long-standing pre-existing symptoms of CMI, including postprandial abdominal pain (abdominal angina), food fear, diarrhoea and weight loss. Indeed, 80% of patients were inappropriately medically treated with proton pump inhibitors, cortisone or antibiotics in the diagnostic phase in a recent series.[12] Current reports do not support the view that the majority of these patients suffer from cachexia at diagnosis, as often stated in textbooks. Weight loss is a consistent finding, however, but a proportion of patients were in fact overweight when they fell ill, decreasing in weight to normal weight at the time of diagnosis.[12] The median body mass index (BMI) was 20.2 kg/m^2 in women and 23.1 kg/m^2 in men at diagnosis in a recent consecutive series,[12] rising to 23.4 kg/m^2 and 25.8 kg/m^2, respectively, 24 months after stenting of the SMA.

The three clinical phases of acute embolic SMA occlusion

Awareness of the three clinical phases of an acute embolic occlusion can lead to an earlier diagnosis:

- Phase 1 is the hyper-peristaltic phase with severe abdominal pain and minimal abdominal findings, forceful bowel emptying (vomiting and/or diarrhoea) and the presence of a source of embolus (e.g. atrial fibrillation).
- Phase 2 is the paralytic phase of bowels with distended and silent abdomen. The pain intensity often decreases.
- Phase 3 is the peritonitis phase with continuous pain, peritonitis, rapid general deterioration and acidosis.

LABORATORY MARKERS (LEVEL 2, GRADE C)

No plasma marker is yet sufficiently accurate to be diagnostic in the acute setting.[13] D-Dimer has been found to be the most consistent highly sensitive early marker, but specificity was low.[14,15] The high sensitivity, approaching 100%, makes it an excellent exclusion test, but many other conditions are associated with high D-dimer values. The early promising results of alfa-glutathione S-transferase as a plasma biomarker could not be reproduced. The results of intestinal fatty acid binding globulin (I-FABP) and D-lactate have been conflicting. The encouraging preliminary results of urinary FABP as an accurate biomarker has to be confirmed in a follow-up study in patients with acute abdomen.[13] In a recent publication, Matsumoto and colleagues reported that plasma I-FABP was much higher among 19 patients with vascular intestinal ischaemia than among 26 patients with non-vascular irreversible intestinal ischaemia.[16] Most importantly, clinicians should be aware of diagnostic pitfalls that may be encountered in patients with acute SMA occlusion such as elevated troponin I and elevated pancreas amylase and normal plasma lactate, which may lead the clinician away from the correct diagnosis.[17]

ENDOSCOPY

Acute on CMI, with an insidious clinical course, may show signs of ischemia in the duodenum and in the right colon on endoscopy, a fact that seems to be virtually unknown to many physicians. *Helicobacter pylori* testing is typically negative. Capsule endoscopy may be helpful to detect chronic ischemic lesions in the small bowel.[12]

CT ANGIOGRAPHY (LEVEL 2, GRADE B)

The major breakthrough for diagnosis of acute (or chronic) SMA occlusion has been the evolution and availability of high-resolution CT around the clock.[18] Reconstruction of images in the sagittal, coronal and transverse planes can be diagnostic. Embolic occlusion often appears as an oval-shaped clot surrounded by contrast in a non-calcified arterial segment located in the middle and distal part of the main stem of the SMA. Thrombotic occlusion usually appears as a clot superimposed on a heavily calcified occlusive lesion at the ostium of the SMA. The presence of vascular pathology precedes the intestinal pathology, which is of crucial importance when the images are studied.[19] In the absence of intestinal findings at CT or peritonitis on clinical examination, patients have likely been diagnosed in time for intestinal revascularization. Patients with impaired renal function or increased creatinine values should undergo CT angiography if there is a suspicion of acute SMA occlusion, without fear of contrast-induced renal failure,[20] to improve their chances of survival.

DIAGNOSIS OF CHRONIC MESENTERIC ISCHEMIA

Diagnosis of CMI is first based upon medical history, CT angiography or magnetic resonance angiography and endoscopy findings. If available, gastric exercise tonometry or 24 hours of gastrointestinal tonometry may be performed in the diagnostic work-up.[21] A less sophisticated method is to use clinical exercise testing, meaning that the abdominal pain is provoked by exercise on a bicycle. Patients with significant or unclear grade of stenosis of the SMA on CT angiography or colour Doppler ultrasound are referred for angiography with pressure measurements across the stenotic lesion(s) and immediately stented if the pressure gradient in mean arterial pressure, aorta minus SMA distal to the occlusive lesion, is ≥10 mmHg. Stenting of the celiac trunk may be performed if there is a significant stenosis and a persistent visceral ischemia after SMA stenting, if recanalization of the SMA fails or if there is a SMA stent occlusion that, if re-intervened, is considered to be at very high risk for distal embolic complications and intestinal infarction. The presence of postprandial abdominal pain before treatment should disappear after successful stenting of the SMA.

TREATMENT OF ACUTE SMA OCCLUSION

Optimal treatment may include both open and endovascular surgery, and patients are best treated in a vascular centre with a hybrid operating room. From preoperative clinical and radiological evaluation, it can be determined whether the patient has peritonitis or not and whether the occlusion is embolic or thrombotic. Laparotomy is indicated if there is peritonitis, unless a palliative approach was decided upon. This aims to assess the extent and severity of intestinal ischemia: colour of the intestines, dilatation and peristaltic motion of the bowel, visible pulsations in the mesenteric arcade arteries and bleeding from cut surfaces are most important to assess. Laparotomy, rather than laparoscopy, is usually safer and quicker to evaluate the visceral organs. Extensive intestinal paralysis with dilated bowel loops may be impossible to evaluate at laparoscopy, even by an expert. Furthermore, even a low grade of intra-abdominal hypertension may become fatal when a large portion of the intestinal tract is gangrenous.[22] In this situation, it is important to optimize the perfusion of the remaining bowel, which often requires open abdomen treatment.[23] Elderly patients with complete transmural infarction of the small bowel up to the mid-transverse colon would need extensive bowel resection that would lead to short bowel syndrome and increased morbidity. Survival in these patients is poor and surgery may be inappropriate for ethical reasons. In the event of bowel perforation, the affected intestinal segment is resected with staples, leaving the reconstruction of the intestines until second-look laparotomy after 18–36 hours.

ACUTE MESENTERIC ARTERIAL REVASCULARIZATION

Acute mesenteric arterial revascularization is done preferably before any bowel surgery. If no vascular surgeon is available, it may be preferable to resect necrotic bowel, close the abdomen and transport the patient to a vascular centre for revascularization. According to the national Swedish registry of vascular procedures, Swedvasc,[24] there has been a steady increase in mesenteric revascularizations for AMI since 2004. In 2009, endovascular treatment surpassed open surgery: 29 endovascular *versus* 24 open revascularizations. In contrast, this shift in treatment modality has not taken place in North America.[25] The 30-day mortality rate in Swedvasc was similar after open *versus* endovascular surgery for embolic occlusions (37% vs. 33%), whereas the mortality rate was significantly higher after open than endovascular treatment for thrombotic occlusions (56% vs. 23%). Of note, no patient had completion angiography after open surgical treatment, whereas completion angiography is part of the procedure after endovascular surgery. There may have been differences in disease severity between the treatment groups, but it remains possible that the endovascular approach is better for thrombotic occlusions in elderly, fragile patients. There is rarely any indication for revascularization of both the SMA and the celiac trunk, and SMA revascularization seems to be more important.

OPEN SMA EMBOLECTOMY

Open SMA embolectomy remains a good treatment option.[26] When laparotomy has been performed in a patient with peritonitis, exposure of the SMA and balloon embolectomy, with a 3- or 4-Fr Fogarty catheter, through a transverse arteriotomy is indicated. The result should be checked by completion angiography of the SMA with anteroposterior and lateral views. Stenosis and dissection at the arteriotomy closure site, residual peripheral embolus in arterial branches not cleared and venous return to the portal vein can all be assessed.

OPEN VASCULAR SURGERY FOR ACUTE AND CHRONIC THROMBOTIC SMA OCCLUSION

Division of the SMA distal to the occlusive lesion and reimplantation into the infrarenal aorta, TEA with patch angioplasty and bypass distal to the occlusive lesion are the open surgical options. If available, the preoperative CT angiography scan can be very useful to determine the source of inflow artery and sites with extensive atherosclerotic lesions are avoided. Bypass with a short graft from the infrarenal aorta to the SMA is the simplest bypass procedure and may be most appropriate in the emergency setting. This solution is seldom possible, however, since patients with thrombosis of the SMA very often have an infrarenal aorta that is heavily calcified, explaining why the orifice of the SMA was stenotic as part of the aortic atherosclerotic disease.

In case of extensive atherosclerotic lesions in the infrarenal aorta, the supraceliac aorta or the common iliac artery (Figure 41.2) may be used as the inflow of the graft. Very often the anterior part of the common iliac artery is possible to use for inflow. Autologous reversed saphenous vein may be the preferred conduit, in case of contamination, and especially in elective supraceliac – SMA bypass. Grafts originating from the infrarenal aorta or the common iliac artery are prone to kinking when the intestines

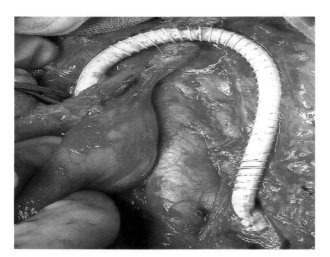

Figure 41.2 Bypass with reinforced PTFE conduit from the left common iliac artery to the superior mesenteric artery due to chronic mesenteric ischaemia.

are moved back into the abdomen after completion of the bypass. Therefore, the preferred graft material is Dacron® or expanded polytetrafluoroethylene reinforced with rings (Figure 41.2) is a good bypass conduit alternative, especially in the emergency setting in a non-contaminated peritoneal cavity, to withstand kinking of the graft. It is important to cover the graft with an omentum flap or in other creative ways, to prevent contact between the graft and the intestines, which may result in graft-enteric fistula.

Endovascular therapeutic options in acute or chronic mesenteric ischaemia

ACCESS TO THE SUPERIOR MESENTERIC ARTERY

The SMA can be reached via the femoral and brachial routes, although sometimes local exposure of the SMA in the abdomen is also needed. Brachial access may be preferable if there is a sharp downward angle between the aorta and the SMA, which is common, or if the ostium of the SMA is calcified. Passage of wires, catheters and introducers may cause dissection of the SMA. If an antegrade approach from the femoral or brachial artery fails, a retrograde approach through the exposed SMA after laparotomy is performed.[27]

ASPIRATION EMBOLECTOMY OF THE SMA

Endovascular aspiration embolectomy is a treatment option in patients without peritonitis.[27-29] The SMA is cannulated as earlier and catheterized using a reverse-curve catheter and a hydrophilic 0.035 in. guidewire, which is passed into the ileocolic branch of the SMA. The wire is then replaced with a stiffer, Jindo or Rosen wire to achieve stability. With the wire in place, typically a 7-Fr, 45 cm introducer with a removable hub (Destination®; Terumo, Tokyo, Japan) is placed proximal to the embolus in the SMA. Inside this, a 6-Fr guiding catheter is introduced into the clot, which is aspirated with a 20 mL syringe as the guiding catheter is withdrawn. The aspiration catheter needs to be stiff in order not to collapse during aspiration. The hub of the introducer is removed to allow clearance of residual clots. Angiography is performed, usually followed by repeated aspirations. An alternative is to use an over-the-wire double-lumen aspiration catheter such as the Export® (Medtronic, Minneapolis, Minnesota, USA), which may allow removal of smaller peripheral clots.

LOCAL SMA THROMBOLYSIS

In cases of incomplete aspiration embolectomy or distal embolization, local thrombolysis is a viable treatment alternative in patients without peritonitis.[27-30] With the introducer placed in the proximal SMA, a multiple side-hole catheter delivering drugs over 10 cm, or a 4-Fr end-hole catheter, is advanced to within the embolus. Local thrombolysis is achieved by administration of recombinant tissue plasminogen activator at a rate of 0.5–1 mg/h, checking status with repeated angiographies once or twice per day. Bleeding complications during local thrombolysis are infrequent and self-limiting. In a recent report,[30] bleeding from the gastrointestinal tract occurred in only one of 34 procedures. Small peripheral residual emboli can be treated conservatively with heparin anticoagulation as the marginal arteries in the mesentery may provide sufficient collateral circulation to the affected intestinal segment.[28] Only 38% of patients needed to undergo check laparotomy after local thrombolysis.[30] Endovascular rheolytic thromboembolectomy may be a supplementary technical method to aspiration thromboembolectomy in cases where thrombolysis is contraindicated (Figure 41.3a through d).

ANTEGRADE RECANALIZATION AND STENTING OF THE SMA

Treatment of underlying stenotic or occlusive lesions is most often achieved during the same procedure, after removal

of a thrombotic clot by aspiration or thrombolysis.[28] The sequence of endovascular intervention *versus* exploratory laparotomy depends on the clinical state of the patient. If femoral access fails, an attempt to cross the occlusive lesion using a brachial approach with a 4-Fr (Headhunter®; Terumo, Tokyo, Japan) catheter may be successful. When eventually a stable 0.035-in. wire has been placed in the ileocolic artery, an introducer is advanced across the atherosclerotic lesion. A balloon-expandable stent is chosen as they have better properties than self-expanding stents to maintain lumen diameter after stent deployment. The balloon-expandable stent is placed at the treatment site, followed by retraction of the protective introducer sheath, thus exposing the stent. The hard, calcified ostial lesion is usually treated with a 7–8 mm diameter stent. Unfavourable artery angulation or a potential risk of arterial dissection at the distal end of the stent is treated by extension with a self-expanding stent into the middle SMA.

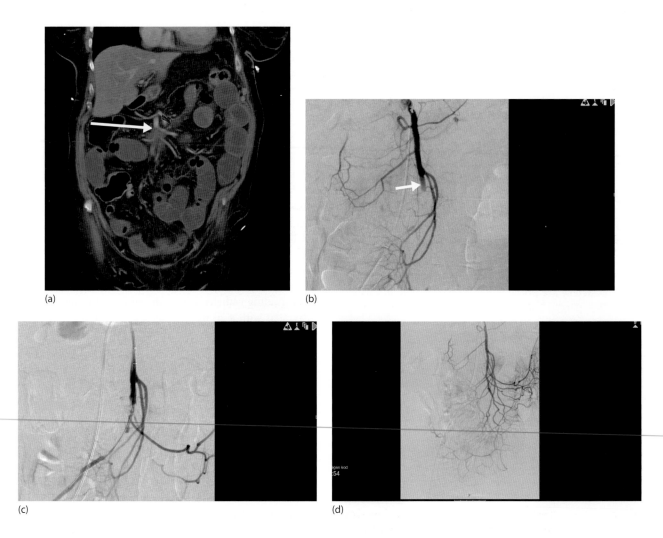

(a)

(b)

(c)

(d)

Figure 41.3 Patient with generalized peritonitis due to acute SMA embolic occlusion. At laparotomy, 2 m of small bowel was resected with staples due to transmural infarction, whereas the other 2 m of the remaining small bowel was found to be ischemic. In accordance with the CT angiography (a), the initial angiography showed an embolic occlusion in the middle part of the main stem of the SMA (b). The white arrows indicate the level of occlusion. Rheolytic thromboembolectomy with the AngioJet® Ultra Thrombectomy System (MEDRAD Inc, PA) was performed (c), followed by repeated aspiration thromboembolectomy (d). At second look, all the intestines were found to be well revascularized, and reanastomosis of the small bowel ends was performed. Recovery was uneventful.[28]

Results after stenting are checked by angiography, as well as with pressure measurement. If there is residual pressure gradient across the stent exceeding 12 mmHg, additional angioplasty and/or stenting is performed. One of the most feared complications is dissection from the SMA ostium into the peripheral branches of the SMA, worsening the intestinal ischaemia further.[28] This complication can be managed at laparotomy by exposure of a peripheral branch in the arterial mesentery (see 'Retrograde recanalization and stenting of the superior mesenteric artery' section), with puncture into the true arterial lumen. The guidewire then has a better chance of following the true lumen into the aorta, establishing through-and-through access with the femoral artery. The dissection is then stented, sometimes into peripheral branches beyond the main trunk of the SMA (Figure 41.4a through c).

RETROGRADE RECANALIZATION AND STENTING OF THE SMA

If brachial access fails, laparotomy and exposure of the SMA is performed for retrograde SMA recanalization and stenting.[27,28] This approach offers the opportunity to inspect the abdominal viscera, to have distal control of the SMA and to avoid bypass surgery in the setting of necrotic bowel (Figure 41.5a through f). The SMA is exposed at the junction of the mesocolon and the small bowel mesentery. A puncture is made in the vessel in its main trunk with a micropuncture needle; the occlusion is often recanalized easily with a 0.018 mm in. guidewire into the aorta. The SMA is clamped distally to avoid distal embolization if there is fresh thrombus at the occlusion site. The proximal SMA lesion is then crossed with a stiff, braided 4-Fr catheter, exchanging for a 260 cm long 0.035 in. hydrophilic

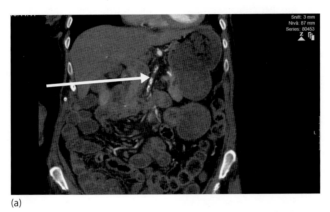

(a)

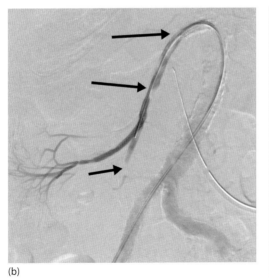

(b)

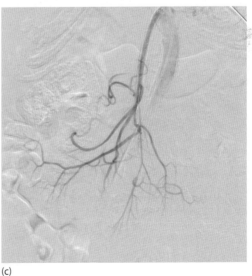

(c)

Figure 41.4 A patient with acute on chronic mesenteric ischaemia who had first undergone an exploratory laparotomy and resection of the distal small bowel and proximal large bowel due to mesenteric ischaemia. Post-operative CT angiography identified a 7 cm long thrombotic occlusion from the origin of the SMA. The arrow indicates the calcified SMA mixed with thrombotic clots (a). Recanalization and stenting of the proximal part of the occlusive SMA lesion was performed but was complicated by a long dissection (multiple black arrows) ending up with an occlusion of the distal part of the SMA (b). Re-exploratory laparotomy was performed and the entire small bowel was ischemic. A peripheral arterial SMA branch was punctured and a guidewire entered the true lumen up to the aorta and snared with devices from a transfemoral approach, creating a through-and-through access. The long dissection was stented extensively from the true lumen from the aorta into a non-dissected site in the ileocolic artery (c). The patient is still alive and has been asymptomatic during the 4 years of follow-up with repeated CT angiographies.

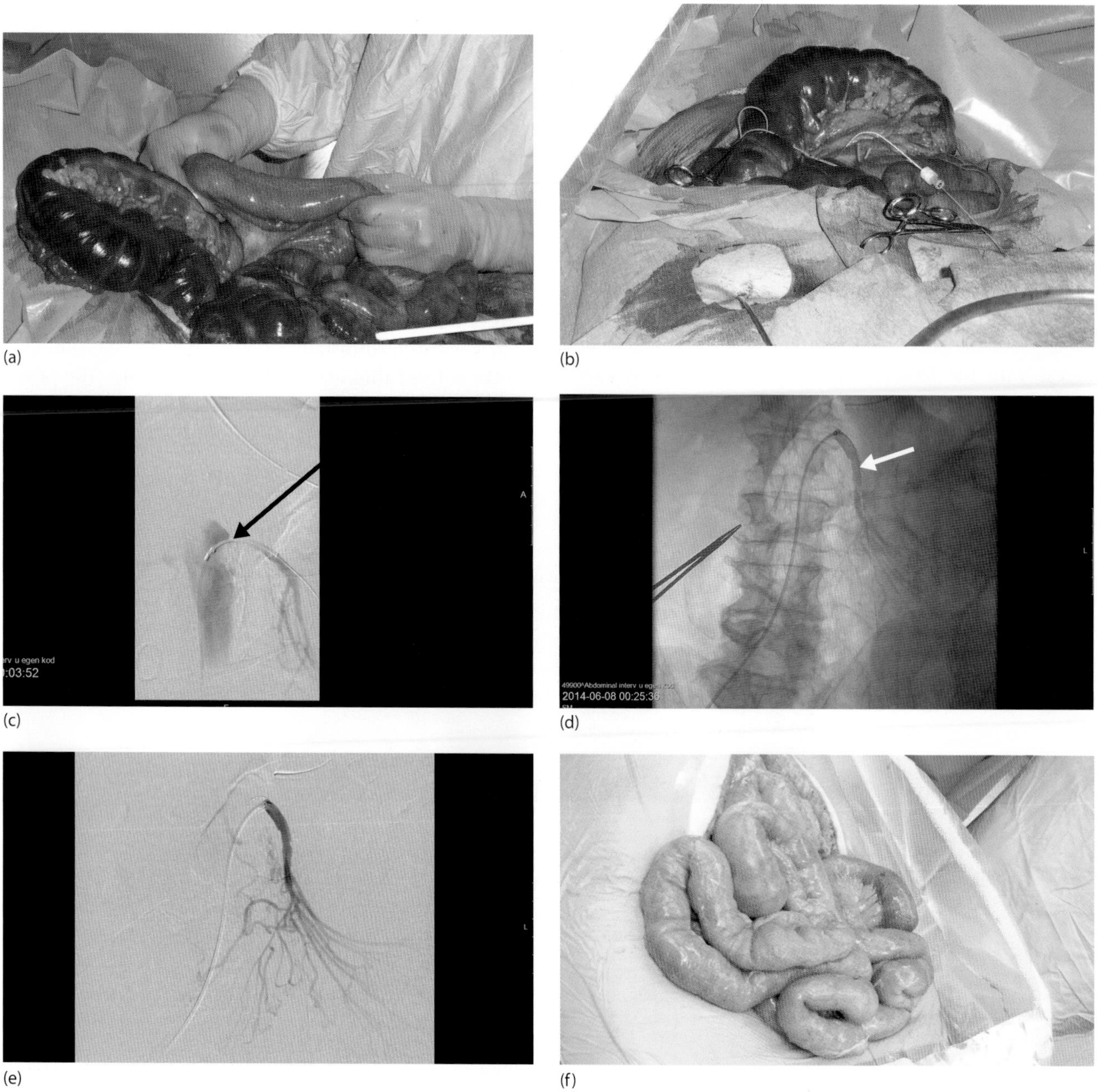

Figure 41.5 A 76-year-old female patient with a history of smoking and chronic obstructive pulmonary disease. She fell ill for 6 months ago with abdominal pain and 13 kg of weight loss. Colonoscopy and gastroscopy were negative. She was admitted with 1 day of worsening of abdominal pain, vomiting and developed generalized peritonitis during her stay. CT angiography showed a thrombotic occlusion of the proximal SMA. Explorative laparotomy was performed after 48 hours of acute symptoms. (a) Extensive bowel ischaemia is shown. Full bowel wall gangrene of the right and transverse colon, variable depths of ischaemia in the ileum and a normal colour but distended proximal jejunum (in between the surgeon's hands) are shown. (b) Through-and-through access was established from the SMA to the right common femoral artery: after exposure of the SMA, thrombectomy was performed with evacuation of fresh thrombus, but poor flow. Needle puncture of the SMA above the suture closure site was performed, followed by easy retrograde recanalization to the aorta with a 0.018 in. guidewire. The guidewire was snared from below and brought out into the introducer from the right groin. (c) The introducer was then easily advanced passed the tight short stenosis at the origin of the SMA (arrow). The stent was advanced to the tip of the introducer, and the introducer was thereafter withdrawn for permitting stent deployment. (d) Frontal angiography shows good flow within the SMA and the branches to the small bowel. The arrow indicates the puncture site in the SMA and entrance of the through-and-through guidewire. (e) Completion frontal digital subtraction angiography. Another 2 m of proximal small bowel was normalized in colour 15 minutes afterwards. Resection of the right and transverse colon and 2 m of small intestine was performed. (f) At second look 40 hours after the first procedure, 3 m of viable small bowel was found, and no additional bowel resections were required, and an ileocolic anastomosis was reconstructed.

guidewire. The wire is snared in the aorta using a snare passed through a brachial or femoral access and then brought out, creating through-and-through access.

A small transverse arteriotomy is then done at the level of the puncture, and an over-the-wire Fogarty balloon is passed into the aorta if thrombectomy is necessary. Thrombectomy is performed over the wire and the SMA inflow evaluated. If thrombectomy is not necessary, no arteriotomy is required. With slight traction on the wire, a 6–7-Fr introducer, Flexor® (Cook Medical; Bloomington, IN, USA) or Destination, is then placed antegrade in the SMA over the through-and-through wire. An appropriate stent can then be placed across the lesion. The access puncture from the 4-Fr catheter in the SMA is treated by manual compression or suture. Antegrade stenting is better than retrograde stenting because the procedure can be performed in a familiar manner with standard devices without exposing the operators to a higher dose of radiation.

OUTCOMES AFTER OPEN *VERSUS* ENDOVASCULAR REVASCULARIZATION FOR ACUTE MESENTERIC ISCAHEMIA (LEVEL 2, GRADE C)

Five non-randomized studies[24,25,31–33] have compared open *versus* endovascular revascularization for AMI (Table 41.2). One retrospective single-centre experience[25] showed no difference in mortality between the two treatments modalities, whereas the other single-centre study showed lower bowel morbidity and mortality after endovascular therapy for acute thrombotic occlusions compared with open surgery.[32] The other three multicentre studies are nationwide reports.[24,31,33] These studies showed a lower frequency of bowel resection and lower short-term[24,31,33] and long-term[24] death rates after endovascular compared with open surgical therapy for acute thrombotic occlusion. The long-term survival at 5 years after endovascular treatment and open vascular surgery was 40% and 30%, respectively.[24] Independent risk factors for decreased long-term survival were short bowel syndrome and age.

TREATMENT OF CHRONIC MESENTERIC ISCHAEMIA (LEVEL 2, GRADE C)

Open surgical and endovascular revascularization are the treatment options for CMI. Endovascular therapy seems to be the best treatment option in vascular centres with expertise in these often elderly and fragile patients due to the minimal invasive nature of the treatment, shorter in-hospital stay, no requirement for intensive care unit, lower costs and better cost-effectiveness.[34] On the other hand, endovascular treatment is associated with high frequencies of restenosis and reinterventions,[35] and thus, follow-up is necessary (see succeeding text). In a retrospective comparative study, covered stents were associated with less restenosis, symptom recurrences and reinterventions, than bare metal stents, in patients undergoing primary interventions or reinterventions for CMI.[36] Patients who are good candidates for open surgery may benefit from a more durable procedure. The Mayo clinic used open surgery in one third of patients treated for CMI 2002–2009, with good results, indicating that there is still a room for open surgical treatment in selected cases.[37]

Radiological follow-up

Patients who have a stent inserted in the SMA after treatment for AMI or CMI need to be followed regularly by either duplex imaging or CT angiography due to the risk of restenosis and the need for reintervention to prevent the serious consequences of stent occlusion.[12]

Arterial hypoperfusion syndromes

Occlusive arterial disease is a more common cause of bowel gangrene than non-occlusive hypoperfusion, yet these syndromes are important to recognize. NOMI is a well established clinical condition affecting patients with low cardiac output, associated with the use of digitalis and/or other vasoactive drugs. Modern pharmacotherapy seems to have decreased the frequency of this condition, but a new clinical situation has occurred with the use of cardiac pump devices, resulting in better survival among patients with low cardiac output but paradoxically a higher risk of NOMI. There are no modern epidemiological data on this condition. An interesting finding in an autopsy series was that 40% of the patients with NOMI had an SMA stenosis,[38] a lesion potentially treatable with stenting. Patients with NOMI are sometimes difficult to transport

Table 41.2   Studies reporting outcomes after open and endovascular revascularization for acute SMA occlusion.

First author	Publication year	Population	Study period	Endovascular or hybrid therapy/all cases (%)	Bowel resection (%)	30-day or in-hospital mortality (%)
Schermerhorn[31]	2009	USA	2000–2006	35 (1857/5237)	41 (2138/5237)	31 (1615/5237)
Block[24]	2010	Sweden	1999–2006	26 (42/163)	51 (80/157)	37 (61/163)
Arthurs[32]	2011	Cleveland, Ohio, USA	1999–2008	80 (56/70)	86 (60/70)	41 (29/70)
Ryer[25]	2012	Rochester, Minnesota, USA	1990–2010	12 (11/93)	41 (38/93)	22 (20/93)
Beaulieu[33]	2014	USA (sample)	2005–2009	24 (165/679)	29 (196/679)	36 (244/679)

to radiology or hybrid suites, in particular if they are connected to cardiac pump devices. If at all possible, however, angiography should be performed to confirm or rule out this treatable condition.[39] The main advantage with angiography is that therapy can be initiated immediately with local administration of continuous vasodilator therapy. If transportation to the endovascular surgical suite is associated with high risk, a duplex scan confirming or ruling out a stenosis can be performed. There are no safe duplex criteria to rule out a stenosis in this particular clinical scenario, however, characterized by a low-flow situation.

Aortic dissection Stanford type A or B can be complicated by mesenteric hypoperfusion, either by compression of the true lumen creating a general hypoperfusion below the diaphragm, which is the most common situation, or by dissection propagating into the SMA.[40] The primary treatment is to perform an open repair with prosthetic graft of the ascending aorta (type A) or a thoracic endovascular aortic repair covering the entry tear (type B), followed by stenting of the SMA and exploratory laparotomy, when required.

A third hypoperfusion syndrome that can complicate trauma, burn injury, pancreatitis and aortic aneurysm repair, among others, is the intra-abdominal hypertension (IAH) that can deteriorate into ACS. The condition is common after ruptured AAA repair; in this clinical situation, a relationship between IAH and colonic ischaemia has been established.[41] In a recent multicentre study,[42] open abdomen treatment was used after approximately 3% of ruptured AAA repairs, compared with less than 1% after elective AAA repair. Definitions and treatment guidelines[43] regarding this condition were updated recently using the evidence-based Grades of Recommendation, Assessment, Development and Evaluation methodology. Treatment of IAH consists of proactive early non-surgical treatment and, whenever necessary, open abdomen treatment.[44]

In the aftermath of arterial or venous occlusive disease, when the patient is hypotensive and has lost part of their bowel, an active treatment of even lesser degrees of IAH may save life and maximize perfusion of the remaining intestinal tract. Thus, open abdomen treatment should be considered after treatment of AMI. Although it has been shown that intestinal ischaemia is a major risk factor for development of enteroatmospheric fistula during open abdomen treatment,[45] closing a tense abdomen is not a good alternative.

Damage-control surgery

Laparotomy after mesenteric revascularization serves to evaluate the possible damage to the visceral organs. Bowel resection and organ removal owing to clear transmural and gall bladder necrosis, respectively, are carried out according to the principles of damage-control surgery.[46] Bowel resections are performed with staples, leaving the creation of anastomoses or stomas until the second- or third-look laparotomy. The abdominal wall can be left un-sutured when repeat laparotomy is planned. In this situation, skin-only closure or temporary abdominal closure with an abdominal VAC® dressing (Kinetic Concepts Inc, TX, USA) may be applied.

VENOUS MESENTERIC VASCULAR DISEASE

Pathogenesis (Level 2, Grade B)

Several conditions are associated with MVT, and these can be divided into three main categories: direct injury, local venous congestion or stasis and thrombophilia. Splenectomy is a risk factor for the development of thrombus propagation from the ligated splenic vein to the portomesenteric venous system. Inflammatory states such as inflammatory bowel disease may lead to peripheral vein thrombosis in the mesentery propagating to central parts of the SMV, and severe acute pancreatitis may lead to MVT but more frequently to splenic vein thrombosis due to its very close proximity to the inflamed pancreas. Obesity was found to be a risk factor in a case–control study.[47] Inherited thrombophilia has been reported up to 55% of patients with MVT.[48] Factor V Leiden mutation (activated protein C resistance) was present in 45% of the patients with MVT in Malmö, Sweden,[48] which was considerably higher than the known prevalence rate of 7% in the background population. Although factor V Leiden mutation is a genetic defect, peripheral venous thrombotic manifestations are frequently delayed until adulthood, even in homozygotes. MVT has been reported to be a common first clinical manifestation of patients with newly diagnosed myeloproliferative disorders such as polycythemia vera or essential thrombocytosis and often occurs before a rise in peripheral blood counts. The JAK2 V617F (Janus-activated kinase gain-of-function substitute of valine to phenylalanine at position 617) mutation is diagnostic of myeloproliferative disorders. Primary cytomegalovirus infection has also been associated with MVT. Neither liver cirrhosis nor abdominal cancer was a risk factor in a population-based case-control study based on autopsies.[47] Synchronous venous thromboembolism in the systemic circulation occurs frequently in patients with MVT, especially pulmonary embolism.[47] There may be an increased risk of MVT following laparoscopic surgery because of venous stasis from increased intra-abdominal pressure, especially in obese patients undergoing Roux-en-Y bypasses, or when there is a more extensive intraoperative mobilization of the mesenteric, portal or splenic vein, and together with the presence of any systemic thrombophilic state, development of MVT seems to be more likely.

The degree of intestinal ischaemia that develops depends on the extent of venous thrombosis within the splanchnic venous circulation and whether there is occlusion and collateral flow. Patients with isolated PVT without peripheral propagation to the superior mesenteric vein are asymptomatic in the majority of cases, 61%, and almost never experience intestinal infarction.[49] In 270 patients with portomesenteric venous thrombosis found at autopsy, 29 of 31 (94%) patients with MVT had intestinal infarction and 0 of 239 (0%) with isolated PVT had intestinal infarction.[50]

Diagnosis

CLINICAL DIAGNOSIS

Patients with symptoms of less than 4 weeks of duration are classified as having acute MVT. Those with symptoms lasting longer than 4 weeks but without bowel infarction, or those with clinically insignificant MVT diagnosed incidentally on abdominal imaging, are classified as having chronic MVT. The majority of patients, above 70%, in two large clinical series,[48,51] have acute MVT.

Acute and particularly chronic MVT is a difficult diagnosis among patients presenting with acute or subacute abdominal pain. Awareness of the disease, a careful risk factor evaluation and positive findings at physical examination should lead the clinician to the diagnosis. The onset of acute MVT is often insidious, and diffuse abdominal pain may be present for days or weeks. Abdominal pain is often, but not always, present at admission.[52] The second most common symptom is nausea/vomiting, whereas diarrohea and lower gastrointestinal bleeding are only present in less than 20% of cases. Typically, a middle-aged patient with a personal or a family history of deep venous thrombosis presents with abdominal pain of a few days' duration, vomiting and abdominal distention, as well as a clearly raised C-reactive protein level. The patient may develop localized peritonitis. With progression to transmural intestinal infarction, peristalsis ceases, and signs of generalized peritonitis occur.

LABORATORY MARKERS (LEVEL 3, GRADE D)

There are no accurate plasma biomarkers for diagnosing intestinal ischaemia. D-Dimer has been reported to be a sensitive but not a specific marker of acute thromboembolic occlusion of the SMA. From a theoretical point of view, we have reason to believe that a normal D-dimer level may be useful to exclude MVT as well. This view is supported by experience from a small series of patients.[48]

Further, because inherited thrombophilic factors are common in MVT, it is recommended that all patients with MVT should be screened for the following inherited disorders: factor V Leiden mutation, prothrombin gene mutation, protein C deficiency, protein S deficiency, JAK2 V617F mutation and antithrombin deficiency. Simultaneously, the patient should be checked for acquired disorders such as lupus anticoagulant and cardiolipin antibodies.[48]

CT VENOGRAPHY (LEVEL 2, GRADE B)

CT of the abdomen, with intravenous contrast injection and imaging in the portal venous phase, is the most important and accurate diagnostic tool. MVT is seldom suspected by the clinician before ordering CT (Figure 41.6). In fact, the

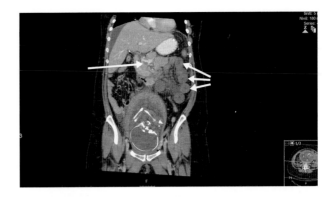

Figure 41.6 A 33-year-old female patient with a history of pulmonary embolism after giving birth to her first child. Coagulation screening showed that she was heterozygous for activated protein C resistance. She was now pregnant with her third child and medicated with low-molecular-weight heparin at deep venous thrombosis prophylaxis dosage of Klexane® 40 mg subcutaneously once a day. When the fetus had a gestational age of 30 weeks, she developed abdominal pain, frequent vomiting, fever and localized peritonitis. CT venography showed mesenteric venous thrombosis extending upwards to the extrahepatic portal vein (long arrow), ascites, small bowel wall oedema (short thick arrows), local small bowel dilatation and adjacent mesenteric oedema. She underwent caesarean section and delivery of the child first, followed by resection of 90 cm of ischemic jejunum and primary bowel anastomosis. Full-dose anticoagulation of low-molecular-weight heparin commenced immediately thereafter. Recovery was uneventful for both the mother and the child.

diagnosis is often first made by the radiologist.[53] In one series, MVT or intestinal ischaemia was suspected before CT in only one patient with congenital portal vein occlusion out of 20 with verified MVT.[53]

CT often demonstrates extensive thrombosis of the portomesenteric system, with extension of thrombosis to at least the extrahepatic portal and splenic veins. Intestinal findings are less common and more subtle. Hence, the radiologist should always examine the mesenteric vessels in cases of an acute or unclear abdomen.

LAPAROSCOPY OR LAPAROTOMY

Explorative laparoscopy or laparotomy will continue to be a necessary diagnostic tool for some patients, especially those presenting with unclear peritonitis, even after CT. In experienced hands, laparoscopy can be the preferred method to assess intestinal viability. Major obstacles for full visualization and macroscopic evaluation of the small intestines are extensive paralysis with bowel dilatation and prior adhesions.

At operation, MVT is characterized by a limited segment of intestinal ischaemia, with oedema, swelling and reddish discoloration of the affected small bowel and its adjacent mesentery and a palpable pulse in the SMA and its branches. In contrast, intestinal ischaemia due to arterial occlusive or non-occlusive disease is often characterized by extensive ischaemia that includes the jejunum, ileum and colon, with patchy cyanosis, reddish black discoloration and no palpable pulsations. MVT can be confirmed during surgery if an infarcted bowel segment is removed. Division of a small part of the adjacent mesentery, without previous vessel ligation, reveals thrombosis within the veins, whereas a pulsatile haemorrhage arises from the arteries. The extent of intestinal infarction is often limited to the jejunum or the ileum.

TREATMENT OF MESENTERIC VENOUS THROMBOSIS (LEVEL 3, GRADE C)

There is a clear trend towards a higher proportion being diagnosed at CT.[52] Therapeutic anticoagulation with a continuous infusion of unfractionated heparin is used for patients treated without surgery as well those diagnosed at operation, using standard monitoring protocols. If necessary, the infusion can be stopped or protamine given to reverse the anticoagulation if urgent repeat laparotomy or second-look laparotomy is indicated.

In one series,[53] CT in the portal venous phase was diagnostic in all 20 patients investigated, and conservative management was possible in 19. Hence, there is seldom need for invasive vascular treatment if the diagnosis is made on CT.

ENDOVASCULAR TREATMENT

There are no studies with comparative data to help establish the indication for endovascular treatment of MVT. Few patients deteriorate during medical treatment; endovascular treatment might be an option for them. A number of endovascular procedures for the treatment of MVT have been developed in recent years, including percutaneous transjugular intrahepatic portosystemic shunting (TIPS) with mechanical aspiration thrombectomy and direct thrombolysis, percutaneous transhepatic mechanical thrombectomy, percutaneous transhepatic thrombolysis, thrombolysis via the SMA and thrombolysis via a surgically placed mesenteric vein catheter. Rapid thrombus removal or dissolution can be achieved by these techniques, especially after TIPS and stent placement to create a low-pressure run-off. Mechanical thrombectomy is performed using a variety of thrombectomy devices and is most effective in cases of acute rather than chronic thrombus. Indirect thrombolytic therapy via the SMA is less effective and more time-consuming, may require longer infusion times and higher doses of thrombolytic agent and is also associated with an increased risk of bleeding. Balloon angioplasty is an alternative technique for clot fragmentation in cases of refractory thrombus and fixed venous stenosis. Aspiration thrombectomy is performed with a stiff, large-diameter (at least 8-Fr), angled catheter connected to a Luer-Lok™ syringe (Bluebird Medical, Göteborg, Sweden) to create a vacuum effect.

Endovascular techniques improve survival, increase patency of the portomesenteric veins, with lower rates of portal hypertension,[54] and have low complication rates, avoiding bowel resection in selected patients. In a series[55] of 16 patients with MVT treated by local thrombolysis, 1 had complete lysis, 11 had partial lysis and 4 had no lysis. Local thrombolysis was associated with bleeding complications in 60% of patients, including intra-abdominal bleeding, bleeding from the access site, perihepatic haematoma, nosebleed and haematuria. Accumulation of blood from the portal vein in the right pleural space, causing right-sided haemothorax, has also been reported during percutaneous transhepatic thrombectomy and thrombolysis, as have deaths from gastrointestinal haemorrhage and sepsis.

PROGNOSIS IN PATIENTS WITH MESENTERIC VENOUS THROMBOSIS (LEVEL 3, GRADE C)

Morbidity rates in cases managed with and without surgery are similar,[52] although it must be recognized that these are different groups of patients. The most common complications following surgery are pneumonia, wound infection, renal failure, sepsis and gastrointestinal bleeding.[51,52] Fortunately, the occurrence of short bowel syndrome after bowel resection for MVT is rare. In a recent series, none of the 12 patients who underwent bowel resection developed short bowel syndrome.[48] The median length of the resected intestinal segment in that series was 0.6 m (range 0.1–2.2 m). The relatively high frequency (23%) of short bowel syndrome in patients with acute MVT in an older study might be attributable to unnecessarily extensive bowel resections or suboptimal pharmacologic therapy.[51] Among patients with MVT, bowel resections should always be conservative. The short-term[56] and 2-year[52] survival rates are comparable between groups undergoing surgery and medical treatment. The survival rate after bowel resection is around 80%.[51,56] Long-term survival in patients with MVT depends largely on the underlying disease, especially the presence of cancer.[48]

MEDICAL TREATMENT IN MESENTERIC VASCULAR DISEASE (LEVEL 3, GRADE C)

Patients who survive after acute mesenteric vascular occlusion need long-term medical treatment. After thrombotic arterial occlusion, patients should have best medical therapy against atherosclerosis, including an antiplatelet agent and a statin. In case of embolic arterial occlusion, lifelong vitamin K antagonist or a new oral anticoagulant is indicated. Patients with MVT also receive anticoagulation for at least 6 months, or lifelong, depending on the underlying cause.

DEFICIENCIES IN CURRENT KNOWLEDGE AND AREAS FOR FUTURE RESEARCH

There are no accurate plasma biomarker for diagnosis of AMI.[13] It is suggested that such a plasma biomarker should preferably arise from the intestinal mucosa and pass the liver metabolism to reach the systemic circulation.

Analysis of a venous blood sample for such a biomarker would increase awareness, shorten time to diagnosis and have a potential to increase survival.

The studies comparing outcomes between endovascular and open vascular surgery suffer from selection bias due to the competence of the vascular surgeons in charge, availability of hybrid room facilities, endovascular staff, material and logistics and maybe also by severity of disease. In analogy with the IMPROVE randomized trial[57] where comparison of outcomes following endovascular or open repair strategy for ruptured AAA was analysed, a randomized controlled trial comparing outcomes following endovascular or open vascular surgical therapy for acute SMA occlusion is warranted.

BEST CLINICAL PRACTICES

- AMI is twice as common than ruptured AAA.
- SMA emboli are associated with synchronous embolism to other arteries, not seldom to the other visceral arteries.
- No need for echocardiography of the heart to detect any remnant cardiac thrombus in survivors. The patient is managed as if there are remnant cardiac thrombus and treated accordingly.
- Symptoms of CMI precedes often acute onset of acute thrombotic occlusion of the SMA.
- In case of suspicion of AMI, CT angiography is the best diagnostic method to visualize the vascular pathology, whereas intestinal lesions are visualized late in the course. CT angiography should be performed despite an elevated serum creatinine due to the low risk of contrast-induced nephropathy and the suspected lethal condition.
- MVT is associated with venous thromboembolism and activated protein C resistance. Survivors should undergo screening for coagulation disorders.

Key points

- An elderly patient with severe abdominal pain and atrial fibrillation should be suspected to have an embolic occlusion of the SMA, and diagnosis should be confirmed or out ruled with CT angiography.
- The patient is best treated in a hybrid room with angiography facilities.
- The result after open SMA embolectomy is best controlled by angiography.
- A conservative approach with anticoagulation is the preferred first choice of therapy in MVT.

DISCLOSURE

The authors declare no conflict of interest.

KEY REFERENCES

1. Acosta S, Ogren M, Sternby NH, Bergqvist D, Björck M. Clinical implications for the management of acute thromboembolic occlusion of the superior mesenteric artery: Autopsy findings in 213 patients. *Ann Surg.* 2005;241:516–522.

   Comprehensive solid data on epidemiology and pathology of acute SMA occlusion.
2. Menke J. Diagnostic accuracy of multidetector CT in acute mesenteric ischemia: Systematic review and meta-analysis. *Radiology.* 2010;256:93–101.

   One of the first reports of the accuracy of CT angiography in acute SMA occlusion.
3. Block TA, Acosta S, Björck M. Endovascular and open surgery for acute occlusion of the superior mesenteric artery. *J Vasc Surg.* 2010;52:959–966.

   Multicenter study with review of each patient reported to the Swedish Vascular Registry, comparing open and endovascular therapy for acute SMA occlusion.
4. Acosta S, Alhadad A, Svensson P, Ekberg O. Epidemiology, risk and prognostic factors in mesenteric venous thrombosis. *Br J Surg.* 2008;95:1245–1251.

   Thorough epidemiological and risk factor data in mesenteric venous thrombosis.
5. Di Minno MN, Milone F, Milone M et al. Endovascular thrombolysis in acute mesenteric vein thrombosis: A 3-year follow-up with the rate of short and long-term sequaele in 32 patients. *Thromb Res.* 2010;126:295–298.

   Long-term results in a large series of endovascular thrombolysis in acute mesenteric venous thrombosis.

REFERENCES

1. Acosta S. Epidemiology of mesenteric vascular disease: Clinical implications. *Semin Vasc Surg.* 2010;23:4–8.
2. Acosta S, Ogren M, Sternby NH, Bergqvist D, Björck M. Clinical implications for the management of acute thromboembolic occlusion of the superior mesenteric artery: Autopsy findings in 213 patients. *Ann Surg.* 2005;241:516–522.
3. Sanna A, Adani GL, Anania G, Donini A. The role of laparoscopy in patients with suspected peritonitis: Experience of a single institution. *J Laparoendosc Adv Surg Techn.* 2003;46:111–116.
4. Rozycki G, Tremblay L, Feliciano D, Joseph R, deDelvia P, Salomone J, et al. Three hundred consecutive emergent celiotomies in general surgery patients. Influence of advanced diagnostic imaging techniques and procedures on diagnosis. *Ann Surg.* 2002;235:681–689.
5. Khan A, Hsee L, Mathur S, Civil I. Damage-control laparotomy in nontrauma patients: Review of indications and outcomes. *J Trauma Acute Care Surg.* 2013;75:365–368.

6. Arenal J, Bengoechea-Beeby M. Mortality associated with emergency abdominal surgery in the elderly. *Can J Surg.* 2003;46:111–116.

7. Weir-McCall J, Shaw A, Arya A, Knight A, Howlett DC. The use of pre-operative computed tomography in the assessment of the acute abdomen. *Ann R Coll Surg Engl.* 2012;94:102–107.

8. Green G, Shaikh I, Fernandes R, Wegstapel H. Emergency laparotomy in octogenarians: A 5-year study of morbidity and mortality. *World J Gastrointest Surg.* 2013;5:216–221.

9. Kolkman JJ, Mensink. Non-occlusive mesenteric ischemia: A common disorder in gastroenterology and intensive care. *Best Pract Res Clin Gastroenterol.* 2003;17:457–473.

10. Brandt LJ, Boley SJ. AGA technical review on intestinal ischemia. American Gastrointestinal Association. *Gastroenterology.* 2000;118:954–968.

11. Batellier J, Kieny R. Superior mesenteric artery embolism: Eighty-two cases. *Ann Vasc Surg.* 1990;4:112–116.

12. Björnsson S, Resch T, Acosta S. Symptomatic mesenteric atherosclerotic disease – lessons learned from the diagnostic workup. *J Gastrointest Surg.* 2013;17:973–980.

13. Acosta S, Nilsson T. Current status on plasma biomarkers for acute mesenteric ischemia. *J Thromb Thrombolysis.* 2012;33:355–361.

14. Acosta S, Nilsson TK, Björck M. Elevated D-dimer level could be a useful early marker for acute bowel ischaemia. A Preliminary Study. *Br J Surg.* 2001;88:385–388.

15. Acosta S, Nilsson TK, Björck M. D-Dimer testing in patients with suspected acute thromboembolic occlusion of the superior mesenteric artery. *Br J Surg.* 2004;91:991–994.

16. Matsumoto S, Sekine K, Funaoka H, Yamazaki M, Shimizu M, Hayashida K, Kitano M. Diagnostic performance of plasma biomarkers in patients with acute intestinal ischemia. *Br J Surg.* 2014;101:232–238.

17. Acosta S, Block T, Björnsson S, Resch T, Björck M, Nilsson T. Diagnostic pitfalls at admission in patients with acute superior mesenteric artery occlusion. *J Emerg Med.* 2012;42:635–641.

18. Menke J. Diagnostic accuracy of multidetector CT in acute mesenteric ischemia: Systematic review and meta-analysis. *Radiology.* 2010;256:93–101.

19. Wadman M, Block T, Ekberg O, Syk I, Elmståhl S, Acosta S. Impact of MDCT with intravenous contrast on the survival in patients with acute superior mesenteric artery occlusion. *Emerg Radiol.* 2010;17:171–178.

20. Acosta S, Björnsson S, Ekberg O, Resch T. CT angiography followed by endovascular intervention for acute superior mesenteric artery occlusion does not increase risk of contrast-induced renal failure. *Eur J Vasc Endovasc Surg.* 2010;39:726–730.

21. Van Noord D, Sana A, Moons LM, Pattynama PM, Verhagen HJ, Kuipers EJ, Mensink PB. Combining radiological imaging and gastrointestinal tonometry:

A minimal invasive and useful approach for the workup of chronic gastrointestinal ischemia. *Eur J Gastroenterol Hepatol.* 2013;25:719–725.

22. Acosta S, Björck M. Modern treatment of acute mesenteric ischemia. *Br J Surg.* 2014;101:e100–e108.

23. Björck M, Wanhainen A. Management of abdominal compartment syndrome and the open abdomen. *Eur J Vasc Endovasc Surg.* 2014;47:279–287.

24. Block TA, Acosta S, Björck M. Endovascular and open surgery for acute occlusion of the superior mesenteric artery. *J Vasc Surg.* 2010;52:959–966.

25. Ryer EJ, Kalra M, Oderich GS et al. Revascularization for acute mesenteric ischemia. *J Vasc Surg.* 2012;55:1682–1689.

26. Yun WS, Lee UK, Cho J, Kim HK, Huk S. Treatment outcome in patients with acute superior mesenteric artery. *Ann Vasc Surg.* 2013;27:613–620.

27. Resch TA, Acosta S, Sonesson B. Endovascular techniques in acute arterial mesenteric ischemia. *Semin Vasc Surg.* 2010;23:29–35.

28. Acosta S, Sonesson B, Resch T. Endovascular therapeutic approaches for acute superior mesenteric artery occlusion. *Cardiovasc Intervent Radiol.* 2009;32:896–905.

29. Heiss P, Loewenhardt B, Manke C et al. Primary percutaneous aspiration and thrombolysis for the treatment of acute embolic superior mesenteric artery occlusion. *Eur Radiol.* 2010;20:2948–2958.

30. Björnsson S, Björck M, Block T, Resch T, Acosta S. Thrombolysis for acute occlusion of the superior mesenteric artery. *J Vasc Surg.* 2011;54:1734–1742.

31. Schmerhorn ML, Giles KA, Hamdan AD, Wyers MC, Pomposelli FB. Mesenteric revascularization: Management and outcomes in the United States, 1988–2006. *J Vasc Surg.* 2009;50:341–348.

32. Arthurs ZM, Titus J, Bannazadeh M et al. A comparison of endovascular revascularization with traditional therapy for the treatment of acute mesenteric ischemia. *J Vasc Surg.* 2011;167:308–311.

33. Beaulieu RJ, Arnaoutakis KD, Aburrhage CJ, Efron DT, Schneider E, Black JH 3rd. Comparison of open and endovascular treatment of acute mesenteric ischemia. *J Vasc Surg.* 2014;59:159–164.

34. Hogendoorn W, Hanink MG, Schlösser FJ, Moll FL, Muhs BI, Sumpio BE. A comparison of open and endovascular revascularization for chronic mesenteric ischemia in a clinical decision model. *J Vasc Surg.* 2014;60:715–725.

35. AbuRahma A, Campbell J, Stone P, Hass S, Mousa A, Srivastava M, Nanjundappa A, Dean S, Keiffer T. Perioperative and late clinical outcomes of 105 percutaneous transluminal stentings of the celiac and superior mesenteric arteries over the past decade. *J Vasc Surg.* 2013;57:1052–1061.

36. Oderich GS, Erdoes LS, Lesar C, Mendes BC, Gloviczki P, Cha S, Duncan AA, Bower T. Comparison of covered stents versus bare metal stents for treatment of chronic atherosclerotic mesenteric arterial disease. *J Vasc Surg.* 2013;58:1316–1323.

37. Ryer E, Oderich G, Bower T, Macedo T, Vrtiska T, Duncan A, Kalra M, Gloviczki P. Differences in anatomy and outcomes in patients treated with open mesenteric revascularization before and after the endovascular era. *J Vasc Surg.* 2011;53:1611–1618.

38. Acosta S, Ogren M, Sternby N-H, Bergqvist D, Björck M. Fatal non-occlusive mesenteric ischaemia: Population-based incidence and risk factors. *J Intern Med.* 2006;259:305–313.

39. Minko P, Stroeder J, Groesdonk H, Graeber S, Klingele M, Buecker A, Schäfers H, Katoh M. A scoring-system for angiographic findings in nonocclusive mesenteric ischemia (NOMI): Correlation with clinical risk factors and its predictive value. *Cardiovasc Intervent Radiol.* 2014;37:657–663.

40. Steuer J, Eriksson MO, Nyman R, Björck M, Wanhainen A. Early and long-term outcome after thoracic endovascular aortic repair (TEVAR) for acute complicated type B aortic dissection. *Eur J Vasc Endovasc Surg.* 2011;41:318–323.

41. Djavani K, Wanhainen A, Valtysson J, Björck M. Colonic ischemia and intra-abdominal hypertension following open surgery for ruptured abdominal aortic aneurysm. *Br J Surg.* 2009;96:621–627.

42. Sörelius K, Wanhainen A, Acosta S, Svensson M, Djavani-Gidlund K, Björck M. Open abdomen treatment after aortic aneurysm repair with vacuum-assisted wound closure and mesh-mediated fascial traction. *Eur J Vasc Endovasc Surg.* 2013;45:588–594.

43. Kirkpatrick A, Roberts DJ, De Waele J et al.; Pediatric Guidelines Sub-Committee for the World Society of the Abdominal Compartment Syndrome. Intra-abdominal hypertension and the abdominal compartment syndrome: Updated consensus definitions and clinical practice guidelines from the World Society of the Abdominal Compartment Syndrome. *Intensive Care Med.* 2013;39:1190–1206.

44. Björck M, Petersson U, Bjarnason T Cheatham ML. Intra-abdominal hypertension and abdominal compartment in non-trauma surgical patients. *Am Surg.* 2011;77:S62–S66.

45. Acosta S, Bjarnason T, Petersson U et al. A multicentre prospective study of fascial closure rate after open abdomen with vacuum and mesh-mediated fascial traction. *Br J Surg.* 2011;98;735–743.

46. Rotondo MF, Schwab CW, McGonigal MD et al. 'Damage control': An approach for improved survival in exsanguinating penetrating abdominal injury. *J Trauma.* 1993;35:375–382.

47. Acosta S, Ögren M, Sternby N-H, Bergqvist D, Björck M. Mesenteric venous thrombosis with intestinal infarction: A population-based study. *J Vasc Surg.* 2005;41:59–63.

48. Acosta S, Alhadad A, Svensson P, Ekberg O. Epidemiology, risk and prognostic factors in mesenteric venous thrombosis. *Br J Surg.* 2008;95:1245–1251.

49. Amitrano L, Guardiascione MA, Scaglione M et al. Prognostic factors in noncirrhotic patients with splanchnic vein thrombosis. *Am J Gastroenterol.* 2007;102:2464–2470.

50. Acosta S, Alhadad A, Verbaan H, Ögren M. The clinical importance in differentiating portal from mesenteric venous thrombosis. *Int Angiol.* 2011;30:71–78.

51. Rhee RY, Gloviczki P, Mendonca CT et al. Mesenteric venous thrombosis: Still a lethal disease in the 1990s. *J Vasc Surg.* 1994;20:688–697.

52. Brunaud L, Antunes L, Collinet-Adler S et al. Acute mesenteric venous thrombosis: Case for nonoperative management. *J Vasc Surg.* 2001;34:673–679.

53. Acosta S, Alhadad A, Ekberg O. Findings in multidetector row CT with portal phase enhancement in patients with mesenteric venous thrombosis. *Emerg Radiol.* 2009;16:477–482.

54. Di Minno MN, Milone F, Milone M et al. Endovascular thrombolysis in acute mesenteric vein thrombosis: A 3-year follow-up with the rate of short and long-term sequaelae in 32 patients. *Thromb Res.* 2010;126:295–298.

55. Hollingshead M, Burke C, Mauro M, Weeks SM, Dixon RG, Jaques PF. Transcatheter thrombolytic therapy for acute mesenteric and portal vein thrombosis. *J Vasc Interv Radiol.* 2005;16:651–661.

56. Morasch M, Ebaugh JL, Chiou AC, Pearce WH, Yao JS. Mesenteric venous thrombosis: A changing clinical entity. *J Vasc Surg.* 2001;34:680–684.

57. IMPROVE Trial Investigators, Powell JT, Sweeting MJ, Thompson MM et al. Endovascular or open repair strategy for ruptured abdominal aortic aneurysm: 30-day outcomes from IMPROVE randomised trial. *Br Med J.* 2014 January 13;348:f7661.

Vascular Disorders of the Upper Extremity and Vasculitis

42

Thoracic outlet disorders

Thoracic outlet compression syndrome and axillary vein thrombosis

MICHAEL S. HONG and JULIE A. FREISCHLAG

CONTENTS

ANATOMY

The normal anatomy of the thoracic outlet includes three spaces through which the neurovascular structures pass. These three spaces consist of the scalene triangle, the costoclavicular space and the pectoralis minor space. Starting proximally, the scalene triangle is bordered by the anterior scalene muscle, the middle scalene muscle and the first rib. The subclavian artery and brachial plexus course through this space. The subclavian vein is anterior to the anterior scalene muscle and instead courses through the costoclavicular space, which is bordered by the anterior scalene muscle, the subclavius muscle and the first rib. The neurovascular structures then pass under the clavicle and continue laterally until the brachial plexus, axillary artery and axillary vein pass through the pectoralis minor space, which is bordered by the pectoralis minor anteriorly and the ribs posteriorly (Figure 42.1).

PATHOPHYSIOLOGY

Thoracic outlet syndrome (TOS) can be caused by multiple factors that affect the anatomy of the three spaces through which the neurovascular structures pass. Some of these causes are congenital, in the case of aberrant structures such as a cervical rib, while other causes are acquired from trauma, repetitive motion or hypertrophy.

Congenital abnormalities include the presence of a cervical rib. Cervical ribs are variable in their extent; some form a complete ring, whereas most are partially present. In the latter group, pathology occurs due to a congenital band that connects the cervical rib to the first rib.

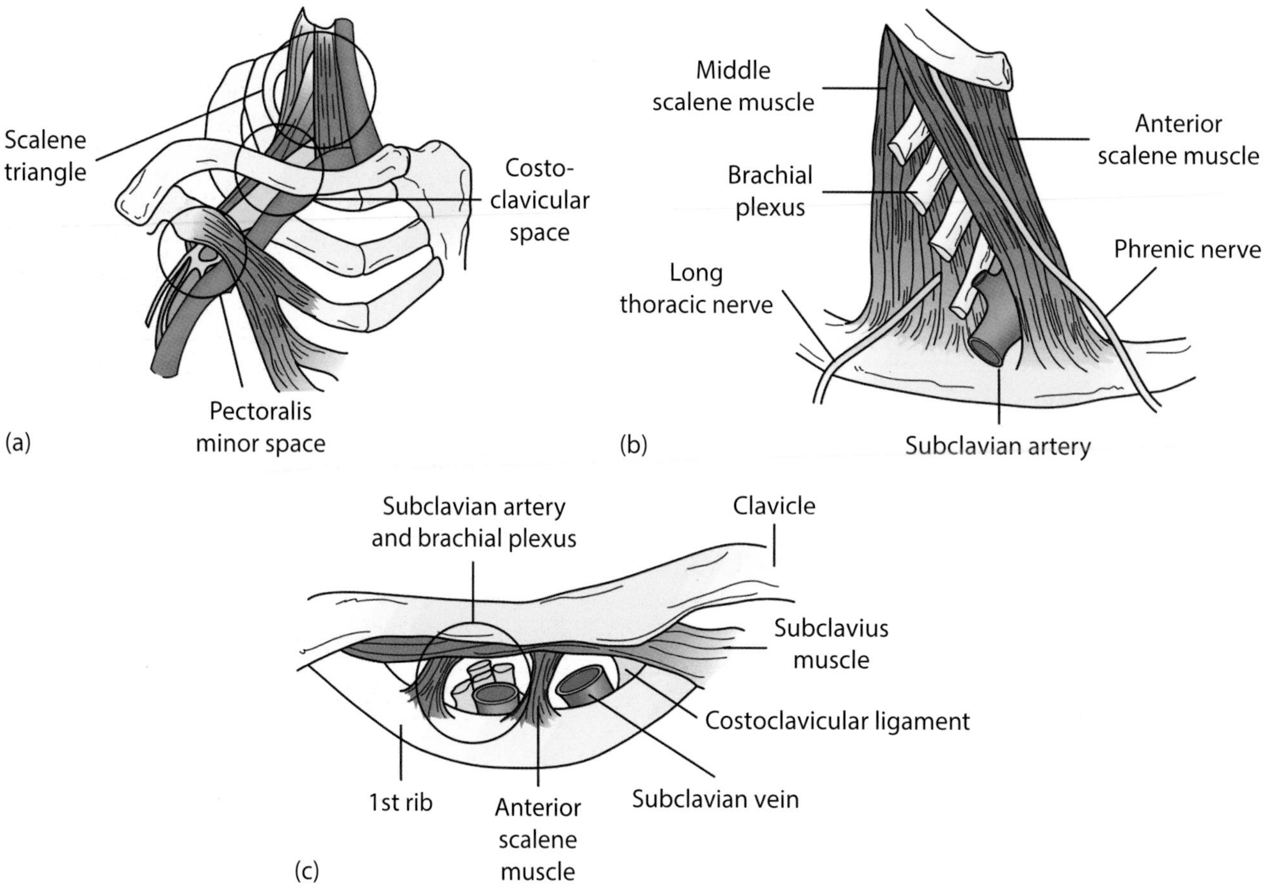

Figure 42.1 The three spaces of the thoracic outlet: (a) the scalene triangle, (b) the costoclavicular space, and (c) the pectoralis minor space. The brachial plexus and subclavian artery passes through the scalene triangle. The subclavian vein passes through the costoclavicular space. All structures pass through the pectoralis minor space.

Neurogenic

Neurogenic thoracic outlet syndrome (nTOS) is the most common, comprising an estimated 95% of all cases of TOS. Most patients with TOS do not have objective brachial plexus or peripheral neuropathies. For this reason, this subset of patients has been previously described as having the 'disputed form' of nTOS. In contrast, a small minority of nTOS patients have objective neurological findings in the C8/T1 nerve distribution and may represent an advanced disease process rather than a unique pathophysiological aetiology.[1] nTOS is often associated with a history of cervical trauma such as a whiplash injury or a clavicular fracture. Whiplash injury is thought to contribute to nTOS by causing stretch and resultant inflammation in the anterior scalene muscle. This inflammation can lead to irritation and sometimes scarring of the associated brachial plexus. In other instances, due to inflammation from chronic repetitive motion or trauma, the anterior scalene muscle becomes spastic and contracts, which serves to narrow the scalene triangle by pulling up on the first rib. In patients with a clavicle fracture, scarring on the clavicle can cause local inflammation and also

externally impinge on the brachial plexus as it exits the scalene triangle. Finally, a small subset of patients have neurogenic symptoms that are attributed to impingement at the pectoralis space, which is termed neurogenic pectoralis minor syndrome.

Venous

Venous thoracic outlet syndrome (vTOS) has variable causes and presentations and comprises approximately 3%–4% of cases of TOS. Some have aberrant insertion of the anterior scalene muscle, whereas others may have an aberrant or inflamed subclavius tendon or even a hypertrophied subclavius muscle. These abnormalities all contribute to narrow or otherwise cause local inflammation near the costoclavicular space and associated subclavian vein. Venous thoracic outlet can present with intermittent external compression without luminal thrombosis, as first described by McCleery.[2] This intermittent compression of the subclavian vein is due to impingement by the subclavius tendon during provocative manoeuvres. In other forms, there may be stenosis, partial thrombosis or occlusion of the vein. The latter form is described as 'effort thrombosis', or Paget–Schroetter syndrome, and is generally found in young athletes who participate in repetitive overhead arm motions, such as baseball pitchers and swimmers. The hypertrophy of the subclavius muscle or tendon decreases the size of the costoclavicular space, leading to subclavian vein impingement and thrombosis.

Arterial

Arterial thoracic outlet syndrome (aTOS) is the least common form of TOS, comprising approximately 1% of all cases. It is commonly associated with bone abnormalities. The most common bone abnormality is a presence of a cervical rib, which is found in over half of aTOS. The cervical rib anteriorly displaces the subclavian artery, causing compression between the first rib and the anterior scalene muscle. Other abnormalities include an anomalous first rib, a fibrocartilaginous band, scar and abnormal healing from a clavicular fracture and, rarely, an enlarged C7 transverse process. Extrinsic compression from these bone abnormalities results in stenosis and post-stenotic dilatation and possible development of a subclavian artery aneurysm. Intimal injury and development of mural thrombus within the aneurysm are potential sources of embolism to the fingers and hand of the affected extremity.

HISTORY

Neurogenic

Patients with nTOS may have a history of cervical trauma such as a whiplash injury or repetitive neck trauma. They report a history of numbness and tingling in the arm or fingers and may also have pain in the neck, shoulder or upper extremity. Weakness of the hand and arm with possible muscle atrophy can also be found in advanced cases. Intermittent hand ischemia can also be found due to vasomotor dysfunction secondary to sympathetic stimulation resulting from brachial plexus inflammation. Those with spasm of the trapezius muscles may also report occipital headaches, which manifest as posterior head and neck pain.

Symptom severity can vary at different times but typically is more pronounced with manoeuvres that cause stretch on the brachial plexus, such as arm abduction and elevation. A common presentation is weakness or clumsiness (loss of dexterity) when performing activities with their hands raised above their shoulder level. Overall, however, symptoms and function in the arm tend to generally worsen with time. Vasospasm, hypersensitivity and allodynia mark the most severe form of progressive neurogenic thoracic outlet symptoms.

Venous

Patients with vTOS are characteristically young and active and present with upper extremity swelling and a history of repetitive arm use such as baseball pitching or swimming. Patients with McCleery syndrome manifest with positional enlargement of the superficial arm veins and bluish discoloration without significant edema. Paget–Schroetter syndrome refers to axillary or subclavian vein thrombosis from repetitive arm motion. Patients with acute vein occlusion typically demonstrate impressive edema and pain of the affected upper arm that is not position dependent.

Arterial

The arterial form is also most likely to be correlated with congenital abnormalities, such as a cervical rib. Patients with aTOS present with evidence of hand ischemia. Early manifestations include arm pain with exertion due to the subclavian artery stenosis. Acute presentations consist of pain, paresthesias and poikilothermia due to thrombosis of the subclavian artery or distal embolization. Those with chronic presentations may report hand weakness, clumsiness or tissue loss. Those with impressive subclavian artery aneurysms may report a pulsatile lump near the clavicle.

PHYSICAL EXAMINATION

The physical exam can be tailored for diagnosis and differentiation of the various aetiologies of TOS. It is important to note that no single test is very sensitive or specific in establishing a diagnosis of TOS, and therefore, the diagnosis must be made after careful evaluation of the entire clinical presentation.

Neurogenic

Patients with nTOS should be assessed both at rest and with provocative manoeuvres. At rest, the distribution and description of symptoms should be noted. Inspection of the hand and upper extremity should be performed, evaluating for evidence of muscular atrophy, particularly in the thenar or hypothenar areas.

The scapula can also be inspected to identify asymmetry. Typically, the ipsilateral shoulder is rotated anterior and downwards due to the effect of the pectoralis minor muscle. This latter finding may identify patients who would benefit from physical therapy to improve their posture.

Peripheral nerve entrapment disorders should be ruled out by eliciting paresthesias with tapping on the median nerve at the wrist, the radial nerve at the extensor forearm or the ulnar nerve at the elbow.

Findings consistent with nTOS include reproduction of the patient's upper extremity paresthesias or direct point tenderness upon palpation of the anterior scalene muscle. In addition, for patients with impingement by the pectoralis minor muscle, symptoms may be reproduced by applying pressure on the area inferior to the coracoid process.

In addition to scalene and pectoralis minor palpation, provocative manoeuvres can also help diagnose nTOS. The elevated arm stress test (EAST) consists of arm abduction with the elbows bent and hands up, followed by opening and closing the fist repeatedly for up to 3 minutes. This manoeuvre can trigger pain or paresthesias typically within the first 60 seconds.

The upper limb tension test seeks to elicit symptoms by causing traction on the brachial plexus through increasingly provocative steps. The test starts by abducting the arms and placing the elbows straight and palms down, then dorsiflexing both wrists and finally tilting the head to the affected side. A positive test results in pain or paresthesias on the ipsilateral side as the wrist dorsiflexion and the contralateral side of the neck flexion.

Finally, the Adson test evaluates arterial impingement by palpating the radial pulse at rest and during a provocative manoeuvre. This manoeuvre is accomplished by abducting and externally rotating the arm, rotating and laterally flexing the neck to the ipsilateral side, and then inhaling deeply. The test is positive when the radial pulse is diminished or absent with the manoeuvre. The main limitation is that a positive test can be seen in up to 50% of normal patients. A positive Adson test should never be used in isolation to justify the diagnosis or treatment of aTOS.

Venous

Physical examination in vTOS should include evaluation for edema or cyanosis of the affected extremity. Depending on the aetiology (Paget–Schroetter vs. McCleery syndrome), the edema may be present at baseline or only with exertion or arm elevation. Those with more chronic presentations may also have evidence of prominent superficial collateral veins in the arm, shoulder or chest wall.

Arterial

For aTOS, a careful pulse exam should be performed at resting position and with provocative manoeuvres. A difference in the blood pressure in either arm may be caused by an otherwise asymptomatic subclavian artery occlusion. Due to anterior displacement of the subclavian artery from the cervical rib, a prominent pulse may be seen or felt superior to the clavicle. The underlying cervical rib may also be palpated, although these are most commonly diagnosed with a chest radiograph. A bruit may be heard under the clavicle in cases of subclavian aneurysms, particularly with provocative manoeuvres which exacerbate

the extrinsic compression of the subclavian artery and therefore exaggerate the stenosis. Patients may also have evidence of distal emboli from a subclavian aneurysm and tissue loss in the fingers from either vasospasm or embolism.

STUDIES

Routine tests for all patients with TOS should include a chest x-ray to evaluate for congenital cervical ribs or elongated C7 transverse process.

Neurogenic

For patients with nTOS, several studies can be performed to rule out other aetiologies of neurogenic pain. A nerve conduction study can be performed to identify carpal or cubital compression syndrome. Although nerve conduction tests are usually negative in nTOS, a positive result can also be due to advanced brachial plexus disease. Patients with a high pre-test probability of non-thoracic outlet aetiologies, such as those with previous history of neck trauma, bilateral symptoms or those over 40 years old, benefit from a cervical spine MRI to rule out cervical spine impingement or foraminal narrowing.

The diagnosis of nTOS can be supported by a positive response to an anterior scalene block with 1% lidocaine, which is typically injected under ultrasound, EMG or CT guidance. Symptoms generally improve immediately, as the lidocaine relieves spasm of the anterior scalene muscle. Because the effects are temporary, lidocaine injection is diagnostic rather than therapeutic. Symptomatic relief with this block helps to differentiate nTOS from other neurogenic aetiologies and also identifies those who are more likely to have a positive result with an operation, particularly in the subset of patients who are over 40 years of age.[3]

Botox has been studied as an alternative to operative management in nTOS. The main drawbacks of Botox are that the effects take several weeks to manifest and wear off after several months.[4] Furthermore, Botox causes inflammation and further scarring of the anterior scalene muscle, which not only inhibits the effectiveness of multiple injections but may also exacerbate the neurogenic symptoms in the long run. In a randomized control trial of 38 patients with a long duration of symptoms, Botox injection to the anterior and middle scalene muscle did not result in clinically or statistically significant improvement in pain or paresthesias at 6 weeks compared to placebo saline injections.[5]

Venous

The primary workup for most cases of vTOS is an upper extremity duplex ultrasound or CT venography to demonstrate thrombosis of the brachial, axillary or subclavian vein. For McCleery syndrome, a duplex can be performed with the arm abducted more than 90° to test for position impingement. In a select group presenting with acute (less than 2 weeks) and severe symptoms, a catheter-based venography with thrombolysis can be diagnostic and therapeutic.

Arterial

It is important to note that upcoming reporting standards for TOS state that aTOS must have objective injury to the subclavian artery (aneurysms, thrombosis, embolization) or symptomatic arm ischemia with arm abduction.

For aTOS, arterial duplex with segmental arterial waveform analysis should be done both at rest and with arm abduction. A positive finding is usually defined as a 50% increase in subclavian artery flow velocity as seen with duplex ultrasound during arm abduction. In severe forms, a loss of distal signals can also be elicited. An arterial duplex is also helpful to identify concomitant arterial and neurogenic TOS in patients with suggestive findings. Likes reported 22 patients successfully treated for concomitant neurogenic and arterial aetiologies. This subset of patients does not respond to physical therapy, unlike most patients with nTOS.[6] Other imaging modalities include a CT scan or MRI for diagnosing arterial aneurysms.

MANAGEMENT

Neurogenic

Once the diagnosis of nTOS is made, physical therapy for no less than 8 weeks should be performed. Over half improve with physical therapy, and this should be the first-line treatment for nearly all suspected cases of nTOS, except in cases of concomitant arterial TOS. Operative intervention should be reserved for those who fail physical therapy and conservative measures.

Preoperative scalene injection with lidocaine can help confirm the diagnosis and predict those who would have a successful 1-year result with surgical decompression and is done for most cases, unless the presentation is very classic for nTOS. Botox injection has had less success in treating symptoms and is generally reserved for patients who are not fit for surgery, due to previous operations in this area, active smoking or prohibitive perioperative risk. In this latter group, an initial treatment must Botox may allow greater participation in physical therapy, but repeated injections decrease efficacy.[3]

Fractures of the clavicle can cause nTOS due to irritation from aberrant scar tissue. In most cases, the clavicle itself need not be repaired or removed. Instead, removal of the first rib with scalenectomy allows the neurovascular structures to lay more inferior and removes the clavicle from possible impingement.

Venous

Patients with McCleery syndrome can proceed to first rib resection and scalenectomy (FRRS). For those with Paget–Schroetter syndrome, the management is more complex. Historically, these patients were managed with elevation and anticoagulation for 3 months. This approach however was associated with recurrent symptoms in up to 85% of patients. Management subsequently shifted to venography and catheter-directed thrombolysis followed by FRRS, either during the same hospitalization or as a staged procedure.[7]

However, Guzzo and others compared the results of patients with subacute or chronic vTOS, managed with preoperative anticoagulation compared to catheter-directed thrombolysis, and found no long-term difference in 1-year patency following FRRS. Furthermore, it was noted that several patients who underwent preoperative thrombolysis were found to be re-occluded prior to FRRS, despite being on anticoagulation.[8] These findings were again reproduced by Taylor and others, who reported that 19% of those who had thrombolysis developed re-occlusion and that long-term post-operative outcomes after FRRS were similar among those who had preoperative thrombolysis and those who did not.[9]

Chang and others previously reported a protocol of preoperative anticoagulation with enoxaparin, FRRS and post-operative venography at 2 weeks. At 2 weeks, based on the venographic findings, anticoagulation is stopped or continued, or balloon venoplasty is performed. Excellent long-term results were recently published by the same group using this protocol and are described later in the chapter.[10]

Therefore, for most patients with vTOS, a reasonable initial approach is a CT venogram or venous duplex to establish the diagnosis, followed by 2 weeks of arm elevation and anticoagulation with enoxaparin. Definitive operative management with FRRS is ideally performed within 2 weeks, as these patients have a risk of re-occlusion if the underlying anatomic cause of the venous thrombosis is not addressed. These patients will then undergo a venogram through the basilic or brachial vein post-operatively to assess for need for venoplasty or continued anticoagulation. The cephalic vein in particular is generally avoided, as the thrombus can sometimes extend laterally past where the cephalic vein drains into the axillary vein. Anticoagulation is continued until there is no significant stenosis. The key benefit of this approach is that patients can receive timely initial treatment prior to referral or transfer to a vascular surgeon for their operative repair.

Arterial

Patients with aTOS should be managed primarily with operative decompression, as conservative management and physical therapy will not improve symptoms, and the delay risks the development of arterial degeneration and complications. There is still some controversy regarding the best operative approach for aTOS; however, Chang and others reported successful management of aTOS via the transaxillary approach in most cases and also found that resection of the cervical rib in addition to the first rib was possible through a single incision.[11]

Arterial reconstruction is reserved for patients with subclavian or axillary aneurysms greater than 2 cm, arterial occlusion or evidence of embolism. When arterial reconstruction in planned, this is best performed through the supraclavicular or infraclavicular approach, which offers more direct access to the artery than the transaxillary approach.

OPERATIVE APPROACH

The two main surgical options for treatment of TOS include the transaxillary and the supraclavicular approach. The transaxillary approach has the advantage of being more cosmetic and potentially less painful and allows for exposure to perform a complete repair for most patients, even in aTOS. In addition, the transaxillary approach may be better for vTOS as the subclavius tendon, first rib and cervical rib can all be removed with this approach.[11] Particular attention should be paid to resection of large portion of the anterior scalene muscle to reduce recurrent symptoms. In aTOS with bony abnormalities, it is important to remove both the cervical rib in addition to the first rib. Overall, there is less dissection involved in the transaxillary approach; however, visualization is reduced.

The supraclavicular approach affords greater exposure of all anatomic structures and allows for complete resection of the anterior and middle scalene muscle. Extensive neurolysis of the brachial plexus can also be performed with this approach. However, it is not clear whether such extensive dissection yields more than a theoretical benefit. The most significant advantage is the ability to perform vascular reconstruction.

Axillary approach to first rib resection and anterior scalenectomy

After general anesthesia, the patient is placed in the lateral decubitus position with an axillary roll and bean bag. The legs are padded. The axilla, chest and neck are prepped and draped. The arm is wrapped with an extremity sleeve to the elbow, followed by two layers of Kerlix. The arm is then placed on a Machleder retractor over four towels and wrapped with a sterile Coban dressing.

The borders of the pectoralis major and latissimus dorsi muscles are marked and serve as the anterior and posterior borders of the incision, respectively. The incision is made just under the hairline and the soft tissue is dissected sharply. The intercostal muscle is seen with the pectoralis major anteriorly and latissimus dorsi posteriorly. The first rib is encountered cephalad and generally

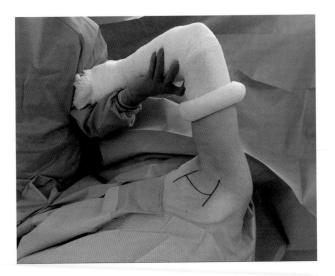

Figure 42.2 The incision is made below the hair line at the axilla. The pectoralis major and latissimus dorsi mark the anterior and posterior borders of the skin incision. (From Sanders RJ and Haug CE, *Thoracic Outlet Syndrome: A Common Sequela of Neck Injuries*, Philadelphia, PA: Lippincott Williams & Wilkins, p. 237, 1991.)

not seen until further blunt dissection is carried superiorly (Figure 42.2).

The intercostal muscle over the first rib is then dissected free with the periosteal elevator. Blunt dissection with the finger can be done to dissect the posterior aspect of the first rib. Care should be taken to avoid passing beyond the first rib, as this can create a tear in the pleura and result in pneumothorax. The scalene triangle can be further developed with blunt dissection. The subclavian vein, anterior scalene muscle and subclavian artery are generally well visualized. The brachial plexus is posterior to the subclavian artery and may not be seen until further dissection is made.

The subclavius muscle is found anterior to the subclavian vein and is typically hypertrophied in the case of Paget–Schroetter syndrome. For patients with neurogenic TOS, the brachial plexus can be stretched and somewhat far from the subclavian artery. These two structures typically become more closely aligned after first rib resection.

Next, the subclavius muscle is cut sharply from the first rib. The anterior scalene muscle is bluntly dissected free and then cut sharply approximately 2–3 cm from its insertion on the first rib while being retracted towards the field with a right angle clamp to avoid inadvertent injury to the subclavian artery. The middle scalene muscle is then dissected free from the posterior aspect of the first rib with the periosteal elevator, staying close to the bone to reduce the risk of injury to the long thoracic nerve, which pierces the middle scalene muscle along its course.

The first rib is then resected as far anterior as possible, taking care to avoid injury to the subclavian vein. Additional rib can be removed with a rongeur to avoid

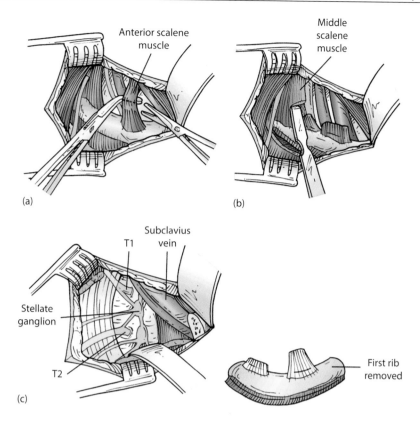

Figure 42.3 (a) The anterior scalene muscle is divided sharply under direct visualization, tented by a right angle clamp to reduce injury to posterior structures. (b) The middle scalene muscle is removed with a periosteal elevator in order to reduce risk of long thoracic nerve injury. (c) The first rib is cut anterior and posteriorly. (Reprinted from *Annals of Vascular Surgery*, 11, Thompson RW and Petrinec D, Surgical treatment of thoracic outlet compression syndromes: diagnostic considerations and transaxillary first rib resection, 315–323, Copyright 1997, with permission from Elsevier.)

recurrent venous TOS. The first rib is resected posteriorly, taking care to avoid injury to the brachial plexus that is generally found deep and posteriorly. The rongeur is used to resect additional bone until it is well posterior to the brachial plexus, in order to reduce the risk of recurrent neurogenic TOS (Figure 42.3).

The wound bed is then filled with saline and Valsalva is performed through the endotracheal tube, to evaluate for bubbles suggestive of a pneumothorax. If a pneumothorax is identified, a small calibre chest tube can be placed.

A chest x-ray is taken post-operatively. A small pneumothorax generally resolves spontaneously and should be confirmed with a repeat x-ray the next day. Patients can sometimes have numbness on the ipsilateral arm from dissection around the brachial plexus, but unless there was a specific injury, these symptoms usually resolve spontaneously within 24 hours.

Supraclavicular approach

After induction with general anesthesia, the patient is positioned in a semi-Fowler position with the head tilted away from the side of dissection. An incision is made cephalad and parallel to the clavicle extending from the sternocleidomastoid muscle to the trapezius. The incision was deepened past the platysma muscle until the anterior scalene fat pad is encountered. The fat pad is reflected away from the internal jugular vein medially and the superior and inferior aspect is ligated. The thoracic duct can usually be identified at this point and should be ligated with silk sutures. Once the fat pad is mobilized, it is retracted laterally to expose the anterior scalene muscle in the brachial plexus and eventually the middle scalene muscle.

The anterior scalene muscle is then dissected free from its surrounding structures such as the subclavian artery and brachial plexus, and care should be taken to preserve the phrenic nerve. Once the vital structures are protected, the anterior scalene muscle is removed in entirety, first by dissecting it sharply from its insertion on the first rib and then by tracing it back to its origin at the cervical spine transverse process.

Next, the middle scalene muscle is exposed by medial retraction of the brachial plexus. The muscle is then removed from the lateral aspect of the first rib to the extent of the long thoracic nerve. During this dissection, abnormalities including the scalene minimus muscle or anomalous fibrous bands near the brachial plexus can also be identified and resected. Similarly, the cervical rib is also identified at this point, and the cervical rib, at its insertion point on the cervical spine, is resected. The anterior aspect of the cervical rib tends to be variable, either free-floating, connected to the first rib with a ligamentous band or fused with the first rib. The anterior aspect can be divided prior to resection of the first rib, unless it is fused. In this latter scenario, the first rib is resected and the cervical rib is removed en bloc.

Once the first rib is freed from the scalene muscles, it is also dissected from the intercostal muscles either with sharp dissection or a periosteal elevator. The first rib is then resected laterally and then anteriorly, with a rongeur used to resect additional bone in either direction.

The supraclavicular approach for TOS offers excellent exposure to the structures in the thoracic outlet and is particularly helpful when arterial reconstruction is anticipated. The improved exposure allows resection of the anterior and middle scalene muscle, thereby reducing the risk of recurrence due to inadequate decompression of the thoracic outlet. In addition, greater access to the brachial plexus allows for neurolysis of fibrous bands, although this should be performed with caution as dissection in itself can cause inflammatory scarring and recurrent symptoms. Rarer anomalies such as a scalene minimus muscle, or accessory phrenic nerve causing impingement on the subclavian vein, can also be more easily identified with the supraclavicular approach compared to the axillary approach. In addition, identification of the thoracic duct is generally easier and can be ligated prior to extensive venous dissection and mobilization of the scalene fat pad. Finally, the cervical rib is also accessible and able to be removed with this approach.

For vTOS, it is particularly important to remove the first rib at the costochondral junction, to reduce the risk of re-impingement of the subclavian vein. Frequently, however, the anterior most aspect of the first rib is difficult to access with the supraclavicular approach, and an infraclavicular approach is also needed for adequate resection.

Another source of impingement on the brachial plexus is passed the scalene triangle, coursing more laterally as it goes posterior to the pectoralis minor muscle in the subcoracoid space. Therefore, a pectoralis minor tenotomy has been advocated by Sanders as an adjunct in treatment of TOS, in selected patients with tenderness on palpation of the pectoralis space, or persistent symptoms after surgery.[12] A vertical incision is made at the deltopectoral groove, the pectoralis major is retracted medially to expose the pectoralis minor muscle, and the pectoralis minor muscle is resected below the coracoid process.

FOLLOW-UP

Follow-up for all causes of TOS should be done at 3, 6, 12 and 24 months after endovascular or surgical treatment. During follow-up, it is important to compare current arm function compared to pre-interventional baseline. The QuickDASH is an 11-item questionnaire that has frequently been used in TOS to track physical function and upper limb symptoms. SF-36 and other measures have been used; however, there is not yet a TOS-specific questionnaire.

For nTOS, post-operative physical therapy is started within 2 weeks after surgery to maintain shoulder mobility. Post-operative physical therapy is essential, as rib resection causes the shoulder to anteriorly rotate, and patients are already deconditioned from long-term symptoms. Therapy should be continued until function is optimized.

For vTOS, enoxaparin is started on post-operative day 3 and continued until a venogram is performed 2 weeks later. If there is no residual stenosis or thrombosis, anticoagulation is stopped. If there is significant stenosis or thrombosis, balloon angioplasty is performed and anticoagulation is continued. If there is occlusion, anticoagulation is continued. Surveillance is performed with imaging at 3-month intervals up to a year, followed by annually thereafter.

For patients with bilateral symptoms, the most symptomatic side is generally treated first. Physical therapy is then continued post-operatively, and the contralateral side is addressed approximately 1 year later. This time frame allows for continued physical therapy, as up to 10% eventually have improvement of their contralateral symptoms. In addition, this time frame allows for recovery of phrenic nerve palsy that may have arisen during resection of the anterior scalene muscle.

RESULTS

Neurogenic

In a large series, 87% with nTOS who fail conservative management with physical therapy have symptomatic benefit from FRRS at 1 year, and this benefit is sustained at a longer follow-up of about 4 years. Factors associated with lower quality of life scores at long-term follow-up include age greater than 40, history of smoking, prior opioid use, co-morbid pain syndromes and those with post-operative complications. Of note, initial positive response to lidocaine scalene block was associated with improved outcomes at 1 year, but not at 4 years. It is suggested that other factors such as smoking, age and comorbid conditions play a more prominent role in the long term.[3,13]

Venous

Operative management of vTOS with FRRS has high success rates with most resuming full activity in 4–6 months, with a long-term patency of 97%.[14,15]

Non-operative management of vTOS after initial catheter-directed thrombolysis had a 23% thrombotic recurrence rate in one series by Lee and others. Those with recurrence tended to be younger (mean age 22 vs. 36 without recurrence). It is important to note that in this study, as well as in other similar studies, the use of a subclavian vein stent was associated with a high rate of thrombosis.[16] In Taylor's study, patients managed conservatively had no long-term improvement in QuickDASH scores, whereas those managed with FRRS had significantly improved scores.

Taken together, those with vTOS are more likely to benefit from FRRS, particularly if they are young and more physically active. Preoperative thrombolysis has a high rate of re-occlusion prior to surgical decompression, and long-term outcomes are not different. Therefore, preoperative anti-coagulation without thrombolysis appears to be sufficient for most cases, and FRRS is crucial for long-term patency. Non-operative management can be considered in select older patients but with less reliable improvement in quality of life. The use of subclavian vein stents are not supported, especially if the costoclavicular space is not decompressed surgically.

Arterial

Results after repair of aTOS are generally excellent with up to 100% long-term success, though embolization and asymptomatic bypass occlusion have been noted in a small minority of cases.[11]

Choice of operative approach

In a report of 538 patients treated with the transaxillary FRRS, Orlando and others reported excellent long-term outcomes. Significant symptom improvement or resolution was noted in about 95% overall, and within this group, 93% of patients with nTOS had markedly improved or fully resolved symptoms, there was a 97% long-term patency rate for vTOS, and a 100% success rate for aTOS. The most common complication was pneumothorax (23%), which was generally treated intraoperatively with a chest tube and removed the next day. Serious complications were rare (all less than 1% each), and no nerve injuries were noted among the 538 patients. The mean length of hospital stay was 1 day.[15]

The supraclavicular approach can also result in excellent outcomes. Hempel and others reported a series of 770 consecutive patients. Twenty per cent had pleural violation, and there was 1 lymphatic leak, and 2 cases of causalgia requiring sympathectomy. There were no cases of phrenic or brachial plexus injuries noted.[17]

Direct comparison of the transaxillary and supraclavicular approach to treatment of TOS is rare. Sheth and others reported the only randomized trial involving 55 patients treated with either transaxillary first rib resection or supraclavicular brachial plexus neuroplasty. In this study, all outcome measures favoured the transaxillary approach. Patients reported significantly less pain on a visual analogue scale, a greater percentage of patients had pain relief, and a greater percentage of patients reported good or excellent outcomes with the transaxillary approach.[18]

DEFICIENCIES IN CURRENT KNOWLEDGE

- Long-term outcomes in nTOS patients who undergo physical therapy without operative intervention.
- Lack of randomized trials for thrombolysis alone for vTOS versus preoperative thrombolysis with FRRS versus FRRS alone.
- Unknown long-term patency of arterial reconstruction and best conduit for arterial bypass.
- Lack of large randomized trial on supraclavicular approach versus transaxillary approach. A concurrent study with Baylor-Dallas and UC-Davis is underway for comparison. A retrospective analysis of the Johns Hopkins experience with both supraclavicular and transaxillary operations over the past 10 years is being analysed.

BEST PRACTICE

- The physical exam should include palpation of the anterior scalene, as well as provocative manoeuvres such as EAST (Grade D).
- Physical therapy is the mainstay of neurogenic thoracic outlet syndrome. Operative management should be reserved for failure of conservative management (Grade B).
- Anterior scalene blocks with lidocaine help diagnose patients with neurogenic thoracic outlet syndrome and can identify those who are likely to have a favourable outcome (Grade C).
- Other causes of neurological symptoms should be investigated with nerve conduction studies and cervical MRI, particularly in patients over 40 years of age (Grade C).
- Perioperative anticoagulation with first rib resection and scalenectomy is the main treatment or venous thoracic outlet syndrome, and thrombolysis does not afford long-term improvement in outcomes (Grade B).
- Subclavian vein stents should be avoided (Grade C).
- Arterial or venous duplex is the main objective test for arterial and venous thoracic outlet syndrome, respectively (Grade D).
- Chest radiograph should be performed on all patients with suspected thoracic outlet syndrome to evaluate for cervical ribs (Grade D).

- The first rib and, if present, the cervical rib should both be resected in cases of arterial thoracic outlet syndrome (Grade C).
- Arterial reconstruction should be performed for cases of arterial embolism, occlusion or aneurysms greater than 2 cm (Grade D).

Key points

- Physical therapy is effective for the majority of patients with neurogenic TOS.
- Preoperative anticoagulation without thrombolysis is sufficient for most cases of venous TOS, and timely first rib resection and scalenectomy are important for long-term venous patency.
- Arterial TOS should be managed operatively.

KEY REFERENCES

1. Finlayson HC, O'Connor RJ, Brasher PM, Travlos A. Botulinum toxin injection for management of thoracic outlet syndrome: A double-blind, randomized, controlled trial. *Pain.* 2011;152(9):2023–2028.

    The only randomized control trial regarding the efficacy of botulinum toxin for management of thoracic outlet syndrome.

2. Lum YW, Brooke BS, Likes K et al. Impact of anterior scalene lidocaine blocks on predicting surgical success in older patients with neurogenic thoracic outlet syndrome. *J Vasc Surg.* 2012;55(5):1370–1375.

    Axillary vs. supraclavicular approach. This paper discusses the diagnostic and possibly prognostic importance of anterior scalene lidocaine blocks and also discusses factors predictive of poor early outcomes.

3. Guzzo JL, Chang K, Demos J, Black JH, Freischlag JA. Preoperative thrombolysis and venoplasty affords no benefit in patency following first rib resection and scalenectomy for subacute and chronic subclavian vein thrombosis. *J Vasc Surg.* 2010;52(3):658–662; discussion 662–663.

    This study supports the use of anticoagulation without thrombolysis and provides evidence against preoperative venoplasty.

4. Sheth RN, Campbell JN. Surgical treatment of thoracic outlet syndrome: A randomized trial comparing two operations. *J Neurosurg Spine.* 2005;3(5):355–363.

    The only randomized trial comparing the two main operative approaches to thoracic outlet syndrome.

5. Chang KZ, Likes K, Demos J, Black JH 3rd, Freischlag JA. Routine venography following transaxillary first rib resection and scalenectomy (FRRS) for chronic subclavian vein thrombosis ensures excellent outcomes and vein patency. *Vasc Endovasc Surg.* 2012;46(1):15–20.

    Describes the recommended protocol for management of venous thoracic outlet syndrome.

REFERENCES

1. Wilbourn AJ. The thoracic outlet syndrome is over-diagnosed. *Arch Neurol.* 1990;47(3):328–330.
2. McCleery RS, Kesterson JE, Kirtley JA, Love RB. Subclavius and anterior scalene muscle compression as a cause of intermittent obstruction of the subclavian vein. *Ann Surg.* 1951;133(5):588–602.
3. Lum YW, Brooke BS, Likes K et al. Impact of anterior scalene lidocaine blocks on predicting surgical success in older patients with neurogenic thoracic outlet syndrome. *J Vasc Surg.* 2012;55(5):1370–1375.
4. Torriani M, Gupta R, Donahue DM. Botulinum toxin injection in neurogenic thoracic outlet syndrome: Results and experience using a ultrasound-guided approach. *Skeletal Radiol.* 2010;39(10):973–980.
5. Finlayson HC, O'Connor RJ, Brasher PM, Travlos A. Botulinum toxin injection for management of thoracic outlet syndrome: A double-blind, randomized, controlled trial. *Pain.* 2011;152(9):2023–2028.
6. Likes K, Rochlin DH, Call D, Freischlag JA. Coexistence of arterial compression in patients with neurogenic thoracic outlet syndrome. *JAMA Surg.* 2014;149(12):1240–1243.
7. Angle N, Gelabert HA, Farooq MM et al. Safety and efficacy of early surgical decompression of the thoracic outlet for Paget-Schroetter syndrome. *Ann Vasc Surg.* 2001;15(1):37–42.
8. Guzzo JL, Chang K, Demos J, Black JH, Freischlag JA. Preoperative thrombolysis and venoplasty affords no benefit in patency following first rib resection and scalenectomy for subacute and chronic subclavian vein thrombosis. *J Vasc Surg.* 2010;52(3):658–662; discussion 662–663.
9. Taylor JM, Telford RJ, Kinsella DC, Watkinson AF, Thompson JF. Long-term clinical and functional outcome following treatment for Paget-Schroetter syndrome. *Br J Surg.* 2013;100(11):1459–1464.
10. Chang KZ, Likes K, Demos J, Black JH 3rd, Freischlag JA. Routine venography following transaxillary first rib resection and scalenectomy (FRRS) for chronic subclavian vein thrombosis ensures excellent outcomes and vein patency. *Vasc Endovasc Surg.* 2012;46(1):15–20.
11. Chang KZ, Likes K, Davis K, Demos J, Freischlag JA. The significance of cervical ribs in thoracic outlet syndrome. *J Vasc Surg.* 2013;57(3):771–775.
12. Sanders RJ, Rao NM. The forgotten pectoralis minor syndrome: 100 operations for pectoralis minor syndrome alone or accompanied by neurogenic thoracic outlet syndrome. *Ann Vasc Surg.* 2010;24(6):701–708.
13. Rochlin DH, Gilson MM, Likes KC et al. Quality-of-life scores in neurogenic thoracic outlet syndrome patients undergoing first rib resection and scalenectomy. *J Vasc Surg.* 2013;57(2):436–443.
14. Chang DC, Rotellini-Coltvet LA, Mukherjee D, De Leon R, Freischlag JA. Surgical intervention for thoracic outlet syndrome improves patient's quality of life. *J Vasc Surg.* 2009;49(3):630–635; discussion 635–637.

15. Orlando MS, Likes KC, Mirza S et al. A decade of excellent outcomes after surgical intervention in 538 patients with thoracic outlet syndrome. *J Am Coll Surg.* 2015;220(5):934–939.

16. Lee JT, Karwowski JK, Harris EJ, Haukoos JS, Olcott Ct. Long-term thrombotic recurrence after nonoperative management of Paget-Schroetter syndrome. *J Vasc Surg.* 2006;43(6):1236–1243.

17. Hempel GK, Shutze WP, Anderson JF, Bukhari HI. 770 consecutive supraclavicular first rib resections for thoracic outlet syndrome. *Ann Vasc Surg.* 1996;10(5):456–463.

18. Sheth RN, Campbell JN. Surgical treatment of thoracic outlet syndrome: A randomized trial comparing two operations. *J Neurosurg Spine.* 2005;3(5):355–363.

43

Raynaud's syndrome and upper extremity small artery occlusive disease

GREGORY J. LANDRY

CONTENTS

INTRODUCTION

All vascular disease specialists encounter occasional patients with fixed or intermittent upper extremity ischemia, a group estimated to comprise about 5% of patients with limb ischemia. A large majority of patients with upper extremity ischemia complaints have only intermittent vasospasm of the hands and fingers, a condition termed Raynaud's syndrome (RS). An estimated 5%–10% of patients with upper extremity ischemia symptoms have severe hand and finger ischemia or digital ischemia ulceration associated with fixed arterial occlusive disease of the palmar and digital arteries. Only a small percentage of these patients develop distal arterial occlusion as a result of potentially correctable arterial obstruction at or proximal to the wrist, including proximal subclavian and innominate atherosclerosis, subclavian aneurysms with or without a coexistent cervical rib, subclavian and upper extremity giant cell arteritis, radiation arteritis and associated disorders. The discussion that follows will focus on both upper extremity vasospasm and fixed arterial occlusive disease of both the large and small arteries of the upper extremities.

RAYNAUD'S SYNDROME

RS defines a clinical condition characterized by episodic digital ischemia occurring in response to cold or emotional stimuli. RS was first described by the French physician Maurice Raynaud in 1862 with the characteristic tricolour change featuring pallor (ischemic phase), cyanosis (deoxygenation phase) and erythema (reperfusion phase) induced by cold or stress. All patients with RS have palmar and digital episodic vasospasm which may be primary (vasospastic RS) associated with normal arteries between attacks or may be secondary (obstructive RS) and associated with fixed palmar and digital arterial obstruction. Uncomplicated primary vasospastic RS does not produce digital ischemic ulceration. All patients with digital ischemic ulceration have one or more of a variety of systemic disease processes, which have as one of their manifestations obstruction of

Table 43.1 Raynaud's syndrome–associated diseases.

Connective tissue diseases
  Progressive systemic sclerosis (scleroderma)
  Systemic lupus erythematosus
  Rheumatoid arthritis
  Sjögren's syndrome
  Mixed connective tissue disease
  Overlap connective tissue disease
  Dermatomyositis and polymyositis
  Vasculitis (small, medium-sized vessel)
Occlusive arterial disease
  Atherosclerosis
  Thromboangiitis obliterans (Buerger's disease)
  Giant cell arteritis
  Arterial emboli (cardiac and peripheral)
  Thoracic outlet syndrome
Occupational arterial disease
  Hypothenar hammer syndrome
  Vibration induced
Drug-induced vasospasm
  Beta-adrenergic blocking drugs
  Vasopressors
  Ergot
  Cocaine
  Amphetamines
  Vinblastine/bleomycin
Myeloproliferative and hematological disease
  Polycythemia rubra vera
  Thrombocytosis
  Cold agglutinins
  Cryoglobulinemia
  Paraproteinemia
Malignancy
Multiple myeloma
  Leukemia
  Adenocarcinoma
  Astrocytoma
Infection
Hepatitis B and C antigenemia
  Parvovirus
  Purpura fulminans

the palmar and digital arteries. These diseases are listed in Table 43.1. Interestingly, the phenotypic presentation of the two groups may be indistinguishable. This section is concerned with the diagnosis, classification and treatment of vasospastic and obstructive diseases of the palmar and digital arteries. The division of patients with upper extremity small artery disease into these two subgroups (vasospastic and obstructive) is somewhat arbitrary, and there is often a continuum of disease between these two categories. However, the subgrouping emphasizes the unique and important diagnostic and therapeutic implications of each of these disorders.

Pathophysiology

RS may be classified as obstructive or vasospastic.

> ### Key point
>
> Differentiating vasospastic from obstructive pathophysiology is a critical point of the diagnostic workup, providing guidance for both prognosis and subsequent treatment.

The episodic attacks of both types of RS classically consist of pallor of the affected part upon cold exposure or emotional stimulation followed by cyanosis and rubor upon rewarming, with full recovery in 15–45 minutes. The hands and fingers are most affected in a large majority of patients, although the toes, cheeks and ears are occasionally involved and the thumbs frequently spared. About 5% of affected patients have primary symptoms in the feet and toes. The initial pallor of an attack is caused by spasm of the digital arteries and arterioles. After a variable period of time, the capillaries and probably the venules dilate in response to both hypoxia and the accumulation of products of anaerobic metabolism. As the arterial spasm relaxes, the initial blood flow into the dilated capillaries rapidly desaturates, causing cyanosis. Finally, rubor results from increasing amounts of the blood entering the dilated capillary bed, and the digits return to normal as the capillaries constrict. Many patients do not demonstrate the classic tricolour changes during a Raynaud's attack and experience cold hands with only pallor or cyanosis. Since these patients may have the same arteriographic and hemodynamic abnormalities encountered in patients with the classic tricolour changes, colour changes are no longer considered essential for diagnosis. The underlying pathophysiology of RS has been the object of investigation for over a century. Raynaud hypothesized that the condition was due to sympathetic nervous system hyperactivity. Hutchinson, in the latter part of the nineteenth century, observed that episodic hand ischemia occurred in association with a variety of disease processes and did not represent the single disease entity suggested by Raynaud. In 1932, Allen and Brown, recognizing the frequency with which other diseases were associated with RS, proposed dividing the syndrome into Raynaud's disease (primary RS), which represented a benign, idiopathic form of vasospasm without any associated disease, and Raynaud's phenomenon (secondary RS), which occurred in association with a systemic disease process. Eventually, a number of investigators observed that classification of patient by the pathophysiologic cause (obstruction vs. vasospasm) made more sense than classification by the presence or absence of an associated disease, as autoimmune disease may be missed at the initial evaluation or present years after the onset of digital vasospastic symptoms. Additionally, evaluation, treatment and response to treatment of patients are better directed by the pathophysiologic classification.

Patients with obstructive RS have considerably decreased digital arterial flow at room temperature, with striking additional decrease with cooling. In these patients, a normal arterial vasoconstrictive response to cold overcomes the diminished baseline arterial pressure and causes complete arterial closure. Abnormally, forceful cold-stimulated arterial constriction is not required to cause digital arterial closure in patients with obstruction RS. Patients with palmar and digital arterial obstruction severe enough to produce a significant decrease in digital artery pressure at rest will have at least some degree of cold-induced RS. Patients with vasospastic RS do not have significant hand or digital artery obstruction and have normal digital blood pressures and flow at room temperature. Arterial closure in these patients is caused by a markedly increased force of cold-induced vasospasm. Lewis, in the 1920s, observed that digital nerve blocks did not prevent vasospasm and concluded that sympathetic nerves were not the source of the vasospastic stimulus. He hypothesized a 'local vascular fault' as the cause of the hyperreactivity to cold observed in the digital arteries in patients with vasospastic RS.

Vasospastic RS is likely a manifestation of altered adrenergic receptor activity. The characterization of alpha1- and alpha2-adrenoceptors has led to an improved understanding of the mechanisms of RS. The alpha1-adrenoceptors are located post-synaptically and, when stimulated, produce vasoconstriction. The alpha2-adrenoceptors are located both pre- and post-synaptically. While stimulation of the presynaptic alpha2-receptors inhibits norepinephrine release and has a vasodilatory effect, stimulation of post-synaptic alpha2-receptors induces vasoconstriction. In patients with RS, the alpha2-receptors play a predominant role, with either increased density or hyperactivity of the post-synaptic alpha2-receptors causing abnormal vasoconstriction.

The endothelial cell also produces factors that cause vessel contraction, such as endothelin (ET)-1, which is a potent vasoconstrictor as well as a promoter of fibroblast and smooth muscle proliferation. Plasma ET-1 levels become elevated in response to the cold exposure, which may suggest an association between the rise in ET-1 levels and cold-induced vasoconstriction. A relative decrease in the level of naturally occurring vasodilating agents has also been hypothesized as the cause of RS. The best studied of these is calcitonin gene–related peptide (CGRP). Patients with scleroderma appear to have a decrease in cutaneous CGRP and respond favourably to CGRP infusion.

Epidemiology

RS is a common disorder with a prevalence in the general population varying greatly with climate and ethnic origin. The exact incidence of RS in the general population is difficult to determine as many people who are troubled by cold sensitivity do not seek medical attention. Surveys in areas with cold, damp climates have estimated a disease prevalence of about 20%–30%. Women comprise 70%–90% of most reported patient groups with RS, except in African-American and Asian populations, where the gender prevalence is equal. Typically, younger women will have vasospastic RS without evidence of associated disease. Some patients will develop an associated disease at a later date. Older males with RS usually have digital artery occlusion, often from arteriosclerosis or autoimmune disease. Select occupational groups have a high prevalence of RS, especially those associated with the use of vibrating tools. In a 14-year study in a community in southern France, the annual incidence of new cases of primary RS was 0.25% with a declining incidence with age.[1]

Associated diseases

The general classification of disorders associated with RS is presented in Table 43.1.

Key point

Up to 1/3 of patients with RS who present without an associated disease will develop an associated disease, most frequently a connective tissue disease (CTD), over time. This points to the need for ongoing surveillance of these patients with periodic reassessment for CTDs.

Many of these conditions may be associated with diffuse obstructive palmar and digital arterial disease, which may be sufficiently severe to produce ischemic ulceration. The possibility that digital gangrene or ulceration may result from intrinsic small artery occlusive disease with normal proximal arteries is often considered only after an extensive evaluation of a patient with hand and finger ischemia fails to reveal proximal arterial obstruction or a cardiac embolic source. The majority of patients seen in our tertiary practice have secondary RS in association with one of the diseases or conditions listed in Table 43.1. That percentage undoubtedly does not apply to minimally symptomatic patients who have never sought medical care; the incidence of coexistent disease in this group is unknown. However, available evidence indicates that the likelihood of coexisting disease in all patients with RS is sufficiently high to warrant a thorough evaluation of each patient, as described later in this chapter.

Large artery occlusive disease proximal to the wrist may result in ischemic finger ulceration, usually in association with digital artery embolization. Although the most frequent symptoms of giant cell arteritis are related to temporal arteritis and polymyalgia rheumatica, the appearance of isolated arm ischemia in older women is sufficiently characteristic of this condition to warrant consideration of this diagnosis even in the absence of other manifestations of the disease. This is especially true in elderly females with bilateral upper extremity ischemic symptoms in the absence of recognized atherosclerotic risk factors. The symptoms may range from cold intolerance to exertional pain to pulselessness and severe ischemia, although tissue loss is uncommon. The erythrocyte sedimentation rate is nearly always elevated and provides a useful screening test. The angiographic features most suggestive of arteritis are

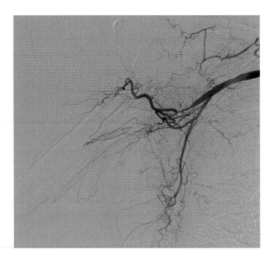

Figure 43.1 Typical angiographic appearance of giant cell arteritis with smooth, tapering stenosis or occlusion of the subclavian, axillary and brachial arteries.

(1) long segments of smooth stenosis interspersed among normal areas, (2) smoothly tapered occlusion, (3) absence of irregular plaques and ulceration and (4) distribution of these abnormalities among the subclavian, axillary and brachial arteries (Figure 43.1).

The most frequent cause of upper extremity ischemia in our practice has been intrinsic small artery occlusive disease of the palmar and digital arteries, most frequently associated with CTDs. Ischemia in these circumstances may progress to fingertip ulceration or gangrene. The most frequently associated disease states encountered in patients with ischemic digital ulceration are the autoimmune or CTDs. All CTDs have an associated arteritis, which may cause progressive obstruction of the small- and medium-sized arteries of the hands and fingers. Scleroderma, particularly with the calcinosis, Raynaud phenomenon, esophageal dysmotility, sclerodactyly, and telangiectasia (CREST) variant, is the autoimmune disease most frequently associated with digital artery obstruction. While most patients with scleroderma develop RS, this symptom may precede recognition of the underlying CTD by years.

Patients who have clinical and serologic evidence of CTD but do not fulfil the criteria for a specific disease diagnosis are classified as having undifferentiated CTD. We apply the term hypersensitivity angiitis to a subset of patients with digital gangrene resulting from intrinsic small artery occlusive disease. These patients are characterized by the precipitous onset of severe ischemia at the tips of multiple fingers without any premonitory signs or symptoms. Immunologic evaluation in this patient group typically fails to reveal any diagnostic serologic abnormalities, while arteriography consistently demonstrates diffuse palmar and digital arterial occlusion.

Buerger's disease is another cause of widespread digital artery occlusions and finger gangrene. It appears to represent a thrombotic arteriopathy occurring mainly in young male smokers and is characterized by the occurrence of segmental thrombotic occlusions in both the upper and lower extremities.

A small number of patients with digital gangrene will be found to have a malignancy. In certain patients, the malignancy-associated ischemia is due to arterial thrombosis, while in others the mechanism appears to be that of an inflammatory arteritis.

PATIENT PRESENTATION

Raynaud's syndrome

Primary vasospastic RS most frequently affects women with symptom onset in the teens or early twenties. Both hands are affected equally, although the thumbs may be spared.

> **Key point**
>
> Thumb involvement is more frequently associated with a connective tissue disorder. In purely vasospastic RS, the thumbs are frequently spared.

Some increased sensitivity of the feet and toes may be elicited, and between 5% and 10% of patients describe primary lower extremity involvement. Conversely, obstructive RS has a 1:1 male-to-female ratio, and most patients are over 40 years of age. The lower extremities are infrequently involved, and there may be only a few involved digits. The asymmetry of digital involvement is an important difference between vasospastic and obstructive RS. Most RS attacks are produced by cold exposure, although about half of these patients describe occasional attacks provoked by emotional stress. The stimulus for an attack may be as mild as walking into an air-conditioned room, getting one's hands wet or picking up a cold glass. In addition to colour changes, attacks may be associated with numbness. Severe pain is rare. Most spontaneous indoor attacks resolve in 5–10 minutes. Most attacks precipitated by outdoor cold exposure terminate only with hand warming.

Digital ulceration/gangrene

In contrast, patients with underlying occlusive disease have little or no reserve and cannot increase digital blood flow with the result that ischemic damage can occur during cold exposure. These patients with secondary RS are more likely to complain of digital pain on rewarming of cold fingers because the blood flow cannot increase to match the increased metabolic activity of the finger. These patients are also more likely to present with digital ulceration or gangrene, with two groups emerging based on their presentation with an acute or chronic history of finger gangrene. Approximately 40% present within several weeks to a few months of the acute onset of digital ischemia. Most of these patients experience the precipitous onset of cyanosis and pain involving the distal portions of multiple fingers, followed in days to several weeks by the development of skin necrosis with a variable amount of tissue loss. Systemic signs and symptoms of CTD are usually absent in these patients. About 60% of patients present with a chronic history of digital gangrene. Patients frequently describe multiple exacerbations and remissions extending over years. Patients in this group are, on average, 5–10 years older than those in the acute group and more likely to have pre-existing RS.

CLINICAL EVALUATION OF THE PATIENT

History and physical examination

The diagnosis of RS is made mainly by clinical findings, based on patient descriptions of self-limiting cold or emotionally induced skin changes as previously described. It is helpful for patients to bring photos of the events due to the rarity of witnessing them in clinic (Figure 43.2). A thorough history should be obtained regarding symptoms of CTD, including arthralgia, dysphagia, skin tightening, xerophthalmia or xerostomia. Symptoms of large-vessel occlusive disease, exposure to trauma or frostbite, smoking and drug history and history of malignancy should also be sought.

Since RS is primarily diagnosed by history, the physical examination in suspected individuals is often normal. Nonetheless, the determination of primary or secondary disease is aided by a focused physical examination. The hands and fingers should be inspected for ulcerations or

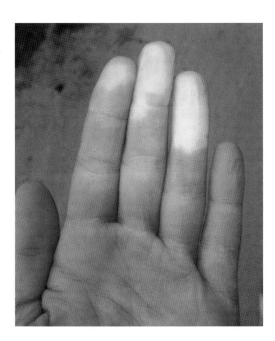

Figure 43.2 Typical clinical appearance of Raynaud's attack.

fingertip hyperkeratotic areas, skin thinning, tightening, sclerodactyly or telangiectasias, all of which may suggest associated autoimmune disease. Splinter hemorrhages under the nails may be a normal finding in manual workers with hand trauma but is also an indicator of distal cholesterol emboli. Pulse examination should include palpation of subclavian, brachial, radial and ulnar arteries. Palpation above the clavicle can determine the presence of a cervical rib and/or aneurysm of the subclavian artery. A palpable thrill indicates high-grade arterial stenosis. Auscultation over large arteries for a bruit, in particular over the sternoclavicular joint and above the clavicle, may identify an arterial stenosis. The Allen test should be performed in every patient with suspected RS to detect the presence of ulnar artery occlusion. A positive reverse Allen test may signify occlusion of the radial artery.

Non-invasive vascular laboratory

The non-invasive vascular laboratory is an important adjunct to the office-based clinical assessment of patients with RS.

> **Key point**
>
> The initial vascular laboratory analysis is performed at room temperature, allowing differentiation between vasospasm vs. obstruction. Patients with vasospasm generally have normal findings at room temperature, while those with obstruction demonstrate significant blunting in one or more fingers. Cold challenge testing is not necessary for diagnosis.

Non-invasive vascular laboratory testing can assist in differentiating between fixed arterial obstruction and pure vasospasm and can provide assessment of the location and severity of the circulatory impairment. To evaluate for large-vessel occlusive arterial disease, segmental blood pressure measurements in the upper extremity can be obtained. Pneumatic cuffs are placed on the brachial, upper elbow and wrist levels, and systolic blood pressures are measured. A pressure differential exceeding 10 mmHg between levels may be significant, indicating proximal occlusive arterial disease.

Measurement of finger systolic pressures is possible by using small digital cuffs applied to the proximal finger and assessment of systolic blood pressure by pulse-volume recording, strain-gauge plethysmography or photoplethysmography. A difference of more than 15 mmHg between fingers or an absolute finger systolic blood pressure of less than 70 mmHg may indicate occlusive disease.[1] The normal finger–brachial index may range from 0.8 to 1.3. The fingers are especially temperature sensitive, and cool fingers can result in falsely low indices. Because the digits have dual arteries, early disease with occlusion of one of the digital arteries cannot be detected by finger pressure measurement if the contralateral artery is open.

Evaluation of digital plethysmographic waveforms is also useful, particularly in identifying obstructive RS. Patients with obstructive RS have blunted waveforms, whereas patients with vasospastic RS have either normal waveforms or a 'peaked pulse' (Figure 43.3). The peaked-pulse pattern, first described by Sumner and Strandness, appears to reflect increased vasospastic arterial resistance.[2]

Cold challenge testing, such as ice water immersion with temperature recovery, is highly sensitive but lacks specificity. A delay in rewarming suggests a vasospasm tendency. Raynaud's patients typically may take more than 10 minutes and sometimes 30 minutes or longer to recover resting finger temperatures compared with less than 10 minutes for normal subjects. The digital blood pressure response to 5 minutes of digital occlusive hypothermia as described by Nielsen and Lassen has proved to be a more accurate method of diagnosis of RS in the vascular laboratory. This method employs a double-inlet plastic cuff for local digital cooling. A cuff that can be sequentially cooled is placed on the proximal phalanx of the test finger, with a cuff maintained at room temperature placed on the proximal phalanx of a reference finger. The test is repeated at several temperatures, and the result is expressed as the percentage drop in finger systolic pressure with cooling. In an evaluation of this test at the Oregon Health & Science University, this test was found to be 87% specific and 90% sensitive for an overall accuracy of 92%.[3] Other non-invasive tests, such as laser Doppler and digital thermography, have minimal clinical use and are mainly used in the research setting.

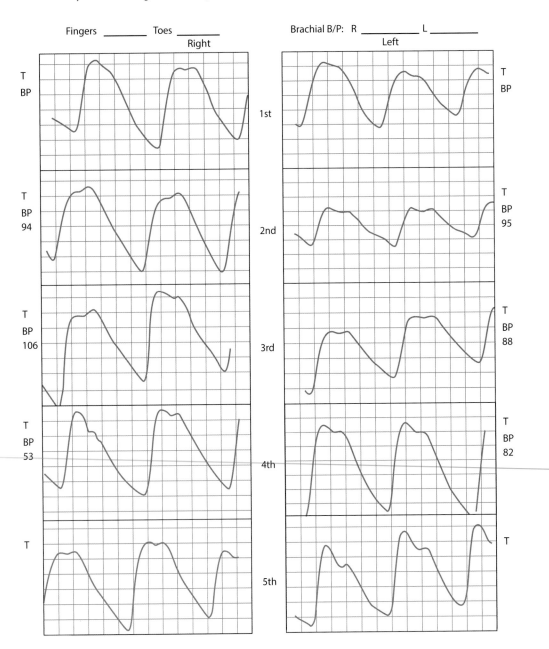

Figure 43.3 Peaked pulse on plethysmography often seen in patients with vasospastic Raynaud's syndrome.

Serologic testing

Serologic studies may help to confirm the diagnosis of CTD and are also useful in screening for occult underlying CTD. Useful screening tests include anti-nuclear antibody and rheumatoid factor. Anti-nuclear antibodies are present in 95% of systemic sclerosis patients. Anti-nuclear antibodies are not specific for scleroderma and can be present in a number of other CTDs – in particular, lupus erythematosus. A positive anti-nuclear antibody raises suspicion but on its own does not make a diagnosis of a CTD. Several autoantibodies are specific for systemic sclerosis. The anticentromere antibody is associated with limited CREST syndrome. Rheumatoid factor is an antibody directed against the Fc region of IgG that has been used as a diagnostic marker for rheumatoid arthritis. As opposed to vasculitis, the erythrocyte sedimentation rate is usually normal in CTDs.

Angiography

The purpose of angiography is not to confirm distal arterial obstruction, which is presumed present in patients with digital gangrene, but to rule out a proximal disease process, such as subclavian artery stenosis or aneurysm, which may be serving as a source of emboli and may be amenable to surgical repair.

Key point

The main purpose for angiography is to rule out a proximal arterial lesion that may be leading to digital ischemia. This is most useful in patients with unilateral hand ischemia where the contralateral hand plethysmography is normal. Angiography is not needed to confirm intrinsic arterial disease in the hand, as this is adequately diagnosed with less invasive measures.

Particularly if the patient's signs and symptoms are unilateral, the diagnosis of isolated distal small artery occlusive disease can be established with certainty only after proximal arterial disease has been angiographically eliminated. Complete angiography has traditionally constituted an integral portion of the evaluation of patients with digital gangrene and has included visualization of the arterial circulation from the aortic arch to the fingertips of both hands. These angiograms are best performed by the transfemoral approach, using magnification technique for the filming of the hand circulation. The angiograms may be obtained before and after cold exposure (cryodynamic angiography) and before and after intra-arterial vasodilators if significant vasospasm is present on the initial films. Arteriography is not indicated in patients with bilateral finger ischemia and a normal upper extremity arterial exam to the wrist. The likelihood of finding bilateral proximal arterial disease in such patients does not appear sufficient to warrant the small risk of arteriography.

TREATMENT

The primary goal of medical therapy is to reduce the frequency and intensity of attacks and to minimize the related morbidity rather than to cure the underlying condition. The treatment will depend on whether the RS is primary or secondary. If it is secondary, it will depend on the underlying disease. The initial treatment of patients with Raynaud's phenomenon includes the following: patient education, general measures to maintain body warmth, avoidance of other triggers and pharmacotherapy.

Patient education and general measures

General measures are often sufficient to control symptoms in patients with primary RS. All patients should be advised on the avoidance of cold exposure and use of hand warming when in a cold environment. Other triggers, such as stress, hand trauma and tobacco, should also be assiduously avoided.

Pharmacologic therapy

While a number of medications are routinely used for vasospasm, there are no currently available drugs that are specifically FDA approved for the treatment of RS. Choosing the one best medication has been difficult owing to a lack of large prospective, randomized, double-blind studies comparing the efficacy of different medications. There is significant placebo effect in published clinical trials ranging from 20% to 40%, an important factor when interpreting the results of uncontrolled trials. Most clinical trials rely on the patient's self-assessment of frequency and severity of RS episodes, and objective confirmation of benefit has been difficult to determine.

Key point

Response to pharmacologic therapy varies from person to person. While calcium channel blockers (CCBs) are typically considered first-line therapy, lack of response to one drug type does not imply lack of response to drugs of a different class. In general, pharmacologic therapy is more effective in vasospastic RS than obstructive RS.

Pharmacologic therapy is indicated for patients whose symptoms do not respond to simple conservative measures. Currently used pharmacologic agents are summarized in Table 43.2.[4]

CALCIUM CHANNEL BLOCKERS

For purely vasospastic RS, CCBs are currently the most prescribed and studied medications. They are divided into

Table 43.2 Medical therapy of Raynaud's syndrome.

Drug class	Drug names	Dosage	Highest level of evidence	Results	Most frequent side effects
CCBs (dihydropyridine)	Nifedipine	10–30 mg po qD-tid	1A	33%–66% reduction in frequency and severity of attacks; most extensively studied medication	Hypotension, flushing, edema, palpitations, dizziness (similar for entire class of drugs)
	Nicardipine	20–50 mg po bid	1A	Mixed results compared to placebo	
	Amlodipine	10 mg po qD	1A	27% reduction in frequency of attacks	
	Felodipine	5–20 mg po qD	1A	Similar to nifedipine in small trial	
	Nisoldipine	5–10 mg po qD	1A	Mixed results improving severity and frequency of attacks	
CCBs (non-dihydropyridine)	Diltiazem	30–120 mg po tid	1A	Some improvement but less efficacious than dihydropyridine class	Fewer side effects than dihydropyridine class
	Verapamil			No proven benefit	
Alpha1-receptor antagonists	Prazosin	1 mg po tid	1A	1–2 fewer attacks per day, decreased duration; modest benefit in secondary RS	Orthostatic hypotension, palpitations
	Terazosin	1 mg po qhs	3C	Not systematically studied	
	Doxazosin	1 mg po qhs	3C		
Renin–angiotensin system mediators (ACE inhibitors)	Captopril	12.5–25 mg po bid-tid	1A	Improved finger blood flow; symptom relief mixed	Dry cough, headache, fatigue, dizziness (similar for entire drug class)
	Enalapril	20 mg po qD	1A	Mixed results in clinical trials	
	Quinapril	80 mg po qD	1A	No clinical benefit	
Renin–angiotensin system mediators (angiotensin II receptor blockers)	Losartan	12.5–50 mg po qD	1A	Up to 50% reduction in severity and frequency of attacks	Dizziness
Serotonin reuptake inhibitors	Fluoxetine	20–40 mg po qD	1A	Significant decrease in severity and frequency of attacks vs. nifedipine	Headaches, nausea, palpitations, lethargy
Phosphodiesterase-5 inhibitors	Sildenafil	50 mg po qD-bid Extended release 100–200 mg qD	1A	Decreased duration and frequency of attacks; improvement of capillary blood flow; benefit primarily in secondary RS	Headache, flushing, nausea, muscle pain, dyspepsia, dizziness (similar for all drugs in this class)
	Tadalafil	20 mg every other day	1A	Decreased frequency and duration of attacks and improved ulcer healing as add on therapy; less beneficial as monotherapy	
	Vardenafil	10 mg po bid	2C	Improved digital blood flow and symptoms in secondary RS	

(Continued)

Table 43.2 (*Continued*)   Medical therapy of Raynaud's syndrome.

Drug class	Drug names	Dosage	Highest level of evidence	Results	Most frequent side effects
Nitrates	Topical nitroglycerin (MQX-503)	0.5 g of gel up to four times a day	1A	Improved Raynaud's condition score; no change in duration or frequency of attacks	Headache, upper respiratory tract infection, dizziness
Prostaglandins	Epoprostenol	1–2 ng/kg/ minute iv	1A	Decreased severity of symptoms in patients with scleroderma and pulmonary hypertension	Flushing, headache, nausea, vomiting, hypotension
	Iloprost	0.5–2 ng/kg/ minute iv or 50 μg po bid		IV form effective in ulcer healing and reducing symptoms; PO form not more effective than placebo	Headache, nausea, vomiting
Endothelin-receptor antagonist	Bosentan	62.5 mg po bid	1A	Decreased new ulcer formation in patients with scleroderma; no effect on healing of existing ulcers	Elevated hepatic transaminases, peripheral edema

two major categories: the dihydropyridines and the non-dihydropyridines. Drugs in the dihydropyridine class (nifedipine, amlodipine, felodipine, nisoldipine and isradipine) are more potent vasodilators than the non-dihydropyridine classes (diltiazem) but also more frequently associated with side effects. Long-acting or sustained-release preparations are preferred. Diltiazem is less potent and consequently has fewer adverse effects but is also less efficacious.[5] Verapamil has more cardiac than peripheral vascular selectivity and is not a good peripheral vasodilator.

Nifedipine is considered by many to be the drug of first choice for RS. A 66% reduction in frequency of attacks has been reported in a multicentre, randomized, controlled trial of 313 patients with primary RS treated with sustained-release nifedipine compared with placebo.[6] Other studies have shown that CCBs reduced frequency of ischemic attacks on average 2.8–5.0 fewer attacks per week and a 33% reduction in severity.[7] Other dihydropyridines have also been used in RS. Amlodipine has a longer half-life, with the theoretical advantage of fewer adverse effects.[8] Nicardipine, felodipine and isradipine have also been shown to be efficacious.

ALPHA1-ADRENERGIC BLOCKERS

Alpha1-adrenergic blockers competitively inhibit postsynaptic alpha-adrenergic receptors, which results in vasodilation of veins and arterioles and a decrease in total peripheral resistance and blood pressure. Prazosin, a selective alpha1-adrenergic antagonist, has been found to be more effective than placebo in the treatment of RS secondary to scleroderma. In a double-blind, placebo-controlled, crossover study of 24 patients, subjective benefit with significant reduction in number and duration of attacks was noted in two-thirds of those patients treated with prazosin

with improvement in finger blood flow assessed during a finger-cooling test.[9]

ANGIOTENSIN-CONVERTING ENZYME INHIBITORS

Captopril has been used most extensively for the treatment of RS. Studies evaluating angiotensin-converting enzyme (ACE) inhibitors have found conflicting results in their ability to improve digit blood flow and reduce both frequency and severity of RS attacks. A recent systematic review analyzed three separate clinical trials that found no significant difference between captopril and placebo. It also reported that patients treated with enalapril had an increase in frequency and duration of attacks when compared to placebo.[10]

ANGIOTENSIN II RECEPTOR BLOCKERS

Losartan is the most commonly used drug in this category. In a randomized controlled study, losartan 50 mg daily was found to be more effective than nifedipine 40 mg daily in reducing the frequency and severity of vasospastic episodes in patients with primary RS and those with secondary RS due to systemic sclerosis following 12 weeks of therapy.[11] Another review concluded that angiotensin II receptor blockers (ARBs) may have some benefits in the treatment of RS, but larger, randomized controlled trials of longer duration are needed to compare the effectiveness of ARBs with conventional treatment.[12]

SELECTIVE SEROTONIN REUPTAKE INHIBITORS

The vasoconstrictive effects of serotonin can be inhibited by fluoxetine, a selective serotonin reuptake inhibitor. There is one study that compared fluoxetine with placebo and fluoxetine showed a reduction in attack frequency and severity of RS.[13]

PHOSPHODIESTERASE-5 INHIBITORS

Sildenafil, tadalafil and vardenafil are selective inhibitors of phosphodiesterase-5 (PDE-5), which increases cGMP, resulting in enhanced cGMP-dependent vasodilatation. PDE-5 inhibitors significantly have been shown to improve Raynaud's condition score and decrease the frequency and duration of RS attacks, including those resistant to traditional vasodilators.[14] Sildenafil improves symptoms, ulcer healing and capillary blood flow in patients with secondary RS.[15,16] Tadalafil and vardenafil have longer half-lives than sildenafil but have been less well studied in RS, although both have demonstrated symptom improvement in small clinical trials.[17,18]

NITRATES

Because of their vasodilating properties on vascular smooth muscle, nitrates have been used for many years in the treatment of RS. Topical nitrates in the form of 2% nitroglycerine ointment or as a transdermal patch can be applied locally to an ischemic finger and have been shown to be effective in the treatment of RS in randomized controlled trials.[19] Several other formulations including sublingual tablets, tape and transdermal patches have been proven to be effective. All forms are limited by side effects, particularly headaches and hypotension.

ENDOTHELIN INHIBITORS

Bosentan is an ET-1 receptor antagonist licensed in Europe to treat pulmonary hypertension and to prevent the onset of new digital ulcers in secondary RS when associated with scleroderma. When used as monotherapy, it has not proven to change rates of ulcer healing nor improve pain or disability.[20] When used in combination with iloprost, it increased fingertip blood perfusion as well as capillary dilation and number.[21]

PROSTAGLANDINS AND ANALOGUES

Prostaglandins and prostacyclins are vasodilators that have been used to treat critical digital ischemia secondary to fixed occlusive disease. Iloprost is a prostacyclin analogue reported to reduce the severity, frequency and duration of RS attacks and promote healing of ischemic ulcers. Multiple studies have shown that intravenous preparations improve ulcer healing and reduce severity of attacks.[22] Oral formulations of iloprost have failed to show any significant improvement for RS or digital ischemia.[23] Epoprostenol has been shown to increase fingertip skin temperature and laser Doppler flow; however, improved blood flow was not sustained in the follow-up period.[24]

Digital ulcers

Treatment of digital ischemic ulceration resulting from palmar and digital artery occlusive disease should be directed at four main points. First, surgically treatable lesions, although rare, must be detected and treated or their presence eliminated by testing, as outlined in the following. Second, elimination or reduction of any associated vasospasm should be attempted by cold avoidance and the elimination of tobacco use. The same vasodilators which are used for vasospastic RS may be helpful. Third, basic wound care is stressed. Gangrenous ulcers should be scrubbed with soap and water twice daily and dressed with dry gauze. Antibiotics appropriate to culture results are used for lesions with surrounding cellulitis. Conservative surgical debridement of necrotic tissue is performed as needed, including removal of protruding phalangeal tips. Formal phalangeal amputation is performed only when an entire digital segment (i.e. total phalanx) is necrotic. Most patients require amputation of a portion or all of the distal phalanx, although occasionally amputation at the midphalangeal level is required. Partial phalangeal amputation has been very effective in controlling ulcer pain. Fourth, medical therapy as appropriate is initiated for the treatment of associated systemic diseases.

Surgical/invasive therapy

Surgical and other invasive therapies are rarely indicated in the management of RS. Most invasive therapies have been reserved for patients with recalcitrant obstructive RS, with the evidence of efficacy primarily limited to case reports and series. A summary of invasive therapies is listed in Table 43.3.[4]

Botulinum toxin A is a neurotoxin causing temporary muscle paralysis at the neuromuscular junction. Several recent case series have described the use of onabotulinum toxin A in the treatment of both vasospastic and obstructive RS.[25,26]

Table 43.3 Surgical/Invasive therapy of Raynaud's syndrome.

Invasive therapy	Highest level of evidence	Results
Botulinum toxin	3D	Improved pain and ulcer healing in small case series
Sympathetic block	3D	Improved ulcer healing in small case series
Thoracoscopic sympathectomy	3C	High recurrence rate in primary RS; improved ulcer healing and pain control in selected patients with secondary RS
Digital sympathectomy	3D	Anecdotal reports of improved pain and ulcer healing
Spinal cord stimulators	3D	Reduced pain and improved ulcer healing in small case series

Thoracic sympathectomy is seldom indicated for RS but may be effective in some patients with critical ischemia of the digits, achieving up to 95% ulcer healing with long-term (>18 months) benefit of 58% in primary RS and 89% in secondary RS.[27] Currently, thoracoscopic sympathectomy has supplanted open cervicothoracic sympathectomy as the technique of choice.

Digital sympathectomy, which involves adventitial stripping of hand and digital arteries, has shown anecdotal success in healing ulcers and improving ischemic pain.[28] Additional invasive treatment modalities that have demonstrated benefit in case reports or small case series include percutaneous sympathetic blockade,[29] transcutaneous nerve stimulation[30] and spinal cord stimulation.[31] In general, these types of treatments are discouraged due to the anecdotal results as well as lack of controlled trials comparing them to other less invasive treatment modalities. They should only be considered in refractory cases with risk for tissue loss.

RESULTS OF TREATMENT

Raynaud's syndrome

Primary vasospastic RS is a benign disorder. Several natural history studies have demonstrated low incidences of finger ulcers or tissue loss in the presence of vasospasm. In longitudinal study from the authors, digital ulcers occurred in 5% of patients initially diagnosed with vasospastic RS when followed for over 10 years,[32] with other epidemiologic studies demonstrating complete remission in 1/3 of patients, suggesting that vasospastic RS may be a transient phenomenon.[1]

Digital ischemia

Complete healing of ischemic finger ulcers without recurrence has been achieved in 90% of patients with ischemic finger ulceration treated with conservative measures. About one-fourth of patients with ischemic finger ulceration require surgical debridement or a conservative amputation before healing, with the healing process occurring over several weeks to months. In the remaining 10% of patients, recurrent tissue loss of ulceration will persist despite optimal conservative care. In our experience, these patients have all had CTD, most commonly scleroderma. We are not able to predict reliably which patients will experience recurrent or persistent ischemic finger ulceration. Obviously, the patient who presents with chronic disease is at higher risk for recurrent problems.

It is extremely important to note that ischemic finger ulceration resulting from intrinsic small artery occlusive disease does not herald an inexorable progression to major tissue loss. Rather, it appears that the natural history of the disorder, regardless of aetiology, is one of short periods of exacerbation followed by long periods of remission with healing and stable, mild symptoms. Appreciation of this basically benign prognosis has major therapeutic implications. It is unclear to what degree treatment with simple wound care and low-dose oral vasodilators has been responsible for the overall good results achieved. This outcome likely reflects the natural history of the condition. Beneficial results claimed for any mode of therapy in past or future studies must be carefully evaluated against this standard.

BEST CLINICAL PRACTICE

- Diagnosis of RS is primarily clinical based on description of patient's symptoms.
- Initial vascular laboratory diagnosis should focus on differentiating vasospastic and obstructive pathophysiology.
- Vast majority of patients are treated conservatively with lifestyle modifications to avoid factors (typically cold and stress) that initiate attacks.
- Pharmacologic treatment, with CCBs typically accepted as first-line treatment, reserved for patients with symptoms refractory to conservative management.
- Digital ulcers also typically managed conservatively, with soap and water scrubs and debridement as needed. Some evidence that the PDE-5 inhibitors can augment ulcer healing. Minor distal phalangectomies are common, but whole digit or major limb amputations are rare.
- More extensive surgical treatment, such as cervicothoracic or digital sympathectomy, has limited role and is largely unproven in controlled trials.

DEFICIENCIES IN CURRENT KNOWLEDGE AND AREAS FOR FUTURE RESEARCH

- Determination of exact pathophysiologic mechanism of vasospasm. While current evidence points towards predominant role of post-synaptic alpha2-receptor, it is not known if this is due to upregulation or overexpression of receptors. Additional factors that interact with these receptors also need to be determined. This would potentially allow more targeted therapy.
- As noted, there are currently no medications approved specifically for treatment of either primary or secondary RS. Since response of existing agents is not consistent for all patients, more refined pharmacologic options are needed.
- Current invasive and surgical therapies are supported mainly by uncontrolled case series. In order for these treatments to gain further credibility, controlled clinical trials are needed.

KEY REFERENCES

1. Landry GJ, Edwards JM, McLafferty RB et al. Long-term outcome of Raynaud's syndrome in a prospectively analyzed patient cohort. *J Vasc Surg.* 1996;23:76.

This longitudinal study of over 1000 patients demonstrated the prognostic utility in subdividing patients into categories based on initial vascular laboratory (vasospastic vs. obstructive) and serologic findings.

2. Carpentier PH, Satger B, Poensin D et al. Incidence and natural history of Raynaud phenomenon: A long-term follow-up (14 years) of a random sample from the general population. *J Vasc Surg*. 2006;44:1023.

This study represents one of the longest prospectively evaluated patient cohorts with RS, demonstrating both its incidence in a general population and the long-term outcomes of RS. It is the first study to clearly demonstrate the transient nature of RS in up to 1/3 of patients.

3. Raynaud's Treatment Study Investigators. Comparison of sustained-release nifedipine and temperature biofeedback for treatment of primary Raynaud phenomenon: Results from a randomized clinical trial with 1-year follow-up. *Arch Intern Med*. 2000;160:1101–1108.

Randomized controlled trial demonstrating the efficacy of CCBs in the treatment of RS. This study also demonstrated the relative lack of efficacy of biofeedback.

4. Fries R, Shariat K, Von Wilmowsky H et al. Sildenafil in the treatment of Raynaud's phenomenon resistant to vasodilatory therapy. *Circulation*. 2005;112:2980–2985.

This randomized controlled trial was the first to demonstrate the efficacy of the PDE-5 inhibitors in treating ulcerations in patients with secondary RS due to scleroderma.

5. Dziadzio M, Denton CP, Smith R et al. Losartan therapy for Raynaud's phenomenon and scleroderma: Clinical and biochemical findings in a 15-week, randomized, parallel-group, controlled trial. *Arthritis Rheum*. 1999;42:2646–2655.

This randomized controlled trial established the angiotensin receptor blocker, losartan, as an alternative to CCBs in the treatment of RS.

REFERENCES

1. Carpentier PH, Satger B, Poensin D et al. Incidence and natural history of Raynaud phenomenon: A long-term follow-up (14 years) of a random sample from the general population. *J Vasc Surg*. 2006;44:1023.
2. Sumner D, Strandness DE. An abnormal finger pulse associated with cold sensitivity. *Ann Surg*. 1972;175:294–298.
3. Gates KH, Tyburczy J, Zupan J et al. The non-invasive quantification of digital vasospasm. *Bruit*. 1984;8:34.
4. Landry GJ. Current medical and surgical management of Raynaud's syndrome. *J Vasc Surg*. 2013;57:1710–1716.
5. Da Costa J, Gomes JA, Espirito Santo J et al. Inefficacy of diltiazem in the treatment of Raynaud's phenomenon with associated connective tissue disease: A double blind placebo controlled study. *J Rheumatol*. 1987;14:858–859.
6. Raynaud's Treatment Study Investigators. Comparison of sustained-release nifedipine and temperature biofeedback for treatment of primary Raynaud phenomenon: Results from a randomized clinical trial with 1-year follow-up. *Arch Intern Med*. 2000;160:1101–1108.
7. Thompson AE, Pope JE. Calcium channel blockers for primary Raynaud's phenomenon: A meta-analysis. *Rheumatology*. 2005;44:145–150.
8. La Civita L, Pitaro N, Rossi M et al. Amlodipine in the treatment of Raynaud's phenomenon. *Br J Rheumatol*. 1993;32(Suppl. 3):524–525.
9. Wollersheim H, Thien T, Fennis J et al. Double-blind, placebo-controlled study of prazosin in Raynaud's phenomenon. *Clin Pharmacol Ther*. 1986;40:219–225.
10. Stewart M, Morling JR. Oral vasodilators for primary Raynaud's phenomenon. *Cochrane Database Syst Rev*. 2012; Issue 7. Art. No.: CD006687.
11. Dziadzio M, Denton CP, Smith R et al. Losartan therapy for Raynaud's phenomenon and scleroderma: Clinical and biochemical findings in a fifteen-week, randomized, parallel-group, controlled trial. *Arthritis Rheum*. 1999;42:2646–2655.
12. Wood HM, Ernst ME. Renin-angiotensin system mediators and Raynaud's phenomenon. *Ann Pharmacother*. 2006;40:1998–2002.
13. Coleiro B, Marshall SE, Denton CP et al. Treatment of Raynaud's phenomenon with the selective serotonin reuptake inhibitor fluoxetine. *Rheumatology*. 2001;40:1038–1043.
14. Roustit M, Blaise S, Allanore Y et al. Phosphodiesterase-5 inhibitors for the treatment of secondary Raynaud's phenomenon: Systematic review and meta-analysis of randomised trials. *Ann Rheum Dis*. 2013;72:1696–1699.
15. Fries R, Shariat K, Von Wilmowsky H et al. Sildenafil in the treatment of Raynaud's phenomenon resistant to vasodilatory therapy. *Circulation*. 2005;112:2980–2985.
16. Herrick AL, Van Den Hoogen F, Gabrielli A et al. Modified-release sildenafil reduces Raynaud's phenomenon attack frequency in limited cutaneous systemic sclerosis. *Arthritis Rheum*. 2011;63:775–782.
17. Shenoy PD, Kumar S, Jha LK et al. Efficacy of tadalafil in secondary Raynaud's phenomenon resistant to vasodilator therapy: A double-blind randomized cross-over trial. *Rheumatology*. 2010;49:2420–2428.
18. Caglayan E, Axmann S, Hellmich M et al. Vardenafil for the treatment of Raynaud phenomenon: A randomized, double-blind, placebo-controlled crossover study. *Arch Intern Med*. 2012;172:1182–1184.
19. Chung L, Shapiro L, Fiorentino D et al. MQX-503, a novel formulation of nitroglycerin, improves the severity of Raynaud's phenomenon. *Arthritis Rheum*. 2009;60:870–877.

20. Matucci-Cerinic M, Denton CP, Furst DE et al. Bosentan treatment of digital ulcers related to systemic sclerosis: Results from the RAPIDS-2 randomised, double-blind, placebo-controlled trial. *Ann Rheum Dis.* 2011;70:32–38.

21. Cutolo M, Ruaro B, Pizzorni C et al. Longterm treatment with endothelin receptor antagonist bosentan and iloprost improves fingertip blood perfusion in systemic sclerosis. *J Rheumatol.* 2014;41:881–886.

22. Torley HI, Madhok R, Capell HA et al. A double blind, randomised, multicentre comparison of two doses of intravenous iloprost in the treatment of Raynaud's phenomenon secondary to connective tissue diseases. *Ann Rheum Dis.* 1991;50:800–804.

23. Wigley FM, Korn JH, Csuka ME et al. Oral iloprost treatment in patients with Raynaud's phenomenon secondary to systemic sclerosis: A multicenter, placebo-controlled, double-blind study. *Arthritis Rheum.* 1998;41:670–677.

24. Kingma K, Wollersheim H, Thien T. Double-blind, placebo-controlled study of intravenous prostacyclin on hemodynamics in severe Raynaud's phenomenon: The acute vasodilatory effect is not sustained. *J Cardiovasc Pharmacol.* 1995;26:388–393.

25. Kalliainen LK, O'Brien VH. Current uses of botulinum toxin A as an adjunct to hand therapy interventions of hand conditions. *J Hand Ther.* 2014;27:85–95.

26. Mannava S, Plate JF, Stone AV et al. Recent advances for the management of Raynaud phenomenon using botulinum neurotoxin A. *J Hand Surg.* 2011;36:1708–1710.

27. Coveliers HME, Hoexum F, Nederhoed JH et al. Thoracic sympathectomy for digital ischemia: A summary of evidence. *J Vasc Surg.* 2011;54:273–277.

28. Balogh B, Mayer W, Vesely M et al. Adventitial stripping of the radial and ulnar arteries in Raynaud's disease. *J Hand Surg.* 2002;27:1073–1080.

29. Han KR, Kim C, Park EJ. Successful treatment of digital ulcers in a scleroderma patient with continuous bilateral thoracic sympathetic block. *Pain Physician.* 2008;11:91–96.

30. Kaada B. Vasodilation induced by transcutaneous nerve stimulation in peripheral ischemia (Raynaud's phenomenon and diabetic polyneuropathy). *Eur Heart J.* 1982;3:303–314.

31. Sibell DM, Colantonio AJ, Stacey BR. Successful use of spinal cord stimulation in the treatment of severe Raynaud's disease of the hands. *Anesthesiology.* 2005;102:225–227.

32. Landry GJ, Edwards JM, McLafferty RB et al. Long-term outcome of Raynaud's syndrome in a prospectively analyzed patient cohort. *J Vasc Surg.* 1996;23:76.

44

Vasculitis and dysplastic arterial lesions

AAMIR S. SHAH, HISHAM S. BASSIOUNY and BRUCE L. GEWERTZ

CONTENTS

The vascular surgeon may occasionally encounter organ or limb ischemia resulting from vasculitic or dysplastic lesions distinct from the much more common atherosclerotic process. This chapter will discuss these unusual disorders and review diagnostic and therapeutic options in the most common lesions.

To aid in clinical differentiation, arteritis may be classified by the size of the involved vessel. One such nomenclature system is adopted from the 2012 Chapel Hill Consensus Conference (CHCC; see Table 44.1 and Figure 44.1).[1] There is, however, substantial overlap among different vasculitides, and the type of vessel involved is merely one of many features that must be assessed before a diagnosis can be rendered. Furthermore, all three major categories of vasculitis can affect any size artery.[1]

The most prominent arteritis involving the aorta and its primary branches is Takayasu's arteritis. Other inflammatory disorders involve medium-sized and small muscular arteries or the arterioles and capillaries and rarely require operative consideration.[2,3] Fibrodysplastic lesions will be discussed separately, as there is minimal, if any, inflammatory component to these lesions.

VASCULITIS AND VASCULITIC DISORDERS

Large vessel lesions

TAKAYASU'S ARTERITIS

Takayasu's arteritis (TA) is a dramatic and unusual disorder involving the aorta and its primary branches. Because of its chronic obliterative nature, it is also called 'pulseless disease' and occlusive thromboarteriopathy. Women are much more frequently affected than men (8:1), although the true incidence and distribution of these lesions remain ill defined. The disease was originally named for the Japanese ophthalmologist who described associated ocular abnormalities in 1908.[4] Perhaps as a consequence of his early observation, the highest incidence appears to be in Asia, especially Japan, although more recent reports have contributed large numbers of patients from Mexico and India. In the United States, there seems to be an increased recognition of this disorder in Caucasians.[5]

A majority of patients (70%) are first affected between 10 and 30 years of age. The precise aetiology remains unknown, although both infections and autoimmune phenomena have been suggested. The association of this disorder with rheumatoid arthritis, ankylosing spondylitis and ulcerative colitis appears to reinforce the latter mechanism. Currently, there is no experimental model for this form of aortitis.

Clinical presentation

The disease process can be broadly divided into two stages: an early phase ('prepulseless') and late phase ('pulseless'). Initial symptoms include generalized malaise and other non-specific indicators such as a skin rash, anorexia, myalgia, weight loss, fatigue and fever. Laboratory examinations at this time may reflect the general inflammatory process. The erythrocyte sedimentation rate (ESR) is nearly always increased and mild hypochromic anemia is evident. Elevated alpha$_2$ and/or gamma fractions are frequently noted.[6] A high prevalence of anti-endothelial cell antibodies (AECAs) has been identified in the sera of

Table 44.1 Definitions of vasculitis.

CHCC2012 name	CHCC2012 definition
Large vessel vasculitis (LVV)	Vasculitis affecting large arteries more often than other vasculitides. Large arteries are the aorta and its major branches. Any size artery may be affected.
Takayasu arteritis (TAK)	Arteritis, often granulomatous, predominantly affecting the aorta and/or its major branches. Onset usually in patients younger than 50 years.
Giant cell arteritis (GCA)	Arteritis, often granulomatous, usually affecting the aorta and/or its major branches, with a predilection for the branches of the carotid and vertebral arteries. Often involves the temporal artery. Onset usually in patients older than 50 years and often associated with polymyalgia rheumatica.
Medium vessel vasculitis (MVV)	Vasculitis predominantly affecting medium arteries defined as the main visceral arteries and their branches. Any size artery may be affected. Inflammatory aneurysms and stenoses are common.
Polyarteritis nodosa (PAN)	Necrotizing arteritis of medium or small arteries without glomerulonephritis or vasculitis in arterioles, capillaries or venules and not associated with anti-neutrophil cytoplasmic antibodies (ANCAs).
Kawasaki disease (KD)	Arteritis associated with the mucocutaneous lymph node syndrome and predominantly affecting medium and small arteries. Coronary arteries are often involved. Aorta and large arteries may be involved. Usually occurs in infants and young children.
Small vessel vasculitis (SVV)	Vasculitis predominantly affecting small vessels, defined as small intra-parenchymal arteries, arterioles, capillaries and venules. Medium arteries and veins may be affected.
ANCA-associated vasculitis (AAV)	Necrotizing vasculitis, with few or no immune deposits, predominantly affecting small vessels (i.e. capillaries, venules, arterioles and small arteries), associated with myeloperoxidase (MPO) ANCA or proteinase 3 (PR3) ANCA. Not all patients have ANCA. Add a prefix indicating ANCA reactivity, e.g. MPO-ANCA, PR3-ANCA, ANCA-negative.
Microscopic polyangiitis (MPA)	Necrotizing vasculitis, with few or no immune deposits, predominantly affecting small vessels (i.e. capillaries, venules or arterioles). Necrotizing arteritis involving small and medium arteries may be present. Necrotizing glomerulonephritis is very common. Pulmonary capillaritis often occurs. Granulomatous inflammation is absent.
Granulomatosis with polyangiitis (Wegener's) (GPA)	Necrotizing granulomatous inflammation usually involving the upper and lower respiratory tract and necrotizing vasculitis affecting predominantly small to medium vessels (e.g. capillaries, venules, arterioles, arteries and veins). Necrotizing glomerulonephritis is common.
Eosinophilic granulomatosis with polyangiitis (Churg–Strauss) (EGPA)	Eosinophil-rich and necrotizing granulomatous inflammation often involving the respiratory tract and necrotizing vasculitis predominantly affecting small to medium vessels and associated with asthma and eosinophilia. ANCA is more frequent when glomerulonephritis is present.
Immune complex vasculitis	Vasculitis with moderate to marked vessel wall deposits of immunoglobulin and/or complement components predominantly affecting small vessels (i.e. capillaries, venules, arterioles and small arteries). Glomerulonephritis is frequent.
Anti-glomerular basement membrane (anti-GBM) disease	Vasculitis affecting glomerular capillaries, pulmonary capillaries or both, with GBM deposition of anti-GBM autoantibodies. Lung involvement causes pulmonary hemorrhage, and renal involvement causes glomerulonephritis with necrosis and crescents.
Cryoglobulinemia vasculitis (CV)	Vasculitis with cryoglobulin immune deposits affecting small vessels (predominantly capillaries, venules or arterioles) and associated with serum cryoglobulins. Skin, glomeruli and peripheral nerves are often involved.
IgA vasculitis (Henoch–Schönlein) (IgAV)	Vasculitis with IgA1-dominant immune deposits, affecting small vessels (predominantly capillaries, venules or arterioles). Often involves skin and gastrointestinal tract and frequently causes arthritis. Glomerulonephritis indistinguishable from IgA nephropathy may occur.
Hypocomplementemic urticarial vasculitis (HUV) (anti-C1q vasculitis)	Vasculitis accompanied by urticaria and hypocomplementemia affecting small vessels (i.e. capillaries, venules or arterioles) and associated with anti-C1q antibodies. Glomerulonephritis, arthritis, obstructive pulmonary disease and ocular inflammation are common.
Variable vessel vasculitis (VVV)	Vasculitis with no predominant type of vessel involved that can affect vessels of any size (small, medium and large) and type (arteries, veins and capillaries).
Behçet's disease (BD)	Vasculitis occurring in patients with Behçet's disease that can affect arteries or veins. Behçet's disease is characterized by recurrent oral and/or genital aphthous ulcers accompanied by cutaneous, ocular, articular, gastrointestinal and/or central nervous system inflammatory lesions. Small vessel vasculitis, thromboangiitis, thrombosis, arteritis and arterial aneurysms may occur.

(Continued)

Table 44.1 (*Continued*) Definitions of vasculitis.

CHCC2012 name	CHCC2012 definition
Cogan's syndrome (CS)	Vasculitis occurring in patients with Cogan's syndrome. Cogan's syndrome characterized by ocular inflammatory lesions, including interstitial keratitis, uveitis and episcleritis, and inner ear disease, including sensorineural hearing loss and vestibular dysfunction. Vasculitic manifestations may include arteritis (affecting small, medium or large arteries), aortitis, aortic aneurysms and aortic and mitral valvulitis.

Source: Adopted by Jennette JC et al., *Arthritis Rheum*, 65(1), 1, 2013.

Notes: 'Large vessel' refers to the aorta and the largest arterial branches directed towards major body regions (e.g. to the extremities and the head and neck). 'Medium vessel' refers to the main visceral arteries and their branches. 'Small vessel' refers to small intra-parenchymal arteries, arterioles, venules and capillaries.

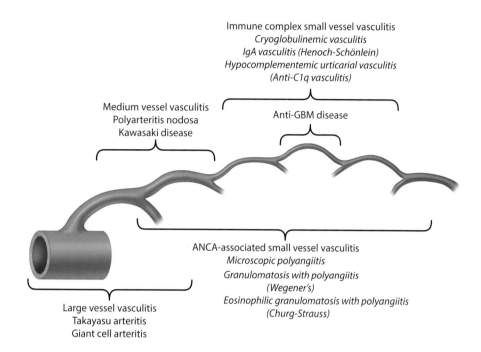

Figure 44.1 Schematic and detailed characterization of vasculitis nomenclature. (Proposed by Jennette JC et al., *Arthritis Rheum*, 65(1), 1, 2013.)

patients with documented TA. Although long-term observations are as yet unavailable, AECAs may present an objective measure of the activity of TA.[7]

After a variable period of time from the onset of vague constitutional symptoms, arterial lesions become evident. A vast majority of patients present during the pulseless stage and predictably demonstrate an absence of one or more peripheral pulses. Symptoms at this time predictably reflect the extremity or organ that is rendered ischemic. Lightheadedness and vertigo are frequent complaints if the aortic arch or extracranial carotid vessels are involved. Emotional instability, 'drop attacks' and headache may also be present, along with more lateralizing signs such as hemiparesis. Ocular symptoms include blurring, diplopia and progressive blindness. A rare symptom is decreasing vision on physical exertion ('visual claudication'). Such ocular complaints can be associated with retinal atrophy or hemorrhage.

Ophthalmoscopic examination may also demonstrate optic atrophy and retinal vein or artery thrombosis.

It has been observed that many of these patients assume a characteristic 'face-down' posture to prevent neck extension, which further compromises carotid or vertebral flow. Extremities with arterial stenoses may manifest exercise-related symptoms; with progression of occlusive lesions, rest pain or tissue loss may occur. Compromise of the external carotid circulation can cause atrophy of the facial muscles as well as ulcerations of the palate, nose or ear. Chronic intestinal or renal ischemia is associated with abdominal aortic involvement.[8]

In 1990, the American College of Rheumatology established diagnostic criteria for TA (see Table 44.2). These criteria were found to have 91% sensitivity and 98% specificity when patients met at least 3 of 6 requirements required to establish the diagnosis.[9]

Table 44.2 The American College of Rheumatology 1990 criteria for the classification of Takayasu arteritis (3 of 6 required to make diagnosis).

Age at disease onset	Symptoms or signs of TA before 40 years of age
Claudication	Upper or lower extremity fatigue with exercise
Diminished brachial pulse	Unilateral or bilateral diminished brachial pulse on examination
Asymmetric brachial blood pressure (BP)	>10 mmHg difference between brachial systolic BP
Bruit	Audible over aorta or either subclavian artery
Angiographic abnormalities	Narrowing or occlusion of aorta, aortic branches or large arteries in upper extremities, usually focal or segmental. Must not be secondary to atherosclerosis, fibromuscular dysplasia or other causes

Source: Arend WP et al., *Arthritis Rheum*, 33(8), 1129, 1990.

Non-invasive vascular tests suggest TA if bilateral upper extremity and extracranial occlusive disease are documented in a patient of appropriate age. Arteriography is most useful in confirming the diagnosis and is essential for planning operative therapy.[10,11]

Arteriography (Figures 44.2 and 44.3) allows classification of TA into four main types based on the distribution of lesions: type I (8% prevalence) is limited to the aortic arch and its primary branches; type II (11% prevalence) includes lesions of the descending thoracic and abdominal aorta; type III (prevalence 65%) extends from the aortic valve to the abdominal aorta (essentially combining types I and II); and type IV (prevalence 15%) comprises lesions with pulmonary artery involvement and any aneurysmal change in any vessel.[8,12,13]

Pathology

The classic gross appearance of TA is a 'tree-bark' surface not dissimilar to that seen in luetic arteritis. Patchy involvement with numerous skip areas is the most common pattern, although some patients present with continuous involvement. Although inflammation is most severe in the adventitia and outer media, TA is truly a pan-arteritis. TA may involve a cell-mediated autoimmune process, with involvement of CD4+, CD8+ T cells and macrophages.[14] The media are infiltrated by lymphocytes, plasma cells and histiocytes. Polymorphonuclear and multinucleated giant cells are consistently observed, especially around the vasa vasorum.

Elastic and smooth muscular components of the media are gradually eroded by this process, and extensive transmural fibrosis is evident. The erosion and destruction of arterial smooth muscle cells may also lead to arterial aneurysmal formation. Additional intimal proliferation may contribute to intimal thrombosis as well as stenotic occlusive lesions.[6,8] It has been demonstrated that TA is

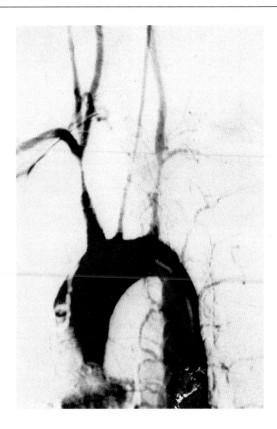

Figure 44.2 Typical distribution of lesions in Takayasu's arteritis (type I) with severe uniform stenoses of the brachiocephalic and left common carotid arteries. Patient presented with syncope and dizziness.

often associated with a hypercoagulable state and thrombus formation,[15] which may also contribute to thrombotic complications allowing arterial reconstructions.

Therapy

Corticosteroids are of some efficacy in this disorder, especially if the disease can be recognized in the prepulseless stage.[16] Other medical therapies have included cytotoxic agents; unfortunately, these drugs are also of questionable benefit. Anti-tumor necrosis factor medications including infliximab have been successfully utilized for treatment in patients with TA who are unable to taper corticosteroid therapy due to vasculitis relapse.[17]

In patients with symptomatic lesions, both open surgical reconstruction and endovascular therapy have been employed with success. Operative therapy is directed towards bypass of involved and occluded vessels.[18] Endovascular therapy with percutaneous transluminal angioplasty (PTA) and stenting has been limited by increased rates of restenosis. If possible, it is recommended to delay intervention until active signs of the disease have resolved. That said, in patients presenting with cerebrovascular insufficiency, this may be impossible. Indicators of quiescence include normalization of markedly elevated ESR and white blood cell counts.

Operative dissection should be confined to the nondiseased portions of the aorta and distal vessels, as the

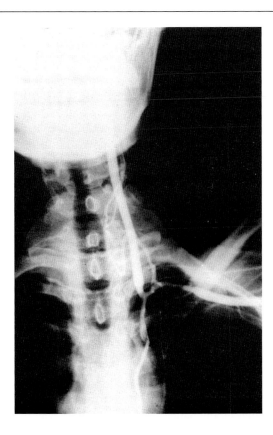

Figure 44.3 Selective injection of left subclavian artery, demonstrating poststenotic dilation of patent vertebral artery. Note restriction of disease to intrathoracic subclavian with normal calibre of left axillary artery.

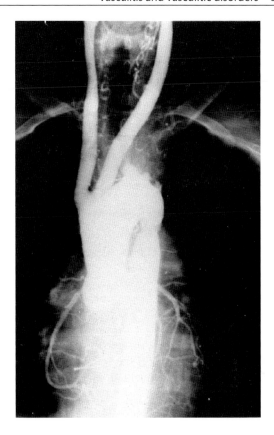

Figure 44.4 Bifurcated graft originates at ascending aorta, with distal anastomoses at carotid bifurcations.

inflammatory nature of the arteritis may predispose to injury of adjacent structures. In general, the disease is limited to the more proximal brachiocephalic vessels; carotid bifurcation disease and axillary involvement are minimal. It is not uncommon for patients to require bilateral carotid revascularization with grafts originating from the ascending aorta. A most versatile procedure is anastomosis of a bifurcated aortic graft to the ascending aorta with limbs to carotid or brachiocephalic vessels. The proximal anastomosis must be tailored obliquely to lie parallel to the ascending aorta so as to avoid kinking or compression when the sternum is closed (Figure 44.4).

Although endarterectomy has been performed on these lesions, clinical experience strongly favours bypass using prosthetic grafts because of the uncertain strength of the inflamed arterial wall after endarterectomy. Even without endarterectomy, the development of pseudoaneurysms at anastomoses remains a problem. Some surgeons routinely buttress suture lines with pledgets or place interrupted sutures at regular intervals along a continuous suture line.[19]

Miyata et al.[20] reported their experience in 91 patients with TA treated surgically over 40 years in 1998. A total of 259 anastomoses were surveyed with a remarkable follow-up of 93% at 30 years. The cumulative incidence of anastomotic aneurysms at 20 years was 12%. Continued systemic inflammation or steroid administration had no apparent influence on formation of anastomotic aneurysm. Instead, anastomotic aneurysms tended to occur after operations for aneurysmal lesions.

Perera and associates recently reported a series of 97 patients treated at a single tertiary centre from 2001 to 2012.[21] Thirty-eight percent of the patients required interventions. The overall success rate (defined as freedom from restenosis or reintervention) was 79% for patients undergoing open surgical reconstruction (27 patients underwent 33 surgical procedures with a mean graft patency of 9.4 years) compared to 52% for 31 endovascular procedures (p = 0.035) with a median follow-up of 6 years. The overall patient survival was 97%. Success rates were significantly improved in both groups of patients if they received preoperative immunosuppression.

Kim and colleagues reported a series of 21 patients with TA who required intervention due to supra-aortic arterial occlusive disease at a single academic institution from 1994 to 2010.[22] During the study period, 9.6% of patients diagnosed with TA required open surgical or endovascular intervention. Endovascular therapy was selected for symptomatic occlusive lesions <5 cm length, with PTA being performed with selective stenting if complications arose during the procedures. For surgical bypasses, the ascending aorta was the preferred site of origin. Surgical bypass was performed in 15 patients with 24 arteries being reconstructed, and 10 patients underwent endovascular intervention with 15 lesions being treated. Anti-inflammatory medications were administered to 48% of patients who had evidence of active disease after intervention. Restenosis or occlusion was significantly higher in the endovascular treatment group compared with the open surgical group with a mean follow-up of 39 months (53% in endovascular group vs. 13% in surgical bypass group; p = 0.01). There were increased perioperative complications in the surgical bypass group including in intracerebral hemorrhage due to cerebral hyperperfusion in 2 patients (13%) but no operative deaths in either group.

A recent retrospective series from the Cleveland Clinic in 2007 reported 75 patients treated for TA from 1992 to 2004.[23] In this study group, 97% of patients had vascular stenosis, 3% had aneurysms only and 8% had both aneurysms and stenosis. Recurrent stenosis occurred in 36% of 44 surgical bypasses at 3 years' follow-up and in 78% of 18 percutaneous angioplasties (PTA) at 3 years' follow-up. Initial disease remission was observed in 93% of patients, but only 28% of patients maintained remission of greater that 6 months after their prednisone dose was tapered to less than 10 mg daily.[23] It has been reported in a small series of patients treated at the Cleveland Clinic that endovascular techniques utilizing stent grafts in favour of uncovered stents may be associated with lower rates of in-stent restenosis.[24]

TEMPORAL ARTERITIS

Temporal arteritis is a giant cell arteritis which may be distinguished from TA on clinical grounds. It is a far more prevalent disorder and nearly always occurs in patients over 50 years of age. While women are affected more commonly than men, the proportion is 2:1, rather than the 8:1 ratio commonly recognized for TA. The incidence of temporal arteritis is surprisingly high, especially in the north central regions of the United States. One series documented a prevalence of 133 cases per 100,000 people aged 50 and over.[25] As with most vascular inflammatory lesions, autoimmune mechanisms are implicated. This is particularly true in temporal arteritis, which is frequently associated with polymyalgia rheumatica.[26,27]

Clinical presentation

In most series, the mean age of onset is roughly 70 years of age. While the onset of symptoms has been classically described as abrupt, more careful histories will often elicit the presence of symptoms for several months before the diagnosis is established. Fatigue, weight loss and fever are characteristic of the disorder. Typical presentations also include headache associated with scalp tenderness over the distribution of the temporal artery. The character of the headache is variable, although this manifestation is often severe and may be misdiagnosed as 'migraine' headache. Fifty percent of patients experience some visual disturbances. The most worrisome presenting symptoms are blindness and diplopia. While visual loss may be partial or complete, it is generally accepted that once established, the deficit is permanent. The mechanism of these visual changes is thought to be ischemia of the retina or optic

nerve associated with arteritis of branches of the ophthalmic or posterior ciliary arteries.[28,29] Ophthalmoscopic examination may occasionally demonstrate central retinal artery occlusion. In the era before the emphasis on early diagnosis and aggressive treatment with steroids, the incidence of permanent visual loss was as high as 60%. More recent series have documented a much lower incidence, approximating 10%–20%.

Other specific complaints include difficulty in mastication or swallowing consistent with ischemia of the facial muscles, tongue and pharynx. Neuropsychiatric symptoms are prevalent and include memory loss, depression and anxiety.[30] While many patients with temporal arteritis have concomitant atherosclerosis, approximately 10%–15% demonstrate nonatherosclerotic large artery occlusive lesions similar to those seen in TA.[31]

Laboratory examinations reflect the non-specific inflammatory process. Most common abnormalities include normochromic normocytic anemia associated with decreased albumin and increased fibrinogen, $alpha_2$ and gamma globulins. The ESR usually remains quite high (100 mm/h) until successful treatment is initiated. In roughly a third of patients, liver function tests are abnormal.[25,32]

The diagnosis of temporal arteritis should be strongly suspected in any patient over the age of 50 who presents with a new onset of headache, visual symptoms or hip and shoulder pain compatible with polymyalgia rheumatica. Physical examination may demonstrate scalp tenderness, although this feature can be quite short-lived.

The most definitive diagnosis procedure is biopsy of the temporal artery; adjacent branches of the external carotid can be sampled if other areas of tenderness are elicited. It is important that an adequate length of temporal artery be exposed and that atraumatic technique be used in removing the specimen. A retrospective review by Ypsilantis and colleagues of 966 temporal artery biopsies between 2004 and 2009 in six hospitals in south-east England revealed patient age, specimen length and ESR value to be predictors of GCA.[33] Positive biopsies were found to have a significantly longer specimen length, with a postfixation length of at least 0.7 cm having the highest predictive value (25% positive with length > 0.7 cm vs. 13% positive for length < 0.7 cm).

In the few patients with suspected large artery involvement, arteriography may be indicated. However, such studies are less useful in this disorder in comparison to their central diagnostic role in TA.[34,35]

The usefulness of colour duplex ultrasonography in patients suspected of having temporal arteritis was examined by Schmidt et al.[36] In 73% of patients with biopsy-confirmed temporal arteritis, ultrasonography showed a dark halo around the lumen of the temporal arteries (Figure 44.5) (see also colour plate). The halos disappeared after a mean of 16 days of treatment with corticosteroids. The authors concluded that in patients with typical clinical signs and demonstration of such an appearance on ultrasonography, it may be possible to make a diagnosis of temporal arteritis and begin treatment without performing a temporal artery biopsy.

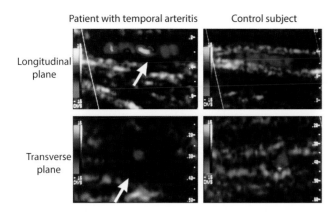

Patient with temporal arteritis   Control subject

Longitudinal plane

Transverse plane

Figure 44.5 Characteristic ultrasound appearance of acute temporal arteritis with 'halo' (lower panel) and turbulent blood flow (upper panel). (From Schmidt WA et al., *N Engl J Med*, 337, 1336, 1997.)

A more recent study reported the sensitivity of this finding to be 82%, with 92% specificity in patients with unilateral disease.[37] The specificity was 100% in patients with bilateral disease, suggesting that confirmatory biopsy may not be necessary in patients with bilateral characteristic colour duplex findings.

Positron emission tomography (PET) may also be a useful diagnostic imaging modality, with a reported 98% specificity, 93% positive predictive value and 80% negative predictive value.[38] The value of PET scan however has been reported to be significantly decreased following the administration of immunosuppressive therapy, with diagnostic accuracy decreasing from 93% to 65%.[39]

It remains controversial whether all patients with polymyalgia rheumatica should be subjected to temporal artery biopsy even if no other symptoms of temporal arteritis are evident. Such 'blind' biopsies yield a 10%–20% incidence of pathologically proven but clinically silent temporal arteritis.[40] In view of this relatively low yield, it may be more appropriate to follow patients with polymyalgia rheumatica closely and to initiate steroid therapy immediately if scalp tenderness or visual changes are noted.

Pathology

The pathologic lesion is best described as a granulomatous inflammation of the media, with varying degrees of fibrocellular intimal proliferation. Mononuclear and polymorphonuclear leukocytes are identified within the media, but lymphocytes and histiocytes predominate. The internal elastic lamina is characteristically necrotic and disrupted. Late in the disease, fibrosis with recanalization of the lumen is often seen. The classic multinucleated or Langhans giant cells are demonstrated in the majority of cases.[41]

Treatment

Once the diagnosis is made by biopsy, temporal arteritis is treated non-surgically. Patients are usually started on 45–60 mg of prednisone per day. An equivalent dose of another steroid preparation can also be administered. Steroid treatment can cause remission in up to 75% of patients.[42] In patients with active visual symptoms, intravenous steroids are appropriate. Most patients respond to treatment quite rapidly; visual changes and scalp tenderness subside within 12–24 hours. Although some authors have suggested that steroid therapy should be reduced after 1 month, the incidence of early relapse is relatively high (approximately 20%), leading many physicians to continue therapy for 1–2 years.[43,44] Additional therapy with methotrexate may reduce relapse as well as allow a decrease in the steroid dosage.[45] Despite its lack of specificity, the ESR is the most reliable test to assess activity of the disease during the gradual tapering of the steroid dose.

THROMBOANGIITIS OBLITERANS

Thromboangiitis obliterans (TAO), also known as Buerger's disease, classically involves the medium- and small-sized arteries of the distal lower extremity and, less commonly, those of the upper extremity.[46] Although it is controversial, most believe that it is a unique clinicopathologic entity distinct from premature atherosclerotic arterial occlusive disease as evidenced by the characteristic anatomic, histopathologic and angiographic features.[47] The prevalence of this disease varies according to the strictness with which the diagnostic criteria are applied. Classic criteria for the disease include (1) most severe involvement in the digital circulation, (2) highest incidence in young males, (3) close association with tobacco dependency and (4) recurrent episodes of superficial thrombophlebitis. Patients with all four of these components represent a most challenging, if extremely small, subgroup of those evaluated for finger or toe ischemia.

Results of therapy are notoriously poor because of the difficulty in moderating the strong tobacco addiction. Although this disease was originally thought to be limited to Jews, additional investigation has revealed a broad incidence across all ethnic groups, with a particularly high prevalence in some Asian countries. Although men are predominantly affected, a larger number of cases have recently been reported in women. This may reflect both improved diagnosis and increased tobacco use by women.[48] The differential diagnosis includes collagen vascular disease, ergot abuse, autoimmune vasculitis, embolic disease, thoracic outlet syndrome or hypothenar 'hammer' syndrome.

Clinical presentation

Patients present with manifestations of recurrent migratory thrombophlebitis and varying degrees of distal limb ischemia. More than 90% are males with a long history of cigarette smoking. It has been suggested that tobacco use in Buerger's disease patients may not be excessive but, rather, that the disease may reflect a specific hypersensitivity to even small or moderate doses of tobacco.[47] When questioned carefully, patients may describe less specific symptoms such as hand or foot claudication, cold sensitivity, dysesthesia, rubor or cyanosis, which predate the development of ischemic lesions of the fingers and toes. True claudication of the major muscle mass of the leg is relatively uncommon (10% of patients). When present, these symptoms occur late in the course of the disease due to progression of proximal disease. Severe digital ischemia is accompanied by severe pain, which often leads to an addictive pattern of analgesic abuse. Migratory superficial thrombophlebitis is observed in one-third to one-half of patients with Buerger's disease and may precede arterial involvement.[49,50]

Shionoya described five clinical criteria which are necessary for diagnosis of TAO: (1) smoking history, (2) onset before the age of 50 years, (3) infrapopliteal arterial occlusive disease, (4) either upper extremity involvement or phlebitis migrans and (5) absence of atherosclerotic risk factors other than smoking.[51]

On examination, radial, ulnar and tibial pulses may be reduced or absent, but popliteal and brachial pulses are generally palpable. Secondary infection of the digital ischemic ulcerations is common, with involvement of the underlying soft tissue and bone (Figure 44.6). Trophic changes of toe- and fingernails may be accompanied by digital clubbing in as many of 50% of patients. The proximal aspects of the limbs and uninvolved digits are, in general, well preserved. Cold sensitivity in the hands can be demonstrated in the majority of patients and is due to multiple occlusive lesions involving the palmar and plantar arches.

The non-invasive vascular laboratory may be quite helpful in diagnosis. Assessment of the patency of the palmar arch and the digital flow patterns can be easily achieved using the continuous-wave Doppler probe. The photoplethysmograph allows documentation of digital pressures.

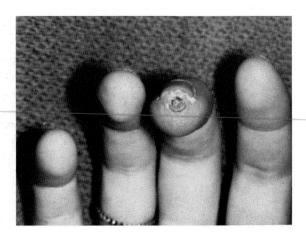

Figure 44.6 Distinctive presentation of Buerger's disease, with erythema and ulceration of the most distal fingertip. Ulcers are typically unresponsive to local care and severely painful. General appearance of fingers is described as 'pruned' with a tapered contour due to wasting of subcutaneous tissue.

The most confusing differential diagnosis is that of peripheral arterial embolization presenting with 'blue toe' or 'blue finger' syndromes. Vegetative cardiac lesions and aneurysmal or ulcerative arterial lesions in the axillary, femoral or popliteal arteries should be investigated. In the absence of echocardiographic documentation of intracavitary cardiac thrombi, arteriography may be useful for diagnostic purposes.

In classic Buerger's disease, multiple segmental occlusions are demonstrated in the medium and small arteries of the forearm and hand, leg and foot. Proximal or intervening arterial segments often appear normal. Importantly, these occlusions and tapered stenoses are not reversible with the intra-arterial administration of vasodilators.

In angiographic studies by Shionoya et al.[52] and Suzuki et al.,[53] bilateral involvement of the infrapopliteal arteries was observed in all patients presenting with the stigmata of Buerger's disease. The anterior and posterior tibial arteries were most commonly involved, with relative sparing of the peroneal artery. Superficial femoral artery involvement was noted in 40% of cases. Distal upper extremity arterial involvement occurs in 10%–15% of cases and is commonly seen in the later stages of the disease. Many arteriographers have described a corkscrew appearance, which is believed to represent both recanalization of previously occluded arteries and enlargement of periadventitial vessels along thrombosed arterial segments. In a few patients, a proximal atherosclerotic lesion may contribute to the distal ischemia.

Pathology

Study of arterial specimens recovered in the acute phase reveals a classic panangiitis with lymphocytes and fibroblasts abundant within a relatively well-preserved arterial wall.[47,50,54] In the acute phase of the disease, primarily macrophages as well as few giant cells are observed in the characteristic intraluminal thrombus with infiltration of CD4(+) and CD8(+) T cells and macrophages in the internal lamina.[55] The role of autoimmunity has also been implicated, with various autoantibodies targeting endothelial cells and blood vessel wall components being associated with active disease.[55]

In later stages of the disease, the vessels are occluded by chronic thrombus, which is highly cellular and composed primarily of fibroblasts. Recanalization of thrombosed arteries and veins is frequently observed. Remarkably, such diseased segments are in direct continuity with normal proximal and distal vessels. Features of atherosclerotic plaque formation are notably absent.

Therapy

Steroid therapy has no place in thromboangiitis obliterans, unlike the other forms of arteritis discussed previously in this chapter. The most specific and useful therapy is complete abstinence from tobacco. Unfortunately, results of even the most rigorous behavioural modification programmes have been discouraging in this group of patients. Their abuse of cigarettes is a true physiologic addiction.

The most crucial surgical therapy is appropriate care of ischemic and gangrenous digits. Cautious applications of tepid soaks and other local therapies are appropriate. Treatment with intravenous antibiotics followed by long-term oral antibiotics is recommended in patients with active ischemic lesions. Although surgical debridement may be complicated by poor wound healing, drainage and removal of infarcted tissue is frequently necessary. Additional modalities of therapy that have been useful include sympathectomy, which is often combined with primary amputation of a single involved digit. The temporary increase in skin blood flow following sympathectomy (2–4 weeks) seems to improve the chances of healing such amputations.

Recent clinical trials in Great Britain and Japan have centred on continuous infusions of prostaglandin, including PGE_1 and PGI_2. In these studies, intra-arterial therapy appears more efficacious than the intravenous route; healing or improvement was noted in 79% of patients in one small series of 29 patients.[56] The benefits of these vasoactive agents, while controversial,[57] are presumably due to dilation of collateral pathways and an anticoagulant effect on the microcirculation. A randomized trial involving 133 patients with TAO comparing iloprost (a synthetic PGI_2 analogue) with low-dose aspirin for 28 days demonstrated increased resolution of ischemic symptoms (63% vs. 28%) and complete ulcer healing (35% vs. 13%) with iloprost therapy.[58]

Other vasodilating agents have not been shown to clearly benefit these lesions. Epidural anesthesia to reduce rest pain, foot dependency and edema may be offered as a temporary measure in periods of acute exacerbation. Hyperbaric oxygen therapy has also been used to minimize pain and promote healing but remains of unproven value.[59] The efficacy of fibrinolytic agents and heparin in limiting the thrombotic process in the acute stage of the disease also remains unclear.

If a proximal atherosclerotic occlusion lesion is demonstrated, bypass or percutaneous angioplasty may be appropriate; unfortunately, such lesions are present in only a small percentage of patients. Amputation is indicated in instances of secondary infection of gangrenous digits or intractable pain. Even if patients do not permanently restrict their tobacco use, abstinence during the first 7–10 days following amputation and other debridement procedures appears to be of some benefit.

Prognosis

In one large series of 193 patients with Buerger's disease, 75% eventually developed digital ischemia, tissue loss or gangrene. Arterial reconstructive surgery was deemed possible in only 17% with suboptimal patency rates of less than 50% during a 1- to 9-year follow-up period.[60,61] Although digital ischemic lesions are common, the amputation rate for major limbs remains less than 5%. Foot salvage can be achieved in the majority of cases with abstinence from smoking, meticulous care of ischemic lesions, selective prostaglandin therapy and sympathectomy.

Bozkurt and colleagues reported a series of 198 patients with TAO treated with sympathectomy in 161 patients and revascularization in 19 patients.[62] Following sympathectomy, the clinical outcome was reported improved in 52%, stable in 28% and diminished in 20% of patients. Among those undergoing surgical bypass, secondary patency was 58% at a mean follow-up of 5.4 years. The limb salvage rate was 96%.

Endovascular therapy has been associated with some success in selected patients. Graziani and associates reported a series of 17 patients with TAO with a mean age of 41.5 years and with critical limb ischemia Rutherford classification grades 3–5 treated with endovascular tibial recanalization.[63] This group reported technical success in 95% of treated limbs and major amputation- free survival of 84% with a mean follow-up of 23 months.[63]

Bone marrow–derived stem cells and progenitor cells are being investigated as a potential therapeutic alternative to promote angiogenesis in patients with peripheral arterial disease not amenable to surgical or endovascular revascularization.[64] A recent meta-analysis and systematic review of the literature examining autologous stem cell therapy for peripheral arterial disease revealed significant improvement in ankle–brachial index, transcutaneous partial pressure of oxygen and ulcer healing versus control groups.[65] Randomized trials are currently ongoing to determine efficacy of stem cell therapy in this patient population.

KAWASAKI'S DISEASE

Kawasaki's disease is a systemic vasculitis of the small- and medium-sized arteries with a unique predilection of the coronary arteries. This acute febrile illness was first described in 1967 by Kawasaki in a group of Japanese schoolchildren who presented with a unique constellation of signs and symptoms including high fever, cervical lymph node enlargement, conjunctivitis and truncal, solar and palmar erythema.[66] Although this was initially thought to be a benign and self-limiting disease, it was soon recognized that sudden unexpected death occurred in about 2% of patients in the subacute phase due to cardiac complications.

Approximately 15%–20% of patients develop coronary artery aneurysms.[67] This complication is most common in the first month of the illness but may appear up to 4 years after initial symptoms. An intense vasculitis that historically resembles infantile polyarteritis nodosa underlies the degeneration of the arterial wall and aneurysm formation. Although rare, abdominal aortic, brachial, axillary, iliac, renal and mesenteric aneurysms have also been reported.

The syndrome is more common in Japan but has been diagnosed worldwide. In the United States, the incidence is rising; 3000 children are diagnosed annually with 80% of these being below 5 years of age.[68] Asians are affected six times more frequently than Caucasians. Outbreaks have seasonal variations and definable case clusters occur at 2- to 3-year intervals.

The aetiology is unknown but has been attributed to innumerable viral and bacterial pathogens. More recently, an inherited defect in T-lymphocyte immunoregulation has been demonstrated in some patients with Kawasaki's disease.[69]

Clinical presentation

The diagnostic criteria for Kawasaki's disease include six principal signs: (1) high-grade fever persisting for at least 5 days; (2) polymorphic rash; (3) conjunctival congestion; (4) oropharyngeal changes, erythema and fissuring of the lips, mucosal injection and strawberry tongue; (5) acute nonpurulent cervical lymphadenopathy; and (6) erythema of the palms and soles, edema of the hands and feet and desquamation of the fingertips. Associated findings also include sterile pyuria with urethritis, transient elevation of the liver enzymes and asymptomatic gallstones; these occur in 7%–30% of patients. Classic laboratory findings include leukocytosis, thrombocytosis and elevation of acute-phase reactants. Complement levels are normal; viral and bacterial cultures as well as antinuclear and rheumatoid factors are usually negative.[70]

Cardiovascular manifestations remain the most disturbing feature of this disease. Based on echocardiographic and angiographic data, the majority of aneurysms involve the coronary arteries and develop during the convalescent phase of the disease, 10–14 days after the onset of fever. Peripheral aneurysms are nearly always associated with coronary involvement. Other cardiac abnormalities include myocarditis, valvulitis and dysrhythmias. The natural history of coronary artery aneurysms has been determined using serial angiography and echocardiography.[67,71,72] It is generally accepted that aneurysms smaller than 8 mm in size eventually regress while those greater than 8 mm are associated with high morbidity and mortality secondary to aneurysm rupture and thrombosis. Male children over 2 years of age who present with fever lasting more than 3 weeks and with persistent elevation of the ESR appear to be more vulnerable to persistent coronary artery aneurysms.[73] The observation that saccular aneurysms are less likely to regress than fusiform aneurysms suggests a more severe medial disruption in the saccular configuration. In a 13-year follow-up study of 594 patients with Kawasaki's disease,[74] 25% developed coronary aneurysms in the acute phase of the disease. It is noteworthy that 55% of these aneurysms apparently regressed, based on arteriographic follow-up. Whether this change in appearance was related to intraluminal thrombosis or true remodelling remains unknown.

Pathogenesis

The predilection of the coronary arteries to aneurysmal degeneration may be related to the additional stresses imposed by the bimodal systolic pressure wave characteristic of the coronary circulation in the presence of a necrotizing inflammation of the media. The fact that both the incidence of aneurysm formation and the morbid consequences have been reduced by the early administration of anti-inflammatory and immunoglobulin therapy would suggest that rapid control of the necrotizing process limits the injury and protects newly proliferating smooth muscle cells. In a study by Barron et al.,[69] an elevated serum level of interleukin-2 receptor was found to be a reliable predictor of the development of aneurysms in 82 children with clinical evidence of Kawasaki's disease.

Diagnosis

Echocardiography is recommended in any patient who satisfies the classic criteria of the disease, and it is useful in detecting coronary arterial involvement. Coronary catheterization is performed only in those children in whom aneurysms are suggested by ultrasound.

Management

Prompt initiation of anti-inflammatory agents such as aspirin and ticlopidine has reduced mortality from 2% to about 0.5%. Intravenous gamma globulin combined with aspirin has been found to dramatically reduce the incidence of coronary artery aneurysms if started within 10 days of the onset of illness.[75] Such therapy may prevent deposition of circulating immune complexes, thereby limiting the vasculitic process. Currently, there is no evidence to suggest that this therapy is effective in regressing chronic coronary aneurysms. Operative treatment with arterial conduit or saphenous interposition grafting is indicated in patients with symptomatic or expanding coronary and peripheral arterial aneurysms.[76]

Ruptures of coronary artery aneurysms are rare but catastrophic events. A recent review of the world literature from 1997 to 2013 revealed 11 reported patients with ruptured coronary aneurysms and only 2 survivors.[77] One of the survivors was a 3-year-old male who underwent coronary artery bypass grafting followed by percutaneous cardiopulmonary support and successful heart transplantation, and the other was a 5-year-old male who underwent bedside pericardial window followed by emergency coronary artery bypass grafting.[77] The authors recommended intravenous immunoglobulin and steroid therapy for the treatment of all patients with severe Kawasaki disease.

Kitamura and colleagues recently reported outstanding long-term outcomes of coronary artery bypass surgery in 114 pediatric patients for Kawasaki disease aged 1–19 years (median 10 years) with a median follow-up of 19 years.[78] The indication for surgery in this series was the presence of angiographic significant obstructive coronary lesions greater than 75% associated with myocardial ischemia. The internal thoracic artery was used in 97% of patients and saphenous vein grafts used in 21% of patients, primarily for lesions not involving the left anterior descending artery. The mean number of bypasses was 1.7 ± 0.8 per patient. The 20-year graft patency was 87% for internal thoracic artery grafts and 44% for saphenous vein grafts. The 25-year survival was 95%. The proximal native coronary artery aneurysmal segment was not ligated due to the concern for coronary hypoperfusion in the immediate post-operative period associated with narrow internal thoracic artery grafts in pediatric patients.

BEHÇET'S DISEASE

Behçet's disease[79] is a rare vasculitis with protean manifestations in the systemic arteries and veins as well as the pulmonary circulation. Venous complications include recurrent episodes of deep venous thrombosis, which occasionally result in vena cava thrombosis. While arterial symptoms are elicited in only 10%–20% of patients, sudden arterial occlusions and aneurysmal ruptures represent a frequent cause of death in this otherwise benign disease.

Clinical presentation

First manifestations of Behçet's disease include relapsing iridocyclitis associated with oral and genital ulcerations. Patients may also present with poorly characterized polyarthritis and neurologic deficits compatible with both central lesions and peripheral neuropathies. Involvement of the gastrointestinal tract is unusual but may result in spontaneous ileal and cecal perforations associated with ulcerative enteritis.[80–82] Abdominal aortic and peripheral aneurysms have been reported, although the frequency of these lesions remains ill defined.[83–85] The highest prevalence of the disease is in the Middle East, the Mediterranean region and Asia.[86] Aneurysm rupture is the most frequent cause of death.[86]

Diagnosis is based on the history of mucosal ulcerations associated with arterial and venous disease in a young patient. Generally, the disease has a predilection for males. This helps distinguish it from TA, which has a distinct female predominance. Genetic and environmental factors have been associated with the pathogenesis of Behçet's disease. The HLA-B51 allele is the strongest associated genetic factor with Behçet's disease.[86]

Physical examination may demonstrate central or peripheral aneurysms and, rarely, absence of peripheral pulses. Ultrasound or computerized tomography (CT) can confirm the impression of aneurysmal dilation. Arteriography is occasionally needed to better delineate the pattern of thoracic aortic involvement; however, such studies should generally be reserved for preoperative evaluation (Figure 44.7).

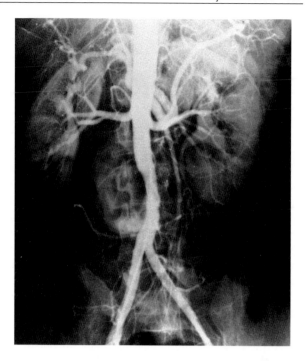

Figure 44.7 Preoperative angiogram in patient with Behçet's disease and abdominal pain demonstrates large infrarenal aneurysm with intraluminal thrombus.

Pathology

The histologic picture is consistent with focal arteriolitis. Lymphocytes and polymorphonuclear leukocytes are widely infiltrated, resulting in fibrinoid necrosis with complete or partial vascular occlusion. This inflammatory process is noted in both the arteries and veins of involved areas.

Aneurysms may appear grossly infected in some patients. While it is impossible to definitively rule out such an aetiology, intraoperative cultures are typically negative and graft infections have not been reported following in situ reconstruction. On occasion, however, it may be impossible to grossly differentiate Behçet's disease aneurysms from true infected aneurysms, and extra-anatomic reconstruction may be appropriate.[87]

Therapy

Patients frequently are first seen for complications of venous thrombosis. Most authors recommend that patients be maintained indefinitely on both support stockings and anticoagulation with warfarin. The need for long-term anticoagulation makes it essential that any complaints of abdominal or back pain be aggressively evaluated as they may herald expansion or rupture of a previously undiagnosed aortic aneurysm.

Due to the heterogeneous clinical manifestations, various biologic and immunosuppressive agents have been used for treatment of Behçet's disease. This includes tumor necrosis factor inhibitors, interleukin-1 beta, interferon alpha, corticosteroids, non-steroidal anti-inflammatory drugs and various immunosuppressive agents.[86] Treatment has been based on few randomized trials, and further investigation will be required to improve therapy.[86]

SMALL AND MEDIUM VESSEL DISEASE

A large number of disorders are incorporated in this classification, including hypersensitivity angiitis, microscopic polyangiitis, granulomatosis with polyangiitis (Wegener's), mixed cryoglobulinemia, eosinophilic granulomatosis with polyangiitis (Churg–Strauss), polyarteritis nodosa and collagen disease vasculitis (see Table 44.1).[1,88] Medium and small vessel vasculitides can be further categorized according to the presence of anti-neutrophil cytoplasm antibodies.[89] The common underlying pathology in necrotizing vasculitis is fibrinoid necrosis of the arterial or venous wall characteristically involving the cutaneous vessels. More than 50% of patients with necrotizing vasculitis will present with palpable purpuric nodules, most frequently on the lower extremities. These cutaneous lesions are usually associated with fever and multiple-system organ involvement.

Digital ischemic ulceration may be the first manifestation of a systemic autoimmune disease.[90,91] The diagnosis is confirmed by skin biopsy. Histologic examination reveals neutrophilic infiltration of the vessel wall, fibrinoid necrosis and dermal hemorrhage.[92] Direct immunofluorescence studies of the lesion demonstrate IgM or IgA, which is commonly associated with Henoch–Schönlein purpura.[93] In two-thirds of patients, the ESR is elevated. Abnormal urine analysis and elevated serum creatinine levels are found in patients with renal involvement.[94] Antinuclear antibody and rheumatoid factor are positive in 10% and 20% of patients, respectively.

The precise aetiology of this group of disorders is dependent on the associated collagen disease and, in general, reflects continuing immune complex damage of the small vessels, especially the postcapillary venules and muscular arterioles. The inciting antigen may be a drug, a virus such as hepatitis B or a tumor antigen. Vascular injury also may be accentuated by external factors such as trauma or hypothermia.

Treatment depends on associated vital organ involvement and whether vasospasm is an important contributing factor to digital ischemia. Cases of necrotizing vasculitis strictly limited to the skin may be treated with local sulfones. Steroids and/or immunosuppressant drugs are indicated if there is evidence of progressive skin involvement, nephropathy or internal organ damage. If cryoglobulins or other circulating proteins are identified, plasmapheresis may be of benefit. Digital vasospasm can be managed with vasodilators such as nifedipine and nicotinamide. In some instances, acute digital ischemia can be temporarily ameliorated by tourniquet-controlled intravenous reserpine injection or a Bier block.[95] At the current time, anti-thrombotic agents are of unproven value.

FIBROMUSCULAR DYSPLASIA

Since the first report of arterial fibrodysplasia in 1938, these lesions have received much attention[96,97] as a cause of renovascular hypertension. Additional reports have focused on the neurologic manifestations of extracranial dysplastic lesions and the occasional case of mesenteric vascular involvement.[98–102] Clinically significant fibromuscular dysplasia (FMD) is most common in women between the ages of 20 and 40 years and can be distinguished from the other lesions discussed previously in this chapter by the lack of a true inflammatory component.

The aetiology of these lesions remains unknown as they are not caused by atherosclerosis or inflammatory vascular disease, although hormonal influences, mechanical stresses and disorders of vascular wall nutrition have been suggested.[103] Genetic factors have also been implicated as the majority of FMD cases have been found to be due to an autosomal-dominant trait with variable penetrance.[104,105]

Clinical presentation

The clinical presentation is dependent on the location of the dysplastic lesion. The United States Registry for Fibromuscular Dysplasia recently reported their findings on 447 patients enrolled from 9 sites in 2012.[106] The majority of patients were female (91%) and the mean age at diagnosis was 52 years. The most common presenting symptoms and clinical signs were hypertension (64%), headache (52%), pulsatile tinnitus (28%), dizziness (26%) and cervical bruit and neck pain (22%).

The distribution of vascular arterial involvement in this registry was the renal artery (79.7%), extracranial carotid artery (74.3%), vertebral artery (36.6%) and mesenteric arteries (26.3%), although nearly any artery in the human body can be affected.[106] With renal artery involvement, the most common clinical presentation is hypertension. Extracranial carotid or vertebral artery involvement can cause stroke, transient ischemic attack or dissection.[107] In the FMD registry, arterial dissections were observed in 19.7% of patients and aneurysms in 17% of patients.[106]

The most frequently affected arterial bed is the main renal artery and its secondary branches (Figure 44.8). Bilateral renal artery involvement has been noted in greater than 35% of patients.[107] Hemodynamically significant stenoses predictably decrease renal perfusion pressure, resulting in hyper-reninemia and activation of the angiotensin–aldosterone axis. Dysplastic renal artery lesions must be investigated in any young patient presenting with diastolic hypertension greater than 100 mmHg.

The incidence of renovascular hypertension is bimodal, with a first peak at 2–4 years of age and a second large peak at 20–40 years. Females predominate

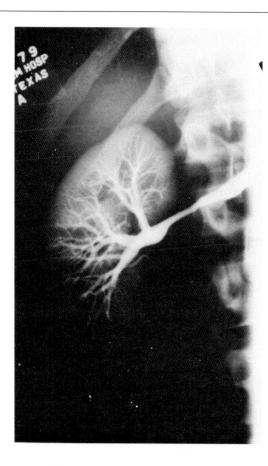

Figure 44.8 Tapered fibrodysplastic lesion of right renal artery extends to bifurcation.

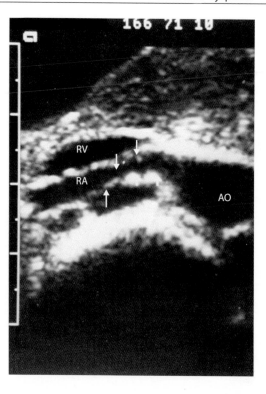

Figure 44.9 Duplex ultrasound of the juxtarenal aorta (AO), right renal artery (RA) and right renal vein (RV). An irregular stenosis is noted in the proximal renal artery.

8:1 in the second group, but this sex predilection is less obvious in pediatric patients.

Physical findings other than hypertension are not very specific. Although flank bruits are classically associated with renal artery stenosis, the specificity and sensitivity of this sign are both low in most clinical series. Intravenous pyelograms (IVPs) may suggest the diagnosis, especially if disparity in renal size, hyperconcentration of dye or ureteral notching from collateral vessels is demonstrated. However, the principal function of an IVP is the exclusion of primary renal parenchymal disease.

Currently, non-invasive examination of renal arterial flow patterns by duplex ultrasonography is evolving as the most suitable screening method for significant renal arterial stenoses. Although B-mode real-time imaging of the renal arteries is possible (Figure 44.9), resolution is often suboptimal. Quantitation of the degree of stenosis currently relies on serial velocity measurements along the renal artery from the aorta to the hilum of the kidney. Barnes[108] and others have demonstrated that a renal/aortic peak systolic velocity ratio of 3.5 or more is indicative of hemodynamically significant renal stenosis greater than 60%. Using these criteria, duplex Doppler ultrasonography carries a specificity rate of 93%–97% and a sensitivity rate of 83%–90% as compared to angiography.[109,110] The examination requires considerable technical expertise and

proper patient preparation. Colour-flow imaging appears to facilitate identification of the juxtarenal aorta, the left renal vein and the origin of the renal arteries. Its value in detecting significant renal arterial stenoses, however, remains to be determined.

Specific diagnosis requires arteriography. Intravenous digital angiography can suffice, although it is usually necessary to perform arterial catheterization with Seldinger technique, which allows selective injections and oblique views. Fibrodysplastic lesions generally spare the proximal portion of the renal artery but extend distally to the major branches of the vessel (Figure 44.10). CT angiography and MR angiography are useful imaging modalities but have limitations because resolution is insufficient to identify renal artery branch vessel involvement.[111]

While renal vein renin ratios and renal systemic renin values are commonly obtained, the diagnostic reliability of these determinations is compromised by bilateral disease and the multiple medications which are usually required to control hypertension. Nonetheless, renal systemic renin values can predict the degree of improvement following successful revascularization.[103,112]

Patients with carotid involvement present with intermittent neurologic deficits often corresponding to the middle cerebral artery distribution. Mechanisms for cerebral ischemia include platelet or thrombotic emboli as well as 'low flow' distal to an obstructing lesion. Non-invasive studies such as duplex scanning may detect these lesions; however, arteriography is usually required for a

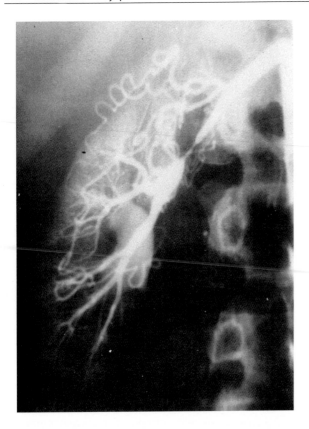

Figure 44.10 Severe stenosis of right renal artery associated with an extensive network of capsular collaterals from adrenal (top) and ureteral (bottom) arteries. The presence of these collateral vessels confirms the hemodynamic significance of the main renal artery lesion.

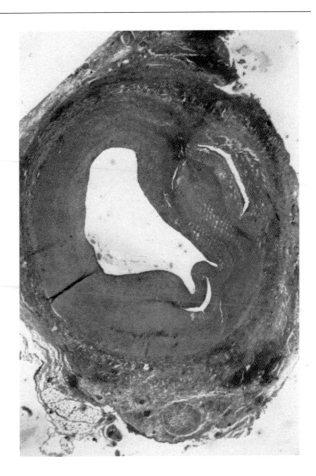

Figure 44.11 A spontaneous dissection compromises the lumen in this renal artery with severe medial fibroplasia. Urgent aortorenal bypass was required.

full definition of the extent of disease. Fibromuscular disease may vary from a localized web at the carotid bifurcation to diffuse involvement of the entire extracranial and intracranial internal carotid artery. These lesions are occasionally associated with subintimal internal carotid artery dissections, distinguished angiographically by an irregular narrowed arterial lumen.

Pathology

Dysplastic lesions are most conveniently classified into four general types[100]: (1) intimal fibroplasia, (2) medial hyperplasia, (3) medial fibroplasia and (4) perimedial dysplasia. Of these, medial fibroplasia accounts for more than 85% of all lesions (Figure 44.11). Gross examination of excised vessels demonstrates a wide range of morphology from focal stenoses to series of stenoses with intervening aneurysmal dilations producing a 'chain of lakes' appearance (Figure 44.12). Intimal fibroplasia constitutes approximately 10% of all FMD.[107] Intimal involvement causes angiographic appearance of focal fibrotic constriction resulting in a concentric stenosis or a long cylindrical narrowing.[107,113]

Histologic examination of medial fibroplasia reveals few intact smooth muscle cells in the media and a marked

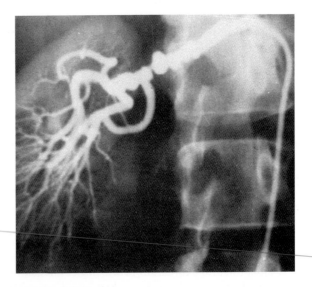

Figure 44.12 Classic 'chain of lakes' appearance with saccular dilations and segmental stenoses.

increase in collagen and ground substance. Disease may be limited to the outer media or extend throughout the entire media, although the intima may be fractured and some degree of intimal fibrosis can be seen. In the medial and intimal lesions, the adventitia is usually spared completely.

Treatment

Indications for operation in patients with renovascular hypertension include the documentation of an appropriate renal artery lesion in an adult with severe hypertension, requiring multiple adrenergic blocking agents for control. Other candidates for surgery in fibrodysplasia include children with severe hypertension and any patient with a documented decrease in renal function.

With the emergence of endovascular techniques, percutaneous balloon angioplasty (PTA) has essentially replaced open surgery as the primary initial therapy.[114] However, long-term results have yet to be clearly documented. Indications for stenting include a significant residual gradient post-PTA and to treat renal artery dissection.[107] Stenting may not be feasible when the distal renal artery and its branches are involved. Surgical revascularization is indicated primarily in patients in whom endovascular therapy is not technically feasible, including aneurysms and failed PTA.[107]

Renal artery lesions can usually be treated quite successfully with aortorenal bypass using autologous vein or artery.[112] In rare instances of distal segmental involvement, ex vivo repair with autotransplantation may be appropriate.[115] In expert hands, perioperative kidney loss is less than 2% and cure or improvement of hypertension can be expected in up to 90% of patients. In a retrospective review from the University of Michigan, Stanley et al.[116] reviewed a 30-year experience (1963–1993) with operative correction of renovascular hypertension in 57 pediatric patients. The most common renal artery pathology was atypical medial–perimedial dysplasia, usually associated with secondary intimal fibroplasia. Aortorenal bypass with autogenous vein was the most prevalent procedure (60%) early in the experience but was infrequently utilized in the last decade of the study. In fact, direct reimplantations of distal vessels into the aorta as well as reimplantation of segmental arteries into adjacent renal arteries accounted for the majority of reconstructions in the modern era.

A meta-analysis and systematic review of hypertensive FMD patients undergoing treatment with PTA or surgical repair was recently published by Trinquart and associates.[117] Forty-seven PTA studies containing 1616 patients were compared with 23 surgical studies with 1014 patients. Cure rates of hypertension with definition of cure being blood pressure < 140/90 mmHg without antihypertensive therapy were 36% after PTA and 54% after surgery. These findings are difficult to interpret due to significant variability among the studies. The authors concluded that both therapies resulted in moderate benefit to patients with FMD and renovascular hypertension. The risk of major complications was less after PTA than surgery (6% vs. 15%).

Cerebrovascular manifestations of carotid artery disease such as transient ischemic attacks or stroke strongly indicate intervention. PTA is the recommended initial primary therapy for patients with symptomatic extracranial cerebrovascular FMD.[118] Intraoperative dilation has generally been replaced by PTA. Surgical therapy is indicated for patients with aneurysms not amenable to endovascular treatment with stent grafts. Operations have included intraoperative dilation, vein graft bypass and extracranial–intracranial (EC–IC) bypass.

Surgical or endovascular therapy is generally not indicated for carotid artery dissections secondary to FMD; the majority of these lesions will resolve with anti-thrombotic therapy alone, despite their ominous appearance on angiography. Evidence supporting anti-thrombotic therapy is the observation that 90% of strokes due to dissection are of thromboembolic aetiology rather than due to hypoperfusion and transcranial Doppler studies demonstrate a high incidence of cerebral microemboli.[119] Intracranial extension of the dissection is a contraindication to anticoagulation.[119]

Treatment with either aspirin or anticoagulants may both be acceptable. Although no large randomized trials comparing these therapies have been performed, a recent prospective trial of patients with spontaneous dissection of the cervical carotid artery compared 202 patients treated with anticoagulants to 96 patients treated with aspirin alone.[120] Seventy percent of the patients in this trial had symptoms of cerebral or retinal ischemia on presentation, 27% had local symptoms (headache, neck pain, cranial nerve palsy, Horner syndrome), and only 3% were asymptomatic. During the 3-month follow-up period, the overall incidence of ischemic events was very low with only 1 patient having an ischemic stroke (ischemic stroke 0.3%); the risk of all neurologic events including TIA or retinal ischemia did not differ significantly between the two groups (5.9% anticoagulation vs 2.1% aspirin). The incidence of hemorrhagic adverse events also did not differ among the groups (2% anticoagulation vs. 1% aspirin). It was noteworthy that new ischemic events occurred more frequently in patients with ischemic symptoms at initial presentation than those patients who were asymptomatic or had only local symptoms at presentation (6.2% vs. 1.1%).

Most authors would advocate treatment for 3–6 months with some form of anticoagulant to allow for the dissection to heal. The majority of carotid and vertebral dissections will resolve with time.[119] It may be helpful to repeat angiography in 3–6 months if the lesion cannot be followed by duplex ultrasound. Magnetic resonance angiography and CT angiography are replacing conventional angiography as the accepted standard in the evaluation of carotid and vertebral artery dissecions.[119]

Intervention with endovascular stent graft placement or surgical therapy is rarely indicated and is limited to patients who experience ischemic symptoms despite adequate anticoagulation.[107,119] In these unusual patients, extra-anatomic reconstruction with an EC–IC bypass may be a prudent option, as distal extension of these lesions into the petrous portion of the carotid artery makes a cervical approach difficult or impossible.

FMD of the mesenteric vessels is unusual and usually involves more than one visceral vessel.[107,121] It can present as occlusive or aneurysmal disease.[121] If acute or chronic intestinal ischemia does result, the operative approach is similar to the treatment of atherosclerotic occlusive lesions although FMD may extend more distally in the mesenteric vessels complicating the distal anastomosis.

FMD involving the coronary arteries is a very infrequent condition.[122] It can result in coronary artery dissection, intramural hematoma, tapered stenosis or increased tortuosity resulting in acute coronary ischemia, myocardial infarction or cardiac dysrhythmias. Treatment is primarily non-operative as these lesions mostly resolve spontaneously.

REFERENCES

1. Jennette JC, Falk RJ, Bacon PA et al. 2012 Revised International Chapel Hill consensus conference nomenclature of vasculitides. *Arthritis Rheum.* 2013;65(1):1–11.
2. Christian CL, Sergent JS. Vasculitis syndromes: Clinical and experimental models. *Am J Med.* 1976;61:385.
3. Fauci AS, Haynes BF, Katz P. The spectrum of vasculitis: Clinical pathologic, immunologic, and therapeutic considerations. *Ann Intern Med.* 1978;89(part I):660.
4. Takayasu M. Case with unusual change of the vessels in the retina. *Acta Soc Ophthalmol.* 1908;12:544.
5. Ask-Upmark E. On the "Pulseless Disease" outside of Japan. *Acta Med Scan.* 1954;149:161.
6. Nakao K, Ikida M, Kimata S. Takayasu's arteritis: Clinical report of eighty-four cases and immunologic studies of seven cases. *Circulation.* 1967;35:1141.
7. Eichhorn J, Sima D, Thiele B, Lindschau C, Turowski A, Schmidt H, Schneider W, Haller H, Luft FC. Anti-endothelial cell antibodies in Takayasu arteritis. *Circulation.* 1996;94:2396.
8. Lupi-Herrera E, Sanchez-Torres G, Marchushamer J et al. Takayasu's arteritis: Clinical study of 107 cases. *Am Heart J.* 1977;93:94.
9. Arend WP, Michel BA, Bloch DA et al. The American college of rheumatology 1990 criteria for the classification of Takayasu arteritis. *Arthritis Rheum.* 1990;33(8):1129–1134.
10. Lande A, Rossi P. The value of total aortography in the diagnosis of Takayasu's arteritis. *Radiology.* 1975;114:297.
11. Gotsman M, Beck W, Schrine V. Selective angiography in arteritis of the aorta and its major branches. *Radiology.* 1967;88:232.
12. Ishikawa KK. Natural history and classification of occlusive thromboartopathy (Takayasu's disease). *Circulation.* 1978;57:27.
13. Lupi-Herrera E, Sanchey G, Horwitz S, Gutierrey E. Pulmonary artery involvement in Takayasu's arteritis. *Chest.* 1975;67:69.
14. Noguchi S, Numano F, Gravanis MB et al. Increased levels of soluble forms of adhesion molecules in Takayasu arteritis. *Int J Cardiol.* 1998;66(Suppl 1):S23–S33.
15. Akazawa H, Ikeda U, Yamamoto K, Kuroda T, Shimada K. Hypercoagulable state in patients with Takayasu's arteritis. *Thromb Hacmost.* 1996;75:712.
16. Alpert HJ. The use of immunosuppressive agents in Takayasu's arteritis. *Med Ann.* DC 1974;43:69.
17. Comarmond C, Plaisier E, Dahan K et al. Anti TNF-alpha in refractory Takayasu's arteritis: Cases series and review of the literature. *Autoimmun Rev.* 2012;11(9):678–684.
18. Bloss RS, Duncan JM, Cooley DA et al. Takayasu's arteritis: Surgical considerations. *Ann Thorac Surg.* 1979;27:574.
19. Kimoto S. The history and present status of aortic surgery in Japan particularly for aortitis syndrome. *J Cardiovasc Surg.* 1979;20:107.
20. Miyata T, Sato O, Deguchi J, Kimura H, Namba T, Kondo K, Makuuchi M, Hamada C, Takagi A, Tada Y. Anastomotic aneurysms after surgical treatment of Takayasu's arteritis: A 40-year experience. *J Vasc Surg.* 1998;27:438.
21. Perera AH, Youngstein T, Gibbs RG et al. Optimizing the outcome of vascular intervention for Takayasu arteritis. *Br J Surg.* 2014 January;101(2):43–50.
22. Kim YW, Kim DI, Park YJ et al. Surgical bypass vs endovascular treatment for patients with supra-aortic arterial occlusive disease due to Takayasu arteritis. *J Vasc Surg.* 2012 March;55(3):693–700.
23. Maksimowicz-MiKinnon K, Clark TM, Hoffman GS. Limitations of therapy and a guarded prognosis in an American cohort of Takayasu arteritis patients. *Arthritis Rheum.* 2007;56(3):1000–1009.
24. Qureshi MA, Martin Z, Greenberg RK. Endovascular management of patients with Takayasu arteritis: Stents versus stent grafts. *Semin Vasc Surg.* 2011 March;24(1):44–52.
25. Huston KA, Hunder GG, Lie JT et al. Temporal arteritis: A 25-year epidemiologic clinical and pathologic study. *Ann Intern Med.* 1978;88:162.
26. Hunde GG, Allen GL. The relationship between polymyalgia rheumatica and temporal arteritis. *Geriatics.* 1973;28:134.
27. Hamilton CR Jr, Shelley WM, Trumulty PA. Giant cell arteritis and polymyalgia rheumatica. *Medicine.* 1971;50:1.
28. Wagner HP, Hollenhorst RW. Ocular lesions of temporal arteritis. *Am J Ophthalmol.* 1958;45:617.
29. Cohen DN, Damaske MM. Temporal arteritis: A spectrum of ophthalmic complications. *Ann Ophthalmol.* 1975;7:1045.
30. Cochran JW, Fox JH, Kelly MP. Reversible mental symptoms in temporal arteritis. *J Nerv Ment Dis.* 1978;6:446.
31. Klein RG, Hunder GG, Stanson AW, Sheps SG. Large artery involvement in giant cell (temporal) arteritis. *Ann Intern Med.* 1975;83:806.
32. Seignalet J, Janbon C, Sany J et al. HLA in temporal arteritis. *Tissue Antigens.* 1977;9:69.

33. Ypsilantis E, Courtney ED, Chopra N et al. Importance of specimen length during temporal artery biopsy. *Br J Surg.* 2011;98(11):1556–1560.

34. Beever DG, Harpur JE, Turk KAD. Giant cell arteritis: The need for prolonged treatment. *J Chronic Dis.* 1973;26:571.

35. Stanson AW, Klein RG, Hunder GG. Extracranial angiographic findings in giant cell (temporal) arteritis. *Am J Roentgenol.* 1976;12:957.

36. Schmidt WA, Kraft HE, Vorpahl K, Volker L, Gronica-Ihle EJ. Color duplex ultrasonography in the diagnosis of temporal arteritis. *N Engl J Med.* 1997;337:1336.

37. Karahaliou M, Vaiopoulos G, Papaspyrou S et al. Colour duplex sonography of temporal arteries before decision for biopsy: A prospective study in 55 patients with suspected giant cell arteritis. *Arthrits Res Ther.* 2006;8(4):R116.

38. Blockman D, Stroobants S, Maes A et al. Positron emission tomography in giant cell arteritis and polymyalgia rheumatica: Evidence for inflammation of the aortic arch. *Am J Med.* 2000;108(3):246–249.

39. Fuchs M, Briel M, Daikeler T et al. The impact of 18F-FDG PET on the management of patients with suspected large vessel vasculitis. *Eur J Nuc Med Mol Imaging.* 2012;39(2):344–353.

40. Pollock M, Blennerhasset JB, Clarke AM. Giant cell arteritis and the subclavian steal syndrome. *Neurology.* 1973;23:653.

41. Mowat AG, Gazleman BL. Polymyalgia rheumatica: Clinical study with particular references to arterial disease. *J Rheumatol.* 1974;1:190.

42. Proven A, Gabriel SE, Orces C et al. Glucocorticoid therapy in giant cell arteritis: Duration and adverse outcomes. *Arthritis Rheum.* 2003;49(5):703–708.

43. Ostberg G. Temporal arteritis in a large necropsy series. *Ann Rheum Dis.* 1971;30:224.

44. Hunder GG, Sheps SG, Allen GL, Joyce JW. Daily and alternate day corticosteroid regimens in treatment of giant cell arteritis: Comparison in a prospective study. *Ann Intern Med.* 1975;82:613.

45. Jover JA, Hernández-García C, Morado IC et al. Combined treatment of giant-cell arteritis with methotrexate and prednisone. A randomized, double-blind, placebo-controlled trial. *Ann Intern Med.* 2001;134(2):106–114.

46. Buerger L. *The Circulatory Disturbances of the Extremities, Including Gangrene, Vasomotor and Trophic Disorders.* Philadelphia, PA: Saunders; 1924.

47. McKusick VA, Harris WS, Oltesen OE et al. Buerger's disease: A distinct clinical and pathologic entity. *J Am Med Assoc.* 1962;181:5.

48. Lie JT. Thromboangiitis obliterans (Buerger's Disease) in women. *Medicine.* 1987;66:65.

49. Shionoya S. Pathology of Buerger's disease clinico-pathologico-angiographic correlation. *Pathol Microbiol.* 1975;43:163.

50. Szilagyi ED, DeRusseo FJ, Elliot JP Jr. Thromboangiitis obliterans: Clinico-angiographic correlations. *Arch Surg.* 1964;88:824.

51. Shionoya S. Diagnostic criteria of Buerger's disease. *Int J Cardiol.* 1998;66(Suppl 1):S243–S245.

52. Shionoya S, Hiari M, Kawai S. Pattern of arterial occlusion in Buerger's disease. *Angiology.* 1982;33:375.

53. Suzuki S, Mine H, Umehara I et al. Buerger's disease (Thromboangiitis Obliterans): An analysis of the arterio-grams of 119 cases. *Clin Radiol.* 1982;33:235.

54. Lie JT. Thromboangiitis obliterans (Buerger's disease) revisited. *Pathol Annu.* 1988;23(part 2):257.

55. Ketha SS, Cooper LT. The role of autoimmunity in thromboangiitis obliterans (Buerger's disease). *Ann N Y Acad Sci.* 2013;1285:15–25.

56. Shionoya, S. Clinical experience with prostaglandin E1 in occlusive arterial disease. *Inter Angio.* 1984;3:99.

57. Schuler JJ, Flanigan DP, Holcroft JW et al. Efficacy of prostaglandin E1 in the treatment of lower extremity ischemic ulcers secondary to peripheral vascular occlusive disease: Results of a prospective randomized double-blind, multicenter clinical trial. *J Vasc Surg.* 1984;1:160.

58. Fiessinger JN, Schafer M. Trial of iloprost versus aspirin treatment for critical limb ischaemia of thromboangiitis obliterans. The TAO Study. *Lancet.* 1990;335(8689):555–557.

59. Sakakibara K, Takahaski H, Kobayashi S. Clinical experience of hyperbaric oxygen therapy (OHP) for chronic peripheral vascular disorders. In: Shiraki D, Matsuoka S, eds. *Hyperbaric Medicine and Underwater Physiology.* Bethesda, MA: Undersea Medical Society; 1983, p. 337.

60. Shionoya S, Ban I, Nakata Y et al. Vascular reconstruction in Buerger's disease. *Br J Surg.* 1976;63:841.

61. Shionoya S. Buerger's disease (Thromboangiitis obliterans). *Rutherford Vasc Surg.* 1989;3:207.

62. Bozkurt AK, Beşirli K, Köksal C et al. Surgical treatment of Buerger's disease. *Vascular.* 2004;12(3):192–197.

63. Graziani L, Morelli L, Parini F et al. Clinical outcome after extended endovascular recanalization in Buerger's disease in 20 consecutive cases. *Ann Vasc Surg.* 2012;26(3):387–395.

64. Lawall H, Bramlage P, Amann B. Treatment of peripheral arterial disease using stem and progenitor cell therapy. *Vasc Surg.* 2011;53(2)445–453.

65. Fadini GP, Agostini C, Avogaro A. Autologous stem cell therapy for peripheral arterial disease meta-analysis and systematic review of the literature. *Atherosclerosis.* 2010;209(1):10–17.

66. Kawasaki T. Acute febrile mucocutaneous syndrome with lymphoid involvement with specific desquamation of the fingers and toes. *Arerugi.* 1967;16:178.

67. Kato H, Koike S, Yamamoto M et al. Coronary aneurysms in infants and young children with acute febrile mucocutaneous lymph node syndrome. *J Pediatr*. 1975;86:892.

68. Rauch AM. Kawasaki syndrome: Critical review of US epidemiology. *Prog Clin Biol Res*. 1987;20:33.

69. Barron K, DeCunto C, Montalvo J et al. Abnormalities of immunoregulation in Kawasaki syndrome. *J Rheumatol*. 1988;15:1243.

70. Leung DY. Immunologic abnormalities in Kawasaki syndrome. *Prog Clin Biol Res*. 1987;20:159.

71. Capannari TE, Daniels SR, Meyer RA et al. Sensitivity, specificity and predictive value of two-dimensional echocardiographic in detecting coronary artery aneurysms in patients with Kawasaki disease. *J Am Coll Cardiol*. 1986;7:355.

72. Yoshikawa J, Tanagihara K, Owaki T et al. Cross-sectional echo-cardiographic diagnosis of coronary artery aneurysms in patients with the mucocutaneous lymph node syndrome. *Circulation*. 1979;59:133.

73. Kato H, Inoue O, Akagi T. Kawasaki disease: Cardiac problems and management. *Pediatr Rev*. 1988;9:209.

74. Kato H, Sugimura T, Akagi T, Sayo N, Hashino K, Maeno Y, Kazue T, Eto G, Yamakawa R. Long-term consequences of Kawasaki disease: A 10–21-year follow-up study of 594 patients. *Circulation*. 1996;94:1379.

75. Newburger JW, Takahashi M, Burns JC et al. The treatment of Kawasaki syndrome with intravenous gammaglobulin. *N Engl J Med*. 1986;315:341.

76. Kitamura S. Surgery for coronary heart disease due to mucocutaneous lymph node syndrome (Kawasaki Disease). In: Shulman ST, ed. *Kawasaki Disease: Proceedings of the Second International Kawasaki Disease Symposium*. New York: Liss, 1987.

77. Miyamoto T, Ikeda K, Ishii Y et al. Rupture of a coronary artery aneurysm in Kawasaki disease: A rare case and review of the literature for the past 15 years. *J Thorac Cardiovasc Surg*. 2014 June;147(6):e67–e69.

78. Kitamura S, Tsuda E, Kobayashi J et al. Twenty-five-year outcome of pediatric coronary artery bypass surgery for Kawasaki disease. *Circulation*. 2009;120(1):60–68.

79. Behcet, H. Über Rezidivierende Aphthose Durch ein Virus Verursachte Geschwure am Mund, am Auge und an den Genitalien. *Dermatol Wochnschr*. 1937;105:1152.

80. Chajet T, Fainaru M. Behcet's disease: Report of 41 cases and a review of the literature. *Medicine*. 1975;54(3):179.

81. James DG. Behcet's syndrome. *N Engl J Med*. 1979;301:431.

82. Lebwohl O, Forde KA, Berdon WE et al. Ulcerative esophagitis and colitis in a pediatric patient with Behcet's syndrome. *Am J Gastroenterol*. 1977;68:550.

83. Enoch BA, Castillo-Olivares JL, Khou TCL et al. Major vascular complications in Behcet's syndrome. *Postgrad Med J*. 1968;44:453.

84. Haim RS, Reshef R, Peleg E, Riss E. Cardiac involvement and superior vena cava obstruction in Behcet's disease. *N Engl J Med*. 1979;301:431.

85. Little AG, Zarins CK. Abdominal aortic aneurysm and Behcet's disease. *Surgery*. 1982;91:359.

86. Saleh Z, Arayssi T. Update on the therapy of Behçet disease. *Ther Adv Chronic Dis*. 2014;5(3):112–134.

87. Ketch LL, Buerk CA, Liechty RD. Surgical implications of Behcet's disease. *Arch Surg*. 1980;115:759.

88. Montgomery H. *Montgomery's Textbook of Dermatopathology*. New York: Harper & Row; 1967, p. 685.

89. Lugmani RA, Suppiah R, Grayson PC et al. Nomenclature and classification of vasculitis – Update on the ACR/EULAR diagnosis and classification of vasculitis study (DCVAS). *Clin Exp Immunol*. 2011;164(Suppl 1):11–13.

90. Baur GM, Porter JM, Bardana EJ et al. Rapid onset of hand ischemia of unknown etiology. *Ann Surg*. 1977;186:184.

91. Porter JM, Taylor LM. Small artery disease of the upper extremity. *World J Surg*. 1983;7:326.

92. Sanchez NP, Van Hale HM, Su WPD. Clinical and histopathologic spectrum of necrotizing vasculitis: Report of findings in 101 cases. *Arch Dermatol*. 1985;121:220.

93. Wall Bake AWL, Lobatto SS, Jonges L et al. IgA antibodies directed against cytoplasmic antigens of polymorpho-nuclear leukocytes in patients with Henoch-Schönlein purpura. *Adv Exp Med Biol*. 1987;216B:1593.

94. Heng MCY. Henoch-Schönlein purpura. *Br J Dermatol*. 1985;112:235.

95. Taylor LM, Rivers SP, Porter JM. Treatment of finger ischemia with Bier block reserpine. *Surg Gynecol Obstet*. 1982;154:39.

96. Fry WJ, Ernest CB, Stanely JC et al. Renovascular hypertension in the pediatric patient. *Arch Surg*. 1973;107:692.

97. Harrison EG, McCormack LJ. Pathologic classification of renal artery disease in renovascular hypertension. *Mayo Clin Proc*. 1971;46:161.

98. Ehrenfeld WK, Wylie EJ. Fibromuscular dysplasia of the internal carotid artery: Surgical management. *Arch Surg*. 1974;109:676.

99. Morris GC Jr, Lechter A, DeBakey ME. Surgical treatment of fibromuscular disease of the carotid arteries. *Arch Surg*. 1968;96:636.

100. Sandok BA, Houser OW, Baker III et al. Fibromuscular dysplasia: Neurologic disorders associated with disease involving the great vessels in the neck. *Arch Neurol*. 1971;24:462.

101. Stanley JC, Fry WJ, Seeger JF et al. Extracranial internal carotid and vertebral artery fibrodysplasia. *Arch Surg*. 1974;109:215.

102. Wylie EJ, Binkley FM, Palubinskas AJ. Extrarenal fibromuscular hyperplasia. *Am J Surg*. 1966;112:149.

103. Stanley JC, Gewertz BL, Bove EL, Fry WJ. Arterial fibrodysplasia: Histopathologic character and current etiologic concepts. *Arch Surg.* 1975;110:561.

104. Mettinger KL, Ericson K. Fibromuscular dysplasia and the brain. I. Observations on angiographic, clinical and genetic characteristics. *Stroke.* 1982;13:46–52.

105. Rushton AR. The genetics of fibromuscular dysplasia. *Arch Intern Med.* 1980;140:233–236.

106. Olin JW, Froehlich J, Gu X et al. The United States registry for fibromuscular dysplasia: Results in the first 447 patients. *Circulation.* 2012;125:3182–3190.

107. Olin JW, Sealove BA. Diagnosis, management, and future developments of fibromuscular dysplasia. *J Vasc Surg.* 2011 March;53(3):826–836.

108. Barnes RW. Utility of duplex scanning of the renal artery. In: Bergan JJ, Yao JST, eds. *Arterial Surgery: New Diagnostic and Operative Techniques.* Orlando, FL: Grune and Stratton; 1988, pp. 351–366.

109. Hansen KJ, Tribble R, Reavis SW et al. Renal duplex sonography: Evaluation of clinical utility. *J Vasc Surg.* 1990;12:227.

110. Kohler TR, Zierler RE, Martin RI et al. Noninvasive diagnosis of renal artery stenosis by ultrasonic duplex scanning. *J Vasc Surg.* 1986;4:450.

111. Das CJ, Neyaz Z, Thapa P et al. Fibromuscular dysplasia of the renal arteries: A radiological review. *Int Urol Nephrol.* 2007;39(1):233–238.

112. Ernst CB, Stanley JC, Marshall FF et al. Autogenous saphenous vein aortorenal grafts: A ten-year experience. *Arch Surg.* 1972;105:855.

113. Begelman SM, Olin JW. Fibromuscular dysplasia. *Curr Opin Rheumatol.* 2000;12(1):41–47.

114. Tyagi S, Kaul UA, Satsangi DK. Percutaneous transluminal angioplasty for renovascular hypertension in children: Initial and long-term results. *Pediatrics.* 1997;99(1):44.

115. Gewertz BL, Stanley JC, Fry WJ. Renal artery dissections. *Arch Surg.* 1977;112:409.

116. Stanley JC, Zelenock GB, Messina LM, Wakefield TW. Pediatric renovascular hypertension: A thirty-year experience of operative treatment. *J Vasc Surg.* 1995;21(2):212.

117. Trinquart L, Mounier-Vehier C, Sapoval M et al. Efficacy of revascularization for renal artery stenosis caused by fibromuscular dysplasia: A systematic review and meta-analysis. *Hypertension.* 2010;56(3):525–532.

118. Olin JW, Pierce M. Contemporary management of fibromuscular dysplasia. *Curr Opin Cardiol.* 2008;23(6):527–536.

119. Schievink WI. Spontaneous dissection of the carotid and vertebral arteries. *N Engl J Med.* 2001 March 22;344(12):898–906.

120. Georgiadis D, Arnold M, von Buedingen HC et al. Aspirin vs anticoagulation in carotid artery dissection: A study of 298 patients. *Neurology.* 2009;72(21):1810–1815.

121. Mertens J, Daenens K, Fourneau I et al. Fibromuscular dysplasia of the superior mesenteric artery – Case report and review of the literature. *Acta Chir Belg.* 2005;105(5):523–527.

122. Michelis KC, Olin JW, Kadian-Dodov D et al. Coronary artery manifestations of fibromuscular dysplasia. *J Am Coll Cardiol.* 2014 September 9;64(10):1033–1046.

Venous and Lymphatic Disorders

45

Natural history and sequelae of deep vein thrombosis

MERYL A. SIMON and JOHN G. CARSON

CONTENTS

INTRODUCTION

Venous thrombosis, including deep vein thrombosis (DVT) and pulmonary embolism (PE), occurs at an annual incidence of about 1 per 1000 adults. Rates increase sharply after around age 45 years and are slightly higher in men than women of older age. Risk factors, other than age, include surgery, hospitalizations, immobility, trauma, pregnancy, hormone use, cancer, obesity and inherited disorders[1] (see Table 45.1). DVT usually starts in the lower extremities, with the calf veins, often extending into the proximal veins. The DVT may subsequently break free to cause pulmonary emboli. Other major outcomes are death, recurrence, post-thrombotic syndrome (PTS) and major bleeding due to anticoagulation. Thrombosis is also associated with impaired quality of life particularly when PTS develops.[2,3] With DVT, death is reported within one month at 6% and 10% for those with PE.[4] The morbidity impact of thrombosis on the elderly appears to be greater, with a steeper rise in the incidence of PE compared to DVT with aging.[1,5] The development of symptoms depends on the extent of thrombosis, the adequacy of collateral vessels and the severity of associated disease.[6,7]

HISTORY

It was Baille who perhaps first noted the importance of 'stasis' or reduced blood flow as a cause of thrombosis, and Rokitansky subsequently reported that thrombosis occurred in a vein at the site of an injury or adjacent to inflammation. Hunter noted the role of inflammation and infection as causes of thrombi. In 1856, German physician Rudolf Virchow's detailed pathological studies postulated that thrombosis may be caused by a slowing or cessation of blood flow (stasis), increased thrombotic potential of the blood (hypercoagulability) and abnormalities in the vessel wall.[8] Today, these findings are referred to as 'Virchow's triad' (Figure 45.1). Oschner and DeBakey reported that DVT was common after surgical operations and advocated its avoidance and treatment by vein ligation or anticoagulants to prevent PE.[9] Homans had previously advocated vein ligation to prevent PE as a consequence of DVT. He also recognized that the post-thrombotic leg was an important cause of venous ulceration.[10] Homans, Bauer and Linton advocated ligation of the deep veins in patients with post-thrombotic limbs to prevent venous reflux and reduce the risk of recurrent venous ulceration.[11,12]

In 1966, John Gay recognized clot and thrombi in the deep veins of many of the limbs he dissected with venous ulcers, and he was also the first person to recognize the importance of the calf-perforating veins and lipodermatosclerosis.[13]

The advent of anticoagulants, retrieval vena caval filters and advancement in pharmacomechanical thrombolysis are the bases for therapy and further discussion.

EPIDEMIOLOGY AND RISK FACTORS

The pathogenesis of DVT is often related to the factors that compromise Virchow's triad: stasis, hypercoagulability and vascular endothelial damage. Over 100 years ago,

Table 45.1   The epidemiology of venous thromboembolism (VTE).

Summary of the epidemiology of first-time VTE	
Variable	**Finding**
Incidence in total population (Assuming >95% Caucasian)	≈70–113 cases/100,000/year[1,2,11–14]
Age	Exponential increase in VTE with age, particularly after age 40 years[1,2,4,7]
25–35 years old	≈30 cases/100,000 persons
70–79 years old	≈300–500 cases/100,000 persons
Gender	No convincing difference between men and women[1,2]
Race/ethnicity	2.5–4-fold lower risk of VTE in Asian-pacific Islanders and Hispanics[9]
Relative incidence of PE vs. DVT	Absent autopsy diagnosis; ≈ 33% PE; 66% DVT[1,10]
	With autopsy; ≈55% PE, 45% DVT[2,6]
Seasonal variation	Possibly more common in winter and less common in summer[24–26]
Risk factors	≈25%–50% "idiopathic" depending on exact definition
	15%–25% associated with cancer; ≈20% following surgery (3 mo.)[2,5,27]
Recurrent VTE	6-month incidence: ≈7% higher rate in patients with cancer[5,28–30]
	Recurrent PE more likely after PE than after DVT[4,10,31]
Death after treated VTE	30 day incidence ≈6% after incident DVT[2,5,10]
	30 day incidence ≈12% after PE[1,32,33]
	Death strongly associated with cancer, age, and cardiovascular disease

Source: Anderson FA Jr and Spencer FA, *Circulation*, 107(23 Suppl. 1), 2003.

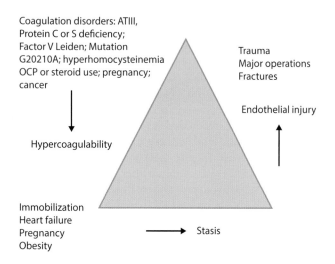

Coagulation disorders: ATIII, Protein C or S deficiency; Factor V Leiden; Mutation G20210A; hyperhomocysteinemia OCP or steroid use; pregnancy; cancer

Trauma
Major operations
Fractures

Endothelial injury

Hypercoagulability

Immobilization
Heart failure
Pregnancy
Obesity

Stasis

Figure 45.1   Coagulation disorders. (From Original artwork created by Meryl Simon, Division of Vascular Surgery, University of California, Davis. Sacramento, CA, 2015.)

Virchow proposed that abnormalities of this triad were found in patients with thrombosis. Factors that exacerbate one of these elements will increase a patient's risk for developing a DVT (see Table 45.2).

Risk factors can be classified as hereditary or acquired. Hypercoagulable states can arise from disorders of the coagulation cascade. This cascade consists of highly regulated proteins that control both the formation and dissolution of thrombus. Understanding this cascade has allowed us to not only identify effective means of thromboembolic treatment but additionally isolate congenital disorders of coagulation.

Table 45.2   Risk factors of venous thromboembolism.

Strong risk factors (odds ratio >10)
    Fracture (hip or leg)
    Hip or knee replacement
    Major general surgery
    Major trauma
    Spinal cord injury
Moderate risk factors (odds ratio 2–9)
    Arthroscopic knee surgery
    Central venous lines
    Chemotherapy
    Congestive heart or respiratory failure
    Hormone replacement therapy
    Malignancy
    Oral contraceptive therapy
    Paralytic stoke
    Pregnancy/postpartum
    Previous venous thromboembolism
    Thrombophilia
Weak risk factors (odds ratio <2)
    Bed rest >3 days
    Immobility due to sitting (e.g. prolonged car or air travel)
    Increasing age
    Laparoscopic surgery (e.g. cholecystectomy)
    Obesity
    Pregnancy/antepartum
    Varicose veins

Source: Anderson FA Jr and Spencer FA, *Circulation*, 107(23 Suppl. 1), 2003.

Deficiencies of the naturally occurring inhibitors of the cascade are some of the more common congenital states.[14]

Anti-thrombin deficiency occurs in 0.2% of the general population and in 0.5%–7.5% of patients presenting with venous thromboembolism (VTE). Even mild levels of anti-thrombin deficiency are associated with venous thrombosis, and over 60% with the deficiency will have an event before the age of 60.

Protein C deficiency is another congenital state associated with venous thrombosis. Activated protein C is a potent anticoagulant, which inactivates factors Va and VIIIa. Deficiency of protein C is also found in about 0.2% of the population and in 2.5%–6% of patients with venous thrombosis. For protein C to function properly, the cofactor protein S must be present. Thus, a deficiency of protein S will present similarly to protein C deficiency.

The most common congenital disorder of coagulation occurs when factor V is resistant to protein C inactivation. This is known as activated protein C resistance or factor V Leiden. Factor V Leiden is present in 5% of the general population and is seen in 10% of patients presenting with venous thrombosis. Fortunately, most patients with factor V Leiden will not experience a thrombotic event, unless additional risk factors, such as post-operative states, come into play.

Another common congenital prothrombotic state is the prothrombin gene mutation G20210A. This mutation is associated with elevated levels of prothrombin at baseline. Approximately 4% of the general population carries this mutation, and it is found in 5%–10% of patients presenting with venous thrombosis.

Hyperhomocysteinemia is an additional risk factor for venous thrombosis and can be congenital or acquired. Hyperhomocysteinemia can be related to a gene mutation or seen in vitamin deficiencies (B6 or B12). Hyperhomocysteinemia can also be associated with arterial thrombotic events.

Many acquired risk factors have been elucidated over the last several decades. Advancing age, male gender, malignancy, obesity, tobacco use, heart failure, immobilization, surgery, trauma and prior thrombotic events make up just some those identified.

Anderson et al. discovered that the three most common risk factors for hospitalized patients were age over 40, obesity and major surgery. In fact, older patients were often found to have more risk factors for DVT than younger patients. Their study reported that 3 or more risk factors were found in 30% of patients over 40, but in only 3% of patients younger than 40.[15] The impact of age on DVT risk is likely multifactorial. VTE is rare in young children. In addition to advancing age being associated with an increased number of risk factors, there is probably a physiologic component as well.

Immobilization after major surgery or trauma is a well-known risk for DVT. Major surgery can encompass abdominal and thoracic procedures, urologic and gynecologic procedures and neurosurgery, but intracranial surgery is often a contradiction to anticoagulation. Lower extremity orthopedic operations carry a particularly high risk for venous thrombosis. Without prophylaxis, about half of all patients undergoing an elective total knee or hip replacement will develop a VTE. Extremity fractures convey a high risk, especially after cast immobilization. For example, tibial fractures carry a VTE rate of 45%, but with only 1/3 being symptomatic.[16] In a study of immobilized trauma, patients were on bed rest for 10 days or longer, a silent DVT was identified in 60%, and in over half of these patients, the thrombi extended above the level of the knee.[17] While assessing risk factors for DVT and PE, Heit et al. found that the risk of VTE was 22-fold higher for patients who had undergone recent surgery, over 12-fold higher for recent trauma and 8-fold higher for any hospitalized or nursing home patient.[18] Prolonged travel has also been associated with DVT formation, and in 1988, this connection was even dubbed the 'economy class syndrome' by Cruickshank et al..[19] Sitting on the edge of a seat for prolonged periods increases stasis by decreasing venous blood flow as well as increasing pressure of the back of calves. In one case-controlled study, investigators found that travel greater than 4 hours in any form represented a risk factor for VTE.[20]

Malignancy and treatment of the disease are well-recognized risk factors for thrombosis. One study found that cancer alone was associated with a 4.1-fold increased risk, while chemotherapy increased that risk to 6.5-fold. Additionally, a VTE may be the first presentation of cancer in a patient. About 10% of patients presenting with an idiopathic VTE are subsequently diagnosed with cancer within 5–10 years, but the majority, >75%, are diagnosed within the first year.[21]

Oral contraceptives create a hypercoagulable state that can also lead to VTE. Dating back to case reports in the 1960s, oral contraception has been identified as an independent risk factor, often quoted with odds ratio of 3–6 times that of non-users.[22] Despite lower doses of the ethinyl estradiol component of more modern contraception, the risk still remains, yet for an otherwise healthy young woman, the absolute risk of VTE is relatively low, about 20–40/100,000 users. For contraceptive use in women with congenital hypercoagulable states, such as protein C or anti-thrombin deficiency, as well as advanced age, the risk becomes much greater. A retrospective family cohort study found that the annual incidence of VTE in deficient women on contraception was 1.64% vs. 0.18% in non-deficient women. They found the risk to be highest for anti-thrombin deficiency, at 2.06%, versus 1.89% for protein C deficiency and 1.01% for protein S deficiency[23] (see Figure 45.2).

Pregnancy is associated with an increased risk of VTE. Fortunately, this risk is low, but PE does remain the leading cause of maternal death after childbirth.[16] DVT risk during pregnancy is likely due to a combination of a hypercoagulable state and increased stasis as the pregnant uterus may impair venous outflow due to external compression.

Inflammatory and autoimmune disorders have been found to be associated with increased thrombosis risk. These patients present with higher VTE rates compared to the general population. Two examples of disease states

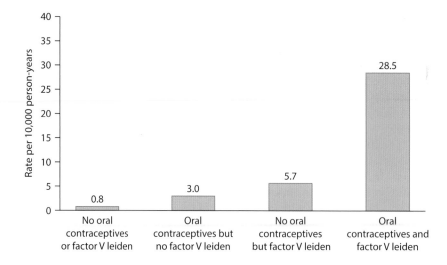

Figure 45.2 Cases of deep-vein thrombosis per 10,000 person-years, according to the use of oral contraceptives and the presence of factor V Leiden. (From Vandenbroucke JP, *N Engl J Med.*, 344, 1527, 2001.)

with higher VTE rates include systemic lupus erythematosus (SLE) and inflammatory bowel diseases (IBDs). In one study that looked at DVT in symptomatic outpatients, SLE was associated with an odds ratio of 4.3 for patients with the disease versus those without.[24] Another reviewed over 13,000 patients with IBD and compared them to matched controls and found that the risk of VTE was 2.6/1000 for IBD patients. Additionally, during times of acute IBD flare, that risk rose to 9/1000.[25]

One risk factor not previously discussed is central venous catheters. Catheters can be life-saving interventions: providing fluids and medications, hemodynamic monitoring or allowing for hemodialysis, but they are not without risk. One study found femoral vein catheterization to be associated with a 25% frequency of lower extremity DVT.[26] The type of central venous catheter plays a role in its own thrombotic risk as well. Catheters made of polyethylene are associated with greater thrombosis than those made of silicon or polyurethane. Thrombosis tends to increase with the greater number of lumens of the catheter, as well as catheter duration, and vascular trauma incurred during placement.[27]

PATHOGENESIS

As discussed previously, a clot may form whenever blood flow is altered. Often, two of the three Virchow's triad factors must come into play for a thrombus to develop. Thrombi are composed primarily of erythrocytes and fibrin, with interspersed platelets and leukocytes. The majority of symptomatic DVTs will begin in the calf veins, but symptoms are often uncommon until there is extension into the proximal veins. In the absence of treatment, 25% of these isolated distal DVTs will extend to involve the proximal veins.[7]

The initial clot will expand – eventually leading to venous occlusion.[28] Once the clot becomes adherent to the vessel wall, the local inflammatory response initiates

thrombus organization with subsequent contraction. The body's natural lysis system will begin to break down the clot, finally leading to vessel recanalization. This process takes time, and duplex scanning with B-mode imaging can depict these processes. The vein segment will proceed from a no-flow state with occlusion, through augmentable flow on distal compression, to continuous flow with partial obstruction, finally returning to phasic flow if and when full patency is regained[29] (see Figures 45.1 and 45.2).

The process of venous thrombus resolution is similar to that of wound healing. Studies with animal models have

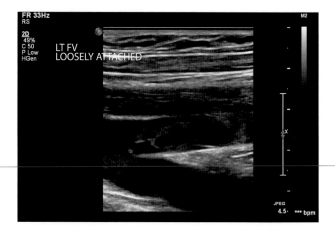

Image 45.1 This is a B-mode image of fresh free-floating thrombus in a left common femoral vein from a 47-year-old man involved in a motorcycle collision. Readmission 3 weeks after trauma discharge with shortness of breath and chest pain. Diagnosed with massive bilateral pulmonary embolism as well as left lower extremity deep vein thrombosis. Underwent pulmonary angiography with angiojet thrombectomy of his right pulmonary artery as well as inferior vena cava filter placement. (Image from University of California, Davis Vascular Laboratory, Sacramento, CA, 2012.)

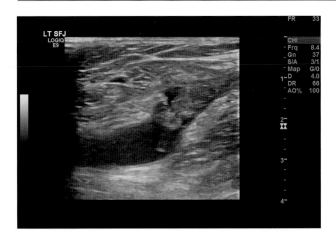

Image 45.2 This is a B-mode image of a woman several days after great saphenous vein (GSV) ablation. It depicts thrombus in the GSV extending into the common femoral vein, also known as endothermal heat-induced thrombosis (EHIT). (Image from University of California, Davis Vascular Laboratory, Sacramento, CA, 2015.)

shown that soon after thrombus formation, neutrophils influx into the vein wall, which are later joined by macrophages, leukocytes and fibroblasts – forming the local inflammatory response phase. The recruited neutrophils not only adhere to the endothelium of the affected vein wall but also migrate through the wall, exposing the basement membrane. This exposure provides a thrombogenic surface, furthering clot formation. Neutrophils and leukocytes will also enter the affected venous segment by means of the vasa vasorum, leading to involvement of all three layers of the vein wall.[30] The monocytes involved in the inflammatory phase likely play a key role in thrombus resolution by expressing plasminogen activators – thus initiating the body's natural thrombolysis pathway. Additionally, monocytes can degrade fibrin in the absence of plasmin. Both of these pathways begin the natural resolution of the thrombus.[31]

Although early in thrombus formation neutrophils play a thrombogenic role, they also likely play a critical role in thrombus resolution. In rat model investigations, neutrophils appeared to help promote fibrinolysis by releasing collagenases, such as metalloproteinases 8 and 9, which actively break down collagen. They also appear to release their own plasminogen activator. Plasminogen activator inhibitor-1 is the chief inhibitor for plasminogen activators, and this is degraded by neutrophil elastase.[32]

Vessel recanalization actually begins quiet rapidly after venous occlusion occurs. One study, using duplex scanning, showed recanalization to occur in as early as seven days after initial presentation. By 3 months, the average residual obstruction was less than 20%. Additionally, 50% of patients showed recanalization of all previously occluded segments. This recanalization opens up channels for venous outflow for the acutely thrombosed extremity.[33] The previously mentioned inflammatory cells

likely play an important role in this spontaneous vessel recanalization.

POST-THROMBOTIC SYNDROME

PTS is the number one long-term complication following DVT. PTS is a form of chronic venous insufficiency and may present with a wide range of symptoms including but not limited to leg heaviness, pain, fatigue, edema, pruritus, varicosities, hyperpigmentation, eczema and even ulceration. Venous claudication may even develop, in which patients describe a bursting sensation with ambulation, due to chronic venous obstruction. One study showed that almost 44% of patients with prior iliofemoral DVT developed venous claudication, and walking was interrupted in 15%.[34] As many as 50% of patients with a DVT may develop PTS sequelae, and about 10% will develop severe PTS, which include venous ulcers. PTS results from a combination of outflow obstruction combined with vein valve damage leading to venous reflux. The end result is venous hypertension.[35] This is a process that evolves over time. PTS is a clinical diagnosis, and treatment should really be focused on prevention of further disease progression and ulcer management if applicable. Unfortunately, PTS may occur even in the face of optimal anticoagulation therapy. Routine use of early thrombolytic therapy in preventing PTS has yet to be proven.[36] Risk factors for the development of PTS include extent of the DVT (such as into the common femoral or iliac vein), severity of residual thrombus at 1 month, prior DVT, obesity, advanced age and female gender.[37] Although DVT treatment will be discussed in another chapter, compression therapy has been found to be key in PTS prevention. A 2004 randomized controlled trial evaluated the efficacy of below-knee compression in preventing PTS in patients with a first-time proximal DVT. They found that long-term compression use (of 2 years) leads to a decrease in the incidence of PTS by almost 50%, as well as decreasing rates from 49% to 26% upon 5-year follow-up. More importantly, the incidence of severe sequelae decreased from 12% to 3.5%.[38] Identifying patients at increased risk for DVT and preventing thrombosis from occurring is primary prevention for PTS occurrence.

DEFICIENCIES IN CURRENT KNOWLEDGE AND AREAS OF FUTURE RESEARCH

- Identification of patients with risk factors who may need anticoagulation without symptoms
- Prevention and treatment of venous valve injury and chronic fibrinolytic changes in deep veins
- Identification of those at risk for developing the PTS
- Identification of the best medical or surgical therapy in the acute stage of DVT with the aim to prevent the PTS

REFERENCES

1. Cushman M. Epidemiology and risk factors for venous thrombosis. *Semin Hematol.* 2007;44(2):62–69.

2. van Korlaar IM, Vossen CY, Rosendaal FR et al. The impact of venous thrombosis on quality of life. *Thromb Res.* 2004;114(1):11–18.

3. Kahn SR, Ducruet T, Lamping DL et al. Prospective evaluation of health-related quality of life in patients with deep venous thrombosis. *Arch Intern Med.* 2005;165(10):1173–1178.

4. Cushman M, Tsai AW, White RH et al. Deep vein thrombosis and pulmonary embolism in two cohorts: The longitudinal investigation of thromboembolism etiology. *Am J Med.* 2004;117(1):19–25.

5. Silverstein MD, Heit JA, Mohr DN et al. Trends in the incidence of deep vein thrombosis and pulmonary embolism: A 25-year population-based study. *Arch Intern Med.* 1998;158(6):585–593.

6. Nicolaides AN, Kakkar VV, Field ES et al. The origin of deep vein thrombosis: A venographic study. *Br J Radiol.* 1971;44(525):653–663.

7. Kearon C. Natural history of venous thromboembolism. *Circulation.* 2003;107(23 Suppl. 1):I22–I30.

8. Virchow RR. *Cellular Pathology.* London, UK: Churchill, 1860.

9. Oschner AD, DeBakey M. Therapy of phlebothrombosis and thrombophlebitis. *Surgeon.* 1939;8(269).

10. Homans J. The aetiology and treatment of varicose ulcers of the leg. *Surg Gynecol Obstet.* 1917;24(300).

11. Bauer G. Division of popliteal vein in the treatment of so-called varicose ulceration. *Br Med J.* 1950;2(4674):318–321.

12. Bauer G. Indications for popliteal vein ligation. *J Cardiovasc Surg (Torino).* 1963;4:18–22.

13. Gay J. On varicose disease of the lower extremities. In: *Lettsomian Lecture.* London, UK: Churchill, 1866.

14. Crowther MA, Kelton JG. Congenital thrombophilic states associated with venous thrombosis: A qualitative overview and proposed classification system. *Ann Intern Med.* 2003;138:128–134.

15. Anderson FA Jr, Wheeler HB, Goldberg RJ et al. The prevalence of risk factors for venous thromboembolism among hospital patients. *Arch Intern Med.* 1992;152(8):1660–1664.

16. Anderson FA Jr, Spencer FA. Risk factors for venous thromboembolism. *Circulation.* 2003;107(23 Suppl. 1):I9–I16.

17. Kudsk KA, Fabian TC, Baum S et al. Silent deep vein thrombosis in immobilized multiple trauma patients. *Am J Surg.* 1989;158(6):515–519.

18. Heit JA, Silverstein MD, Mohr DN et al. Risk factors for deep vein thrombosis and pulmonary embolism: A population-based case-control study. *Arch Intern Med.* 2000;160(6):809–815.

19. Cruickshank JM, Gorlin R, Jennett B. Air travel and thrombotic episodes: The economy class syndrome. *Lancet.* 1988;2(8609):497–498.

20. Ferrari E, Chevallier T, Chapelier A et al. Travel as a risk factor for venous thromboembolic disease: A case-control study. *Chest.* 1999;115(2):440–444.

21. Lee AY, Levine MN. Venous thromboembolism and cancer: Risks and outcomes. *Circulation.* 2003;107(23 Suppl. 1):I17–I21.

22. Vandenbroucke JP, Rosing J, Bloemenkamp KW et al. Oral contraceptives and the risk of venous thrombosis. *N Engl J Med.* 2001;344(20):1527–1535.

23. van Vlijmen EF, Brouwer JL, Veeger NJ et al. Oral contraceptives and the absolute risk of venous thromboembolism in women with single or multiple thrombophilic defects: Results from a retrospective family cohort study. *Arch Intern Med.* 2007;167(3):282–289.

24. Cogo A, Bernardi E, Prandoni P et al. Acquired risk factors for deep-vein thrombosis in symptomatic outpatients. *Arch Intern Med.* 1994;154(2):164–168.

25. Grainge MJ, West J, Card TR. Venous thromboembolism during active disease and remission in inflammatory bowel disease: A cohort study. *Lancet.* 2010;375(9715):657–663.

26. Trottier SJ, Veremakis C, O'Brien J et al. Femoral deep vein thrombosis associated with central venous catheterization: Results from a prospective, randomized trial. *Crit Care Med.* 1995;23(1):52–59.

27. Rooden CJ, Tesselaar ME, Osanto S et al. Deep vein thrombosis associated with central venous catheters – a review. *J Thromb Haemost.* 2005;3(11):2409–2419.

28. Mammen EF. Pathogenesis of venous thrombosis. *Chest.* 1992;102(6 Suppl.):640S–644S.

29. van Ramshorst B, van Bemmelen PS, Hoeneveld H et al. Thrombus regression in deep venous thrombosis. Quantification of spontaneous thrombolysis with duplex scanning. *Circulation.* 1992;86(2):414–419.

30. Wakefield TW, Strieter RM, Wilke CA et al. Venous thrombosis-associated inflammation and attenuation with neutralizing antibodies to cytokines and adhesion molecules. *Arterioscler Thromb Vasc Biol.* 1995;15(2):258–268.

31. Humphries J, McGuinness CL, Smith A et al. Monocyte chemotactic protein-1 (MCP-1) accelerates the organization and resolution of venous thrombi. *J Vasc Surg.* 1999;30(5):894–899.

32. Varma MR, Varga AJ, Knipp BS et al. Neutropenia impairs venous thrombosis resolution in the rat. *J Vasc Surg.* 2003;38(5):1090–1098.

33. Killewich LA, Bedford GR, Beach KW et al. Spontaneous lysis of deep venous thrombi: Rate and outcome. *J Vasc Surg.* 1989;9(1):89–97.

34. Delis KT, Bountouroglou D, Mansfield AO. Venous claudication in iliofemoral thrombosis: Long-term effects on venous hemodynamics, clinical status, and quality of life. *Ann Surg.* 2004;239(1):118–126.

35. Kahn SR, Comerota AJ, Cushman M et al. The post-thrombotic syndrome: Evidence-based prevention, diagnosis, and treatment strategies: A scientific statement from the American Heart Association. *Circulation*. 2014;130(18):1636–1661.

36. Prandoni P, Kahn SR. Post-thrombotic syndrome: Prevalence, prognostication and need for progress. *Br J Haematol*. 2009;145(3):286–295.

37. Kahn SR, Shrier I, Julian JA et al. Determinants and time course of the postthrombotic syndrome after acute deep venous thrombosis. *Ann Intern Med*. 2008;149(10):698–707.

38. Prandoni P, Lensing AW, Prins MH et al. Below-knee elastic compression stockings to prevent the post-thrombotic syndrome: A randomized, controlled trial. *Ann Intern Med*. 2004;141(4):249–256.

46

Pathophysiology of chronic venous disease

SESHADRI RAJU

CONTENTS

INTRODUCTION

Chronic venous disease (CVD) has been recognized since antiquity, a millennium before arterial disease. Paradoxically, the pathophysiology of cardiac and arterial disease is much better understood than many aspects of CVD. An impediment to progress is the sheer weight of enormous accumulated literature steeped in dogma that has retarded a rational approach. A comprehensive classification of the polymorphous disease – a necessity for methodical research – has emerged only recently. Considerable progress has occurred since, coincidentally, with emergence of newer imaging techniques to explore the disease. Yet, much remains poorly understood. The pathophysiology of the disease is presented herein based on the framework of the *c*linical stage, *e*tiology, *a*natomy and *p*athology (CEAP) classification.

CLINICAL STAGE, ETIOLOGY, ANATOMY AND PATHOLOGY CLASSIFICATION

Clinical stages

A simplified version of the CEAP classification is shown in Table 46.1.[1] Various components of the classification allow for over 1000 potential combinations. However, many potential combinations do not occur in practice, and some occur more frequently. Common clinical patterns are shown in Table 46.2 – although the clinical class in the CEAP classification is based in order of clinical severity. Clinical progression does occur stepwise in

the hierarchy in many patients, but some patients present with advanced disease apparently without progressing through preceding clinical stages. Longitudinal level 1 studies are lacking for better understanding of disease progression.

Etiology

The etiology of CVD can be divided into 'primary' (non-thrombotic), secondary (post-thrombotic) and congenital causes. Congenital anomalies of the venous segments such as agenesis and valve dysplasia can lead to obstructive and reflux CVD disease, respectively. They are thought to represent about 5% of all CVD pathologies. The relative prevalence of primary and secondary CVD is variably reported from large centres. Prevalence estimates are imprecise because complete thrombus resolution may obscure the original pathology. Primary obstruction (May–Thurner syndrome) is known to result in secondary thrombosis, further complicating analysis.

The majority of varices are primary in origin with variable genetic, hormonal and degenerative influences that predispose to it. Recent evidence indicates that reflux-mediated inflammation of valve cusps may lead to aberration of collagen synthesis from an excess of metalloproteinases resulting in abnormal wall structure – a heterogeneous vein with hypertrophied inelastic segments interspersed with atrophied portions results typical of varices.[2,3] Valve damage including complete dissolution may occur.

Varices increase with age and are more common in women. Like other venous pathologies, they occur more

Table 46.1 Clinical stage, etiology, anatomy and pathology classification: summary.

Clinical	Etiologic	Anatomic	Pathophysiologic
C0: no visible or palpable signs of venous disease	**Ec:** congenital	**As:** superficial veins	**Pr:** reflux
C1: telangiectasies or reticular veins	**Ep:** primary	**Ap:** perforator veins	**Po:** obstruction
C2: varicose veins	**Es:** secondary (post-thrombotic)	**Ad:** deep veins	**Pr,o:** reflux and obstruction
C3: edema	**En:** no venous cause identified	**An:** no venous location identified	**Pn:** no venous pathophysiology identifiable
C4a: pigmentation or eczema			
C4b: lipodermatosclerosis or atrophic blanche			
C5: healed venous ulcer			
C6: active venous ulcer			
S: symptomatic			
A: asymptomatic			

Table 46.2 Common clinical patterns in chronic venous insufficiency (CVI).

Clinical pattern	Symptoms and presentation
Varices	
Uncomplicated	Cosmetic or health concerns or both.
With local symptoms	Pain is confined to the varices and is not diffuse.
With local complications	Superficial thrombophlebitis, internal rupture with hematoma or external rupture through a 'pinpoint' ulcer.
Complex varicose disease	Diffuse limb pain, ankle swelling, skin changes or ulcer.
Venous hypertension syndrome	Severe orthostatic venous pain; patients are often young or middle-aged; other features of CVI are minimal or absent.
Venous leg swelling	Other features of CVI may be absent or variable; swelling may be bilateral. Iliac vein obstruction is common.
Complex multisystem venous disease	Clinical features of advanced CVI (i.e. pain, swelling, stasis dermatitis) or ulceration present in varying combinations. Multisystem involvement with combined obstruction reflux involvement.

commonly in the left lower limb. Older 'ascending' and 'descending' theories of varix formation resulting from successive valve failures from perforators or sapheno-femoral junction are now discounted based on the finding that varices are polycentric in origin in the limb.[4]

Anatomy

Anatomically, the disease may involve the superficial venous system, the perforator system, the deep system or frequently all three in advanced disease.[5] Isolated perforator incompetence without involvement of superficial and/or deep system is very rare in symptomatic patients.[6] Valves occur infrequently above the inguinal ligament. Valves in the iliac vein and the common femoral vein can be found in about 20% and 50% of limbs, respectively, and are thought to play a role in saphenous reflux.[6,7] In reflux of the great saphenous vein, the sapheno-femoral

valve is commonly involved. In about 10%, the valve is competent with reflux entering the vein through a perforator or tributary (escape point) lower down. Valves become more frequent in distal deep venous segments and are most numerous in the crural veins, teleologically designed to protect against the increased orthostatic venous pressure because of the gravity component.[8] This design is functionally useful only with calf pump contraction when valves close to maintain the lowered pressure in the calf. The lower pressure prevails for up to 20 seconds or more before recovery through arterial inflow. The foot pump also ejects venous volume, arguably priming the calf pump through foot perforators (many are avalvular) for sequential action during walking.[9] The thigh muscles, though more bulky than in the calf, play only an accessory role. Reflux obviously short-circuits this pressure reduction arrangement. Clinical focus has centred on refluxive valves in the femoro-popliteal segments which can be repaired to induce remission of symptoms. Controversy persists if more distal valves, particularly the popliteal valve, are not functionally more important in guarding the all-important calf pump from venous hypertension.[10] Clinical experience in repair of the more distal valves is limited, and level I evidence to support the notion of the popliteal valve in its 'gatekeeper' function is lacking. Reflux in the superficial system also compromises the calf pump due to premature refilling of the calf pump through perforators. Perforator valves are designed to prevent outward flow from the deep system into superficial veins, but bidirectional flow has been observed in perforators near the ankle in normal individuals.[11] Because of this observation and also because consistent hemodynamic improvement has not been demonstrated after perforator interruption procedures, controversy surrounds the utility of such procedures.[10] The issue is far from settled, as perforator ablation directly underneath the ulcer has been clinically useful in healing the ulcer in several studies.[12,13]

Pathology

Primary CVD has hitherto mainly focused on valve reflux. The cause of primary valve reflux is degenerative, resulting in lax and redundant valve cusps.[14] Abnormal collagen and elastin synthesis from inflammation of the cusps may originate and amplify this cycle.[2,3] Modern imaging techniques such as intravascular ultrasound have now established that an obstructive element in the iliac vein is frequently present in symptomatic CVD patients of the primary variety (Figure 46.1).[15]

Most post-thrombotic diseases are now known to be associated with a combination of obstruction and reflux.[16] The obstruction is a result of inadequate resolution of thrombus which quickly organizes into fibrotic tissue evolving into obstructive trabeculae. The term 'chronic thrombus' is a misnomer – the initial thrombus has turned into non-dissolvable fibrous tissue in a few weeks after onset. Post-thrombotic reflux results from entrapment or varying degrees of damage to the valve cusps; in some cases, the valve may survive thrombus resolution, but the intense mural and perivenous post-thrombotic fibrosis may result in valve station restriction resulting in relative valve cusp redundancy and reflux (Figure 46.2).[17] The inflammatory cascade that involves the venous segment after a thrombotic insult has not been fully appreciated.[18,19]

Relative importance of obstruction and reflux

It is now clear that most patients (≥80%) with advanced CVD whether primary or secondary in origin have a combination of obstruction and reflux in the deep system. An

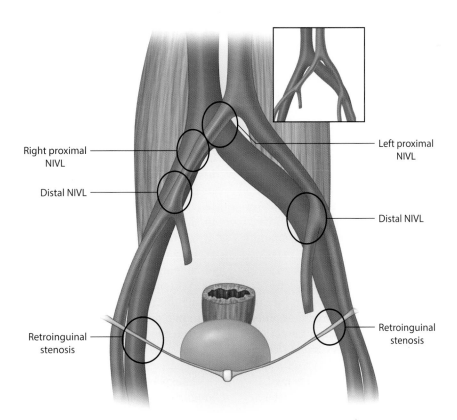

Right proximal NIVL

Distal NIVL

Retroinguinal stenosis

Left proximal NIVL

Distal NIVL

Retroinguinal stenosis

Figure 46.1 Sites of obstruction in iliac veins on IVUS examination. They generally occur behind arterial crossover points or the inguinal ligament. These lesions occur on both sides and in all age groups.

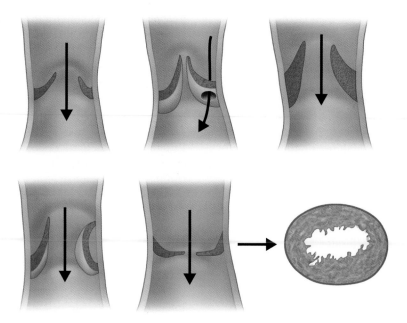

Figure 46.2 Mechanism of post-thrombotic reflux. Various degrees of valve cusp damage result in reflux. In some cases, valve cusps are relatively undamaged, but become redundant and refluxive due to valve station fibrosis and restriction.

unsolved problem is the relative importance of obstruction and reflux in these subsets with combined pathologies. Success with anti-reflux procedures such as valve reconstruction is now well documented in large series of primary as well as post-thrombotic disease.[20,21] Because of the high prevalence of obstruction in these subsets, it is certain that a significant proportion of patients in the reported series had undiagnosed underlying obstruction. Similarly, excellent symptom remission has been reported with stent correction of iliac vein stenosis in patients with known associated severe reflux that remained uncorrected.[22] It appears that partial correction of venous pathology in advanced CVD can lead to symptom remission even though residual obstruction or reflux remains uncorrected.

A related puzzle is the well-documented fact that ≈30% of the general population appear to have significant obstruction of the iliac-caval segments but remain asymptomatic.[23,24] Yet, the ubiquitous lesion is even more prevalent in symptomatic patients and its correction leads to relief of symptoms.[15] A plausible explanation is that the obstructive element behaves as a permissive pathology remaining silent until additional insult of trauma, thrombosis, infection or reflux precipitates symptoms. Many such permissive pathologies occur in human disease. Carotid stenosis and ureteric obstruction that may remain silent until additional insults unmask the lesions are parallel examples.

Conductance in venous conduits

The importance of resistance and conductance (its reciprocal) in the arterial system is well known. Resistance is inversely proportional to the *fourth power* of the radius, explaining why arterioles are the major contributor to peripheral resistance. A reduction in radius of a vessel by 1/2 will not halve the flow but result in a flow reduction (conductance) of 1/16 the original flow under the same pressure gradient. The exponential change in flow related to calibre is relevant in venous hemodynamics as well as both in reflux and collateral flow. Because of the low velocities, the Reynolds number is low. Any turbulence related to stenosis or reflux is transient and Poiseuille flow characteristics predominate. For example, a refluxive saphenous vein of a given size carries reverse flow much less than its maximum potential indicated by its size, probably because of the relative small calibre of re-entry perforators. A refluxive saphenous vein 6 mm in size will require 81 re-entry perforators each 2 mm in size to equal its conductance. Reflux limitation likely occurs in perforator reflux as well. Only a small fraction of calf pump flow will escape through a refluxive perforator if the main femoro-popliteal pathway is open because of the discrepancy in size (by 3–4 X). Saphenous flow draining refluxive perforators have normal pressures. Clinical effects of perforator reflux must depend on other factors such as shear and not on pressure overloading of the superficial system.

The exponential reduction in conductance with size also limits collateral flow. A total of 256 collaterals each 4 mm in size will be required to equal the flow of a 16 mm common iliac vein under the same pressure gradient. This explains why many patients with iliac vein obstruction and seemingly profuse collaterals remain symptomatic. When the

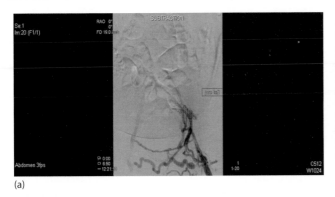

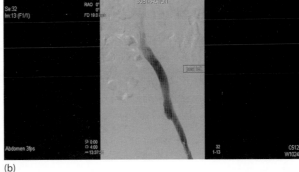

(a)   (b)

Figure 46.3 Chronic total occlusion of the common iliac vein (a) with collaterals. Collaterals disappear when a stent is inserted, opening up a lower resistance pathway for venous outflow (b).

iliac vein lesion is stented opening a large outflow pathway, the collaterals promptly disappear (Figure 46.3).

Collaterals

The process of collateral formation in the venous system is poorly understood. Collaterals can be demonstrated on venography only in about a third of patients with iliac vein obstruction.[15] The higher viscosity of contrast which retards flow rate is only a partial explanation. Many other factors in collateral formation such as shear rate, intra-abdominal pressure and valves in tributary collaterals remain to be explored.

There is regional variation in collateral formation and function. After femoral vein occlusion, the profunda femoris vein rapidly enlarges, often reaching the size of the femoral vein.[25] It is often mistaken for the native femoral vein because of anatomic similarity (Figure 46.4). The profunda femoris is the embryologic axial vein later replaced by the femoral vein to take on this role. A high-resistance connection between the two persists at the popliteal level. The connection is visible as early as a few hours after onset of femoral vein occlusion and rapidly enlarges in a few months to replace femoral vein flow. An axially transformed profunda femoris vein can be found in some patients without symptoms. Valve orientation favouring profunda collateral flow may explain its rapid development.

Such natural collaterals based on embryologic development also appear to occur in occlusions of the inferior vena cava (IVC).[26] An absent IVC is an occasional incidental finding on imaging studies carried out in asymptomatic patients for other reasons. The azygos and hemiazygos veins enlarge to provide collateral flow, sometimes giving the appearance of 'double' IVC (Figure 46.5). Curiously, one of the two azygos systems is often inadequate as ≈70% of patients with IVC occlusion present with unilateral symptoms. The ipsilateral iliac vein appears to be the key for symptom production, as most collaterals in IVC occlusions arise from this location. Some patients presenting

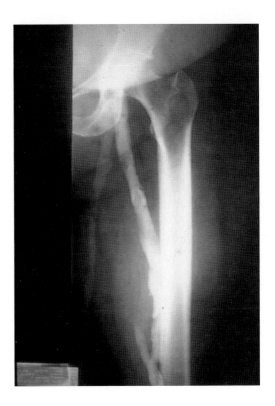

Figure 46.4 Axial transformation of profunda femoral vein, which connects with the popliteal vein near the knee. Note the remnant stump of the occluded femoral vein above the profunda/popliteal junction.

with extensive iliac-caval thrombosis have an underlying absent IVC as the initiating cause. This becomes apparent when the iliac segments are cleared of thrombus but the IVC remains occluded after lysis. A subset of these patients becomes asymptomatic after clearance of the iliac vein despite the occluded IVC.

Collateralization is relatively poor in iliac vein occlusions compared to the femoral and IVC occlusions. It is rarer to find patients with chronic occlusions of the iliac vein without symptoms. Collateralization is through

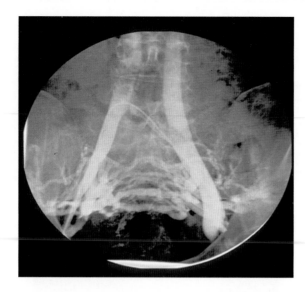

Figure 46.5 Venogram of a 'double' inferior vena cava. The appearance is due to stenosis or occlusion of the main inferior vena cava and the enlargement of hemiazygys-a natural collateral.

tributaries arising from uninvolved iliac-femoral segments below the occlusion. These may include femoral, pudendal, hypogastric, transpelvic and ascending lumbar collaterals depending upon the level of iliac occlusion. In all instances, these are not 'natural' collaterals, as flow in these tributaries has to reverse against valves.

Hemodynamics of obstruction and reflux

There is a fundamental difference between arterial and venous stenosis in clinical impact.[27] The critical element in arterial stenosis is downstream perfusion which may not be affected until stenosis exceeds 70% of normal lumen in many arterial beds. The critical element (relevant to symptom production) is not perfusion but upstream (peripheral) venous pressure. In experimental models, as little as 10% stenosis begins to raise the pressure in the periphery. The critical degree of iliac vein stenosis is influenced by intra-abdominal pressure.

Overall lower limb flow is generally not diminished in most cases of chronic iliac vein obstruction but there is peripheral venous hypertension due to flow through higher resistance collaterals. A simplistic analogy is river flow going over a dam. The flow is the same as before but a reservoir (congestion) forms behind the dam. After stent correction of iliac vein obstruction, overall flow does not increase, but there is decompression of the limb veins with faster velocity due to reduction in their calibre from the decongestion.

In venous obstruction, there is chronic elevation of resting venous pressure. In reflux, resting pressures are normal but duration of pressure reduction during ambulation

is abbreviated. The relative importance of these two types of aberrations is unknown.

The pathophysiology of reflux is not well understood and sometimes misunderstood. It is often stated that reflux defeats 'column segmentation'. It can be shown in a simple experimental model that reflux does not transmit column pressure until after the reflux ceases.[28] If the column pressure is immediately transmitted with onset of reflux, reflux will stop immediately as the pressure gradient inducing the reflux will vanish. It is more appropriate to say that reflux shortens the *duration* of column segmentation. With calf pump action, ejection takes place simultaneously through superficial and deep veins, the popliteal valve closes and the veins below collapse. There is a steep pressure reduction in the collapsed veins below the closed popliteal valve, while the popliteal pressure above the valve remains unchanged with minor undulations. The duration of low pressure in the calf pump is 20 seconds or more until refill from arterial inflow restores the pressure. Reflux results in premature refilling of the calf pump shortening the pressure recovery time (VFT); often, the extent of pressure reduction in the calf is also less leading to the term 'ambulatory venous hypertension' for this premature pressure recovery. Other aspects of calf pump function besides reflux can also result in ambulatory venous hypertension (see later).

Clinical measurement of obstruction and reflux

It has been difficult to measure the degree of obstruction for clinical use. Pressure-based techniques such as arm/foot pressure differential, reactive hyperemia test, outflow fraction measurement and resistance calculation from flow measurements have proven to be unreliable, cumbersome or insensitive. A feasible approach in iliac vein stenosis is morphological measurement of outflow lumen at its narrowest point by accurate imaging or intravascular planimetry. This is based on the assumption that an outflow lumen approximating normal anatomy is necessary for maintenance of normal peripheral venous pressure. As postcapillary venous pressure is nearly the same in individuals, any reduction from 'normal' will result in peripheral venous hypertension. The percentage stenosis should be calculated based on deviation from normal but not on comparison to the immediate adjacent segment as is the custom in arterial stenosis. This is because long diffuse lesions, first described by Rokitanski, are common in iliac vein segments.[29] They often occur in association with focal lesions. Baseline nominal values for normal luminal areas are 200 mm², 150 mm² and 125 mm² for the common iliac, external iliac and common femoral veins, respectively. These are based on diameters of 16, 14 and 12 mm, respectively. In practice, most symptomatic patients with advanced CVD have area stenosis of >50% (median ≈70%).[30] Lesser degrees of stenosis ranging from 30% to 50% are found in about 20% of limbs; many of these have membranous echolucent lesions only detectable by balloon waste intraoperatively.

Clinical measurement of reflux is even more problematic. Original hopes for valve closure time (VCT) – reflux duration – as a measure of reflux has not been borne out.[31] VCT is currently used as a threshold to define qualitative reflux in the superficial, deep and perforator systems. One second is generally used for the femoral and saphenous veins. For perforators, 400 milliseconds is recommended and the perforator should also have a minimum size of 3 mm is for the reflux to be considered significant. Peak velocity of reflux has good clinical correlation but is still not good enough for routine clinical use.[32] Reflux severity can be clinically graded according to the distal extent of the reflux column (Kistner grading). Developed for use with descending venography, the method is now used with duplex, which has fewer false positives than with contrast. Reflux extending to below the knee or ankle (axial reflux) is considered severe.[33] The number of individual valve segments involved, one each for the saphenous vein, short saphenous vein, femoral vein, profunda femoral vein, popliteal vein and perforators (maximum score 6), can be used to assign a reflux segment score. This method correlates with reflux severity better than other methods of measuring reflux.[5] Such measures, while useful to a certain, they cannot be used in isolation as the end point of reflux is the calf pump whose functional status must be taken into account. The intrinsic components of the calf pump are capacitance, wall compliance, ejection volume and residual volume (Figure 46.6).[34] Ejection fraction and residual volume fraction are derivative parameters. Compensatory mechanisms in the calf pump can buffer reflux by increasing capacitance and/or ejection volume. Calf pump dysfunction may be present without reflux. Even a relatively small volume of reflux may be detrimental if the calf pump is compromised with poor capacitance, decreased compliance or reduced ejection. Often, a combination of these abnormalities is present. Air plethysmography (APG) and ambulatory venous pressure measurement can together provide a comprehensive evaluation of calf pump function.[5] APG can also provide a measure of reflux (venous filling index) and arterial inflow (occlusion plethysmography). Arterial inflow may be increased in arteriovenous malformations and in some cases of CVD. Ambulatory venous pressure measure is considered the gold standard as an index of global calf pump function.

Microvascular injury

Most but not all cases with advanced CVD clinical stages are associated with ambulatory venous hypertension. In earlier clinical stages such as CEAP clinical classes I-2, ambulatory venous hypertension may be absent. Furthermore, it has been observed that limb varicosities may recede and become less prominent after saphenous ablation even though the erect resting venous pressure should have remained unchanged due to the dominant gravity component.[35] There is strong experimental evidence to suggest that reflux-induced shear may release nitrous oxide and other cytokines with vasodilator effects.[36] This is a plausible explanation for the receding of varices after elimination of reflux.

An inflammatory microvascular injury has emerged as the central theme in the genesis of CVD supplanting earlier theories.[2,37] While the details may change with expanding research in this field, the basic elements are clear. The phenomenon is initiated by abnormal shear which includes reverse shear (reflux) or no shear (stasis). This is based on the observation that endothelial cells are the most stable with steady forward flow. Reverse flow, local turbulence or absence of flow allows expression of a cascade of cytokine-mediated inflammation. Leukocytes adhere

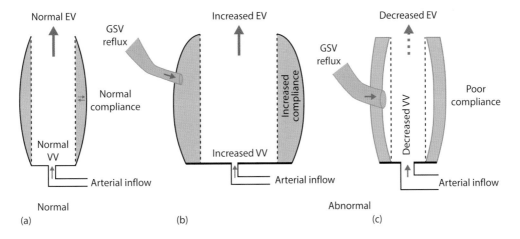

Figure 46.6 Cath-pump mechanics: compliance, capacitance, and ejection volume control residual volume and ambulatory venous pressure (a). GSV reflux can be compensated by an increase in these cath-pump parameters (b). If the GSV reflux is massive and/or the cath-pump mechanics are compromised, ambulatory venous pressure hypertension may occur. Increased arterial inflow into the limb (e.g. AV Fistula) can also result in ambulatory venous hypertension (c).

to the endothelium, damage the glycocalyx and escape into the tissues. Edema, inflammation, lipodermatosclerosis and fibrosis result from a combination of cytokine and tissue factors. Ulcer formation with abnormal vascularization in the area is the final end point. The process has a positive feedback with self-amplification. Valve damage and vein wall abnormalities augment and sustain the process in a vicious cycle. Many elements of this process, such as leukocyte trapping and aberrations of cytokine, enzyme and tissue factors in the circulation of CVD limbs, have been documented in clinical studies.

Deficiencies in current knowledge and areas for future research

Major elements of the pathophysiology of CVD remain obscure. Clinical practice has largely evolved empirically, often aided by emerging technology such as venous stenting. Clinical results from these empirical clinical approaches have yielded intriguing results that set the stage for targeted further enquiry. Knowledge of microcirculatory abnormalities in CVD is rapidly evolving and is likely to change in details with ongoing work.

Key points

- The CEAP classification provides the necessary framework for systematic understanding of clinical stage, etiology, anatomy and pathology.
- Most perforator reflux is associated with superficial and/or deep reflux. Selective ablation of perforators beneath the ulcer bed may heal the ulcer.
- Many aspects of reflux itself are poorly understood. Currently, there is not a good way to quantitate reflux in a precise way.
- Reflux may initiate shear-related valve damage, vasodilatation, microvascular injury leading to edema, tissue damage and ulceration.
- Reflux does not defeat column segmentation per se but shortens the duration of ambulatory pressure recovery.
- The effect of reflux cannot be considered in isolation as calf pump function can compensate for it or make it worse if calf pump is compromised.
- Calf pump abnormalities may be present without reflux.
- The importance of venous obstruction has been recognized only recently.
- Clinical experience with stent correction of venous obstruction has produced intriguing findings. Particularly, stent correction alone appears to relieve symptoms despite the presence of uncorrected severe reflux.
- The interrelationship between obstruction and reflux remains to be fully explored.
- Currently, assessment of obstruction severity depends on morphological methods solely.
- Criteria for determination of 'critical' venous stenosis are different from arterial stenosis. In veins, elevation of upstream pressure rather than downstream perfusion as in arteries is the critical element.

KEY REFERENCES

1. Raju S, Neglen P. Clinical practice. Chronic venous insufficiency and varicose veins. *N Engl J Med.* 2009;360(22):2319–2327.
2. Bergan JJ, Schmid-Schonbein GW, Smith PD, Nicolaides AN, Boisseau MR, Eklof B. Chronic venous disease. *N Engl J Med.* 2006;355(5):488–498.
3. Neglen P, Raju S. A rational approach to detection of significant reflux with duplex Doppler scanning and air plethysmography. *J Vasc Surg.* 1993;17(3):590–595.
4. Myers KA, Ziegenbein RW, Zeng GH, Matthews PG. Duplex ultrasonography scanning for chronic venous disease: Patterns of venous reflux. *J Vasc Surg.* 1995;21(4):605–612.
5. O'Donnell TF. The role of perforators in chronic venous insufficiency. *Phlebology.* 2010;25(1):3–10.
6. Gabriel V, Jimenez JC, Alktaifi A et al. Success of endovenous saphenous and perforator ablation in patients with symptomatic venous insufficiency receiving long-term warfarin therapy. *Ann Vasc Surg.* 2012;26(5):607–611.
7. Raju S, Neglen P. High prevalence of nonthrombotic iliac vein lesions in chronic venous disease: A permissive role in pathogenicity. *J Vasc Surg.* 2006;44(1):136–143; discussion 144.
8. Raju S, Darcey R, Neglen P. Unexpected major role for venous stenting in deep reflux disease. *J Vasc Surg.* 2010;51(2):401–408; discussion 408.
9. Raju S, Mark W Jr, Jones T. Quantifying saphenous reflux. *J Vasc Surg: Venous Lym Dis.*; in press.

REFERENCES

1. Raju S, Neglen P. Clinical practice. Chronic venous insufficiency and varicose veins. *N Engl J Med.* 2009;360(22):2319–2327.
2. Bergan JJ, Schmid-Schonbein GW, Smith PD, Nicolaides AN, Boisseau MR, Eklof B. Chronic venous disease. *N Engl J Med.* 2006;355(5):488–498.
3. Pappas PJ, Lal BK, Ohara N, Saito S, Zapiach L, Duran WN. Regulation of matrix contraction in chronic venous disease. *Eur J Vasc Endovasc Surg.* 2009;38(4):518–529.
4. Labropoulos N, Giannoukas AD, Delis K et al. Where does venous reflux start? *J Vasc Surg.* 1997;26(5):736–742.
5. Neglen P, Raju S. A rational approach to detection of significant reflux with duplex Doppler scanning and air plethysmography. *J Vasc Surg.* 1993;17(3):590–595.
6. Myers KA, Ziegenbein RW, Zeng GH, Matthews PG. Duplex ultrasonography scanning for chronic venous disease: Patterns of venous reflux. *J Vasc Surg.* 1995;21(4):605–612.
7. Ludbrook J. Primary great saphenous varicose veins revisited. *World J Surg.* 1986;10(6):954–958.

8. Gooley NA, Sumner DS. Relationship of venous reflux to the site of venous valvular incompetence: Implications for venous reconstructive surgery. *J Vasc Surg.* 1988;7(1):50–59.

9. White JV, Katz ML, Cisek P, Kreithen J. Venous outflow of the leg: Anatomy and physiologic mechanism of the plantar venous plexus. *J Vasc Surg.* 1996;24(5):819–824.

10. O'Donnell TF. The role of perforators in chronic venous insufficiency. *Phlebology.* 2010;25(1):3–10.

11. Sarin S, Scurr JH, Smith PD. Medial calf perforators in venous disease: The significance of outward flow. *J Vasc Surg.* 1992;16(1):40–46.

12. Gabriel V, Jimenez JC, Alktaifi A et al. Success of endovenous saphenous and perforator ablation in patients with symptomatic venous insufficiency receiving long-term warfarin therapy. *Ann Vasc Surg.* 2012;26(5):607–611.

13. Masuda EM, Kessler DM, Lurie F, Puggioni A, Kistner RL, Eklof B. The effect of ultrasound-guided sclerotherapy of incompetent perforator veins on venous clinical severity and disability scores. *J Vasc Surg.* 2006;43(3):551–556; discussion 556–557.

14. Kistner RL. Surgical repair of the incompetent femoral vein valve. *Arch Surg.* 1975;110(11):1336–1342.

15. Raju S, Neglen P. High prevalence of nonthrombotic iliac vein lesions in chronic venous disease: A permissive role in pathogenicity. *J Vasc Surg.* 2006;44(1):136–143; discussion 144.

16. Johnson BF, Manzo RA, Bergelin RO, Strandness DE, Jr. Relationship between changes in the deep venous system and the development of the postthrombotic syndrome after an acute episode of lower limb deep vein thrombosis: A one- to six-year follow-up. *J Vasc Surg.* 1995;21(2):307–312; discussion 313.

17. Raju S, Fredericks RK, Hudson CA, Fountain T, Neglen PN, Devidas M. Venous valve station changes in "primary" and postthrombotic reflux: An analysis of 149 cases. *Ann Vasc Surg.* 2000;14(3):193–199.

18. Downing LJ, Strieter RM, Kadell AM et al. Neutrophils are the initial cell type identified in deep venous thrombosis induced vein wall inflammation. *ASAIO J.* 1996;42(5):M677–M682.

19. Henke PK, Varma MR, Moaveni DK et al. Fibrotic injury after experimental deep vein thrombosis is determined by the mechanism of thrombogenesis. *Thromb Haemost.* 2007;98(5):1045–1055.

20. Kistner RL, Eklof B, Masuda EM. Deep venous valve reconstruction. *Cardiovasc Surg.* 1995;3(2):129–140.

21. Raju S, Fredericks RK, Neglen PN, Bass JD. Durability of venous valve reconstruction techniques for "primary" and postthrombotic reflux. *J Vasc Surg.* 1996;23(2):357–366; discussion 366–367.

22. Raju S, Darcey R, Neglen P. Unexpected major role for venous stenting in deep reflux disease. *J Vasc Surg.* 2010;51(2):401–408; discussion 408.

23. May R, Thurner J. The cause of the predominantly sinistral occurrence of thrombosis of the pelvic veins. *Angiology.* 1957;8(5):419–427.

24. Negus D, Fletcher EW, Cockett FB, Thomas ML. Compression and band formation at the mouth of the left common iliac vein. *Br J Surg.* 1968;55(5):369–374.

25. Raju S, Fountain T, Neglen P, Devidas M. Axial transformation of the profunda femoris vein. *J Vasc Surg.* 1998;27(4):651–659.

26. Raju S, Hollis K, Neglen P. Obstructive lesions of the inferior vena cava: Clinical features and endovenous treatment. *J Vasc Surg.* 2006;44(4):820–827.

27. Raju S, Kirk O, Davis M, Olivier J. Hemodynamics of 'critical' venous stenosis and stent treatment. *J Vasc Surg: Venous Lym Dis.*; in press.

28. Raju S, Fredericks R, Lishman P, Neglen P, Morano J. Observations on the calf venous pump mechanism: Determinants of postexercise pressure. *J Vasc Surg.* 1993;17(3):459–469.

29. Raju S, Davis M. Anomalous features of iliac vein stenosis that affect diagnosis and treatment. *J Vasc Surg: Venous Lym Dis.*; in press.

30. Raju S, Oglesbee M, Neglen P. Iliac vein stenting in postmenopausal leg swelling. *J Vasc Surg.* 2011;53(1):123–130.

31. Rodriguez AA, Whitehead CM, McLaughlin RL, Umphrey SE, Welch HJ, O'Donnell TF. Duplex-derived valve closure times fail to correlate with reflux flow volumes in patients with chronic venous insufficiency. *J Vasc Surg.* 1996;23(4):606–610.

32. Neglen P, Egger JF 3rd, Olivier J, Raju S. Hemodynamic and clinical impact of ultrasound-derived venous reflux parameters. *J Vasc Surg.* 2004;40(2):303–310.

33. Danielsson G, Eklof B, Grandinetti A, Lurie F, Kistner RL. Deep axial reflux, an important contributor to skin changes or ulcer in chronic venous disease. *J Vasc Surg.* 2003;38(6):1336–1341.

34. Raju S, Mark W Jr, Jones T. Quantifying saphenous reflux. *J Vasc Surg: Venous Lym Dis.*; in press.

35. Schanzer H. Endovenous ablation plus microphlebectomy/sclerotherapy for the treatment of varicose veins: Single or two-stage procedure? *Vasc Endovasc Surg.* 2010;44(7):545–549.

36. Pascarella L, Schonbein GW, Bergan JJ. Microcirculation and venous ulcers: A review. *Ann Vasc Surg.* 2005;19(6):921–927.

37. Adamson RH, Sarai RK, Altangerel A, Clark JF, Weinbaum S, Curry FE. Microvascular permeability to water is independent of shear stress, but dependent on flow direction. *Am J Physiol Heart Circ Physiol.* 2013;304(8):H1077–H1084.

47

Endovenous and surgical management of varicose veins

Techniques and results

JUAN CARLOS JIMENEZ

CONTENTS

INTRODUCTION

Recent population studies have estimated the prevalence of varicose veins to be greater than 20% in the adult Western population with approximately 5% presenting with signs of advanced chronic venous insufficiency.[1] For close to a century, treatment of chronic venous insufficiency and varicose veins consisted of a variety of open surgical techniques performed in the operating room under general anesthesia. Over the past decade, a variety of novel endovenous and surgical techniques have been developed which have shifted management to the ambulatory and clinical setting with improved patient outcomes and minimal morbidity.

ENDOVENOUS THERMAL ABLATION OF THE GREAT AND SMALL SAPHENOUS VEINS

Current invasive management of symptomatic varicose veins is now primarily performed in the outpatient and ambulatory settings largely due to the development of endovenous thermal ablation. The two distinct modalities used are radiofrequency ablation (RFA) and endovenous laser ablation (EVLT). With both techniques, a catheter probe with a heating element at its tip is introduced percutaneously into the vein using ultrasound guidance (Figure 47.1a and b). The heating element causes direct thermal injury to the adjacent vein wall, resulting in damage to the endothelium, denaturation of medial collagen and fibrotic and thrombotic occlusion of the vein.[1]

The Food and Drug Administration (FDA) approved RFA in 1999 for treatment of the incompetent great saphenous vein (GSV). Laser ablation was first reported by Bone et al. in 2001 following successful clinical application of a diode laser for the treatment of varicose veins.[1] It is also FDA approved for the same indication. These procedures are routinely performed in the outpatient and/or clinical setting with less post-operative pain and morbidity compared with saphenous ligation and stripping.[2] Preoperative duplex ultrasonography should be performed for all patients to assess the size, anatomic course and duration of reflux time and to assess patients' eligibility for this procedure. Patients with axial veins, which are too small

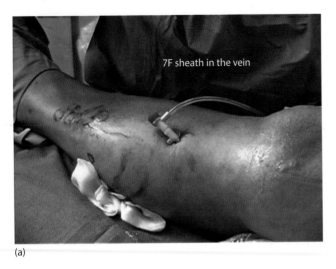

7F sheath in the vein

(a)

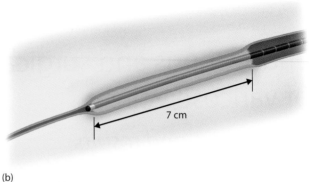

7 cm

(b)

Figure 47.1 (a) Percutaneous placement of a sheath in the great saphenous vein for introduction of a thermal ablation catheter. (b) Thermal heating element at the tip of a radiofrequency ablation catheter.

(<2 mm) or too large (>15 mm), are likely better candidates for traditional surgical high ligation and stripping. Other factors, which may exclude patients from endovenous thermal ablation, include tortuosity, saphenous veins that are too superficial and prior occlusion of the deep venous system. Duplex ultrasound should ensure patency of the deep venous system prior to endovenous closure of the saphenous veins.

The technique for both laser ablation and RFA is similar with small variations. The affected leg is prepped and draped in sterile fashion and intraoperative duplex ultrasound is used to access the GSV at the level of the knee using a micropuncture needle and wire. The patient should be placed in reverse Trendelenburg position at this time in order to dilate the vein maximally for venipuncture. A smaller profile sheath (4F) can be used for introduction of most laser ablation catheters, while most current RFA catheters require placement of a 7F sheath. We position the catheter 2–3 cm caudal to the saphenofemoral junction based on real-time ultrasound measurements. A tumescent solution consisting of 100–300 mL of 445 mL of 0.9 N saline, 50 mL of 1% lidocaine with 1:100,000 epinephrine and 5 mL of 8.4% sodium bicarbonate is injected using a spinal needle to the perivenous tissues surrounding the saphenous vein deep to the saphenous fascia. The tumescent anesthesia is used to compress the vein around the catheter, in addition to cooling the tissues surrounding the vein being treated to prevent the spread of thermal energy. Once the vein is completely surrounded with tumescent fluid (confirmed with ultrasound), the patient is placed in Trendelenburg position for treatment. With laser ablation, the laser fibre is withdrawn at a rate of 1–2 mm/s for the first 10 cm and 2–3 mm/s for the remaining distance. For optimal treatment, 50–80 J/cm energy is delivered when using the 810 nm diode laser.[1] With RFA, treatment is performed to 120°C at 20 second

intervals over a catheter length of either 3 or 7 cm, depending on the catheter chosen. The 3 cm treatment length is used when the access site is in the mid- or proximal thigh, and sufficient length from the saphenofemoral junction cannot be achieved with the 7 cm catheter. We generally treat the segment of the vein closest to the saphenofemoral junction with two 20 second treatments. The catheter and sheath are then withdrawn and pressure is held at the access site until hemostasis is achieved.

The technique for ablation of the small saphenous vein (SSV) is similar and the preferred puncture site is in the distal leg at the level of the ankle. Because of the proximity of the sural nerve to the SSV, care should be taken to inject sufficient tumescent solution to the perivenous tissues to avoid thermal injury. Because increased anatomic variability of the SSV and the saphenopopliteal junction has been well described, accurate localization of the saphenopopliteal junction should be ensured by the operating surgeon using ultrasonography.[3]

Our protocol for post-operative care includes placing sterile folded abdominal (ABD) pads along the length of the treated vein and wrapping of the leg with 4 and 6 in. ACE wraps from the foot to the groin. Patients are instructed to elevate the leg at home and keep the wrap in place for 24–48 hours. Frequent (but not excessive) ambulation is encouraged. Post-operative duplex ultrasound is performed 1–3 days post-procedure to rule out the presence of endovenous heat-induced thrombus (EHIT), a rare but potentially morbid complication.

Results

The use of endovenous thermal ablation has been validated in the peer-reviewed literature as safe and effective treatment for symptomatic saphenous vein reflux. Nordon and colleagues demonstrated excellent results with both RFA and laser ablation of the GSV in their patient cohort.[4] In their series, 159 patients were randomized to either RFA (n = 79) or EVLT (n = 80). Immediate post-operative vein occlusion was 100% for both groups, and, at 3 months, occlusion was 97% for RFA and 96% for EVLT. RFA was associated with less immediate post-operative pain and bruising. Quality of life was assessed using the Aberdeen Varicose Vein Questionnaire and EQ-5D and was similar at 3 months for both groups. No patients sustained post-operative infections requiring antibiotics and the incidence of skin burn, paresthesia and thrombophlebitis was 2% for each independent complication. No deep venous thrombosis (DVT) or pulmonary embolus was noted post-operatively. In this cohort, the median time to return to work was 7 days in the EVLT group and 9 days in the RFA group.

Another randomized comparison study was performed by Gale and colleagues between EVLT with a 810 nm wavelength laser and RFA to the GSV.[5] In this study, 118 patients were randomized to either RFA (n = 46) or EVLT (n = 48). Laser treatment was associated with more frequent early bruising; however, at 1 year, there was no difference between the two treatments. Overall quality of life improved for both groups at 1 year. Of note, the recanalization rate was noted to be significantly higher in the RFA group at 1 year (24% for RFA vs. 4% for EVLT). However, it should be noted that the RFA device (ClosurePLUS, VNUS Medical Technologies, Sunnyvale, CA) used in this cohort was the older generation device, which has subsequently been replaced on the market with the ClosureFast (Covidien/Medtronic, Minneapolis, MN, USA) device.

Rasmussen and colleagues also performed a randomized trial with 5-year follow-up comparing EVLT with high ligation and stripping of the GSV.[6] In their series, 137 patients were randomized to either EVLT (980 nm bare fibre) or high ligation and stripping. Venous clinical severity scores and quality of life improved in both groups with no difference between the groups at 5 years. Clinical recurrence of symptoms was also similar in both groups.

Complications

Serious complications from endovenous thermal ablation of the saphenous vein are rare. Localized pain and bruising overlying the treated vein are well-recognized clinical sequelae of treatment, and most patients resolve these symptoms 1–4 weeks post-operatively. Other potential complications include paresthesias, hematoma, skin burns, thrombophlebitis, vein recanalization, neuralgia and hyperpigmentation.

The development of post-operative DVT also referred to as 'endovenous heat-induced thrombus' has been associated with this procedure, and all patients should undergo post-operative duplex scan 24–72 hours post-procedure to rule out the presence of EHIT (Figure 47.2). In a recent series from our institution, 500 consecutive patients underwent RFA of the GSV and 13 patients (2.6%) experienced thrombus bulging into the femoral vein or adherent to its wall, which required treatment with anticoagulation.[7] No patients developed occlusive femoral DVT. All of the patients had thrombus retraction to the level of the saphenofemoral junction in an average of 16 days following treatment with anticoagulation, and no patients developed pulmonary embolism (PE) in this cohort. We developed a classification system and treatment algorithm for management of EHIT based on its location relative to the femoral vein. There was a significantly higher rate of proximal thrombus extension in patients with a history of prior DVT and in patients with a GSV diameter greater than 8 mm. We also demonstrated similar results following RFA of the SSV.[8] In our series, 80 patients underwent RFA of the SSV and 2 patients (2.5%) developed EHIT with extension into the popliteal vein requiring treatment with anticoagulation. Similarly, no occlusive DVTs were noted and a corresponding classification system and treatment algorithm were also developed for the SSV.

The natural history of EHIT appears to be more benign than that of primary DVT, and treatment with anticoagulation for 1–2 weeks resolves the thrombus in the majority of patients. Nonetheless, pulmonary embolus

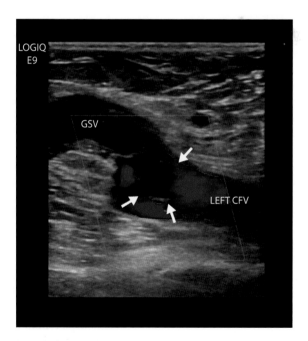

Figure 47.2 Duplex ultrasound demonstrates the presence of endovenous heat-induced thrombus extending into the common femoral vein lumen following endovenous thermal ablation.

following development of EHIT has been reported.[9] We recommend post-operative duplex be performed 24–72 hours following endothermal saphenous ablation, and perform this testing in all patients during the post-operative period.

PERFORATOR VEINS

In patients with healed or active venous ulceration, the initial recommended treatment, aside from compression therapy, is ablation of the incompetent axial veins directed to the bed of the ulcer.[10] In patients with persistent perforator vein reflux following successful ablation of axial reflux, endovenous thermal techniques (RFA and EVLT) may be used. These techniques are preferable to open surgery due to the risk of complications from incisions in areas of compromised skin.

The technique for perforator ablation is similar for both RFA and laser ablation. The patient should undergo preoperative duplex ultrasonography to locate and map the pathologic perforator veins in the ulcer bed. At our institution, we use the ClosureRFS system (Covidien/Medtronic, Minneapolis, MN). The affected leg is prepped and draped in sterile fashion and the patient should be placed in reverse Trendelenburg position. Intraoperative duplex is used to localize the optimal puncture site, directly above the perforator vein. An 11-blade scalpel is used to perform a small stab incision overlying the perforator, and the stylet from the RFS catheter is advanced at a 45° angle to the junction of the perforator vein and the fascia. The wall of the vein should be punctured at the level of or immediately below the fascia. Once the location of the catheter is confirmed, the stylet is removed and blood return through the proximal end of the catheter confirms placement within the vein lumen. At this point, a 25 g needle is used to inject 1% lidocaine to generously infiltrate the perivenous tissues at the level of the fascia. The patient is then placed in Trendelenburg position and the vein is treated with radiofrequency energy for 1 minute at each quadrant, while impedance and temperature are kept within the therapeutic range (<400 ohms and at 85°C, respectively). An additional ablation may be performed in the segment of vein above the fascia. The catheter is removed and the leg is dressed with a three- or four-layer compression dressing. Post-operative duplex is confirmed at the next wound care visit to confirm closure of the treated vein and to rule out DVT of the adjacent calf veins.

Results

The evidence for primary perforator ablation in the absence of superficial venous disease in patients with venous ulceration is supportive, but not as clear as saphenous vein ablation.[10] The most recent guidelines of the Society for Vascular Surgery and the American Venous Forum suggest ablation of the 'pathologic' perforating veins in addition to standard compression therapy to aid in venous ulcer healing and to prevent recurrence.[10] This recommendation is not made based on level 1 evidence since there is no randomized controlled trial which has evaluated isolated perforator interruption on ulcer healing or recurrence.

At our institution, we perform perforator ablation in patients with either healed or active venous ulcers following correction of incompetent axial and tributary reflux in addition to compression therapy. Lawrence and colleagues demonstrated excellent ulcer healing rates with radiofrequency perforator ablation in patients with recalcitrant venous ulcers.[11] In this study, 75 ulcers with 86 associated perforator veins were treated with ablation in 45 patients. Although initial success of perforator ablation was only 59%, repeat ablation was 90% successful and 71% had eventual successful perforator closure. When at least one perforator vein closed and no major complications were noted, 90% of ulcers healed.[11] Of patients who healed their ulcers, healing occurred at a mean of 138 days.

In another series by Harlander-Locke and colleagues, also from our institution, we performed 140 consecutive endovenous ablation procedures (74 superficial and 66 perforator) on 110 venous ulcers in 88 limbs.[12] Following ablation, healing rates were noted to significantly improve, and after 6 months, 76.3% of patients healed at a mean of 142 ± 14 days. Of the healed ulcers, only four patients with six ulcers (7.1%) recurred.

Abdul-Haqq and colleague compared EVLT of the GSV and perforator vein ablation with EVLT of the GSV alone in a series of 95 patients with venous ulcers.[13] Seventy-eight patients were treated with EVLT of the GSV alone. In patients who had combined GSV perforator vein reflux, the healing rate for patients treated with ablation to both incompetent veins was 71% compared to 33% in patients who underwent GSV ablation alone. This study suggested that all patients with venous ulcers should be routinely examined for both axial and perforator reflux and treatment of incompetent at both levels should be strongly considered.

Complications

In our study, the most common complication of perforator ablation is failure to close the perforator following a single ablation. Initial success following thermal perforator ablation was 58%. However, repeat ablation was 90% successful with 71% of patients eventually achieving vein closure.[11] Other reported complications include paresthesias,[14] DVT,[15] puncture-site infections, hyperpigmentation and scarring.[16] In our experience with perforator ablation in patients receiving long-term warfarin therapy, three hematomas were noted which resolved with conservative measures.[17]

SCLEROTHERAPY

Liquid sclerotherapy was first described almost a century ago for the treatment of spider and reticular veins (measuring <3 mm).[1] In the mid-1990s, Cabrera described the technique of mixing polidocanol with 'physiologic' gas to prepare a foam which could be used to treat larger diameter veins.[1] The mechanism of action includes the destruction of venous endothelial cells, exposure of subendothelial collagen fibres and formation of a fibrotic obstruction.[1] Frequently used sclerosing agents include polidocanol, sodium tetradecyl sulfate (STS), sodium morrhuate, glycerin and hypertonic saline.

The technique of foam sclerotherapy has been popularized by Tessari and colleagues and involves mixing one part sclerosant with 4–5 parts air using two syringes through a 3-way stopcock.[18] Although room air is most frequently used for this technique, carbon dioxide and oxygen may also be used primarily in order to reduce the risk of nitrogen embolization, a gas much more slowly resorbed.[19] Although the maximum volume of foam sclerosant, which should be used, continues to be debated, injection of more than 10 mL has been associated with more than a threefold increased risk for deep venous occlusion.[20] Ultrasound guidance can be used to assist with venipuncture and to monitor the progress of foam injected into the vein. The leg should be elevated prior to vein injection, mainly to reduce the volume of foam required. This technique can be performed for axial, tributary and perforator veins. Compression bandaging or graduated compression is routinely used following treatment. There is minimal quality evidence concerning the optimal length of compression following this procedure.[21]

Results

The peer-reviewed literature demonstrates good outcomes with use of foam sclerotherapy, with and without ultrasound guidance, for treatment of varicose veins. However, long-term occlusion rates appear to be inferior to EVLT and surgery.[22] A recent randomized trial compared EVLT, conventional surgery (high ligation and stripping) and ultrasound guided foam sclerotherapy (UGFS) for treatment of primary GSV reflux.[22] A total of 240 consecutive patients were randomized to one of the three groups and all treatments demonstrated improvement in quality-of-life questionnaires. Ultrasound-guided sclerotherapy (UGS) was noted to have significantly lower success (occlusion) rates at 1 year compared with the other modalities. The complication rates were low and comparable in all groups.

Another randomized trial by Shadid and colleagues compared UGFS with high ligation and stripping of the GSV.[23] In this study, 230 patients underwent UGFS and 200 underwent GSV stripping. At 2 years, clinical recurrence of symptoms was similar in both groups; however, the presence of reflux in the treated vein was significantly higher in the UGFS group than the surgical group (35% vs. 21%, respectively). Hospital costs were significantly lower for the UGFS group.

A meta-analysis by van den Bos et al. reviewed 64 eligible studies and assessed 12,320 limbs, which underwent EVLT, RFA, UGFS and surgical ligation and stripping.[24] Pooled success rates were highest following EVLT (94%), followed by RFA (84%), high ligation and stripping (78%) and foam sclerotherapy (77%).

With regard to the SSV, authors have also demonstrated good results.[25] In a recent study by Darvall and colleagues, 86 patients underwent UGFS for treatment of SSV incompetence and varicose veins.[25] At 1, 6 and 12 months, technical success rates were 100%, 91% and 91%, respectively. Of the 8 technical failures which occurred, only 3 required additional treatment. Immediate and sustained improvements in quality-of-life measurements were noted in the majority of patients.

Recently, a new commercially available microfoam sclerosant (Varithena®, BTG International Inc, West Conshohocken, PA, USA) has been made available in the United States with FDA approval. This endovenous microfoam solution consists of polidocanol foam with a low nitrogen gas mixture compared with conventional foam prepared at the bedside using the Tessari method.[26] Other advantages include smaller bubble size and increased stability. Regan and colleagues demonstrated no evidence of cerebral or cardiac microinfarction in patients with right to left shunts following treatment with microfoam sclerotherapy, despite 60 patients having detectable middle cerebral artery detected by transcranial Doppler.[27] The rate of DVT was relatively high (7.3%) compared with previous trials of endovenous microfoam ablation.[27] Further investigation is required to determine the long-term safety and efficacy of this relatively novel compound; however, postprocedural risk for embolic sequelae appears lower than conventional foam.

The most recent guidelines for the treatment of varicose veins from the Society for Vascular Surgery and the American Venous Forum recommend endovenous thermal ablation over foam sclerotherapy for the treatment of axial vein reflux.[1] Large, randomized controlled trials comparing long-term saphenous occlusion rates with foam sclerotherapy and other modalities are required before foam sclerotherapy can be recommended as primary treatment for saphenous vein insufficiency.

PERFORATOR SCLEROTHERAPY

Current Society for Vascular Surgery (SVS) practice guidelines recommend against selective treatment of incompetent perforator veins in patients with simple varicose veins (CEAP Class C_2) based on level 1 evidence. They recommend treatment of 'pathologic' perforating veins with outward flow of ≥500 ms duration, with a diameter of ≥3.5 mm and located beneath healed or open venous ulcers.[1] Recommended techniques for treatment include subfascial endoscopic perforator surgery (SEPS), UGS or thermal ablation based on Grade 2C evidence.[1]

Endovenous treatment of incompetent perforator veins has gained popularity due to its minimally invasive nature and is supported by mostly nonrandomized data in the peer-reviewed literature. It is an alternative to open perforator ligation, SEPS and endovenous ablation. A main advantage of this approach is decreased trauma to the overlying skin, which is frequently chronically diseased. Masuda and colleagues demonstrated significant clinical improvement in patients with chronic venous insufficiency using UGS.[28] In their study, 80 limbs were treated with UGS using sodium morrhuate (5%). The authors noted that 98% of incompetent perforators were successfully closed at the time of treatment and that 75% of limbs demonstrated persistent closure and remained clinically improved at a mean follow-up of 20.1 months. A significant reduction in venous clinical severity and disability scores was also measured in the majority of patients. No cases of DVT were observed. Perforator recurrence occurred mostly in patients with ulceration.

Kiguchi and colleagues identified factors that influence perforator thrombosis following sclerotherapy for venous ulcers in the absence of axial reflux.[29] Over a 2-year period, 73 venous ulcers were treated in 62 patients with either STS or polidocanol foam. At a mean follow-up of 30.2 months, 52% of ulcers healed and the average thrombosis rate was 54%. The vein closure rate in patients who healed their ulcer was 69% compared with 41% in patients with non-healing ulcers. Male gender and warfarin therapy were identified as negative predictors of vein thrombosis. Complete perforator vein thrombosis was predictive of ulcer healing, while a large initial ulcer area was a negative predictor. Predictors of increased ulcer recurrence were hypertension and increased follow-up time. DVT was noted in 3% of patients treated.

Complications of sclerotherapy

Most complications reported following sclerotherapy are minor and may include localized pain, hyperpigmentation, itching and allergic reactions to the sclerosant.[1] Life-threatening complications are rare (<0.01%) but have been reported following this procedure. These may include death, anaphylactic reaction, DVT, PE, stroke and skin necrosis.[1] Neurologic complications from gas bubble embolization are concerning and may be more common in patients with a patent right to left cardiac shunt, larger gas bubble size, prolonged immobilization and higher volumes of sclerosant used in single sessions (>12 cc). Strokes, seizures and transient ischemia attacks have been reported.[27] Because a patent foramen ovale is present in 25%–30% of adults, a significant percentage of patients may be exposed to arterial gas embolization and providers should be aware of the potential risks.[27] Potential treatment options for this complication include 100% oxygen and possibly urgent hyperbaric therapy.[1]

NEWER ENDOVENOUS MODALITIES

Mechanochemical endovenous ablation

The ClariVein® infusion system (Vascular Insights, Quincy, MA, USA) received FDA approval in 2008 and utilizes a percutaneously introduced catheter with a rotating tip which induces endothelial damage while infusing liquid sclerosant simultaneously resulting in vein fibrosis.[30] The catheter does not utilize generated thermal energy and does not require tumescent anesthesia. One advantage over EVLT and RFA may be decreased thermal-induced neuralgias, especially in the GSV and SSV. Ultrasound-guided puncture of the saphenous vein is performed and a 4F sheath is placed using Seldinger technique. The catheter is introduced through the sheath and is positioned 2 cm caudal to the saphenofemoral junction. It is then connected to a motorized unit, which unsheathes the distal end of the wire to expose the dispersion tip. The catheter is then activated and the rotating tip is steadily withdrawn at a rate of 2 mm/s. Liquid sclerosant is simultaneously infused through the tip. Duplex ultrasound is used to rule out DVT and a compression wrap is placed from the foot to the ankle.

Because this device is relatively new, level 1 evidence is not available. However, early reports suggest less postoperative pain, faster recovery and earlier return to work compared with RFA of the GSV.[31,32] In one recent study, 68 patients with GSV reflux were treated with either RFA or mechanochemical endovenous ablation (MOCA) (van Eekeren, 2013). Patients treated with MOCA reported significantly less post-operative pain compared with the RFA group. The mean time for work resumption was 3.3 days for the MOCA group vs. 5.6 days for the RFA group (p = 0.2). At 6 weeks, both groups reported an improved change in health status and improved quality of life. No patients experienced DVT, pulmonary embolus or skin burns. Hematomas (6%), induration (12%) and hyperpigmentation (9%) were notable minor complications.

Bishawi and colleagues also demonstrated high occlusion rates with significant clinical improvement following MOCA. They treated 126 patients with this technique and adjunct procedures were performed in 11% of patients. Closure rates were 100%, 98% and 94% at 1 week, three months and six months, respectively. No cases of DVT were noted and complications encountered were hematoma (1%), ecchymosis (9%) and thrombophlebitis (10%).

CYANOACRYLATE EMBOLIZATION

Another recently described treatment modality is injection of cyanoacrylate adhesive (CA) directly into the GSV under ultrasound guidance. Morrison et al. described their technique in their recent randomized study.[33] The authors used a novel delivery system (VenaSeal, Sapheon Inc, Morrisville, NC, USA) to inject CA directly into the vein under ultrasound guidance.

A 5F sheath is placed into the vein and a catheter is positioned 5 cm caudal to the saphenofemoral junction. No tumescent anesthesia was required. The GSV is compressed proximally with the ultrasound probe and two injections of 0.10 mL of CA were given 1 cm apart at this location, followed by a 3 minute period of local compression. The injections are then repeated followed by 30 second compression sessions which are performed until the entire length of the targeted segment is treated. Compression bandages were applied for 48 hours of continued use post-operatively and for 4 additional days during waking hours.

A recent randomized trial assigned 108 patients to undergo cyanoacrylate embolization (CAE) and 114 patients to RFA. Three-month closure rates were 99% for CAE and 96% for RFA. Post-operative pain was mild and similar between groups and less ecchymosis was present in the CAE group at day 3. The authors concluded that CAE was noninferior to RFA for treatment of incompetent GSV's at 3 months following treatment. No DVT or pulmonary emboli were noted in the study. No major complications were reported. Other early reports suggest similar favourable outcomes with the use of CAE.[34,35]

OPEN SURGICAL TECHNIQUES

Ligation and stripping of the saphenous veins

High ligation and division with or without stripping of the saphenous veins was the most common surgical technique performed prior to the advent of endovenous ablation. This technique was first described by Keller in 1905.[1] Currently, this operation has been largely relegated to patients who are poor candidates for endovenous therapy. These indications include aneurysmal or tortuous saphenous veins. Thermal ablation of very superficial saphenous veins (located superior to the saphenous fascia) risks the possibility of burn injury to the skin, and surgical removal of the vein may be preferred in these patients. Prior ablation or thrombophlebitis of the vein may also prevent proper placement of endoluminal catheters and may be easier treated with open surgery.

The most recent SVS Consensus Guidelines suggest high ligation and inversion stripping of the GSV to the level of the knee.[1] Due to the proximity of the saphenous nerve to the GSV below the knee, this portion of the vein should not be stripped. The technique of GSV ligation involves exposure of the saphenofemoral junction via surgical incision. Intraoperative ultrasound aids in accurate localization of the saphenofemoral junction (SFJ) and allows for smaller incisions to be made. Ligation of the saphenous vein is performed flush to the SFJ with silk suture to avoid formation of a reservoir adjacent to the femoral vein susceptible to thrombus formation.

A Codman stripper is introduced through the GSV through exposure at the level of the knee. The stripper is passed to the level of the SFJ and the vein is transected at this level (Figure 47.3a). Tumescent anesthesia (using a spinal needle) is commonly injected to the perivenous tissue surrounding the entire GSV in the thigh to minimize discomfort and post-operative bleeding. The mushroom tip of the stripper is then secured and the vein is invaginated and removed through the knee incision (Figure 47.3b and c). A compression dressing is placed from the foot to the groin similar to the post-operative dressing used following endovenous ablation.

Stripping of the SSV should be performed with caution because of potential damage to the sural nerve. The most recent SVS Consensus Guidelines recommend high ligation of the SSV at the knee crease, about 3–5 cm distal to the saphenopopliteal junction, with selective invagination stripping of the incompetent portion of the vein.[1]

Results of high ligation and stripping

High ligation and stripping of the GSV have demonstrated good outcomes in patients with symptomatic varicose veins. In their randomized trial comparing endovenous ablation to high ligation and stripping of the GSV, Rasmussen and colleagues demonstrated no significant difference at 5 years in venous clinical severity and quality-of-life scores.[6] Other studies have demonstrated similar safety and efficacy using this technique.[6,36]

Open stripping has been associated with increased perioperative pain and a longer return to normal activities compared with endovenous techniques.[37] Lurie and colleagues reported that the mean time to normal activities was significantly longer following ligation and stripping (3.89 days) compared with endovenous ablation (1.15 days) in their randomized comparison.[37] Rautio and colleagues also demonstrated significantly shorter sick leaves and cost savings following analysis of lost working days with endovenous ablation compared with GSV stripping.[38]

Complications

Wound complications have been reported between 3% and 10%, with wound infection rates between 1.5% and 16% in the current literature.[1] Factors influencing the development of wound-related complications include elevated body mass index, smoking and the absence of perioperative antibiotic prophylaxis.[39] Other potential complications include bleeding, post-operative neuralgia, bruising and a recurrence of symptoms. Direct injury to the common femoral artery and vein is rare but can cause severe morbidity if not recognized promptly.[40] Of note, although routine post-operative duplex is not commonly performed following vein stripping (compared with RFA and EVLT), DVT rates following open venous surgery have been reported in up to 5% of patients.[41]

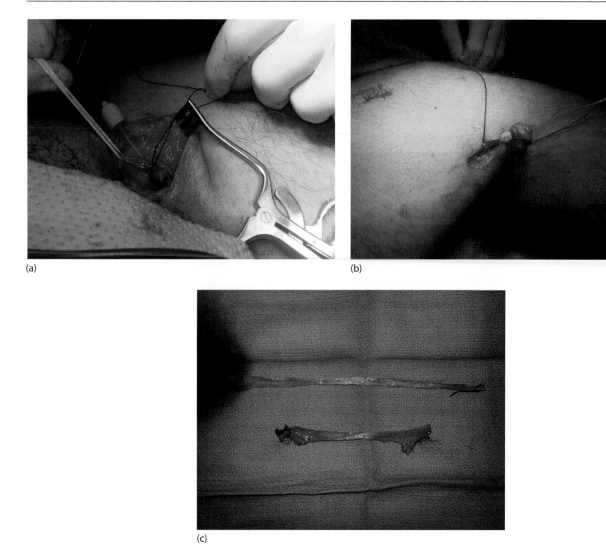

(a)

(b)

(c)

Figure 47.3 (a–c) Introduction of a Codman stripper into the great saphenous vein (GSV) following cutdown of the knee. The GSV in the thigh is invaginated and removed following injection of tumescent anesthesia.

AMBULATORY (STAB) PHLEBECTOMY

Stab phlebectomy is a well-established technique for removal of varicose veins through small incisions. Prior to the operation, the patient is asked to stand for several minutes and the surgeon marks the varicose veins with a marking pen. The operation may or may not be performed with injection of tumescent anesthetic solution. At our institution, we use subcutaneous 1% lidocaine injected subcutaneously at the level of the vein. A 1.0–1.5 mm stab incision is made in the transverse direction and extended through the skin and subcutaneous tissue. A phlebectomy hook is then inserted in to the subcutaneous tissue to ensnare the vein and exteriorize it through the stab incision. We use small mosquito clamps to grasp the vein and use them to elevate the vein to a maximal length prior to vein avulsion (Figure 47.4a and b). Direct pressure is placed following vein removal until hemostasis is achieved. Folded sterile gauze and compression wraps are used post-operatively. We do not routinely obtain post-operative duplex ultrasounds following stab phlebectomy, unless GSV ablation is performed concomitantly.

At our institution, we routinely use both RFA and/or mechanochemical ablation of the saphenous veins with concomitant phlebectomy and have reported excellent outcomes using this approach.[42] In our series, we performed 1000 consecutive thermal saphenous ablations and 500 ambulatory phlebectomy procedures for chronic venous insufficiency. Concomitant phlebectomy was performed in 355 patients with RFA. Additionally, 145 limbs required later-staged phlebectomy for persistent symptoms after RFA alone. The majority of patients in the entire cohort had successful relief of their symptoms (86.7%). No post-operative DVT was noted; however, one patient did develop post-operative pulmonary embolus despite a negative post-operative ultrasound. This patient was treated successfully with anticoagulation without long-term sequelae.

Transilluminated powered phlebectomy (Trivex, InaVein, Lexington, MA, USA) is a technique, which uses a continuous tumescent irrigation with transillumination in

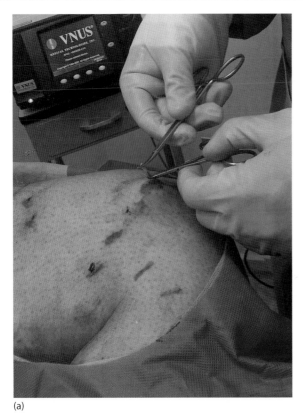
(a)

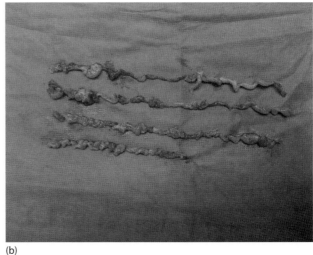
(b)

Figure 47.4 (a) Technique of ambulatory (stab) phlebectomy for removal of branch varicose veins. (b) A significant number of branch varicose veins can be removed using the ambulatory phlebectomy technique.

conjunction with an oscillating vein resector. Good results have been reported with this technique; however, its main disadvantage is the need for general, spinal or epidural anesthesia.[43] A modified stab phlebectomy technique using transillumination and tumescence without the powered oscillator has also been described with excellent outcomes.[44]

REFERENCES

1. Gloviczki P, Comerota AJ, Dalsing MC et al. The care of patients with varicose veins and associated chronic venous diseases: Clinical practice guidelines of the Society for Vascular Surgery and the American Venous Forum. *J Vasc Surg.* 2011;53:2S–48S.
2. Subramonia S, Lees T. Randomized clinical trial of radiofrequency ablation or conventional high ligation and stripping for great saphenous varicose veins. *Br J Surg.* 2010;97:328–336.
3. Kerver AL, van der Ham AC, Theeuwes HP et al. The surgical anatomy of the small saphenous vein and adjacent nerves in relation to endovenous thermal ablation. *J Vasc Surg.* 2012;56:181–188.
4. Nordon IM, Hinchliffe RJ, Brar R et al. A prospective double-blind randomized controlled trial of radiofrequency versus laser treatment of the great saphenous vein in patients with varicose veins. *Ann Surg.* 2011;254:876–881.
5. Gale SS, Lee JN, Walsh ME et al. A randomized controlled trial of endovenous thermal ablation using the 810-nm wavelength laser and the ClosurePLUS radiofrequency ablation methods for superficial venous insufficiency of the great saphenous vein. *J Vasc Surg.* 2010;52:645–650.
6. Rasmussen L, Lawaetz M, Bjoern L et al. Randomized clinical trial comparing endovenous laser ablation and stripping of the great saphenous vein with clinical and duplex outcome after 5 years. *J Vasc Surg.* 2013,58:421–426.
7. Lawrence, PF, Chandra A, Wu M et al. Classification of proximal endovenous closure levels and treatment algorithm. *J Vasc Surg.* 2010;52:388–393.
8. Harlander-Locke M, Jimenez JC, Lawrence PF et al. Management of endovenous heat-induced thrombus using a classification system and treatment algorithm following segmental thermal ablation of the small saphenous vein. *J Vasc Surg.* 2013;58:427–431.
9. Sufian S, Arnez A, Lakhanpai S. Case of the disappearing heat-induced thrombus causing pulmonary embolism during ultrasound evaluation. *J Vasc Surg.* 2012;55:529–531.
10. O'Donnell TF, Passman MA, Marston WA et al. Management of venous leg ulcers: Clinical practice guidelines of the Society for Vascular Surgery and the American Venous Forum. *J Vasc Surg.* 2014;60:3S–59S.

11. Lawrence PF, Alkraifi A, Rigberg D et al. Endovenous ablation of incompetent perforating veins is effective treatment for recalcitrant venous ulcers. *J Vasc Surg.* 2011;54:737–742.

12. Harlander-Locke M, Lawrence PF, Alkaifi A, Jimenez JC, Rigberg D, Derubertis B. The impact of ablation of incompetent superficial and perforator veins on ulcer healing rates. *J Vasc Surg.* 2012;55:454–464.

13. Abdul-Haqq R, Almaroof B, Chen BL et al. Endovenous laser ablation of great saphenous vein and perforator veins improves venous stasis ulcer healing. *Ann Vasc Surg.* 2013;27:932–939.

14. Boersma D, Smulders DL, Bakker OJ et al. Endovenous laser ablation of insufficient perforating veins: Energy is the key to success. *Vascular.* 2016;24:144–149.

15. Chehab M, Dixit P, Anypas E et al. Endovenous laser ablation of perforating veins: Feasibility, safety and occlusion rate using a 1,470-nm laser and bare tip fiber. *J Vasc Interv Radiol.* 2015;26:871–877.

16. Spiliopoulos S, Theodosiadou V, Sotiriadi A et al. Endovenous ablation of incompetent truncal veins and their perforators with a new radiofrequency system. Mid-term outcomes. *Vascular.* 2015;23:592–598.

17. Gabriel V, Jimenez JC, Alktaifi A et al. Success of endovenous saphenous and perforator ablation in patients with symptomatic venous insufficiency receiving long-term warfarin therapy. *Ann Vasc Surg.* 2012;26:607–611.

18. Tessari L, Cavezzi A, Frullini A. Preliminary experience with a new sclerosing foam in the treatment of varicose veins. *Dermatol Surg.* 2001;27:58–60.

19. Simka M. Principles and technique of foam sclerotherapy and its specific use in the treatment of venous leg ulcers. *Int J Low Extrem Wounds.* 2011;10:138–145.

20. Myers KA, Jolley D. Factors affecting the risk of deep venous occlusion after ultrasound-guided sclerotherapy for varicose veins. *Eur J Vasc Endovasc Surg.* 2008;36:602–605.

21. El-Sheikha J, Carradice D, Nandhra S et al. Systematic review of compression following treatment for varicose veins. *Br J Surg.* 2015;102:719–725.

22. Biemans AA, Kockaert M, Akkersdijk GP et al. Comparing endovenous laser ablation, foam sclerotherapy, and conventional surgery for great saphenous varicose veins. *J Vasc Surg.* 2013;58:727–34.

23. Shadid N, Ceulen R, Nelemans P et al. Randomized clinical trial of ultrasound-guided foam sclerotherapy versus surgery for the incompetent great saphenous vein. *Br J Surg.* 2012;99:1062–1070.

24. Van den Bos R, Arends L, Kockaert M et al. Endovenous therapies of lower extremity varicosities: a meta-analysis. *J Vasc Surg.* 2009;49:230–239.

25. Darvall KA, Bate GR, Silverman SH et al. Medium-term results of ultrasound-guided foam sclerotherapy for small saphenous varicose veins. *Br J Surg.* 96:1268–1273.

26. Carugo D, Ankrett DN, Zhao X et al. Benefits of polidocanol endovenous microfoam (Varithena®) compared with physician compounded foams. *Phlebology.* 2016;31:283–295.

27. Regan JD, Gibson KD, Rush JE et al. Clinical significance of cerebrovascular gas emboli during polidocanol endovenous ultra-low nitrogen microfoam ablation and correlation with magnetic resonance imaging in patients with right to left shunt. *J Vasc Surg.* 2011;53:131–138.

28. Masuda EM, Kessler DM, Lurie F et al. The effect of ultrasound-guided sclerotherapy of incompetent perforator veins on venous clinical severity and disability scores. *J Vasc Surg.* 2006;43:551–556.

29. Kiguchi MM, Hager ES, Winger DG et al. Factors that influence perforator thrombosis and predict healing with perforator sclerotherapy for venous ulceration without axial reflux. *J Vasc Surg.* 2014;59:1368–1376.

30. Van Eekeren RR, Hillebrands JL, van der Sloot K et al. Histological observations one year after mechanochemical endovenous ablation of the great saphenous vein. *J Endovasc Ther.* 2014;21:429–433.

31. Van Eekeren RR, Boersma D, Konjin V et al. Postoperative pain and early quality of life after radiofrequency ablation and mechanochemical endovenous ablation of incompetent great saphenous veins. *J Vasc Surg.* 2013;57:445–450.

32. Bootun R, Lane T, Dharmarajah B et al. Intra-procedural pain score in a randomized controlled trial comparing mechanochemical ablation to radiofrequency ablation: The Multicentre Venefit versus ClariVein® for varicose veins trial. *Phlebology.* 2016;31:61–65.

33. Morrison N, Gibson K, McEnroe S et al. Randomized trial comparing cyanoacrylate embolization and radiofrequency ablation for incompetent great saphenous veins (VeClose). *J Vasc Surg.* 2015;61:985–944.

34. Proebstle TM, Alm J, Dimitri et al. Twelve-month follow up of the European multicenter study on cyanoacrylate embolization of incompetent great saphenous veins [abstract]. *J Vasc Surg: Venous Lym Dis.* 2014;105–106.

35. Almeida JI, Javier JJ, MacKay E et al. First human use of cyanoacrylate adhesive for treatment of saphenous vein incompetence. *J Vasc Surg: Venous Lym Dis.* 2013;174–180.

36. MacKenzie RK, Allan PL, Ruckley CV et al. The effect of long saphenous vein stripping on deep venous reflux. *Eur J Vasc Endovasc Surg.* 2004;28:104–107.

37. Lurie F, Creton D, Eklof B et al. Prospective randomized study of endovenous radiofrequency obliteration (closure procedure) versus ligation and stripping in a selected patient population (EVOLVeS Study). *J Vasc Surg.* 2003;207–214.

38. Rautio T, Ohinmaa A, Perala J et al. Endovenous obliteration versus conventional stripping operation in the treatment of primary varicose veins: A randomized controlled trial with comparison of the costs. *J Vasc Surg.* 2002;35:958–965.

39. Mekako AI, Chetter IC, Coughlin PA et al. Randomized clinical trial of co-amoxiclav versus no antibiotic prophylaxis in varicose vein surgery. *Br J Surg.* 2010;97:29–36.

40. Rudstrom H, Bjorck M, Bergqvist D. Iatrogenic vascular injuries in varicose vein surgery: A systematic review. *World J Surg.* 2007;31:228–233.

41. Van Rij AM, Chai J, Hill GB et al. Incidence of deep vein thrombosis after varicose vein surgery. *Br J Surg.* 2004;91:1582–1585.

42. Harlander-Locke M, Jimenez JC, Lawrence PF et al. Endovenous ablation with concomitant phlebectomy is a safe and effective method of treatment for symptomatic patients with axial reflux and large incompetent tributaries. *J Vasc Surg.* 2013;58:166–172.

43. Passman M. Transilluminated powered phlebectomy in the treatment of varicose veins. *Vascular.* 2007;15:262–268.

44. Lawrence PF, Vardanian AJ. Light-assisted stab phlebectomy: Report of a technique for removal of lower extremity varicose veins. *J Vasc Surg.* 2007;46:1052–1054.

48

Deep vein thrombosis
Prevention and management

ANDREA T. OBI and THOMAS W. WAKEFIELD

CONTENTS

EPIDEMIOLOGY

Venous thromboembolism (VTE) includes deep vein thrombosis (DVT) and pulmonary embolism (PE). VTE affects up to 900,000 patients per year and results in 300,000 deaths per year. The incidence has remained constant since the 1980s and may be increasing in frequency as VTE risk increases with age.[1] VTE is a common cause of emergency department visits, accounting for 175 of every 100,000 visits by individuals aged >60 years in the United States.[2] VTE has been identified as a major threat to the safety of hospitalized patients.[3] In 2008, the US Surgeon General's Call to Action for VTE prevention was published, advocating for development of evidence-based practices for VTE screening and prevention.[4] This resulted in advancements in the prevention, diagnosis and treatment of VTE.

VTE represents a commonly encountered post-operative complication for the practising vascular surgeon. Among patients receiving a lower extremity amputation, the reported rate of VTE is 9.4%–13.2%.[5,6] VTE occurs in 2.4% of patients undergoing open aortic surgery. This rate increases with each increasing risk factor (to a maximum of 8% with ≥4 risk factors): operative time ≥ 5 hours, chronic steroid use, preoperative dyspnea, body mass index (BMI) ≥ 30, post-operative pneumonia, post-operative mechanical ventilation >48 hours or return to operating room within 30 days.[7] Among patients undergoing all types of outpatient surgery, saphenofemoral ligation and other venous procedures represented the highest risk for VTE (adjusted odds ratios [ORs] 13.2 and 15.6).[8]

RISK FACTORS

Risk factors for VTE include both acquired and genetic factors. Acquired factors include older age, surgery, malignancy, trauma, immobilization, oral contraceptives and hormone replacement therapy, pregnancy and puerperium, cardiac disease, neurologic disease, obesity and the development of antiphospholipid antibodies. Genetic factors include antithrombin deficiency; protein C and protein S deficiency; factor V Leiden, prothrombin 20210A gene variant, blood group non-O, fibrinogen and plasminogen abnormalities; elevated levels of clotting factors; and elevation in plasminogen activator inhibitor-1 (PAI-1). Work-up for hypercoagulability (including testing for the conditions noted in the previous sentence) may be indicated when a patient presents with an idiopathic VTE, has a strong family history of VTE, has multiple recurrences of VTE, has VTE in unusual locations or has VTE at an early age. Although the levels of evidence vary by condition between 1B/1C–2B/2C, indiscriminate testing for heritable thrombophilia in unselected patients with a first episode of DVT is not recommended (at 1B level of evidence).[9] Hematologic diseases associated with VTE include heparin-induced thrombocytopenia (HIT), disseminated intravascular coagulation, antiphospholipid antibody syndrome, thrombotic thrombocytopenic purpura, hemolytic uremic syndrome and myeloproliferative disorders.

Multiple weight-based scoring systems exist to predict the risk of VTE in the hospitalized patient. The aggregate risk score is associated with a percentage risk of VTE, which can be utilized to assign appropriate thromboprophylaxis regimen. The 2005 Caprini score is currently the most widely utilized and well-validated risk assessment model among surgical patients (Figure 48.1).[10] Based on our own institutional data, implementation of mandatory risk assessment of surgical patients with the 2005 Caprini risk model resulted in 50% decrease of in-hospital VTE over a 4-year period (Moote and Wakefield 2014, unpublished data).

Without prophylaxis, surgical procedures may have a VTE prevalence of up to 80%.[11] Historically, trials comparing no perioperative VTE prophylaxis to prophylaxis methods ranging from stockings and sequential compression devices (SCDs) or any form of anticoagulation showed that each prophylactic modality could decrease the risk of VTE at least 2–3-fold.[12,13] For this reason, every patient undergoing surgery should have some form of prophylaxis unless it is a minor or ambulatory procedure and the patient has no other VTE risk factors other than the procedure.[13]

There is no evidence to support the use of IVC filters for perioperative or trauma-related PE prophylaxis.

Whether based on a category or risk score, most at-risk patients who undergo major surgical procedures or suffer significant trauma should receive prophylaxis with an anticoagulant unless they have a high bleeding risk; in these cases, SCDs are recommended until the bleeding risk subsides. In high-risk VTE cases (such as in spine injury and hip replacement), stronger pharmacological agents (LMWH, pentasaccharides or warfarin) plus SCDs are recommended for prophylaxis, while unfractionated heparin, SCDs and aspirin alone are not

effective prophylaxis. In surgical procedures where the bleeding risk outweighs the benefit of an anticoagulant (such as certain neurologic and vascular procedures), mechanical prophylaxis usually suffices. These include graduated compression stockings and SCDs. These devices need to be on patient's limbs and working, requiring surveillance for compliance.[14]

PATHOPHYSIOLOGY

Although Virchow's triad of stasis, vein injury and hypercoagulability has defined the events that predispose to DVT formation since the mid-nineteenth century, the inflammatory response at the level of the vein wall, in relation to thrombogenesis, is increasingly becoming appreciated.[15] The inflammatory response determines both the ultimate resolution of the thrombosis and the fibrosis of the vein wall and vein valves leading to post-thrombotic syndrome.[16–19]

DIAGNOSIS

Deep venous thrombosis

The diagnosis of DVT must be made with duplex ultrasound imaging and laboratory testing, because history and physical examination is frequently inaccurate. Patients often present with a dull ache or pain the calf or legs. Conditions that may be confused with DVT include, muscle strain, muscle contusion, lymphedema, and systemic problems such as cardiac, renal or hepatic abnormalities. Systemic problems usually lead to bilateral edema. The most common physical finding is edema, and Wells has classified patients into a scoring system. Characteristics that score points in the Wells system include active cancer, paralysis or paresis, recent plaster immobilization of the lower extremity, being recently bedridden for 3 days or more, localized tenderness along the distribution of the deep venous system, swelling of the entire leg, calf swelling that is at least 3 cm larger on the involved side than on the noninvolved side, pitting edema in the symptomatic leg, collateral nonvaricose superficial veins and a history of previous DVT.[20] With extensive proximal iliofemoral DVT, swelling, cyanosis and dilated superficial collateral veins may become very significant.

Duplex ultrasound imaging has become the gold standard for the diagnosis of DVT (Figure 48.2 and Table 48.1) over the past 20–25 years. Duplex imaging includes both a B-mode image and Doppler flow pattern, thus the name. Duplex imaging demonstrates sensitivity and specificity rates greater than 95% for the diagnosis of DVT.[21] According to the Grade criteria for the strength of medical evidence, duplex ultrasound is given 1B level of evidence.[22] Even for calf vein DVT where concern has been expressed for the accuracy of duplex imaging, this technique is acceptable in symptomatic patients. Advantages of duplex

Thrombosis risk factor assessment

Patient's Name:_____ Age:_____ Sex:_____ Wgt:_____ lbs

Choose All That Apply

Each Risk Factor Represents 1 Point
- Age 41–60 years
- Minor surgery planned
- History of prior major surgery
- Varicose veins
- History of inflammatory bowel disease
- Swollen legs (current)
- Obesity (BMI >30)
- Acute myocardial infarction (<1 month)
- Congestive heart failure (<1 month)
- Sepsis (<1 month)
- Serious lung disease incl. pneumonia (<1 month)
- Abnormal pulmonary function (COPD)
- Medical patient currently at bed rest
- Leg plaster cast or brace
- Other risk factors

Each Risk Factor Represents 3 Points
- Age over 75 years
- Major surgery lasting 2–3 hours
- BMI >50 (venous stasis syndrome)
- History of SVT, DVT/PE
- Family history of DVT/PE
- Present cancer or chemotherapy
- Positive Factor V Leiden
- Positive Prothrombin 20210A
- Elevated serum homocysteine
- Positive Lupus anticoagulant
- Elevated anticardiolipin antibodies
- Heparin-induced thrombocytopenia (HIT)
- Other thrombophilia
  Type_____

Each Risk Factor Represents 2 Points
- Age 60–74 years
- Major surgery (>60 minutes)
- Arthroscopic surgery (>60 minutes)
- Laparoscopic surgery (>60 minutes)
- Previous malignancy
- Central venous access
- Morbid obesity (BMI >40)

Each Risk Factor Represents 5 Points
- Elective major lower extremity arthroplasty
- Hip, pelvis or leg fracture (<1 month)
- Stroke (<1 month)
- Multiple trauma (<1 month)
- Acute spinal cord injury (paralysis) (<1 month)
- Major surgery lasting over 3 hours

For Women Only (Each Represents 1 Point)
- Oral contraceptives or hormone replacement therapy
- Pregnancy or postpartum (<1 month)
- History of unexplained stillborn infant, recurrent spontaneous abortion (≥3), premature birth with toxemia or growth-restricted infant

Total Risk Factor Score   ☐

Please see Following Page for Prophylaxis Safety Considerations Revised May 16, 2006

Prophylaxis Regimen

Total Risk Factor Score	Incidence of DVT	Risk Level	Prophylaxis Regimen	Legend
0–1	<10%	Low Risk	No specific measures; early ambulation	ES – Elastic Stockings
2	10–20%	Moderate Risk	ES or IPC or LDUH, or LWMH	IPC – Intermittent Pneumatic Compression
3–4	20–40%	High Risk	IPC or LDUH, or LMWH alone *or* in combination with ES or IPC	LDUH – Low Dose Unfractionated Heparin
5 or more	40–80% 1–5% mortality	Highest Risk	Pharmacological: LDUH, LMWH*, Warfarin*, or Fac Xa* alone *or* in combination with ES or IPC	LMWH – Low Molecular Weight Heparin

Prophylaxis Safety Considerations: Check box if answer is 'YES'

Anticoagulants: Factors Associated with Increased Bleeding
- ☐ Is patient experiencing any active bleeding?
- ☐ Does patient have (or has had history of) heparin-induced thrombocytopenia?
- ☐ Is patient's platelet count < 100,00/mm^3?
- ☐ Is patient taking oral anticoagulants, platelet inhibitors (e.g. NSAIDS, Clopidigrel, Salicylates)?
- ☐ Is patent's creatinine clearance abnormal? If yes, please indicate value_____

If any of the above boxes are checked, the patient may not be a candidate for anticoagulant therapy and you should consider alternative prophylactic measures.

Intermittent Pneumatic Compression (IPC)
- ☐ Does patient have severe peripheral arterial disease?
- ☐ Does patient have congestive heart failure?
- ☐ Does patient have an acute superficial/deep vein thrombosis?

If any of the above boxes are checked, then patient may not be a candidate for intermittent compression therapy and you should consider alternative prophylactic measures.

Figure 48.1 Caprini risk factor thrombosis assessment tool. (Reprinted with permission from Wakefield T and Henke P, *Complications in Surgery*, 2nd ed. Lippincott Williams & Wilkins, Philadelphia, PA, 2011, p. 353.)

imaging include the fact that it is painless, requires no contrast, can be repeated and is safe to perform during pregnancy. Importantly, duplex can also identify other causes of a patient's symptoms. Additional tests available for making the diagnosis include magnetic resonance imaging (MRI) (especially good for assessing central pelvic vein and inferior vena cava thrombosis) and spiral computed tomographic (CT) imaging (especially with chest imaging during examination for PE).

A single complete negative duplex scan is accurate enough to withhold anticoagulation with minimal long-term adverse thromboembolic complications.[23] For a complete test, this requires all venous segments of the leg have been imaged and evaluated. If the duplex scan is unavailable or indeterminate owing to edema or other technical issues, treatment may be based on factors such as biomarkers, with the duplex repeated in 24–72 hours when swelling has decreased. Combining clinical characteristics with a biomarker for thrombosis (D-dimer assay) can decrease the number of duplex scans necessary.[20] Although clinical characteristics and D-dimer levels are useful to rule out thrombosis, the converse is not true due to the relative low specificity of D-dimer for diagnosis of VTE. There is no combination of biomarkers and clinical presentation that can rule in the diagnosis as of today. Work is ongoing to establish new biomarkers based on the inflammatory response to DVT involving P-selectin (sPSel).[16] We have demonstrated that combining two variables, sPSel with Wells score (clinical pretest probability of DVT), establishes the diagnosis of DVT.[17] Furthermore, in order to rule in DVT, sPSel (≥90 ng/mL) combined with Wells score (≥2) showed a better PPV (91%) than D-dimer (≥500 ng/mL) combined with Wells score (≥2), which was 69%, thus for the first time suggesting a biomarker and clinical evaluation that can establish the diagnosis of DVT.[16]

Pulmonary embolism

The diagnosis of PE has included ventilation–perfusion (V/Q) scanning and pulmonary angiography. However, the most current techniques include spiral CT imaging and MRI. CT imaging demonstrates excellent specificity and sensitivity. The sensitivity of isolated chest CT imaging is increased when clinical analysis is added and when adding lower extremity imaging to the chest scan.[18] In a study which defined the role of CT as compared to other techniques for diagnosis, results from the PIOPED II study demonstrate that if the clinical presentation and spiral CT imaging results are concordant, therapies can be safely recommended. However, if clinical presentation and spiral CT imaging are discordant and do not support each other, other confirmatory tests are necessary to be assured of the diagnosis. For the diagnosis of PE, spiral CT imaging is given a 1A level of evidence. MRI and V/Q imaging are useful alternative techniques for these situations where discordant results are obtained, and pulmonary angiography if an intervention is planned.[24]

TREATMENT

Standard therapy for venous thromboembolism

The traditional treatment of VTE is systemic anticoagulation, which reduces the risk of PE, thrombus extension and recurrence. Because VTE recurrence is higher if anticoagulation is not therapeutic in the first 24 hours, immediate anticoagulation should occur. For PE, this usually means anticoagulation and then diagnostic testing. For DVT, since duplex imaging is rapidly obtained, testing precedes anticoagulation. Recurrent DVT can still occur in up to one-third of patients over an 8-year period, even with appropriate anticoagulant therapy.[19]

Heparin/LMWH

Unfractionated heparin or low-molecular-weight heparin (LMWH) is given for 5 days, during which time oral anticoagulation with vitamin K antagonists (usually warfarin) is begun as soon as anticoagulation is therapeutic.

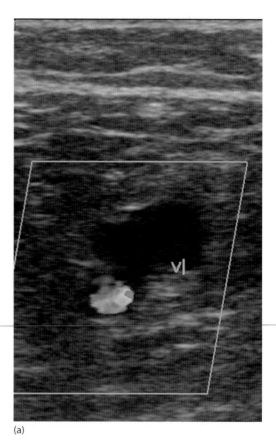

(a)

Figure 48.2 DVT, as assessed by duplex ultrasound. (a) Acute DVT of the right popliteal vein. Note the dilated vein with lack of intraluminal echoes. *(Continued)*

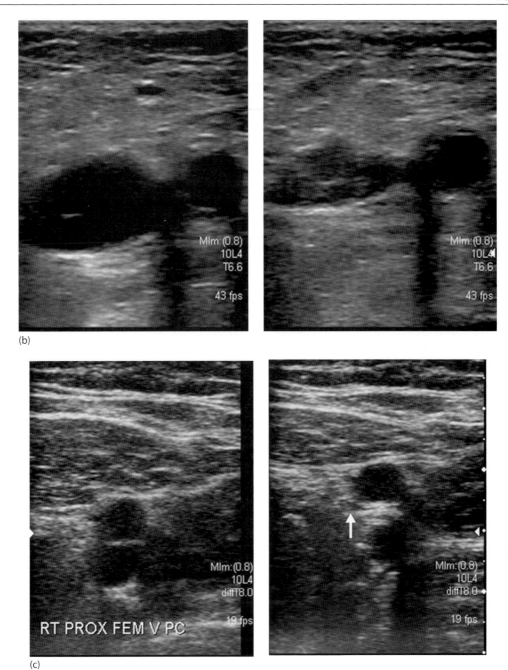

(b)

(c)

Figure 48.2 (*Continued*) DVT, as assessed by duplex ultrasound. (b) Subacute DVT of the left common femoral vein, without and with compression. Note the chronic echoes in a dilated vein, when the vein is compressed in the right panel. (c) Chronic DVT of the right femoral vein, without and with compression. Note the chronic echoes in the vein indicated by the white arrow.

Table 48.1 Features of acute and chronic deep vein thrombosis.

Acute DVT	Chronic DVT	Subacute DVT
Vein enlarged compared to adjoining artery	Vein small compared to adjoining artery	Characteristics from both acute and chronic present
Lack of intraluminal echoes	Intraluminal echoes present	
Lack of significant collaterals	Presence of significant collaterals	

It is recommended that the international normalized ratio (INR) be therapeutic for 2 consecutive days before stopping heparin or LMWH.[25]

LMWH, derived from the lower molecular weight range of standard heparin, has become the standard treatment. LMWH is preferred because it is administered subcutaneously, requires no monitoring (except in certain circumstances such as renal insufficiency or morbid obesity) and it is associated with lower bleeding. This allows for home administration. Additionally, LMWH demonstrates less direct thrombin inhibition and more factor Xa inhibition and the half-life of LMWH is dose independent, and it is given in a weight-based fashion. Certain LMWHs decrease indices of chronic venous insufficiency compared to standard therapy when used over an extended period. In a study of 480 patients, the LMWH tinzaparin for 12 weeks was superior to warfarin regarding treatment satisfaction, signs and symptoms of postthrombotic syndrome and the incidence of leg ulcers.[26] Although the reason for this fact is not known, it suggests that there are pleiotropic effects of LMWH or that more consistent anticoagulation is accomplished. LMWH is now preferred over standard unfractionated heparin for the initial treatment of VTE with a level of evidence given 2B (according to the 2012 ACCP guidelines).[27]

Warfarin

Warfarin (Coumadin) should be started after anticoagulation is therapeutic to prevent warfarin-induced skin necrosis. For standard unfractionated heparin, this requires therapeutic activated partial thromboplastin time, while for LMWH, this assumes an appropriate weight-based dose of LMWH has been administered and allowed to circulate. Warfarin causes inhibition of protein C and S before factors II, IX and X, leading to potential paradoxical hypercoagulability at therapy initiation. The goal for warfarin dosing is an INR between 2.0 and 3.0.

New anticoagulants (factor Xa and factor IIa inhibitors)

Fondaparinux (Arixtra), a synthetic pentasaccharide that has an antithrombin sequence identical to heparin, targets factor Xa (Figure 48.3). Fondaparinux has been approved for the treatment of DVT and PE; for thrombosis prophylaxis in patients with total hip replacement, total knee replacement and hip fracture in patients undergoing abdominal surgery, and in general medical patients.[29] Fondaparinux is administered subcutaneously and has a 17-hour half-life; its dosage is based on body weight. It exhibits no endothelial or protein binding and importantly does not produce thrombocytopenia. However, no antidote is readily available. In a meta-analysis involving more than 7000 patients, there was more than a 50% risk reduction using fondaparinux beginning 6 hours after surgery compared to LMWH beginning 12–24 hours after surgery.[28] Major

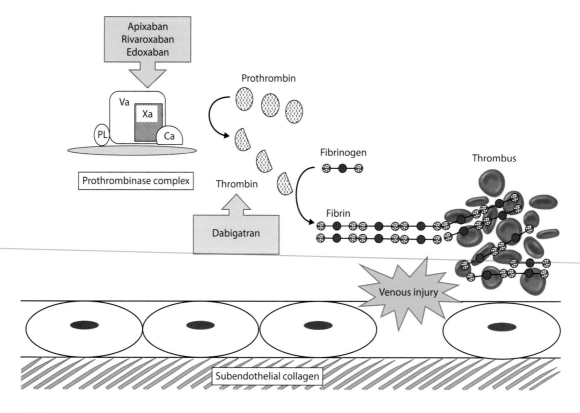

Figure 48.3 Mechanism of action of new anticoagulants. (Modified with permission from Knepper J et al., *J Vasc Surg: Venous Lym Dis*, 1(4), 419, 2013.)

bleeding was increased, while critical bleeding was not increased.[29] For the treatment of VTE, fondaparinux was found equal to LMWH for DVT, and for PE, it was found equal to standard heparin.[29,30] Fondaparinux has also been found to be effective for the treatment of superficial thrombosis over a 45-day course of treatment, and it has been given a level of evidence of 2B for the treatment of superficial thrombophlebitis.[27,31]

Dabigatran targets active factor II (factor IIa), whereas rivaroxaban, apixaban and edoxaban target activated factor X (factor Xa) (Figure 48.3). Dabigatran etexilate is FDA approved for stroke and systemic embolization prevention in patients with atrial fibrillation and for the treatment of DVT and PE in patients who have been treated with another anticoagulant for 5–10 days. Rivaroxaban is FDA approved for VTE prophylaxis in patients undergoing hip or knee replacements, for stroke and systemic embolization prevention in patients with atrial fibrillation and for VTE treatment. The Einstein trial evaluated rivaroxaban compared to standard anticoagulation in the treatment of acute DVT.[32] Rivaroxaban, as monotherapy, was found statistically noninferior to standard therapy, without increased bleeding. Additionally, the Einstein group added a continued treatment group compared to placebo for an additional 6–12 months. Extended rivaroxaban showed a significant decrease in recurrent VTE without an increase in major bleeding compared to placebo. A similar finding with PE has been found.[33] Apixaban is currently FDA approved for the prevention of complications of atrial fibrillation, for the prophylaxis of DVT following hip or knee replacement surgery, for the treatment of DVT/PE and for reduction in the risk of recurrence of DVT/PE. Apixaban as extended treatment of VTE was investigated compared to placebo. After initial treatment, an additional 12 months of apixaban therapy was compared to placebo. A significant decrease in the rate of VTE without increase in bleeding was found.[34] Finally, edoxaban has also shown promise in treatment of DVT and has recently been approved by FDA for prevention of stroke and non-central-nervous system systemic embolization in patients with nonvalvular atrial fibrillation, and for treating DVT and PE in patients who have been treated with a parenteral anticoagulant for 5 to 10 days.[35] Problems with these new agents include the inability at the present time to reliably reverse their anticoagulant effects, the paucity of data available regarding bridging of these agents when performing other procedures and no reliable way to measure levels if these agents fail. Although many questions remain unanswered, these agents demonstrate great promise.

Duration of treatment

The duration of anticoagulation depends on a number of factors including the risk of thrombosis at presentation, the presence of continuing risk factors for thrombosis, the type of thrombosis (idiopathic or provoked), the number of times thrombosis has occurred, the status

of the veins when stopping anticoagulation and the level of D-dimer measured approximately 1 month after stopping warfarin (Figure 48.4).[27,36] The recommended duration of anticoagulation after a first episode of VTE is 3 months for both proximal and distal thrombi.[27] After a second episode of VTE, the usual recommendation is prolonged warfarin unless the patient is very young at the time of presentation or there are other mitigating factors. Factors that increase the rate of VTE recurrence include homozygous factor V Leiden and prothrombin 20210A mutation, protein C or protein S deficiency, antithrombin deficiency, antiphospholipid antibodies and cancer (unless resolved). In these circumstances, long-term warfarin is usually recommended. Heterozygous factor V Leiden and prothrombin 20210A do not carry the same risk for recurrence as their homozygous counterparts, and the length of oral anticoagulation is shortened for these conditions.[37]

Regarding idiopathic DVT, in those with a low bleeding risk, the recommended length of treatment is extended therapy for more than 3 months. A statistically significant advantage to resuming warfarin if the D-dimer assay is elevated over an average 1.4-year follow-up (OR 4.26; p = 0.02) has been described and confirmed by a meta-analysis. Criteria that have been described for discontinuing anticoagulation are given a level of evidence of 1B to 2B, depending on the clinical situation. In addition, there is growing evidence that in certain circumstances, such as active cancer, the use of LMWH is superior to warfarin for long-term treatment, at least when given over a 6-month period of time.[27] Regarding the new oral anticoagulants, there is not enough data to know if they are indicated in cancer patients.

Complications

Bleeding is the most common complication of anticoagulation. With standard heparin, bleeding occurs over the first 5 days in approximately 10% of patients. Another potentially devastating complication is HIT, which occurs in 0.6%–30% of patients. Although historically morbidity and mortality have been high, it has been found that early diagnosis and appropriate treatment have decreased these rates. HIT usually begins 3–14 days after heparin starts, although it can occur earlier if the patient has been exposed to heparin in the past. A heparin-dependent antibody binds to platelets and activates them with the release of procoagulant microparticles leading to both arterial and venous thromboses and thrombocytopenia.[38]

Both bovine and porcine unfractionated heparin and LMWH have been associated with HIT, although the incidence and severity of the thrombosis appear to be less with LMWH. Even small exposure to heparin, such as heparin coating on indwelling catheters, can cause the syndrome. The diagnosis should be suspected with a 50% or greater drop in platelet count, when the platelet count falls below

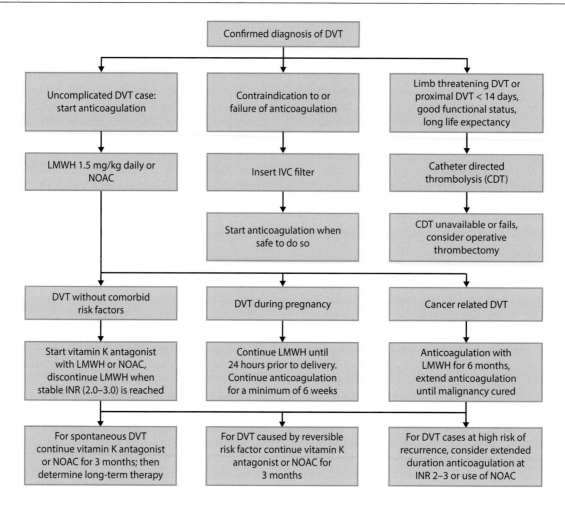

Figure 48.4 DVT treatment algorithm.

100,000 µL or when thrombosis occurs during heparin or LMWH therapy.[39] HITTS is HIT associated with episodes of thrombosis.

The enzyme-linked immunosorbent assay (ELISA) detects the antiheparin antibody in the plasma. This test is highly sensitive put poorly specific. The serotonin release assay is another test that can be used, and this test is more specific but less sensitive than the ELISA test. Often, a combination of both tests gives the best diagnostic accuracy.

When the diagnosis is made, heparin must be stopped. Warfarin should not be given until an adequate alternative anticoagulant is given and established and until the platelet count has normalized (or at least returned to 150,000). Because LMWHs demonstrate high cross-reactivity with standard heparin antibodies, they cannot be substituted for standard heparin in patients with HIT. The direct thrombin inhibitor argatroban has been approved by FDA as an alternate agent. Fondaparinux (Arixtra) has also been found effective for treatment of HIT in many cases, but it is not FDA approved for this indication. The use of these alternative agents is given either a 2C or 1C level of evidence according to the 2012 ACCP guidelines.

NONPHARMACOLOGICAL TREATMENTS

The severity of postthrombotic syndrome after proximal DVT can be decreased by the use of compression stockings.[40] Additionally, walking with good compression does not increase the risk of PE, whereas significantly decreases the incidence and severity of the postthrombotic syndrome.[41] The use of strong compression and early ambulation after DVT treatment can significantly reduce the pain and swelling resulting from the DVT and carries a 1A level of evidence. However, a recent multicentre randomized trial has suggested that stockings do not prevent post-thrombotic syndrome after a first proximal DVT.[42] This large randomized study, brings to light the fact that no adequate medical therapy exists for prevention of PTS in modern day healthcare.

AGGRESSIVE THERAPIES FOR VENOUS THROMBOEMBOLISM

For DVT treatment, the goals are to prevent extension or recurrence of DVT, prevent PE and minimize the late sequelae of thrombosis, namely, chronic venous insufficiency called the postthrombotic syndrome. Standard anticoagulants accomplish the first two goals but not the third goal. The postthrombotic syndrome occurs in up to 30% of patients after DVT, even higher if ipsilateral recurrent DVT, and in an even higher percentage of patients with iliofemoral level DVT.[19] More aggressive therapies for extensive thrombosis are indicated.

Experimentally, prolonged contact of the thrombus with the vein wall increases damage.[15] The thrombosis initiates an inflammatory response in the vein wall that can lead to valvular dysfunction and vein wall fibrosis. Thus, removing the thrombus should be an excellent solution to decrease this interaction, although it may not eliminate the pathophysiology. For example, the longer a thrombus is in contact with a vein valve, the more chance that valve will no longer function.[43]

Venous thrombectomy has proved superior to anticoagulation over 6 months to 10 years as measured by venous patency and prevention of venous reflux.[44] Catheter-directed thrombolysis has been employed in many nonrandomized studies and in small, randomized trials was more effective than standard therapy. Quality of life was improved with thrombolysis. Results are optimized further by combining catheter-directed thrombolysis with mechanical devices.[45,46] These devices include the AngioJet rheolytic catheter and the EKOS ultrasound-accelerated catheter. These devices hasten thrombolysis, decrease the amount of thrombolytic agent needed and thus decrease bleeding potential.

Additionally, the use of venous stents for iliac venous obstruction has been shown to decrease the incidence of postthrombotic syndrome and chronic venous insufficiency.[47] To evaluate the role of aggressive therapy in proximal iliofemoral venous thrombosis, a study has been approved by the National Institutes of Health to compare catheter-directed pharmacomechanical thrombolysis to standard anticoagulation for significant iliofemoral venous thrombosis. This study, the Attract Trial, will evaluate anatomic, physiologic and quality-of-life end points.

For PE, evidence exists that thrombolysis is indicated when there is hemodynamic compromise from the embolism.[48] Consensus does not exist on whether thrombolysis should be used in situations in which there is no hemodynamic comprise but there is evidence of right heart dysfunction or there are positive biomarkers. Future studies will address these situations.[49]

INFERIOR VENA CAVA FILTERS

Traditional indications for the use of IVC filters include a contraindication to anticoagulation, a complication of anticoagulation or failure of anticoagulation. Protection from PE is greater than 95% using cone-shaped, wire-based permanent filters in the IVC.[50] Recently, indications have expanded to the presence of free-floating thrombus tails, prophylactic use when the risk for anticoagulation is excessive and when the risk of PE is thought to be high and to allow the use of perioperative epidural anesthesia.

IVC filters can be either permanent or retrievable. If a retrievable filter is left, then it becomes a permanent filter; the long-term fate of these filters has yet to be defined adequately. Most filters are placed in the infrarenal location in the IVC. However, they may be placed in the suprarenal or the superior vena cava position. Indications for the suprarenal placement include pregnancy or patient of childbearing age, or previous device failure filled with thrombus. Although some have suggested that sepsis is a contraindication to the use of filters, sepsis has not been found to be contraindication because the trapped material can be sterilized with intravenous antibiotics.

Filters may be inserted under x-ray guidance or using ultrasound techniques, either external ultrasound or intravascular ultrasound. Other than two randomized prospective studies on the use of IVC filters as treatment of DVT (which is not how filters are traditionally used), evidence for the use of filters is rated at a 2C grade.[51] This randomized study, suggesting that filters may lead to a higher incidence of DVT, has been the catalyst for the development of retrievable IVC filters.

UNIQUE CIRCUMSTANCES

Upper extremity thrombosis

Upper extremity venous thrombosis is found most frequently in the subclavian vein followed by the axillary and brachial veins. Thrombosis is primary (approximately 20%) when related to thoracic outlet obstruction, Paget–Schroetter syndrome (so-called effort-related thrombosis) or idiopathic. Thrombosis is secondary (approximately 80%) when related to catheters and lines, surgery or trauma, pregnancy or the use of oral contraceptive pills and cancer. Patients present with arm discomfort, edema, dilated venous collateral and discoloration. However, when associated with catheters, most patients are asymptomatic. The main complications, although less frequent than with lower extremity DVT, include PE (6%), recurrence at 12 months (2%–5%) and postthrombotic syndrome (5%).[52] If there is mortality, it usually relates to underlying malignancy or other medical problems. As with lower extremity DVT, the diagnosis is most often made by duplex ultrasound imaging (sensitivity/specificity rates greater than 95%). Duplex cannot evaluate certain locations well such as behind the clavicle, while for central locations, CTV or MRV may be most effective.

Therapy depends on aetiology. Spontaneous thrombosis is most frequently treated with anticoagulation for 3 months. Catheter- or line-associated thrombosis is treated with anticoagulation with catheter removal if the catheter is no longer needed or anticoagulation leaving the catheter in place if still needed.[27] If the catheter must remain in place for ongoing medical therapy, it is recommended that anticoagulation be continued for the duration that the catheter remains in place. For those patients presenting with venous thrombosis of recent onset, extensive swelling and functional arm impairment, catheter-directed thrombolysis may be indicated. For thrombosis associated with thoracic outlet compression, catheter-directed thrombolysis or pharmacomechanical thrombolysis followed by thoracic outlet decompression is most applicable.[53] Thrombosis of superficial veins or those distal to the brachial vein (such as basilic or cephalic) do not require treatment with anticoagulation and should be treated as superficial thrombophlebitis.

Phlegmasia

Massive iliofemoral DVT may result in the development of phlegmasia alba dolens (white swollen leg) or phlegmasia cerulea dolens (blue swollen leg). Venous gangrene may occur if the phlegmasia is not aggressively treated as the arterial inflow becomes obstructed due to the effects of the venous hypertension.[54] As an alternative explanation, arterial emboli or spasm may occur and contribute to the pathophysiology. The skin blisters and the toes on the limb may turn black. Venous gangrene is often associated with an underlying malignancy and is always preceded by phlegmasia cerulea dolens. Venous gangrene is associated with significant morbidity including amputation rates of 20%–50%, PE rates of 12%–40% and mortality rates of 25%–40%. The reversible phase of ischemic venous occlusion may lead to irreversible changes of gangrene and tissue loss in 40%–60% of patients, unless it is treated aggressively.[55] Aggressive therapies may include both venous thrombectomy and thrombolysis. In a recent meta-analysis of 62 patients, systemic heparin was used in 87%, angioplasty in 8%, angioplasty with stenting in 7%, catheter-directed thrombolysis in 23%, fasciotomy in 16%, venous thrombectomy in 29% and venous bypass in 2%. With this treatment, the overall outcome was improvement in 60%, major amputation in 14% and mortality in 26%. The highest mortality was seen in those managed with surgical thrombectomy (22%), and the highest rate of amputation was noted in those treated with fasciotomy.[55] We do not favour fasciotomy in this situation, as it makes further anticoagulation therapy and certainly thrombolytic therapy problematic. As a general rule, if the patient does not respond to initial extremity elevation, fluid resuscitation and aggressive systemic anticoagulation (usually within the first 6 hours), then catheter-directed thrombolysis with pharmacomechanical assist should be the first-line therapy, while surgical venous thrombectomy is reserved for patients who have contraindications to thrombolysis.[56]

Superficial vein thrombophlebitis

The clinical diagnosis of superficial vein thrombophlebitis (SVT) usually is made with the presence of pain, a firm palpable cord with inflammation, tenderness, surrounding erythema and edema.[57] Duplex ultrasound of the affected extremity should be performed due to the high incidence of concomitant DVT.[57] A thrombophilia work-up may be indicated in selected patients (those with recurrent primary SVT, a strong family history and concomitant DVT). Screening including mammography, colonoscopy and chest x-ray for underlying diseases, including malignancy or vasculitis, should be performed if indicated.[57]

Treatment of SVT should be based on location of the thrombus, the presence or absence of concomitant DVT and any associated infectious process. When SVT coexists with DVT, the treatment is the same as for the DVT. In a recent prospective epidemiologic study including 844 patients with symptomatic SVT, approximately 25% had concomitant DVT upon enrollment. Of the 600 patients without DVT followed up for 3 months, an additional 58 (10%) developed thromboembolic complications including 3 (0.5%) PE, 15 (2.8%) DVT, 18 (3.3%) extension and 10 (1.9%) recurrence of SVT. These events occurred despite anticoagulant treatment with LMWH 374 (63%) at therapeutic and 216 (37%) prophylactic dose for 10–17 days.[58]

If the thrombus extends toward the level of the saphenofemoral junction, several difference approaches have been followed. These include ligation and/or stripping, elastic support, nonsteroidal anti-inflammatory drugs (NSAIDs) to reduce pain and inflammation and heparin (unfractionated heparin or LMWH) followed by oral anticoagulant therapy. SVT in either the GSV or SSV may have the greatest risk for extension into the deep venous system and thus requires aggressive anticoagulant therapy.[59] However, other locations may be associated with a lower risk of extension, thus requiring less aggressive therapy such as compression and NSAIDs.[60] Treatment for SVT in tributaries and the distal GSV includes ambulation, warm soaks, compression and NSAIDs.[61,62] If a patient has risk factors for extension to DVT, then pharmacological treatment at the prophylactic dose of LMWH for 4 weeks may be appropriate.[60] In patients with SVT of at least 5 cm of length and at least 3 cm distal to the saphenofemoral junction, daily treatment for 45 days for patients with fondaparinux or prophylactic LMWH is recommended (evidence grade 2B).[31] In those with SVT treated with anticoagulation, the recommendation is for fondaparinux 2.5 mg daily over a prophylactic dose of LMWH (evidence grade 2C).[27]

Among studies that have been completed, LMWH has been compared with saphenofemoral disconnection for the treatment of proximal great saphenous vein SVT in a prospective, randomized clinical study.[63] Eighty-four consecutive patients with proximal thrombophlebitis alone were divided into two groups treated with saphenofemoral disconnection under local anesthesia with a short hospital stay (n = 45) or enoxaparin (1 mg/kg bid) on an outpatient basis for 4 weeks (n = 39). Thirty patients in each group completed the study with follow-up at 1, 3 and 6 months. In the surgical group 2 patients (6.7%) developed complications of the surgical wound, 1 (3.3%) developed thrombophlebitis recurrence, and 2 (6.7%) suffered non-fatal PE over 6 months. In the medical group, there was no progression of the thrombosis to the deep venous system or

PE, two cases (6.7%) of minor bleeding noted and three cases (10%) of thrombophlebitis recurrence. Even though the study found no statistically significant difference between the two groups, the LMWH group showed a significant socio-economic advantage and confirmed the efficacy of LMWH treatment. Twenty-four studies involving 2469 patients were included in a Cochrane Review.[60] Both LMWH and NSAIDs significantly reduced SVT extension or recurrence by about 70% compared to placebo, while surgical treatments improved local relief from pain. Surgical treatment with ligation of the great saphenous vein at the saphenofemoral junction allows for superior symptomatic relief of pain, while medical management with anticoagulants appears superior for minimizing complications and preventing subsequent DVT/PE.[64]

ENDOVENOUS HEAT-INDUCED THROMBOSIS

Endovenous heat-induced thrombosis (EHIT) is a condition in which there is a tail of thrombus that extends from the part of the great saphenous vein that has been closed with heat, either with laser or radiofrequency ablation. The incidence of EHIT ranges in general from approximately 2%–8%, depending on the series and the technique of ablation. There are two classification systems about EHIT, one by Kabnick classes 1–4 and a second system from Lawrence (levels 1–6). In the first system, the four classes are[65,66]:

- *Class 1*: Venous thrombosis to the superficial–deep junction (i.e. saphenofemoral junction or saphenopopliteal junction, but not extending into the deep system)
- *Class 2*: Non-occlusive venous thrombosis, with an extension into the deep system of a cross-sectional area of less than 50%
- *Class 3*: Non-occlusive venous thrombosis into the deep venous system, with an extension into the deep system of a cross-sectional area of more than 50%
- *Class 4*: Occlusive DVT of the common femoral vein

In the second system, levels are described[67]:

- *Level 1*: Thrombus below the level of the epigastric vein
- *Level 2*: Closure with thrombus extension flush with the orifice of the epigastric vein
- *Level 3*: Closure with thrombus extension flush with the saphenofemoral junction
- *Level 4*: Closure with thrombus bulging into the common femoral vein
- *Level 5*: Closure with proximal thrombus extension adherent to the adjacent wall of the common femoral vein past the saphenofemoral junction
- *Level 6*: Closure with proximal thrombus extension into the common femoral vein, consistent with a DVT

EHIT appears to be a different pathophysiologic entity than DVT. It appears to display ultrasound characteristics of chronicity earlier than does DVT, and it tends to regress much more rapidly than DVT. It is also rarely associated with PE. As such, its treatment is different than that for DVT and its treatment is driven by the anatomical class or level. In the Kabnick system, class 1 EHIT is totally benign and can be ignored for the most part; for classes 2 EHIT, duplex follow-up may be indicated but no pharmacological treatment is recommended; class 3 is usually treated with 1 week of anticoagulation and then duplex follow-up, while class 4 is treated as DVT.[65] In the Lawrence system, patients with level 1 or 2 closure undergo no further management, patients with level 3 are managed with both observation and repeat duplex imaging or with LMWH, patients with level 4 are treated uniformly with LMWH until the thrombus retracts flush with or into the GSV and then no further anticoagulation is given, patients with level 5 are treated with outpatient LMWH, which is used until the thrombus retreats to level 3, while for level 6, patients are treated with LMWH and Coumadin for 3 months.[67] A similar classification system has been developed for the small saphenous vein with level A closure (thrombus extending ≥1 mm caudal to the saphenopopliteal junction [SPJ]), level B closure (thrombus flush with or <1 mm with the popliteal vein), level C closure (thrombus extending into the popliteal vein) and level D closure (entire popliteal vein involved). In this system, level A closures are ignored, level B closures return for a repeat ultrasound in 1 week to assess for progression, level C closures are managed with LMWH until the thrombus retracts to level A or B and level D closures are managed as a DVT.[68]

Splanchnic thrombosis

Splanchnic thrombosis occurs most commonly in the setting of cirrhosis, solid organ cancer and abdominal infection or inflammation, although nearly a third of cases may be idiopathic.[69] The main benefit of treatment of symptomatic thrombosis is to decrease risk of bowel and splenic infarct and is given a grade 1B recommendation by the ACCP guidelines. Anticoagulation can decrease progression and recurrence of thrombosis with acceptable bleeding risk in this patient population.[27] However, data regarding treatment of incidentally discovered asymptomatic thrombosis are lacking. Treatment might be considered if thrombosis is acute, extends on serial imaging and is associated with malignancy and the patient is a good risk candidate for anticoagulation. Chronic changes such as cavernous transformation of portal vein usually indicate that the anticoagulation will be of minimal benefit.

Cancer associated

Malignancy increases the risk of developing VTE up to 7-fold compared to the general population.[70] Certain cancers (such as stomach and pancreas) and active chemotherapy predispose a greater risk of thrombosis. The increased risk is multifactorial: tumor cell release of microparticles and tissue factor, oncogene-driven expression of hemostatic proteins, activation of neutrophils and release of neutrophil extracellular traps have all been implicated. Primary prevention of VTE in cancer patients undergoing abdominal or pelvic surgery with 4 weeks of LMWH is recommended by the ACCP (grade 1B). In a randomized controlled trial, major VTE events were significantly reduced (RR reduction, 82.4%; 95% CI, 21.5%–96.1%; p = 0.01) in patients receiving extended duration prophylaxis.[71]

Treatment of acute VTE in patients with malignancy should be limited to LMWH as recommended by both the ACCP and American Society of Clinical Oncology Guidelines (grade 2B). Use of LMWH over VKAs has been demonstrated to decrease the risk of recurrent VTE at 6 months to 1 year (8% vs. 16% in the oral anticoagulant group [HR, 0.48; p = 0.002]), without a significant difference in major (6% vs. 4%) or minor bleeding rates (14% vs. 19%).[72] Active malignancy confers a high risk of recurrent VTE over the course of the patient's lifetime, about 15% risk per year. Additionally, the risk of death from VTE is higher 10-fold among patients with cancer compared to those without.[73] Therefore, most patients benefit from extended duration anticoagulation, unless at exceptionally high risk for bleeding (grade 1B).[27] Consideration of cessation of anticoagulation could be given under circumstances such as (1) VTE that occurred in the setting of reversible risk factor (such as surgery), (2) isolated calf DVT without proximal extension, (3) cancer that responded to therapy and (4) cancer that remained localized and has not metastasized.[27]

Pregnancy associated

Pregnancy increases risk of VTE 4- to 5-fold secondary to physiologic and anatomic changes. VTE is a leading cause of maternal death (10%) in developed countries.[74] Treatment with VKAs should be avoided, as they cross the placenta, can lead to fetal bleeding and are teratogenic if given beyond 6 weeks. The most common birth defect associated with VKAs is midface hypoplasia and stippled epiphysis. On the contrary, neither heparin nor LMWH crosses the placenta. LMWH in particular has a low rate of bleeding complications, a lower rate of HIT and a lower rate of osteoporosis than heparin and is preferred in the treatment of pregnancy-associated VTE (grade 1B).[75] No trials have evaluated the duration of anticoagulation in pregnant women with VTE. However, the risk of PE is highest in the post-partum period (43%–60%); therefore, it is recommended that patients undergo a similar duration as non-pregnant patients, a minimum of 3 months, including 6-week post-partum therapy (grade 2C).[75]

FUTURE DIRECTIONS

Aptamers, selectins and venous thrombosis

Aptamers are oligonucleotides that have high affinity and specificity in binding ligands (e.g. proteins) such as cytokines, proteases, kinases, cell surface receptors and cell adhesion molecules, including selectins. Aptamers fold into stable scaffolds for molecular recognition interactions (van der Waals, hydrogen bonding, electrostatic interactions), which drive high-affinity target binding. Aptamers have short or long half-lives depending upon whether an acute or chronic response is necessary. They have a low risk of toxicity and do not cause an immunologic response when administered.[76] In a baboon study, prophylaxis and treatment with an anti-P-selectin aptamer (ARC5692) showed 80% and 73% vein lumen reopening, respectively, after complete occlusion, compared to 13% in the control group and 42% in an LMWH-treated group, as demonstrated by magnetic resonance venography and confirmed by conventional venography and ultrasonography. Also, P-selectin inhibition accelerated thrombus resolution with no bleeding complications. In addition, GMI-1070, a pan-selectin antagonist, has been shown to effectively inhibit selectin-dependent adhesion of sickle red blood cells and leukocytes to endothelial cells in a mouse model of sickle cell disease.[77,78] Since the selectin cell adhesion process in sickle cell disease and DVT initiation is similar, this pan-selectin inhibitor and others appear to be a promising future treatment option to be investigated for DVT.

DEFICIENCIES IN CURRENT KNOWLEDGE AND AREAS FOR FUTURE RESEARCH

1. What is the definitive role of coagulation testing in the work-up of VTE?
2. What is the role of platelets in the pathophysiology of VTE?
3. How does one perform risk assessment for outpatient venous surgery?
4. How reliable is soluble P-selectin for ruling in the diagnosis of DVT?
5. What is the best alternative test to spiral CT imaging for the diagnosis of PE?
6. How well does LMWH prevent the development of chronic venous insufficiency?
7. What is the best medical treatment for HIT and EHIT?
8. Can the new oral anticoagulant agents be used effectively in cancer patients?
9. Which patients should qualify for more aggressive therapy who present with iliofemoral DVT?
10. When is fondaparinux essential to the treatment of superficial venous thrombosis?

11. Can one use either a P-selectin or E-selectin inhibitor for the treatment of DVT?
12. Do IVC filters really cause an increase in venous thrombosis?

BEST CLINICAL PRACTICE

Prophylaxis

- All patients should undergo an assessment of their risk for VTE on admission to the hospital, and appropriate prophylaxis then administered depending on their risk.

Diagnosis

- The gold standard for diagnosis of VTE is duplex ultrasound imaging for DVT and spiral CT imaging for PE.

Treatment

- LMWH has become the standard treatment for VTE. It is preferred due to better safety and improved outcomes.
- The INR goal for treatment of VTE with warfarin is between 2.0 and 3.0.
- No effective treatment definitively and reliably prevents PTS, although compression stockings decrease symptoms of pain and swelling.
- Thrombolysis is indicated in patients with massive PE leading to hemodynamic compromise.
- Aggressive therapies should be offered to patients with significant iliofemoral venous thrombosis and significant symptoms with a good life expectancy.
- IVC filters should be used for a contraindication to anticoagulation, a complication of anticoagulation or failure of anticoagulation.

Unique circumstances

- Thrombosis associated with a line does not mandate the line be removed if it is still needed and anticoagulation can be administered.
- Massive iliofemoral DVT can lead to limb-threatening gangrene. Aggressive pharmacomechanical catheter-directed thrombolysis is indicated if patient fails to respond to initial limb elevation, compression and anticoagulation.
- The optimal treatment of superficial vein thrombosis ≥5 cm in length is with 2.5 mg daily of fondaparinux for 45 days.

- Symptomatic splanchnic thrombosis should be treated with anticoagulation.
- Treatment of VTE in the setting of active malignancy should consist of extended duration LMWH.
- Pregnancy-associated VTE should be treated with anticoagulation throughout the pregnancy and for at least 6 weeks postpartum.

Key points

Prophylaxis

- Assessment can be based on broad categories of patient types and procedure types or based on individual assessment.

Diagnosis

- Risk prediction with clinical likelihood estimates and biomarkers can rule out the diagnosis of DVT and PE, but not rule in the diagnosis.

Treatment

- New oral anticoagulants dabigatran, rivaroxaban, apixaban, and edoxaban are FDA approved for the treatment of VTE. Currently, there is no reliable method to measure anticoagulant effect and no reversal agent available, except for the recent FDA approval of an agent for dabigatran.
- Suprarenal IVC filter placement is indicated in pregnancy or infrarenal IVC filter failure.
- The duration of anticoagulant treatment depends on the risk of thrombosis at presentation, the presence of continuing risk factors for thrombosis, the type of thrombosis, the level of D-dimer measured 1 month after stopping anticoagulation and the status of the veins when stopping anticoagulation.
- HIT should be suspected when platelet count falls below 100,000 or >50% drop. Confirmatory tests are HIT ELISA and serotonin release assay.

Unique circumstances

- EHIT occurs when the great and/or small saphenous vein has been closed with laser or radiofrequency ablation and requires less aggressive therapy than true DVT.
- The risk of death from VTE is 10-fold higher in cancer patients compared to the general population.
- Pregnancy-induced VTE is a leading cause of maternal death. Treatment with vitamin K antagonists should be avoided.

KEY REFERENCES

1. Bahl V, Hu HM, Henke PK, Wakefield TW, Campbell DA Jr, Caprini JA. A validation study of a retrospective venous thromboembolism risk scoring method. *Ann Surg.* 2010;251:344–350.

2. Kearon C, Kahn SR, Agnelli G, Goldhaber S, Raskob GE, Comerota AJ. Antithrombotic therapy for venous thromboembolic disease: American college of chest physicians evidence-based clinical practice guidelines (8th edition). *Chest.* 2008;133:454S–545S.

3. Wakefield TW, Myers DD, Henke PK. Mechanisms of venous thrombosis and resolution. *Arterioscler Thromb Vasc Biol.* 2008;28:387–391.

4. Decousus H, Prandoni P, Mismetti P, Bauersachs RM, Boda Z, Brenner B, Laporte S, Matyas L, Middeldorp S, Sokurenko G, Leizorovicz A. Fondaparinux for the treatment of superficial-vein thrombosis in the legs. *N Engl J Med.* 2010;363:1222–1232.

5. Enden T, Haig Y, Kløw NE et al.; CaVenT Study. Long-term outcome after additional catheter-directed thrombolysis versus standard treatment for acute ilio-femoral deep vein thrombosis (the cavent study): A randomised controlled trial. *Lancet.* 2012;379:31–38.

REFERENCES

1. Heit JA. The epidemiology of venous thromboembolism in the community. *Arterioscler Thromb Vasc Biol.* 2008;28:370–372.

2. Yusuf HR, Tsai J, Siddiqi AEA, Boulet SL, Soucie JM. Emergency department visits by patients with venous thromboembolism 1998–2009. *J Hosp Adm.* 2012;1:1–8.

3. Pannucci CJ, Obi A, Alvarez R, Abdullah N, Nackashi A, Hu HM, Bahl V, Henke PK. Inadequate venous thromboembolism risk stratification predicts venous thromboembolic events in surgical intensive care unit patients. *J Am Coll Surgeons.* 2014;218:898–904.

4. Wakefield TW, McLafferty RB, Lohr JM, Caprini JA, Gillespie DL, Passman MA. Call to action to prevent venous thromboembolism. *J Vasc Surg.* 2009;49:1620–1623.

5. Struijk-Mulder MC, van Wijhe W, Sze YK, Knollema S, Verheyen CC, Buller HR, Fritschy WM, Ettema HB. Death and venous thromboembolism after lower extremity amputation. *J Thromb Haemost.* 2010;8:2680–2684.

6. Bandeira FC, Pitta GB, Castro AA, Miranda F Jr. Postoperative incidence of deep vein thrombosis after major lower extremity amputation. *Intl Angiol.* 2008;27:489–493.

7. Scarborough JE, Cox MW, Mureebe L, Pappas TN, Shortell CK. A novel scoring system for predicting postoperative venous thromboembolic complications in patients after open aortic surgery. *J Am Coll Surg.* 2012;214:620–626; discussion 627–628.

8. Pannucci CJ, Shanks A, Moote MJ et al. Identifying patients at high risk for venous thromboembolism requiring treatment after outpatient surgery. *Ann Surg.* 2012;255:1093–1099.

9. Baglin T, Gray E, Greaves M, Hunt BJ, Keeling D, Machin S, Mackie I, Makris M, Nokes T, Perry D. Clinical guidelines for testing for heritable thrombophilia. *Br J Haematol.* 2010;149:209–220.

10. Bahl V, Hu HM, Henke PK, Wakefield TW, Campbell DA Jr, Caprini JA. A validation study of a retrospective venous thromboembolism risk scoring method. *Ann Surg.* 2010;251:344–350.

11. Geerts WH, Bergqvist D, Pineo GF, Heit JA, Samama CM, Lassen MR, Colwell CW. Prevention of venous thromboembolism: American college of chest physicians evidence-based clinical practice guidelines (8th edition). *Chest.* 2008;133:381S–453S.

12. Gallus AS, Hirsh J. Prevention of venous thromboembolism. *Semin Thromb Hemost.* 1976;2:232–290.

13. Scurr J, Coleridge-Smith P, Hasty J. Regimen for improved effectiveness of intermittent pneumatic compression in deep venous thrombosis prophylaxis. *Surgery.* 1987;102:816–820.

14. Epstein NE. Efficacy of pneumatic compression stocking prophylaxis in the prevention of deep venous thrombosis and pulmonary embolism following 139 lumbar laminectomies with instrumented fusions. *J Spinal Disord Tech.* 2006;19:28–31.

15. Wakefield TW, Myers DD, Henke PK. Mechanisms of venous thrombosis and resolution. *Arterioscler Thromb Vasc Biol.* 2008;28:387–391.

16. Vandy FC, Stabler C, Eliassen AM, Hawley AE, Guire KE, Myers DD, Henke PK, Wakefield TW. Soluble p-selectin for the diagnosis of lower extremity deep venous thrombosis. *J Vasc Surg Venous Lym Dis.* 2013;1:117–125.

17. Ramacciotti E, Blackburn S, Hawley AE, Vandy F, Ballard-Lipka N, Stabler C, Baker N, Guire KE, Rectenwald JE, Henke PK, Myers DD, Wakefield T. Evaluation of soluble p-selectin as a marker for the diagnosis of deep venous thrombosis. *Clin Appl Thromb Hemost.* 2011;17(4):425–431.

18. Stein PD, Fowler SE, Goodman LR et al. Multidetector computed tomography for acute pulmonary embolism. *N Engl J Med.* 2006;354:2317–2327.

19. Prandoni P, Lensing AW, Cogo A, Cuppini S, Villalta S, Carta M, Cattelan AM, Polistena P, Bernardi E, Prins MH. The long-term clinical course of acute deep venous thrombosis. *Ann Intern Med.* 1996;125:1–7.

20. Wells PS, Anderson DR, Rodger M, Forgie M, Kearon C, Dreyer J, Kovacs G, Mitchell M, Lewandowski B, Kovacs MJ. Evaluation of d-dimer in the diagnosis of suspected deep-vein thrombosis. *N Engl J Med.* 2003;349:1227–1235.

21. Fowl RJ, Strothman GB, Blebea J, Rosenthal GJ, Kempczinski RF. Inappropriate use of venous duplex scans: An analysis of indications and results. *J Vasc Surg.* 1996;23:881–885; discussion 885–886.

22. Bates SM, Jaeschke R, Stevens SM et al., American College of Chest P. Diagnosis of DVT: Antithrombotic therapy and prevention of thrombosis, 9th ed: American college of chest physicians evidence-based clinical practice guidelines. *Chest.* 2012;141:e351S–e418S.

23. Schellong SM, Schwarz T, Halbritter K, Beyer J, Siegert G, Oettler W, Schmidt B, Schroeder HE. Complete compression ultrasonography of the leg veins as a single test for the diagnosis of deep vein thrombosis. *Thromb Haemost.* 2003;89:228–234.

24. Stein PD, Chenevert TL, Fowler SE, Goodman LR, Gottschalk A, Hales CA, Hull RD, Jablonski KA, Leeper KV, Naidich DP. Gadolinium-enhanced magnetic resonance angiography for pulmonary embolisma multicenter prospective study (pioped iii). *Ann Intern Med.* 2010;152:434–443.

25. Bates SM, Ginsberg JS. Treatment of deep-vein thrombosis. *N Engl J Med.* 2004;351:268–277.

26. Hull RD, Pineo GF, Mah AF, Brant R. A randomized trial evaluating long-term low-milecular-weight heparin therapy out-of-hospital versus warfarin sodium comparing the post-phlebitic outcomes at three months. *Blood.* 2001;98:447A.

27. Kearon C, Akl E, Comerota A, Prandoni P, Bounameaux H, Goldhaber S, Nelson M, Wells P, Gould M, Dentali F. Antithrombotic therapy for VTE disease: Antithrombotic therapy and prevention of thrombosis: American college of chest physicians evidence-based clinical practice guidelines. *Chest.* 2012;141:e419S–e494S.

28. Turpie AG, Bauer KA, Eriksson BI, Lassen MR. Fondaparinux vs enoxaparin for the prevention of venous thromboembolism in major orthopedic surgery: A meta-analysis of 4 randomized double-blind studies. *Arch Intern Med.* 2002;162:1833–1840.

29. Buller HR, Davidson BL, Decousus H et al. Fondaparinux or enoxaparin for the initial treatment of symptomatic deep venous thrombosis: A randomized trial. *Ann Intern Med.* 2004;140:867–873.

30. Buller HR, Davidson BL, Decousus H et al. Subcutaneous fondaparinux versus intravenous unfractionated heparin in the initial treatment of pulmonary embolism. *N Engl J Med.* 2003;349:1695–1702.

31. Decousus H, Prandoni P, Mismetti P, Bauersachs RM, Boda Z, Brenner B, Laporte S, Matyas L, Middeldorp S, Sokurenko G. Fondaparinux for the treatment of superficial-vein thrombosis in the legs. *N Engl J Med.* 2010;363:1222–1232.

32. Einstein Investigators. Oral rivaroxaban for symptomatic venous thromboembolism. *N Engl J Med.* 2010;363:2499–2510.

33. Einstein P. Oral rivaroxaban for the treatment of symptomatic pulmonary embolism. *N Engl J Med.* 2012;366:1287–1297.

34. Agnelli G, Buller HR, Cohen A, Curto M, Gallus AS, Johnson M, Porcari A, Raskob GE, Weitz JI. Apixaban for extended treatment of venous thromboembolism. *N Engl J Med.* 2013;368:699–708.

35. Hokusai-VTE Investigators. Edoxaban versus warfarin for the treatment of symptomatic venous thromboembolism. *N Engl J Med.* 2013;369:1406–1415.

36. Palareti G, Cosmi B, Legnani C et al. D-dimer testing to determine the duration of anticoagulation therapy. *N Engl J Med.* 2006;355:1780–1789.

37. Gabriel F, Portolés O, Labiós M, Rodríguez C, Cisneros E, Vela J, Nuñez M, RIETE Investigators. Usefulness of thrombophilia testing in venous thromboembolic disease: Findings from the riete registry. *Clin Appl Thromb Hemost.* 2013;19:42–47.

38. Greinacher A, Michels I, Mueller-Eckhardt C. Heparin-associated thrombocytopenia: The antibody is not heparin specific. *Thromb Haemost.* 1992;67:545–549.

39. Alving BM. How I treat heparin-induced thrombocytopenia and thrombosis. *Blood.* 2003;101:31–37.

40. Prandoni P, Lensing AW, Prins MH, Frulla M, Marchiori A, Bernardi E, Tormene D, Mosena L, Pagnan A, Girolami A. Below-knee elastic compression stockings to prevent the post-thrombotic syndrome: A randomized, controlled trial. *Ann Intern Med.* 2004;141:249–256.

41. Aschwanden M, Labs KH, Engel H, Schwob A, Jeanneret C, Mueller-Brand J, Jaeger KA. Acute deep vein thrombosis: Early mobilization does not increase the frequency of pulmonary embolism. *Thromb Haemost.* 2001;85:42–46.

42. Kahn SR, Shapiro S, Wells PS et al. Compression stockings to prevent post-thrombotic syndrome: A randomised placebo-controlled trial. *The Lancet.* 2014;383:880–888.

43. Meissner MH, Manzo RA, Bergelin RO, Markel A, Strandness DE Jr. Deep venous insufficiency: The relationship between lysis and subsequent reflux. *J Vasc Surg.* 1993;18:596–605; discussion 606–598.

44. Juhan CM, Alimi YS, Barthelemy PJ, Fabre DF, Riviere CS. Late results of iliofemoral venous thrombectomy. *J Vasc Surg.* 1997;25:417–422.

45. Enden T, Haig Y, Kløw NE et al.; CaVenT Study. Long-term outcome after additional catheter-directed thrombolysis versus standard treatment for acute iliofemoral deep vein thrombosis (the cavent study): A randomised controlled trial. *Lancet.* 2012;379:31–38.

46. Baekgaard N, Broholm R, Just S, Jørgensen M, Jensen LP. Long-term results using catheter-directed thrombolysis in 103 lower limbs with acute iliofemoral venous thrombosis. *Eur J Vasc Endovasc Surg.* 2010;39:112–117.

47. Raju S, Darcey R, Neglén P. Unexpected major role for venous stenting in deep reflux disease. *J Vasc Surg.* 2010;51:401–408.

48. Marti C, John G, Konstantinides S, Combescure C, Sanchez O, Lankeit M, Meyer G, Perrier A. Systemic thrombolytic therapy for acute pulmonary embolism: A systematic review and meta-analysis. *Eur Heart J.* 2015;36:605–614.

49. Meyer G, Vicaut E, Danays T et al. Fibrinolysis for patients with intermediate-risk pulmonary embolism. *N Engl J Med.* 2014;370:1402–1411.

50. Greenfield LJ, Proctor MC. Current status of inferior vena cava filters. *Ann Vasc Surg.* 2000;14:525–528.

51. Prepic SG. Eight-year follow-up of patients with permanent vena cava filters in the prevention of pulmonary embolism the prepic (prévention du risque d'embolie pulmonaire par interruption cave) randomized study. *Circulation.* 2005;112:416–422.

52. Kucher N. Deep-vein thrombosis of the upper extremities. *N Engl J Med.* 2011;364:861–869.

53. Thompson RW. Comprehensive management of subclavian vein effort thrombosis. *Sem Interv Radiol.* 2012;29:44.

54. Perkins JM, Magee TR, Galland RB. Phlegmasia caerulea dolens and venous gangrene. *Br J Surg.* 1996;83:19–23.

55. Chinsakchai K, ten Duis K, Moll FL, de Borst GJ. Trends in management of phlegmasia cerulea dolens. *Vasc Endovasc Surg.* 2011;45:5–14.

56. Comerota AJ, Paolini D. Treatment of acute iliofemoral deep venous thrombosis: A strategy of thrombus removal. *Eur J Vasc Endovasc Surg.* 2007;33:351–360; discussion 361–352.

57. Blattler W, Schwarzenbach B, Largiader J. Superficial vein thrombophlebitis – Serious concern or much ado about little? *Vasa.* 2008;37:31–38.

58. Decousus H, Quere I, Presles E et al. Superficial venous thrombosis and venous thromboembolism: A large, prospective epidemiologic study. *Ann Intern Med.* 2010;152:218–224.

59. Blumenberg RM, Barton E, Gelfand ML, Skudder P, Brennan J. Occult deep venous thrombosis complicating superficial thrombophlebitis. *J Vasc Surg.* 1998;27:338–343.

60. DiNisio M, Wichers IM, Middeldorp S. Treatment for superficial thrombophlebitis of the leg. *Cochrane Database Syst Rev.* 2008;3.

61. Samlaska CP, James WD. Superficial thrombophlebitis. I. Primary hypercoagulable states. *J Am Acad Dermatol.* 1990;22:975–989.

62. Verlato F, Zucchetta P, Prandoni P, Camporese G, Marzola MC, Salmistraro G, Bui F, Martini R, Rosso F, Andreozzi GM. An unexpectedly high rate of pulmonary embolism in patients with superficial thrombophlebitis of the thigh. *J Vasc Surg.* 1999;30:1113–1115.

63. Lozano FS, Almazan A. Low-molecular-weight heparin versus saphenofemoral disconnection for the treatment of above-knee greater saphenous thrombophlebitis: A prospective study. *Vasc Endovascular Surg.* 2003;37:415–420.

64. Sullivan V, Denk PM, Sonnad SS, Eagleton MJ, Wakefield TW. Ligation versus anticoagulation: Treatment of above-knee superficial thrombophlebitis not involving the deep venous system. *J Am Coll Surg.* 2001;193:556–562.

65. Dexter D, Kabnick L, Berland T, Jacobowitz G, Lamparello P, Maldonado T, Mussa F, Rockman C, Sadek M, Giammaria L. Complications of endovenous lasers. *Phlebology.* 2012;27:40–45.

66. Kabnick L, Berland T. Endothermal heat induced thrombosis (ehit). *VEITH Symposium – 38th Annual Vascular and Endovascular Issues, Techniques and Horizons,* New York, 2011.

67. Lawrence PF, Chandra A, Wu M, Rigberg D, DeRubertis B, Gelabert H, Jimenez JC, Carter V. Classification of proximal endovenous closure levels and treatment algorithm. *J Vas Surg.* 2010;52:388–393.

68. Harlander-Locke M, Jimenez JC, Lawrence PF, Derubertis BG, Rigberg DA, Gelabert HA. Endovenous ablation with concomitant phlebectomy is a safe and effective method of treatment for symptomatic patients with axial reflux and large incompetent tributaries. *J Vasc Surg.* 2013;58:166–172.

69. Ageno W, Riva N, Schulman S, Bang SM, Sartori MT, Grandone E, Beyer-Westendorf J, Barillari G, Di Minno MN, Dentali F, group Is. Antithrombotic treatment of splanchnic vein thrombosis: Results of an international registry. *Semin Thromb Hemost.* 2014;40:99–105.

70. Timp JF, Braekkan SK, Versteeg HH, Cannegieter SC. Epidemiology of cancer-associated venous thrombosis. *Blood.* 2013;122:1712–1723.

71. Kakkar VV, Balibrea JL, Martinez-Gonzalez J, Prandoni P, Group CS. Extended prophylaxis with bemiparin for the prevention of venous thromboembolism after abdominal or pelvic surgery for cancer: The canbesure randomized study. *J Thromb Haemost.* 2010;8:1223–1229.

72. Lee AY, Levine MN, Baker RI, Bowden C, Kakkar AK, Prins M, Rickles FR, Julian JA, Haley S, Kovacs MJ. Low-molecular-weight heparin versus a coumarin for the prevention of recurrent venous thromboembolism in patients with cancer. *N Engl J Med.* 2003;349:146–153.

73. Prandoni P, Lensing AW, Piccioli A, Bernardi E, Simioni P, Girolami B, Marchiori A, Sabbion P, Prins MH, Noventa F, Girolami A. Recurrent venous thromboembolism and bleeding complications during anticoagulant treatment in patients with cancer and venous thrombosis. *Blood.* 2002;100:3484–3488.

74. Berg CJ, Callaghan WM, Syverson C, Henderson Z. Pregnancy-related mortality in the united states, 1998 to 2005. *Obstet Gynecol.* 2010;116:1302–1309.

75. Bates SM, Greer IA, Middeldorp S, Veenstra DL, Prabulos AM, Vandvik PO, American College of Chest Physicians. VTE, thrombophilia, antithrombotic therapy, and pregnancy: Antithrombotic therapy and prevention of thrombosis, 9th ed:

American college of chest physicians evidence-based clinical practice guidelines. *Chest.* 2012; 141:e691S–e736S.

76. Keefe AD, Schaub RG. Aptamers as candidate therapeutics for cardiovascular indications. *Curr Opin Pharmacol.* 2008;8:147–152.

77. Gutsaeva DR, Parkerson JB, Yerigenahally SD, Kurz JC, Schaub RG, Ikuta T, Head CA. Inhibition of cell adhesion by anti-p-selectin aptamer: A new potential therapeutic agent for sickle cell disease. *Blood.* 2011;117:727–735.

78. Chang J, Patton JT, Sarkar A, Ernst B, Magnani JL, Frenette PS. Gmi-1070, a novel pan-selectin antagonist, reverses acute vascular occlusions in sickle cell mice. *Blood.* 2010;116:1779–1786.

79. Wakefield T, Henke P. *Complications in Surgery*, 2nd ed. Philadelphia, PA: Lippincott Williams & Wilkins, 2011, p. 353.

80. Knepper J, Horne D, Obi A, Wakefield TW. A systematic update on the state of novel anticoagulants and a primer on reversal and bridging. *J Vasc Surg: Venous Lym Dis.* 2013;1(4):419.

49

Surgical management, lytic therapy and venous stenting

ANTHONY J. COMEROTA and MAXIM E. SHAYDAKOV

CONTENTS

INTRODUCTION

It has been 10 years since the previous edition of this chapter was published. The past decade was marked by progressive advancement of theoretical and practical management of acute venous thrombosis. Important fundamental and clinical studies offer data which are reflected in clinical practice guidelines.[1-7] An update of the evidence for the endovascular treatment of acute deep venous thrombosis (DVT) will help guide clinicians in the safe and effective management of acute DVT, especially acute iliofemoral DVT (IFDVT).

Although thrombolytic therapy is not widely adopted for DVT treatment, we will review the rationale supporting early thrombus removal in selected patients. This chapter will focus on contemporary catheter-based techniques for acute IFDVT and treatment of postthrombotic iliofemoral obstruction. Generally accepted criteria for patient selection, treatment evaluation, techniques of lytic therapy and postoperative follow-up will be reviewed. Clinical trials providing the risks and benefits of interventional treatment of IFDVT will be discussed. A concise overview of published guidelines is included. Principles of therapeutic thrombolysis using catheter-based lytic therapy to improve outcomes in patients with less commonly seen venous thrombotic disorders (Paget–Schroetter syndrome, Budd–Chiari syndrome, superior vena cava [SVC] thrombosis) are included with approaches based upon our experience and available literature.

Venous stenting is an effective option to restore patency to obstructed segments of the central venous system in patients with residual venous lesions following catheter-directed thrombosis (CDT) for acute DVT, obstructive lesions in patients with postthrombotic syndrome (PTS) and those with symptomatic iliac vein compression. Venous stenting will be discussed and the published experience summarized.

RATIONALE FOR THROMBUS REMOVAL IN PATIENTS WITH ILIOFEMORAL DVT

Acute DVT of the lower extremity is a spectrum of diseases from asymptomatic muscular calf vein thrombosis to the extensive proximal thrombosis of the iliofemoral and vena caval segments. Occasionally, venous hypertension will be so severe that venous pressure exceeds the critical closing pressure of capillaries putting patients at risk for venous gangrene. The natural history of venous thrombosis is determined by its anatomic location, relevant risk factors and thrombus burden. This diversity of clinical presentation, natural history and prognosis suggests that an individual approach to DVT treatment based on the specific benefits/risks ratio for each patient is most appropriate.

A combination of anticoagulation, early ambulation and compression is the most commonly used treatment strategy, which is appropriate for the majority of patients with DVT. Although our observation suggests that appropriate compression is underutilized in most patients, early anticoagulation is strongly recommended for all patients with confirmed DVT.[2]

The goal of conventional anticoagulation is to prevent propagation and embolization and allow the patient's intrinsic fibrinolytic system to lyse, clot and recanalize the thrombosed vein. Spontaneous recanalization occurs to a certain extent in half of patients 6 months after an acute DVT episode, with a greater likelihood of recanalization in patients with isolated calf vein thrombosis. In patients with a large burden of thrombus, recanalization is unlikely. When early spontaneous lysis occurs, preservation of valve function is likely[8]; however, prognostic indicators of spontaneous thrombus resolution are unavailable.

PTS is a common consequence in patients with DVT involving the popliteal veins and more proximal veins, in which early and complete recanalization is not achieved. PTS develops in approximately 50%–60% of these patients within 2 years. The pathophysiology of PTS is ambulatory venous hypertension, defined as a failure of venous pressure to appropriately decrease in response to calf muscle contraction during exercise. The components of ambulatory venous hypertension are endoluminal obstruction, venous valve reflux and calf pump muscle dysfunction.

The risk of PTS is influenced by the location of the clot. The highest postthrombotic venous pressures are found in patients who had IFDVT.[9] A recent prospective observational study of patients treated with anticoagulation alone for their acute DVT found that IFDVT was the strongest predictor for severe PTS.[10] Other investigators reported that more than 40% of patients had venous claudication within 5 years following IFDVT.[11] Within the same time frame, 15% of patients developed venous ulcers.[12] This high postthrombotic morbidity after anticoagulation alone for IFDVT is the basis for the strategy of early thrombus removal to prevent luminal obstruction and preserve valve function in these patients.[13]

The role of good compression therapy in patients with acute DVT is well established. Randomized controlled trials (RCTs) demonstrated that 30–40 mmHg ankle gradient compression stockings were effective in reducing PTS by 50% within 2 years of follow-up.[14,15] An earlier randomized trial did not find any difference between below-the-knee to above-the-knee compression for PTS prevention, while thigh-length compression therapy was found to be less tolerated.[16] A recently published meta-analysis of 5 RCTs demonstrated the significantly lower incidence of PTS in patients treated with compression therapy (n = 338) compared with controls (n = 324), 26% versus 46%, respectively (95% CI, 0.44–0.67; p < 0.001).[17] Early mobilization and compression with inelastic bandages or compression stockings improved early outcomes of acute proximal DVT, reducing limb edema and pain without increasing the risk of PE.[18] A multicentre

placebo-controlled, randomized trial of compression stockings to prevent PTS after proximal DVT (the S.O.X. Trial) was recently reported. After 2 years of follow-up of 410 patients treated with knee-length class II elastic compression stockings and 396 randomized to placebo stockings, there was no difference in the onset or severity of PTS (14.2% vs. 12.7%, respectively; HR 1.13, 95% CI 0.73–1.76; p = 0.58).[19] Unfortunately, there were numerous flaws in this study. Patients did not receive personal instruction on the use of the stockings, and 3 days of use per week was considered good compliance; according to patient self-reporting, the majority of patients could not distinguish if they were wearing therapeutic or placebo stockings. This last finding is particularly disturbing considering the difficulty most individuals (even young, healthy patients) have in applying 30–40 mmHg compression hose. It raises the question whether the majority of patients were wearing their compression stockings at all. The 56% of patients who admitted using their stockings for ≥3 days/week is likely overestimated.

Early ambulation with good compression is recommended for all DVT patients to decrease the risk of PTS (1C).[2] We suggest that all patients with proximal DVT wear knee-length compression stockings (class III, 30–40 mmHg) unless contraindicated. This is supported by the American Heart Association's (AHA's) 2011 guidelines (IB).

Although eliminating the large thrombus burden and restoring unobstructed venous drainage reduces PTS in patients with IFDVT, there are other benefits.[20–22] Patients with iliofemoral thrombosis have a twofold higher risk of venous thromboembolism (VTE) recurrence than patients with infrainguinal venous thrombosis (11.8% vs. 5.2%).[20] A meta-analysis of 11 RCTs revealed a strong correlation between clot burden and VTE recurrence after anticoagulation alone (r = 0.81, p = 0.005).[22] A prospective study of 313 patients with proximal DVT treated with conventional short-term anticoagulation revealed a 2.4× higher risk for VTE recurrence in patients with persistent luminal obstruction.[21] This body of clinical evidence forms the basis for the rationale for a strategy of thrombus removal, particularly in patients with acute IFDVT, in order to reduce thrombus burden, alleviate acute symptoms, prevent PTS and potentially avoid VTE recurrence.

Patients with both acute and chronic venous diseases limited to the infrainguinal venous system caudad to the profunda femoris vein often have controllable symptoms and acceptable long-term sequelae following routine anticoagulation, particularly if the popliteal vein is not involved.[23] The femoral vein from the adductor canal to the junction of the profunda femoris vein has been harvested for arterial and venous reconstructions with minimal long-term morbidity. Less than one-third of patients develop edema in the 3 years after femoral vein harvesting for reconstructive surgery,[24] with no patients suffering from significant symptoms. Likewise, ligation of the femoral vein caudad to the profunda results in minimal venous morbidity.[25] We have used femoral ligation or other means of obliteration as an effective treatment option in patients with severely symptomatic femoral vein incompetence. It is therefore not surprising that isolated femoral vein thrombosis results in minimal patient morbidity. Isolated calf vein (distal) thrombosis results in less postthrombotic morbidity when these patients are treated with proper anticoagulation. A recent prospective study demonstrated a 7% risk of proximal propagation and a 6% risk of PE in high-risk patients with isolated distal DVT.[26] Although it may be reasonable to treat certain patients with infrainguinal DVT with an initial strategy of thrombus removal, such as those with distal popliteal vein thrombosis involving the confluence of the calf veins, current guidelines recommend conventional anticoagulation (1C).[5]

THROMBOLYTIC THERAPY

Mechanism of action of thrombolytic drugs

Cross-linked fibrin polymer is the scaffold of acute venous thrombosis. Fibrinolysis is based upon the activation of plasminogen to produce plasmin, which breaks down polymerized fibrin. In addition to fibrin, clotting factors are also broken down which increases the risk of bleeding when plasminogen is systemically activated.

Plasminogen is a zymogen produced by the liver. In its native form plasminogen contains a glutamic acid residue at the N-terminus (Glu-plasminogen) and circulates in plasma in a closed conformation resistant to its main activators – tissue plasminogen activator (tPA), urokinase plasminogen activator (uPA), kallikrein factor XIa and factor XIIa. During the process of thrombus amplification, circulating Glu-plasminogen binds to polymerized fibrin becoming Lys-plasminogen which amplifies its ability to bind with plasminogen activators to produce plasmin. It was established long ago that the basic mechanism of thrombolysis is the activation of fibrin-bound plasminogen (within the thrombus).[27] This forms the scientific basis for the intraclot delivery of plasminogen activators, which has been validated in numerous clinical studies.

Currently available thrombolytic agents are plasminogen activators:

- Tissue plasminogen activators (tPA): alteplase (rtPA, Activase), reteplase (Retavase) and tenecteplase (TNK-tPA)
- Urokinase (uPA, Abbokinase)
- Streptokinase: natural streptokinase (SK) and anistreplase (Eminase)

The enzymatic activity of tPA is insignificant without fibrin, and tPA action is highly fibrin specific. On the contrary, uPA, SK and anistreplase activate both fibrin-bound and circulating plasminogen to a much greater extent. The mechanism action of tPA has potential to more effectively lyse clot with reduced bleeding risk.

Proteolytic cleavage of the native Glu-plasminogen by plasmin results in the truncated protein and Lys77-plasminogen, which possesses both higher affinity for

fibrin and more binding sites for plasminogen activators, thereby increasing their catalytic activity. This positive feedback amplifies plasminogen-to-plasmin conversion on the surface of fibrin. CDT takes advantage of this physiologic self-acceleration mechanism by means of delivering the plasminogen activator directly within the thrombus saturated with fibrin-bound Lys-plasminogen.

Antifibrinolytic proteins maintain physiologic balance of the coagulation/fibrinolysis system, plasminogen activator inhibitor-1 (PAI-1) and α2-antiplasmin. α2-antiplasmin rapidly inactivates circulating plasmin neutralizing its activity in milliseconds, while plasmin bound to fibrin is protected from such rapid degradation. PAI-1 concentration is the main determinant of circulating tPA level, which declines exponentially as a function of active PAI-1.[28] Therefore, when infused systemically, a high concentration of the plasminogen activator is required to supersaturate circulating PAI-1 and α2-antiplasmin. The intrathrombus administration of thrombolytic agents offers much better plasminogen activator/PAI-1 ratio and prevents plasmin from degradation by circulating antiplasmins. This provides an enormous clinical advantage, allowing a lower dose of thrombolytic agent without loss of lytic potential.

Progress of experimental pharmacology has led to the development of thrombolytic drugs, which are currently under investigation. This is a new class of agents, which possess a direct activity to degrade fibrin, without intermediate plasminogen activation. Human plasmin derived from pooled plasma is being evaluated in phase II–III clinical trials. Potential advantages of direct thrombolytics (plasmin) are instantaneous inactivation by antiplasmin and alpha-2 macroglobulin when it is ultimately released into the systemic circulation and potentially more rapid lytic action.

Appropriate time frame for thrombolysis

The chance for successful thrombolysis decreases with thrombus age.[29] A clear cut-off on the timeline for CDT for DVT has not been established, although most protocols advise treatment within 2–3 weeks of symptom onset.

The addition of mechanical techniques to CDT has been shown to improve overall success, reduce treatment times and reduce rtPA dose. According to the Society of Interventional Radiology's and the Cardiovascular and Interventional Radiological Society of Europe's 2009 guidelines, endovascular treatment of DVT 14–28 days may be reasonable in patients with moderate to severe symptoms and low risk of bleeding.[3] Clinical improvement in patients with longer-term symptomatic IFDVT after pharmacomechanical thrombolysis (PMT) and ultrasound-accelerated thrombolysis has been observed.[30,31]

The recommended duration of DVT symptoms prior to CDT ranges from 19 to 21 days in clinical guidelines:

- 14 days, ACCP 8th (2B)
- 14 days, AVF 2008 (2B)

- 14 days, SVS/AVF 2012 (2C)
- 14 days, National Institute for Health and Clinical Excellence (NICE) 2012
- 21 days, AHA 2011 (IIIB)
- Not stated, EVF 2013
- Considered CDT for *subacute or chronic* DVT, SIR/CIRSE 2009

Clinical experience

SYSTEMIC THROMBOLYSIS

Systemic thrombolysis is reviewed here for completeness, but is essentially of historical interest. It has been replaced by the intrathrombus delivery of plasminogen activators. Early attempts of thrombolytic therapy for acute DVT used systemic intravenous infusion of plasminogen activators. This simple method of drug delivery resulted in significant dilution of the fibrinolytic agent in the plasma volume, with a high dose required for lytic effect resulting in substantial systemic plasminogen activation. Systemic administration of the thrombolytic drug had poor intraclot penetration and insufficient lytic response in many patients. However, the lessons learned from the systemic thrombolytic therapy of DVT inspired subsequent achievements in the field. Randomized trials performed more than 25 years ago reported >50% lysis of deep venous clot in 28%–58% of patients with systemic rtPA infusion compared to the minimal, if any, lytic effect observed with heparin.[32,33] Thrombus dissolution correlated with a lower incidence of PTS in these reports. A randomized trial performed 10 years later compared results of anticoagulation with heparin versus a systemic or *regionally* administered thrombolytic agent infused via the dorsal pedal vein for acute DVT treatment in 250 patients.[34] One year after treatment, deep vein patency was 52% in the conventional anticoagulation group compared to 64%–74% after thrombolysis (p < 0.05). PTS occurred with less frequency after lytic therapy (57% vs. 83%, p < 0.001). However, 6% of patients suffered major bleeding and 4.5% had PE. The infusion of a thrombolytic agent through the dorsal pedal vein failed to demonstrate any additional benefit in that study. A subsequent randomized trial also demonstrated little benefit from this approach.[35]

To estimate an average effect of systemic thrombolysis, we performed a pooled analysis of 13 studies that compared anticoagulation with systemic lytic therapy for acute DVT. The diagnosis was established with ascending phlebography, which was repeated to assess the results of systemic thrombolysis. Eighty-two per cent of patients in the anticoagulation group had no phlebographic evidence of recanalization or demonstrated extension of thrombus. In the patients treated with thrombolytic therapy, 45% had significant and an additional 18% had partial clearing of the clot. Unfortunately, publications did not differentiate between iliofemoral and femoral–popliteal DVTs (Table 49.1).

These studies helped to clarify the effect of successful lysis on preservation of vein valve function. In a long-term RCT reported by Jeffery et al., patients with acute DVT who initially enjoyed successful lysis by systemic streptokinase infusion demonstrated better overall lower extremity venous haemodynamics 5–10 years after treatment. An incompetent popliteal vein valve was found in only 9% of patients after successful thrombolysis, but in 77% of those who failed to lyse (p < 0.001).[36]

Although systemic thrombolysis is simple and might be effective in some patients, it failed to demonstrate adequate thrombus dissolution in the majority of cases. The increased risk of major bleeding of 3.5× that of anticoagulation alone[32] essentially eliminated systemic therapy as a treatment option for patients with acute DVT.

CATHETER-DIRECTED THROMBOLYSIS

The first application of transcatheter thrombolytic drug infusion for iliofemoral venous thrombosis was reported by Okrent in 1991.[37] Successful uneventful lysis was achieved after 68 hours of continuous urokinase infusion in a 29-year-old woman with extensive IFDVT.[37] At the dawn of CDT, a number of observational studies were published with positive and encouraging results. Today CDT is supported by a high level of evidence.

Bjarnason et al. prospectively evaluated 77 patients (87 limbs) treated with CDT with urokinase for IFDVT during a 5-year period.[38] Technical success was determined by thrombus location: 86% for iliac segments and 63% for femoral veins. The success rate was significantly higher in patients with less than 21 days of symptom duration compared to those with a longer duration of symptoms, 85% versus 42%, respectively. The 1-year secondary patency rate after catheter-directed urokinase infusion was 78% for iliac and 51% for femoral venous segments. Major bleeding complications occurred in 7% of patients.[38]

The North American Venous Registry is the largest single database to date, comprising 473 patients with acute DVT treated with thrombolytic therapy.[50] In this prospective registry, 313 clinical cases of symptomatic DVT (303 limbs in 287 patients) treated with catheter thrombolysis with urokinase were analyzed. IFDVT was present in 71% of cases (221/312), extending into the inferior vena cava (IVC) in 21% (46/221). The age of the DVT was ≤10 days in 66% patients and >10 days in 16%. The remaining 19% of patients had acute symptoms superimposed on chronic disease. Complete lysis determined by venography was achieved in 31% of patients and more than 50% lysis in another 52%. Patients with longer duration of symptoms had a lower success rate. One-year primary patency was higher in patients with IFDVT than with femoral–popliteal lesion (64% vs. 47%, p < 0.01). The degree of initial lysis was found to be the strongest predictor of long-term patency. Two deaths resulted from PE and intracranial haemorrhage. Overall mortality was <0.5%. Major bleeding complications occurred in 11% of patients, most often at the catheter puncture site. Symptomatic PE occurred in 0.5% of cases.

Table 49.1 Review of studies of catheter-directed thrombolysis for acute deep vein thrombosis.

Author (year)	Total no. of patients (limbs)	Intervention	Results			Complications			
			Significant/ complete resolution (%)	Partial resolution (%)	No resolution (%)	Bleeding		PE	Death due to Rx (%)
						Minor (%)	Major (%)		
Semba et al. (1994)[39]	21 (27)	CDT with UK, angioplasty/stenting for residual stenosis	18 (72)	5 (25)	2 (8)	1 (4)	0 (0)	None	None
Semba et al. (1996)[40]	32 (41)	CDT with UK, angioplasty/stenting for residual stenosis	21 (32)	9 (28)	2 (6)	0 (0)	0 (0)	None	None
Verhaeghe et al. (1997)[41]	24	CDT with rtPA, stenting for residual stenosis	19 (79)	5 (21)	0 (0))	0 (0)	6 (25)	None	None
Bjarnason et al. (1997)[38]	77 (87)	CDT with UK, angioplasty, stenting, thrombectomy, bypass for residual stenosis	69 (793)	0 (0)	18 (21)	11 (14)	5 (6)	1	None
Mewissen et al. (1999)[50]	287 (312)	CDT with UK, stenting for residual stenosis; systemic lysis (n = 6)	96 (31)	162 (52)	54 (17)	15 (28)	54 (11)	6	2 (<1)
Comerota et al. (2000)[51]	54	CDT with UK or rtPA, thrombectomy for residual stenosis	14 (26)	28 (52)	6 (11)	8 (15)	4 (7)	1	None
Horne et al. (2000)[42]	10	CDT with rtPA	9 (90)	1 (10)	0 (0)	3 (30)	None	2 (20)	None
Kasirajan et al. (2001)[61]	9	CDT with UK, rtPA or rPA	7 (78)	1 (11)	1 (11)	NA	NA	NA	NA
AbuRahma et al. (2001)[43]	51	CDT with UK or rtPA, stents/18	15 (83)	NR	NR	3 (17)	2 (11)	None	None
		Hep/33	1 (3)	NR	NR	3 (9)	2 (6)	2 (6)	None
Vedantham et al. (2002)[60]	20 (28)	CDT with UK, rtPA or rPA, thrombectomy, stenting	23 (82)	NR	NR	None	3 (14)	None	None
Elsharawy et al. (2002)[52]	35	CDT with SK, angioplasty, stent/18	13 (72)	5 (28)	0 (0)	None	None	None	None
		Hep/17	2 (12)	8 (47)	7 (41)	None	None	None	None
Castaneda et al. (2002)[44]	15	CDT with rPA	15 (100)	NR	NR	None	None	None	None
Grunwald et al. (2004)[45]	74 (82)	CDT with UK, tPA or rPA, angioplasty, stenting	54 (73)	26 (32)	NR	6 (8)	4 (5)	None	None
Laiho et al. (2004)[46]	32	CDT with rtPA/16	8 (50)	5 (31)	NR	4 (25)	2 (13)	2 (13)	None
		systemic lysis with rtPA/16	5 (31)	8 (50)	NR	6 (38)	1 (6)	5 (31)	None
Sillesen et al. (2005)[47]	45	CDT with rtPA, angioplasty, stenting	42 (93)	NR	NR	4 (8)	None	1 (2)	None
Jackson et al. (2005)[48]	28	CDT with UK or rPA, stenting	5 (18)	20 (72)	NR	2 (7)	None	None	None
Ogawa et al. (2005)[70]	24	CDT with UK/10	0 (0)	10 (100)	None	None	None	None	None
		CDT with UK + IPC/14	5 (36)	9 (64)	None	None	None	None	None
Kim et al. (2006)[49]	37 (45)	CDT with UK/23	21 (81)	3 (11)	2 (8)	1 (4)	2 (7)	1 (4)	None
		CDT + PMT/14	16 (84)	3 (16)	None	None	1 (5)	1 (5)	None
Lin et al. (2006)[62]	93 (98)	CDT with rPA, rtPA or UK, angioplasty, stenting/46	32 (70)	14 (30)	5 (11)	2 (4)	1 (2)	None	None
		PMT with rPA, rt-PA or UK, angioplasty, stenting/52	39 (75)	13 (25)	4 (8)	2 (4)	None	None	None

Source: Comerota AJ, Gravett MH, *J Vasc Surg*, 46(5), 1065, November 2007. With permission.

Abbreviations: CDT, catheter-directed thrombolysis; Hep, heparin; IPC, intermittent pneumatic compression; rPA, PMT, pharmacomechanical thrombolysis; rtPA, recombinant tissue plasminogen activator; tPA, tissue plasminogen activator; UK, urokinase.

Patients with IFDVT treated with CDT who were enrolled in the National Venous Registry were asked to complete a health-related quality of life questionnaire. Questionnaires were also administered to a cohort-controlled group of patients with IFDVT who were eligible for CDT but were treated with anticoagulation alone because of physician preference. Patients treated with CDT reported better overall physical functioning (p = 0.046), less stigma (p = 0.033), less health distress (p = 0.022) and fewer postthrombotic symptoms (p = 0.006) compared to patients treated with anticoagulation alone. Improved quality of life directly correlated with phlebographically successful lysis (p = 0.038). Patients who had failure of CDT had the same quality of life as those treated with anticoagulation alone.[51]

The first clinical trial of CDT for IFDVT was performed in 35 patients randomized to either CDT with streptokinase or anticoagulation alone, the primary efficacy end points being patency and vein valve function.[52] Patients treated with CDT had a significantly higher immediate- and long-term venous patency and better valve function. After 6 months, 72% of patients treated with thrombolysis maintained patency of the iliofemoral venous segment, compared to only 12% after conventional anticoagulation (p < 0.001). Unfortunately, these investigators did not assess patients for postthrombotic morbidity; however, one would not expect PTS to occur in patients with patent veins with functional valves.

Baekgaard et al.[53] reported 101 consecutive patients (103 limbs) with acute IFDVT who were treated with CDT. Patients who were ≤60 years old with a first episode of IFDVT of less than 14 days from symptom onset were included. The Kaplan–Meier survival analysis demonstrated patent deep veins with competent valves in 82% of treated limbs 6 years after the CDT only. Three cases of early rethrombosis (3%) and three cases of late rethrombosis (3%) were reported. The incidence of major bleeding was less than 1%.

The CaVenT trial recently reported the long-term outcomes of CDT for IFDVT treatment.[54] This multicentre, open-label, RCT assigned 209 patients with first-time IFDVT to conventional anticoagulation or CDT treatment groups. Knee-length compression stockings (class II) were prescribed for both groups during follow-up, with approximately a 50% compliance rate. Thrombolysis was performed with alteplase infusion at a dose of 0.01 mg/kg/hour. After 2 years of follow-up, the prevalence of PTS according to the Villalta score was 41.1% (95% CI 31.5–51.4) in the CDT group and 55.6% (95% CI 45.7–65.0) in patients treated with anticoagulation only (p = 0.047). Absolute risk reduction of PTS was 14.4% (95% CI 0.2–27.9). There was a direct correlation of iliofemoral occlusion and PTS. Likewise, the benefit of CDT on reducing PTS was directly related to the patency of the iliofemoral veins (Table 49.2). There was a 3.3% risk of major bleeding; no PE or cerebral haemorrhage related to CDT was observed.

The seventh edition of the ACCP guidelines (ACCP 7th, 2004) did not include any strategy for thrombus

Table 49.2 CaVenT data.

End point	Additional CDT (N = 90)	Anticoagulation only (N = 99)	p-value
Iliofemoral patency at 6 months	58 (66%)	45 (47%)	0.012
Iliofemoral patency at 24 months	37 (41%)	55 (56%)	0.047

Note: Primary outcomes of iliac vein patency and postthrombotic syndrome in the CaVenT trial.

removal of DVT. The guidelines 4 years later (ACCP 8th, 2008) included a number of recommendations regarding a strategy of thrombus removal and recognized that IFDVT patients were a clinically important subset. It was suggested that surgical thrombectomy and CDT may be options for acute (<14 days) IFDVT in patients with good functional status, life expectancy of more than 1 year and low risk of bleeding in order to alleviate acute symptoms and prevent PTS (2C-thrombectomy, 2B-CDT). CDT was preferred to open thrombectomy for patients with low risk of bleeding (2C). Unfortunately, the last edition of the ACCP guidelines (ACCP 9th, 2012) offers an update of anticoagulation management of DVT, but does not address strategies of thrombus removal. This should not be mistakenly interpreted as a loss of evidence supporting CDT, as the 2012 ACCP guidelines emphasized the methodologic quality of studies to drive recommendations. Hence, almost all recommendations and suggestions for treatment in VTE patients were downgraded and there is no 1A recommendation for any treatment for acute VTE. The AVF guidelines[2] suggest CDT for patients with IFDVT and less than 14 days of symptom duration to reduce acute symptoms and decrease risk of PTS (2B).

In 2009, SIR together with CIRSE issued guidelines for appropriate utilization of endovascular techniques for DVT treatment. The list of indications included phlegmasia cerulea dolens; acute and subacute IVC thrombosis; acute (<14 days), subacute (14–28 days) and chronic (>28 days) IFDVT; and acute femoral–popliteal DVT.[3]

The AHA issued guidelines for PE, IFDVT and chronic thromboembolic pulmonary hypertension treatment in 2011. For the first time, the term *thromboreductive strategy* was mentioned in national guidelines, calling attention to the morbidity of large-volume, persistent clots. Compared to previous guidelines, CDT was strongly recommended for IFDVT associated with a limb-threatening presentation (IC) and has finally been considered reasonable as a first-line treatment strategy to prevent PTS in patients with iliofemoral disease (IIaB). Other indications are clinical deterioration (IIaB) and rapid thrombus propagation (IIaC) on the background of adequate anticoagulation. DVT >21 days and a high risk of bleeding are contraindications for CDT according to the AHA (IIIB).

The 2012 practice guidelines of the SVS and AVF[5] suggest early thrombus removal in patients with a first episode of acute IFDVT, ≤14 days of symptom duration, low risk of bleeding and who are ambulatory with acceptable life expectancy (2C). Thrombus removal is also strongly indicated in patients with severe limb-threatening symptoms (1A). In selected patients, CDT is a first-line strategy of thrombus removal (2C).

The NICE 2012 guidelines recommend CDT for symptomatic IFDVT with symptoms less than 14 days, good functional status, at least 1 year of life expectancy and low risk of bleeding. The EVF 2013 guidelines[7] recognize the importance of a strategy of thrombus removal in patients with IFDVT and recommend CDT for acute IFDVT (level of evidence: moderate) without further specifications of patient-related or disease-related factors. In summary, most of the current guidelines suggest CDT for IFDVT although marked distinctions exist in appropriate timing, class of recommendation and the level of evidence between them.

Bleeding complications occur with contemporary CDT despite the high fibrin affinity of tPA and its precise catheter-directed delivery. However, with the current *low-dose* infusion of 1 mg/hour or less, bleeding complications have substantially diminished. tPA can escape into the circulation, bind to plasminogen contained within small haemostatic plugs in areas of vessel wall injury and subsequently induce bleeding.

A concern which limits the wide adoption of CDT is the safety of thrombolysis in high-risk patients, specifically pregnant women and cancer patients. A retrospective cohort of 178 consecutive patients with acute iliofemoral or brachiosubclavian DVT (202 limbs) demonstrated the same efficacy and safety of lytic therapy for patients with and without cancer. Major bleeding occurred in 4.9% of cancer patients compared to 3.4% in non-cancer patients (p = 0.6924), while PE was reported with the same frequency (1.6% vs. 1.7%, p = 0.9999).[55] Our experience of active thrombus removal in 13 pregnant women with acute IFDVT demonstrated both efficacy and safety, avoiding PTS with a low recurrence rate.[56] With appropriate low-molecular-weight heparin (LMWH) prophylaxis, the course of subsequent pregnancies was shown to be uneventful.[57]

According to published data, early rethrombosis occurs in 6%–25% of patients after CDT, with a pooled mean of 20%.[3] This appears to be high and likely occurs as a result of inadequate lysis which leaves a large volume of residual thrombus, inadequate inflow or outflow and uncorrected venous lesions or inadequate post-lysis anticoagulation.

PHARMACOMECHANICAL THROMBOLYSIS

The risk of major bleeding after CDT drip techniques, high rates of incomplete lysis, long treatment times, high cumulative doses of lytic agents and prolonged ICU and hospital stays have stimulated advances in endovascular techniques.

Several devices were developed to eliminate thrombus using minimally invasive approaches. Rotational devices such as Trerotola (Arrow International, PA, United States) and Amplatz (Microvena, MN, United States) rely on a spinning helix that fragments the clot. Rheolytic thrombectomy, AngioJet (Possis, MN, United States), is based on the Bernoulli principle which breaks down thrombus by the pressure gradient created by high-speed saline jet. Isolated segmental pharmacomechanical thrombolysis (ISPMT) is achieved using the Trellis Infusion System (Covidien, Mansfield, MA). This innovative system consists of two occluding balloons with an intervening spiral catheter which spins at 3000 RPMs after a small dose of plasminogen activator is injected into the occluded segment. The fragmented and lysed thrombus is then aspirated and repeat phlebography performed. The EndoWave Infusion Catheter System (EKOS Corp, Bothell, WA) uses a multiple side-hole catheter with a retrievable ultrasound core emitting high-frequency, low-energy ultrasound during infusion of a plasminogen activator. The addition of ultrasound waves separates fibrin strands allowing better penetration of the rtPA into the thrombus, thereby accelerating thrombolysis.[58,59]

Vedantham studied the effectiveness of endovascular mechanical thrombectomy using different devices (Amplatz, AngioJet, Trerotola and Oasis) in 28 limbs.[60] Based upon a venography scoring system, catheter thrombectomy alone removed only 26% of thrombus, while administration of plasminogen activator reduced thrombus load by 62% (p = 0.006). A small series of patients (n = 17) treated with rheolytic thrombectomy with the AngioJet catheter demonstrated that only 24% had >90% clot removal. The addition of CDT improved the success rate.[61]

A retrospective cohort study of 98 patients with symptomatic DVT compared CDT (n = 46) with CDT and rheolytic thrombectomy (n = 52).[62] Similar overall rates were observed. Importantly, patients in the PMT group underwent fewer venograms (p < 0.001) and had significantly shorter intensive care unit and hospital lengths of stay and lower overall cost of care (p < 0.01).

Several studies compared CDT with ISPMT. A retrospective analysis of ISPMT in 19 consecutive patients with acute proximal DVT demonstrated more than 50% lysis in 95% of cases with the median administered dose of tPA of 13.4 mg and mean treatment time of 91 minutes. No major complications were reported.[63] A retrospective review of 43 patients was published by Martinez.[64] Twenty-one consecutive patients (27 limbs) were treated with CDT and 22 consecutive patients (25 limbs) with ISPMT plus CDT. The addition of ISPMT increased immediate success of lytic therapy by 20% (60% vs. 80%; p = 0.0016), with a concomitant 39% decrease in dose of plasminogen activator. Improved success, shorter treatment times (55.4 vs. 23.4 hours; p < 0.0001) and lower doses of rtPA (59.3 vs. 33.4 mg; p = 0.0009) were the main advantages of additional ISPMT. There were no differences in bleeding complications (5% in both groups).

A concern frequently expressed is that mechanical devices cause valve damage. Vogel et al. studied this issue.[65] They reported outcomes of CDT by the drip technique (n = 20), rheolytic thrombolysis using AngioJet catheter (n = 14) and isolated PMT with the Trellis device (n = 35) in 54 patients (61 limbs) with IFDVT. By the end of the follow-up (44 months), the rate of deep valve incompetence assessed by venous duplex was similar in patients after CDT and PMT, 65% and 53%, respectively (p = 0.42). Thus, no adverse effect of PMT on long-term valve function was noticed.[65] An important incidental observation was the 35% incidence of deep vein valve reflux in the contralateral, noninvolved leg.

PMT is recommended by the EVF 2013 as an initial therapy for IFDVT (low evidence). The AVF 2008 suggests PMT as a preferable method compared to CDT because of a shortened treatment time (2B). The ACCP 8th and SVS/AVF 2012 support this statement but with lower levels of evidence (2C). To date, there is no evidence that PMT is a preferable treatment method because of better long-term outcomes. However, there is a growing tendency of combining CDT with endovascular thrombectomy to shorten treatment time and reduce dose of lytic agent.

Our current approach to patients with symptomatic IFDVT is to access their ipsilateral popliteal vein to treat their proximal thrombus and access their distal position tibial vein to treat their popliteal and distal thrombus (Figure 49.1). Using current techniques, patency can be restored with expected short- and long-term benefits.

The promising Acute Venous Thrombosis: Thrombus Removal with Adjunctive Catheter-directed Thrombolysis trial is currently in progress to clarify the best treatment for patients with iliofemoral and femoral–popliteal vein thrombosis. This is an NIH-funded, multicentre, randomized, open-label, assessor-blinded, parallel, two-arm, iliofemoral versus femoral–popliteal stratified, controlled clinical trial. Six hundred ninety-two patients have been randomized to catheter-based thrombolysis (with or without PMT) plus anticoagulation or anticoagulation alone. The primary study outcome is the cumulative incidence of PTS 24 months after treatment. In addition to the important issues this study may address lies the question, 'Is thrombus removal better than anticoagulation alone for PTS prevention?' This question addresses factors facing both IFDVT patients and those with femoral–popliteal DVT. Other important targets are quality of life, risks and cost-effectiveness and how thrombus removal affects recurrence.

The benefit of ultrasound-accelerated thrombolysis in patients with DVT was studied in a multicentre registry. Parikh et al. reported using the EKOS system in 53 patients with DVT. Lytic effect was achieved in 91% of patients (complete 70%, partial 21%). In 3.8% of cases, major bleeding occurred.[66] Important limitations of this report were different DVT locations, where only 60% of patients had lower extremity DVT; various thrombolytic agents used; and different times from symptom onset, with only 47% of patients having acute DVT (<14 days).

The DUTCH CAVA trial will elucidate the role of ultrasound-accelerated endovascular thrombolysis by randomizing patients with acute IFDVT to use accelerated lysis versus anticoagulation alone.

Patient selection, preoperative evaluation and risk assessment

Patients presenting with a swollen, painful lower extremity, especially when the swelling extends to the inguinal ligament, should be suspected of having IFDVT. The diagnosis is usually confirmed with duplex ultrasound which has a high sensitivity (97%) and specificity (94%).[67] The most specific finding of acute DVT on duplex ultrasound is noncompressibility of the veins. Other helpful sonographic findings include visible intraluminal echogenic material, absence of spontaneity and respiratory phasicity of venous blood flow, filling defect on colour flow imaging and increased vein diameter. It is important to establish whether the thrombus extends into the vena cava and whether the contralateral iliofemoral segment is involved. The proximal extent of thrombus can be evaluated by spiral CT venography of the abdomen and pelvis, gadolinium-enhanced magnetic resonance venography and conventional contrast phlebography.

Although PE is a potential complication of endovascular treatment of DVT, procedure-related symptomatic PE is infrequent if the vena cava does not contain clot. About 50% of patients with iliofemoral thrombosis have asymptomatic pulmonary emboli at the time of DVT diagnosis.[64] Some may develop pleuritic symptoms days later. In some cases, physicians might mistakenly attribute pleuritic symptoms to a new PE and conclude that the patient had failed anticoagulation. In cases such as this, knowledge of the asymptomatic PE would be helpful.

Testing patients for heredity thrombophilia is not helpful for patient care. The purpose of thrombophilia testing is to assess patient risk for recurrent venous thrombosis. Since patients with extensive DVT and unprovoked DVT have an inherently higher risk of recurrence than that imposed by hereditary thrombophilia, the presence of an existing thrombophilia will not alter patient care. On the other hand, the absence of a thrombophilia may give the physician and a patient a false sense of security, which leads to under treatment of the patient. However, first-degree female relatives of child bearing potential should be evaluated for hereditary thrombophilia, especially factor V Leiden and prothrombin gene mutation. If positive, these women would require VTE prophylaxis during future pregnancy.[68]

Technique of CDT

Initial therapeutic anticoagulation with intravenous UFH, LMWH or fondaparinux and long leg compression wraps are applied once the diagnosis is confirmed. Patients are permitted to ambulate until CDT has begun. CDT is not required as an emergency and is usually begun on the next business day. Our preferred approach is via ultrasound-guided access to the ipsilateral popliteal vein. In patients with bilateral disease (which usually involves the vena cava), catheters are placed via both popliteal veins, with one being advanced into the vena cava. It is advantageous to integrate pharmacomechanical techniques to speed clot resolution. Our preference is the use of the Trellis catheter to debulk iliofemoral thrombus, power pulse spray to saturate the remaining thrombus with the plasminogen activator and ultrasound-accelerated

thrombolysis to more rapidly lyse residual thrombus and lyse distal clot. If the distal popliteal and tibial veins appear thrombosed, a second infusion catheter is placed into the posterior tibial vein at the ankle and advanced cephalad through the popliteal vein. Alternative access via the femoral vein in the thigh or a retrograde approach from the jugular vein has been used with success.

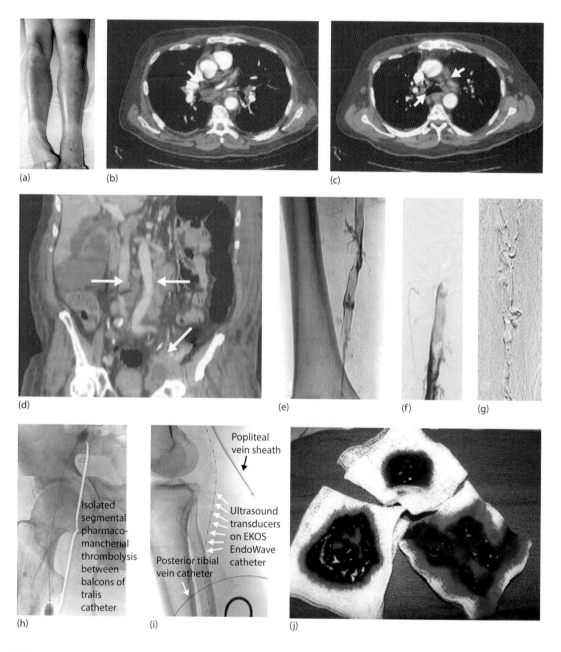

Figure 49.1 A 65-year-old white man was referred with phlegmasia cerulea dolens of his left leg (a) 36 hours after major abdominal laparotomy. Venous duplex demonstrated clot in the posterior tibial veins extending to the external iliac vein. A contrast-enhanced CT scan of the chest, abdomen and pelvis was performed and demonstrated asymptomatic pulmonary emboli (b) and mediastinal (c), retroperitoneal (c, arrows) and pelvic lymphadenopathy (d, arrows). The extensive thrombus was demonstrated by a catheter phlebogram of the femoral vein (e) and (f) and the silhouette of the calf thrombus (g) by the catheter in the posterior tibial vein at the ankle. The bulk of the thrombus from the proximal popliteal vein to the common iliac vein was treated with the Trellis catheter via an ultrasound-guided popliteal vein approach (h). The clot in the posterior tibial and popliteal veins was treated with the EKOS EndoWave system (i). Liquefied and fragmented thrombus resulting from isolated segmental pharmacomechanical thrombolysis was aspirated via the Trellis catheter (j).

(Continued)

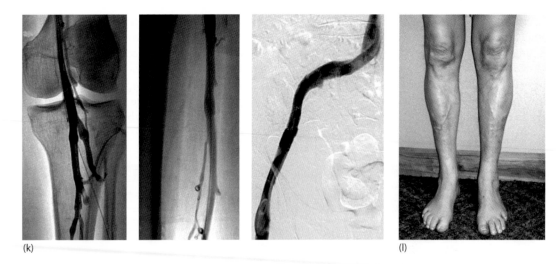

(k)   (l)

Figure 49.1 (*Continued*) A completion phlebogram shows successful elimination of thrombus and stenting of the compressed iliac vein (k). A 16-month follow-up photo demonstrates a normal lower extremity (l) which has patent veins with normal valve function.

During lytic infusion through the catheter, we infuse UFH at a dose of 500 IU/hour through the sheath. This reduces the risk of thrombosis distal to the infusion catheter and reduces the risk of rethrombosis. Thrombolytic therapy is commonly started with a high-pressure bolus injection of a small volume of concentrated plasminogen activator (1–6 mg) to rapidly penetrate and saturate the thrombus. This approach of initial thrombus 'lacing' before continuous infusion has been shown to achieve better intraclot distribution of the plasminogen activator.[69]

Recombinant tissue plasminogen activators (alteplase, reteplase and tenecteplase) are the most commonly used for CDT, with rtPA being the most popular. There are no comparative data suggesting that one agent is more effective, although most of the experience is with rtPA. An important modification of the CDT technique is increasing the volume of lytic solution with a decrease of the dose of plasminogen activator, thereby reducing rtPA concentration. We commonly use a concentration of 1 mg rtPA contained within 50–100 cc of saline. The larger volume is preferable. The goal is to activate the thrombus with the rtPA solution which appears to accelerate lysis compared to higher dose lower volume infusions.

During CDT, intermittent pneumatic compression (IPC) is applied to the calf of the involved limb. Ogawa et al.[70] reported improved efficacy of lysis when IPC cuffs were applied during lytic infusion. Repeat phlebograms are performed approximately every 12 hours to monitor lytic success.

Some clinicians follow the fibrinogen level as an indicator of the risk of bleeding using the threshold of 100 to temporarily discontinue the infusion. This approach is based on the observations of the STILE trial,[71] where depletion of fibrinogen was found to be a predictor of bleeding complication with catheter-based thrombolysis

for acute arterial ischemia ($p < 0.01$). While a drop in fibrinogen is an obvious marker of systemic activation of the fibrinolytic system and induced coagulopathy, the correlation between bleeding risk and plasma fibrinogen level is not precise, but can give an overall impression of relative bleeding risk.

Routine use of vena caval filters is not recommended. A randomized trial of 396 patients with proximal DVT who could receive therapeutic anticoagulation was randomized to filter versus non-filter. There was no survival advantage, although filter patients had fewer PEs and more DVTs. If a patient has a free floating segment of thrombus in the IVC, we recommend that an IVC filter be placed to reduce the risk of procedural-related PE. In most instances, a retrievable filter will be used and removed immediately after the procedure. To reduce the risk of rethrombosis, UFH is infused through the sheath at a dose of 500 units per hour.

Following lysis, a completion phlebogram is performed. Grading the degree of lysis according to the SIR/CIRSE 2009 guidelines will lend objectivity to treatment outcome. The long-term benefit of successful thrombus removal cannot be overstated. Patients will have markedly reduced postthrombotic morbidity,[72] and the patients will possibly face less risk of recurrent DVT.[73]

Persistent iliofemoral lesions increase the risk of recurrent thrombosis. Single plane phlebography inadequately evaluates the iliofemoral veins. Intravascular ultrasound is the most sensitive technique to quantify the degree of residual stenosis, its location and its response to treatment.[74,75]

Adequate therapeutic anticoagulation following CDT is important to avoid rethrombosis. Lozier et al.[76] reported increased PAI-1 following CDT, which indicates a prothrombotic state. Our preference is to infuse a therapeutic dose UFH for 12–24 hours through the sheath after thrombolysis is completed. This ensures that supratherapeutic heparin levels are in the target vein. Heparin binds to residual thrombus and endothelial and subendothelial tissue, which should significantly reduce the likelihood of rethrombosis. Subsequently, patients are converted to oral anticoagulation for long-term treatment (ACCP 8th IC, AVF/SVS-1A).

SURGICAL THROMBECTOMY

Operative venous thrombectomy, when properly performed, is an effective and durable technique. A randomized trial of operative venous thrombectomy versus anticoagulation reported significant short- and long-term benefits in patients randomized to thrombectomy.[77] A detailed review of operative thrombectomy is beyond the scope of this chapter. The principles and surgical technique of contemporary venous thrombectomy have been previously reported.[78,79] With the significant advances in endovascular techniques, the need for open surgery has substantially diminished. Surgical thrombectomy is reserved for patients with acute IFDVT who have contraindications to any degree of lytic therapy or in instances where catheter-based therapy is unavoidable. Most clinical practice guidelines support this with low to moderate level of evidence.[1]

VENOUS STENTING

The first experience with venous stenting was reported by Berger in 1995 for treatment in a patient with May–Thurner syndrome.[80] A year later, Nazarian and coworkers retrospectively analyzed a 4-year experience using Gianturco, Palmaz and Wallstents in a variety of locations in 55 patients. Primary, primary-assisted and secondary 4-year patency rates were 59%, 63% and 72%, respectively.[81] Such reporting of cumulative results in a variety of venous locations is of little help to clinicians, as intrinsic outcomes for different venous beds vary. Iliofemoral venous stents are associated with durable outcomes if there is good inflow and good outflow and if the stent is of large diameter.

Currently used intravascular stents are categorized into three basic types:

1. *Balloon-expandable stents* – These stents are rigid and require the use of a balloon catheter for insertion and deployment within the diseased vessel segment. The Palmaz stent (Johnson & Johnson Interventional Systems Co., Warren, NJ) is the most commonly used stent of this type.
2. *Self-expanding stents* – These stents are compressed into a smaller-diameter introducer sheath and released into the diseased vein by withdrawing the sheath while holding the stent in place. The inherent memory of the stent wire determines its expansile force. Wallstent (Schneider, Minneapolis, MN.) and Zilver (Cook,

Bloomington, Ind.) stents are such examples of self-expanding stent systems.
3. *Thermal-expanding stents (S.M.A.R.T. Control Stent System, Cordis Corp., NJ)* – These stents are made of nickel–titanium alloy and based on its unique property of thermal recovery at bloodstream temperature.

Venous stents have been used to support the patency of a stenotic or occluded vein. Venus stents have been used for a variety of indicators including iliocaval stenosis or occlusive venous thoracic outlet syndrome, venous stenosis of haemodialysis access, SVC syndrome and Budd–Chiari syndrome.

Obstruction of iliofemoral venous segment

Iliocaval and iliofemoral segment stenting is an important part of endovascular treatment of residual stenotic venous disease for managing patients with acute and chronic thrombotic obstruction. This residual stenosis may be caused by organized intraluminal thrombus or external compression of the left iliac vein by the overriding right common iliac artery (May–Thurner syndrome), collagenous intraluminal obstruction or a scarred and thickened vein wall. Thirty-two to forty-eight of patients with IFDVT have a residual stenotic lesion after lytic therapy that requires adjunctive stenting.[50,82] A single-centre prospective study randomized 74 patients with more than 50% residual stenosis of the iliac vein into a stenting group (n = 45) or control group (n = 29).[82] A significantly higher long-term patency rate was found at last follow-up visit (6–24 months) in patients who underwent endovascular treatment (87.5% vs. 29.6%, p < 0.05). Venous clinical severity score considerably differed between groups (0.69 ± 0.23 vs. 7.57 ± 0.27, p < 0.001).[82] Meng's study confirmed the observations of the National Venous Registry, which showed that iliac stenting improved 1-year patency of the iliofemoral venous segment after CDT for DVT (74% vs. 53%, p < 0.001).[50] National guidelines indicate that it is reasonable to perform balloon angioplasty and stenting to correct underlying or residual iliac vein obstruction: ACCP 8th (2C), AHA (IIaC) and SVS/AVF (2C), whereas the AHA guidelines indicate that residual obstruction of common femoral vein may be treated by balloon angioplasty alone (IIaC).

Chronic central postthrombotic obstruction is often associated with severe morbidity. Percutaneous balloon angioplasty and stenting is an effective treatment for patients with chronic iliofemoral obstruction and used for symptom relief and quality of life improvement. Retrospective studies have shown favourable primary (71%–83%), assisted primary (89%–90%) and secondary (93%–95%) patency rates.[83–85] The largest experience was reported by Neglen et al.[86] Nine hundred eighty-two consecutive femoroiliocaval obstructions were treated endovascularly from 1997 to 2005. At 3 years, primary, assisted primary and secondary cumulative patency rates were 79%, 100% and 100% when treated for nonthrombotic disease and 57%, 80% and 86% when postthrombotic patients were treated. Patients treated for postthrombotic occlusions had the poorest results. In-stent restenosis occurred in 10% of postthrombotic lesions and 1% of non-thrombotic stenosis during follow-up.[86]

Technical aspects are important. An appropriately large-diameter stent and insuring good inflow and outflow from the treated segment are most important. A 12–14 mm stent in the external iliac or a 14–18 mm stent in common iliac is adequate in most cases. Most postthrombotic patients require stenting of the entire segment from the cephalad common femoral to common iliac vein/venacaval junction. Stents have been safely placed across the inguinal ligament; however, self-expanding stainless steel stents appear to function best in this location.[87] Although conventional anticoagulation is used following these procedures, a systematic review failed to find benefit of antithrombotic therapy on the long-term outcomes of iliofemoral stenting.[88] Since the mechanism of failure is thrombosis, we believe all patients should be treated with anticoagulation after stenting. The proper duration of anticoagulation, proper agent and proper dose remain to be determined.

All stents placed in the venous system in the United States are used off-label. Two ongoing trials of venous stents will likely lead to FDA approval for venous indications. The VIRTUS study (Veniti Vici Venous Stent System, Veniti Inc.) and the VIVO study (Zilver Vena Venous Self-Expanding Stent, Cook Medical Inc.) are evaluating the safety and efficiency of stents for the treatment of iliofemoral venous obstruction.

DVT of upper extremity

The initial epidemiological reports of DVT published more than 25 years ago indicated that the incidence of upper extremity DVT was 2.03 per 100,000 people annually.[89] Recent studies found that thrombosis of deep veins of upper extremity has increased to 4.4%–10.9% of all DVT cases.[90,91] Expanded use of indwelling central venous catheters, pressure lines and pacemakers and implanted defibrillators contributes to this. An indwelling central venous catheter is the strongest independent predictor of secondary upper extremity DVT (OR 7.3; 95% CI 5.8–9.2).[90] Other important causes of secondary thrombosis are intravenous drugs, trauma, cancer and several systemic diseases (CHF, uraemia, etc.).

Primary upper extremity DVT is a separate condition, which has attracted the attention of clinicians since James Paget described a spontaneous thrombosis of the subclavian vein in 1875. Primary axillosubclavian vein thrombosis has been historically referred to by many terms including idiopathic or spontaneous subclavian thrombosis, effort-induced thrombosis and Paget–Schroetter syndrome. This condition is also known as venous thoracic outlet syndrome, which is compression of the subclavian vein between the clavicle and the first rib, with additional narrowing by hypertrophy of the subclavius and anterior scalene muscles since this obstructs the venous inlet to the thorax *venous thoracic outlet* is a misnomer. Positional narrowing of the costoclavicular space from extensive shoulder abduction is the most common mechanism. Various congenital anomalies also may be responsible for the primary disease: exostosis of the first rib, anomalous or hypertrophied subclavius or anterior scalene muscle or fibromuscular bands. Although the process of venous injury is not well understood, it is thought that the repetitive external compression of subclavian vein and subluxation of the shoulder during vigorous exercise and sport activities causes intimal tears and venous wall damage coupled with compromised venous outflow leading to acute axillosubclavian thrombosis.

The typical patient with primary axillosubclavian DVT is a healthy young person living an active life and is often involved in various exercise or sports activities leading to forceful shoulder hyperabduction or external rotation (baseball, volleyball, swimming, football or body building). The right upper extremity is most commonly involved, most likely because the right arm is frequently the most vigorously used.

The proximal location of the upper extremity thrombosis is responsible for the most striking clinical manifestation and the worst prognosis. Axillosubclavian vein thrombosis is the upper extremity equivalent of IFDVT. Distal propagation of the subclavian thrombus to the axillary vein compromises important collaterals leading to progressive venous hypertension of the upper extremity. Patients with axillosubclavian vein thrombosis typically present with sudden onset of heaviness, swelling, pain and cyanosis of the affected extremity.

Colour Doppler ultrasound is the first step to establish a diagnosis of upper extremity DVT. Gadolinium-enhanced MRI is commonly used for central vein visualization. Contrast venography remains the best diagnostic test, but is usually reserved for patients who will undergo CDT. A chest CT scan is valuable to exclude mass lesions and exclude cervical ribs or to establish the presence of foreign intraluminal material (catheter or wire).

Compared to IFDVT, the natural history of upper extremity DVT is more favourable, most likely due to the lower venous pressures in the upper extremity. According to the US prospective DVT Registry Database, PE complicates upper extremity DVT much less frequently than the lower extremity (3% vs. 16%; $p < 0.001$).[90] PTS is also less commonly seen after upper extremity DVT. A systematic review reported the incidence of PTS as high as 15% (7%–46%) based on seven studies.[92] However, there is no generally adopted scoring system for the evaluation of postthrombotic symptoms of the upper extremity similar to the validated Villalta score for the leg.

There are no randomized trials regarding management of axillosubclavian DVT. Observational and retrospective studies constitute the evidence for patient management. An evolution of treatment strategy for Paget–Schroetter syndrome has been reported covering 294 consecutive patients (312 limbs) over a 30-year experience. Prior to 1980, patients were treated with anticoagulation alone (n = 35). Sixty percent developed postthrombotic symptoms after returning to work. Because of these unsatisfactory results, the treatment strategy was modified to thrombolysis and early surgical decompression. This approach resulted in 89% of patients enjoying an active lifestyle and returning to work within 6 weeks. The remaining 241 patients followed were treated in a similar fashion. Clinical success was achieved in 95% of patients (189/199) who were treated within 6 weeks of symptom onset. Thrombolysis failed in all patients who were treated more than 6 weeks after DVT onset. In 57% (24/42), spontaneous recanalization occurred with a good clinical result. Moderate to severe postthrombotic symptoms were reported by 61% of patients with chronic occlusion (11/18).

Angioplasty with stenting prior to first rib resection is often associated with stent compression and fracture. Decompression of the thoracic outlet should precede stenting of the subclavian vein, if it is required. Stenting after initial thrombolysis without surgical decompression is a risk factor of disease recurrence (p = 0.05).[93]

The management of Paget–Schroetter syndrome has undergone significant evolution. A multidisciplinary approach which offers catheter-based thrombolytic therapy to restore venous, surgical decompression of venous thoracic outlet syndrome via first rib resection and percutaneous transluminal angioplasty has had increased acceptance. However, experience has shown that most patients who become asymptomatic following CDT will not require first rib resection.[94] If patients remain symptomatic because of residual subclavian vein compression, or if recurrent thrombosis occurs, lysis followed by first rib resection is recommended. We have now developed and follow the algorithm illustrated in Figure 49.2.[95]

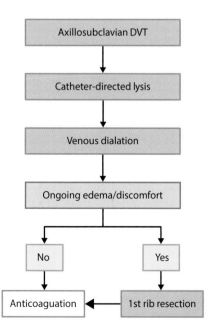

Figure 49.2 Algorithm for the management of patients with acute venous thrombosis outlet syndrome.

Venous stenosis of haemodialysis access

Approximately 300,000 individuals in the United States receive haemodialysis for the end-stage renal disease. Vascular access is the lifeline for these patients. Stenoses or occlusions complicating arteriovenous fistulas and prosthetic arteriovenous grafts frequently occur at the site of venous anastomosis or adjacent to the venous anastomosis due to neointimal hyperplasia. Another serious problem with haemodialysis access is central vein stenosis often caused by the indwelling venous haemodialysis catheters. Thrombosis of the haemodialysis access site is the common final event.

Traditional methods of venous stenosis management are surgical graft revision with vein patch angioplasty or graft extension, percutaneous angioplasty, stenting and finally abandonment of the access site. According to the Kidney Disease Outcomes Quality Initiative Clinical Practice Guidelines of 2006, there is no evidence supporting the endovascular approach over conventional surgery, and a haemodialysis access with >50% stenosis should be treated with either percutaneous intervention or open surgical revision at the surgeon's discretion. Transluminal angioplasty and stenting is the preferred treatment for patients with central vein stenosis which is associated with a good secondary patency rate.

Although stenting was initially assumed to be more effective than angioplasty alone, RCTs failed to demonstrate a benefit of bare metal stents over balloon angioplasty.[96] Endovascular stenting is helpful in treating patients with failed percutaneous balloon angioplasty. Vorwerk et al. demonstrated that self-expandable stents improve technical success of intervention for failing haemodialysis grafts, when balloon angioplasty alone was insufficient. Their cumulative haemodialysis access patency rate was 77% at 2 years.[97]

The technical success of percutaneous balloon angioplasty for venous stenosis of haemodialysis access is reasonable, but transient, as there is a high recurrence rate. The incidence of restenosis is especially high in central veins, with 2-year patency as low as 6%.[98]

The latest multicentre prospective trial randomly assigned 190 patients with prosthetic haemodialysis graft stenosis to balloon angioplasty alone or balloon angioplasty plus an expanded polytetrafluoroethylene endovascular stent graft. Patency of the access at 6 months was greater after the stent graft compared to balloon angioplasty (51% vs. 23%, p < 0.001), with a lower incidence of restenosis and reinterventions.[99] Additional studies are required to clarify the role of stent grafts to prolong the life of haemodialysis access due to prevention of neointimal hyperplasia.

Quality improvement guidelines of the Society of Interventional Radiology indicate that stenting of haemodialysis access is reasonable for peripheral lesions which fail to restore patency after angioplasty, if surgery is difficult or contraindicated, for central vein lesion that either failed angioplasty or reoccluded in 3 months after a successful attempt and for vein rupture during angioplasty.[100]

Budd–Chiari syndrome

The classic triad of abdominal pain, ascites and tender hepatomegaly describes the Budd–Chiari syndrome. This clinical presentation is attributable to hepatic venous outflow obstruction causing increased intrahepatic pressure and portal hypertension. IVC webs, myeloproliferative disorders and oral contraceptive use are associated aetiologies. The natural history of hepatic vein thrombosis is variable ranging from asymptomatic to acute illness with a fatal outcome. Thrombotic occlusion of only one hepatic vein is usually well tolerated.

The medical management of Budd–Chiari syndrome is based on diuretics to control the ascites and anticoagulation to correct an underlying coagulopathy. The success of conservative treatment is determined by the severity and progression of the underlying disease. The goal of surgical management is to relieve severe portal and intrahepatic hypertension. Transjugular intrahepatic portosystemic shunting (TIPS) has been effective in patients with Budd–Chiari syndrome. Operative approaches include side-to-side portocaval, splenorenal and mesocaval shunts. A cohort of 124 patients with severe Budd–Chiari syndrome treated with TIPS demonstrated high 1- and 5-year transplantation-free survival, 88% and 78%, respectively.[101] PTFE-covered stents have been reported to have improved outcomes over bare metal stents.[102] Percutaneous transluminal venous angioplasty has been used with favourable results in selected patients with membranous obstruction of the IVC and the right hepatic vein. Stent use is increasing as a means to improve the result of angioplasty alone.

Hepatic venous occlusion leads to severe congestion, liver cell atrophy and impaired regeneration. Progressive hepatic failure occurs in some, and liver transplantation is the treatment of last resort for these patients. A multicentre European study included 248 patients who underwent orthotopic liver transplantation for Budd–Chiari syndrome and demonstrated excellent results. Overall patient survival was 76% at 1 year, 71% at 5 years and 68% at 10 years. Recurrence was responsible for 44% of the late deaths.[103]

Superior vena cava syndrome

SVC syndrome represents symptoms and clinical signs resulting from either SVC endoluminal obstruction or external compression by intrathoracic pathology. In most cases, SVC syndrome is not considered a life-threatening condition and does not require emergent care.[104–107] SVC syndrome develops in 10% of patients with right-sided intrathoracic tumour.[108]

The classic pentad of SVC syndrome comprises the following:

- Swelling of the neck, face and eyelids
- Swelling of the upper extremities
- Superficial venous collaterals on the neck and chest wall
- Headache
- Conjunctival injection

Cough and dyspnea are commonly seen in patients with SVC syndrome, but may represent the underlying pulmonary or mediastinal process rather than hypertension in the SVC system. Patients with severe stenosis or occlusion of SVC below the azygos vein inflow frequently manifest with respiratory distress and/or central nervous system depression and have more profound symptoms and worse survival rates.[109]

There is an increased incidence of thrombotic SVC lesions due to cardiac implantable devices and central vein catheters.[110,111] A pooled analysis revealed 104 reports of symptomatic SVC obstruction following implantation of a pacemaker or cardioverter–defibrillator.[112] Pacemaker wires lead to SVC stenosis in up to 14% of patients.[113] In some cases, non-malignant SVC syndrome may be associated with fibrosing mediastinitis.[114,115]

A contrast-enhanced CT scan of the chest is the best diagnostic tool for patients with SVC syndrome to determine the aetiology, location and extent of obstruction. The rapidity of onset and clinical scenario should easily distinguish between acute and chronic SVC syndrome. Formal catheter-based venography is part of the procedure for definitive correction.[109,116]

Patients with chronic SVC syndrome often have primary lung malignancy or mediastinal metastatic disease which accounts for the majority of SVC cases.[110,111,117,118] Contemporary treatment of patients with chronic SVC obstruction is guided by the severity of symptoms, causative disease and overall life expectancy. The average life expectancy of patients with malignant SVC syndrome is 6 months.[119] Management for an underlying cancer is usually the basis of treatment in this group.[106] Non-small cell bronchogenic carcinoma is the most common cause of symptomatic SVC obstruction, existing in 1.7% of these patients.[118] The SVC also may be compressed or invaded by small cell lung cancer, non-Hodgkin lymphoma, thymic neoplasms or mediastinal metastatic disease.[111,116] Duration of SVC obstructive symptoms does not appear to influence the outcome in patients with malignant SVC syndrome.[104–106] ACCP 2007 guidelines for palliative care in lung cancer emphasize that every patient with SVC obstructive symptoms should undergo histologic/cytologic evaluation before the initiation of treatment (grade 1C).[120]

Malignant caval obstructions with only mild or moderate symptoms are commonly treated with nonsurgical methods such as radiation and chemotherapy to shrink the tumour and decrease its mass effect. A systematic review demonstrated that palliative radiation improves symptoms of SVC obstruction in two thirds of patients with lung cancer.[118] ACCP 2007 recommends chemotherapy as the first line of treatment for patients with small cell lung cancer (grade 1C). A randomized trial failed to demonstrate the benefit of additional radiotherapy in patients with small cell lung cancer for managing their SVC syndrome.[120] Patients with non-small cell carcinoma have better palliation after stent placement with or without radiation therapy (ACCP 2007, 1C).

The problem of conventional treatment of lung cancer complicated by SVC syndrome is that tumour shrinkage requires time and symptomatic relief is not always obtained. Based on the systematic review of 759 patients, SVC stenting relieved symptoms in 95% of patients, while only 60%–77% improved after radiotherapy/chemotherapy.[118] Severely symptomatic patients with clinical signs of cerebral edema or respiratory failure may need a prompt relief of SVC hypertension. The symptomatic relief after endovascular treatment occurs quite rapidly.[121–123] Venous stents are used to prevent recurrent SVC occlusion. Radiation therapy (n = 25) and stenting with self-expandable stents (n = 76) were compared in a prospective trial by Nicholson et al. Stenting of SVC was found to be better palliative care for patients with malignant SVC obstruction, providing them with significantly more rapid symptom relief and lower symptom recurrence (p < 0.001).[124] The overall clinical success of SVC stenting is 80%–100%.[116,118]

Different stent types were used to restore and maintain SVC patency.[123,125–127] A recent prospective study demonstrated the advantage of covered stents over bare metal stents for malignant obstruction.[128] There was no observed benefit for bilateral brachiocephalic stent placement in patients with malignant SVC obstruction. It has been shown that bilateral stenting increases stent occlusion rate (p < 0.05) and leads to increased complications (p = 0.039).[129] Thrombolysis may be performed to decrease the degree of stenosis and simplify stent deployment.[116,130] However, a systematic review demonstrated that additional thrombolytic therapy increases post-stenting morbidity without any additional benefit.[118]

The first step in the treatment of patients with catheter-related SVC thrombosis is to remove the catheter and initiate systemic anticoagulation. Percutaneous balloon angioplasty has been successfully used for benign SVC obstructions.[131,132] A retrospective analysis of outcomes for 70 patients with non-malignant SVC syndrome after open surgical repair (n = 42) and stenting (n = 28) demonstrated similar outcomes in 4-year follow-up with significantly lower periprocedural morbidity in the endovascular treatment group. Assisted primary and secondary patency was higher after stenting compared with angioplasty alone (p = .02).[133] Limited data suggest that an SVC stent may be safely placed over pacemaker/cardioverter–defibrillator wires,[134] but prophylactic placement of a pacing wire should be considered in certain patients to prevent potentially dangerous arrhythmias should pacemaker malfunction occur.

In patients with thrombotic SVC obstructions, catheter-directed thrombolytic therapy is effective.[130,135] A successful case of ultrasound-directed thrombolysis with subsequent stenting in a patient with catheter-related SVC thrombotic occlusion was reported recently.[136] Steroids have been used to alleviate SVC obstructions caused by lymphoma.[110,118]

Open SVC reconstructive surgery with a PTFE graft, autologous spiral saphenous vein graft and femoral vein or extra-anatomical jugular-to-femoral bypass has been effective to treat benign SVC obstruction with good long-term results.[137–139] Endovascular treatment is associated with higher rate of reinterventions.[137] Thus, CIRSE guidelines consider benign SVC syndrome as a relative contraindication for stenting, which is associated with the high estimated risk of long-term stent occlusion.[116] Endovascular treatment is an attractive strategy for any vascular stenosis, short, segmental lesions which should be treated with an appropriately sized stent. Randomized trials are needed to compare long-term outcomes after endovascular and conventional interventions in patients with benign SVC obstructions. However, they are unlikely to be performed because of the relatively small numbers of patients and the increasing skill of interventionalists.

SUMMARY

Percutaneous transluminal angioplasty with endoluminal stenting is the preferred treatment for patients with chronic venous outflow obstruction of the central veins and correction of central venous outflow stenosis after catheter-based or open surgical techniques of thrombus removal. Catheter-directed, pharmacomechanical and ultrasound-accelerated thrombolysis substantially improves outcomes of patients treated for acute central vein thrombosis. Randomized trial data are now available supporting this approach. A nationwide database indicates progressive acceptance of these catheter-based approaches.[140] Further standardization and implementation of national practice guidelines are important.

ACKNOWLEDGEMENT

The authors thank Shakela Watkins, MA, for her expert assistance in the preparation of this chapter.

REFERENCES

1. Kearon C, Kahn SR, Agnelli G, Goldhaber S, Raskob GE, Comerota AJ. Antithrombotic therapy for venous thromboembolic disease: American College of Chest Physicians Evidence-Based Clinical Practice Guidelines (8th Edition). *Chest.* 2008 June;133(6 Suppl.):454S–545S.
2. Gloviczki P. *Handbook of Venous Disorders: Guidelines of the American Venous Forum.* 3rd ed. London, UK: Hodder Arnold, 2009.
3. Vedantham S, Thorpe PE, Cardella JF et al. Quality improvement guidelines for the treatment of lower extremity deep vein thrombosis with use of endovascular thrombus removal. *J Vasc Interv Radiol.* 2009 July;20(7 Suppl.):S227–S239.
4. Jaff MR, McMurtry MS, Archer SL et al. Management of massive and submassive pulmonary embolism, iliofemoral deep vein thrombosis, and chronic thromboembolic pulmonary hypertension: A scientific statement from the American Heart Association. *Circulation.* 2011 April 26;123(16):1788–1830.

5. Meissner MH, Gloviczki P, Comerota AJ et al. Early thrombus removal strategies for acute deep venous thrombosis: Clinical practice guidelines of the Society for Vascular Surgery and the American Venous Forum. *J Vasc Surg.* 2012 May;55(5):1449–1462.

6. Holbrook A, Schulman S, Witt DM et al. Evidence-based management of anticoagulant therapy: Antithrombotic therapy and prevention of thrombosis, 9th ed: American College of Chest Physicians Evidence-Based Clinical Practice Guidelines. *Chest.* 2012 February;141(2 Suppl.):e152S–e184S.

7. Nicolaides AN, Fareed J, Kakkar AK et al. Prevention and treatment of venous thromboembolism – International consensus statement. *Int Angiol.* 2013 April;32(2):111–260.

8. Meissner MH, Manzo RA, Bergelin RO, Markel A, Strandness DE Jr. Deep venous insufficiency: The relationship between lysis and subsequent reflux. *J Vasc Surg.* 1993 October;18(4):596–605.

9. Labropoulos N, Volteas N, Leon M et al. The role of venous outflow obstruction in patients with chronic venous dysfunction. *Arch Surg.* 1997 January;132(1):46–51.

10. Kahn SR, Shbaklo H, Lamping DL et al. Determinants of health-related quality of life during the 2 years following deep vein thrombosis. *J Thromb Haemost.* 2008 July;6(7):1105–1112.

11. Delis KT, Bountouroglou D, Mansfield AO. Venous claudication in iliofemoral thrombosis: Long-term effects on venous haemodynamics, clinical status, and quality of life. *Ann Surg.* 2004 January;239(1):118–126.

12. Akesson H, Brudin L, Dahlstrom JA, Eklof B, Ohlin P, Plate G. Venous function assessed during a 5 year period after acute ilio-femoral venous thrombosis treated with anticoagulation. *Eur J Vasc Surg.* 1990 February;4(1):43–48.

13. Comerota AJ, Aldridge SC, Cohen G, Ball DS, Pliskin M, White JV. A strategy of aggressive regional therapy for acute iliofemoral venous thrombosis with contemporary venous thrombectomy or catheter-directed thrombolysis. *J Vasc Surg.* 1994 August;20(2):244–254.

14. Brandjes DP, Buller HR, Heijboer H et al. Randomised trial of effect of compression stockings in patients with symptomatic proximal-vein thrombosis. *Lancet.* 1997 March 15;349(9054):759–762.

15. Prandoni P, Lensing AW, Prins MH et al. Below-knee elastic compression stockings to prevent the post-thrombotic syndrome: A randomized, controlled trial. *Ann Intern Med.* 2004 August 17;141(4):249–256.

16. Kearon C, Akl EA, Comerota AJ et al. Antithrombotic therapy for VTE disease: Antithrombotic therapy and prevention of thrombosis, 9th ed: American College of Chest Physicians Evidence-Based Clinical Practice Guidelines. *Chest.* 2012 February;141(2 Suppl.):e419S–e494S.

17. Musani MH, Matta F, Yaekoub AY, Liang J, Hull RD, Stein PD. Venous compression for prevention of postthrombotic syndrome: A meta-analysis. *Am J Med.* 2010 August;123(8):735–740.

18. Partsch H, Blattler W. Compression and walking versus bed rest in the treatment of proximal deep venous thrombosis with low molecular weight heparin. *J Vasc Surg.* 2000 November;32(5):861–869.

19. Kahn SR, Shapiro S, Wells PS et al. Compression stockings to prevent post-thrombotic syndrome: A randomised placebo-controlled trial. *Lancet.* 2014 March 8;383(9920):880–888.

20. Douketis JD, Crowther MA, Foster GA, Ginsberg JS. Does the location of thrombosis determine the risk of disease recurrence in patients with proximal deep vein thrombosis? *Am J Med.* 2001 May;110(7):515–519.

21. Prandoni P, Lensing AW, Prins MH et al. Residual venous thrombosis as a predictive factor of recurrent venous thromboembolism. *Ann Intern Med.* 2002 December 17;137(12):955–960.

22. Hull RD, Marder VJ, Mah AF, Biel RK, Brant RF. Quantitative assessment of thrombus burden predicts the outcome of treatment for venous thrombosis: A systematic review. *Am J Med.* 2005 May;118(5):456–464.

23. Shull KC, Nicolaides AN, Fernandes e Fernandes J et al. Significance of popliteal reflux in relation to ambulatory venous pressure and ulceration. *Arch Surg.* 1979 November;114(11):1304–1306.

24. Wells JK, Hagino RT, Bargmann KM et al. Venous morbidity after superficial femoral-popliteal vein harvest. *J Vasc Surg.* 1999 February;29(2):282–289.

25. Masuda EM, Kistner RL, Ferris EB III. Long-term effects of superficial femoral vein ligation: Thirteen-year follow-up. *J Vasc Surg.* 1992 November;16(5):741–749.

26. Singh K, Yakoub D, Giangola P et al. Early follow-up and treatment recommendations for isolated calf deep venous thrombosis. *J Vasc Surg.* 2012 January;55(1):136–140.

27. Alkjaersig N, Fletcher AP, Sherry S. The mechanism of clot dissolution by plasmin. *J Clin Invest.* 1959 July;38(7):1086–1095.

28. Chandler WL, Trimble SL, Loo SC, Mornin D. Effect of PAI-1 levels on the molar concentrations of active tissue plasminogen activator (t-PA) and t-PA/PAI-1 complex in plasma. *Blood.* 1990 September 1;76(5):930–937.

29. Lin PH, Chen C, Surowiec SM, Conklin B, Bush RL, Lumsden AB. Evaluation of thrombolysis in a porcine model of chronic deep venous thrombosis: An endovascular model. *J Vasc Surg.* 2001 March;33(3):621–627.

30. Dasari TW, Pappy R, Hennebry TA. Pharmacomechanical thrombolysis of acute and chronic symptomatic deep vein thrombosis: A systematic review of literature. *Angiology.* 2012 February;63(2):138–145.

31. Dumantepe M, Tarhan A, Yurdakul I, Ozler A. US-accelerated catheter-directed thrombolysis for the treatment of deep venous thrombosis. *Diagn Interv Radiol.* 2013 May;19(3):251–258.

32. Goldhaber SZ, Meyerovitz MF, Green D et al. Randomized controlled trial of tissue plasminogen activator in proximal deep venous thrombosis. *Am J Med.* 1990 March;88(3):235–240.

33. Turpie AG, Levine MN, Hirsh J et al. Tissue plasminogen activator (rt-PA) vs heparin in deep vein thrombosis. Results of a randomized trial. *Chest.* 1990 April;97(4 Suppl.):172S–175S.

34. Schweizer J, Kirch W, Koch R et al. Short- and long-term results after thrombolytic treatment of deep venous thrombosis. *J Am Coll Cardiol.* 2000 October;36(4):1336–1343.

35. Schwieder G, Grimm W, Siemens HJ et al. Intermittent regional therapy with rt-PA is not superior to systemic thrombolysis in deep vein thrombosis (DVT) – A German multicenter trial. *Thromb Haemost.* 1995 November;74(5):1240–1243.

36. Jeffrey P, Immelman E, Amoore J. Treatment of deep vein thrombosis with heparin or streptokinase: long-term venous function assessment. In *Proceedings of the Second International Vascular Symposium,* London, UK, 1986. Abstract S20.3.

37. Okrent D, Messersmith R, Buckman J. Transcatheter fibrinolytic therapy and angioplasty for left iliofemoral venous thrombosis. *J Vasc Interv Radiol.* 1991 May;2(2):195–197.

38. Bjarnason H, Kruse JR, Asinger DA et al. Iliofemoral deep venous thrombosis: Safety and efficacy outcome during 5 years of catheter-directed thrombolytic therapy. *J Vasc Interv Radiol.* 1997 May;8(3):405–418.

39. Semba CP, Dake MD. Iliofemoral deep venous thrombosis: Aggressive therapy with catheter-directed thrombolysis. *Radiology.* 1994;191:487–494.

40. Semba CP, Dake MD. Catheter-directed thrombolysis for iliofemoral venous thrombosis. *Semin Vasc Surg.* 1996;9:26–33.

41. Verhaeghe R, Stockx L, Lacroix H, Vermylen J, Baert AL. Catheter-directed lysis of iliofemoral vein thrombosis with use of rt-PA. *Eur Radiol.* 1997;7:996–1001.

42. Horne MK III, Mayo DJ, Cannon RO III, Chen CC, Shawker TH, Chang R. Intraclot recombinant tissue plasminogen activator in the treatment of deep venous thrombosis of the lower and upper extremities. *Am J Med.* 2000;108:251–255.

43. AbuRahma AF, Perkins SE, Wulu JT, Ng HK. Iliofemoral deep vein thrombosis: Conventional therapy versus lysis and percutaneous transluminal angioplasty and stenting. *Ann Surg.* 2001;233(6):752–760.

44. Castaneda F, Li R, Young K, Swischuk JL, Smouse B, Brady T. Catheter-directed thrombolysis in deep venous thrombosis with use of reteplase: Immediate results and complications from a pilot study. *J Vasc Interv Radiol.* 2002;13:577–580.

45. Grunwald MR, Hofmann LV. Comparison of urokinase, alteplase, and reteplase for catheter-directed thrombolysis of deep venous thrombosis. *J Vasc Interv Radiol.* 2004;15:347–352.

46. Laiho MK, Oinonen A, Sugano N, Harjola VP, Lehtola AL, Roth WD et al. Preservation of venous valve function after catheter-directed and systemic thrombolysis for deep venous thrombosis. *Eur J Vasc Endovasc Surg.* 2004;28:391–396.

47. Sillesen H, Just S, Jorgensen M, Baekgaard N. Catheter-directed thrombolysis for treatment of ilio-femoral deep venous thrombosis is durable, preserves venous valve function and may prevent chronic venous insufficiency. *Eur J Vasc Endovasc Surg.* 2005;30:556–562.

48. Jackson LS, Wang XJ, Dudrick SJ, Gersten GD. Catheter-directed thrombolysis and/or thrombectomy with selective endovascular stenting as alternatives to systemic anticoagulation for treatment of acute deep vein thrombosis. *Am J Surg.* 2005;190:864–868.

49. Kim HS, Patra A, Paxton BE, Khan J, Streiff MB. Adjunctive percutaneous mechanical thrombectomy for lower-extremity deep vein thrombosis: Clinical and economic outcomes. *J Vasc Interv Radiol.* 2006;17:1099–1104.

50. Mewissen MW, Seabrook GR, Meissner MH, Cynamon J, Labropoulos N, Haughton SH. Catheter-directed thrombolysis for lower extremity deep venous thrombosis: Report of a national multicenter registry. *Radiology.* 1999 April;211(1):39–49.

51. Comerota AJ, Throm RC, Mathias SD, Haughton S, Mewissen M. Catheter-directed thrombolysis for iliofemoral deep venous thrombosis improves health-related quality of life. *J Vasc Surg.* 2000 July;32(1):130–137.

52. Elsharawy M, Elzayat E. Early results of thrombolysis vs anticoagulation in iliofemoral venous thrombosis. A randomised clinical trial. *Eur J Vasc Endovasc Surg.* 2002 September;24(3):209–214.

53. Baekgaard N, Broholm R, Just S, Jorgensen M, Jensen LP. Long-term results using catheter-directed thrombolysis in 103 lower limbs with acute iliofemoral venous thrombosis. *Eur J Vasc Endovasc Surg.* 2010 January;39(1):112–117.

54. Enden T, Haig Y, Klow NE et al. Long-term outcome after additional catheter-directed thrombolysis versus standard treatment for acute iliofemoral deep vein thrombosis (the CaVenT study): A randomised controlled trial. *Lancet.* 2012 January 7;379(9810):31–38.

55. Kim HS, Preece SR, Black JH, Pham LD, Streiff MB. Safety of catheter-directed thrombolysis for deep venous thrombosis in cancer patients. *J Vasc Surg.* 2008 February;47(2):388–394.

56. Herrera S, Comerota AJ, Thakur S et al. Managing iliofemoral deep venous thrombosis of pregnancy with a strategy of thrombus removal is safe and avoids post-thrombotic morbidity. *J Vasc Surg.* 2014 February;59(2):456–464.

57. Jorgensen M, Broholm R, Baekgaard N. Pregnancy after catheter-directed thrombolysis for acute ilio-femoral deep venous thrombosis. *Phlebology.* 2013 March;28(Suppl. 1):34–38.

58. Francis CW, Blinc A, Lee S, Cox C. Ultrasound accelerates transport of recombinant tissue plas-minogen activator into clots. *Ultrasound Med Biol.* 1995;21(3):419–424.

59. Braaten JV, Goss RA, Francis CW. Ultrasound revers-ibly disaggregates fibrin fibers. *Thromb Haemost.* 1997 September;78(3):1063–1068.

60. Vedantham S, Vesely TM, Parti N, Darcy M, Hovsepian DM, Picus D. Lower extremity venous thrombolysis with adjunctive mechanical thrombectomy. *J Vasc Interv Radiol.* 2002 October;13(10):1001–1008.

61. Kasirajan K, Gray B, Ouriel K. Percutaneous AngioJet thrombectomy in the management of extensive deep venous thrombosis. *J Vasc Interv Radiol.* 2001 February;12(2):179–185.

62. Lin PH, Zhou W, Dardik A et al. Catheter-direct thrombolysis versus pharmacomechanical throm-bectomy for treatment of symptomatic lower extremity deep venous thrombosis. *Am J Surg.* 2006 December;192(6):782–788.

63. O'Sullivan GJ, Lohan DG, Gough N, Cronin CG, Kee ST. Pharmacomechanical thrombectomy of acute deep vein thrombosis with the Trellis-8 isolated thrombolysis catheter. *J Vasc Interv Radiol.* 2007 June;18(6):715–724.

64. Martinez Trabal JL, Comerota AJ, LaPorte FB, Kazanjian S, Disalle R, Sepanski DM. The quan-titative benefit of isolated, segmental, phar-macomechanical thrombolysis (ISPMT) for iliofemoral venous thrombosis. *J Vasc Surg.* 2008 December;48(6):1532–1537.

65. Vogel D, Walsh ME, Chen JT, Comerota AJ. Comparison of vein valve function following pharmacomechanical thrombolysis versus simple catheter-directed throm-bolysis for iliofemoral deep vein thrombosis. *J Vasc Surg.* 2012 November;56(5):1351–1354.

66. Parikh S, Motarjeme A, McNamara T et al. Ultrasound-accelerated thrombolysis for the treat-ment of deep vein thrombosis: Initial clinical experi-ence. *J Vasc Interv Radiol.* 2008 April;19(4):521–528.

67. Zierler BK. Ultrasonography and diagnosis of venous thromboembolism. *Circulation.* 2004 March 30;109(12 Suppl. 1):I9–I14.

68. Bates SM, Greer IA, Middeldorp S, Veenstra DL, Prabulos AM, Vandvik PO. VTE, thrombo-philia, antithrombotic therapy, and pregnancy: Antithrombotic therapy and prevention of throm-bosis, 9th ed: American College of Chest Physicians Evidence-Based Clinical Practice Guidelines. *Chest.* 2012 February;141(2 Suppl.):e691S–e736S.

69. Diamond SL, Anand S. Inner clot diffusion and permeation during fibrinolysis. *Biophys J.* 1993 December;65(6):2622–2643.

70. Ogawa T, Hoshino S, Midorikawa H, Sato K. Intermittent pneumatic compression of the foot and calf improves the outcome of catheter-directed thrombolysis using low-dose urokinase in patients with acute proximal venous thrombosis of the leg. *J Vasc Surg.* 2005 November;42(5):940–944.

71. The STILE investigators. Results of a prospective ran-domized trial evaluating surgery versus thromboly-sis for ischemia of the lower extremity. The STILE trial. *Ann Surg.* 1994 September;220(3):251–266.

72. Comerota AJ, Grewal N, Martinez JT et al. Postthrombotic morbidity correlates with residual thrombus following catheter-directed thrombolysis for iliofemoral deep vein thrombosis. *J Vasc Surg.* 2012 March;55(3):768–73.

73. Aziz F, Comerota AJ. Quantity of residual throm-bus after successful catheter-directed thrombolysis for iliofemoral deep venous thrombosis correlates with recurrence. *Eur J Vasc Endovasc Surg.* 2012 August;44(2):210–213.

74. Neglen P, Raju S. Intravascular ultrasound scan evaluation of the obstructed vein. *J Vasc Surg.* 2002 April;35(4):694–700.

75. Murphy EH, Broker HS, Johnson EJ, Modrall JG, Valentine RJ, Arko FR, III. Device and imaging-spe-cific volumetric analysis of clot lysis after percutane-ous mechanical thrombectomy for iliofemoral DVT. *J Endovasc Ther.* 2010 June;17(3):423–433.

76. Lozier JN, Cullinane AM, Nghiem K, Chang R, Horne MK III. Biochemical dynamics relevant to the safety of low-dose, intraclot alteplase for deep vein throm-bosis. *Transl Res.* 2012 September;160(3):217–222.

77. Plate G, Eklof B, Norgren L, Ohlin P, Dahlstrom JA. Venous thrombectomy for iliofemoral vein thrombosis – 10-year results of a prospective ran-domised study. *Eur J Vasc Endovasc Surg.* 1997 November;14(5):367–374.

78. Comerota AJ, Gale SS. Technique of contemporary iliofemoral and infrainguinal venous thrombec-tomy. *J Vasc Surg.* 2006 January;43(1):185–191.

79. Comerota AJ, Aziz F. Acute deep venous throm-bosos: Surgical and interventional treatement. In: Cronenwett J, Johnston K, eds. *Rutherford's Vascular Surgery.* 8th (1) ed. Philadelphia, PA: Elsevier Saunders, 2014, p. 792.

80. Berger A, Jaffe JW, York TN. Iliac compression syn-drome treated with stent placement. *J Vasc Surg.* 1995 March;21(3):510–514.

81. Nazarian GK, Austin WR, Wegryn SA et al. Venous recanalization by metallic stents after fail-ure of balloon angioplasty or surgery: Four-year experience. *Cardiovasc Intervent Radiol.* 1996 July;19(4):227–233.

82. Meng QY, Li XQ, Jiang K et al. Stenting of iliac vein obstruction following catheter-directed thromboly-sis in lower extremity deep vein thrombosis. *Chin Med J (Engl).* 2013;126(18):3519–3522.

83. Hartung O, Loundou AD, Barthelemy P, Arnoux D, Boufi M, Alimi YS. Endovascular management of chronic disabling ilio-caval obstructive lesions: Long-term results. *Eur J Vasc Endovasc Surg.* 2009 July;38(1):118–124.

84. Titus JM, Moise MA, Bena J, Lyden SP, Clair DG. Iliofemoral stenting for venous occlusive disease. *J Vasc Surg.* 2011 March;53(3):706–712.

85. Kurklinsky AK, Bjarnason H, Friese JL et al. Outcomes of venoplasty with stent placement for chronic thrombosis of the iliac and femoral veins: Single-center experience. *J Vasc Interv Radiol.* 2012 August;23(8):1009–1015.

86. Neglen P, Hollis KC, Olivier J, Raju S. Stenting of the venous outflow in chronic venous disease: Long-term stent-related outcome, clinical, and hemodynamic result. *J Vasc Surg.* 2007 November;46(5):979–990.

87. Neglen P, Tackett TP Jr, Raju S. Venous stenting across the inguinal ligament. *J Vasc Surg.* 2008 November;48(5):1255–1261.

88. Eijgenramm P, ten Cate H, ten Cate-Hoek AJ. Venous stenting after deep venous thrombosis and antithrombotic therapy. *Rev Vasc Med.* 2014 September;2(3):88–97.

89. Lindblad B, Tengborn L, Bergqvist D. Deep vein thrombosis of the axillary-subclavian veins: Epidemiologic data, effects of different types of treatment and late sequelae. *Eur J Vasc Surg.* 1988 June;2(3):161–165.

90. Joffe HV, Kucher N, Tapson VF, Goldhaber SZ. Upper-extremity deep vein thrombosis: A prospective registry of 592 patients. *Circulation.* 2004 September 21;110(12):1605–1611.

91. Munoz FJ, Mismetti P, Poggio R et al. Clinical outcome of patients with upper-extremity deep vein thrombosis: Results from the RIETE Registry. *Chest.* 2008 Janaury;133(1):143–148.

92. Elman EE, Kahn SR. The post-thrombotic syndrome after upper extremity deep venous thrombosis in adults: A systematic review. *Thromb Res.* 2006;117(6):609–614.

93. Lee JT, Karwowski JK, Harris EJ, Haukoos JS, Olcott C. Long-term thrombotic recurrence after nonoperative management of Paget-Schroetter syndrome. *J Vasc Surg.* 2006 June;43(6):1236–1243.

94. Sajid MS, Ahmed N, Desai M, Baker D, Hamilton G. Upper limb deep vein thrombosis: A literature review to streamline the protocol for management. *Acta Haematol.* 2007;118(1):10–18.

95. Tsekouras N, Comerota AJ. Current trends in the treatment of venous thracic outlet syndrome: A comprehensive review. *Interv Cardiol.* 2014;6(1):103–115.

96. Beathard GA. Gianturco self-expanding stent in the treatment of stenosis in dialysis access grafts. *Kidney Int.* 1993 April;43(4):872–877.

97. Vorwerk D, Guenther RW, Mann H et al. Venous stenosis and occlusion in haemodialysis shunts: Follow-up results of stent placement in 65 patients. *Radiology.* 1995 April;195(1):140–146.

98. Glanz S, Gordon DH, Lipkowitz GS, Butt KM, Hong J, Sclafani SJ. Axillary and subclavian vein stenosis: Percutaneous angioplasty. *Radiology.* 1988 August;168(2):371–373.

99. Haskal ZJ, Trerotola S, Dolmatch B et al. Stent graft versus balloon angioplasty for failing dialysis-access grafts. *N Engl J Med.* 2010 February 11;362(6):494–503.

100. Aruny JE, Lewis CA, Cardella JF et al. Quality improvement guidelines for percutaneous management of the thrombosed or dysfunctional dialysis access. *J Vasc Interv Radiol.* 2003 September;14(9 Pt 2):S247–S253.

101. Garcia-Pagan JC, Heydtmann M, Raffa S et al. TIPS for Budd-Chiari syndrome: Long-term results and prognostics factors in 124 patients. *Gastroenterology.* 2008 September;135(3):808–815.

102. Hernandez-Guerra M, Turnes J, Rubinstein P et al. PTFE-covered stents improve TIPS patency in Budd-Chiari syndrome. *Hepatology.* 2004 November;40(5):1197–1202.

103. Mentha G, Giostra E, Majno PE et al. Liver transplantation for Budd-Chiari syndrome: A European study on 248 patients from 51 centres. *J Hepatol.* 2006 March;44(3):520–528.

104. Schraufnagel DE, Hill R, Leech JA, Pare JA. Superior vena caval obstruction. Is it a medical emergency? *Am J Med.* 1981 June;70(6):1169–1174.

105. Ahmann FR. A reassessment of the clinical implications of the superior vena caval syndrome. *J Clin Oncol.* 1984 August;2(8):961–969.

106. Gauden SJ. Superior vena cava syndrome induced by bronchogenic carcinoma: Is this an oncological emergency? *Australas Radiol.* 1993 November;37(4):363–366.

107. Cohen R, Mena D, Carbajal-Mendoza R, Matos N, Karki N. Superior vena cava syndrome: A medical emergency? *Int J Angiol.* 2008;17(1):43–46.

108. Baker GL, Barnes HJ. Superior vena cava syndrome: Etiology, diagnosis, and treatment. *Am J Crit Care.* 1992 July;1(1):54–64.

109. Stanford W, Jolles H, Ell S, Chiu LC. Superior vena cava obstruction: A venographic classification. *Am J Roentgenol.* 1987 February;148(2):259–262.

110. Ostler PJ, Clarke DP, Watkinson AF, Gaze MN. Superior vena cava obstruction: A modern management strategy. *Clin Oncol (R Coll Radiol).* 1997;9(2):83–89.

111. Rice TW, Rodriguez RM, Light RW. The superior vena cava syndrome: Clinical characteristics and evolving etiology. *Medicine (Baltimore).* 2006 January;85(1):37–42.

112. Riley RF, Petersen SE, Ferguson JD, Bashir Y. Managing superior vena cava syndrome as a complication of pacemaker implantation: A pooled analysis of clinical practice. *Pacing Clin Electrophysiol.* 2010 April;33(4):420–425.

113. Korkeila P, Nyman K, Ylitalo A et al. Venous obstruction after pacemaker implantation. *Pacing Clin Electrophysiol*. 2007 February;30(2):199–206.

114. Davis AM, Pierson RN, Loyd JE. Mediastinal fibrosis. *Semin Respir Infect*. 2001 June;16(2):119–130.

115. Bays S, Rajakaruna C, Sheffield E, Morgan A. Fibrosing mediastinitis as a cause of superior vena cava syndrome. *Eur J Cardiothorac Surg*. 2004 August;26(2):453–455.

116. Uberoi R. Quality assurance guidelines for superior vena cava stenting in malignant disease. *Cardiovasc Intervent Radiol*. 2006 May;29(3):319–322.

117. Parish JM, Marschke RF Jr, Dines DE, Lee RE. Etiologic considerations in superior vena cava syndrome. *Mayo Clin Proc*. 1981 July;56(7):407–413.

118. Rowell NP, Gleeson FV. Steroids, radiotherapy, chemotherapy and stents for superior vena caval obstruction in carcinoma of the bronchus: A systematic review. *Clin Oncol (R Coll Radiol)*. 2002 October;14(5):338–351.

119. Chen JC, Bongard F, Klein SR. A contemporary perspective on superior vena cava syndrome. *Am J Surg*. 1990;207–211.

120. Kvale PA, Selecky PA, Prakash UB. Palliative care in lung cancer: ACCP evidence-based clinical practice guidelines (2nd edition). *Chest*. 2007 September;132(3 Suppl.):368S–403S.

121. Irving JD, Dondelinger RF, Reidy JF et al. Gianturco self-expanding stents: Clinical experience in the vena cava and large veins. *Cardiovasc Intervent Radiol*. 1992 September;15(5):328–333.

122. Rosch J, Uchida BT, Hall LD et al. Gianturco-Rosch expandable Z-stents in the treatment of superior vena cava syndrome. *Cardiovasc Intervent Radiol*. 1992 September;15(5):319–327.

123. Hennequin LM, Fade O, Fays JG et al. Superior vena cava stent placement: Results with the Wallstent endoprosthesis. *Radiology*. 1995 August;196(2):353–361.

124. Nicholson AA, Ettles DF, Arnold A, Greenstone M, Dyet JF. Treatment of malignant superior vena cava obstruction: Metal stents or radiation therapy. *J Vasc Interv Radiol*. 1997 September;8(5):781–788.

125. Elson JD, Becker GJ, Wholey MH, Ehrman KO. Vena caval and central venous stenoses: Management with Palmaz balloon-expandable intraluminal stents. *J Vasc Interv Radiol*. 1991 May;2(2):215–223.

126. Edwards RD, Cassidy J, Taylor A. Case report: Superior vena cava obstruction complicated by central venous thrombosis – Treatment with thrombolysis and Gianturco-Z stents. *Clin Radiol*. 1992 April;45(4):278–280.

127. Stock KW, Jacob AL, Proske M, Bolliger CT, Rochlitz C, Steinbrich W. Treatment of malignant obstruction of the superior vena cava with the self-expanding Wallstent. *Thorax*. 1995 November;50(11):1151–1156.

128. Gwon DI, Ko GY, Kim JH, Shin JH, Yoon HK, Sung KB. Malignant superior vena cava syndrome: A comparative cohort study of treatment with covered stents versus uncovered stents. *Radiology*. 2013 March;266(3):979–987.

129. Dinkel HP, Mettke B, Schmid F, Baumgartner I, Triller J, Do DD. Endovascular treatment of malignant superior vena cava syndrome: Is bilateral wallstent placement superior to unilateral placement? *J Endovasc Ther*. 2003 August;10(4):788–797.

130. Kee ST, Kinoshita L, Razavi MK, Nyman UR, Semba CP, Dake MD. Superior vena cava syndrome: Treatment with catheter-directed thrombolysis and endovascular stent placement. *Radiology*. 1998 January;206(1):187–193.

131. Sherry CS, Diamond NG, Meyers TP, Martin RL. Successful treatment of superior vena cava syndrome by venous angioplasty. *Am J Roentgenol*. 1986 October;147(4):834–835.

132. Capek P, Cope C. Percutaneous treatment of superior vena cava syndrome. *Am J Roentgenol*. 1989 January;152(1):183–184.

133. Rizvi AZ, Kalra M, Bjarnason H, Bower TC, Schleck C, Gloviczki P. Benign superior vena cava syndrome: Stenting is now the first line of treatment. *J Vasc Surg*. 2008 February;47(2):372–380.

134. Slonim SM, Semba CP, Sze DY, Dake MD. Placement of SVC stents over pacemaker wires for the treatment of SVC syndrome. *J Vasc Interv Radiol*. 2000 February;11(2 Pt 1):215–219.

135. Fine DG, Shepherd RF, Welch TJ. Thrombolytic therapy for superior vena cava syndrome. *Lancet*. 1989 May 27;1(8648):1200–1201.

136. Kumar B, Hosn NA. Images in clinical medicine. Superior vena cava syndrome. *N Engl J Med*. 2014 September 18;371(12):1142.

137. Kalra M, Gloviczki P, Andrews JC et al. Open surgical and endovascular treatment of superior vena cava syndrome caused by nonmalignant disease. *J Vasc Surg*. 2003 August;38(2):215–223.

138. Schifferdecker B, Shaw JA, Piemonte TC, Eisenhauer AC. Nonmalignant superior vena cava syndrome: Pathophysiology and management. *Catheter Cardiovasc Interv*. 2005 July;65(3):416–423.

139. Dhaliwal RS, Das D, Luthra S, Singh J, Mehta S, Singh H. Management of superior vena cava syndrome by internal jugular to femoral vein bypass. *Ann Thorac Surg*. 2006 July;82(1):310–312.

140. Bashir R, Zack CJ, Zhao H, Comerota AJ, Bove AA. Comparative outcomes of catheter-directed thrombolysis plus anticoagulation vs anticoagulation alone to treat lower-extremity proximal deep vein thrombosis. *JAMA Intern Med*. 2014 September;174(9):1494–1501.

141. Comerota AJ, Gravett MH. Iliofemoral venous thrombosis. *J Vasc Surg*. 2007 November;46(5):1065–1076.

Vascular Trauma

50

Thoracic and abdominal vascular trauma

NAVEED SAQIB, JOSEPH DUBOSE and ALI AZIZZADEH

CONTENTS

INTRODUCTION

Thoracic and abdominal vascular injuries are much less common compared to vascular injuries involving peripheral vessels. The majority of thoracic and abdominal vascular injuries are caused by penetrating trauma, including gunshot and stab wounds, and iatrogenic injuries. Injury to the aorta, great vessels, visceral vessels, pulmonary veins and vena cava can also occur following blunt trauma, typically secondary to high-impact motor vehicle collisions. The severity of penetrating injury is directly proportional to the kinetic energy transferred to the tissue by the penetrating object. Penetrating trauma can create lateral wall defects with free bleeding or hematomas, partial or complete transection with free bleeding or thrombosis and blast effects with intimal flaps and secondary thrombosis. In blunt trauma, injury is caused by local compression or rapid deceleration.

The thoracic vascular injuries and abdominal vascular injuries are summarized in separate sections in this chapter, with special emphasis on thoracic aortic injury (TAI). Significant progress has been made over the last two decades in the diagnosis and treatment of thoracic and abdominal vascular injuries. These advances have significantly improved the outcomes of patients with life-threatening vascular trauma. This paradigm shift includes the widespread use of computed tomography angiography (CTA) for diagnosis, aggressive blood pressure control, delayed repair for stable patients, adoption of endovascular repair as the treatment modality of choice for anatomically suitable candidates and medical management of minimal aortic injuries.

THORACIC VASCULAR TRAUMA

Thoracic vascular trauma includes injuries to the aorta, intrathoracic segment of the great vessels, superior and inferior vena cava (SVC and IVC), major veins at the thoracic inlet, intercostal arteries and internal mammary artery. Thoracic vascular injuries account for 15%–20% of all vascular injuries treated in level 1 trauma centres receiving large numbers of penetrating injuries.

Thoracic aortic injury

Traumatic TAI is the second most common cause of death due to blunt force. It is implicated as cause of mortality in up to one-third of all automobile accident deaths, the majority (80%) of which occur prior to hospital arrival.[1] Despite this frequency among motor vehicle deaths, the public health issue of TAI has been underappreciated.

The mechanism of TAI is likely related to a complex combination of both relative motion of the structures within the thorax and local loading of the tissues, as either a result of the anatomy or the nature of the impact. The interaction of these forces has been shown to have the greatest impact at the level of the aortic isthmus, found to be the site most characteristically involved in TAI due to blunt mechanisms.

Reports postulate that differences in retropleural fixation between the transverse arch and descending thoracic aorta, upward displacement of the heart by sternal compression, increased intraluminal hydrostatic pressure or a congenital weakness of tissues at the isthmus explains this common location for injury. Among published series, however, motor vehicle collisions remain the leading cause. In our own experience with 175 patients with TAI, this injury is most commonly associated with motor vehicle crash (78%), followed by motorcycle crash (9%), automobile vs. pedestrian crash (7%), falls (5%), bicycle crash (1%) and sporting injury (parachute, 1 patient).[2]

CLINICAL PRESENTATION

High clinical suspicion in patients with high-energy impact is required to identify and diagnose patients with TAI. The clinical presentation of TAI is variable and depends on the severity of the injury. Patients may be asymptomatic or complain of pain in the chest or radiating to the neck, back or shoulder and have associated multiple traumas. Hemodynamics may range from normotensive to hemorrhagic shock, with hypotension being a common sign.[2]

DIAGNOSTIC MODALITIES

The initial diagnostic test of choice is the plain chest x-ray, which has a number of findings that are suggestive – but not confirmatory – of the diagnosis. A supine anteroposterior chest radiograph should be obtained routinely in trauma patients. Radiographic findings suggestive of penetrating great vessel injury include a large hemothorax; foreign bodies or their trajectory close to the great vessels; a confusing trajectory, which may indicate a migrating intravascular course; or a 'missing' missile, suggesting embolization. Radiographic findings suggestive of blunt injury to the thoracic aorta include fractures of the sternum, scapula, clavicle, first rib or multiple left-sided ribs. Indirect mediastinal clues include obliteration of the aortic knob, depression of the left main stem bronchus, loss of the paravertebral pleural stripe, an apical pleural cap, deviation of a nasogastric tube and lateral displacement of the trachea at the T4 level. Pathologic widening of the mediastinum is defined as more than 8 cm at the level of the aortic knob or a mediastinum-width-to-chest-width ratio exceeding 25% and has a reported sensitivity of 81%–100% and a specificity of 60%.[3]

CTA has emerged as a mainstay of evaluation for TAI, with a documented sensitivity (95%–100%) and concomitant high-negative predictive value (99%–100%) following trauma, indicating that few patients with TAI will be missed.[4,5] Unfortunately, false positives do occur, particularly in low-grade injuries. In an examination of patients undergoing traditional angiogram after CTA, Bruckner and colleagues noted that CTA had an appreciably low specificity of 40% and a positive predictive value of only 15%.[6] Despite these findings, the majority of studies have validated the utilization of CTA after trauma due to the high sensitivity and ability to exclude TAI with very high negative predictive value when CTA is utilized in this setting.

Among patients with equivocal diagnosis following CTA, additional studies can be utilized to confirm or exclude TAI after trauma. Traditional angiography and transesophageal echocardiogram are both well-established means of further investigation that continue to be utilized actively at many centres. Intravascular ultrasound (IVUS) has also shown considerable promise in this regard.[7] IVUS allows avoidance of contrast administration, which is required for traditional angiographic confirmation, and has demonstrated an improved sensitivity over angiography in the published experience by our own group.[8] For this reason, we advocate for the use of IVUS in potential TAI patients in whom traditional angiography is being considered to confirm or exclude TAI diagnosis.

SPECTRUM OF INJURY, CLASSIFICATION AND GRADING

Several groups continue to study the characterization of TAI into useful classifications that can then be utilized to guide optimal therapy. While alternative approaches have been suggested, the most widely utilized system for grading presently employed was reported by Azizzadeh et al.[8] and has been adopted by the Society of Vascular Surgery (SVS) in the clinical practice guidelines for TAI management. According to this consensus definition, TAI is classified into four categories, depending on the extent of aortic wall disruption (Figures 50.1 and 50.2). Grade I injuries present with an intimal tear; grade II have an intramural hematoma; grade III have an aortic pseudoaneurysm; and grade IV have free rupture of the aorta.[8,9]

MANAGEMENT

Medical management

Grade I injuries are medically managed among patients without contraindication to the required anti-impulse blood pressure control. We utilize beta-blockade, initially in an intensive care setting, followed by CTA in 6 weeks to confirm healing or stability of lesion (Grade C recommendation). Patients with grade II and grade III injuries are also treated with optimal medical management prior to definitive intervention.

Some centres have reported their experience with medical management of grade II injuries. Osgood et al.[10] reported non-operative treatment of 49 patients with grade I and II injuries. These investigators found that only 5% of these lesions advanced in grade on serial imaging. Successful medical management of patients with TAI requires patient compliance with oral anti-impulse medications as well as the follow-up imaging protocols. Furthermore, the presence of associated injuries may play a role in the selection of conservative therapy over intervention or vice versa. There remains a significant need for additional study to establish the natural history grade II injuries as well as the relative risk of medical management vs. thoracic endovascular aneurysm repair (TEVAR) in this cohort.

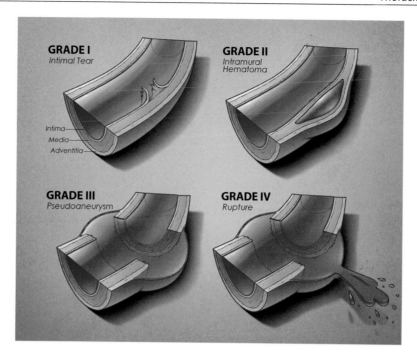

Figure 50.1 Classification of traumatic aortic injury (TAI) based on extent of aortic wall disruption into 4 grades.

Thoracic endovascular aneurysm repair

In recent years, TEVAR has emerged as the primary treatment for TAI among amenable patients surviving to reach treatment, gradually replacing traditional open repair (OR) (level 1 evidence). Among patients

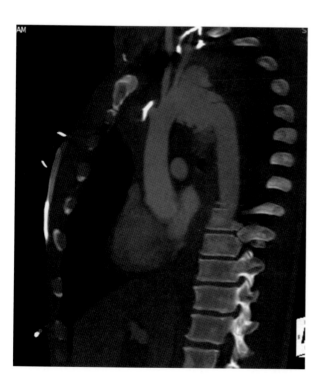

Figure 50.2 Computed Tomography Angiography (CTA) of thorax revealing Grade 3 traumatic aortic injury.

with severe blunt thoracic injury, the use of TEVAR has been associated with improved morbidity and mortality compared to traditional OR approaches. Several recent meta-analyses have documented these results, demonstrating improved short-term outcomes with TEVAR compared to OR.[7–13] In a 2011 analysis of the accumulated literature, the Clinical Practice Guidelines from the SVS suggested that 'endovascular repair be performed preferentially over open surgical repair or non-operative management'.[14]

While prompt repair of TAI is preferred, we have adopted selective delayed repair consistent with the recommendations proposed by the Eastern Association for the Surgery of Trauma (EAST) Practice Work Group.[11] In this fashion, 'delayed' repair is defined as intervention occurring beyond 24 hours from the time of admission. This approach is commonly required among trauma patients requiring treatment of more immediately life-threatening injuries, such as laparotomy or emergent craniotomy – a common occurrence among the severely injured cohort.[9–12,16] The subsequent timing of definitive repair is then individualized for the specific patient through a multi-disciplinary decision-making process involving inputs from cardiothoracic/vascular surgery, the trauma team and other key stakeholders as required. Currently, we perform urgent repair in grade II and III injuries. Grade IV injuries are transported expeditiously to the operating room for emergent repair.

Once the optimal timing of intervention for the individual patient has been established, endovascular repair has emerged as the mainstay of subsequent definitive TAI treatment. Select patients with unsuitable anatomy or other confounding factors may continue to require open surgical repair via techniques previously described by our group.[11] The evolution in endovascular technologies occurring over the last decade or more, however, has afforded that TEVAR can be safely and effectively be performed in the majority of patients with TAI.

The first endovascular device approved by the US Food and Drug Administration (FDA) for the treatment of thoracic aortic aneurysms was the Thoracic Aortic Graft (TAG) (W.L. Gore & Associates Inc., Flagstaff, AZ) in 2005.[17,18] Our initial 'off-label' utilization of this device for the purpose of TEVAR for TAI, beginning in September of that year, has previously been reported. The initial capabilities of this device limited TEVAR application to patients with a minimum aortic diameter of 23 mm. The approval of smaller diameter devices, including Talent (Medtronic, Santa Rosa, CA) and TX2 (Bloomington, IN) in 2008 made TEVAR feasible for a broader range of patients when employed in 'off-label' utilization. The subsequent introduction and FDA approval for TAI treatment of two additional devices, CTAG (W.L. Gore) and Valiant (Medtronic), have increased the tools available for definitive treatment of these injuries by effective endovascular means.

The subsequent evolution in standard of care has led to the employment of TEVAR as the treatment modality of choice for the majority of anatomically suitable patients with TAI. The early research results of the American Association for the Surgery of Trauma Thoracic Aortic Injury Study Group[12] followed by subsequent work by multiple groups, including our own,[9–13] have demonstrated that appropriately selected patients undergoing TEVAR have improved outcomes compared to those traditionally attributed to open means of repair.

Our technique for endovascular repair of TAI has been described previously.[9] In summary, all endovascular procedures are performed under general anesthesia in a hybrid operating room equipped with fixed imaging equipment (Axiom, Siemens Medical, Malvern, PA). Intraoperatively, the abdomen and bilateral groins are prepped in standard fashion. An arch aortogram is performed through femoral access and the location of the injury is confirmed. The cerebrovascular anatomy is evaluated based on the arch angiogram, especially if left subclavian artery coverage is planned. IVUS is used selectively based on the discretion of the attending surgeon. The patient is anticoagulated using a weight-based heparin protocol if there are no contraindications. Otherwise, a smaller dose of heparin (3000–5000 units) is administered.

The thoracic device is selected based on CT images according to the manufacturer's sizing recommendations. Measurements are made based on 2D, thin-cut axial CT scans with intravenous contrast. The device is delivered and deployed using standard technique, without any pharmacological adjunct; extension pieces may be deployed as indicated. The subclavian artery is covered as needed to obtain a proximal landing zone or gain better apposition with the lesser curvature of the aortic arch. We maintain a policy of selective delayed subclavian artery revascularization for such

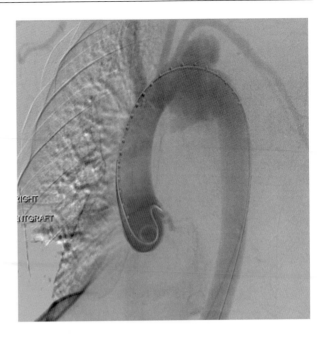

Figure 50.3 Digital subtracted angiography of thoracic aorta (pre-stent placement) reveals Grade 3 traumatic aortic injury.

cases. Post-deployment balloon angioplasty is performed selectively when incomplete apposition of the graft at the proximal landing zone is noted. The heparin is then reversed with protamine. Postoperatively, patients are returned to the surgical-trauma intensive care unit and discharged following stabilization of their other injuries. The diagnostic and completion angiogram of a patient with a grade III TAI is shown in Figures 50.3 and 50.4.

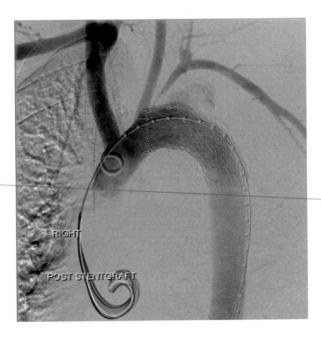

Figure 50.4 Completion digital subtracted angiography reveals stent graft repair of TAI with Zone 2 deployment of thoracic endograft.

Postoperative management

The hemodynamic state of the patient is closely monitored following the procedure, and meticulous care is provided for any other trauma they have experienced. We are vigilant for any of the complications that can arise following aortic trauma, including bleeding, infection and neurologic changes. Barring other major trauma or complications, most patients with endovascular aortic repair will be discharged from the hospital within 3–7 days. Long-term data on durability and major complications are limited to less than 10 years, as widespread adoption of TEVAR did not occur until the mid-2000s. As a result, our follow-up surveillance includes clinical examination and CT at 1, 6 and 12 months, and yearly thereafter.

Current data suggest that in comparison to OR, TEVAR may reduce early death, paraplegia, renal insufficiency, transfusions, reoperation for bleeding, cardiac complications, pneumonia and length of hospital stay.[12–15] However, there are risks associated with endovascular repair, including device migration or malfunction, endoleak, retrograde dissection and access vessel rupture. The continued advancement of device technology specific to utilization for TAI, however, continues to decrease the complications associated with TEVAR in this setting.[17] Common factors implicated in complications related to TEVAR include excessive oversizing and tight curvature of the aortic arch among select victims of TAI.

RESULTS AND OUTCOMES

Murad and colleagues have previously conducted a review commissioned by the SVS to evaluate and compare different modalities (non-operative, OR and TEVAR) for treatment of patients with TAI.[14] This systematic review is comprised of 7768 patients from 139 previously published studies. The study determined that the non-operative approach is associated with highest mortality rate (non-operative 46%; OR 19% and TEVAR 9%; p < 0.01). In their review, they noted that TEVAR was associated with a lower mortality (relative risk 0.61; 95% CI 0.46–0.80) and decreased rates of spinal cord ischemia (relative risk 0.34; 95% CI 0.16–0.74), end-stage renal disease and systemic and graft infections as compared to previously reported OR series. However, TEVAR resulted in increased secondary interventions for graft-related complications.

In a subsequent report by Dake et al., investigators reported a multicentre observation study commissioned by the SVS Outcomes Committee – a group that included ad hoc members from the American Association for Thoracic Surgery, Society of Thoracic Surgeons and Society for Interventional Radiology. In this limited study of 60 patients with TAI, the 30-day all-cause mortality was 9.1% and 1-year cumulative mortality was 14.4%, with the majority of deaths (multi-organ trauma) occurring during the initial 30 days. There were only two additional deaths in 1-year follow-up. While 20% of the patients (12/60) experienced more than one major adverse event during the first 30 days, only 3.6% of patients (2/55) experienced major adverse events thereafter. There were no secondary endovascular or open aortic reinterventions required in the first year post-TEVAR. This report highlights the early and midterm effectiveness of TEVAR and also absence from the need for early secondary aortic interventions (open or endovascular).

In 2012, Celis et al.[18] reinforced the superiority of TEVAR outcomes as compared to OR while also highlighting the need for continued surveillance of these patients. In this limited, 10-year, single-institution experience of 91 patients presenting with TAI, 41 underwent OR. The operative mortality was lower in the TEVAR group (6% vs. 19.5%, p = .06) but did not reach statistical significance in this small study. Over a mean follow-up interval of 24 months, stent graft complications occurred in eight patients (8/50, 16%). Early stent graft–related complications occurred in two patients (4%), with late stent graft–related complications occurring in six (12%). Both early stent graft–related and late stent graft–related complications were asymptomatic graft collapse identified incidentally on postoperative radiological studies. A secondary endovascular intervention was required in four patients (8%) and open conversion was required for a single patient with aorto-esophageal fistula and physiologic coarctation of the aorta (4%). Delayed left subclavian revascularization was required in only two patients (4%).

The experience at our level 1 urban trauma centre correlates the trends and outcomes reported elsewhere. In our reported 15-year, single-institution experience,[2] 338 patients with TAI were identified in the institutional trauma registry between 1997 and 2012. Of the 338 patients, 175 patients (52%) required thoracic aortic repair with 29 (17%) ORs with cross-clamp, 77 (44%) ORs with distal aortic perfusion and 69 (39%) repairs with TEVAR. Early mortality for all TAI patients was 41% (139/338). TEVAR patients had 4% mortality rate as compared to 17% in the OR group. In TEVAR patients, 1- and 5-year survival rates were 92% and 87%, respectively. In ORs, 1-, 5-, 10- and 15-year survival rates were 76%, 75%, 72% and 68%, respectively.

A more recent report of our TAI outcomes, spanning a period from 2005 to 2012, has documented sustained improved outcomes over traditionally reported OR techniques and lower device-related complications as device capabilities continue to evolve and experience is accumulated. In this report of 82 consecutive patients, we noted a technical success rate of 100% and in-hospital mortality, stroke and paraplegia rates of 5.0%, 2.4% and 0%, respectively. Associated survival was 95% at 30 days, 88% at 1 year, 87% at 2 years and 82% at 5 years.[19] These findings, considered in cohort with our prior report, demonstrate that fixed and total costs of TEVAR are not increased compared to OR, clearly favour the continued utilization of TEVAR as the treatment of choice for anatomically suitable victims of TAI. In summary, the current body of evidence supports the preferential use of TEVAR over OR techniques for anatomically suitable candidates requiring repair of TAI. The short-term and midterm outcomes of TEVAR appear favourable, but the long-term durability of the current devices remains to be determined.

Ascending aortic and transverse aortic arch injury

The exact incidence of ascending aorta and transverse arch rupture is unknown, due to the lethality of these injuries, but is uncommon. A widened mediastinum and cardiac tamponade are frequently associated with ascending aortic ruptures. Repair of these injuries requires a median sternotomy, cardiopulmonary bypass and systemic heparinization (Figure 50.5). Management of the aortic tear may be primary or with an interposition graft. Special attention should be paid to the status of the aortic valve. Similarly, injuries to the aortic arch may require hypothermic circulatory arrest and associated antegrade and retrograde cerebral perfusion techniques. Survival depends primarily on the severity of associated injuries.[19]

Trauma to innominate vessels

PENETRATING TRAUMA TO INNOMINATE VESSELS

Penetrating trauma to the innominate artery requires exposure through medial sternotomy and mobilization of overlying left innominate vein for repair. If a high emergency room anterolateral thoracotomy has already been performed, partial median sternotomy may be necessary to obtain complete exposure of the artery. Lateral arteriorrhaphy is the preferred technique; however,

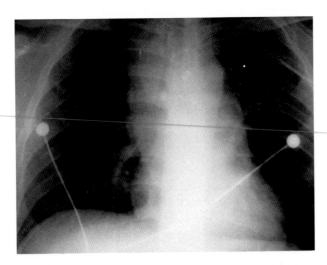

Figure 50.5 Widening of superior mediastinum in modestly hypotensive patient with parasternal stab wound. Through-and-through injury to ascending aorta was repaired through a median sternotomy.

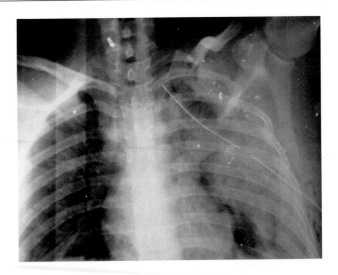

Figure 50.6 Large hemothorax in profoundly hypotensive patient with missile traversing the superior mediastinum and injuring the left innominate vein, left subclavian vein, left clavicle, and left first rib.

ascending aorta to innominate prosthetic bypass is the most common form of repair. The survival rate after penetrating injuries to innominate artery is approximately 85%.

Penetrating injuries to the left innominate vein occur three times more than those to the right innominate vein. Ligation has been the treatment in 80% of the patients with penetrating wounds (Figure 50.6).

BLUNT TRAUMA TO INNOMINATE VESSELS

Rupture of the innominate artery is the second most common TAI following blunt trauma. Innominate artery injuries are repaired via a median sternotomy with a right cervical extension when necessary. Blunt injury typically involves the base of the innominate artery, and this is most expeditiously repaired with a bypass from the ascending aorta to the distal innominate artery, followed by oversewing of the innominate stump. Division of the innominate vein is occasionally required for exposure, and shunts or cardiopulmonary bypass is often not required. Avoidance of the injured area until completion of the bypass leads to a technically easier repair.[20]

Trauma to intrathoracic left common carotid artery

The surgical approach to injuries of the proximal left carotid artery requires a median sternotomy with a left cervical extension, if needed. Repair with bypass graft repair is preferred over an end-to-end reanastomosis for injuries involving the proximal left carotid artery.[20]

The management of a carotid injury in the setting of neurologic deficit is controversial. If the patient presents soon after injury, revascularization (open or endovascular) is recommended because hypotension (rather than ischemic infarct) is the most likely cause of morbidity.

Traumatic carotid lesions have recently been managed with endovascular techniques. An endovascular approach is especially useful for lesions when proximal and distal vascular control are challenging may result in increased morbidity – near the base of the skull. The goal of endovascular therapy is the elimination of a fistula, aneurysm or stenosis while preserving native flow to the brain. There have been multiple reports on the successful management of traumatic carotid injuries with endovascular techniques. However, the use of stents introduces new considerations, such as the probability of in-stent thrombosis/late occlusion. The administration of postprocedural medications, such as aspirin and clopidogrel, can minimize the incidence of in-stent thrombosis.

Trauma to subclavian vessels

Injuries to the subclavian vessels are mostly due to penetrating trauma. Preoperative imaging in stable patients with CTA helps in appropriate incision planning in subclavian vascular injuries.

The safest incision in a stable patient with right subclavian artery injury is via median sternotomy with right supraclavicular extension. Exposure of the entire subclavian artery and vein can be obtained by subperiosteal or complete removal of the medial two-thirds of clavicle (without including the sternoclavicular joint) and division of anterior scalene muscle.

Proximal control of left-sided subclavian injuries can be obtained via a left anterolateral thoracotomy. A separate supraclavicular incision can be used for distal control. These two incisions can be connected with a sternotomy to facilitate exposure. This incision should be used sparingly because of reports of postoperative 'causalgia' neurologic symptoms. In addition, the second or third portion of the subclavian artery can usually be exposed without the need for clavicular resection or sternotomy (Figures 50.7 and 50.8).

Endovascular approaches to innominate, intrathoracic carotid and subclavian arterial injuries have been described in both blunt and penetrating trauma. The long-term results of this approach are not known, but it can be an attractive option in a multi-trauma patient as a damage control manoeuvre until the patient is ready for definitive repair.[21,22]

Trauma to pulmonary hilum

PENETRATING TRAUMA

Penetrating injuries to the pulmonary hilum usually result in prehospital exsanguination. On rare occasions, anterolateral thoracotomy (fifth intercostal space) performed in the emergency room and cross-clamping of the entire hilum will allow for transport of the patient to the

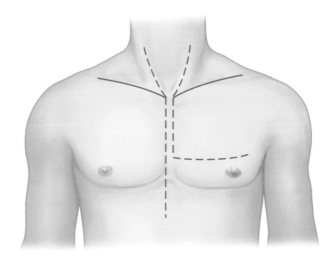

Figure 50.7 Cervicothoracic incisions used for repair of injuries to the innominate artery or veins, common carotid arteries or subclavian arteries or veins. (Courtesy of Baylor College of Medicine, Houston, TX, 1980.)

operating room. Injury to multiple structures in the hilum is treated with emergent pneumonectomy. Individual hilar structures can be ligated separately or en bloc stapling using a 55 or 90 mm stapler with 3.5 mm stapler can be used alternatively. A 50% survival rate after emergent pneumonectomy has been reported (Figure 50.9).

BLUNT TRAUMA

Pulmonary vascular injuries are rare in blunt trauma. In a series of 585 fatal traffic accidents, the thoracic aorta was involved in 46 patients and the pulmonary veins in 5 patients. Sudden deceleration may cause tears at the points of anatomic fixation, such as the junction of the pulmonary veins and the left atrium. Massive hemothorax on presentation or continued chest tube output more than 200 mL/hour should prompt consideration of thoracotomy. When filled with blood, the pleural space may generate modest positive pressure, impeding further bleeding and acting as a blood reservoir. The abrupt institution of closed-suction drainage of the pleural space may induce a rapid loss of intravascular volume in such situations. Therefore, in the setting of a large hemothorax, physicians must be prepared for a rapid thoracotomy if hemodynamic instability ensues following chest tube placement with substantial output. Following thoracotomy, pulmonary venous bleeding can usually be controlled by digital pressure and hilar clamping, if needed. Careful attention to the presence of air in the left atrium must be maintained at all times when dealing with lacerations of the pulmonary veins. Injuries to the pulmonary veins may be accompanied by cardiac, pulmonary arterial and bronchial injuries. Some of these injuries may remain undiagnosed during the initial treatment period, resulting in the development of chronic sequelae, including arteriovenous fistulae and pseudoaneurysms, necessitating subsequent repair.

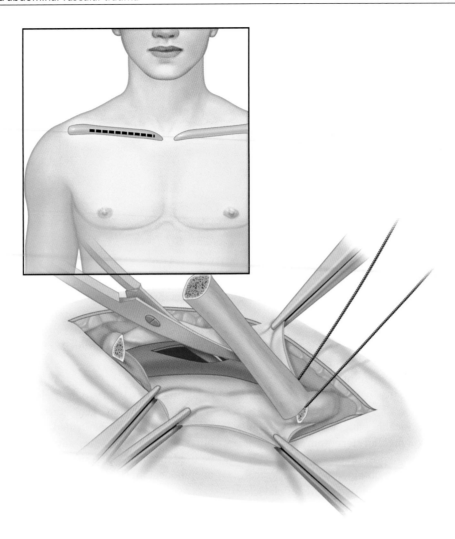

Figure 50.8 Excision of the medial clavicle (not including the sternoclavicular joint) will improve exposure of the second and third portions of the subclavian artery. (Courtesy of Baylor College of Medicine, Houston, TX, 1985.)

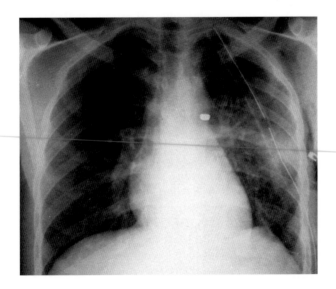

Figure 50.9 Proximity of missile to the great vessels in superior mediastinum of asymptomatic patient. At thoracotomy, missile was found to be tamponading perforation of main pulmonary artery.

Trauma to superior vena cava and inferior vena cava

The cavae are fixed at the pericardial reflections and are vulnerable to sheer forces of blunt trauma at these locations. Rapid deceleration and a mobile heart can cause lacerations of both the SVC and IVC. Downward deceleration of the liver may result in IVC laceration and the Valsalva effect with sudden abdominal compression may cause caval rupture. Associated retrohepatic IVC and hepatic vein injuries are not uncommon. Blunt trauma resulting in SVC or IVC injuries is rare. Penetrating injuries to the cavae are more common, but their location is not predictable.

Diagnostic evaluation of caval injuries should follow the advanced trauma life support protocol, with a chest radiograph followed by surgeon-performed subxiphoid echocardiography in the trauma resuscitation unit. CTA can identify pericardial fluid, but the test of choice is ultrasound, either transthoracic or transesophageal. Repair of these injuries can be done without cardiopulmonary bypass. However, with extensive injuries to the SVC, IVC or retrohepatic vena cava, atrial–caval shunts and cardio-pulmonary bypass with femoral venous drainage may be necessary. Stenosis must be avoided when repairing the cavae. Native or bovine pericardial patch angioplasty should be used liberally to prevent difficult problems, such as SVC syndrome, IVC occlusion or stenosis. Endovascular repair with stent grafts have been reported, but long-term outcomes are unknown.

ABDOMINAL VASCULAR TRAUMA

Abdominal vascular trauma includes injuries to the vessels in four separate areas of the retroperitoneum:

1. *Zone I*: Midline retroperitoneum includes the *supramesocolic area* (suprarenal abdominal aorta, celiac artery, proximal superior mesenteric artery, proximal renal artery and superior mesenteric vein) and the *inframesocolic area* (infrarenal abdominal aorta and infrahepatic IVC).
2. *Zone II*: Upper lateral retroperitoneum (renal artery and vein).
3. *Zone III*: Pelvic retroperitoneum (iliac artery and vein).
4. *Portal–retrohepatic area* (portal vein, hepatic artery, retrohepatic vena cava).

Any retroperitoneal hematoma in Zone I is generally explored. Zone II hematomas secondary to penetrating trauma are explored, and Zone II hematoma secondary to blunt trauma can be managed non-operatively, unless there is expanding hematoma or an additional injury requiring operation. Zone III hematomas secondary to penetrating trauma are explored. Surgical exploration of a pelvic hematoma (Zone III) is discouraged.

Zone I: Midline supramesocolic vascular injuries

The midline retroperitoneum (Zone I) is anatomically divided into supramesocolic zone and inframesocolic zone by the attachment of the transverse mesocolon. Retroperitoneum superior to and beneath the transverse mesocolon contains the suprarenal abdominal aorta, celiac artery, proximal superior mesenteric artery, proximal renal arteries and proximal superior mesenteric vein.

Proximal vascular control is obtained by aortic clamp in descending thoracic aorta or supraceliac abdominal aorta. After performing midline laparotomy, the left lobe of the liver is mobilized, gastro-hepatic ligament is incised to gain access to the lesser sac. Care should be taken to identify and preserve aberrant left hepatic artery is gastro-hepatic ligament. The esophagus is identified and preserved. The left crus of diaphragm is transected at the 2 o'clock position to permit exposure of the distal descending aorta through the aortic hiatus and to ensure adequate application of the proximal aortic clamp. Temporary control with application of aortic compression device can be performed to allow resuscitation in unstable patients.

A hematoma in this zone is approached by medial visceral rotation on the left side 'Mattox manoeuvre'. White line of Toldt is incised by cautery or a pair of scissors and extended around the splenic flexure of the colon and the left-sided abdominal viscera, including the left colon, left kidney, spleen, tail of pancreas and fundus of the stomach.

Distal control of the diaphragmatic or proximal visceral abdominal aorta may require ligation and division of the celiac axis.

Repair of injuries of the suprarenal abdominal aorta can be performed primarily with 3-0 or 4-0 polypropylene suture in a transverse direction. Extensive injuries require patch angioplasty or repair with Dacron graft. Aggressive fluid resuscitation and bicarbonate is administered to the patient prior to release of the clamps on the suprarenal aorta in the patients with hemorrhagic shock.[23–25]

Injuries to the celiac artery are ligated. The injured superior mesenteric artery is usually repaired with prosthetic graft. Ligation of superior mesenteric artery is not well tolerated, as collateral circulation from the celiac artery and inferior mesenteric artery is often inadequate to maintain viability of the small bowel and right colon in the trauma patient in hemorrhagic shock. Control of the proximal superior mesenteric artery is obtained via the Mattox manoeuvre, while exposure of retropancreatic injuries may mandate complete transection of the neck of the pancreas. Distal injuries are approached through the base of the transverse mesocolon or mesentery. Lateral repair of the superior mesenteric artery is performed with 5-0 polypropylene suture. With destruction of the proximal artery, ligation is performed at the origin of the vessel on the visceral aorta, and aorto-mesenteric bypass with saphenous vein or prosthetic graft is performed to restore flow. Control of bleeding and placement of temporary intraluminal shunt is recommended in patients with profound shock, hypothermia, metabolic acidosis and coagulopathy.[28]

Injuries to the proximal renal artery are often associated with injures to the visceral abdominal aorta, and survival rates are poor.

The superior mesenteric vein injury at its junction with the splenic and portal veins is exposed by transection of the neck of the pancreas. Distal injuries of superior mesenteric vein are identified at the base of the mesentery of the small bowel. These injuries can be repaired with lateral venorrhaphy utilizing 5-0 polypropylene suture. Ligation of superior mesenteric vein is performed when venorrhaphy or repair cannot be performed and is tolerated if patient is hydrated aggressively.

Zone I: Midline inframesocolic vascular injuries

The midline retroperitoneum inferior to the transverse mesocolon contains the infrarenal abdominal aorta and the infrarenal IVC. The abdominal aorta is the second most common injured vessel in cases of abdominal vascular injury. In a review of 302 abdominal vascular injuries, the aorta was involved in 63 cases (21%) only surpassed by IVC injuries (25%). The most common cause of abdominal aortic injury (AAI) is penetrating injury. The incidence of AAI in stab wounds is lower as compared to gunshot wounds and is reported to be 1.5% (8 out of 529 patients).[24]

AAI can range from free rupture, contained hematoma, pseudoaneurysm, focal dissection, aortocaval fistula or focal mural hematoma.[24–29] Blunt AAI can be classified similar to TAI into grade I (intimal injury), grade II (intramural hematoma), grade III (pseudoaneurysm) and grade IV (free rupture). Authors[30] have proposed additional classification of abdominal aortic based on the location into Zone I (from diaphragmatic hiatus to SMA), Zone II (SMA to renal artery origin) and Zone III (infrarenal aorta).

A patient with a hematoma or hemorrhage from this area should have initial proximal control of the supraceliac abdominal aorta by technique explained in the preceding section. A more caudal proximal control at infrarenal or suprarenal aortic segment can be obtained afterward.

Repair with lateral aortorrhaphy is possible in most cases due to the relative healthy aorta and limited injury in the trauma population. In patients with high-velocity missiles, the extent of the injury may not be fully appreciated by visual inspection, and care must be taken not to leave behind devitalized tissue. In such cases and other extensive aortic wall injuries, a prosthetic graft repair may be needed. In cases where enteric spillage is encountered along with extensive aortic injury, it is recommended that enteric spillage is controlled and peritoneum is washed out prior to use of prosthetic graft. Although suboptimal, several reports do not consider the presence of enteric spillage a contraindication for the use of prosthetic graft for aortic repair in trauma. Acute renal failure, intraoperative blood loss, morbidity of associated injuries, pulmonary failure, pulmonary infections, graft infections, aortoenteric fistulae and incisional hernia have all been reported complications with open surgical repair of aortic injuries.

Endovascular aortic repair traditionally has a limited role in most AAIs. In select cases with CT diagnosis of a blunt trauma distant from the visceral branches, it offers definitive management without increased morbidity and mortality of OR. Endovascular treatment of the selected traumatic vascular injuries is particularly promising for restoring continuity of the lumen, closing aortocaval fistula and isolating the pseudoaneurysm that would otherwise require extensive surgical procedures in a critically ill patient.[25]

We have treated patients with limited infrarenal traumatic aortic dissection, focal traumatic pseudoaneurysm or traumatic aortocaval fistula at our institution with placement of abdominal endografts or covered stent grafts. Clinicians from other institutions have similarly reported efficacy of endovascular repair in setting of blunt trauma to infrarenal abdominal aorta.

If there is not an injury to the aorta, then an injury to the infrarenal IVC should be suspected in cases with midline hematoma in inframesocolic segment. The hematoma over an injured IVC frequently fills the right paracolic gutter, elevates the right colon and leaks through its mesentery medially. The infrarenal IVC can be exposed through the retroperitoneum in the midline. However, most trauma surgeons perform right medial visceral rotation (Cattell–Braasch manoeuvre; mobilize the retroperitoneal duodenum and right colon medially) to expose the entire cava from the liver to the iliac veins.

An isolated anterior or lateral perforation of the IVC is grabbed with a forceps or Allis clamp and a Satinsky vascular clamp and repaired primarily. When extensive hemorrhage precludes visualization of the perforation, sponge-stick compression or application of vascular clamps above and below the presumed area of injury is indicated. Simultaneous cross-clamping of the infrarenal abdominal aorta at the time of IVC clamping decreases the risk of hypotension secondary to loss of preload. Isolated perforations are repaired in a transverse direction with continuous 5-0 polypropylene suture frequently with two rows of sutures to ensure hemostasis. The posterior wall of the IVC is then mobilized to rule out a second perforation. The perforation in the posterior wall can be repaired via transluminal exposure by extending the length of the anterior perforation.

Narrowing usually results when primary repair is used on large wounds of the IVC. Reconstruction of the narrowed area with a prosthetic patch cavoplasty is indicated only in hemodynamically stable patients without a coagulopathy or hypothermia. This narrowing or even surgical ligation of the infrarenal IVC is well tolerated in young trauma patients if their circulating volume is maintained and if both lower extremities are wrapped and elevated for the first 7–10 postoperative days.

Injuries to the IVC at the confluence of the iliac veins are often difficult to visualize. For this reason, division of the right common iliac artery and mobilization of the overlying aortic bifurcation to the left may be necessary to complete the venous repair, followed by reanastomosis of the artery.

Injury to IVC at the confluence of renal veins requires silastic loops for control of both renal veins with clamp or sponge-stick control of the infrarenal and suprarenal cava before performing the repair.

Zone II: Lateral perirenal vascular injuries

Injury to the renal artery, renal vein, both, or the kidney should be suspected when a hematoma or hemorrhage is present in lateral retroperitoneum. In the patient who has suffered blunt abdominal trauma and with a normal IVP, renal arteriogram, or CT of the kidneys, open exploration of the perirenal hematoma at a subsequent laparotomy is avoided. In the absence of preoperative CT screening, all perirenal hematomas found in patients with penetrating wounds are explored and repaired.

Proximal control of supraceliac abdominal aorta and then the proximal renal arteries is performed prior to entering a perirenal hematoma secondary to penetrating wound. On the right side, mobilization of the duodenum will be necessary before the renal vein can be controlled.

In situations where there is active hemorrhage from a perirenal hematoma, midline control of the main vessels is too time consuming and direct control at the renal hilum is recommended instead of proximal control. The kidney is quickly mobilized out of the retroperitoneum, and a vascular clamp is applied to the renal hilum under direct view.

Repair of the injured renal artery after penetrating trauma is rarely attempted due to presentation with hypotension and presence of multiple injuries. Techniques of repair that have been suggested but rarely utilized include bypass grafting from the aorta or hepatic artery on the right and transposition of the splenic artery on the left. In the hypotensive patient with multiple intra-abdominal injuries, injury to the renal artery or both hilar vessels and a normal contralateral kidney on intraoperative palpation, nephrectomy is the procedure of choice.

Portal vein, hepatic veins, retrohepatic inferior vena cava injury

Portal vein injuries are accompanied with associated hepatic artery and bile duct injuries and have high mortality rates. Proximal control with surgeon's fingers or clamp is performed by clamping the gastroduodenal ligament (Pringle manoeuvre).

After obtaining proximal control, careful dissection is performed to dissect and identify the portal vein, hepatic artery and bile duct. The portal vein is exposed by mobilizing the common bile duct to the left and stripping the lymphatic tissue off the right posterolateral aspect of the vessel. Injury of the segment of the portal vein beneath the neck of the pancreas necessitates division of the pancreas between noncrushing clamps. Lateral repair of the portal vein is performed using a continuous 5-0 polypropylene suture. Standard techniques of repair with patch or interposition graft are performed for more extensive injuries. Ligation for severe injuries is compatible with survival; however, it is reserved for the inpatients with hypothermia, acidosis and coagulopathy.

Injuries to the hepatic artery are treated with ligation rather than repair because of multiple associated visceral and vascular injuries in the right upper quadrant. Necrosis of hepatic parenchyma under mattress sutures naturally increases if the common hepatic artery or hepatic artery to the injured lobe is ligated.

Penetrating wounds of the hepatic veins or retrohepatic vena cava or avulsions of the hepatic veins from blunt trauma are all rare but extremely lethal. Right upper quadrant or liver hemorrhage uncontrolled by the Pringle manoeuvre suggests hepatic veins of retrohepatic IVC injuries. Most patients are hypotensive on admission and are found to have a massive retrohepatic hematoma extending to the infrahepatic area at laparotomy.

If the hematoma is stable after penetrating or blunt trauma and there is no rupture with associated free bleeding into the peritoneal cavity, many experienced trauma surgeons will opt to leave the hematoma intact. In patients with profound hypotension and active hemorrhage from the retrohepatic area, initial attempts to obtain hemostasis are performed with insertion of perihepatic packs for compression or an attempt at repair. The packs are left in place, and damage control laparotomy with open abdominal wound vac is performed whenever packs successfully control hemorrhage and the patient has hypothermia, a metabolic acidosis and a coagulopathy before a repair has been started.

Failure of the packs to control retrohepatic hemorrhage mandates an attempt at repair using the following procedures:

1. *Direct lateral approach after mobilization of the overlying hepatic lobe*: This approach is useful in children and in selected adults with side perforations or avulsions of hepatic veins.
2. *Total hepatic vascular isolation*: Cross-clamping of the suprarenal aorta, hepatoduodenal ligament, suprarenal infrahepatic IVC and suprahepatic vena cava isolates the liver but often worsens hypotension in the hypovolemic patients.
3. *Extensive hepatotomy to expose the injured cava*: An extensive hepatotomy should be utilized only by surgeons with significant experience in hepatic trauma.
4. *Insertion of an atriocaval shunt*: Atriocaval shunting using a #36 thoracostomy tube or #8 endotracheal tube has been the most widely used approach in patients where packing alone cannot attain hemostasis.

DAMAGE CONTROL APPROACH

When intraoperative hypothermia (34°C), metabolic acidosis (pH 7.1–7.2) or a coagulopathy (prothrombin time and/or partial thromboplastin time 50% of normal) occurs, a 'damage control' operative approach is indicated.

With thoracic vascular injuries, this would include temporary intraluminal shunting rather than a complex or prolonged repair of the common carotid or subclavian artery, ligation of major venous injuries and placement of wound vac with intention to return for definite repair after resuscitation.

In the abdomen, this would include temporary intraluminal shunting rather than a complex or prolonged repair of the superior mesenteric or common or external iliac artery, ligation of major venous injuries (with the exception of the suprarenal IVC) and abdominal wound vac placement. Vascular reconstruction, visceral resection or repair and attempted closure of the midline incision are the goals at this first reoperation.

CONCLUSION

Significant progress has been made over the last decade in the management of TAI. Individualized treatment decisions, with multi-disciplinary input, are required to insure optimal outcomes following TAI. The current body of evidence supports the preferential use of TEVAR over OR techniques for anatomically suitable candidates requiring repair of TAI. In these cases, meticulous case planning can help avoid potential complications of TEVAR.

The short-term and midterm outcomes of TEVAR appear favourable, but the long-term durability of the current devices is unknown. Adherence to the surveillance regimen is necessary to detect long-term complications. There remains a considerable need to determine the long-term natural history of TEVAR among patients treated for TAI.

REFERENCES

1. Teixeira PG, Inaba K, Barmparas G, Georgiou C, Toms C, Noguchi TT, Rogers C, Sathyavagiswaran L, Demetriades D. Blunt thoracic aortic injuries: An autopsy study. *J Trauma.* 2011 January;70(1):197–202.

2. Estrera AL, Miller CC 3rd, Salinas-Guajardo G, Coogan SM, Charlton-Ouw KM, Safi HJ, Azizzadeh A. Update on blunt thoracic aortic injury: 15-year single-institution experience. *J Thorac Cardiovasc Surg.* 2013 March;145(3 Suppl.):S154–S158.

3. Mirvis SE, Bidwell JK, Buddemeyer EU et al. Value of chest radiography in excluding traumatic aortic rupture. *Radiology.* 1987;163:487–493.

4. Gavant ML, Menke PG, Fabian T, Flick PA, Graney MJ, Gold RE. Blunt traumatic aortic rupture: Detection with helical CT of the chest. *Radiology.* 1995;197:125–133.

5. Wicky S, Capasso P, Meuli R, Fischer A, Segesser L, Schnyder P. Spiral aortography: An efficient technique for the diagnosis of traumatic aortic injury. *Eur Radiol.* 1998;8:828–833.

6. Bruckner BA, DiBardino DJ, Cumbie TC et al. Critical evaluation of chest computed tomography scans for blunt descending thoracic aortic injury. *Ann Thorac Surg.* 2006;81:1339–1346.

7. Azizzadeh A, Valdes J, Miller CC 3rd, Nguyen LL, Estrera AL, Charlton-Ouw K, Coogan SM, Holcomb JB, Safi HJ. The utility of intravascular ultrasound compared to angiography in the diagnosis of blunt traumatic aortic injury. *J Vasc Surg.* 2011 March;53(3):608–614.

8. Azizzadeh A, Keyhani K, Miller CC 3rd, Coogan SM, Safi HJ, Estrera AL. Blunt traumatic aortic injury: Initial experience with endovascular repair. *J Vasc Surg.* 2009 June;49(6):1403–1408.

9. Lee WA, Matsumura JS, Mitchell RS, Farber MA, Greenberg RK, Azizzadeh A, Murad MH, Fairman RM. Endovascular repair of trauma traumatic thoracic aortic injury: Clinical practice guidelines of the Society for Vascular Surgery. *J Vasc Surg.* 2011 January;53(1):187–192.

10. Osgood MJ, Heck JM, Rellinger EJ et al. Natural history of grade I-II blunt traumatic aortic injury. *J Vasc Surg.* 2014;59:334–342.

11. Nagy K, Fabian T, Rodman G, Fulda G, Rodriguez A, Mirvis S. Guidelines for the diagnosis and management of blunt aortic injury: An EAST Practice Management Guidelines Work Group. *J Trauma.* 2000 June;48(6):1128–1143.

12. Demetriades D, Velmahos GC, Scalea TM et al. Blunt traumatic thoracic aortic injuries: Early or delayed repair – Results of an American Association for the Surgery of Trauma prospective study. *J Trauma.* 2009 April;66(4):967–973.

13. Demetriades D, Velmahos GC, Scalea TM et al. Operative repair or endovascular stent graft in blunt traumatic thoracic aortic injuries: Results of an American Association for the Surgery of Trauma multicenter study. *J Trauma.* 2008;64:561–570; discussion 570–571.

14. Murad MH, Rizvi AZ, Malgor R, Carey J, Alkatib AA, Erwin PJ, Lee WA, Fairman RM. Comparative effectiveness of the treatments for thoracic aortic transection. *J Vasc Surg.* 2011 January;53(1):193–199.e1–21.

15. Azizzadeh A, Ray HM, DuBose JJ et al. Outcomes of endovascular repair for patients with blunt traumatic aortic injury. *J Trauma Acute Care Surg.* 2014 February;76(2):510–516.

16. Martinelli O, Malaj A, Gossetti B, Bertoletti B, Bresadola L, Irace L. Outcomes in the emergency endovascular repair of blunt thoracic aortic injuries. *J Vasc Surg.* 2013 September;58(3):832–835.

17. Farber MA, Giglia JS, Starnes BW, Stevens SL, Holleman J, Chaer R, Matsumuara JS. Evaluation of the redesigned conformable GORE TAG thoracic endoprosthesis for traumatic aortic transection. *J Vasc Surg.* 2013 September;58(3):651–658.

18. Celis RI, Park SC, Shukla AJ et al. Evolution of treatment for traumatic thoracic aortic injuries. *J Vasc Surg.* 2012 July;56(1):74–80.

19. Azizzadeh A, Charlton-Ouw KM, Chen Z et al. An outcome analysis of endovascular versus open repair of blunt traumatic aortic injuries. *J Vasc Surg.* 2013 January;57(1):108–114; discussion 115.

20. Symbas PJ, Horsley WS, Symbas PN. Rupture of the ascending aorta caused by blunt trauma. *Ann Thorac Surg.* 1998;66(1):113–117.

21. Mattox KL. Approaches to trauma involving the major vessels of the thorax. *Surg Clin North Am.* 1989;69(1):77–91.

22. Dubose JJ, Rajani R, Gilani R, Arthurs ZA, Morrison JJ, Clouse WD, Rasmussen TE; Endovascular Skills for Trauma and Resuscitative Surgery Working Group. Endovascular management of axillo-subclavian arterial injury: A review of published experience. *Injury.* 2012;43(11):1785–1792.

23. Asensio JA, Forno W, Roldan G et al. Abdominal vascular injuries: Injuries to the aorta. *Surg Clin North Am.* 2001;81:1395–1416.

24. Asensio TA, Chahwan S, Hanpeter D et al. Operative management and outcomes of 302 abdominal vascular injuries. *Am J Surg.* 2000;180:524–534.

25. White R, Donayre C, Walot I et al. Endograft repair of an aortic pseudo-aneurysm following gunshot wound injury: Impact of imaging on diagnosis and planning of intervention. *J Endovasc Ther.* 1997;4:344–351.

26. Tucker S Jr, Row VL, Rao R et al. Treatment options for traumatic pseudoaneurysms of paravisceral abdominal aorta. *Ann Vasc Surg.* 2005;19:613–618.

27. Inaba K, Kirkpatrick W, Finkelstein AJ et al. Blunt abdominal aortic trauma with association with thoracolumbar spine fractures. *Injury.* 2001;35:385–389.

28. Accola KD, Feliciano DV, Mattox KL et al. Management of injuries of suprarenal aorta. *Am J Surg.* 1987;154:613–618.

29. Loh SA, Maldonado TS, Rockman CB et al. Endovascular solutions to arterial injury due to posterior spine surgery. *J Vasc Surg.* 2012 May;55(5):1477–1481.

30. Shalhub S, Starnes BW, Tran NT et al. Blunt abdominal aortic injury. *J Vasc Surg.* 2012;55:1277–1285.

51

Thoracic outlet and neck trauma

DAVID L. GILLESPIE and ADAM DOYLE

CONTENTS

INTRODUCTION

Trauma is the fourth leading cause of all civilian deaths in the United States and the leading cause of death among children and adults under age 45.[1] Many victims have multiple injuries involving major vascular structures. Major injury to thoracic outlet and neck vascular structures can occur in virtually any environment, but the greatest incidence occurs in urban areas, where violence is endemic. Although victims of trauma frequently have multiple injuries, wounds of major vessels are the sole cause or the major contributing cause of many of the deaths. Penetrating trauma in combination with an increase in high-energy road traffic accidents has resulted in an increase in major vascular trauma.[2] Outcomes after vascular trauma in terms of survival have been reported to be better in urban areas than in rural.[2] This difference is thought to be due to several factors, but mostly related to prolonged transfer times in the rural setting.

In most situations, there is a little difficulty in ascertaining that the patient has a serious injury. Many of these people have multiple wounds, and a careful assessment of all injuries is required in order to establish priorities of care. This is particularly true of penetrating wounds of the brachiocephalic vessels, because not only is hemorrhage a threat but the interruption of blood flow to the brain may also produce serious neurological problems. Blunt or penetrating injuries to the great vessels can present in the acute setting as exsanguination or, in the chronic setting, as a fistula or post-traumatic aneurysm.

Traditional surgical techniques in combination with modern theories on resuscitation and operative strategy have resulted in increased rates of survival. In addition, the sum of the advances in the diagnosis and management is the result of the increasing quality of computed tomography angiography (CTA) in diagnosing injuries, multiplanar reconstructions for operative planning and the availability of endovascular stent grafts. The development of endovascular therapies has been rapid over the last few years and has provided clinicians with more options for the treatment of life-threatening vascular injuries. This method of management in general is more rapid and less morbid than open repair of vascular injuries. This chapter will focus on the management of patients with thoracic outlet and neck vascular trauma and includes a review of all the elements of pre- and perioperative care.

ETIOLOGY

Major vascular wounds can occur in any environment, but the greatest incidence is seen in urban areas where violence is endemic. Penetrating trauma caused by knives and bullet wounds is more common than blunt trauma, although in some cases, vascular wounds resulting from blunt trauma can be more difficult to diagnose and treat. Certain varieties of blunt trauma are particularly likely to result in vascular injury: steering wheel injuries, deceleration forces, falls and crushing blows to the chest and root of the neck can be followed by serious vascular wounds.

Most penetrating injuries are caused by stabbing or bullets traveling at a low velocity, and the damage is mainly confined to the wound tract. Knife wounds usually cause punctures, lacerations and occasionally transactions, while bullets are more likely to sever the artery. The blast effect of high-velocity missiles may cause widespread damage because the cavitation produced by a missile traveling at 150,023,000 ft/s is capable of damaging vessels remote from the wound tract. When such a blast cavity collapses, a suction effect is generated, which can draw surface structures such as bits of skin, clothing or dirt along the wound tract.

A high-velocity bullet or metal fragment can produce a great deal of tissue damage, especially if it strikes bone and all of the bullet's energy is dissipated in the target. Moreover, splinters of bone may become secondary missiles and injure other structures. Such widespread damage may not be suspected on initial inspection because there may be only small entrance and exit wounds.

PHYSICAL EXAMINATION

The diagnosis of thoracic outlet and neck injuries begins with a history and physical examination. Physical examination and determination of hard signs of vascular injury predict those patients with significant injuries that could benefit from immediate exploration.[3] Examination of the neck and thorax must be prompt and thorough as there are many of these injuries that can be rapidly lethal. Vital signs should be obtained, including bilateral arm pressures, on arrival and at regular intervals thereafter. As soon as the patient is exposed, the anterior chest should be observed for deformity, ecchymosis or penetrating injury. Asymmetry provides insight into possible ongoing pathology. A deviated trachea can be the sign of a developing tension pneumothorax, hemothorax or great vessel injury. Palpation of the anterior chest can demonstrate crepitus, tenderness and fractures that were not readily apparent. Auscultation can demonstrate decreased breath sounds suggestive of a possible hemo-/pneuom-/hemopneumothorax. These findings should be followed with the immediate placement of a tube thoracostomy to decompress the hemithorax. The patient should be turned while maintaining cervical control and the posterior thorax examined. Once a rapid and thorough examination

is completed, routine laboratory tests should be drawn and sent to the lab when IV access is established. In stable patients, radiologic imaging can be performed safely, but should not delay required care when indicated.

ZONES OF THE NECK

Injuries to the neck have been notoriously difficult to manage. A clear anatomic division of the neck into zones has allowed a selective approach to penetrating neck trauma. Zone I lies below the cricoid cartilage, and zone III lies above the angle of the mandible. Zone II lies between zones I and III and has classically been managed with immediate operative exploration and direct evaluation of the aerodigestive tract and the carotid and jugular vessels. Vascular injuries may be associated with injuries of other anterior mediastinal structures including other great vessels, the esophagus or the trachea. These structures should be inspected and repaired if necessary. It should be noted that if adjacent structures are injured and repaired, the repairs must be separated with local tissue flaps and drained appropriately. Failing to cover and drain adjacent repairs can lead to potentially fatal complications such as anastomotic dehiscence and exsanguination, fistula formation and uncontrolled leaks.[4,5]

The diagnostic and therapeutic approach for the management of cervical vascular injuries is dictated by their relative location to the anatomic landmarks used to describe the location of vascular injury. By clinical examination, it may be difficult to determine if injuries in zones I and III have damaged major vascular structures such as the carotid artery. In these situations, if the patients are hemodynamically stable, further imaging is very useful. In selected patients with penetrating injuries in zone II who have no neurological deficit, operation may be performed without further imaging, although preoperative arteriography is helpful in the management of these patients as well. If there is a neurological deficit, a careful imaging study that includes intracranial imaging is required. Some of these patients may have cerebral thromboembolism that will not respond to the repair of cervical arterial wounds.

CONTROL OF HEMORRHAGE

Surgeons should have a good understanding of what exposure is required to control massive hemorrhage. Once the anatomy of the injury has been defined, definitive exposure should be obtained. Initial control of hemorrhage is achieved by a hasty prep, wide surgical exposure and digital occlusion within the wound bed until the patient can be transported to the operating room (OR) where formal control and exposure are obtained.[6] If local control is adequate, further surgical exploration and subsequent blood loss should be delayed until adequate resuscitation is initiated. When the injured vessel is exposed, a clamp should be applied as long as doing so will not exacerbate the existing injury. One must resist the temptation to explore an expanding hematoma prior to obtaining proximal and distal control. Details relating to surgical technique can be found in the following section on surgical exposures.

DIAGNOSTIC IMAGING

Chest x-ray

Chest x-ray is the best and most common initial radiographic evaluation of the chest. The results of this test are rapidly available and can help to direct care. This study is best performed in the upright position. In the setting of penetrating trauma, radiolucent markers should be placed overlying the skin defects. Major vascular injury is suggested by the presence of hemothorax, foreign body proximity to the great vessels or an unusually positioned or missing foreign body suggesting possible missile embolization. In the setting of blunt trauma, the most reliable radiographic finding associated with blunt aortic injury is the loss of the aortic knob contour. Injuries to the innominate artery should be suspected if a widened mediastinum is noted at the thoracic outlet with accompanying leftward tracheal deviation.

Computed tomography angiography

The diagnosis of blunt and penetrating vascular trauma in the modern trauma centre is changing. In the hemodynamically stable trauma patient, conventional angiography has been the gold standard for the diagnosis of vascular injury. In stable patients, an early use of screening CTA is the best test of choice and highly recommended for the evaluation of injuries to the great vessels and thoracic aorta.[7] This test has been shown to accurately identify the presence of an aortic transection, allowing the initiation of aggressive beta-blockade and evaluation and timing of therapeutic options. The quality of available computed tomography (CT) scanners has grown exponentially in recent years. In addition, the scans provide an early baseline of patient anatomy for comparison if non-operative management is going to be attempted and delineates associated injuries. Modern software can provide adequate 3D reconstruction to aid in operative planning and the possibility for endovascular repair.[8] The presence of metallic fragments or external fixators was not found to affect the imaging quality obtained by multidetector CTA studies in vascular trauma.[9]

The use of CTA in the diagnosis of adult neck and extremity injuries has proven highly sensitive and specific (80% and 100%, respectively) in multiple reports.[10,11] In a study of pediatric vascular injury, CTA was shown to have a sensitivity of 100% and specificity of 93% in detecting vascular injuries in penetrating trauma. CTA had a sensitivity of 88% and specificity of 100% in detecting vascular injuries in blunt trauma. These results yielded an overall accuracy in detecting vascular injury for penetrating and blunt trauma of 95% and 97%, respectively.[7]

Identifying penetrating cardiac injuries in hemodynamically stable patients can be more difficult. A recent retrospective review from Kings County Hospital in New York reported excellent negative predictive value using a combination of transthoracic echocardiography and chest CT in the screening of stable patients with a suspected penetrating cardiac injury.[12] If identified by non-invasive means, penetrating cardiac injury warrants sternotomy and exploration.

Catheter angiography

Catheter angiography is now rarely performed as a first-line test in patients with suspected thoracic vascular injury. CTA offers accurate screening without the embolic risk associated with selective angiography of the great vessels.[13] As a result, most injuries are detected with this less invasive modality. However, catheter angiography remains the gold standard for diagnosis of suspected injuries to the innominate, intrathoracic carotid and subclavian arteries as well as for the diagnosis of possible blunt thoracic aortic injuries. Aortography should be performed if there are either physical signs or radiographic findings suggestive of thoracic vascular injury. Most often, catheter angiography is now performed intraoperatively as routine care during endovascular or hybrid repair of vascular injuries.

Re-evaluation and operative planning

Early surgical planning based on patient condition is essential. Urgent operative repair is required for any injury resulting in hemodynamic instability, massive or ongoing hemorrhage or a rapidly expanding hematoma on radiographic studies. Rapid surgical planning and effective communication with the OR personnel are essential. Information regarding patient condition and urgency for an OR, patient and table positioning, need for special or preferred instruments, the basic operative plan, body areas to prepare and other details concerning arteriography or vein harvest should be conveyed to the OR staff and anesthetic team as early on as possible.

SURGICAL MANAGEMENT OF VASCULAR TRAUMA

General principles

The severity and distribution of a vascular injury are largely dependent upon the mechanism of the traumatic insult. The accurate diagnosis of active hemorrhage versus interrupted perfusion with or without subsequent ischemia becomes the cornerstone of management decisions. Penetrating trauma is often associated with vessel laceration and/or transection and may result in vascular thrombosis, active bleeding, arteriovenous fistula and/or pseudoaneurysm. Proper operative management is determined by rapid control of exsanguinating hemorrhage in an abbreviated initial operative intervention, followed by interval resuscitation, correction of physiologic imbalances and a scheduled return to the OR.[6] Only when the aforementioned are successful can the patient be expected to survive a more elaborate and time-consuming vascular repair. This concept of surgical care, known as damage control surgery (DCS), has enhanced the survival of severely injured patients in urban trauma centres. The essence of DCS is to achieve and conclude an operative procedure before the physiologic 'point of no return' is reached.[14] DCS was demonstrated to improve survival in critically injured patients who had suffered massive bleeding.[15] Combining the concepts of DCS with a resuscitation strategy that quickly restores physiology may allow patients to survive major operations required to repair thoracic vascular injuries. The benefits of early rapid infusion of blood products, high plasma ratios and minimal crystalloid should be considered in vascular reconstructions of severely injured patients. Results from the most current conflicts have shown a reduction in mortality from previous wars possibly due to the near uniform application of DCS and DCR principles.[16]

Management of traumatic vascular injuries can offer special challenges to experienced surgeons in peacetime and in combat. Patients with hemodynamic instability with undiagnosed injuries should be placed in the supine position, receive preoperative broad spectrum antibiotics and be prepped and draped from the neck to the knees, with the most appropriate surgical approach dictated by the anatomy of their injury. A rapid initial intraoperative assessment of the injury and the patient's hemodynamic and physiologic status will help direct the overall goal of the operation in the direction of damage control or definitive repair. Thoracic damage control can be approached by either abbreviated thoracotomy restoring survivable physiology or rapid definitive repair.[17] All devitalized tissue should be excised and irrigated under low pressure, with careful evaluation of muscle tissue for viability. The injured segment of artery or vein should be debrided back to normal tissue as attempts to avoid this step can result in disastrous complications. The level of contamination in the wound should be assessed. Conduit choice can be simplified to saphenous vein for vessels of 5 mm and under and polytetrafluoroethylene (PTFE) for vessels greater than 5 mm.[17] When injuries are identified to major deep or collecting venous structures, if the patient is not in extremis, they should be repaired to avoid the long-term morbidity associated with ligation.[18] Completion assessment following repair are performed using physical examination, handheld Doppler or arteriography. Palpable pulses or Doppler signals should be monitored post-operatively to assess continued patency.

Surgical exposures

There is a robust body of knowledge on the operative management of thoracic vascular trauma in both civilian and military from around the world.[19–35] In today's environment, knowledge of how to perform surgical exposures that allow rapid control of vascular structures is extremely important. The decreasing volume of open vascular surgery makes it even more important that the surgeon be familiar with surgical anatomy and various exposures of the vascular tree.

There are three main areas of exposure of vascular injuries to the chest. The decision of which exposure to use will depend upon the surgeon making some observations while examining the patient. In general, the incisions for exposure are placed to obtain proximal vascular control to the site of injury. Through this/these incision/s, you can obtain proximal control of the injured vessel before exposing the arterial injury. Injuries to the chest however require the surgeon to use their judgment and decide whether the injury involves the proximal left subclavian artery or not. This is usually evident either by the trajectory of the missile or the presence of a hematoma in the left supraclavicular area. Anatomically, the left subclavian artery originates from the distal aortic arch and descends in the posterior mediastinum. This makes vascular control of the proximal left subclavian very difficult through a median sternotomy. Therefore, if the surgeon feels that proximal control of the left subclavian is necessary, a left anterior thoracotomy through the third intercostal space is needed. Otherwise, a median sternotomy is the surgical approach of choice for injuries of the heart, ascending aorta, transverse aortic arch, the main pulmonary artery, innominate vein and intrathoracic vena cava. For injuries to the great vessels, a median sternotomy can be used with the appropriate cervical extension incision.

Median sternotomy

Median sternotomy is the preferred method of exposure for suspected injuries to the ascending aorta, heart, SVC/IVC, pulmonary hilum, innominate artery or vein and right or left common carotid artery origins. An incision is made in the midline of the sternum (Figure 51.1). The sternum is exposed from the sternal notch to the xiphoid. At the ends of the sternum, the dissection is performed bluntly exposing the sternal notch and the subxiphoid area. The anesthesiologist is asked to hold ventilation, and the sternum is divided using a sternal saw. Alternatively, the sternum may be divided using a Lipshke knife. The sternum is retracted using a Finochietto retractor. The surgeon should look for a hematoma obscuring the great vessels in the superior mediastinum. The hematoma should be explored in an attempt to identify the left innominate vein. This left innominate vein is a key landmark in the identification

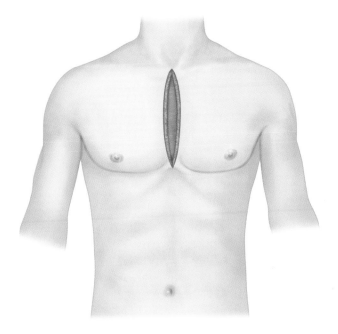

of the location of the great vessels. If visualization is obscured due to hematoma, the surgeon may open the pericardium in order to find the aortic root. By tracing the aorta as it ascends from the heart, one can identify the great vessels safely. The left innominate vein may be ligated and divided or retracted so as to give the surgeon greater visibility of the innominate and carotid arteries (Figure 51.2). Proximal control of injuries

to these vessels can usually be achieved at their take-off from the aortic arch using a vascular clamp. This incision may be combined with a left or right supraclavicular incision for distal vascular control and facilitating arterial repair. After obtaining proximal and distal control of the vascular injury, a decision is made whether the injury can be repaired with lateral suture or patch angioplasty or needs interposition grafting (Figures 51.3 and 51.4).

Anterior thoracotomy

As stated previously, if the surgeon suspects injury to the left subclavian artery and there is a need to obtain proximal control at the aortic arch, an anterior thoracotomy is the incision of choice (Figure 51.5). With the patient in a supine position, an incision is made in the third interspace of the anterior surface of the left chest. The intercostal musculature is divided on the cephalad aspect of the rib to avoid injury to the intercostal neurovascular bundle. After entering the left chest, a Finochietto retractor is inserted between the ribs to improve exposure. The surgeon should ask the anesthesiologist to stop ventilating the left lung. The left lung is then retracted inferiorly and the surgeon should focus his attention medially and cephalad to identify the aortic arch. With a combination of sharp and blunt dissection, the aortic arch and the left subclavian origin are exposed. Proximal control of the left subclavian is achieved using a straight vascular clamp. The surgeon should attempt to identify and protect the vagus nerve as it crosses the aortic arch proximal to the take-off of the left subclavian. Once proximal control is obtained, attention is then turned to the supraclavicular region and the subclavian artery is then exposed to obtain distal control.

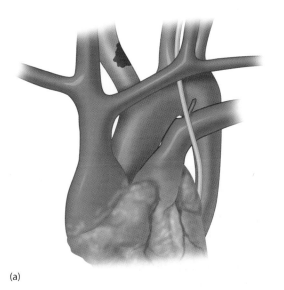

(a)

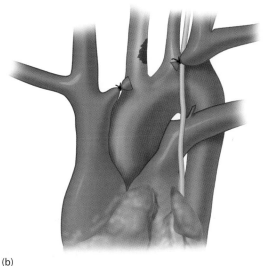

(b)

Figure 51.2 Division of the left innominate vein to improve exposure to proximal innominate artery injury through median sternotomy incision. (a) Before ligation, (b) after ligation and division of the left innominate vein. (From Gillespie D, The management of upper extremity arterial trauma, in Pearce WH et al., eds., *Vascular Surgery in the Endovascular Era*, Greenwood Academic, Evanston, IL, 2008, pp. 457–467.)

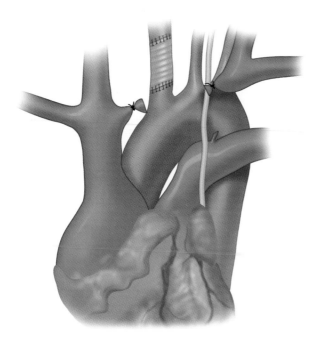

Figure 51.3 Repair of innominate artery injury using prosthetic interposition graft. (From Gillespie D, The management of upper extremity arterial trauma, in Pearce WH et al., eds., *Vascular Surgery in the Endovascular Era*, Greenwood Academic, Evanston, IL, 2008, pp. 457–467.)

Supraclavicular approach

The supraclavicular incision is very useful but requires a knowledgeable surgeon to avoid serious injury to important surrounding structures. It is not a surgical exposure to be taken lightly. The surgeon should also think twice about using this exposure if a large hematoma exists as exposure is the key to avoiding collateral injury. If there is significant hematoma in this area, obtaining distal control of the subclavian using an infraclavicular incision more laterally may be more appropriate.

To obtain supraclavicular control of the injured subclavian injury, an incision is made one fingerbreadth above the clavicle. The incision is carried down to the level of the platysma and it is divided using electrocautery. Exposure is maintained using self-retaining retractors. The scalene fat pad is identified and divided along its inferior and lateral margins. After retracting the scalene fat pad medially, the surgeon should attempt to identify the phrenic nerve as it crosses this region from lateral to medial on the anterior surface of the anterior scalene muscle. Once identified, it is retracted laterally by a vessel loop being cautious not to subject it to undo traction. The anterior scalene muscle is identified and divided from its insertion onto the first rib. The surgeon may need to remove a segment of this muscle to improve exposure of the underlying subclavian artery. Caution should also be used not to put undo traction on the brachial plexus where the roots exit the neck and run laterally to form the cords and innervate the arm. A segment

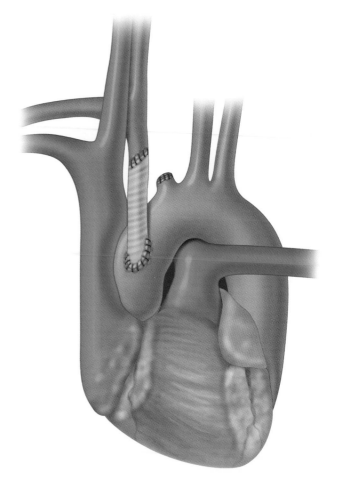

Figure 51.4 Repair of innominate artery injury using aorto-innominate bypass. (From Gillespie D, The management of upper extremity arterial trauma, in Pearce WH et al., eds., *Vascular Surgery in the Endovascular Era*, Greenwood Academic, Evanston, IL, 2008, pp. 457–467.)

of the subclavian artery should be able to me mobilized so as to allow vascular control. Most branches of the subclavian artery can be ligated with the exception of the vertebral artery. This artery should lie at the most medial and cephalad portion of the subclavian artery adjacent from the internal mammary artery. Again the surgeon should exercise caution along the medial aspect of this exposure where the thoracic duct on the left or large lymphatics on the right side reside (Figure 51.6a).

Once the subclavian artery is exposed, the surgeon can consider various methods of repair including lateral suture, ligation and bypass, interposition graft, patch angioplasty or subclavian transposition. The surgeon must consider the extent of injury, the overall status of the patient and the need or availability of conduits to perform the operation. In general there is no difference in long-term patency rate in the subclavian position whether vein or prosthetic is used. Prosthetic is usually larger than the patient's native vein and may be more resistant to infection in the short term. In this case, I usually prefer an 8 mm PTFE externally supported graft (Figure 51.7b). If no conduit is available, the

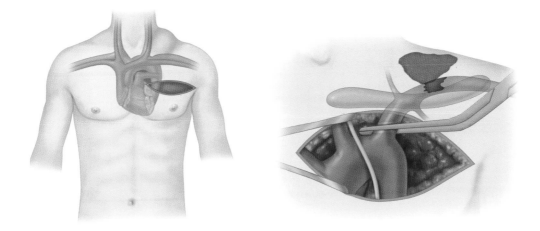

Figure 51.5 Left anterior thoracotomy to obtain proximal control of the left subclavian artery. (From Gillespie D, The management of upper extremity arterial trauma, in Pearce WH et al., eds., *Vascular Surgery in the Endovascular Era*, Greenwood Academic, Evanston, IL, 2008, pp. 457–467.)

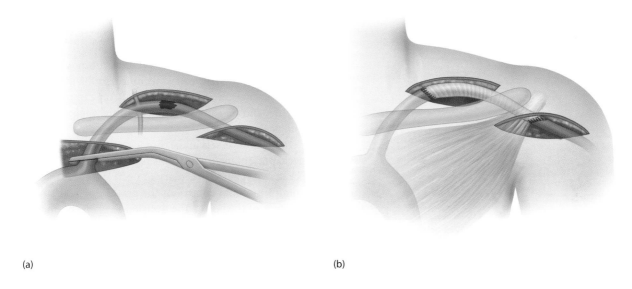

(a)   (b)

Figure 51.6 (a) Supraclavicular exposure of the subclavian injury after left anterior thoracotomy to obtain proximal control. (b) Prosthetic graft interposition repair of subclavian artery injury. (From Gillespie D, The management of upper extremity arterial trauma, in Pearce WH et al., eds., *Vascular Surgery in the Endovascular Era*, Greenwood Academic, Evanston, IL, 2008, pp. 457–467.)

surgeon can consider subclavian artery transposition to the proximal common carotid artery.

Subclavian to carotid transposition is performed by exposing the ipsilateral common carotid through the medial aspect of this same incision (Figure 51.7). The subclavian artery is divided proximal to the vertebral artery. The subclavian artery stump is oversewn using a double suture technique both over and over and vertical mattress. Attention is turned to the exposed common carotid artery taking care to avoid injury to the vagus nerve. No cerebral protection is normally used when operating on the common carotid arteries. As long as the patient has no known carotid disease, the rich collateral network from the external to the internal carotid artery (ICA) should suffice. After obtaining proximal and distal

control, an incision is made in the lateral side of the common carotid and enlarged using a 3–4 mm arterial punch. The subclavian artery is then turned up to and an end-to-side anastomosis is performed using a running 6-0 Prolene suture.

Claviculectomy may be used as an alternate method of exposing distal subclavian artery injuries (Figure 51.8). This exposure has been reported to be associated with minimal blood loss and permits direct repair of complex injuries of the subclavian artery and veins.[37,38] The procedure is relatively straightforward. An incision is made directly over the clavicle. The dissection is carried down to the level of the periosteum using electrocautery. The periosteum is divided longitudinally along the axis of the clavicle. A Gigli saw or equivalent is used to transect the clavicle medially

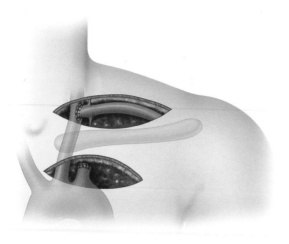

Figure 51.7 Subclavian carotid transposition repair of proximal subclavian injury. (From Gillespie D, The management of upper extremity arterial trauma, in Pearce WH et al., eds., *Vascular Surgery in the Endovascular Era*, Greenwood Academic, Evanston, IL, 2008, pp. 457–467.)

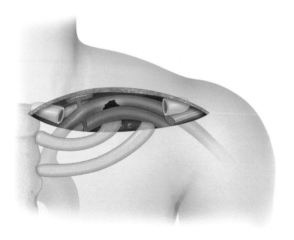

Figure 51.8 Claviculectomy for subclavian artery exposure. (From Gillespie D, The management of upper extremity arterial trauma, in Pearce WH et al., eds., *Vascular Surgery in the Endovascular Era*, Greenwood Academic, Evanston, IL, 2008, pp. 457–467.)

and laterally. This may be more expedient and less morbid than attempting to remove the entire clavicle at the sternum. The underlying scalenus anticus muscle is identified and divided as it inserts on the first rib. The subclavian artery should then be easily exposed and controlled.

Infraclavicular incision

This exposure is normally used either to assist in repairing[39] distal subclavian artery injuries or to gain control of the proximal axillary artery as it exits the thoracic outlet (Figure 51.6). An incision is made about 1 cm inferior to the clavicle over the lateral aspect of the deltopectoral groove. The fibres of the pectoralis major are split and the dissection is carried down to the level of the axillary artery. Arterial control can be obtained at this level to provide distal control of subclavian artery injuries or proximal control of vascular injuries more lateral in the arm. The insertion of the pectoralis major and minor can be preserved or divided to provide more exposure as needed. The surgeon should exercise caution to preserve the adjacent axillary nerve and vein.

OPEN MANAGEMENT OF VASCULAR INJURIES

Brachiocephalic vascular injuries

Most wounds of the cervical vessels and the thoracic outlet are caused by penetrating trauma,[2–5] and the common carotid artery is usually involved, the left more than the right. Special problems are encountered in these patients when there is a vascular injury and a neurological deficit; there may also be wounds of the pharynx, esophagus, trachea and major nerves. The neurological deficit associated with some of these injuries presents a unique and often perplexing problem. Unless technical problems occur during resuscitation and repair, the outcome in most patients will depend on the extent of the initial preoperative neurological deficit (MOP).

Injuries of vessels in the thoracic outlet, at the base of the neck, present major problems regarding surgical exposure, because it may be necessary to open the chest in order to obtain proximal control of the great vessels arising from the arch of the aorta. The decision to open the chest early can be an important part of management. There are a number of vital structures in this area, and the danger of combined injuries of large arteries and veins is apparent. Wounds to vessels in these two areas are considered separately because of the technical requirements (MOP).

Subclavian artery/innominate and venous injury

Subclavian and innominate vascular injuries can present with signs of injury in the thorax, thoracic outlet, cervical or upper extremity. In stable patients, preoperative arteriography greatly improves planning.

The innominate and right subclavian artery injuries are best exposed through a median sternotomy with a right cervical extension incision if needed. Blunt injuries classically involve the proximal innominate artery, and proximal control needs to be obtained at the level of the transverse aortic arch. Simple penetrating injuries to the innominate artery can be closed with running 4-0 polypropylene, but most injuries will require an ascending aorta to distal innominate artery bypass preformed prior to opening and exploring the hematoma and area of injury.

The left subclavian artery is best approached through a combined anterolateral thoracotomy with a separate supraclavicular incision. As a last resort, if better exposure is still required, a 'trap-door' thoracotomy can be performed with the addition of a median sternotomy. The repair of this vessel usually requires a lateral arteriorrhaphy or graft interposition fashioned in an end-to-side manor as a standard end-to-end anastomosis cannot usually be performed. Of note, the subclavian artery is easy to injure, so care should be taken when handling and dissecting this vessel to avoid further blood loss.

CAROTID INJURIES

It is helpful to divide patients with injuries to the carotid arteries into three groups for evaluation: group I, the first and largest group, contains those patients who have injuries of the common and ICA but who have no neurological deficit,[6] group II patients have a mild neurological deficit, and group III patients have a severe neurological deficit, which includes coma and hemiplegia.

A significant number of these patients have other injuries, such as closed-head trauma, which can especially distort the diagnostic picture. Such combined problems are particularly confusing when the indications for surgery are being considered – a precise neurological evaluation is mandatory before an operation is begun. The results of most studies strongly support surgical repair of all penetrating carotid artery injuries in patients who have either no neurological deficit or only a mild one; thus, all the patients in groups I and II would undergo repair of isolated carotid artery wounds.[6–9] This decision is easy to reach when the artery is bleeding briskly, but it may be more difficult to decide what to do when there is a complete carotid artery occlusion without neurological symptoms or occlusion plus a profound stroke. In such a situation, technical problems encountered during surgery could conceivably produce additional brain damage, although in the reported experience, this has been rare.[10–12]

Failure to visualize an artery with arteriograms does not always mean that the vessel is occluded. A very slow flow of blood through a small channel may not be visualized even with good arteriographic techniques, but rapid-sequence CT scanning or nuclear magnetic resonance studies can often clarify such situations. These studies will be especially important in patients who have sustained blunt trauma and in whom there may be hyperextension injuries of the distal ICA. In this situation, the ICA is forcibly stretched over the transverse process of C3 and the body of C2, a mechanism of injury that causes multiple transmural tears that predispose to thromboembolic events. Until a neurological problem appears in these patients, there may be little evidence of carotid artery injury. If such a lesion is untreated, it is likely to progress to complete occlusion, sometimes with extension of the clot into the cerebral arteries, producing a massive stroke.[13] Thromboembolism may supervene; middle cerebral artery emboli have been observed in such patients.

Those signs and symptoms that suggest arterial injury of vessels in the extremities apply equally to the neck, but unfortunately the cervical arteries are not directly accessible for examination of pulses, especially in patients with blunt trauma. Jernigan and Gardner[17] have described features suggesting that the patient has sustained blunt trauma to the carotid artery. There may be very few signs of injury in these people, because less than half of the patients will have superficial evidence of blunt trauma. Unless these patients present with neurological symptoms, blunt trauma to the carotid artery may not be apparent for several hours or much longer in some cases. Preoperative arteriograms are needed in these situations to expose such injuries, and arteriography should be used liberally in patients who have blunt or penetrating trauma to the neck and thoracic outlet.[18] Most major arterial wounds caused by penetrating trauma can be detected by examination, but adjunctive diagnostic studies such as ultrasound and arteriography can be helpful. Arteriograms in trauma patients are usually obtained for one of three reasons: to detect injuries not exposed by other means, to exclude the need for operation when no other indications exist and to plan the operation, especially when special techniques are needed (MOP).

Carotid artery/jugular injury

Surgical exploration of *zone I vascular injuries* requires a median sternotomy. An alternate technique for proximal carotid exposure and control has been described using a neck incision and placement of a Satinsky clamp in the superior mediastinum;[40] however, we favour a median sternotomy as it provide maximal exposure and control. Uncontrollable hemorrhage will continue into the thorax until exposure is attained as most of the proximal vessels are noncompressible. Depending on the patient's clinical course and the availability of a vascular surgeon, proximal control of the great vessels may be performed from a femoral approach with balloon occlusion. Alternatively, if the vessel can be visualized from a cervical approach but is not secured with a vascular clamp, a compliant balloon can be passed retrograde for temporary proximal control. Once the vessel is properly exposed, the balloon can be replaced with the appropriate vascular clamp.

Once initial exposure is obtained, local manual pressure provides adequate hemostasis as more formal proximal and distal control is attained. Depending on the extent of the injury identified, the artery can be repaired primarily with interrupted polypropylene suture, saphenous or PTFE patch angioplasty, interposition reversed saphenous or PTFE, ligation and transposition, ligation and bypass or ligation alone. Saphenous vein is preferred over PTFE due to increased patency rates.[41]

In patients with *penetrating zone II carotid artery injuries* that have an associated neurologic deficit or coma, immediate operative repair is indicated and offers the best and possibly only chance of recovery.[42] Patients presenting with a preoperative GCS of less than 8 are likely to have adverse outcomes regardless of the management of the carotid injury.[43] If the duration of symptoms has been three or more hours or has an established deep coma, emergent head CT should be obtained. If the results of the head CT demonstrate an ischemic infarct, revascularization is contraindicated as has been shown to have a substantial risk of causing a hemorrhagic transformation of the ischemic region.[44]

Patients who have carotid artery injuries and continued prograde blood flow are candidates for surgical repair.[6] A patient who has complete occlusion of the ICA as a result of blunt trauma, who is not bleeding and who has a severe neurological deficit accompanied by coma and hemiplegia may be best treated by non-operative techniques or by ligation of the ICA if operation is required for other reasons. The complete removal of thrombus in these situations is often difficult, and leaving behind residual clots may predispose to embolization, which extends the neurological damage.

With isolated carotid wounds, extensive monitoring is not usually required, but a radial arterial line is helpful for measurements for arterial blood pressure and blood-gas tensions. General anesthesia, hypercapnia and some neurological wounds interfere with cerebral autoregulation, and cerebral blood flow will then respond directly to changes in systemic arterial pressure. The maintenance of normal blood pressure is an important concept in the correct management of these situations. As in almost all cases of cervical trauma, the induction of anesthesia must be accomplished gently to prevent the dislodgment of tamponading clots, which might cause recurrence of bleeding or embolize into the intracranial circulation.[16] A variety of anesthetic agents are effective and safe; the final choice rests with the anesthesiologist. But drugs that are likely to cause hypotension are not desirable and should be avoided. Endotracheal intubation is required in these patients, and preoperative knowledge of laryngeal nerve function is essential; if this information is not known before the patient reaches the OR, the vocal cords can be directly inspected during tracheal intubation. If the wound has not been accurately identified by preoperative arteriography, wide surgical exposure will be needed for exploration. The neurovascular structures are reached through the customary carotid incision made along the anterior border of the sternomastoid muscle, approaching the artery slightly from the anterolateral aspect to initially obtain control of the common carotid artery proximal to the area of suspected injury. Once the arterial wound is exposed, gentle digital pressure will usually control bleeding without clamping the vessel, thus minimizing the time of carotid artery occlusion. Injuries of the external carotid artery are usually clamped and repaired or ligated as indicated, and unless there is evidence that the external carotid artery is functioning as a major cerebral collateral, it often is sacrificed. It is usually neither grafted nor shunted during repair.

Once the bleeding is controlled, the ICA backflow is assessed. Brisk, pulsatile backflow is usually evidence of adequate cerebral perfusion, but measurements of carotid artery stump pressures may be helpful. It has been suggested that back pressures greater than 70 mmHg indicate adequate cerebral perfusion; thus, such patients do not require additional support of cerebral circulation during the period of carotid artery occlusion necessary for repair.[1,12,16] Moreover, if the pressures are above 70 mmHg, the distal carotid cannot be cleared of clots and ligation is necessary; these pressures should be adequate to prevent major stroke unless thromboembolism supervenes.

If the pressures are low or the backflow from the ICA is scanty and shunts are selected, a variety of techniques may be used, but the simple inlying straight-tube shunt is readily available. Unless the patient has multiple injuries or has injuries of the eye or central nervous system or has multiple fractures, most surgeons use systemic heparin when shunts are in place. However, it would seem more important to heparinize the patients if the distal carotid artery was filled with a stagnant pool of blood. Most studies of shunting and intraoperative heparinization during the repair of carotid artery injuries have failed to delineate clearly the need for and results of these maneuvers.[6–8]

In the repair of arterial injuries, standard vascular techniques are used, but because of the importance of securing a smooth intimal surface in the carotid artery, resection and anastomosis are favoured. This is especially important with blunt trauma because the wall damage is likely to be extensive. After resection, a repair without tension is required or an interposition graft is needed. Customarily, the saphenous vein is chosen to restore continuity in the carotid artery. If the defect in the proximal ICA is small, the distal external carotid can be ligated and this vessel substituted for the origin of the ICA, as illustrated in Figure 75.5. If, because of low pressures or scanty backflow, a shunt is selected and a graft is also needed, the graft can be placed over the shunt prior to insertion; the shunt is then removed just before the anastomosis is completed, as shown in Figure 75.6.

Penetrating injuries of the ICA in zone III at the base of the skull is very difficult to expose, but division of the digastric muscle, resection of the styloid process and, on occasion, temporary anterior subluxation of the mandible usually will permit visualization of the carotid as it enters the skull. Lacerations at the carotid foramen that are too high to allow the placement of a vascular clamp distally can be controlled by inserting a balloon-tipped catheter through a separate incision in the artery and then advancing the catheter beyond the laceration and gently inflating the balloon to control soft Fogarty catheters with attached three-way stopcocks, or special balloon occlusion catheters can be used for the carotid artery (these catheters are already in use so there is no need to design new ones).

Blunt carotid injuries are generally caused by an injury mechanism that is associated with combined rotation and either hyperflexion or hyperextension of the neck. Delayed recognition of an occult vascular injury can have disastrous consequences and has been associated with a mortality rate of up to 50%.[45] Patients presenting with physical exam findings worrisome for blunt neck trauma, such as a seatbelt sign, should undergo formal angiographic evaluation of their neck vasculature with either conventional 4 vessel angiography or in most cases multiplanar CTA.[13,46] Most of these lesions can be treated with anticoagulation alone if not contraindicated; however, if there are concurrent symptoms and the lesion is surgically accessible, patients may benefit from exploration and repair.[46] One review of blunt carotid injuries found that all patients could be managed successfully with anticoagulation alone.[47]

Small intimal-based flaps with minimal or no dissection are best managed with antiplatelet therapy or observation with transcranial Doppler examination for embolic potential. Nonocclusive dissections are known to resolve in 70% of patients with anticoagulation therapy alone, with the latter 30% developing pseudoaneurysms. Once pseudoaneurysms develop, they can be the source of thromboembolic events and should be repaired electively. Unfortunately, patients who sustain blunt carotid injuries typically have associated closed-head injuries, solid organ injuries or pelvic fractures that prevent the use of early anticoagulation.[48]

VERTEBRAL ARTERY INJURIES

Wounds of the vertebral arteries are rare; these vessels, which enter the bony canal at the C6 level and exit at C2, are apparently protected from many injuries. In the past, without preoperative arteriograms, vertebral artery damage was probably undetected unless discovered because of bleeding during exploration. Treatment consisted of proximal ligation, packing and, on rare occasions, direct exposure and suture ligation.[11,12,15]

Since preoperative arteriography is now employed more frequently to assess the damage accurately and to evaluate the collateral circulation, more vertebral artery wounds will probably be discovered.[12] Direct repair, even in the bony canal, is possible with modern vascular techniques. A penetrating injury to a dominant or single vertebral artery should be considered for repair. Continued bleeding and the late development of a false aneurysm or arteriovenous fistula are serious complications of such wounds. Traumatic occlusion of a small vertebral artery in a patient with normal connections into the circle of Willis is not likely to cause serious problems and usually can be left alone. In such circumstances, treatment at operation customarily would be ligation only; therefore, the patient can be spared a rather difficult surgical exposure. With multiple injuries (carotid and vertebral), carotid repair is more important; if the patient has the more common cerebral vascular architecture, this should suffice.[1,16] In some patients, the vertebral artery may be occluded by a percutaneously placed balloon to control bleeding (*MOP*).

ENDOVASCULAR MANAGEMENT OF THORACIC OUTLET AND NECK VASCULAR TRAUMA

General principles of endovascular management of vascular trauma

Thoracic vascular trauma carries a high mortality rate.[48] The utility of endovascular techniques in the management of penetrating thoracic trauma is limited to patients presenting with hemodynamic stability, and the foundation for the repair of these injuries should rely on standard open surgical approaches.[48] Visionaries in vascular surgery first conceptualized the use of stent grafts in the treatment of vascular disease in 1969,[49] with the first case report in 1991.[50] In a series of papers in the early 1990s, Marin and Veith describe a series of patients in whom covered stents had been fashioned and successfully deployed for the treatment of vascular trauma.[30,51,52]

The early mortality benefit of endovascular therapy for elective vascular procedures has led centres of excellence to adopt these techniques for emergent aortic repair. Endovascular techniques when applied in the correct setting have the potential to minimize the physiologic burden placed on patients who have very little physiologic reserve. Modern techniques and technology have become more accessible and there is no longer a reliance on homemade covered stent grafts as they are not commercially available. As a result, the majority of pseudoaneurysms are treated with self-expanding covered stents for both blunt and penetrating trauma.[53-57] Covered stent grafts have expanded the possible treatment options for vessel injury, and potential roles are well described in the literature.[58-60] There is a large body of literature regarding the management of acute traumatic vascular injuries involving traditional open surgical techniques.

The application of endovascular technology to the management of penetrating and blunt traumatic vascular injuries represents an exciting and significant advance in modern trauma centres and has been used with increasing frequency for the management of vascular trauma. The diagnosis and management of vascular injuries have rapidly evolved with innovative imaging technology. Catheter-based applications have been used frequently in trauma patients, mostly by surgeons previously familiar with basic access techniques and static film arteriography.[24,58] Specialized training in the last decade has integrated catheter skills to the point that modern management of traumatic vascular injuries can often incorporate sophisticated endovascular therapies. These concepts were originally promoted in urban trauma centres.[52] The endovascular management of vascular trauma seems particularly appealing in the management of blunt truncal injuries, especially in the setting of severe concomitant brain and lung injuries. Utilization of these techniques to stabilize patients in extremis or in serving as a bridge to definitive repair in a controlled setting represents an attractive adjuvant and/or alternative to conventional surgery alone with the potential to lower morbidity and mortality rates. It is of extreme importance that experienced providers perform these procedures in an environment capable of supporting such complex interventions. A variety of devices must be readily available for use in addition to easy access to the imaging technology required to make endovascular interventions possible. In setting where these circumstances cannot be met, such complex interventions have the potential of causing harm and should not be performed.

In unstable patients, there are few options other than immediate exploration, but because of the fibrous attachments surrounding the subclavian vessels, injuries frequently result in contained extrapleural hematoma that may extend into the supraclavicular fossa. If time allows, CTA can be invaluable for identifying the location of injury and evaluating the mediastinum. Benefits of placement of an occlusion balloon in the proximal end of the damaged vessel include control of hemorrhage and ability to perform angiography. However, endovascular techniques may be used as an adjunct to support the standard open repair of these injuries. Zone I injuries with hard signs of vascular injury may have an enlarging hematoma at the thoracic inlet, high output from a chest tube or shock. These injuries notoriously involve the great vessels. Immediate control involves a high anterior thoracotomy, sternotomy or clavicular resection to obtain adequate proximal control. Once the patient is prepared in the OR, an occlusion balloon can be used from the groin to provide endoluminal proximal control of the great vessels allowing conduct of a surgical exposure in a more controlled fashion to ensue. With an occlusion balloon in place, arteriography can locate the injury and allow for further operative planning. After the injury is exposed, a vascular clamp may be place in relief to the occlusion balloon if exposure is adequate.

There should be concern about the unknown long-term outcome of covered stents trauma as minimal long-term follow-up data are available. Stent grafts placed in the thoracic vascular trauma have the possibility for compression and collapse. This raises concern about long-term patency in the young trauma population; it is imperative to follow these patients for late complications. Alternatively, at a later date when the hematoma and edema have resolved, the stent can be explanted with a formal open repair; this approach would ideally reduce the potential for iatrogenic nerve injury in the acute setting and delay open repair. Finally, patients can be longitudinally followed and complications addressed as they arise. Endovascular therapy in thoracic vascular trauma offers a less invasive, rapid treatment and has the added benefit of avoiding the added stress of open surgery that may otherwise make repair unsurvivable in some.

Carotid injuries

In patients with soft signs of vascular injury and hemodynamic stability, a full preoperative workup can be completed. Imaging studies can reveal intimal flaps, dissection, pseudoaneurysm, transection or intramural hematoma.

Operative repair of these lesions has been shown to reduce mortality and stroke rates for both penetrating and blunt traumas when compared to observation or ligation.[42] The natural history of nonocclusive dissections appears to be resolution in about two-thirds of patients, but approximately one-third will go on to develop pseudoaneurysms and can be a source of thromboembolic disease.[61,62] Many of these lesions are amenable to endovascular treatment, and while there is not a comparative study of endovascular repair to open, there are several case series demonstrating feasibility and safety with successful interventions.

Symptomatic traumatic dissections of the carotid in patients that have a contraindication to anticoagulation have been successfully treated with carotid stent placement.[63,64] Thrombosis and thromboembolic events remain a concern after endovascular management of carotid trauma, but this appears to be a rare event. The results of small numbers of case series are difficult to interpret due to the low number of patients and limited follow-up, but it appears that adjuvant anticoagulation in the form of, at a minimum, one antiplatelet agent for at least 6 weeks is required for stent patency. As a result, patients who have contraindications to anticoagulation may have limited patency when compared to traditional open repair.

Axillary and subclavian artery injury

Managing injuries to the thoracic outlet often require incisions that have the potential for profound morbidity. Many injuries in this location are fortunately contained hematomas that allow for definitive diagnosis and a tempered approach to treatment. This period of stability creates a window where successful planning and execution of endovascular interventions can occur. There are several reports in the literature of successful management of supra-aortic trunk injury to the innominate, carotid and subclavian arteries without the need to perform thoracotomy or sternotomy.[59,65,66] A review of the literature finds an ever increasing number of reports on the use of endovascular techniques for the management of upper extremity trauma.[24,30,58,66–74] This is especially important for injuries to the subclavian artery where exposure is difficult, time consuming and potentially morbid. The first report of this application is attributed to Marin et al.[30] In this article, the authors state that patency up to 14 months was achieved (mean follow-up 6.5 months) with these stented grafts. They found that the use of stented grafts appears to be associated with decreased blood loss, a less invasive insertion procedure, reduced requirements for anesthesia and a limited need for an extensive dissection in the traumatized field. More recently, this method of management has been used to treat more devastating military injuries both for acute trauma[68] and for the management of pseudoaneurysms diagnosed late.[24] Interestingly, these stent grafts have also been reported to be used for the management of concomitant subclavian vein injuries in Iraq.

Vascular access is obtained either at the common femoral or brachial artery in a standard fashion. After placement of a 5 Fr short sheath for access, a diagnostic arteriogram is obtained. When performed from a femoral approach, a guidewire is placed into the aorta and followed by a 4 Fr pigtail catheter. The catheter is advanced to the root of the aorta to perform a diagnostic arch aortogram. Using a digital subtraction C-arm and a power injector with an injection protocol of 20/40 at 900 psi, the study is obtained. Either the innominate artery or left subclavian artery is selected. If unable to select using the pigtail catheter, the surgeon can choose another catheter such as 4 Fr angled glide catheter. Once selected, an injection protocol of 3/6 should demonstrate the site of the traumatic arteriotomy.

If approached from a retrograde approach, the initial step after obtaining access is crossing the lesion. With placement of a sheath in the brachial artery, there is often arm with no antegrade flow. As a result, diagnostic angiography is performed with low volumes of contrast as in the lower extremity. At our institution, runs are performed through the sidearm of the introducer sheath at volumes of 3 cc/second for a total volume of 6 cc of ½ strength contrast. If inadequate images are obtained, either full strength of larger volumes can be used. If contrast extravasated, further imaging and interventions can be severely hindered. At this point, it should be noted that the surgeon has no proximal control. Often these lesions do take some effort to cross and occasionally the wire will enter into extraluminal planes. The benefit of the retrograde approach is more control over catheters and wires as the working distance is significantly shorter. When the lesion is crossed, catheters and wires should be exchanged in the standard fashion to build a sturdy endovascular platform as a basis for intervention.

Placement of a covered stent across this injury should provide adequate control and allow stabilization of the patient. Preplacement measurements are made in an attempt to preserve the vertebral artery and not cross the sternoclavicular or acromio-clavicular joints. We typically will use a 6–8 × 24–50 cm Viabahn™ (Gore) or Fluency™ (BARD) stent graft. The delivery catheter length on these stent grafts is often limiting 80–110 cm; therefore, brachial artery access is preferred. Heparinization of the patient at 50–100 units/kg can be considered if the patient is stable and has a single injury. If, however, the patient has multisystem injury, is coagulopathic or has suffered large blood loss, no anticoagulation is given. The selected device is delivered to the zone of injury over the wire and a final positioning digital subtraction arteriogram is obtained. Once placement is confirmed, the device is delivered and a completion arteriogram is performed. On occasion to insure more accurate placement and collateral vessel preservation one could consider using two shorter stent grafts and overlapping them (Figure 51.9).

The results of a multicentre trial that evaluated the use of commercially available covered stents in the treatment of first-order branch arteries support the use of this technology when compared to open surgery.[59] A limiting factor for this study was that the etiology of injury that prompted the use of stents in this study is not similar to that reported in prior reports on vascular trauma, with 78% the result of iatrogenesis. In this study, 29% of the injuries treated were subclavian. With the placement of a covered stent graft, 85% of patients had avoided the OR at 1 year of follow-up. The results of this study should be interpreted with caution as the etiology of vascular injury is very different from that of true vascular trauma, and as the results are likely not translatable to real-world vascular trauma.

Post-operative care

Patients should be followed indefinitely for the development of complications. Bypasses should receive routine surveillance, as secondary interventions may be needed

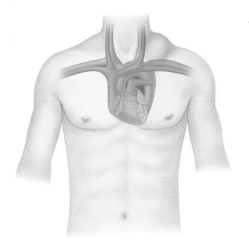
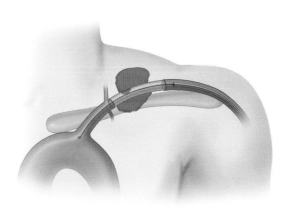

Figure 51.9 Endovascular approach using covered stent to exclude injury to left subclavian artery. (From Gillespie D, The management of upper extremity arterial trauma, in Pearce WH et al., eds., *Vascular Surgery in the Endovascular Era*, Greenwood Academic, Evanston, IL, 2008, pp. 457–467.)

in the future. Special attention should be placed on observation of the potential for infection-related complications that can range from graft thrombosis to rupture and death. In addition, pseudoaneurysm formation can be the source of thromboembolism. Most of these complications can be identified and intervened upon prior to complication.

CONCLUSION

The incidence trauma in the United States continues to increase. The development of catheter-based techniques for the treatment of vascular injuries has been revolutionary. While current reports show these techniques to be successful acutely, there are relatively little long-term data on the use of covered stents for the treatment of vascular injuries. In addition, the widespread use of endovascular therapies for the treatment of innominate vein or artery injuries has not been reported. Finally, the widespread availability of stent grafts and radiographic equipment for the use in emergency situations is still in the process of evolving. As such, even in the era of endovascular surgery, vascular surgeons must maintain their familiarity with open approaches to repairing vascular injuries. Our profession must remain vigilant and provide the best care for the vascularly injured patient that we can. This will only come about by recognizing vascular trauma as a priority for both training and maintenance of both open and endovascular surgical skill sets.

REFERENCES

1. Rice DP, MacKenzie EJ, Jones AS et al. Cost of injury in the United States: A report to Congress. Institute for Health and Aging, University of California and Injury Prevention Center, The Johns Hopkins University, Baltimore, MD, 1989.
2. Gupta R, Rao S, Sieunarine K. An epidemiological view of vascular trauma in Western Australia: A 5-year study. *ANZ J Surg.* 2001;71(8):461–466.
3. Demetriades D, Charalambides D, Lakhoo M. Physical examination and selective conservative management in patients with penetrating injuries of the neck. *Br J Surg.* 1993;80(12):1534–1536.
4. Feliciano DV, Bitondo CG, Mattox KL et al. Combined tracheoesophageal injuries. *Am J Surg.* 1985;150(6):710–715.
5. Symbas PN, Hatcher CR Jr., Vlasis SE. Esophageal gunshot injuries. *Ann Surg.* 1980;191(6):703–707.
6. Fox CJ, Gillespie DL, Cox ED et al. Damage control resuscitation for vascular surgery in a combat support hospital. *J Trauma.* 2008;65(1):1–9.
7. Hogan AR, Lineen EB, Perez EA et al. Value of computed tomographic angiography in neck and extremity pediatric vascular trauma. *J Pediatr Surg.* 2009;44(6):1236–1241; discussion 1241.
8. Scaglione M, Pinto A, Pinto F et al. Role of contrast-enhanced helical CT in the evaluation of acute thoracic aortic injuries after blunt chest trauma. *Eur Radiol.* 2001;11(12):2444–2448.
9. White PW, Gillespie DL, Feurstein I et al. Sixty-four slice multidetector computed tomographic angiography in the evaluation of vascular trauma. *J Trauma.* 2010;68(1):96–102.
10. Conrad MF, Patton JH Jr., Parikshak M et al. Evaluation of vascular injury in penetrating extremity trauma: Angiographers stay home. *Am Surg.* 2002;68(3):269–274.
11. Lineen EB, Faresi M, Ferrari M et al. Computed tomographic angiography in pediatric blunt traumatic vascular injury. *J Pediatr Surg.* 2008;43(3):549–554.
12. Burack JH, Kandil E, Sawas A et al. Triage and outcome of patients with mediastinal penetrating trauma. *Ann Thorac Surg.* 2007;83(2):377–382; discussion 382.
13. Ofer A, Nitecki SS, Braun J et al. CT angiography of the carotid arteries in trauma to the neck. *Eur J Vasc Endovasc Surg.* 2001;21(5):401–407.
14. Fox CJ, Starnes BW. Vascular surgery on the modern battlefield. *Surg Clin North Am.* 2007;87(5):1193–1211, xi.
15. Rotondo MF, Schwab CW, McGonigal MD et al. 'Damage control': An approach for improved survival in exsanguinating penetrating abdominal injury. *J Trauma.* 1993;35(3):375–382; discussion 382–383.
16. Beekley AC, Watts DM. Combat trauma experience with the United States Army 102nd Forward Surgical Team in Afghanistan. *Am J Surg.* 2004;187(5):652–654.
17. Goaley TJ, Dente CJ, Feliciano DV. Torso vascular trauma at an urban level I trauma center. *Perspect Vasc Surg Endovasc Ther.* 2006;18(2):102–112.
18. Quan RW, Adams ED, Cox MW et al. The management of trauma venous injury: Civilian and wartime experiences. *Perspect Vasc Surg Endovasc Ther.* 2006;18(2):149–156.
19. Adar R, Schramek A, Khodadadi J et al. Arterial combat injuries of the upper extremity. *J Trauma.* 1980;20(4):297–302.
20. Andreev A, Kavrakov T, Karakolev J et al. Management of acute arterial trauma of the upper extremity. *Eur J Vasc Surg.* 1992;6(6):593–598.
21. Bongard F, Dubrow T, Klein S. Vascular injuries in the urban battleground: Experience at a metropolitan trauma center. *Ann Vasc Surg.* 1990;4(5):415–418.
22. Diamond S, Gaspard D, Katz S. Vascular injuries to the extremities in a suburban trauma center. *Am Surg.* 2003;69(10):848–851.
23. Fitridge RA, Raptis S, Miller JH et al. Upper extremity arterial injuries: Experience at the Royal Adelaide Hospital, 1969 to 1991. *J Vasc Surg.* 1994;20(6):941–946.
24. Fox CJ, Gillespie DL, O'Donnell SD et al. Contemporary management of wartime vascular trauma. *J Vasc Surg.* 2005;41(4):638–644.

25. Graham JM, Feliciano DV, Mattox KL et al. Management of subclavian vascular injuries. *J Trauma.* 1980;20(7):537–544.

26. Graham JM, Mattox KL, Feliciano DV et al. Vascular injuries of the axilla. *Ann Surg.* 1982;195(2):232–238.

27. Hyre CE, Cikrit DF, Lalka SG et al. Aggressive management of vascular injuries of the thoracic outlet. *J Vasc Surg.* 1998;27(5):880–884; discussion 884–885.

28. Katras T, Baltazar U, Rush DS et al. Subclavian arterial injury associated with blunt trauma. *Vasc Surg.* 2001;35(1):43–50.

29. Lin PH, Koffron AJ, Guske PJ et al. Penetrating injuries of the subclavian artery. *Am J Surg.* 2003;185(6):580–584.

30. Marin ML, Veith FJ, Panetta TF et al. Transluminally placed endovascular stented graft repair for arterial trauma. *J Vasc Surg.* 1994;20(3):466–472; discussion 472–473.

31. Nanobashvili J, Kopadze T, Tvaladze M et al. War injuries of major extremity arteries. *World J Surg.* 2003;27(2):134–139.

32. Pillai L, Luchette FA, Romano KS et al. Upper-extremity arterial injury. *Am Surg.* 1997;63(3):224–227.

33. Rich NM, Hobson RW, Jarstfer BS et al. Subclavian artery trauma. *J Trauma.* 1973;13(6):485–496.

34. Sturm JT, Dorsey JS, Olson FR et al. The management of subclavian artery injuries following blunt thoracic trauma. *Ann Thorac Surg.* 1984;38(3):188–191.

35. Weber MA, Fox CJ, Adams E et al. Upper extremity arterial combat injury management. *Perspect Vasc Surg Endovasc Ther.* 2006;18(2):141–145.

36. Gillespie D. The management of upper extremity arterial trauma. In: Pearce WH, Matsumura JS, Yao JST, eds. *Vascular Surgery in the Endovascular Era.* Evanston, IL: Greenwood Academic; 2008, pp. 457–467.

37. Buscaglia LC, Walsh JC, Wilson JD et al. Surgical management of subclavian artery injury. *Am J Surg.* 1987;154(1):88–92.

38. George SM Jr., Croce MA, Fabian TC et al. Cervicothoracic arterial injuries: Recommendations for diagnosis and management. *World J Surg.* 1991;15(1):134–139; discussion 139–140.

39. Wall MJ Jr., Granchi T, Liscum K et al. Penetrating thoracic vascular injuries. *Surg Clin North Am.* 1996;76(4):749–761.

40. Feliciano DV. Management of penetrating injuries to carotid artery. *World J Surg.* 2001;25(8):1028–1035.

41. Becquemin JP, Cavillon A, Brunel M et al. Polytetrafluoroethylene grafts for carotid repair. *Cardiovasc Surg.* 1996;4(6):740–745.

42. Ramadan F, Rutledge R, Oller D et al. Carotid artery trauma: A review of contemporary trauma center experiences. *J Vasc Surg.* 1995;21(1):46–55; discussion 55–56.

43. Teehan EP, Padberg FT Jr., Thompson PN et al. Carotid arterial trauma: Assessment with the Glasgow Coma Scale (GCS) as a guide to surgical management. *Cardiovasc Surg.* 1997;5(2):196–200.

44. Murray JA, Demetriades D, Asensio JA. Carotid injury: Postrevascularization hemorrhagic infarction. *J Trauma.* 1996;41(4):760–762.

45. Rozycki GS, Tremblay L, Feliciano DV et al. A prospective study for the detection of vascular injury in adult and pediatric patients with cervicothoracic seat belt signs. *J Trauma.* 2002;52(4):618–623; discussion 623–624.

46. Biffl WL, Moore EE, Offner PJ et al. Blunt carotid and vertebral arterial injuries. *World J Surg.* 2001;25(8):1036–1043.

47. Fabian TC, Patton JH Jr., Croce MA et al. Blunt carotid injury. Importance of early diagnosis and anticoagulant therapy. *Ann Surg* 1996;223(5):513–522; discussion 522–525.

48. Arthurs ZM, Sohn VY, Starnes BW. Vascular trauma: Endovascular management and techniques. *Surg Clin North Am.* 2007;87(5):1179–1192, x–xi.

49. Dotter CT. Transluminally-placed coilspring endarterial tube grafts. Long-term patency in canine popliteal artery. *Invest Radiol.* 1969;4(5):329–332.

50. Volodos NL, Karpovich IP, Troyan VI et al. Clinical experience of the use of self-fixing synthetic prostheses for remote endoprosthetics of the thoracic and the abdominal aorta and iliac arteries through the femoral artery and as intraoperative endoprosthesis for aorta reconstruction. *Vasa Suppl.* 1991;33:93–95.

51. Marin ML, Veith FJ, Panetta TF et al. Percutaneous transfemoral insertion of a stented graft to repair a traumatic femoral arteriovenous fistula. *J Vasc Surg.* 1993;18(2):299–302.

52. Marin ML, Veith FJ. Clinical application of endovascular grafts in aortoiliac occlusive disease and vascular trauma. *Cardiovasc Surg.* 1995;3(2):115–120.

53. Coldwell DM, Novak Z, Ryu RK et al. Treatment of posttraumatic internal carotid arterial pseudoaneurysms with endovascular stents. *J Trauma.* 2000;48(3):470–472.

54. Duane TM, Parker F, Stokes GK et al. Endovascular carotid stenting after trauma. *J Trauma.* 2002;52(1):149–153.

55. Ellis PK, Kennedy PT, Barros D'Sa AA. Successful exclusion of a high internal carotid pseudoaneurysm using the Wallgraft endoprosthesis. *Cardiovasc Intervent Radiol.* 2002;25(1):68–69.

56. McNeil JD, Chiou AC, Gunlock MG et al. Successful endovascular therapy of a penetrating zone III internal carotid injury. *J Vasc Surg.* 2002;36(1):187–190.

57. Wyers MC, Powell RJ. Management of carotid injuries in a hostile neck using endovascular grafts. *J Vasc Surg.* 2004;39(6):1335–1339.

58. Starnes BW, Arthurs ZM. Endovascular management of vascular trauma. *Perspect Vasc Surg Endovasc Ther.* 2006;18(2):114–129.

59. White R, Krajcer Z, Johnson M et al. Results of a multicenter trial for the treatment of traumatic vascular injury with a covered stent. *J Trauma.* 2006;60(6):1189–1195; discussion 1195–1196.

60. Lin PH, Bush RL, Zhou W et al. Endovascular treatment of traumatic thoracic aortic injury – Should this be the new standard of treatment? *J Vasc Surg.* 2006;43 Suppl A:22A–29A.

61. Duke BJ, Ryu RK, Coldwell DM et al. Treatment of blunt injury to the carotid artery by using endovascular stents: An early experience. *J Neurosurg.* 1997;87(6):825–829.

62. Pretre R, Kürsteiner K, Reverdin A et al. Blunt carotid artery injury: Devastating consequences of undetected pseudoaneurysm. *J Trauma.* 1995;39(5):1012–1014.

63. Cohen JE, Ben-Hur T, Rajz G et al. Endovascular stent-assisted angioplasty in the management of traumatic internal carotid artery dissections. *Stroke* 2005;36(4):e45–e47.

64. Kerby JD, May AK, Gomez CR et al. Treatment of bilateral blunt carotid injury using percutaneous angioplasty and stenting: Case report and review of the literature. *J Trauma.* 2000;49(4):784–787.

65. Becker GJ, Benenati JF, Zemel G et al. Percutaneous placement of a balloon-expandable intraluminal graft for life-threatening subclavian arterial hemorrhage. *J Vasc Interv Radiol.* 1991;2(2):225–229.

66. Patel AV, Marin ML, Veith FJ et al. Endovascular graft repair of penetrating subclavian artery injuries. *J Endovasc Surg.* 1996;3(4):382–388.

67. Aerts NR, Poli de Figueiredo LF, Burihan E. Emergency room retrograde transbrachial arteriography for the management of axillosubclavian vascular injuries. *J Trauma.* 2003;55(1):69–73.

68. Clouse WD, Rasmussen TE, Perlstein J et al. Upper extremity vascular injury: A current in-theater wartime report from Operation Iraqi Freedom. *Ann Vasc Surg.* 2006;20(4):429–434.

69. Danetz JS, Cassano AD, Stoner MC et al. Feasibility of endovascular repair in penetrating axillosubclavian injuries: A retrospective review. *J Vasc Surg.* 2005;41(2):246–254.

70. Dinkel HP, Eckstein FS, Triller J et al. Emergent axillary artery stent-graft placement for massive hemorrhage from an avulsed subscapular artery. *J Endovasc Ther.* 2002;9(1):129–133.

71. McArthur CS, Marin ML. Endovascular therapy for the treatment of arterial trauma. *Mt Sinai J Med.* 2004;71(1):4–11.

72. Ohki T, Veith FJ, Kraas C et al. Endovascular therapy for upper extremity injury. *Semin Vasc Surg.* 1998;11(2):106–115.

73. Ohki T, Veith FJ, Marin ML et al. Endovascular approaches for traumatic arterial lesions. *Semin Vasc Surg.* 1997;10(4):272–285.

74. Valentin MD, Tulsyan N, James K. Endovascular management of traumatic axillary artery dissection – A case report and review of the literature. *Vasc Endovascular Surg.* 2004;38(5):473–475.

52

Vascular injuries of the extremities

W. DARRIN CLOUSE

CONTENTS

INTRODUCTION

Injuries to the blood vessels in the extremities continue to present significant challenges to surgeons. As with other vascular injuries, there is a severity spectrum depending upon mechanism, anatomic location, temporal circumstances, care available and concomitant injuries. Laceration, complete and partial transection, contusion with or without secondary wall/intimal defect, secondary aneurysm, pseudoaneurysm, arteriovenous fistula, tapered lesions and external compression in the perivascular space may all be at play from blunt, penetrating, blast or combined mechanism. How to manage each particular incident of extremity vascular injury can be quite different depending on these features. As the spectrum noted earlier evolves, repair and management become more complicated. Life-threatening hemorrhage may occur. Tissue ischemia, particularly as it is prolonged, may lead to ischemic neuropathy/plexopathy, compartment syndromes and muscular contracture or necrosis. Associated direct injuries to the nerves, bones and soft tissues may also contribute to pain and dysfunction and ultimately dictate the fate of the limb. Efforts pursuing limb salvage in order to restore vascular integrity and neuromuscular function may fail. In some instances, secondary amputation after salvage attempt is required either in the acute setting or in the chronic phase after injury. Furthermore, primary amputation as initial treatment is a consideration in instances where salvage will provide less functionality than amputation, or where the physiologic insult will be poorly tolerated and might be life-threatening. Heroic efforts focused on reconstruction, and limb salvage alone does not necessarily provide superior quality of life for all patients.

Today, advancements in modern imaging technologies, progress in critical care and hemostasis, acceptance of damage control principles and the revolution in endovascular therapies have provided a contemporary perspective on extremity injuries. Recent large-scale military conflict (Operation Iraqi Freedom [OIF] and Operation Enduring Freedom [OEF]) has yet again provided impetus and experience inspiring concentrated study and reflection on extremity vascular injury in both civilian and military settings. Along with the experiences and principles of the past, these newer insights have provided a platform for revisiting extremity vascular injury recognition, diagnosis and management. The aim of this chapter is to review long-standing principles, as well as contemporary discussions, surrounding the treatment approach to traumatic vascular injury in the extremities attentive to optimizing repair success and limb salvage. It is recognized that the presentation, population and trauma care structure make high-quality evidence difficult to provide for vascular injury. The discussions herein emanate from several small level 2 case–control retrospective studies, animal basic experimental studies and level 3 (observational analysis) and level 4 (expert opinion) literature. Thus, recommendations that were given are from the author's assimilation of data, participation in these studies and clinical experience in Iraq, Afghanistan and level I trauma centres across the United States (grades C and D).

EPIDEMIOLOGY, AMPUTATION AND MORTALITY

Civilian

Within civilian series, the overall rate of vascular injury remains low representing a mere 1%–4% of injured patients.[1,2] The extremities have long been known to be the location most often affected by vascular injury accounting for 40%–80% of arterial injuries identified depending upon the circumstances of the reported series.[1–3] Extremity injury appears to occur relatively equally in the upper and lower extremities with perhaps a slight increase in upper extremity injury recently.[1–6] Mortality from extremity vascular injury, even in isolated cases, can approach 5%–10% depending upon the vessels injured.[3,5,7–12] Kauvar and colleagues queried the National Trauma Data Bank (NTDB) from January 2002 to December 2005 and identified 651 isolated lower extremity vascular injuries and found a mortality of 2.8% with amputation occurring in 6.5%.[12] The more proximal the arterial injury, the higher the mortality as common femoral artery (CFA) injuries led to an 8% mortality. Mortality was significantly higher with injury to common femoral and superficial femoral arteries compared to popliteal and distal vessels (4.8% vs. 1.4%; p = 0.02) (Figure 52.1a). Nearly 80% of deaths were from penetrating injury. On the other hand, amputation occurred more commonly with injury to the popliteal and tibial arteries compared to the femoral arteries (8.3% vs. 4.1%; p = 0.03). Amputation occurred twice as often when the mechanism of injury was blunt (9.1% vs. 5.1%; p = 0.05) (Figure 52.1b).

Recent meta-analysis of almost 3200 lower extremity vascular injuries reported factors associated with secondary amputation after arterial repair.[13] Based upon which factors were delineated within subsets of this cohort, significant prognostic factors heightening amputation risk were soft tissue injury (26% vs. 8%; OR 5.8), compartment syndrome (28% vs. 6%; OR 5.1), multiple arterial injuries (18% vs. 9%; OR 4.9) and ischemia over 6 hours (24% vs. 5%; OR 4.4). Mechanism of injury was also significant as blast and blunt injuries led to amputation more than penetrating injury (19% vs. 15% vs. 5%, respectively). Age over 55 was also an important characteristic as was

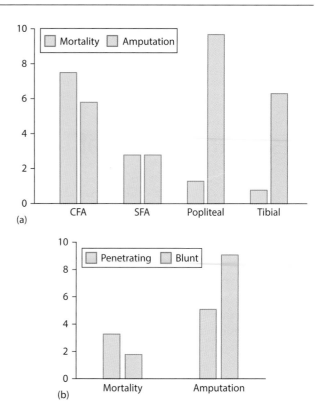

Figure 52.1 (a) Mortality rates and amputation rates by anatomic injury level in isolated lower extremity arterial injuries. (b) In these patients, mortality and amputation rates by general mechanism of injury. (From Kauvar DS et al., *J Vasc Surg*, 53, 1598, 2011.)

the central proximity of injury. Secondary amputation occurred in 18% of iliac, 14% of popliteal and 10% of tibial injuries, while femoral artery injuries led to amputation in only 4%. While most of these factors are indeed what is appreciated on an experiential level across trauma centres, this helps provide perspective on just the impact these features may have.

Injuries to upper extremity arteries in the civilian setting less commonly lead to death or amputation.[3,5,7] The more proximal the injury, the higher the risk of amputation or death. Tan and colleagues queried the NTDB investigating over 8000 civilian extremity arterial injuries to compare lower extremity (LE) and upper extremity (UE) outcomes.[5] They describe LE injury more commonly resulting from blunt mechanisms and UE injury more likely penetrating in nature. LE injury was independently associated with increased mortality (OR 2.2; p < 0.0001) and risk for amputation (OR 4.3; p < 0.0001). This relationship was maintained when stratified by type of mechanism. Blunt mechanism portended higher mortality and amputation (Figure 52.2). Overall, mortality was 2.2% in UE injuries versus 7.7% in those of the LE (p < 0.0001). Amputation occurred in 7.8% of LE injuries compared to only 1.3% of UE arterial injuries (p < 0.0001).

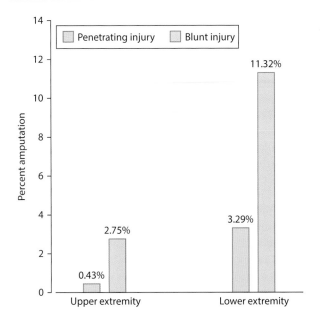

Figure 52.2 Comparative amputation rates by upper and lower extremity arterial injury stratified by mechanism of injury. (From Tan TW et al., *Vasc Endovasc Surg*, 45, 592, 2011.)

Military

Rates of vascular injury during military operations have been a point of interest throughout documented history. Modern assessment began when DeBakey and Simeone reported an identified arterial injury rate of 0.96% in World War II.[14] Accounts from the Korean War cited rates of 1%–3%.[15] Recent data show the rate of vascular injury during war appears to have increased from 2% to 3% of battle-related injuries during the Vietnam War to 4%–12% during the Wars in Iraq and Afghanistan.[16,17] Over 2004–2006 in Balad, Iraq, using a cohort of 6800

casualties with nearly 350 vascular injuries, we documented an incidence of vascular injury (4.8%), the accompanying operative mortality (4.3%) and early amputation rate (6.6%).[18,19] Extremity injuries accounted for 75% of vascular reconstructions performed. This was significantly expanded by White et al. who, using the tools of the Joint Theater Trauma System/Joint Theater Trauma Registry (JTTS/JTTR), were able to more precisely describe this apparent augmentation in vascular injury rates.[17] Between January 2002 and September 2009, over 13,000 battle-related injuries occurred in US troops. Of these, 12% had identified vascular injuries documented and 9% underwent operative intervention for these injuries. Extremity vascular injury accounted for 79% of identified injuries with distal arterial injury in the forearm or tibial vessels accounting for 40%. Only 12% of injuries were in the torso and 8% cervical (Figure 52.3). This clear temporal uptick in vascular injury identification is most likely due to modern casualty care strategy and tactics with better battlefield evacuation, forward surgical assets and newer diagnostic modalities.[18,19]

Improvised explosive devices (IEDs) and gunshot wounds have produced the majority of documented vascular injuries. Similar to reports since World War II, nearly 70% are injured by explosive fragmentation and 30% by gunshot wounds.[17,20] Most are young (mean age, 24 years [19–64]), and over 95% are men.[20] We have reported observed differences in the proportion of extremity and truncal vascular injury between US forces and the local population. Extremity injury was higher amongst US casualties (81% vs. 70%; p = 0.02) and truncal vascular injury more frequent in the local population (4 vs. 13%; p = 0.004) indicating that body armouring technologies do reduce central injury.[18]

Upper extremity injuries should not be underestimated during conflict. They often entail significant transfusion

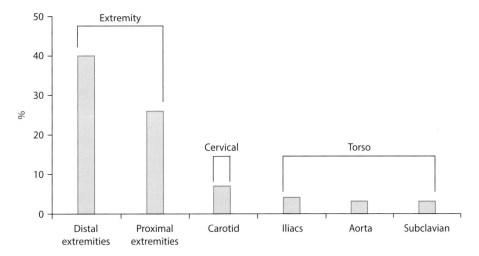

Figure 52.3 Distribution of identified vascular injury in US forces during Operation Iraqi Freedom and Operation Enduring Freedom noting the high prominence of extremity injury. (From White JM et al., *Ann Surg*, 253, 1184, 2011.)

requirements and require special technical considerations, such as creative graft tunnelling, due to the degree of wounding in an overall smaller area of tissue. Although lower extremity vascular injury occurs more frequently during armed conflict, upper limb loss has been suggested to be more substantial than previously documented and found in civilian injury. This may be related to poor tissue coverage, infection, graft thrombosis and modern mechanism.[21,22]

DIAGNOSTIC CONSIDERATIONS

The principles of initial limb evaluation and examination remain the constant cornerstone of assessment. In 2011, the Western Trauma Association (WTA) Guidelines further solidified the accepted algorithm in assessment of extremity injury (Figure 52.4).[23] Hard signs of vascular injury are widely discussed and recognizable. Absent pulses, active bleeding, clinically evident ischemia, expanding hematomas and palpable thrills or audible bruits are clear indications for further assessment and intervention. When more subtle or 'soft' signs of vascular injury are present, a more structured thought process of assessment is needed. These soft signs may include asymmetric/diminished pulse

exam, a history of hemorrhage, stable hematoma, neurologic deficits or wound proximity and character whereby vascular injury may have occurred. Continuous wave Doppler utilization with ankle–brachial indices (ABIs), or arm contralateral brachial index in upper extremity injuries, can be invaluable. Reduction of bony injury with restoration of length should be done prior to pulse exam and ABI. An ABI of less than 0.9 is highly suggestive of injury and is a quick and simple tool. Studies have indicated sensitivities of 80%–97% for arterial injury, but specificities in the 40%–100% range due to a noteworthy false positive rate.[24–27] However, negative predictive values are well over 80%. Thus, if no hard signs are present but either soft signs are present or injury is suspected, a critical pulse examination and ABI performance are indicated. In those with a normal exam and ABI, observation is appropriate, while reduction in ABI below 0.9 indicates the need for further localization and imaging. Some minor injuries may not be recognized by ABI, yet these are generally rare.[25–27] Minor injuries infrequently evolve and rarely declare themselves by clinical deterioration. Only 1%–2% of those with minimal or soft signs and normal examination come to operation for an unrecognized injury.[28,29] Indeed, in those with wounds in proximity to major axial arteries but no pulse or perfusion abnormalities and no signs of vessel injury,

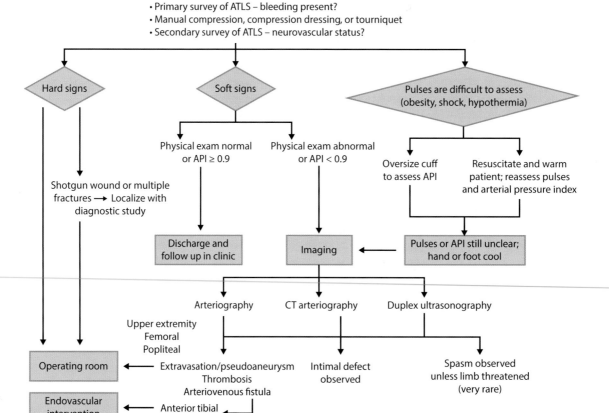

Figure 52.4 This general evaluation algorithm of extremity vascular injury currently espoused by the Western Trauma Association indicates the importance of pulse examination and ankle–brachial index in initial assessment of the injured extremity. (From Feliciano DV et al., *J Trauma*, 70, 1551, 2011.)

the occurrence of occult findings on imaging is 10%–12% with only 1.4% ultimately proceeding to need for intervention.[29] In assessing 300 patients with penetrating extremity injury, proximity wound and otherwise normal physical exam and ABI, Conrad and colleagues found no missed injuries in 51% of the cohort with follow-up available between 1 and 48 months.[30] These descriptive reports plainly support no further assessment in patients with normal examination and ABI.

Computed tomographic angiography (CTA) has largely replaced catheter-based angiography in the diagnosis and definition of arterial and venous injury in the extremity. Sensitivities and specificities of over 90% have been reported (Figures 52.5 and 52.12a).[31–33] It is quickly performed in minutes after presentation with most patients requiring CT for other indications in today's trauma environment. CTA provides information on soft tissue and bony injuries as well. It can be particularly helpful when several levels of injury are suspected, viz., blunt injury or multiple penetrating injuries. It is relatively inexpensive compared to angiography, and its performance over the last two decades in this fashion has created familiarity with its use. Limitations include dependence on proper bolus timing, poor luminal definition in those with atherosclerosis and significant arterial calcification and artefact with foreign bodies and metal fragments including bullets or projectiles. Indeed, a remaining indication for initial diagnostic catheter-based arteriography in extremity injury is the limb with multiple retained metallic fragments over a large region such as shotgun blasts with requirement for anatomic imaging. Arteriography has principally been relegated to performance as part of endovascular therapy.

Duplex ultrasound (DUS) has been shown to be a reasonable first-line diagnostic modality.[34–36] However, it has a broader range of sensitivity and specificity than CTA. It is user dependent and does not afford the degree of definition of inflow, outflow and extent of injury that CTA provides.[37] It is also limited anatomically and can only be realistically considered in evaluation beyond the junctional zones of the thoracic inlet and lower pelvis. Yet, it does have some decidedly useful applications in extremity injury. Minimal vascular injuries such as intimal flaps, pseudoaneurysms, arteriovenous fistulas and nonspecific narrowings ('spasm') can be further physiologically defined and serially imaged with duplex. In this regard, DUS has an additional adjunctive surveillance role.

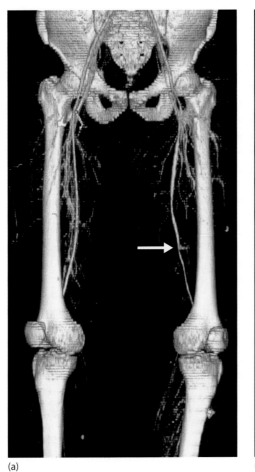
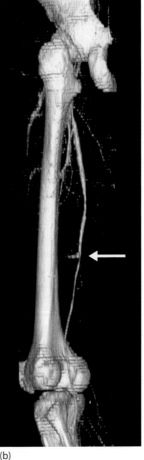

(a)   (b)

Figure 52.5 Computed tomographic angiography reconstruction showing inline bilateral lower extremity arterial flow with partial transection and hemorrhage from a mid-left superficial femoral artery (SFA) wound (a, white arrow) and a left posterolateral view showing the injury (b, white arrow) and patent SFA and trifurcation vessels.

Another arena where DUS may be helpful diagnostically is knee dislocation and assessment of the popliteal artery. These injuries carry a 10%–40% risk of popliteal artery injury. Pulse exam and ABI performance are, of course, first-line assessment, and duplex is easy and quick to assess this focal area after reduction.[38–40] However, as noted earlier, the anatomic benefits of CTA are apparent if repair is needed. Duplex's role in most centres is relegated to confirmation of normalcy, recognition and surveillance of minor injury, or when hardware makes CT impractical or uninterpretable.

GENERAL CONSIDERATIONS

There are several general topics that should be considered in treating a patient with an extremity vascular injury. Technical topics include the utility of tourniquets in initial care, damage control resuscitation (DCR) approach, the proper role for shunting techniques, vein repair, conduit selection, wound management as well as the impact of fasciotomy. Finally, putting the vascular injury into perspective in the multiply injured extremity or a severely injured patient is critical.

Tourniquet use

Use of tourniquets in modern-day civilian trauma has not been systematically endorsed, but the effectiveness of tourniquets has been recently demonstrated in the combat environment. This has led to some provocative dialogue in the trauma community. Early application of tourniquets in OIF/OEF has proven effective and life-saving in patients with extremity injuries.[41] In 2009, Kragh and colleagues reported on application of an extremity tourniquet in casualties in Iraq.[42] Amongst 2838 civilian and military casualties with major limb trauma, survival amongst 232 (8%) casualties with emergency tourniquet use was investigated. Casualties were evaluated for shock and prehospital versus emergency department (ED) tourniquet placement. There were 31 deaths (13%). Tourniquet use when shock was absent was strongly associated with survival (90% vs. 10%; p < 0.001). Prehospital tourniquets were applied in 194 casualties, of which 22 died (11% mortality), whereas 38 patients had ED application, of which 9 died (24% mortality; p = 0.05). The authors concluded that tourniquet use overall and particularly prehospital use were strongly associated with survival in major limb injury. A small percentage (1.7%) experienced nerve palsy at the level of application, but no amputations resulted from tourniquet use. In another evaluation of use in combat over a 4-year period by Israeli Defense Forces, 110 tourniquets were applied to all extremity injuries. The 35 applied to the upper extremities were effective in controlling hemorrhage in 94% of the injuries as compared to 74% of tourniquets applied to the lower extremity injuries.[43] Neurologic complications developed in seven limbs (6%).

Currently, the most commonly used tourniquet is a windlass design such as the Combat Applied Tourniquet and Special Operations Forces Tactical Tourniquet. A pneumatic compression tourniquet called the Emergency and Military Tourniquet is also available. The initial effectiveness of these three tourniquets as compared to others was established in a study where volunteers who self-applied one of these three tourniquets had consistently complete distal occlusion as assessed by Doppler.[44] Recent data from Davidson and the group at Oregon Health and Science University indicate that with tourniquet occlusion of the CFA in human subjects, there remained 25%–35% residual arterial perfusion via collaterals as measured by contrast-enhanced ultrasound perfusion imaging.[45] This information is obviously encouraging and supportive as renewed civilian interest in tourniquet applications is appearing.

Although historical apprehension for the use of tourniquets in the prehospital setting exists, recent developments have shown they can serve as an important adjunct to preventing hemorrhage and saving lives.[46] Yet, it remains difficult to generalize these data to settings outside of military combat where extensive training efforts and rapid medical transport create familiarity and a unique environment likely contributing to success.[47] While widespread recommendation for prehospital tourniquet use may be somewhat premature in the civilian environment, use seems rational and prudent with apparent risk low using these commercially available devices with a goal of removal as soon as feasible. With these newer experiences and products, it seems likely tourniquet use will be further studied and incorporated into civilian care systems in some way.

Damage control resuscitation in extremity injury

Initial experience in OIF, with an absence of component therapy capability, elucidated and revisited advantages of warm whole blood in vascular injury.[48] Later during OIF, our military medical forces further embraced the concept of DCR and helped define how component therapy could be made most effective. Guidelines called for early transfusion of blood products, warmed and infused rapidly. Massive transfusion (>10 units/24 hours) was not uncommon for casualties with extremity vascular injury. It became relatively standard for the first four units of type O PRBCs and four units of AB plasma to be given in the emergency room and continued in a 1:1 ratio.[49] Large theatre-wide studies were performed and emphasized the utility of this 1:1 strategy as well as platelet and fibrinogen transfusion added to the 1:1 strategy.[50] Beneficial use of balanced component replacement in hemorrhage scenarios, including major extremity injury, has become common now in today's civilian trauma settings.

Recombinant factor VIIa was initially used with warm whole blood quite frequently, but selectively in Iraq and Afghanistan in those with coagulopathy. Anecdotally, this worked quite well, and thrombotic

Table 52.1 Damage control resuscitation versus standard crystalloid-based resuscitation in those with extremity vascular injury.

Variable	Group 1 (DCR) (n)	DCR Δ	p	Group 2 (n)	No DCR Δ	p
OR time (minutes)	273 ± 99 (16)			266 ± 89 (24)		0.83
Systolic blood pressure	144 ± 27 (15)	39	0.001*	124 ± 28 (24)	14	0.11
Diastolic blood pressure	78 ± 13 (15)	18	0.005*	65 ± 17 (24)	1	0.93
Heart rate	90 ± 14 (15)	−38	<0.001**	105 ± 26 (24)	−12	0.07
Temperature (°F)	98.5 ± 0.7 (14)	−0.09	0.86	98.4 ± 1.01 (20)	−0.3	0.19
pH	7.39 ± 0.06 (14)	0.12	0.013*	7.32 ± 0.08(17)	0.02	0.34
Base deficit	0.14 ± 2.8 (14)	7.36	<0.001**	4.53 ± 3.9 (17)	2.72	0.09
Hb (g/dL)	11.3 ± 2.3 (14)	2.3	0.014*	9.3 ± 1.7 (24)	−2.1	0.007*
INR	1.0 ± 0.35 (13)	0.3	0.009*	1.5 ± 0.37 (24)	0.1	0.14

Source: Fox CJ et al., *J Trauma*, 64(2 Suppl), S99, 2008.

Notes: Physiologic improvements noted in those undergoing DCR. Data are mean ± SD unless otherwise specified. Δ, comparison of physiologic differences from ED arrival (Table 52.1) to ICU admission. Vitals signs and lab studies were taken immediately at ICU admission. p-values are derived from standard paired *t*-tests, (*p < 0.05, **p < 0.001) except OR time, which used standard *t*-test.

Abbreviations: Hb, hemoglobin; INR, international normalized ratio; DCR, damage control resuscitation; ED, emergency department; ICU, intensive care unit.

complications were not increased in those with vascular grafts.[51,52] Although benefit in hemorrhage therapy was noted, newer experiences with recombinant factor VIIa expressed concern for thromboembolic risk with use in many bleeding scenarios, and enthusiasm has tempered.[53] Both retrospective registry data and prospective multi-institutional analysis indicate tranexamic acid (TXA) reduces mortality and bleeding in hemorrhaging trauma patients.[54–56] Its specific role in extremity vascular injury remains undefined.

This hemostatic component-based resuscitation strategy, along with damage control surgery refinements and experience, as well as avoidance of crystalloid fluid dependence, has increased the effectiveness of systemic management of extremity vascular injuries (Table 52.1).[52] Capability to quickly restore physiologic derangements, particularly coagulopathy and acidemia, has been recognized. Thus, resuscitation strategies now have in many instances shifted the threshold of performing 'life-saving' amputations to expecting limb salvage following an appropriate resuscitation. It cannot be overemphasized that DCR has played a major role in the acknowledged survival advantages in Iraq and Afghanistan compared to prior US conflicts. Thus, resuscitative strategy and focus is important in the treatment of extremity vascular injury and should be pursued.

Temporary vascular shunting

Temporary intravascular shunts can allow for rapid restoration of distal limb perfusion when immediate vascular reconstruction is not possible (Figure 52.6). This may be due to delays involving orthopedic fixation, wound debridement and definition, vein harvest, lack of clinical expertise at the initial treating facility or addressing

more life-threatening injuries. The use of intravascular shunting has been specifically applied as a method to stabilize and temporize peripheral vascular injuries, avoid vascular reconstructions in austere environments with limited resources and time and allow for restitution and preservation of extremity perfusion during transport to definitive care. Further, shunting has been used during mass casualty events and during damage control in those with significantly adverse physiology or concomitant injuries.[57] As such, robust, descriptive evaluations of use in extremity vascular injury during OIF and OEF have been performed.[58–60] The utility of rapidly restoring perfusion when other injuries take precedence or when adverse physiology demands also plays a particularly germane role

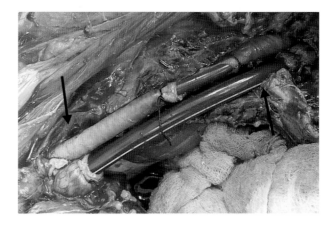

Figure 52.6 Arterial and venous shunting of proximal superficial femoral artery and femoral vein in major multimechanistic injury to the right upper thigh. Note the difference in color, vasa vasorum presence, and apparent viability of the artery at the two locations (black arrows).

in civilian injury. Patency reports for temporary shunts have refuted the obligatory need for systemic anticoagulation for maintenance.[61,62]

The potential role for temporary vascular shunting (TVS) in both civilian and contingency arenas has been recognized for decades. Its use was well described before recent conflicts. However, the contemporary theatre environment and care structure has highlighted its value and effectiveness. Chambers et al. reported the use of 27 temporary vascular shunts in a US Marine Forward Resuscitative Surgical System during OIF. Six (22%) of the shunts clotted during transport, but did not impact early limb outcome.[58]Another Navy report from OIF illustrated similar results with 96% shunt patency and 100% early limb salvage. The mean time to arrival at definitive level III care was 5 hours, 48 minutes. It ranged from 3 hours, 40 minutes to 10 hours, 49 minutes indicating the relative importance of reperfusion abilities forward.[60] We chronicled descriptive data from the Balad Vascular Registry (BVR) demonstrating that shunts placed for proximal vascular injuries (at or proximal to the knee or elbow) had a significantly greater patency (86%, $n = 22$) than shunts placed in distal vascular injuries (distal to the knee or elbow) (12%, $n = 8$).[59] However, no difference in early limb viability was identified between the groups (95% and 88%, respectively; p = NS). Thus, failure of the distal shunts did not result in decreased limb viability. Our experience with shunt use in 126 femoropopliteal arterial injuries in OIF between 2004 and 2007 specifically described 43% were shunted from forward and 93% were patent on arrival to us with only two (4.7%) shunts dislodged during evacuation.[63] Stability for transport was confirmed.

In 2009, Gifford presented our longer-term outcome analysis in a case-controlled, propensity matching fashion with a time-to-event analysis portraying temporary vascular shunting's impact on freedom from amputation using data collected from the JTTR, including the BVR, and the Walter Reed Vascular Registry (WRVR) from 2003 to 2007.[64] Cases and controls consisting of 64 and 61 extremity arterial injuries, respectively, had a mean follow-up of 22 months. While the shunted group showed significant higher mean injury severity scores when compared to the control group (18 vs. 15, p = 0.05), after propensity score adjustment, use of TVS suggested a reduced risk of amputation, but was not statistically significant (RR = 0.47; 95% CI [0.18–1.19]; p = 0.11) (Table 52.2). Similar freedom from amputation was identified in both shunted and nonshunted extremities after definitive reconstruction (78% vs. 77%; p = 0.5), but relative, graduated improvement in limb salvage with shunting as the severity of extremity injury increased was noted (Figure 52.7).

Several case series describing use of TVS in the civilian arena have also been communicated.[62,65–69] These series report similar results and considerations regarding the use of shunts and corroborate potential benefits. Animal study evidence, both physiologic and histologic, in support of venous shunting in combined arterial/venous extremity injuries is scant but available. The generally

Table 52.2 Multivariate proportional hazards regression modelling for factors independently affecting time to amputation in 125 extremity arterial injuries (64 shunted, 61 unshunted).

Proportional hazards model			
Effect	Relative risk	95% CI	p-value
TVS group[a]	0.47	(0.18,1.19)	0.11
MESS score (5–7)[b]	3.46	(0.97,12.36)	0.06
MESS score (8–12)[b]	16.37	(3.79,70.79)	<0.001
Venous repair[c]	0.2	(0.04,0.99)	0.05
Associated bone injury	5.01	(1.45,17.28)	0.01

Source: Gifford SM et al., *J Vasc Surg*, 50(3), 549, 2009.

Note: Propensity score adjustment was used to account for the differences noted in the comparison of the TVS and control group concerning Injury Severity Score and level 2 care.

Abbreviations: *CI*, confidence interval; *MESS*, Mangled Extremity Severity Score; *TVS*, temporary vascular shunting.

[a] Compared with no shunting control group.

[b] Compared with MESS of 1–4.

[c] Compared with venous ligation where venous injury was present.

beneficial effects in these experiments speak to the potential of venous repair.[70,71] However, controversies regarding the use and theoretic benefit of venous shunts as well as therapeutic, or pharmacologic, shunting remain to be further studied and defined, along with the proper posture of shunting during transport in civilian settings.

Shunting's potential drawbacks of unrecognized iatrogenic vessel injury, or necessity for more extensive repair owing to securing mechanisms, seem negligible overall. Even when faced with primary vascular injury at the time of definitive management, the author finds that initial shunt use can be quite effective in providing time for operative planning and optimization. Arterial injury identification, thrombectomy, regional heparin and perhaps intra-arterial vasodilators with temporary shunt placement provide reperfusion and time. This simple strategy may create an environment for a more precise and durable final revascularization with improved neuromuscular outcome.

One cannot divorce the concept of TVS from the discussion of the ischemic interval prior to repair and its impact on outcome. Traditional surgical teaching, based upon simple muscle histology evidence, promulgated 6 hours as the ischemic threshold beyond which functional recovery was likely not possible.[72,73] However, a new porcine model has provided more scientifically rigorous assessment. Our initial model reported by Gifford describing the biochemical effects of various temporal profiles of ischemia confirmed TVS reversed ischemia.[74] Utilizing this model and allowing for survival, Burkhardt studied neuromuscular recovery by electromyography and modified Tarlov functional scores.[75] Just under 5 hours of ischemia was identified as the breakpoint after which neuromuscular recovery was worse than initial ligation at 14 days after injury. This was then taken one step further and Hancock showed that

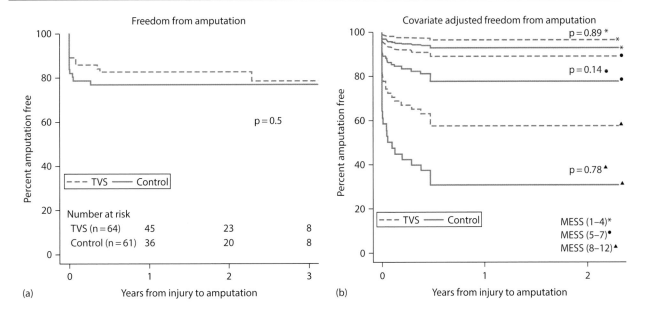

Figure 52.7 (a) Freedom from amputation in shunted versus matched unshunted extremity arterial injury cohorts showing no difference in long-term outcome but no detriment to shunting. (b) Graduated, relative benefit of shunting as the severity of extremity injury worsens. (From Gifford SM et al., *J Vasc Surg*, 50, 549, 2009.)

this threshold was reduced even further, to 3 hours of ischemia, with 35% hemorrhage and class III shock.[76] Exactly how this animal model reflects the physiology of human traumatic ischemia is not certain, but it seems clear 6 hours of ischemia is indeed an extreme regarding the functional recovery potential of the limb, and it is likely less. Further, the clinical physiology and shock status of the patient is, as one would anticipate, important and may reduce this threshold.

Vein repair

The optimal management of extremity venous injury remains a controversial topic. Ligation of the named veins of the extremity can be performed in austere conditions, when another life-threatening injury takes precedence, or when the patient's physiology will not allow extended operation with relatively low acute morbidity. It has been previously recommended that venous injuries ideally should be repaired when the patient's condition permits.[77] Extremity venous repair gained prominence during the Vietnam War with Rich reporting 377 venous injuries, in which 124 (32.9%) were repaired.[78] Lateral suture was the most common repair performed (*n* = 106) followed by end-to-end anastomosis (*n* = 10), vein interposition graft (*n* = 5) and vein patch graft (*n* = 3). It was noted in this report, and further emphasized later from the Vietnam Vascular Registry (VVR), that concern for thromboembolic complications did not materialize as was historically expected with venous repair. Rich went on to also suggest that extremity venous repair may be important to limb salvage, and although many repairs fail, a major proportion of these may recanalize without higher risk.[79–82] How

recanalization relates to meaningful venous return and later insufficiency has not been defined. It was the work of Rich and Hobson that identified the negative impact of proximal femoral venous ligation on arterial flow in a canine model which formed the foundation of the venous shunting and repair mindset.[83] This also established the premise that vein repair might facilitate arterial flow and serve as an important component in arterial reconstruction durability.

In another large, more recent, military series, Quan et al. retrospectively reviewed 82 patients with 103 venous injuries.[84] While a majority of patients (63%) were treated with ligation, no significant difference in postoperative thromboembolic complications was seen between the group that had ligation and the group that underwent venous repair. In 2009, Gifford, in our reported cohort-matched shunting evaluation, identified venous repair as independently protective against amputation (RR = 0.2; 95% CI [0.04–0.99], p = 0.05) during evaluation of 125 combat extremity vascular injuries (Table 52.2).[64]

Civilian series evaluating extremity venous repair are small, descriptive and without consensus. These have indicated a significant early repair thrombosis rate, but have confirmed recanalization with generally low morbidity rates in civilian environments.[85–87] There has been no identifiable difference in outcomes with repair versus ligation or formal associations with amputation based upon management. Smith and co-workers reported that in 20 major extremity venous injury repairs, patency at 72 hours was 55% but increased to 85% at 6 weeks with little morbidity.[85] Meyer et al. reported 34 patients with venous injury (26 lower extremity, 8 upper extremity) and showed 61% early patency for all venous repairs with a 40% early patency for interposition vein grafts.[86] Nypaver and colleagues reviewed longer-term follow-up (mean 49 months; range 6–108 months) for 32 patients who had venous reconstruction and found long-term patency to be 90% as determined by duplex ultrasound.[87] Yet, in 74 patients with extremity venous injury, Yelon and Scalea concluded that ligation was a safe and reasonable option as no differences in outcomes were identified between the 44 ligated and the 30 repaired.[88] Finally, Timberlake and Kerstein reported on 322 patients with venous injury. While 239 were combined arterial and venous injuries, 83 injuries were isolated venous. With mean follow-up of 34 months, only four patients (1.2%) had long-term edema.[77] All four had arterial and venous injury at the popliteal level. This seems to speak to the wide variability in civilian extremity trauma severity and mechanism. Arguments against venous repair surround time required, difficulty in repair, the patient's associated injuries and general condition and unidentified long-term benefit.

These thoughts have collectively led to the author's relatively aggressive stance to repair veins particularly in the proximal limb and in confluence veins where larger veins represent watershed areas of venous drainage such as in the axillosubclavian venous segment, common femoral vein or a single popliteal vein. Contemplative of Rich's Vietnam work, our initial OIF reports characterized a 60%–70% repair rate for identified extremity venous injury.[18,63] Duplicate venous systems can be present and should be identified and sought in these areas. For instance, a duplicate popliteal venous system can be present in up to 30%–40% of individuals (Figure 52.8). Extremity vein repair should also be heavily considered in instances where there is multi-mechanistic injury resulting in a soft tissue defect likely to compromise venous collateral network return. Rich, in his experimental work, suggested each limb has many collateral venous channel networks, and these

are important in limb drainage when the main axial channel is disrupted.[81] With extensive soft tissue injury, these are also compromised, and repair's significance is likely more robust. In these instances, it is the author's observation that maintenance or re-establishment of the main axial venous outflow is important in quality limb salvage. The caveat, of course, is that the patient should be in a physiologic state in which repair can be tolerated and no other life-threatening injuries should take precedence. Ligation is logical and appropriate in this situation. As noted, the role of venous shunting is undefined but intriguing.[71] The general goals of venous repair are acute decompression of the injured limb, to permit venous collateral development or maturation, enhance arterial repair durability and reduce edema and long-term postphlebitic changes.

Conduit selection

Primary repair and interposition grafting are the technical open methods used in most arterial repairs.[7,8,11,18,63,89] This likely represents the spectrum of injury from minor iatrogenic to major acquired traumatic. In the latter, the use of interposition and bypass grafts accounts for the majority of needed repair. The decision for and knowledge of proper conduit use is therefore essential. Autogenous venous conduit should generally be procured from an uninjured extremity so as not to further disrupt venous return. This is usually the great saphenous vein. However, for shorter interposition grafts, a single segment of arm vein is acceptable. Also, should the injury in the extremity not lead to substantial soft tissue injury and no associated axial venous injury is present, a short segment of ipsilateral great saphenous vein, or superficial arm vein in upper extremities, can be considered preferably. When

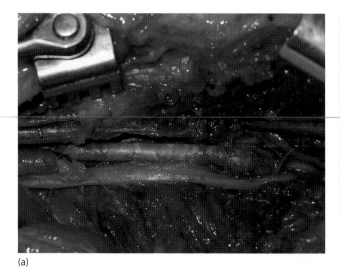

(a)

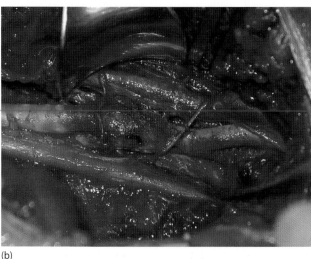

(b)

Figure 52.8 (a) Reconstruction of left trifurcation penetrating injury by below-knee popliteal to tibioperoneal trunk vein graft. Note the intact tibial nerve and ligated popliteal vein. (b) By retraction at the level of the distal anastomosis, intact duplicate popliteal vein is identified and this patient did not undergo vein repair.

multiple extremities are involved, autogenous vein harvest from the extremity with the least amount of injury is proper. Occasionally, femoral vein, internal jugular vein or hypogastric artery may be rational. We have also used both venous and arterial conduits from other limbs primarily amputated.

The use of prosthetic grafts for reconstruction of military extremity vascular trauma has been consistently discouraged.[90] In a report from the VVR, only four (0.4%) patients with arterial injuries were managed using prosthetic graft interposition grafts.[91] The importance of autogenous conduit for contaminated war wounds has also been encouraged and emphasized in OIF/OEF. Amongst 301 arterial injuries in OIF, only 8 (2.7%) were repaired using a prosthetic graft and 3 of these were in the abdomen or chest.[18]

Vertrees and colleagues underscored the need for surgical judgment in knowing when a prosthetic graft may be useful. As of 2010, the WRVR only had 17 (4.6%) casualties who had undergone emergent vascular reconstruction using polytetrafluoroethylene (PTFE) grafts. Despite a prosthetic graft being emergently placed into large contaminated soft tissue wounds, 79% of these prosthetic grafts were patent in the short term. This strategy allowed for patient stabilization, transport to stateside facility and elective rather than emergent revascularization with remaining autologous (arm or leg) vein. There were no prosthetic graft disruptions or amputations performed because of prosthetic graft failure. The authors concluded for complex repairs, when autologous conduit is limited, a temporary prosthetic graft followed by staged, definitive autogenous reconstruction may be a reasonable option.[92] Recently, Watson and colleagues performed a small, retrospective cohort-matched study assessing PTFE ($n = 25$) versus autogenous vein ($n = 24$) in arterial injury in the JTTR. Mean follow-up was over 5 years. While PTFE in the carotid–subclavian domain performed equal to vein, PTFE in the extremity performed poorly. 8-year freedom from complication was significantly worse for prosthetic (77% vs. 31%; p = 0.044). These PTFE failures were evenly distributed amongst thrombosis, infection and restenosis and were distributed throughout the follow-up timeframe. Autogenous failure did not occur after the first few months.[93]

Civilian literature has also espoused the use of PTFE prosthetic as a reasonable alternative.[94,95] This is most logical and successful in proximal larger vessels for appropriate size match in low-impact injuries with little soft tissue injury. Patency in PTFE grafts for extremity vascular injury, generally however, has not been encouraging. In a recent meta-analysis of almost 1200 lower extremity injuries repaired by interposition grafts, the use of PTFE was associated with a nearly twofold higher risk of secondary amputation (OR 1.88; CI 0.55–5.83, p = 0.88).[13] This likely reflects two features of extremity injury grafting. Available data indicate autogenous conduit is preferred, particularly in high-impact, high-velocity injuries, leading to major soft tissue destruction. Yet, even in this considerable number of patients, statistical superiority was not realized indicating that when clinical reasoning dictates, PTFE can logically be used.

Fasciotomy

The standard indications for fasciotomy in extremity injury include ischemia over 4 hours, significant blast, soft tissue or crush injury, patient evacuation scenarios and inability of the patient to subjectively participate in examination (i.e. head injury). In reality, fasciotomies are best done whenever they are considered and remain an integral component of the surgical treatment of extremity vascular injury. The argument for selective fasciotomies stems from small series touting long-term pain and reduction in calf pump efficiency. However, the flaw in this logic is noted by recent assessments of delayed fasciotomy and missed release. Ritenour and colleagues reported on 336 US combat wounded undergoing fasciotomy for major limb trauma.[96] They found those with fasciotomies needing revision had significantly more muscle excision and higher overall mortality (20% vs. 6%; p < 0.01). Further, they noted statistically significant increases in muscle excision, amputation (31% vs. 15%; p < 0.01) and mortality (19% vs. 5%; p < 0.01) if fasciotomies were performed after evacuation, or delayed, than if done in theatre. This theme was reiterated by Farber et al. who recently reviewed outcomes of civilian patients with fasciotomies and lower extremity arterial injury repair in the NTDB.[97] Compared to those who had fasciotomies accomplished beyond 8 hours of repair, those within 8 hours of repair had a significantly lower amputation rate (8.5% vs. 24.6%; p < 0.001), infection rate (6.6% vs. 14.5%; p = 0.028) and shorter hospital stay (18.5 ± 20.7 days vs. 24.2 ± 14.7 days, p = 0.007). On multivariate analysis, early fasciotomy was protective against amputation (OR 0.26, 95%CI 0.14–0.50; p < 0.0001) and led to a 23% shorter stay (p = 0.01).

Two-incision lower extremity compartment release is recommended. Via the medial incision, the posterior superficial compartment is opened with initial fascial incision. The posterior deep compartment is entered by release of the fibrous attachment of the soleus on the tibia for its length. The lateral incision is performed two to three fingerbreadths lateral to the tibial edge. The anterior compartment is opened by fascial incision in this plane. Either the lateral compartment is entered via separation of the intercompartmental septum as viewed in the anterior compartment or it may be entered separately by posterior retraction of the skin and subcutaneous tissue of the incision to expose the lateral compartment external fascia. The skin incisions should be generous and fascia of these compartments separated from just below the knee to the ankle.

Upper extremity fasciotomy can be more complex. Performance of upper extremity fasciotomy should begin medially in the arm and become sinusoidal from medial to lateral at the antecubital fossa incorporating the bicipital aponeurosis. Extension must be sufficiently lateral to open the fascia over the extensor wad. Rarely, a second dorsal fasciotomy incision over the dorsal wad extensor muscles is necessary. Gentle incision back to the volar fascia will help to also release this aspect (Figure 52.9). Depending upon the severity of soft tissue damage and mechanism, this may need to be lengthened into a concomitant carpal tunnel release. In instances with penetrating trauma, the injury itself may provide partial compartment release.

Wound management

Contemporary wound care strategies and definitive reconstructive surgery for casualties with vascular injury have also influenced limb salvage rates. Large cavitary wounds require continual assessment and periodic debridement of devitalized tissue to ensure grafts remain covered with healthy tissue. The use of closed negative pressure wound therapy has advanced the practice of closing deep soft tissue wounds to achieve sufficient muscle coverage.

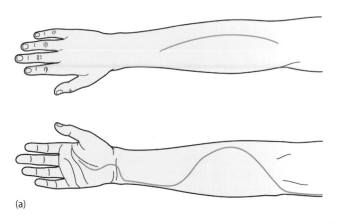

(a)

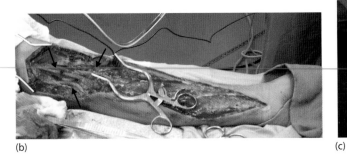

(b)

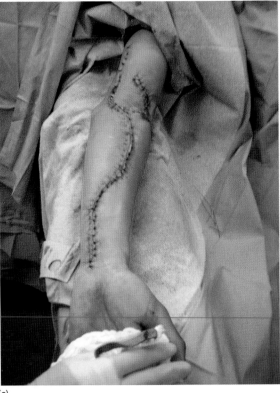

(c)

Figure 52.9 (a) Incision lines for performance of upper extremity fasciotomy with mid-medial arm proceeding to S-shaped antecubital fossa incision opening bicipital aponeurosis and then laterally the extensor muscle were back medially to the forearm muscles and finally through a carpal tunnel release if necessary. A separate dorsal incision to further release the extensor muscles can be created if required. (b) Upper extremity fasciotomy in a penetrating blast injury requiring brachial artery reversed vein graft (upper right arrow) and basilic vein interposition vein graft (lower arrow). The confused but intact median nerve is also seen (upper left arrow). (c) Delayed primary closure of upper extremity fasciotomy wounds and the superior blow out wound in the upper arm after serial debridement, washout and negative pressure therapy in the patient from (b).

Negative pressure wound therapy has advanced the ability to close wounds that previously would require amputation, and the impact of this technology is now used every day in every trauma environment and cannot be underemphasized. Some benefits of negative pressure therapy include wound splinting, perfusion enhancement, stimulation of cell division, wicking of edema and lymph, decreasing bacteriophilic exudate and down-regulation of adverse molecular regulators.[98] Peck and colleagues reported on 134 extremity vascular injuries with extensive soft tissue wounds, 57% of which underwent early delayed primary closure, confirming the effective use of the VAC device with vascular reconstruction (Figure 52.9b and c).[99] For wounds that cannot be closed easily, repeated debridements, wound washouts and changes of the VAC can properly prepare the site for a split-thickness skin graft. Early complications did occur, some requiring alternative revascularization routing. Wound infection occurred in 3.7%, anastomotic disruption in 3%, and graft thrombosis in 4.5%, with amputation and mortality rates of 3% and 1.5%, respectively. Thus, a closure strategy must evolve as promptly as feasible, and prudent use of extra-anatomic graft routing in large defects must be contemplated and prepared for. Finally, definitive reconstructive surgery has also expanded horizons and demonstrated the effectiveness of both local rotational and microvascular free tissue transfers to salvage extremity wounds in those with vascular injury.[100] This should be considered and expertise sought early in the patient's management should this be potentially relevant.

The extremity with multiple system injury ('mangled')

A mangled extremity is defined as a complex injury involving soft tissue, bone, nerve and vasculature. Determining which patients and mangled extremities will benefit from aggressive attempts at limb salvage, or which would be better served with primary amputation in the early stages of management, can be challenging. Exhaustive efforts at limb salvage in severely injured patients may result in misdirection of care, whereas premature extremity amputation may preclude optimal functional outcome.

Scoring systems have been developed to take into consideration concomitant injuries, as well as the degree and nature of the bony, soft tissue, nerve and vessel features of extremity injury. These systems are designed to assist the surgeon in decision making during the early phases of mangled limb management and also provide a mechanism to do comparative retrospective study of extremity injury.[101,102] Application of different scoring systems such as the Mangled Extremity Severity Score (MESS), Mangled Extremity Syndrome Index (MESI), Predictive Salvage Index and Limb Salvage Index has been evaluated regarding ability to predict limb salvage and long-term functional outcome.[101–107]

The most robust validation studies of mangled extremity scores focused on the lower extremity, and caution was proposed in applying MESS to upper extremity injury by the original authors Johansen et al. (Table 52.3).[102] Recommendations against its relevance for upper extremities are found.[107] Yet the simplicity of determining the four clinical variables in MESS has resulted in its application in upper extremities. Slauterbeck et al. reported on 43 mangled upper extremities and found all 9 arms with a MESS of greater than or equal to 7 were primarily amputated, whereas a score of less than 7, found in 34 upper extremities, resulted in salvage.[106] Durham et al. also retrospectively evaluated the application of limb salvage scores independently for both upper and lower mangled extremities and concluded MESS and MESI both decently predicted limb salvage.[105] Interestingly, these authors concluded that these scores did not accurately predict functional outcome, iterating limb viability and function are related but not identical.

In Iraq, using a combination of 17 upper and 43 lower extremity injuries, Rush and colleagues suggested a MESS of 7 or greater predicted limb loss.[108] In our propensity-adjusted multivariate analysis of 64 shunted versus 61 matched unshunted arterial extremity injuries with nearly 2-year mean follow-up, Gifford confirmed the seeming fidelity of MESS.[64] This case–control study included 35 upper extremities along with 90 lower extremity injuries. Proportional hazards modelling showed significant prediction of amputation using MESS (MESS 5–7 [RR 3.5; 95% CI 0.97–12.4; p = 0.06] and MESS 8–12 [RR16.4; 95% CI 3.79–70.98; p < 0.001]) (Table 52.2).

Table 52.3 Mangled extremity severity score.

Variable	Injury assessment	Points
Skeletal	Low energy (stab; simple fracture; 'civilian' GSW)	1
	Medium energy (open or multiple fxs, dislocation)	2
	High energy (close-range shotgun or 'military' GSW; crush injury)	3
	Very high energy (above + gross contamination; soft tissue avulsion)	4
Limb ischemia	Pulse reduced or absent but perfusion intact	1[a]
	Pulseless; paresthesias; diminished capillary refill	2[a]
	Cool; paralyzed; insensate; numb	3[a]
Shock	SBP always > 90mm Hg	0
	Transient hypotension	1
	Persistent hypotension	2
Age (years)	<30	0
	30–50	1
	>50	2

Source: Adapted from Johansen K et al., *J Trauma*, 30, 568, 1990.
[a] Score doubled for ischemia time >6 hours.

The general sentiment regarding mangled extremity scores suggests they serve as an objective reminder of subjective clinical experience. They provide cues to the nuances leading to either limb salvage or limb loss in significantly injured extremities and provide a broad framework. Yet, their clear and unquestioned use as an indicator of whether an extremity should be primarily amputated in the acute setting remains to be proven. The expertise and opinion of the evaluating surgeon remains most essential in management approach.

NONOPERATIVE MANAGEMENT

As indicated earlier, when identified extremity arterial injuries are minimal and there is no diminution in distal perfusion, observation is considered. These lesions are clinically silent. They include intimal flaps and defects, tapered narrowings and small pseudoaneurysms and arteriovenous fistulas. This discussion has become even more relevant due to the continual significant improvements in arterial imaging techniques leading to more sensitive recognition of these injuries. The WTA has substantiated the institution of nonoperative management of these lesions as appropriate (Figure 52.4).[23] However, it is not new. The description of nonoperative management was initially voiced in World War I more out of necessity than strategy. Since development of arterial surgical techniques, a selective nonoperative approach has continued to be discussed and validated and parallels the development and availability of arteriography. Of these lesions, 85%–90% resolve, and in available series, no intervention has been required after 3 months.[23-29] This now mature, small body of descriptive literature, including animal intimal injury models, has indicated that the most benign of these lesions are small intimal flaps and nonspecific taperings (i.e. spasm in otherwise normal vessels) which heal at rates well over 90%.[109-111] It has been suggested that intimal flaps producing over 75% luminal stenosis are more problematic.[112] Aspirin in minimal lesions appears beneficial and improves patency.[113] Small pseudoaneurysms (<5 mm) also spontaneously heal but may require intervention in up to 30%–40%. Arteriovenous fistulas, which are least common, may also spontaneously close when small (<5 mm). Initial nonoperative surveillance is appropriate. Larger ones are probably best served with repair.

When considering all patients with penetrating extremity injury, no hard signs of arterial injury and normal perfusion, only 1%–2% will ultimately re-present with an arterial injury maturing to a point requiring repair, thus reinforcing the passive nature of these occult lesions.[29] How endovascular intervention may impact these minimal injuries is unclear and must be considered on a case-by-case basis. When repair is pursued, endovascular methods logically may simplify this technically. Given the historical rates of resolution and the complication profile of endovascular therapies, this decision is likely to remain left to clinical intuition. Key to nonoperative management of identified arterial minimal injury is duplex surveillance monitoring, and ongoing clinical assessment recognizing follow-up is many times easier stated than accomplished in this population. Nonoperative management may be considered in young children if ischemia is not critical and distal flow can be documented.[114] In newborns and infants, nonoperative management is preferred. Systemic antithrombotic therapy, topical vasodilators and plastic covers on the limb to augment vasodilation and flow are logical options. In the severely injured patient with poor prognosis or a prohibitive risk, a nonoperative approach to asymptomatic or non-hemorrhaging lesions can be considered.

OPERATIVE MANAGEMENT

Operative conduct in extremity vascular injury remains seated upon the foundational aspects of vascular surgery.[115] Proper proximal and distal control is paramount. Depending upon injury location, active hemorrhage may require digital control from an assistant, or placement of an available windlass tourniquet or pneumatic tourniquet to prevent exsanguination. The patient should be placed on a fluoroscopically compatible table to allow for endovascular control and angiography. Today, utilizing hybrid, fixed imaging operating rooms permits the full management option spectrum of open surgical and endovascular therapeutics allowing for comprehensive flexibility. Prepping and draping should be circumferential with extension extended contiguously onto the torso to allow for any conceivable control option. Other extremities in which autogenous conduit may be harvested should be prepared. Not uncommonly, to avoid as much thermal loss as possible, prepping widely with sterile sheets placed over areas until or if they are required is prudent.

Wide exposure of the injured vessel with local control is accompanied by assessment of surrounding soft tissue. Once local control is achieved, release of more global control, if utilized, should be a priority to diminish ischemia. Debridement of devitalized tissue with an eye to reconstruction coverage is necessary. Revascularization is usually able to be accomplished in an anatomic way, but in extensive injury with severe tissue destruction and debridement, creative graft tunnelling in septal planes may be needed and is essential. Prior to repair, vessel debridement should also be performed. While it is easy to say this should be done to 'healthy' vessel, this is sometimes difficult and subjective. In the author's experience, the colour of the vessel is key (Figure 52.6). Arterial appearance should be bright with red vasa vasorum indicating their patency. When the artery is opened, the intima should not only be intact, but moist and tan, not hemorrhagic, contused or gray. More debridement is usually safer than too little within reason. Debridement for venous repair is more challenging as these veins usually have some element of thrombosis, but similar principles should apply with normal-appearing intima and external features after preparation.

Systemic use of heparin should be considered when other injuries do not afford undue risk. In isolated injuries, standard doses can normally be given. Graduated use based upon other injuries is reasonable, and in those with systemic use contraindicated, regional heparin saline is particularly important. The general approach to arterial injury repair should include gentle Fogarty balloon thromboembolectomy proximally and distally starting for just a few centimetres looking for strong, thrombus-free inflow and patent outflow. Too vigorous of embolectomy can cause irritation and spasm. Regional heparin should be instilled after judgment of distal and proximal patency to avoid mobilizing thrombus. Vasodilators such as nitroglycerine should be both considered topically and instilled into the inflow and outflow. In low-velocity, penetrating trauma, with laceration, primary repair or patch angioplasty is occasionally feasible. With blunt injury, gunshot wounds or extensive blast injury, interposition or bypass grafting is the correct construct. Post-repair antiplatelet therapy should be utilized unless contraindicated due to other injuries. The size, quality and reactivity of arteries in children require a specific comment. These features make them quite difficult to adequately repair. Should repair be necessary, liberal use of topical and infused vasodilators can be useful. Interrupted anastomoses are important to allow for radial growth of the vessels (Figure 52.10). The great saphenous vein can be a reasonable conduit, but femoral vein, internal jugular vein and hypogastric artery are important considerations.

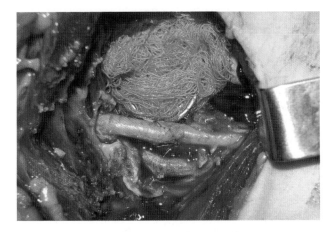

Figure 52.10 This interrupted 7-0 Prolene spatulated anastomosis after vessel mobilization was performed for primary repair of the proximal superficial femoral artery (4 mm) in a 9-year-old for penetrating blast transection. Interrupted anastomoses in children allow for radial arterial growth over time.

Vein repair, when performed, is initiated by Esmarch bandage exsanguination of the elevated distal limb with the distal aspect of the vein widely free and open without occluding control in order to clear distal thrombus as possible. Gentle thromboembolectomy with Fogarty balloons smaller than the veins is helpful in catching strands of thrombus. Regional heparin should be instilled. Depending upon mechanism and destruction, primary repair, patch angioplasty, interposition grafting or panel grafting can be performed (Figure 52.11). It is difficult to gauge what the allowable size mismatch is for venous repair. The author's tact in repair has been to accept up to a 50% decrease in diameter using interposition grafts, as long as the distended autogenous graft diameter is 5 mm or more. Anything less requires panel grafting. Spiral grafting is described but requires more time and is more technically demanding to fashion appropriately and secure. A panel graft allows for placement in situ with appropriate tension to assist construction when each panel is first secured to the proximal and distal ends of the vein. Panel grafting much more than 10 cm of venous defect is simply too time demanding in these acute situations to be normally justifiable. The author has tended to repair venous injury prior to arterial repair when (1) TVS normalizes distal flow with either palpable pedal pulses or brisk continuous wave Doppler signals; (2) the extremity injury is isolated, or there are only minor concomitant injuries; (3) autogenous conduit is adequate and generous; and (4) there is substantial soft tissue injury (Figure 52.11c). This latter scenario often leads to rapid tissue edema and venous oozing with significant ongoing blood loss. Restoration of venous outflow prior to definitive arterial reconstruction can impressively reduce oozing and the appearance of venous congestion.

The use of inferior vena cava (IVC) filters in venous repair or ligation is debated with no clear consensus, but is justifiably important when other injuries preclude antithrombotic use. To this end, the proper antithrombotic regimen indicated with extremity venous repair or ligation is also debated. It would make sense that in isolated extremity injury, anticoagulants should be considered. When concomitant injuries preclude this, the maximal antiplatelet regimen reasonable should be instituted as soon as feasible. When combined arterial and venous injuries occur, low-intensity antiplatelet therapy, such as aspirin, with anticoagulants should be contemplated. These obviously must be tempered with the degrees of soft tissue injury, neuraxial injury or cavitary injury. However, as noted earlier Quan and colleagues have recently reconfirmed that the incidence of clinically important pulmonary embolism after either venous repair or ligation in combat injuries with selective use of antithrombotic regimens is less than 5%.[84] Elevation and compression postoperatively are essential. Identified major nerve injuries can be repaired either early or in a delayed fashion depending upon wound and mechanism, but discussion regarding this disposition is essential during operative management.

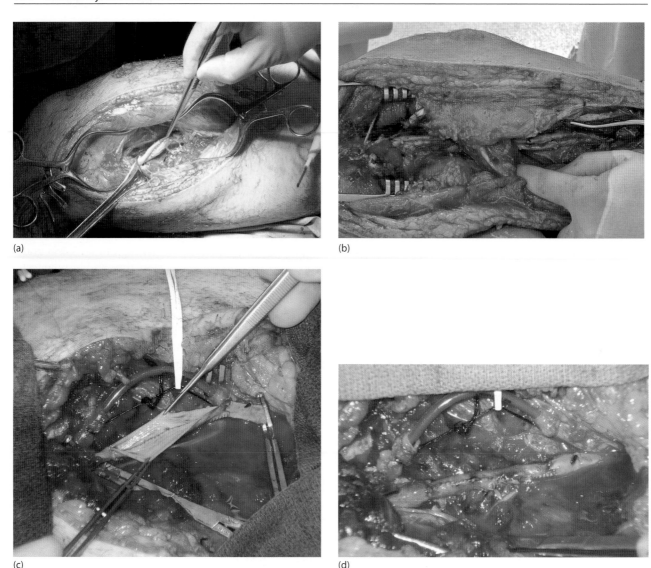

Figure 52.11 Constructs of extremity vein repair. (a) Saphenous vein patch on the above-knee popliteal vein after interposition reverse vein grafting of the above-knee popliteal artery. (b) Interposition vein grafts of the popliteal artery and vein throughout the entire above-knee and below-knee portions with preservation of the medial head of the gastrocnemius. (c) Creation of a panel vein graft with two panels of great saphenous vein to repair the proximal femoral vein. (d) Note the arterial shunt in place after completion of the panel venous graft. In this patient there was an isolated extremity vascular injury. Pulses returned after shunting, and vein repair was performed first.

Upper extremity

SUBCLAVIAN ARTERY INJURIES

Subclavian artery injuries are rare. They account for less than 8% of upper extremity arterial injury and 2% of all arterial injuries. The right subclavian artery origin can be exposed via a median sternotomy. Further mid-portion exposure may require a clavicular extension with or without clavicular resection. The origin of the left subclavian artery is in a more posterior location on the aortic arch and is exposed through a left anterolateral thoracotomy. The left subclavian artery can be controllable through a median sternotomy with a supraclavicular or cervical extension, but is more classically described with origin control in an anterolateral thoracotomy and separate supraclavicular exposure as the former exposure is deep and can be challenging. A scapular/shoulder roll can be quite helpful. When exposure is difficult, particularly in large, muscular individuals, the clavicle can be resected in a subperiosteal fashion to aid exposure.

When the goal is to expose the mid-portion of the subclavian artery in stable patients, a combined supraclavicular/infraclavicular two-incision technique has also been described, but in the authors' experience, a single-incision approach with subperiosteal clavicular resection used liberally with or without contemporaneous reconstruction of the clavicle seems most expeditious and flexible. The distal subclavian artery and proximal axillary artery are potentially treatable from a two-incision approach, but injury management may require a lateral clavicular resection, again with or without bony replacement.

Dissection in the area of the subclavian artery and vein should be performed with care given the abundance of adjacent nerve structures at risk for inadvertent injury. Aside from the brachial plexus and vagus nerve, the phrenic nerve sits on the anterior scalene muscle and should be identified and avoided. The anterior scalene muscle can be divided sharply once phrenic nerve identification occurs. Care must be taken to avoid the thoracic duct on the left and right lymph duct as they enter the jugulo-subclavian venous confluence. The abundance of collaterals around the shoulder and neck may allow for ligation of the subclavian artery in emergency situations with the upper extremity remaining viable. Temporary shunting, however, may be considered and in the author's opinion provides a better expeditious alternative to ligation with delayed reconstruction possible. Tension-free repair of the subclavian artery cannot be overemphasized as the vessel is relatively thin and delicate. Due to this, primary repair and patch angioplasty are challenging. If these are entertained, use of pledgets can be helpful. Prosthetic material can be used as an interposition graft for these larger, more proximal great vessel and upper extremity reconstructions. Autologous conduit such as saphenous vein, panelled saphenous vein, internal jugular vein or even femoral vein can be entertained depending upon size, length, injury and patient considerations. In more extensive injuries, ligation and revascularization using bypass with inflow based more proximally from the ascending aorta, innominate artery or common carotid may also be an option.

AXILLARY ARTERY INJURIES

Axillary artery injury occurs slightly more frequently than subclavian injury but is still rare compared to more distal vessels. It represents 2%–8% of upper extremity and 2%–3% of arterial injury. Sterile preparation of the ipsilateral neck, chest, supraclavicular fossa and circumferential arm is essential in order to fully prepare for optimal exposure and ease repair.

An infraclavicular incision made two fingerbreadths below and parallel to the clavicle will allow for access to the proximal axillary artery. Again, a scapular/shoulder roll can be useful. The clavipectoral fascia is next divided through the superior aspect of this incision opening a space which allows visualization of the proximal most axillary artery. Identification and division of the pectoralis minor muscle through this exposure is frequently necessary to show the entire axillary artery. Exposure of the subclavian artery as discussed may also be required for more proximal axillary artery injuries. Precise clamping is essential given the proximity to the axillary vein and brachial plexus.

Most axillary artery injuries require interposition grafting. Wide mobilization with side branch division for primary repair disrupts collateral flow, and the author avoids it. Conduit concerns are similar to subclavian injury.

BRACHIAL ARTERY INJURIES

The brachial artery is frequently injured and represents 14%–30% of arterial injuries and up to 60% of those in the upper extremity. Proximal control can often be obtained by manual compression of the brachial artery against the humerus should ongoing hemorrhage be present. However, brachial artery contraction and local thrombosis after development of hematoma is not uncommon. A wide prep and drape including the ipsilateral neck and chest should be performed in case more proximal exposure is required. Access to the hand and wrist for palpation and Doppler interrogation of radial and ulnar arteries is also an important consideration in draping.

A longitudinal incision is made in the palpable groove on the medial side of the upper arm between the biceps and the triceps. This incision can be extended proximally and distally as needed. With retraction of the pectoralis muscles, exposure as high as the distal axillary artery is possible. The close proximity of the basilic vein, median nerve and ulnar nerve to the artery should serve as reminders to perform the dissection with care and avoid excessive retraction. The basilic vein should be preserved if possible, and ligation of side branches can aid with mobilization to allow for easier retraction. Distally, the bicipital aponeurosis must be divided to expose the brachial artery. The median nerve will be located just lateral to the artery proximal in the arm with the ulnar nerve medial. The median nerve crosses the brachial artery distally in the arm and will lie medial and deep to the artery in the antecubital fossa.

Brachial artery injuries resulting from low-velocity mechanisms may be repaired primarily if there is not a segment of devitalized artery. Injuries resulting from higher velocity mechanisms with or without soft tissue involvement, as well as blunt injuries, require a more extensive reconstruction. With any anastomosis on the brachial artery, spatulation is necessary to avoid narrowing. In some instances, an interrupted suture technique can be useful given the relative small size of the artery and its tendency to spasm. Injuries to the brachial artery which occur distal to the profunda brachii origin may or may not present with critical ischemia depending upon the type of injury and the amount of associated damage to the collateral circulation from soft tissue wound or fracture.

RADIAL AND ULNAR ARTERY INJURIES

Forearm vascular injuries account for the majority of upper extremity arterial injury. Typically, control of forearm hemorrhage can be obtained with direct pressure or tourniquet. The proximal portion of the arm, hand and fingers should be prepped and draped in a circumferential manner in order to allow for adequate proximal and distal control and adequate operative exposure and assessment of the radial and ulnar arteries.

An S-shaped incision over the antecubital fossa will allow for proximal exposure of both the radial and ulnar arteries. Identifying the brachial artery as described earlier and then tracing it distally may aid in identifying the ulnar and radial arteries. The radial artery follows the medial border of the brachioradialis muscle, and the medial groove of this muscle can be used as a landmark to make an incision in the mid-forearm. In the distal wrist, the radial artery can be exposed by a longitudinal incision slightly lateral to the artery.

The ulnar artery dives deep to the pronator teres slightly beyond the bifurcation and remains deep to the flexor muscles of the proximal forearm before emerging to a more superficial position in the midpoint of the arm, which makes proximal exposure more difficult. A longitudinal incision is made on the medial side of the arm about four fingerbreadths distal to the medial epicondyle, and the artery can be identified between the flexor carpi ulnaris and flexor digitorum superficialis. In the wrist, the ulnar artery can be exposed through a longitudinal incision on the radial side of the flexor carpi ulnaris muscle in order to avoid the ulnar nerve, which runs medial to the ulnar artery.

Typically, the management of forearm artery injury is dependent upon whether or not there is a satisfactory continuous wave Doppler signal at the wrist and/or in the hand. Should a reasonable signal be present with the injured vessel occluded, ligation is a viable alternative. With simple lacerations, primary repair using fine, permanent sutures is also reasonable. Vasodilators may be needed. Spatulation is required because of the small size of the vessel. Interrupted technique is useful. In significant forearm injuries with critical ischemia, vein graft interposition or bypass based from the more proximal brachial artery may be necessary. For reconstructions at the wrist, it may be helpful to have a hand surgeon present. Conduits for wrist/hand level reconstruction can include forearm or foot vein as well as various other autogenous arterial conduits.[116]

Lower extremity

FEMORAL ARTERY INJURIES

The femoral arteries are the most commonly injured lower extremity arteries accounting for 25%–50% in both civilian and military series. The superficial femoral artery (SFA) is injured most frequently. Control for CFA injuries can be accomplished in several ways. First, if the patient is not doing well with ongoing hemorrhage or growing hematoma, it may be most expeditious to perform a lower laparotomy and control the distal external iliac artery in the abdomen. Alternatively, if time allows but the groin morphology is obscure, retroperitoneal exposure of the distal external iliac artery for control is reasonable. This can either be accomplished by extending the traditional longitudinal incision over the groin obliquely onto the abdomen and entering the retroperitoneum with fascial incision parallel to the external oblique fibres or via a separate oblique lower abdominal incision. If the patient is stable and the situation permits, consideration for standard, longitudinal femoral exposure with control at the inguinal ligament can be appropriate if the mechanism is stab or puncture and the groin is stable. If there is any concern for any reason, more extensive exposure and control is encouraged rather than needing to seek further proximal control after hemorrhage control is less stable.

Use of self-retaining retractor systems can be essential. The author prefers the pediatric OMNI system, but others can suffice. Selective iliac endovascular balloon control from the contralateral femoral artery or the arm can also be performed. Nonselective resuscitative endovascular balloon aortic control can be considered in unstable patients, but should be replaced by open control or selective iliac balloon control as soon as possible. Endovascular control is particularly useful when the clinical situation requires manual hemorrhage control in the groin. When the injury is proximal, division of the inguinal ligament has been espoused. This can be frequently avoided with endovascular control, or peritoneal or retroperitoneal exposures. These allow for broader control away from the femoral artery, which makes repair easier with the extent of hematoma and edema in the groin.

Repair of CFA injuries requires judgment. Arterial debridement followed by primary repair, or autogenous or prosthetic patch angioplasty can be performed when injuries are less extensive. These should not narrow the artery's original diameter. In more extensive injuries, interposition grafts are necessary. Autogenous saphenous vein interposition, prosthetic grafts and femoral vein, internal jugular vein, arm vein or panel vein grafts can be considered. Proximal basilic vein is often a good option. It can be formidable to determine if simple vein interposition is adequate in the CFA. As the vein will enlarge over time, it has been the author's practice to accept vein sizes of at least two-thirds the normal CFA size, which is mostly in the 5–8 mm range. Salvage of the femoral bifurcation allowing flow into not only the SFA but also the profunda femoris artery (PFA), the major collateral supply to the limb, is important, and repair should be purposeful in this regard. This can be accomplished with bevelling of the femoral bifurcation, reimplantation of the PFA origin onto the graft or the SFA or separate bypass graft to the PFA. In damage control scenarios, separate parallel TVS from the EIA to the SFA and PFA has been used with a well-planned full revascularization after resuscitation. Isolated SFA injury is largely repairable with GSV or prosthetic. PFA injuries can be ligated if necessary.

POPLITEAL ARTERY INJURIES

The popliteal artery is injured frequently and accounts for some 12%–25% of lower extremity arterial injuries. Combined popliteal venous injury is not uncommon and occurs in 30%–60% of injuries (Figure 52.11b). The tibial nerve is involved in 10%–30% irrespective of the clinical mechanism. This milieu establishes popliteal artery injury as the arterial level carrying the highest risk of amputation in the extremities.[3] Surgical approach to the popliteal vessels is usually through a medial approach, which can utilize both traditional above- and below-knee incisions. This provides the freedom to expose further proximally or distally as needed. Proximal control may be at the common femoral or SFA level should above-knee popliteal artery control be impractical. The posterior approach should be reserved only for patients who are physiologically normal and in whom the injury is isolated. Injury should be focal with little soft tissue injury. The prone position limits the overall systemic care of the trauma patient. The posterior approach may be more applicable in focal injury evolution late after injury event in a more elective situation. Occasionally, mostly in later, chronic scenarios or in cases of major tissue destruction or infection, the lateral approach to the popliteal artery can be useful. Above the knee, the incision is made at the posterior aspect of the iliotibial band with dissection between the vastus lateralis muscle anteriorly and the biceps femoris posteriorly. Below the knee, resection of the proximal fibula is required with protection of the common peroneal nerve. With the fibular periosteum retracted anteriorly, the vessels are found anterior to the gastrocsoleus complex. The lateral soleal arch must be divided.

With the medial approach, most injuries can be defined and exposed. Yet, some 5 cm of retrogeniculate artery is inaccessible and, when injured, must simply be ligated above and below with bypass performed (Figure 52.11b). Late problems, such as bleeding or false aneurysm formation, in this segment due to residual branch flow are not reported but are ostensibly possible. With soft tissue injury, edema and hematoma, exposure becomes more difficult and increases the length of this poorly exposable area. In many multisystem injuries, proper exposure and repair requires external fixation devices to either be loosened and then repositioned after vascular repair or simply accomplished after vascular repair. It can be difficult to appropriately estimate graft length in these circumstances. A helpful method to address this is to expose and control the injury and shunt and then allow proper reduction and placement of the external fixator pins. If necessary, measure the projected length of graft needed when reduced. Then, loosen, repair the vessel, and re-reduce appropriately and secure. This requires multidisciplinary team coordination. Leg exsanguination with tourniquet control can be considered in limbs with minimal deformity, and no major bony or soft tissue injury, but in the author's experience, is rarely utilized.

TIBIAL ARTERY INJURIES

Tibial artery injuries represent 25%–40% of lower extremity arterial injuries. The surgical approach to the tibial arteries is standard. The mid-distal anterior tibial artery (ATA) is approached through an incision two to three fingerbreadths lateral to the anterior tibial edge. It is identified on the interosseous membrane in the raphe lateral to the anterior tibialis muscle and medial to the extensor digitorum longus and extensor hallucis longus muscles. The posterior tibial artery (PTA) is approached medially via an incision one to two fingerbreadths posterior to the medial border of the tibia. Proximally, it runs underneath

the soleal arch, and this should be divided after identification of the below-knee popliteal artery taking care to stay superficial to the arteries. The origin of the ATA is just distal to the soleal arch attachment. The tibioperoneal trunk and its bifurcation can be identified with distal dissection from the arch providing exposure of the proximal PTA. Distal to this the PTA is found between the soleus and the flexor digitorum longus muscle and posterior to the flexor tendon just at and above the medial malleolus. The peroneal artery is more challenging and is usually approached medially with further dissection anterior to the posterior tibial vessels and nerve in the raphe behind the tibialis posterior. The lateral approach to the peroneal with excision of the fibula is rarely used in traumatic injury. These incisions, in standard positions, allow for simultaneous four-compartment fasciotomy.

Similar to the forearm arterial injuries, the redundant perfusion to the foot allows for simple ligation of identified injuries should reasonable perfusion be appreciated. Continuous wave Doppler examination, or on-table duplex, can be invaluable in determining tibial vessel patency and perfusion with ligation. The experiential dictum that one tibial vessel in continuity with the foot is acceptable should be followed. Patients with tibial-level injury frequently have other injuries or reasons to be in shock making clinical assessment difficult. Further, tibial reconstruction for traumatic injury is quite challenging and time consuming, thus making selection of those who need revascularization thought-provoking and vital. Tibial reconstruction should only be pursued in true critical ischemia without viable distal perfusion, in those who do not have significant other life-threatening injuries and have a reasonable salvage potential with little soft-tissue loss or foot deformities. We have recently shown statistically that this selective posture toward tibial injury repair results in similar amputation-free survival in those receiving tibial bypass versus those not and is a reasonable stance.[117] When otherwise normal, these muscular arteries can easily develop spasm and resuscitation after addressing other life-threatening injuries with vigilant reassessment is prudent without hard indication of disruption. Anecdotally, the author has operated on open infrageniculate injuries and been nearly unable to identify the tibial arteries due to this process. Yet, 12–24 hours later, a palpable pulse is present with a warm foot in a vessel not intervened upon. Because of spasm and the points earlier, it is wise to perform end-to-side anastomoses proximally to maintain axial flow to any vessels remaining inline distal.

ENDOVASCULAR TREATMENT

Application of endovascular techniques in the diagnosis and treatment of vascular trauma has become common. Yet, addressing arterial injury with endovascular methods remains relatively rare today as it is utilized in less than 8% of injuries.[118] For obvious reasons, aortic and torso injuries have been the focus, while the majority of reports delineating extremity use involve the junctional zones. Several descriptions of endovascular therapies during conflict in Iraq and Afghanistan can be found in the literature. We have documented development and successful implementation of endovascular capability in a level III surgical facility from 2004 to 2007 during OIF.[119] During this period, 150 catheter-based procedures were performed including covered stenting of extremity axial arterial injury.

Catheter-based techniques offer advantages in both acute vessel injuries and less urgent traumatic sequelae such as arteriovenous fistula and pseudoaneurysm particularly in junctional zones as they avoid operative dissection. Furthermore, use of covered stents is becoming recognized as a feasible alternative in definitive management in both penetrating and blunt traumas.[120,121] These should be sized in a similar way to that of age-related vascular disease; however, the generally healthy arteries in trauma are smaller than atherosclerotic vessels, and more like 20%–30% oversizing may be needed for self-expanding devices. Even in the presence of hard signs of vascular injury (pulsatile bleeding, absent distal pulses, expanding hematoma, bruit or thrill) and hemodynamic instability, patients now may be considered for emergent endovascular repair or control in the operating room. Endovascular management requires endovascular expertise is available and the operating room is capable of timely endovascular proficiency. Today, as fixed hybrid operating room technology with state-of-the-art imaging becomes more commonplace, this is more and more realistic. Endovascular capability facilitates rapid stabilization with balloon occlusion control followed by any open or endovascular methodology and allows for open conversion if necessary. In stable patients, today's use of non-invasive anatomic imaging, usually CTA, allows for injury definition and endovascular treatment planning.

Upper extremity

Control and definitive endovascular management of axillosubclavian artery injuries is arguably the arena in which there is the most experience currently (Figure 52.12). These may require femoral access, retrograde ipsilateral brachial access or both. Passing the wire under fluoroscopic guidance across vessel disruption from either the retrograde femoral or brachial approach may be challenging. Because of the shorter distance from the access site to the injury, many prefer the retrograde brachial approach. Directional catheters, balloon centering guidance as well as combined femoral and brachial access with snare capture of the wire through the injury are techniques used to achieve wire access across the upper extremity vessel injury. Endovascular control and repair allows the surgical team to address other life-threatening injuries, avoiding the time and morbidity of median sternotomy, thoracotomy or junctional zone open exposure.

Either self-expanding or balloon expandable covered stents have been effective in managing select innominate and axillosubclavian injuries. In contrast, bare metal stents have been more commonly reported with treatment of small dissections or intimal flaps. One multicentre trial evaluating use of the self-expanding Wallgraft Endoprosthesis (Boston Scientific, Natick, MA) for the treatment of 62 iliac, femoral or subclavian arterial injuries showed the endoprosthesis achieved exclusion of the injury in 93.5% of cases and 90% of the subclavian artery injuries.[120] Freedom from bypass was achieved in 100% of the subclavian injuries. Overall early mortality was 6.5%, but no procedure-related mortalities were reported, and the most common post-procedure complication involved stenosis or occlusion. While the data support use of endovascular management of arterial injury, most procedures in this series were performed for iatrogenic injury (78%) and comparison of this study population with major accidental traumatic vascular injuries should be done with caution.

du Toit and colleagues reported 57 patients with penetrating subclavian artery injury that underwent stent graft repair during a 10-year period.[121] One patient in this series died due to other injuries, and 3 (5%) developed early, non–limb-threatening stent graft occlusion. Complete follow-up data were available for 16 patients at a mean of 61 months (range 8–104 months), which showed that 5 patients had claudication and >50% in-stent stenosis on arteriogram. These patients were successfully treated with balloon angioplasty. Three additional asymptomatic patients in the follow-up cohort had stent occlusion, but did not require reintervention. There are also multiple case reports exhibiting use of endografts in the setting of upper extremity arterial trauma. Hershberger et al. reviewed 195 studies published between 1995 and 2007 and suggested the overall treatment success rate for supradiaphragmatic arterial injury was 96%.[122] When all reports reviewing endovascular treatment of innominate (n = 7), subclavian (n = 91) and axillary (n = 12) artery injuries were assessed, technical success rates were 85.7%, 96.7% and 100%; peri-procedural morbidities were 0%, 12.1% and 8.3%; and mortalities were 0%, 3% and 0%, respectively, for each segment. The infrequent complications that were reported following endovascular repair of upper extremity vascular injury in these reports included access site pseudoaneurysm, arm claudication and stent fracture and thrombosis.

While short-term durability has been suggested to be equivocal to operative repair, long-term durability of endovascular stents in upper extremity traumatic injuries has not been completely defined. Current results described are encouraging. Specifically, patency rates appear to be acceptable with few reports describing need to revascularize following upper extremity stent graft occlusion. Although the possibility of infection remains a legitimate concern, there is no suggestion that use of today's covered stents in trauma patients poses an undue risk. In our review of available literature on

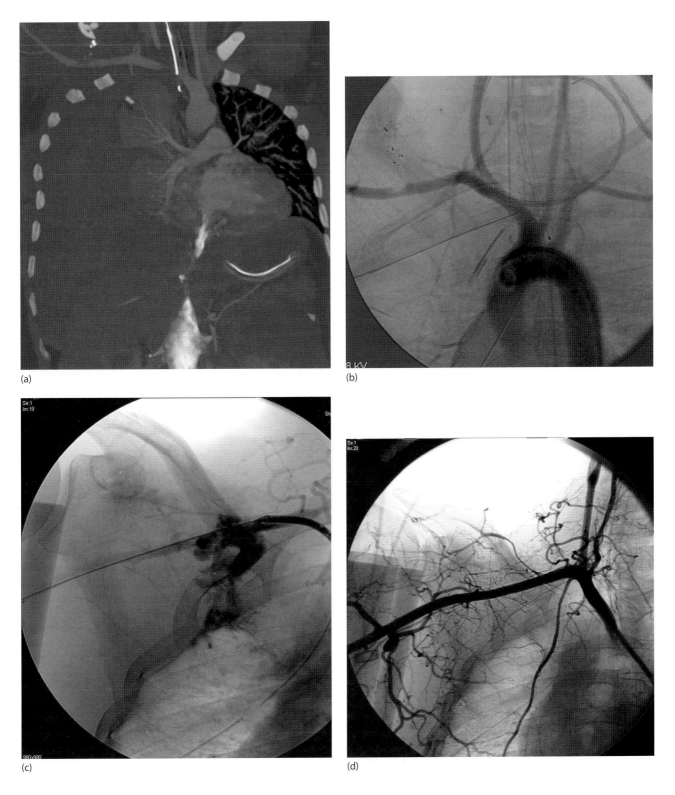

(a)

(b)

(c)

(d)

Figure 52.12 (a) Coronal computed tomographic angiography reconstruction showing injury to the right distal subclavian artery–proximal axillary artery after low-velocity gunshot wound in a 32-year-old woman. (b) Aortogram identifying the injury. (c) Selective subclavian arteriography after selection from a retrograde femoral approach with stiff wire access and sheath placement showing clear extravasation. (d) Completion arteriography after placing an 8 mm × 50 mm self-expanding covered stent indicating exclusion of injury with normal arterial flow.

axillosubclavian arterial injury handled with endovascular repair, of 160 cases no infections were noted, 3% underwent open conversion and 8.5% required reintervention.[123] Thus, use of endovascular stenting does not preclude either future open repair or catheter-based reintervention. Longer follow-up periods and experiences are needed before definitive durability of these interventions can be appreciated. Reports describing endovascular intervention for successful management of brachial artery transection are appearing.[124] Whether this technique becomes widely applicable remains to be seen.

Lower extremity

Description of lower extremity arterial endovascular repair is much less mature than that of the upper extremity. As early as 1994, lower extremity trauma has been approached with endovascular methods when Marin and the Montefiore group in New York described three patients with home-made stent grafts in the SFA location for pseudoaneurysms and arteriovenous fistulas.[125] However, since then most communications are case reports with many describing embolization of branch vessel bleeding and fewer axial endografts. As noted earlier, White and co-workers described use of axial stent grafts at the femoral and iliac levels.[120] Early exclusion failures were most common in the femoral artery, and early mortality was not endograft related. Exclusion success at 1 year was 91.3% for iliac arteries but only 62.3% at the femoral level. No femoral failure required reintervention. Recent assessment of lower extremity arterial injury at a level I trauma centre from 2005 to 2010 indicated endovascular methods for repair of infrainguinal arterial injury occurred in four femoral-level injuries representing only 7.5% of injuries.[11] An initial report from the multicenter Prospective Observational Vascular Injury Treatment Registry describing over 500 arterial injuries at 13 trauma centres over 1 year indicated only 3 endovascular interventions in the lower extremity.[118] Practice Guidelines on lower extremity arterial injury from the Eastern Association for the Surgery of Trauma were provided in 2012, and they decried the lack of series and data describing stent grafting for axial vessel injury.[126] They recommended case-by-case selection. The general technical approach to arterial injury in the lower extremity is similar to that of the upper extremity. The caveat being combined antegrade and retrograde access for transection traversal is more difficult, or may be simply contraindicated. Infrageniculate injuries can be approached via a contralateral, retrograde 'up and over' method or percutaneous or open antegrade access. Proximal extremity injuries may be approached from brachial access. More information is unmistakably needed in order to better define the rolls and outcomes of endovascular repair of axial lower extremity arterial injury. At this point, feasibility and safety are discernable.

BEST CLINICAL PRACTICE

- Full pulse exam and ABI in all injured extremities. If both arms are injured, use an uninjured extremity pressure for reference. Any index less than 0.9 must be further investigated.
- CTA is the most comprehensive and accurate noninvasive diagnostic imaging in extremity vascular injury.
- Hard signs of vascular injury mandate immediate intervention.
- In minimal injuries without diminution of distal perfusion, nonoperative management is rational and suitable.
- Open repair, open repair with endovascular balloon control or endovascular management are all appropriate options in extremity injury.
- Fasciotomies should be performed with any concern for complicated reperfusion or significant fracture/soft tissue injury.
- Wound management with negative pressure therapy and creative soft tissue coverage of vascular reconstruction can be successful. Extra-anatomic routes may be considered.
- Antiplatelet therapy for arterial injury and anticoagulants for vein injury should be strongly considered, but use is frequently dictated by concomitant injuries.

Key points

- The extremities are the most common location of vascular injury.
- In lower extremity vascular injury, mortality is higher the more proximal the injury. Amputation risk is highest in the popliteal tibial location and with blunt mechanism.
- In upper extremity vascular injury, mortality and amputation risk are highest more proximally.
- Temporary vascular shunts provide early restoration of perfusion during preparation for definitive vascular repair and in damage control.
- Vein repair should be considered in those without physiologic compromise, with adequate conduit and in injury in major confluence areas and can impact limb salvage.
- Distal forearm and tibial injuries may be ligated with discernable collateral flow.
- Endovascular repair is feasible in upper and lower extremities and can be definitive.

DEFICIENT AREAS FOR FUTURE RESEARCH

- Ischemic tolerance of extremity tissues based on injury, mechanism and shock
- Physiologic and clinical impact of venous shunting and repair
- Physiologic and clinical impact of various agents for therapeutic shunting

- Tourniquet use for extremity vascular injury in civilian care structures
- Use of temporary shunting for transport in civilian care structures
- Appropriate clinical markers identifying primary amputation indication
- Endovascular therapy durability in extremity vascular injury

REFERENCES

1. Loh SA, Rockman CB, Chung C, Maldonado TS, Adelman MA, Cayne NS, Pachter HL, Mussa FF. Existing trauma and critical care scoring systems underestimate mortality among vascular trauma patients. *J Vasc Surg.* 2011;53:359–366.

2. Perkins ZB, De'Ath HD, Aylwin C, Brohi K, Walsh M, Tai NRM. Epidemiology and outcome of vascular trauma at a British Major Trauma Centre. *Eur J Vasc Endovasc Surg.* 2012;44:203–209.

3. Barmparas G, Inabe K, Talving P, David JS, Lam L, Plurad D, Green D, Demetriades D. Pediatric vs adult vascular trauma: A National Trauma Databank review. *J Pediatr Surg.* 2010;45:1404–1412.

4. Mattox KL, Feliciano DV, Burch J, Beall AC, Jordan GL, DeBakey ME. Five thousand seven hundred sixty cardiovascular injuries in 4459 patients. Epidemiologic evolution 1958 to 1987. *Ann Surg.* 1989;209:698–705.

5. Tan TW, Joglar FL, Hamburg NM, Eberhardt RT, Shaw PM, Rybin D, Doros G, Farber A. Limb outcome and mortality in lower and upper extremity arterial injury: A comparison using the National Trauma Data Bank. *Vasc Endovasc Surg.* 2011;45:592–597.

6. Worni M, Scarborough JE, Gandhi M, Pietrobon R, Shortell CK. Use of endovascular therapy for peripheral arterial lesions: An analysis of the National Trauma Data Bank from 2007 to 2009. *Ann Vasc Surg.* 2013;27:299–305.

7. Franz RW, Skytta CK, Shah KJ, Hartman JF, Wright ML. A five-year review of management of upper-extremity arterial injuries at an urban level I trauma center. *Ann Vasc Surg.* 2012;26:655–664.

8. Asensio JA, Kuncir EJ, Garcia-Nunez LM, Petrone P. Femoral vessel injuries: Analysis of factors predictive of outcomes. *J Am Coll Surg.* 2006;203:512–520.

9. Mullenix PS, Steele SR, Andersen CA, Starnes BW, Salim A, Martin MJ. Limb salvage and outcomes among patients with traumatic popliteal vascular injury: An analysis of the National Trauma Data Bank. *J Vasc Surg.* 2006;44:94–100.

10. Dorlac WC, DeBakey ME, Holcomb JB, Fagan SP, Kwong KL, Dorlac GR, Schreiber MA, Persse DE, Moore FA, Mattox KL. Mortality from isolated civilian penetrating extremity injury. *J Trauma.* 2005;59:217–222.

11. Franz RW, Shah KJ, Halaharvi D, Franz ET, Hartman JF, Wright ML. A 5-year review of management of lower extremity arterial injuries at an urban level I trauma center. *J Vasc Surg.* 2011;53:1604–1610.

12. Kauvar DS, Sarfati MR, Kraiss LW. National trauma databank analysis of mortality and limb loss in isolated lower extremity vascular trauma. *J Vasc Surg.* 2011;53:1598–1603.

13. Perkins ZB, Yet B, Glasgow S, Cole E, Marsh W, Brohi K, Rasmussen TE. Meta-analysis of prognostic factors for amputation following surgical repair of lower extremity vascular trauma. *Br J Surg.* 2015;102:436–450.

14. DeBakey ME, Simeone FA. Battle injuries of the arteries in World War II: An analysis of 2,471 cases. *Ann Surg.* 1946;123:534–579.

15. Hughes CW. Arterial repair during the Korean War. *Ann Surg.* 1958;147:555–561.

16. Rich NM, Baugh JH, Hughes CW. Acute arterial injuries in Vietnam: 1,000 cases. *J Trauma.* 1970;10:359–369.

17. White JM, Stannard A, Burkhardt GE, Eastridge BJ, Blackbourne JH, Rasmussen TE. The epidemiology of vascular injury in the wars in Iraq and Afghanistan. *Ann Surg.* 2011;253:1184–1189.

18. Clouse WD, Rasmussen TE, Peck MA, Eliason JL, Cox MW, Bowser AN, Jenkins DH, Smith DL, Rich NM. In-theater management of vascular injury: 2 years of the Balad Vascular Registry. *J Am Coll Surg.* 2007;204:625–632.

19. Rasmussen TE, Clouse WD, Jenkins DH, Peck MA, Eliason JL, Smith DL. Echelons of care and the management of wartime vascular injury: A report from the 332nd EMDG/Air Force Theater Hospital, Balad Air Base, Iraq. *Perspect Vasc Surg Endovasc Ther.* 2006;18:91–99.

20. Fox CJ, Patel B, Clouse WD. Update on wartime vascular injury. *Perspect Vasc Endovasc Ther.* 2005;41:638–644.

21. Clouse WD, Rasmussen TE, Perlstein J, Sutherland MJ, Peck MA, Eliason JL, Jazerevic S, Jenkins DH. Upper extremity vascular injury: A current in-theater wartime report from Operation Iraqi Freedom. *Ann Vasc Surg.* 2006;20:429–434.

22. Weber MA, Fox CJ, Adams E, Rice RD, Quan R, Cox MW, Gillespie DL. Upper extremity arterial combat injury management. *Perspect Vasc Surg Endovasc Ther.* 2006;18:141–145.

23. Feliciano DV, Moore FA, Moore EE, West MA, Davis JW, Cocanour CS, Kozar RA, McIntyre RC. Evaluation and management of peripheral vascular injury. Part I. Western Trauma Association Critical Decisions in Trauma. *J Trauma.* 2011;70:1551–1556.

24. Weaver FA, Yellin AE, Bauer M, Oberg J, Ghalambor N, Emmanuel RP, Applebaum RM, Pentecost MJ, Shorr RM. Is arterial proximity a valid indication for arteriography in penetrating extremity trauma? A prospective analysis. *Arch Surg.* 1990;125:1256–1260.

25. Schwartz MR, Weaver FA, Bauer M, Siegel A, Yellin AE. Refining the indications for arteriography in penetrating extremity trauma: A prospective analysis. *J Vasc Surg.* 1993;17:116–122.

26. Johansen K, Lynch K, Paun M, Copass M. Non-invasive vascular tests reliably exclude occult arterial trauma in injured extremities. *J Trauma.* 1991;31:515–522.

27. Nassoura ZE, Ivatury RR, Simon RJ, Jabbour N, Vinzons A, Stahl W. A Reassessment of Doppler pressure indices in the detection of arterial lesions in proximity penetrating injuries to the extremities: A prospective study. *J Am Emerg Med.* 1996;14:151–156.

28. Dennis JW, Frykberg ER, Crump JM, Vines FS, Alexander RH. New perspectives on the management of penetrating trauma in proximity to major limb arteries. *J Vasc Surg.* 1990;11:85–93.

29. Dennis JW, Frykberg ER, Veldenz H, Huffman S, Menawat S. Validation of nonoperative management of occult vascular injuries and accuracy of physical examination alone in penetrating extremity trauma: 5-to10-year follow-up. *J Trauma.* 1998;44:243–253.

30. Conrad MF, Patton JH, Parikshak M, Kralovich KA. Evaluation of vascular injury in penetrating extremity trauma: Angiographers stay home. *Am Surg.* 2002;68:269–274.

31. Patterson BO, Holt PJ, Cleanthis M, Tai N, Carrell T, Loosemore TM for London Vascular Injuries Working Group. Imaging vascular trauma. *Br J Surg.* 2012;99:494–505.

32. Rieger M, Mallouhi A, Tauscher T, Lutz M, Jaschke WR. Traumatic arterial injuries of the extremities: Initial evaluation with MDCT angiography. *Am J Roentgenol.* 2006;186:656–664.

33. Inaba K, Branco B, Reddy S, Park JJ, Green D, Plurad D, Talving P, Lam L, Demetriades D. Prospective evaluation of multidetector computed tomography for extremity vascular trauma. *J Trauma.* 2011;70:808–815.

34. Knudson MM, Lewis FR, Atkinson K, Neuhas A. The role of duplex ultrasound arterial imaging in patients with penetrating extremity trauma. *Arch Surg.* 1993;128:1033–1038.

35. Fry WR, Smith RS, Sayers DV, Henderson VJ, Morabito D, Tsai EK, Harness JK, Organ CH. The success of duplex ultrasonographic scanning in diagnosis of extremity vascular proximity trauma. *Arch Surg.* 1993;128:1368–1372.

36. Bynoe RP, Miles WS, Bell RM, Greenwold DR, Sessions G, Haynes JL, Rush DS. Noninvasive diagnosis of vascular trauma by duplex ultrasonography. *J Vasc Surg.* 1991;14:346–352.

37. Bergstein JM, Blair JF, Edwards J, Towne JB, Wittman DH, Aprahamian C, Quebbeman EJ. Pitfalls in the use of color-flow duplex ultrasound for screening of suspected arterial injuries in penetrated extremities. *J Trauma.* 1992;33:395–402.

38. Peskun CJ, Levy BA, Fanelli GC, Stannard JP, Stuart MJ, MacDonald PB, Marx RG, Boyd JL, Whelan DB. Diagnosis and management of knee dislocations. *Physic Sports Med.* 2010;38:101–111.

39. Medina O, Arom A. Vascular and nerve injury after knee dislocation. *Clin Orthop Relat Res.* 2014;472:2621–2629.

40. Miranda FE, Dennis JW, Veldenz HC, Dovgan PS, Frykberg ER. Confirmation of the safety and accuracy of physical examination in the evaluation of knee dislocation for injury of the popliteal artery: A prospective study. *J Trauma.* 2002;52:247–252.

41. Kragh JF Jr., Walters TJ, Baer DG, Fox CJ, Wade CE, Salinas J, Holcomb JB. Practical use of emergency tourniquets to stop bleeding in major limb trauma. *J Trauma.* 2008;64:S38–S50.

42. Kragh JF Jr., Walters TJ, Baer DG, Fox CJ, Salinas J, Holcomb JB. Survival with emergency tourniquet use to stop bleeding in major limb trauma. *Ann Surg.* 2009;249:1–7.

43. Lakstein D, Blumenfeld A, Sokolov T, Lin G, Bssorai R, Lynn M, Ben-Abrham R. Tourniquets for hemorrhage control on the battlefield: A 4-year accumulated experience. *J Trauma.* 2003;54:S221–S225.

44. Walters TJ, Wenke JC, Kauvar DS, McManus JG, Holcomb JB, Baer DG. Effectiveness of self-applied tourniquets in human volunteers. *Prehosp Emerg Care.* 2005;9:416–422.

45. Davidson BP, Belcik JT, Mott BH, Landry G, Lindner JR. Quantification of residual limb skeletal muscle perfusion with contrast-enhanced ultrasound during application of a focal junctional tourniquet. *J Vasc Surg.* 2016;63(1):148–153.

46. Kotwal RS, Montgomery HR, Kotwal BM, Champion HR, Butler FK Jr., Mabry RL, Cain JS, Blackbourne LH, Mechler KK, Holcomb JB. Eliminating preventable death on the battlefield. *Arch Surg.* 2011;146(12):1350–1358.

47. Moore FA. Tourniquets: Another adjunct in damage control? *Ann Surg.* 2009;249:8–9.

48. Spinella PC, Perkins JG, Grathwohl KW, Beekley AC, Holcomb JB. Warm fresh whole blood is independently associated with improved survival for patients with combat-related traumatic injuries. *J Trauma.* 2009;66 (4 Suppl):S69–S76.

49. Borgman MA, Spinella PC, Perkins J, Grathwohl KW, Repine T, Beekley AC, Sebesta J, Jenkins D, Wade CE, Holcomb JB. The ratio of blood products transfused affects mortality in patients receiving massive transfusions at a combat support hospital. *J Trauma.* 2007;63:805–813.

50. Pidcoke HF, Aden JK, Mora AG, Borgman MA, Spinella PC, Dubick MA, Blackbourne LH, Cap AP. Ten-year analysis of transfusion in Operation Iraqi Freedom and Operation Enduring Freedom: Increased plasma and platelet use correlates with improved survival. *J Trauma Acute Care Surg.* 2012;73:S445–S452.

51. Fox CJ, Mehta SG, Cox ED, Kragh JF Jr., Salinas J, Holcomb JB. Effect of recombinant factor VIIa as an adjunctive therapy in damage control for wartime vascular injuries: A case control study. *J Trauma*. 2009;66 (4 Suppl):S112–S119.

52. Fox CJ, Gillespie DL, Cox ED et al. The effectiveness of a damage control resuscitation strategy for vascular injury in a combat support hospital: Results of a case control study. *J Trauma*. 2008;64:S99–S107.

53. Kandane-Rathnayake RK, Willis CD, Bourke BM, Cameron PA, McCall P, Phillips LE. Investigation of outcomes following recombinant activated FVII use for refractory bleeding during abdominal aortic aneurysm repair. *Eur J Vasc Endovasc Surg*. 2013;45:617–625.

54. Morrison JJ, DuBose JJ, Rasmussen TE, Midwinter MJ. Military application of tranexamic acid in trauma emergency resuscitation (MATTERs) study. *Arch Surg*. 2012;147:113–119.

55. Morrison JJ, Ross JD, DuBose JJ, Jansen JO, Midwinter MJ, Rasmussen TE. Association of cryoprecipitate and tranexamic acid with improved survival following wartime injury: Findings from the MATTERs II study. *JAMA Surg*. 2013;148: 218–225.

56. CRASH-2 Trial Collaborators. Effects of tranexamic acid on death, vascular occlusive events, and blood transfusion in trauma patients with significant haemorrhage (CRASH-2): A randomised, placebo-controlled trial. *Lancet*. 2010;376:23–32.

57. Hancock H, Rasmussen TE, Walker AJ, Rich NM. History of temporary intravascular shunts in the management of vascular injury. *J Vasc Surg*. 2010;52:1405–1409.

58. Chambers LW, Green DJ, Sample K, Gillingham BL, Rhee P, Brown C, Narine N, Uecker JM, Bohman HR. Tactical surgical intervention with temporary shunting of peripheral vascular trauma sustained during Operation Iraqi Freedom: One unit's experience. *J Trauma*. 2006;61:824–830.

59. Rasmussen TE, Clouse WD, Jenkins DH, Peck MA, Eliason JL, Smith DL. The use of temporary vascular shunts as a damage control adjunct in the management of wartime vascular injury. *J Trauma*. 2006;61:8–15.

60. Taller J, Kamdar JP, Greene JA, Morgan RA, Blankenship CL, Dabrowski P, Sharpe RP. Temporary vascular shunts as initial treatment of proximal extremity vascular injuries during combat operations: The new standard of care at Echelon II facilities? *J Trauma*. 2008;65:595–603.

61. Dawson DL, Putnam AT, Light JT, Ihnat DM, Kissinger DP, Rasmussen TE, Bradley DV. Temporary arterial shunts to maintain limb perfusion after arterial injury: An animal study. *J Trauma*. 1999;47:64–71.

62. Granchi T, Schmittling Z, Vasquez J, Schreiber M, Wall M. Prolonged use of intraluminal arterial shunts without systemic anticoagulation. *Am J Surg*. 2000;180:493–497.

63. Woodward EB, Clouse WD, Eliason JL, Peck MA, Bowser AN, Cox MW, Jones WT, Rasmussen TE. Penetrating femoropopliteal injury during modern warfare: Experience of the Balad Vascular Registry. *J Vasc Surg*. 2008;47:1259–1265.

64. Gifford SM, Aidinian G, Clouse WD et al. Effect of temporary shunting on extremity vascular injury: An outcome analysis from the Global War on Terror vascular injury initiative. *J Vasc Surg*. 2009;50:549–555.

65. Nichols JG, Svoboda JA, Parks SN. Use of temporary intraluminal shunts in selected peripheral arterial injuries. *J Trauma*. 1986;26:1094–1096.

66. Reber PU, Patel AG, Sapio NL, Ris HB, Beck M, Kniemeyer HW. Selective use of temporary intravascular shunts in coincident vascular and orthopedic upper and lower limb trauma. *J Trauma*. 1999;47:72–76.

67. Sriussadaporn S, Pak-art R. Temporary intravascular shunt in complex extremity vascular injuries. *J Trauma*. 2002;52:1129–1133.

68. Johansen K, Bandyk D, Thiele B, Hansen ST Jr. Temporary intraluminal shunts: Resolution of a management dilemma in complex vascular injuries. *J Trauma*. 1982;22:395–402.

69. Subramanian A, Vercruysse G, Dente C, Wyrzykowski A, King E, Feliciano DV. A decade's experience with temporary intravascular shunts at a civilian level I trauma center. *J Trauma*. 2008;65:316–326.

70. Gifford SM, Propper BW, Burkhardt GE, Clouse WD, Spencer JR, Rasmussen TE. Venous ligation in extremity vascular injury leads to an increase in muscle damage and edema in an animal model. Paper presented at: Uniformed Services University of Health Sciences Annual Trauma Day; August 2010.

71. Oliveira Goes AM, Campos Viera Abib S, Seixas Alves MT, Silva Ferreira SV, Andrade MC. To shunt or not to shunt? An experimental study comparing temporary vascular shunts and venous ligation as damage control techniques for vascular trauma. *Ann Vasc Surg*. 2014;28:710–724.

72. Malan E, Tattoni G. Physio- and anatomo-pathology of acute ischemia of the extremities. *J Cardiovasc Surg*. 1963;4:212–225.

73. Labbe R, Lindsay T, Walker PM. The extent and distribution of skeletal muscle necrosis after graded periods of complete ischemia. *J Vasc Surg*. 1987;6:152–157.

74. Gifford SM, Eliason JL, Clouse WD, Spencer JR, Burkhardt GE, Propper BW, Dixon PS, Zarzabal LA, Gelfond JA, Rasmussen TE. Early versus delayed restoration of flow with a temporary vascular shunt reduces circulating markers of injury in a porcine model. *J Trauma*. 2009;67:259–265.

75. Burkhardt GE, Gifford SM, Propper BW, Spencer JR, Williams K, Jones L, Sumner N, Cowart J, Rasmussen TE. The impact of ischemic intervals on neuromuscular recovery in a porcine (Sus scrofa) survival model of extremity vascular injury. *J Vasc Surg*. 2011;53:165–173.

76. Hancock HM, Stannard A, Burkhardt GE, Williams K, Dixon P, Cowart J, Spencer JR, Rasmussen TE. Hemorrhagic shock worsens neuromuscular recovery in a porcine model of hind limb vascular injury and ischemia-reperfusion. *J Vasc Surg.* 2011;53:1052–1062.

77. Timberlake GA, Kerstein MD. Venous injury: To repair or ligate, the dilemma revisited. *Am Surg.* 1995;61:139–145.

78. Rich NM, Hughes CW, Baugh JH. Management of venous injuries. *Ann Surg.* 1970;171 171:724–730.

79. Rich NM. Principles and indications for primary venous repair. *Surgery.* 1982;91:492–496.

80. Rich NM, Collins GJ, Andersen CA, McDonald PT. Autogenous venous interposition grafts in repair of major venous injuries. *J Trauma.* 1977;17:512–520.

81. Rich NM. Management of venous trauma. *Surg Clin North Am.* 1988;68:809–821.

82. Rich NM, Hobson RW II, Collins GJ, Andersen CA. The effect of acute popliteal venous interruption. *Ann Surg.* 1976;183:365–368.

83. Hobson RW II, Howard EW, Wright CB, Collins GJ, Rich NM. Hemodynamics of canine femoral venous ligation: Significance in combined arterial and venous injuries. *Surgery.* 1973;74:824–829.

84. Quan RW, Gillespie DL, Stuart RP, Chang AS, Whittaker DR, Fox CJ. The effect of vein repair on the risk of venous thromboembolic events: A review of more than 100 traumatic military venous injuries. *J Vasc Surg.* 2008;47:571–577.

85. Smith LM, Block EFJ, Buechter KJ, Draughn DC, Watson D, Hedden W. The natural history of extremity venous repair performed for trauma. *Am Surg.* 1999;65:116–120.

86. Meyer J, Walsh J, Schuler J, Barrett J, Durham J, Eldrup-Jorgensen J, Schwarcz T, Flanigan DP. The early fate of venous repair after civilian vascular trauma: A clinical, hemodynamic and venographic assessment. *Ann Surg.* 1987;206:458–462.

87. Nypaver TJ, Schuler JJ, McDonnell P et al. Long-term results of venous reconstruction after vascular trauma in civilian practice. *J Vasc Surg.* 1992;16:762–768.

88. Yelon JA, Scalea TM. Venous injuries of the lower extremities and pelvis: Repair versus ligation. *J Trauma.* 1992;33:532–538.

89. Hafez HM, Woolgar J, Robbs JV. Lower extremity arterial injury: Results of 550 cases and review of risk factors associated with limb loss. *J Vasc Surg.* 2001;33:1212–1219.

90. Rich NM, Hughes CW. The fate of prosthetic material used to repair vascular injuries in contaminated wounds. *J Trauma.* 1972;12:459–467.

91. Rich NM, Baugh JH, Hughes CW. Significance of complications associated with vascular repairs performed in Vietnam. *Arch Surg.* 1970;100:646–651.

92. Vertrees A, Fox CJ, Quan RW, Cox MW, Adams ED, Gillespie DL. The use of prosthetic grafts in complex military vascular trauma: A limb salvage strategy for patients with severely limited autologous conduit. *J Trauma.* 2009;66:980–983.

93. Watson JDB, Houston R IV, Morrison JJ, Gifford SM, Rasmussen TE. A retrospective cohort comparison of expanded polytetrafluoroethylene to autologous vein for vascular reconstruction in modern combat casualty care. *Ann Vasc Surg.* 2015;29:822–829.

94. Shah DM, Leather RP, Corson JD, Karmody AM. Polytetrafluoroethylene grafts in the rapid reconstruction of acute contaminated peripheral vascular injuries. *Am J Surg.* 1984;148:229–233.

95. Feliciano DV, Mattox KL. Five-year experience with PTFE grafts in vascular wounds. *J Trauma.* 1985;25:71–82.

96. Ritenour A, Dorlac W, Fang R, Woods T, Jenkins DH, Flaherty SF, Wade CE, Holcomb JB. Complications after fasciotomy revision and delayed compartment release in combat patients. *J Trauma.* 2008;64 (2 Suppl):S153–S162.

97. Farber A, Tan TW, Hamburg NM, Kalish JA, Joglar F, Onigman T, Rybin D, Doros G, Eberhardt RT. Early fasciotomy in patients with extremity vascular injury is associated with decreased risk of adverse limb outcomes: A review of the National Trauma Data Bank. *Injury.* 2012;43:1486–1491.

98. Leininger BE, Rasmussen TE, Smith DL, Jenkins DH, Coppola C. Experience with wound VAC and delayed primary closure of contaminated soft tissue injuries in Iraq. *J Trauma.* 2006;61:1207–1211.

99. Peck MA, Clouse WD, Cox MW, Bowser AN, Eliason JL, Jenkins DH, Smith DL, Rasmussen TE. The complete management of extremity vascular injury in a local population: A wartime report from the 332nd Expeditionary Medical Group/Air Force Theater Hospital, Balad Air Base, Iraq. *J Vasc Surg.* 2007;45:1197–1204.

100. Casey K, Sabino J, Jessie E, Martin BD, Valerio I. Flap coverage outcomes following vascular injury and repair: Chronicling a decade of severe war-related extremity trauma. *Plast Reconstr Surg.* 2015;135:301–308.

101. Gregory RT, Gould RJ, Peclet M, Wagner JS, Gilbert DA, Wheeler JR, Snyder SO, Gayle RG, Schwab W. The mangled extremity syndrome (M.E.S.): A severity grading system for multisystem injury of the extremity. *J Trauma.* 1985;25:1147–1150.

102. Johansen K, Daines M, Howey T, Helfet D, Hansen ST Jr. Objective criteria accurately predict amputation following lower extremity trauma. *J Trauma.* 1990;30:568–573.

103. Bonanni F, Rhodes M, Lucke JF. The futility of predictive scoring of mangled lower extremities. *J Trauma.* 1993;34:99–104.

104. Bosse MJ, MacKenzie EJ, Kellam JF et al. A prospective evaluation of the clinical utility of the lower-extremity injury-severity scores. *J Bone Joint Surg Am.* 2001;83:3–14.

105. Durham RM, Mistry BM, Mazuski JE, Shapiro M, Jacobs D. Outcome and utility of scoring systems in the management of the mangled extremity. *Am J Surg.* 1996;172:569–573.

106. Slauterbeck JR, Britton C, Moneim MS, Clevenger FW. Mangled extremity severity score: An accurate guide to treatment of the severely injured upper extremity. *J Orthop Trauma.* 1994;8:282–285.

107. Togawa S, Yamami N, Nakayama H, Mano Y, Ikegami K, Ozeki S. The validity of the mangled extremity severity score in the assessment of upper limb injuries. *J Bone Joint Surg Br.* 2005;87:1516–1519.

108. Rush RM Jr., Kjorstad R, Starnes BW, Arrington E, Devine JD, Andersen CA. Application of the Mangled Extremity Severity Score in a combat setting. *Mil Med.* 2007;172:777–781.

109. Stain SC, Yellin AE, Weaver FA, Pentecost MJ. Selective management of nonocclusive arterial injuries. *Arch Surg.* 1989;124:1136–1140.

110. Frykberg ER, Vines FS, Alexander RH. The natural history of clinically occult arterial injuries: A prospective evaluation. *J Trauma.* 1989;29:577–583.

111. Neville RF, Padberg FT, DeFouw D, Hernandez J, Duran W, Hobson RW II. The arterial wall response to intimal injury in an experimental model. *Ann Vasc Surg.* 1992;6:50–54.

112. Neville RF, Hobson RW II, Watanabe B, Yasuhara H, Padberg FT, Duran W, Franco CD. A prospective evaluation of arterial intimal injuries in an experimental model. *J Trauma.* 1991;31:669–675.

113. Hernandez-Maldonado JJ, Padberg FT, Teehan E, Neville RF, DeFouw D, Duran WN, Hobson RW II. Arterial intimal flaps: A comparison of primary repair, aspirin, and endovascular excision in an experimental model. *J Trauma.* 1993;34:565–570.

114. Lazarides MK, Georgiadis GS, Papas TT, Gardikis S, Maltezos C. Operative and nonoperative management of children aged 13 years or younger with arterial trauma of the extremities. *J Vasc Surg.* 2006;43:72–76.

115. Feliciano DV, Moore EE, West MA, Moore FA, Davis JW, Cocanour CS, Scalea TM, McIntyre RC. Western Trauma Association Critical Decisions in Trauma: Evaluation and management of peripheral vascular injury, part II. *J Trauma Acute Care Surg.* 2013;75:391–397.

116. McClinton MA. Reconstruction for ulnar artery aneurysm at the wrist. *J Hand Surg Am.* 2011;36:328–332.

117. Burkhardt GE, Cox MW, Clouse WD, Porras C, Gifford SM, William K, Propper BW, Rasmussen TE. Outcomes of selective tibial artery repair following combat-related extremity injury. *J Vasc Surg.* 2010;52:91–96.

118. DuBose JJ, Savage SA, Fabian TC et al. The American Association of the Surgery of Trauma PROspective Observational Vascular Injury Treatment (PROOVIT) registry: Multicenter data on modern vascular injury diagnosis, management and outcomes. *J Trauma Acute Care Surg.* 2015;78:215–223.

119. Rasmussen TE, Clouse WD, Peck MA, Bowser AN, Eliason JL, Cox MW, Woodward EB, Jones WT, Jenkins DH. Development and implementation of endovascular capabilities in wartime. *J Trauma.* 2008;64:1169–1176.

120. White R, Krajcer Z, Johnson M, Williams D, Bacharach M, O'Malley E. Results of a multicenter trial for the treatment of traumatic vascular injury with a covered stent. *J Trauma.* 2006;60:1189–1196.

121. du Toit DF, Lambrechts AV, Stark H, Warren BL. Long-term results of stent graft treatment of subclavian artery injuries: Management of choice for stable patients? *J Vasc Surg.* 2008;47:739–743.

122. Hershberger RC, Aulivola B, Murphy M, Luchette FA. Endovascular grafts for treatment of traumatic injury to the aortic arch and great vessels. *J Trauma.* 2009;67:660–671.

123. DuBose JJ, Rajani R, Gilani R, Arthurs ZA, Morrison JJ, Clouse WD, Rasmussen TE. Endovascular management of axillo-subclavian arterial injury: A review of published experience. *Injury.* 2012;43:1785–1792.

124. Carrafiello G, Lagana D, Mangini M, Fontana F, Chiara R, Filippo P, Carlo P, Piffaretti G, Fugazzola C. Percutaneous treatment of traumatic upper-extremity arterial injuries: A single-center experience. *J Vasc Interv Radiol.* 2011;22:31–39.

125. Marin ML, Veith FJ, Panetta TF, Cynamon J, Sanchez LA, Schwartz ML, Lyon RT, Bakal CW, Suggs WD. Transluminally placed endovascular stented graft repair for arterial trauma. *J Vasc Surg.* 1994;20:466–473.

126. Fox N, Rajani R, Bokhari F, Chiu WC, Kerwin A, Seamon MJ, Skarupa D, Frykberg E. Evaluation and management of penetrating lower extremity arterial trauma: An Eastern Association for the Surgery of Trauma practice management guideline. *J Trauma Acute Care Surg.* 2012;73:S315–S320.

Compartment Syndrome, Vascular Access, Malformations and Transplantation

53

Compartment syndrome

CAROLINE A. YAO, DAVID A. KULBER, GEOFFREY S. TOMPKINS and JONATHAN R. HIATT

CONTENTS

INTRODUCTION

Acute compartment syndrome (ACS) is defined alternatively as a condition in which (1) increased pressure within a limited space compromises the circulation and function of tissues within that space or (2) high pressure within a closed fascial space reduces capillary blood perfusion below a level necessary for tissue viability. Chronic or exertional compartment syndrome is characterized by pain and sometimes loss of nerve function that recurs with exercise and abates upon discontinuation of exercise.

Contracture is a complication of compartment syndrome resulting from muscle necrosis of the distal segments of a limb. Crush syndrome, an extreme form of compartment syndrome, results from severe blunt trauma or prolonged compression of skeletal muscle, leading to myonecrosis.

HISTORICAL CONSIDERATIONS

The consequences of compartmental ischemia were first described by Richard von Volkmann in 1881. Volkmann's ischemic contracture in the forearm was attributed to arterial insufficiency and venous stasis resulting from tight bandaging of an injured extremity. In 1906, Hildebrand speculated that hydrostatic fluid transudation caused increased pressure and compromise of the circulation in the condition he termed 'Volkmann's ischemic contracture'. John B. Murphy advocated fasciotomy in 1914, attributing compartmental ischemia to increased intracompartmental pressure.[1]

The importance of vascular injury was recognized and investigated. In 1926, Jepson reported the value of early, preventative fasciotomy in an animal model using bandages to cause venous occlusion. Increased experience with arterial injuries during World War II led Foisie and Griffiths to speculate on the etiologic role of arterial spasm in the newly recognized entity of lower extremity ACS. In 1966, Seddon was first to fully describe lower extremity compartment syndromes and their clinical importance. Clinical and laboratory studies have supported the unified concept that compartment syndrome and Volkmann's contracture are related entities resulting from increased intracompartmental pressure and ischemia of compartmental tissue.

PATHOPHYSIOLOGY

Most investigators agree that the principal abnormality causing ACS is an increase in intracompartmental pressure producing ischemia of muscles and nerves. Critical factors that influence the magnitude of neuromuscular damage include the level of intracompartmental pressure, duration of increased pressure, local changes that impair the restoration of blood flow and tolerance for ischemia. Because of the complex mechanisms involved in compartment syndrome, there remains a debate about the absolute levels of compartment pressure that result in neuromuscular damage.

Microcirculation

Capillary blood flow is regulated by a gradient between arterial and venous pressure (A-V gradient). Factors acting to decrease the A-V gradient that may cause compartmental ischemia include increased venous pressure, arteriolar closure, impaired capillary flow, vasospasm and increased capillary permeability.

Venous capillary closure is a mechanical effect dependent only upon immediately surrounding tissue pressure. The critical closure theory proposes that arterioles may close under tissue pressure less than the mean arterial pressure (MAP).[2] The degree of arteriolar closure at a given tissue pressure depends upon vessel size, level of vasomotor tone and intravascular pressure.

The 'no-reflow' phenomenon suggests that swollen cells cause compression of the vascular lumen. Injured capillary endothelium may cause intraluminal narrowing by forming intravascular blebs. Trapping of red blood cells in the narrowed capillaries also contributes to impaired flow. Vasospasm may result from injury when traction upon an artery stretches its media and stimulates contraction. Also, increased intracompartmental pressure itself has been found to induce arterial spasm by a nonsympathetically mediated antidromic reflex.

In ischemic tissues, adenosine triphosphate is converted to adenosine monophosphate, which is catabolized to hypoxanthine. When oxygen is reintroduced into hypoxic tissue, the rapid reduction of hypoxanthine to xanthine produces an excess of reactive oxygen species (ROS). ROS damage cell membranes through lipid peroxidation and activate neutrophils. Increased capillary permeability ensues, leading to transcapillary fluid leakage and ultimately further increases in intracompartmental pressures. Neutrophils potentiate cellular damage via protease release from azurophilic, specific, gelatinase and secretory granules.

Ischemia also activates the complement system by causing expression of an ischemia antigen on cellular surfaces that induces IgM antibody binding. C1 binding-mediated complement activation results in the formation of C3a and C3b, which ultimately stimulate the membrane attack complex to mediate release of prostaglandin E2 from macrophages, leukotriene B4 from neutrophils, thromboxane B2, prostanoids, interleukin-1 and ROS. Cytokine signalling via IL-1, IL-6, thromboxane A2 and TNF also mediate ischemia–reperfusion cellular injury. Level 2 evidence reports that more muscle damage occurs from 3 hours of partial ischemia than from total ischemia due to the effects

Table 53.1 Critical tissue ischemic times at normothermia.

Muscle	4 hours
Nerve	8 hours
Fat	13 hours
Skin	24 hours
Bone	4 days

Source: Steinau HU, *Major Limb Replantation and Postischemia Syndrome: Investigation of Acute Ischemia-induced Myopathy and Reperfusion Injury*, Springer Verlag, New York, 1988.

of reperfusion injury.[1] Ischemia tolerance varies among different tissues, as summarized in Table 53.1.

Compartmental pressure

Resting intracompartmental pressure in humans is 4 ± 4 mmHg,[3] with normal capillary pressures ranging from 17 to 40 mmHg.[4] In canine histological studies, the lowest level of pressure reported to cause muscle necrosis was 30 mmHg maintained for 8 hours. The conduction velocity in the canine peroneal nerve showed a significant decline at 30 mmHg and complete conduction block at 50 mmHg.[5]

In animal models, local blood flow begins to decrease significantly at tissue pressures in the 40–50 mmHg range and approaches zero at the 60–80 mmHg range or when externally applied pressure is less than 20–30 mmHg below the MAP.[6] In a clinical series by Matsen, no patient with a pressure measured at less than 45 mmHg showed residual sequelae of compartmental syndrome, while all patients who had a maximum pressure greater than 55 mmHg developed significant losses of neuromuscular function.[7] Due to large individual variations in tolerance of elevated intracompartmental pressure, it has been difficult to define a critical pressure warranting surgical decompression. To diagnose ACS, many clinicians now rely on the difference between the mean arterial and compartmental pressures (ΔP) instead of absolute tissue pressures.

Duration of the elevation of pressure is as important as the absolute level of pressure in the pathogenesis of compartment syndromes. Tissue pressures that are tolerated initially may ultimately produce neuromuscular damage if allowed to persist for extended periods.

ETIOLOGY

The causes of compartment syndrome may be classified as intrinsic or extrinsic (Table 53.2). Intrinsic causes increase the compartment's content volume. Extrinsic causes decrease the compartment's volume.

Traumatic injuries of muscle, bone and soft tissues account for the majority of intrinsic causes, with routine traffic accidents and sports injuries being the most common sources of injury. Fractures cause approximately 70% of all ACS cases. Level 3 data show that tibial shaft

Table 53.2 Causes of acute compartment syndromes.

Extrinsic
  Mechanical constriction (casts, dressings, pneumatic trousers)
  Surgical closure of fascial defects
  Environmental injuries (frostbite, burns)
Intrinsic
  Edema
    Ischemia reperfusion (vascular injury, thrombosis/embolism, tourniquet)
    Limb compression–immobilization (drug overdose, positioning during general anesthesia)
  Hemorrhage
    Trauma (vessel, bone, soft-tissue injuries)
    Bleeding disorders
    Anticoagulant therapy

fractures account for 40% of all compartment syndromes and half of the fractures that produce lower extremity ACS; upper extremity compartment syndrome tends to be associated with distal radius fractures. Men under 35 years of age are at particular at risk for developing compartment syndrome after bony or soft tissue injuries.[8] Arterial injuries cause 30% of compartment syndromes, while severe venous injuries cause 14%.[9] Reperfusion injury after significant periods of ischemia is another cause of ACS. Extrinsic causes include casts, bandages, thermal injuries and frostbite.

Case reports identify a wide variety of additional causes, including tumours, hemophilia and other bleeding disorders, lithotomy positioning during surgery, intra-aortic balloon pulsation, transaxillary arteriograms, pneumatic antishock trousers, snakebites, closed intramedullary nailing, drug abuse, ruptured Baker's cyst, systemic capillary leak syndrome and exercise.

Key points

- Ischemic time: muscle < nerve < fat < skin.
- Identify whether ACS is extrinsic or intrinsic to guide treatment.
- Consider duration of increased compartment pressure along with absolute and relative compartment pressures.

DIAGNOSIS

Physical examination

ACUTE COMPARTMENT SYNDROME

Areas at risk for compartment syndrome include not only common sites such as the forearm and the leg but also less common sites such as the buttocks, thighs, feet, deltoids and hands. The prompt diagnosis and management of ACS requires a high degree of suspicion, repeated documented examinations at frequent intervals, additional studies when indicated and treatment based on available information without unnecessary and potentially hazardous delay and observation. In one series, clinical grounds alone were sufficient to identify 16 of 21 patients in need of treatment. Residual neuromuscular deficits occurred only in the five patients who underwent delayed fasciotomies. Spontaneous pain and turgid swelling were the most common clinical findings; pain on passive flexion/extension, hypoperfusion and paresthesias were also noted in some patients.[10]

The clinical diagnosis of ACS is suggested by the presence of a number of subjective and variable signs and symptoms. These include pain, motor deficits, sensory abnormalities and swelling.

Pain is a common clinical finding. Patients often complain of pain out of proportion to the external physical findings. However, pain may be an unreliable sign given high levels of variability and the presence of additional injuries that may produce masking or distracting pain. Pain may be worsened by passive stretch of the muscles in the involved compartment(s), but level 2 evidence shows that pain in response to passive flexion/extension was an unreliable sign of ACS. Hypoesthesia was found to be a more dependable marker.[11]

Sensory abnormalities of the nerves coursing through the affected compartment(s), both subjective and measured, are considered by many authors to be the most reliable physical signs of compartmental ischemia. The subjective changes reported may range from paresthesia to hypoesthesia to anesthesia. Recommended neurologic tests include two-point discrimination, pinprick, light touch and vibratory sensation. However, hypoesthesia is one of the last clinical findings to develop and cannot be used as an early indicator.

Motor weakness presenting as paresis and paralysis in the muscles of the involved compartment is often difficult to interpret in the acute setting. Because nerve tissue is less sensitive to ischemia than the muscle, purely ischemic weakness or deficits appear later in the course of compartment syndrome than do other signs of ischemia. Paresthesias and paralysis are late findings after compartment syndrome has been present for 4 or more hours. As motor deficits are an indication of irreversible damage to the muscle and nerve in the compartment, patients who experience motor deficits rarely achieve a full functional recovery.

Palpation of a tense compartment is uniformly recognized as a crucial sign in the diagnosis of ACS. A tense compartment is an easily observed measure of increased intracompartmental pressure that may be elicited independently of the patient's neurological status or level of consciousness. While a tense compartment may distinguish ACS from acute arterial insufficiency and peripheral nerve injury (Table 53.3), clinicians must keep in mind that a tense compartment is not a consistent finding. Additionally, the deep posterior compartment of the leg is difficult to assess using palpation, given its depth.

Table 53.3 Features distinguishing clinical entities.

	Compartment syndrome	Arterial occlusion	Neurapraxia
Tense compartment	+	−	−
Pain with stretch	+	+	−
Paresthesia or anesthesia	+	+	+
Paresis or paralysis	+	+	+
Pulse intact	+	−	+

Source: Enst CB and Kaufer H, *J Trauma*, 11, 365, 1971.

While assessment of distal arterial pulses is important, a number of clinical series have shown that peripheral pulses and capillary refill may remain intact in patients with compartment syndrome because tissue damage occurs before compartmental pressure exceeds the arterial pressure. The presence of raised erythematous patches and bullae containing serosanguineous fluid may also be useful in diagnosing ACS. The differential diagnosis of ACS includes arterial injury, nerve injury, osteomyelitis, tenosynovitis, cellulitis and thrombophlebitis. Certain features distinguish these entities (Table 53.3).

CHRONIC EXERTIONAL COMPARTMENT SYNDROME

Chronic exertional compartment syndrome (CECS) occurs when a fascial compartment cannot accommodate the volume increase associated with exertional muscle contraction and swelling. Compartment volume can increase by as much as 20% as a result of increased capillary hydrostatic and interstitial osmotic pressures. Athletes, military personnel and active young men are often afflicted and experience chronic pain. CECS occurs most often in the leg bilaterally, usually in the anterior and deep posterior compartments. Reports of the condition have also been documented in forearms (gymnasts and climbers) and feet (runners). CECS can also occur after acute and/or chronic venous insufficiency and blunt extremity trauma.

Patients typically complain of aching, tightness and cramping of the leg that worsens with activity in the distribution of the involved compartment. They may experience neurologic symptoms, including numbness, tingling or weakness corresponding to the affected compartment. Many patients do not seek medical care for CECS because symptoms abate between periods of exercise, and the diagnosis may be missed because physical examinations are normal. In patients who are symptomatic at the time of exam, muscle herniation may be identified by a palpable fullness and tenderness in the involved compartment. Neurologic deficits also may be detectable during routine examination.

Stress fractures may raise clinical suspicion for adjacent CECS. Additionally, anabolic steroids may increase risk of CECS by inducing muscular hypertrophy and decreased fascial elasticity. Myofascial scarring, venous hypertension and post-traumatic soft tissue inflammation are other contributory conditions. The differential diagnosis includes conditions that cause lower extremity pain exacerbated by exercise, such as vascular insufficiency, tendonitis, myositis, periostitis, stress fracture, superficial peroneal nerve entrapment and effort-induced rhabdomyolysis.[13]

The diagnosis of CECS requires the measurement of compartment pressures before, during and after exercise. Patients with CECS may have compartment pressures as high as 80 mmHg at rest. Level 1 evidence recommends measuring compartment pressures 1 minute after exercise and finds that pressures over 27.5 mmHg (the highest reported value for controls) along with a strong clinical history are highly suggestive of CECS. Early stage CECS often presents with lower compartment pressures. Clinicians should suspect the diagnosis in patients with an appropriate clinical history whose compartment pressures rise only to 30–40 mmHg with exercise but show a delay of more than 10 minutes in returning to normal levels after exercise.[13] Table 53.4 summarizes best practices for diagnosing CECS.

> **Key points**
>
> - Classic signs of ACS include pain with stretch, paresthesias, paresis/paralysis, diminished pulses and a tense compartment; individual signs may not be diagnostic.
> - Consider chronic exertional compartment syndrome in a young, highly active patient with a history of pain and swelling induced by activity and possible stress fractures.
> - Pressure monitoring is necessary in patients who are non-compliant or with compromised cognition.

Table 53.4 Principles for diagnosing chronic exertional compartment syndrome.

Maintain a high level of suspicion for CECS in athletes, military personnel and active young men.

Radiographs to detect adjacent stress fractures may aid in the diagnosis of CECS.

Classic symptoms of CECS include recurrent aching, tightness, cramping, numbness, tingling or weakness in a compartment that worsens with activity.

CECS is highly likely in patients with compartment pressures >27.5mmHg after 1 minute of exercise (Grade A).

CECS is also likely in patients whose compartment pressures rise to 30–40 mmHg with exercise and take more than 10 minutes to return to normal after exercise (Grade B).

Measuring and monitoring techniques

ACUTE COMPARTMENT SYNDROME

Elevated interstitial pressure is one of the earliest signs of ACS. While the measurement of increased tissue pressures will suggest the diagnosis in its early stages, all available clinical data should be considered in making a final diagnosis.

Pressure monitoring is required in patients who are unresponsive, uncooperative or unable to adequately communicate (e.g. intoxicated, intubated, too young). Monitoring is also indicated in cases of peripheral or central nerve injury, multiple injuries or indeterminate clinical findings.[11]

While the absolute level of pressure at which fasciotomy is indicated has not been definitively established, accepted values are generally below 30 mmHg. Recent recommendations also advocate interpreting compartment pressures in the context of the diastolic and MAPs, such that fasciotomy may be indicated when compartment pressures are within 30 mmHg of the diastolic blood pressure.[14]

A number of factors should be considered when interpreting compartmental pressure data, including the clinical setting, the type of catheter system and the recognition that actual compartment pressure is the sum of all internal and external components (dressings, armboards and limb positioning).[11] With the advent of more advanced compartment pressure measuring devices, clinicians must have a high level of suspicion before using them, as Level 2 evidence suggests that one-time compartment measurements have a 35% false-positive rate.[15] Table 53.5 outlines best clinical practices for diagnosing ACS.

Catheter systems

NEEDLE MANOMETER[16]

The needle manometer advocated by Whitesides is the oldest catheter technique (Figure 53.1). Pressure is applied through a syringe into the IV tubing until tissue pressure

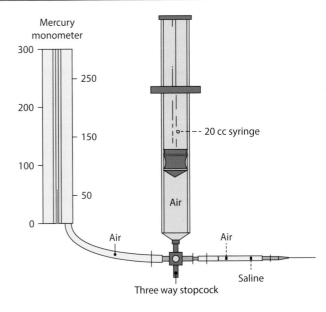

Figure 53.1 Needle manometer for intracompartmental pressure measurement.

is overcome, and the saline meniscus is observed to move as fluid enters the muscle compartment. This pressure is then read from the manometer as tissue pressure. This device cannot be used for continuous monitoring.

INFUSION[7]

The infusion technique proposed by Matsen measures the pressure required to maintain a slow (0.7 mL/day) saline infusion into the muscle compartment being studied. This method measures tissue resistance and can be used for continuous monitoring for several days.

WICK CATHETER[3]

Fibrils of polyglycolic acid suture protrude from the bore of the catheter, acting as a wick to provide more surface area for fluid equilibration and to prevent ball-valve obstruction of the catheter. This permeation of the wick permits contact with a large volume of tissue fluid. Interstitial fluid pressure is transmitted into a catheter filled with sterile, heparinized saline. The advantages of the wick system include accuracy and reproducibility greater than those obtained with the needle manometer method in comparison studies.

SLIT CATHETER[17]

The slit catheter, described by Rorabeck, employs a 20 cm polyethylene tube with 3 mm symmetrical slits cut in its end, which is connected via tubing to a plastic transducer dome. This technique was found to be as accurate as the wick catheter in immediate measurement and more accurate than the wick catheter or needle manometer for continuous measurement over 24 hours. Slit catheters are more accurate than straight or side-port needles, with Level 3 evidence showing a sensitivity of 94% and specificity of 98% for detecting ACS in patients with tibial diaphyseal fractures over 24 hours of

Table 53.5 Best clinical practice for diagnosis of acute compartment syndrome.

A tense compartment and pain are highly variable signs of ACS, while sensory and motor deficits are late findings. Clinicians must maintain a high level of clinical suspicion given a patient's history and overall medical assessment (Grade [B]).

Measure compartment pressures if clinical evidence is insufficient or equivocal.

When direct measurements are clinically necessary, the slit catheter is preferred given high sensitivity and specificity for detection of compartment pressures predict ACS (Grade [B/C]).

Consider prophylactic fasciotomy when diagnosis is delayed beyond 6 hours or if mechanism of injury is high energy, crush or at risk for reperfusion (Grade [B]).

continuous monitoring. Catheter-diagnosed ACS in this study was defined as a <30 mmHg difference in intracompartmental and diastolic pressure, and confirmed ACS was defined as muscle escape or muscle colour change at fasciotomy.[18]

SOLID-STATE TRANSDUCER INTRACOMPARTMENTAL CATHETER[19]

The solid-state transducer intracompartmental (STIC) catheter, designed by the McDermott group, requires heparinized saline around the tip but has its transducer within the catheter tip so that it is automatically equilibrated with compartment testing. The STIC catheter is easier to equilibrate, insert, maintain and interpret. It also was reported to be more sensitive than the wick catheter, registering pressure fluctuations occurring with movement of the patient's toes.

Supplemental studies, new technologies and areas for future research

Nerve stimulation and conduction studies may be useful in unconscious or uncooperative patients or in patients where neurapraxia and paralysis are difficult to differentiate. Electromyography has been helpful in evaluating the extent of muscle necrosis and neurogenic paresis. It can also detect nerve entrapment, a frequent complication of Volkmann's contracture.

Non-invasive studies are used with increasing frequency in the diagnosis of compartment syndrome. These include vascular studies, ultrasonography and spectroscopy techniques.

Vascular studies such as ankle–brachial index and duplex studies may quantify the degree of ischemia and demonstrate decreased venous filling and distorted compartmental architecture caused by swelling or hematoma. Ultrasonography and pulse-phase-locked loops detect intramuscular pressures using fascial movements in response to arterial pulsations. These tests can be conducted serially to trend pressures, especially in early stages of ACS.

Nuclear magnetic resonance (MR) spectroscopy has been used in animal models to determine diminution of blood flow severe enough to cause cellular metabolic derangements. Thallium-201 SPECT imaging (stress testing) may be useful in diagnosing and localizing CECS. Near-infrared spectroscopy detects oxygenation 2–3 cm below the skin to monitor for intracompartmental hypoxia, making the technology best suited to detect compartment syndrome in superficial compartments. Level 2 animal studies show its effectiveness in detecting muscle ischemia despite severe hypotension and hypoxemia, as may be present in critically injured and unstable patients.[20] MR may detect edematous changes during early ACS, but its use is often impractical in trauma settings due to the time commitment of the scan compared to the emergent nature of ACS. MR has a larger role in the diagnosis of CECS with a 90% sensitivity and 63% specificity.[13]

Case example

A 25-year-old man is brought by ambulance to the emergency room after a motor vehicle collision where he was the driver. Initial trauma assessment shows his injuries to include a tibial plateau fracture of the left leg, the side of impact from the accident. Pulses in the leg are palpable, sensation throughout his leg is normal, and he is able to activate all muscle groups. The surgeon notes gross swelling and extreme tenderness at the location of the fracture. Given the crush trauma to the left leg combined with a tibial fracture and pain that may mask compartment syndrome, the surgeon remains vigilant with follow-up exams.

The patient's right leg remains swollen, firm and tender to palpation 30 minutes later. The surgeon uses a wick catheter to measure compartment pressures, which are 22 mmHg. Diastolic pressure is 65. The surgeon continues to physically examine the patient and check compartment pressures every 30 minutes. One hour later, the physical exam is unchanged but the compartment pressure is 32 with diastolic pressure of 60. The surgeon takes the patient to the operating room for a four-compartment lower leg fasciotomy.

TREATMENT OF ACUTE COMPARTMENT SYNDROME

Systemic derangements of oxygenation and fluid volume must be corrected at the outset. Attention should then be directed to the position of the limb and to the dressings. The affected limb should be stabilized and elevated to the level of the heart to minimize venous congestion while preserving arterial inflow. Bandages, splints and casts should be inspected and loosened or split if necessary to increase blood flow.

Fasciotomy

SURGICAL PRINCIPLES

Fasciotomy remains the definitive treatment of compartment syndrome. Indications for fasciotomy[11] include (1) compartmental pressure greater than 30 mmHg or within 30 mmHg of the diastolic blood pressure[14] and associated with signs of compartmental ischemia such as nerve dysfunction or muscle weakness, (2) prolonged coma with compression of the limb, (3) major soft-tissue or orthopedic injury and (4) vascular injuries and operations in which arterial inflow is diminished or absent, significant ischemia occurs before revascularization (6 hours) or arterial and venous injuries coexist. Prophylactic fasciotomy is used for elective tibial operations such as tibial osteotomy, leg lengthening and tibial bone grafts.

Fasciotomy prior to arterial repairs in shotgun wounds or crush injuries is recommended. Stabilization of fractures before vascular repair avoids disruption of anastomoses. Because fasciotomy converts a closed fracture into an open one, rigid external fixation should be applied. Use of an indwelling arterial shunt avoids ischemia of the distal extremity during fracture reduction and fixation, after which the definitive vascular repair may be done.

Prompt and liberal use of fasciotomy will minimize ischemic damage and diminish the chance of complications. Favourable functional results have generally been reported only if the operation is performed with 4–6 hours following onset of signs and symptoms. Debridement of muscle is kept to a minimum because it is extremely difficult to assess tissue viability macroscopically. It has been recommended that no muscle be excised within the first 72 hours after injury. This approach avoids debridement of marginally viable muscle with the potential for regeneration.[21] The only exception is crush syndrome, where necrotic muscle must be removed to minimize systemic derangements.

Epimysiotomy, or incision of the fibrous muscle sheath, is recommended for any muscle not showing rapid revascularization after fasciotomy. This is often required in the buttock and deltoid compartments, where fascial and epimysial fibres blend.

WOUND CARE

Wounds are usually packed open, and the limb is splinted. Primary closure can be attempted if post-fasciotomy compartment pressures return to noncritical levels. Contracture is inhibited by active and passive range-of-motion exercises. Wound closure is performed after 3–7 days, by either delayed primary skin closure or split-thickness skin grafting. Split-thickness grafting often leaves an insensate, aesthetically unpleasant result. The shoelace technique may be used to achieve delayed primary closure without the need for a skin graft and has been shown to be a low-cost strategy that improves likelihood for primary closure.[22]

Newer vacuum or negative pressure dressings have gained popularity in recent years, but level 2 evidence does not support improved healing times with this technology.[22] Vacuum dressings also add significant costs compared to traditional dressings. Several devices that facilitate mechanical closing of fasciotomy wounds have been marketed in recent years, with level 3 evidence showing decreased length of hospital stay and possible benefits for primary closure.[23] Higher-level evidence is needed to demonstrate superiority of different closure techniques.

OUTCOME

Factors affecting outcome include the underlying atherosclerotic disease, anemia and hypovolemia. Infection is the principal complication of fasciotomy and may result in amputation and death. However, Rush has reported a minimal incidence of wound infection in a series of open fasciotomies and has emphasized that persistent ischemia and systemic disease are the usual causes of morbidity and mortality.[24] Other complications of fasciotomy include reduction in active muscle strength, chronic neuropathy and leg swelling.

Reperfusion injury from release of products of muscle necrosis into the systemic circulation may follow fasciotomy or arterial repair. Hyperkalemia, acidosis and myoglobinuric renal failure may result from myonecrosis.

Post-fasciotomy hemorrhage is a stubborn problem seen occasionally in patients who required the procedure for intracompartmental bleeding. These patients often have systemic bleeding disorders, such as hematologic malignancy or thrombocytopenia of other etiologies. Consultation from an experienced hematologist should be obtained.

Adjunctive therapy and areas for future research

Free radical scavengers have been shown to reduce skeletal muscle necrosis after reperfusion injury. In the animal model, Bulkley demonstrated a significant decrease in compartment pressures after reperfusion in animals treated with free radical scavengers.[25] Ricci similarly found a significant reduction of muscle injury by using free radical scavengers in reperfusion injury, but there was no preservation of normal neuromuscular function.[26] Level 2 evidence in animal models has found that vitamin C and antioxidants administered before fasciotomy preserved muscular function and decreased the influx of toxic inflammatory mediators.[27]

Hypertonic mannitol has been shown in animal models to lower interstitial pressure by osmotic diuresis and scavenging of free oxygen radicals. Level 2 data in 186 patients show that hypertonic mannitol may have a protective effect, decrease the need for fasciotomy and minimize neuromuscular dysfunction in patients with ischemia–reperfusion injuries.[28]

TREATMENT OF CHRONIC COMPARTMENT SYNDROME

Fasciotomy is the definitive treatment of chronic compartment syndrome. For a thorough workup, the patient should have plain radiographs and a technetium bone scan to search for stress fractures or other pathology. The duration of symptoms is a factor in the decision to operate, and while there is no consensus on a minimum duration, most experts discourage surgical intervention when symptoms have been present for less than 1 year. Although symptoms from chronic compartment syndrome may temporarily improve with rest, physiotherapy and anti-inflammatory medications, most authors report failure of non-operative management in true chronic compartment syndrome.

Results from fasciotomy vary depending on the population. Bilateral fasciotomies, frequently the subcutaneous type, are often required. Turnipseed found that patients treated by open fasciotomy instead of subcutaneous fasciotomy had fewer early postoperative wound complications and late recurrences.[29] Level 2 data in 611 patients treated with fasciotomy showed return to full activity in 28% and recurrence in 45%.[30]

COMPARTMENT SYNDROMES OF THE LOWER EXTREMITY

Anatomy

COMPARTMENTS OF THE LEG (ANTERIOR, LATERAL, DEEP, SUPERFICIAL)

The anterior compartment is most prone to developing compartment syndrome. Its fascial boundaries are the crural fascia anteriorly, intermuscular septum laterally (separating the lateral compartment) and interosseous membrane between tibia and fibula posteriorly. The muscles of the anterior compartment are dorsiflexors (tibialis anterior, extensor digitorum brevis, extensor hallucis longus and peroneus tertius) and are innervated by the deep peroneal nerve, whose cutaneous distribution is the web space between the great and second toe. The vascular supply is from the anterior tibial artery. The neurovascular bundle is bounded by the tibialis anterior, extensor hallucis longus and interosseous membrane.

The lateral or peroneal compartment is the second most frequently involved in compartment syndromes. Its boundaries are the crural fascia anteriorly and laterally, the anterior intermuscular septum and fibula medially and the posterior intermuscular septum separating the superficial posterior intermuscular compartment posteriorly. The muscle contents of the lateral compartment (peroneus longus and brevis) are innervated by the superficial peroneal nerve, whose cutaneous distribution is primarily the mid-dorsal aspect of the foot. There are no major vessels in this compartment.

Of the two posterior compartments, the deep posterior is more frequently involved in compartment syndrome. This compartment is bounded by the tibia, interosseous membrane and fibula anteriorly and the transverse intermuscular septum separating the superficial compartment posteriorly. The muscles of the deep compartment are the tibialis posterior, flexor digitorum longus and flexor hallucis longus. These are innervated by the tibial nerve, which emerges from the compartment and gives rise to the medial and lateral plantar nerves of the foot, and the medial calcaneal nerve. The posterior tibial vessels course with the tibial nerve in a neurovascular bundle just deep to the transverse intermuscular septum.

The superficial compartment is covered posteriorly by the crural fascia and is bounded anteriorly by the transverse intermuscular septum. The muscles of the compartment, the gastrocnemius, soleus and plantaris, are unique in receiving innervation from the tibial nerve, which travels outside of their compartment. The only nerve within the superficial compartment is the sural, which supplies the cutaneous region over the lateral dorsum of the foot and the lateral malleolar region via its lateral calcaneal branch. The only vascular structures are branches of the peroneal and posterior tibial vessels.

COMPARTMENTS OF THE FOOT

The foot is described classically as having four compartments (medial, central, lateral and interosseous); however, injection studies have demonstrated at least nine compartments.[31] Communication has been demonstrated to exist between the deep posterior compartment of the leg and the calcaneal compartment of the foot, thus explaining the development of deep posterior compartment syndromes in patients with calcaneal and talar fractures.[32]

OTHER COMPARTMENTS

The gluteal, iliacus–psoas and anterior and posterior thigh compartments may be affected by compartment syndrome, but only in rare cases.

Fasciotomy techniques: Leg

SUBCUTANEOUS (CLOSED) FASCIOTOMY

The subcutaneous or limited skin incision fasciotomy has been used to treat chronic compartment syndromes but has only limited utility in the treatment of ACS. The method of Detmer for the anterior compartment involves scissor stripping of the fascia through three transverse incisions, leaving the compartment widely open as verified by finger inspection. Advocates of this technique deem it to be the preferred treatment for selected cases with only moderate swelling and propose that its advantages include avoidance of large infection-prone skin defects which might become infected, delay healing time or require skin grafts for closure. The weakness of subcutaneous fasciotomy is that the skin itself may become the limiting envelope in extremity swelling. It also does not provide adequate decompression of all muscle compartments.

FIBULECTOMY FASCIOTOMY

Transfibular fasciotomy with fibulectomy is intended to provide better exposure for more thorough decompression than is achieved by closed fasciotomy. Extensive fibular resection may be accomplished through a single extensive posterolateral incision allowing access to all muscle compartments and neurovascular structures from the popliteal fossa to the ankle. It has been reported that fibulectomy is of particular importance in the patient who has sustained significant venous injury, where avoidance of a medial incision or multiple incisions is crucial to minimize interruption of venous drainage.

There are several drawbacks to this procedure. It requires extensive muscle stripping and dissection under regional or general anesthesia, eliminating it as a bedside procedure. Also, the potential exists for vascular damage because branches of anterior tibial and peroneal vessels crossing the lower third of the fibula must be ligated. Because of these and other complications, fibulectomy is rarely warranted.

PARAFIBULAR FASCIOTOMY (FIGURES 53.2 AND 53.4a)

The parafibular approach, described by Matsen,[7] is used to decompress all four compartments if an ACS develops in any one of them. A single incision is made from the neck of the fibula to the lateral malleolus, and the lateral compartment is then opened. Retraction of the anterior skin exposes the anterior compartment fascia, which is then opened with care to avoid the superficial peroneal nerve. The posterior skin is retracted to expose and open the fascia of the superficial compartment. The final step is to retract the lateral compartment anteriorly and to release the soleus from the fibular shaft and retract it posteriorly, exposing the deep posterior compartment fascia, which is then opened.

DOUBLE-INCISION FASCIOTOMY (FIGURES 53.3 AND 53.4b)

The double-incision fasciotomy was originally described by Mubarak and Owen[33] and has been modified. The anterolateral incision extends 20–25 cm midway between

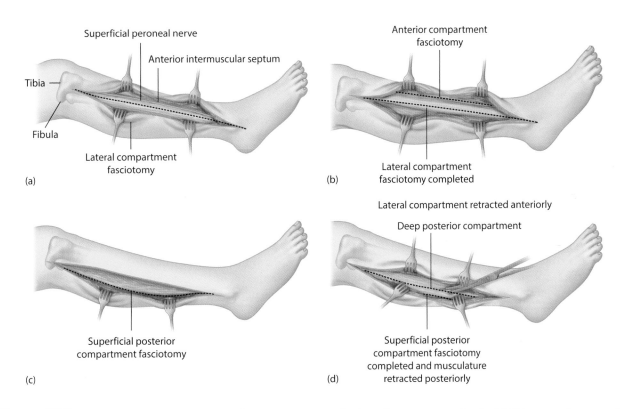

Figure 53.2 Parafibular fasciotomy. (a) Lateral incision exposing the lateral compartment fascia. (b) Skin retraction exposing anterior compartment fascia. (c) Superficial posterior compartment exposed. (d) Exposure and incision of the deep posterior compartment fascia.

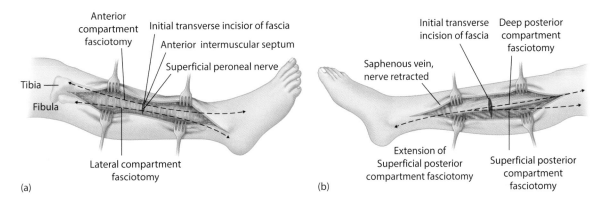

Figure 53.3 Double-incision fasciotomy. (a) Anterolateral skin incision, exposure of septum and superficial peroneal nerve and anterior and lateral compartment fascial incisions. (b) Posteromedial skin incision, exposure of posterior intermuscular septum and superficial and deep compartment fascial incisions.

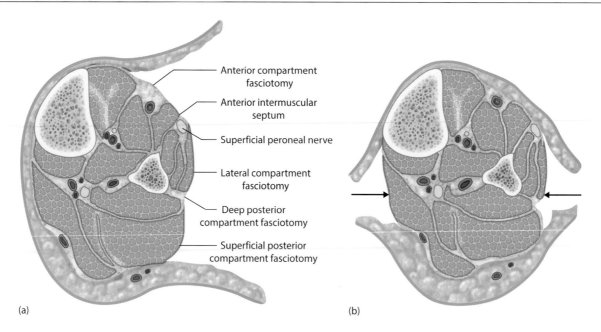

Figure 53.4 Techniques seen in cross section: (a) parafibular fasciotomy and (b) double-incision fasciotomy.

the fibular shaft and the tibial crest, approximately over the anterior intermuscular septum. Skin edges are undermined proximally and distally to allow visualization of most of the compartment fascia. A transverse incision is made in the fascia to identify the anterior intermuscular septum and to locate the superficial peroneal nerve in the lateral compartment adjacent to the septum. The anterior compartment is then opened with scissors, proceeding proximally toward the patella and distally toward the great toe. The lateral compartment fasciotomy is made in line with the fibular shaft, directing the scissors toward the proximal and distal fibular landmarks. The fasciotomy thus remains posterior to the superficial peroneal nerve.

The second, posteromedial incision is 20–25 cm in length and is placed 2 cm posterior to the posterior margin of the tibia, avoiding injury to the saphenous nerve and vein. Skin flaps are raised, and the saphenous structures are retracted anteriorly. Another transverse fascial incision is used to identify the posterior intermuscular septum between superficial and deep posterior compartments. The tendon of the flexor digitorum longus in the deep compartment and the Achilles tendon in the superficial compartment are identified. The superficial compartment fasciotomy is carried as far proximally as possible, and then distally behind the medial malleolus. The deep compartment is next opened from distal to proximal beneath the soleus. If the soleus attaches distally to more than half of the tibia, it should be released.

Fasciotomy techniques: Foot

DORSAL INCISION

The dorsal approach for fasciotomy, described by Mubarak and Owen,[34] is performed by making two longitudinal

incisions placed medial to the second and lateral to the fourth metatarsals, thus creating a wide bridge of the skin. Dissection is carried down to the bone longitudinally with minimal subcutaneous disruption. Once the bone is encountered, further longitudinal dissection is performed in each interosseous space, reaching the medial and lateral compartments.

MEDIAL INCISION

The long plantar-medial incision provides access to all fascial compartments. The incision follows the length of the inferior surface of the first metatarsal and enters the medial compartment between the metatarsal and the abductor hallucis muscle. Retraction of the abductor hallucis muscle permits access to the other compartments by gentle blunt dissection, as described by Myerson.[35]

COMPARTMENT SYNDROMES OF THE UPPER EXTREMITY

Anatomy

VOLAR COMPARTMENT

The flexor or volar compartment of the forearm is bounded by antebrachial fascia anteriorly, medially and laterally and by radius, interosseous membrane and ulna posteriorly. In the distal aspect of this compartment, the superficial muscles palmaris longus, flexor carpi ulnaris and flexor carpi radialis are separated from the remaining structures by a thin fascia. In the proximal volar compartment are the lacertus fibrosus of the biceps and pronator teres; the distal edge is the transverse carpal ligament. The muscular contents of the compartment are the superficial muscles named above and the deep group: flexor digitorum superficialis and profundus, flexor pollicis longus and pronator quadratus. Principal motor supply to these muscles is the median nerve, with the ulnar nerve contributing to half of the flexor digitorum profundus. The compartment contains both radial and ulnar arteries before the former exits beneath the thumb abductors to form the dorsal arch, and the latter travels into the palm to form the superficial palmar arch.

DORSAL COMPARTMENT

The dorsal compartment is also bounded medially, laterally and posteriorly by antebrachial fascia. Ulna, radius and interosseous membrane form its anterior border. Muscles in the dorsal compartment include extensor carpi ulnaris, extensor digitorum communis, abductor pollicis longus and extensor pollicis longus and brevis. The motor nerve to these muscles is the posterior interosseous branch of the radial.

OTHER COMPARTMENTS

The third compartment of the forearm, the so-called mobile wad, is composed of brachioradialis and extensors carpi radialis longus and brevis. Other compartments in the upper extremity include the deltoid, biceps and triceps.

THE HAND

The palm consists of hypothenar and thenar compartments as well as four dorsal and three volar interosseous compartments. The finger is enclosed in tight investing fascia of the skin at the flexor creases. Isolated compartment syndrome of the hand is rare and is often associated with injury to the forearm and wrist. The carpal tunnel should also be released at the time of fasciotomy.

Fasciotomy techniques: Arm

Incisions for decompression of the upper limb, particularly the forearm, should be made with anticipation of the possible need for later tendon transfers should muscle infarction become progressive despite decompression. Volar decompression is performed through a single incision beginning proximal to the antecubital fossa, extending to the midpalm and including a carpal tunnel release. In cases of median nerve dysfunction, three areas where compression may occur should be explored, including the lacertus fibrosus (always released during fasciotomy), the proximal edge of pronator teres and the proximal flexor digitorum superficialis. The dorsal compartment is decompressed through a longitudinal incision over the dorsal forearm, shorter than the volar incision, and skin edges are undermined proximally and distally. The entire length of the dorsal fascia should be incised.

It has been recommended that pressure in the dorsal compartment should be measured prior to and after volar decompression, and fasciotomy should be performed if compartment pressure exceeds 30 mmHg. The 'mobile wad' does not normally require decompression, but if necessary, it can be decompressed through a volar curvilinear incision.[36]

Compartment syndromes of the hand most often are the result of crush injuries or burns. Treatment of subsequent post-traumatic contracture may be challenging and complex.

ABDOMINAL COMPARTMENT SYNDROME

When abdominal pressure becomes elevated to pathological levels, abdominal compartment syndrome may occur. Abdominal compartment syndrome is associated with the following clinical signs: (1) elevated ventilatory pressures, (2) elevated central venous pressure, (3) decreased urine output, (4) massive abdominal distension (5) and reversal of these derangements with abdominal decompression.

Pathophysiology

Major pathophysiological effects are associated with increased intra-abdominal pressure (IAP). The abdominal wall becomes stiffer, and compliance falls in a linear fashion. Venous return is diminished because of decreased IVC flow and elevation of the diaphragm. Diaphragmatic elevation produces increased ventricular filling pressures and decreased cardiac compliance, hindering return of blood to the heart. Visceral blood flow declines linearly with increasing IAP. Perfusion of mesenteric arteries, intestinal mucosa and liver tissue are diminished, with resultant visceral ischemia, which may be quantified using gastric tonometry. Renal blood flow, glomerular filtration rate and urine output are diminished. Oliguria is a hallmark of abdominal compartment syndrome and occurs as a consequence of decreased cardiac output and compression of the aorta, renal arteries and veins, but not of the ureter. The thoracic cavities are compressed by the abdominal distension, and lung compliance falls. Elevated ventilatory pressures, like oliguria, are hallmarks of the syndrome. Pulmonary artery pressures and pulmonary vascular resistance are increased. Arterial blood gas derangements include hypoxemia, hypercarbia and acidosis.

Hemodynamic changes also are marked. Cardiac output is depressed because of markedly diminished stroke volumes, despite compensatory tachycardia. Preload is decreased because of decreased venous return and increased intrathoracic pressure, and afterload is increased because of elevated systemic vascular resistance. Central venous and pulmonary capillary wedge pressures also are increased.

Etiology

Causes of abdominal compartment syndrome may be acute and chronic. Acute causes are spontaneous, postoperative, traumatic and iatrogenic. Acute and chronic causes are listed in Table 53.6. Mortality of abdominal compartment syndrome is as high as 50% in collected

Table 53.6 Causes of abdominal compartment syndrome.

Acute	Chronic
Peritonitis	Ascites
Intra-abdominal abscess	Tumours
Ileus or intestinal obstruction	Pregnancy
Ruptured abdominal aortic aneurysm	Peritoneal dialysis
Intra-abdominal bleeding	
Tight abdominal closure	
Abdominal packing	
Mesenteric vascular occlusion	
Pneumoperitoneum	

Table 53.7 Types of abdominal compartment syndrome defined.

Primary	ACS due to a direct intra-abdominal or retroperitoneal process that frequently requires early intervention, surgical or radiological.
Secondary	ACS that does not originate from the abdomino-pelvic region.
Tertiary	ACS redevelops following previous surgical or medical treatment for primary or secondary ACS.

Source: Cheatham ML, *Intensive Care Med*, 33(6), 951, 2007.

reports of critically ill patients, though early detection may decrease this rate.[37]

Most cases of abdominal compartment syndrome occur in association with major trauma, with or without a major vascular injury. Multifactorial mechanisms are responsible for post-traumatic abdominal compartment syndrome. These mechanisms include hypoperfusion of the viscera with hemorrhagic shock; large-volume fluid resuscitation; sepsis; tight abdominal closures, sometimes with packing, in patients who have undergone exploratory laparotomy; the use of positive-pressure ventilation; hypothermia; and acidosis. The contents of the abdominal compartment may be increased markedly with swollen intestines, ongoing coagulopathic hemorrhage and the use of packs for tamponade of bleeding surfaces. Types of abdominal compartment syndrome are defined in Table 53.7.

Diagnosis

IAP, usually expressed in millimetres of mercury (mm Hg), is 0 in normal adults and 5–7 in critically ill adults,[38] though obesity has systematically increased baseline IAP.[37] In 2006, an international consensus group of multidisciplinary critical care specialists at the World Congress on Abdominal Compartment Syndrome developed guidelines for defining, treating and preventing the syndrome. Table 53.8 shows the grades of intra-abdominal hypertension (IAH) and abdominal compartment syndrome as defined by the World Congress.

Table 53.8 Intra-abdominal pressure classifications.

Intra-abdominal hypertension	
Grade I	12–15 mmHg
Grade II	16–20 mmHg
Grade III	21–25 mmHg
Abdominal Compartment syndrome	Sustained > 20 mmHg associated with new organ dysfunction/failure

Source: Cheatham ML, *Intensive Care Med*, 33(6), 951, 2007.

Table 53.9 Best clinical practice.

Measure IAP at end expiration in the complete supine position after ensuring that abdominal muscle contractions are absent (Grade B).

IAP may be measured at the bedside using a maximal instillation volume of 25 mL of sterile saline (Grade B).

Abdominal perfusion pressure most accurately assesses abdominal blood flow. A goal of 50–60 mmHg should be the clinician's resuscitation goal (Grade B).

IAP should be measured at end expiration in the complete supine position after ensuring that abdominal muscle contractions are absent.[38] IAP may be measured using direct and indirect techniques. The most commonly used direct technique is the electronic insufflator system, used for measurement of the pressures produced with carbon dioxide pneumoperitoneum for laparoscopic operations.

With indirect techniques, pressures are measured across the wall of an intra-abdominal structure via an indwelling device. Bladder pressure is used most commonly today. The bladder serves as a passive diaphragm and bladder pressures have been shown to correlate with IAP for pressures ranging from 5 to 70 mm Hg. Operationally, the indwelling bladder catheter is connected to manometer system, and IAP may be measured at the bedside using a maximal instillation volume of 25 mL of sterile saline. Table 53.9 summarizes the recommendations from this section.

Treatment

Abdominal perfusion pressure (APP) is the difference between mean arterial and IAPs. As different levels of IAP will cause end-organ dysfunction in different people, APP most accurately assesses abdominal blood flow. level 2 data show that differences in APP are associated with patient survival, and Level 3 data show survival benefit to maintaining APP above 50 mmHg.[39] Additional level 2 data show APP ≥60 as an appropriate resuscitation goal.[40]

Surgical abdominal decompression is the cornerstone of treatment. Prior to decompression, aggressive resuscitation is directed to restore intravascular volume and maximize oxygen delivery to end organs. Coagulation defects and hypothermia also should be corrected. Invasive hemodynamic monitoring and large-bore vascular access are essential.

Several paradigms for fluid resuscitation exist, and experts have not reached a consensus on a preferred method. Supportive diuresis and renal replacement therapies may be necessary for volume control in the patients with renal failure.[38]

Adequate sedation/analgesia in ventilated patients and neuromuscular blockade may decrease Grade I or Grade II IAH but are unlikely to reverse more severe IAH or ACS. The World Congress recommends a brief trial of neuromuscular blockade for mild to moderate IAH only, given the risk of prolonged neuromuscular blockade. Head of bed elevation above 20° also contributes to increased IAP (multicentre level 2 data), which must be balanced with the risk of aspiration.[41]

Despite medical intervention, clinical deterioration marked with worsening anuria, ventilatory dysfunction and hemodynamic instability warrants urgent abdominal decompression to reach therapeutic goals. The effects of surgical decompression are dramatic, with immediate improvement in cardiac, respiratory and renal function.

Options for abdominal closure at the time of decompression include open packing, skin closure, prosthetic closure or temporary dressings. Open packing has risks of fistulization, evisceration and massive fluid loss. Skin may be closed over open fascia using sutures or towel clips, but this technique creates risk for recurrent compression. Prosthetic closures are done with various types of prosthetic mesh, which are often expensive. Temporary abdominal closure with vacuum-assisted dressings have gained popularity, while some surgeons prefer the use of a sterilized, open 3 litre irrigation bag, sutured to the fascia or skin.

Abdominal reclosure is performed 4–7 days following decompression. Surgical options include definitive closure of the abdominal wall at this time, or a staged closure with mesh or skin grafts may be chosen. If the closure is staged, definitive closure is performed at a minimum of 3–6 months postoperatively.

Areas for future research

Prospective, randomized studies regarding critical APP and target APP for resuscitation are required. Nasogastric/colonic decompression and intestinal motility agents may potentially decrease IAP, but no adequate trials have tested these treatments.

Ultrasound- or CT-guided percutaneous catheter decompression of ACS caused by intra-abdominal fluid, air, abscess or blood has gained attention in recent years, given the morbidity of surgical decompression. Level 2 and 3 evidence has shown successful resolution of abdominal compartment syndrome using non-invasive techniques.

KEY REFERENCES

1. Mubarak SJ. Acute compartment syndromes: Diagnosis and treatment with the aid of wick catheter. *J Bone Joint Surg.* 1978;60A:1091–1095.
2. McQueen MM, Court-Brown CM. Compartment monitoring in tibial fractures. The pressure threshold for decompression. *J Bone Joint Surg Br.* 1996;78(1):99–104.
3. Rorabeck CH. Compartmental pressure measurements: An experimental investigation using the slit catheter. *J Trauma.* 1981;22:446–449.
4. Cheatham ML, Malbrain ML, Kirkpatrick A et al. Results from the international conference of experts on intra-abdominal hypertension and abdominal compartment syndrome. II. Recommendations. *Intensive Care Med.* 2007;33(6):951–962.

REFERENCES

1. Labbe R, Lindsay T, Walker PM. The extent and distribution of skeletal muscle necrosis after graded periods of complete ischemia. *J Vasc Surg.* 1987;6(2):152–157.
2. Steinau HU. *Major Limb Replantation and Postischemia Syndrome: Investigation of Acute Ischemia-Induced Myopathy and Reperfusion Injury.* New York: Springer Verlag;1988.
3. Mubarak SJ. Wick catheter techniques for measurement of intramuscular pressure: A new research and clinical tool. *J Bone Joint Surg.* 1976;58A:1016–1020.
4. Hamlin C. Compartment syndrome in the upper extremity. *Emerg Med Clin North Am.* 1985;3(2):283–291.
5. Hargens AR. Quantitation of skeletal muscle necrosis in a model compartment syndrome. *J Bone Joint Surg.* 1981;63A:631–636.
6. Matsen FA. Physiological effects of increased tissue pressure. *Int Orthop.* 1979;3:237–244.
7. Matsen FA. Diagnosis and management of compartmental syndromes. *J Bone Joint Surg.* 1980;62A:286–291.
8. McQueen MM, Gaston P, Court-Brown CM. Acute compartment syndrome. Who is at risk? *J Bone Joint Surg Br.* 2000(82):200–203.
9. Patman RD, Thompson JE. Fasciotomy in peripheral vascular surgery. *Arch Surg.* 1970;101:663–672.
10. Rollins DL, Bernhard VM, Towne JB. Fasciotomy. *Arch Surg.* 1981;116:1474–1481.
11. Mubarak SJ. Acute compartment syndromes: Diagnosis and treatment with the aid of wick catheter. *J Bone Joint Surg.* 1978;60A:1091–1095.
12. Enst CB, Kaufer H. Fibulectomy-fasciotomy: An important adjunct in the management of lower extremity arterial trauma. *J Trauma.* 1971;11:365–380.

13. Aweid O, Del Buono A, Malliaras P, Iqbal H, Morrissey D, Maffulli N, Padhiar N. Systematic review and recommendations for intracompartmental pressure monitoring in diagnosing chronic exertional compartment syndrome of the leg. *Clin J Sport Med*. 2012;22(4):356–370.

14. McQueen MM, Court-Brown CM. Compartment monitoring in tibial fractures. The pressure threshold for decompression. *J Bone Joint Surg Br*. 1996;78(1):99–104.

15. Whitney A, O'Toole RV, Hui E et al. Do one-time intra-compartmental pressure measurements have a high false-positive rate in diagnosing compartment syndrome? *J Trauma Acute Care Surg*. 2014;76(2):479–483.

16. Whitesides TE. Tissue pressure measurement as a determinant for the need for fasciotomy. *Clin Orthop*. 1975;113:4351.

17. Rorabeck CH. Compartmental pressure measurements: An experimental investigation using the slit catheter. *J Trauma*. 1981;22:446–449.

18. McQueen MM, Duckworth AD, Aitken SA, Court-Brown CM. The estimated sensitivity and specificity of compartment pressure monitoring for acute compartment syndrome. *J Bone Joint Surg Am*. 2013;95(8):673–677.

19. McDermott AGP. Monitoring dynamic anterior compartment pressures during exercise. A new technique using the STIC catheter. *Am J Sports Med*. 1982;10:83–89.

20. Arbabi S, Brundage SI, Gentilello LM. Near-infrared spectroscopy: A potential method for continuous, transcutaneous monitoring for compartmental syndrome in critically injured patients. *J Trauma*. 1999;47(5):829–833.

21. Sanderson RA. Histological response of skeletal muscle to ischemia. *Clin Orthop*. 1975;113:27–35.

22. Kakagia D, Karadimas EJ, Drosos G, Ververidis A, Trypsiannis G, Verettas D. Wound closure of leg fasciotomy: Comparison of vacuum-assisted closure versus shoelace technique. A randomised study. *Injury*. 2014;45(5):890–893.

23. Matt SE, Johnson LS, Shupp JW, Kheirbek T, Sava JA. Management of fasciotomy wounds—Does the dressing matter? *Am Surg*. 2011;77(12):1656–1660.

24. Rush DS, Frame SB, Bell RM, Berg EE, Kerstein MD, Haynes JL. Does open fasciotomy contribute to morbidity and mortality after acute lower extremity ischemia and revascularization? *J Vasc Surg*. 1989;10(3):343–350.

25. Perler BA, Tohmeh AG, Bulkley GB. Inhibition of the compartment syndrome by the ablation of free radical-mediated reperfusion injury. *Surgery*. 1990;108(1):40–47.

26. Ricci MA, Graham AM, Corbisiero R, Baffour R, Mohamed F, Symes J. F. Are free radical scavengers beneficial in the treatment of compartment syndrome after acute arterial ischemia? *J Vasc Surg*. 1989;9(2):244–250.

27. Kearns SR, Daly AF, Sheehan K. Oral vitamin C reduces the injury to skeletal muscle caused by compartment syndrome. *J Bone Joint Surg Br*. 2004;86(6):906–911.

28. Shah DM, Bock DE, Darling RC, Chang BB, Kupinski AM, Leather RP. Beneficial effects of hypertonic mannitol in acute ischemia-reprefusion injuries in humans. *Cardiovasc Surg*. 1996;4:97–100.

29. Turnipseed W, Detmer DE, Girdley F. Chronic compartment syndrome. An unusual cause for claudication. *Ann Surg*. 1989;210(4):557–562.

30. Waterman BR, Laughlin M, Kilcoyne K, Cameron KL, Owens BD. Surgical treatment of chronic exertional compartment syndrome of the leg: Failure rates and postoperative disability in an active patient population. *J Bone Joint Surg Am*. 2013;95(7):592–596.

31. Manoli A. Compartment syndromes of the foot: Current concepts. *Foot Ankle*. 1990;10:340–344.

32. Myerson MS, Berger BI. Isolated medial compartment syndrome of the foot: A case report. *Foot Ankle Int*. 1996;17:183–185.

33. Mubarak SJ, Owen CA. Double incision fasciotomy of the leg for decompression in compartment syndromes. *J Bone Joint Surg*. 1977;59A:184–187.

34. Mubarak SJ, Owen CA. Compartmental syndrome and its relation to the crush syndrome: A spectrum of disease. *Clin Orthop*. 1975;113:81–89.

35. Myerson MS, Berger BI. Diagnosis and treatment of compartment syndrome of the foot. *Orthopedics*. 1990;13:711–717.

36. Gelberman RH, Garfin SR, Hergenroeder PT, Mubarak SJ, Menon J. Compartment syndromes of the forearm: Diagnosis and treatment. *Clin Orthop Relat Res*. 1981;(161):252–261.

37. Atema JJ, van Buijtenen JM, Lamme B, Boermeester MA. Clinical studies on intra-abdominal hypertension and abdominal compartment syndrome. *J Trauma Acute Care Surg*. 2014;76(1):234–240.

38. Cheatham ML, Malbrain ML, Kirkpatrick A et al. Results from the international conference of experts on intra-abdominal hypertension and abdominal compartment syndrome. II. Recommendations. *Intensive Care Med*. 2007;33(6):951–962.

39. Cheatham ML, White MW, Sagraves SG, Johnson JL, Block EF. Abdominal perfusion pressure- a superior parameter in the assessment of intra-abdominal hypertension. *J Trauma*. 2000;49:621–626.

40. Malbrain ML. Abdominal perfusion pressure as a prognostic marker in intra-abdominal hypertension. In: Vincent JL, ed. *Yearbook of Intensive Care and Emergency Medicine*. Berlin/Heidelberg/New York: Springer, 2002, p. 792–814.

41. Cheatham ML, De Waele JJ, De Laet I et al. The impact of body position on intra-abdominal pressure measurement: A multicenter analysis. *Crit Care Med*. 2009;37(7):2187–2190.

54

Principles of vascular access surgery

SAMUEL ERIC WILSON, JUAN CARLOS JIMENEZ and ROBERT BENNION

CONTENTS

From the beginning, the full potential of hemodialysis for the long-term treatment of patients with chronic renal failure was limited by the lack of a means for repeated access to the vascular system. At the outset, it was necessary for repeated cutdowns to be made on an artery and vein for each dialysis, following which the vessels were ligated. The duration of a course of dialysis was, therefore, limited to the treatment of acute renal failure. W. J. Kolff, the designer of the first practical dialysis machine, observed in 1944 that 'when a preparation of the arteries was necessary (all veins being ruined) very persistent hemorrhages arose from the subcutaneous tissue owing to the heparin.... After the 12th dialysis became a failure, the artery being damaged, the urea percentage of the blood rapidly rose to 640 mg% whereupon death followed'.[1]

Scribner, Dillard and Quinton (an internist, a surgeon and an engineer, respectively) in 1960 introduced the first successful apparatus for provision of reasonably long-term cannulation of an artery and vein using an external Silastic shunt.[2] This was widely adopted over the succeeding 6 years, up to the time Cimino and coworkers[3] reported their success, in 1966, with the autologous, subcutaneous arteriovenous (AV) fistula. This 'arterialized' superficial arm vein could be repeatedly cannulated, and it has stood the test of time, remaining today as the best method for provision of long-term vascular access.

As is shown in Figure 54.1, the number of incident (newly reported) ESRD cases in 2012 was 114,813.[4] After a yearly increase in this number over three decades from 1980 through 2010, it now appears to have plateaued or declined slightly, with the number of incident ESRD cases lower in both 2011 and 2012 than in 2010.

By the end of 2012, there were 636,905 prevalent cases of ESRD in the United States, an increase of 3.7% from the prior year (Figure 54.2).[4] The percentage growth in 2011 and 2012 were the lowest over the last three decades. The size of the prevalent dialysis population (hemodialysis and peritoneal dialysis) increased to 3.8% in 2012, reaching 449,342, and is now 57.4% higher than in 2000. The size of the transplant population rose to 3.6% in 2012, reaching 186,303 patients, and is now 77.7% higher than in 2000.[4]

In addition, the availability of vascular access is also an important consideration in the treatment of patients needing long-term administration of anticancer medication and other drugs, for total parenteral nutrition and for the treatment of patients by means of plasmapheresis.

PHYSIOLOGY OF ARTERIOVENOUS FISTULAS

An AV fistula has local and systemic, hemodynamic and non-hemodynamic effects. These vary, depending on whether the fistula is acute or chronic, and are modified by the anatomical configuration of the fistula, and by how far proximally or distally, it is situated on the vascular tree.

A fistula may be formed directly between an adjacent artery and vein or, if these vessels are separated, by connecting them with a conduit limb of variable diameter or length. When the connecting limb is very short, as

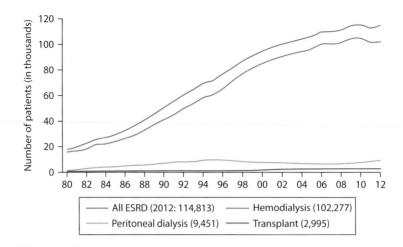

Figure 54.1 Trends in the number of incident cases of ESRD, in thousands, by modality, in the US population, 1980–2012.

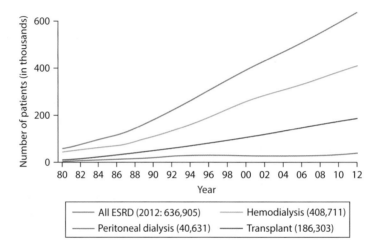

Figure 54.2 Trends in the number of prevalent cases of ESRD, in thousands, by modality, in the US population, 1980–2012.

in a Cimino fistula, the flow through the fistula, when plotted in relation to the fistula diameter, increases following a sigmoid curve with increasing diameter of the fistula.[5] There is little flow through the fistula until its diameter exceeds 20% of that of the proximal artery. From then onward, flow increases rapidly with small changes in fistula diameter until the diameter reaches 75% of the proximal arterial diameter. Following that, there are only small increases in flow with increasing fistula diameter.

In all fistulas, the direction of blood flow in both the proximal artery and vein is normal. With small fistulas (by definition, these have a diameter of less than 75% of the proximal arterial lumen), the blood flow in the distal vein and artery is in the normal direction. However, this is usually reversed in large fistulas (diameter greater than 75% of the arterial lumen).

Fistulas that are to be utilized for therapeutic purposes are constructed so that they are of the large variety. This ensures the greatest blood flow and decreases the likelihood of fistula clotting. Fistulas formed between the radial artery and a vein have blood flow rates of 150–500 mL/min. Grafts attached to larger arteries such as the femoral or axillary have flow rates of 500–1500 mL/min through them.

When a fistula is opened, there is a fall in peripheral resistance, which leads to a decrease in the proximal fistula artery pressure and which is compensated for by an increase in cardiac output. Proximal arterial flow then increases, and, accompanying this, there is an increase in proximal venous outflow that is not accompanied by a significant rise in central venous pressure because of the large capacity of the venous system.

The highest blood pressure in the distal artery is usually only about two-thirds of systemic pressure, which is higher than that at the fistula opening. Therefore, flow is often retrograde in the distal artery. Valves in the veins direct blood flow centrally and result in an initially high peripheral venous pressure. 'Arterialization' of the veins leads to dilation and valvular incompetence, which may cause distal venous hypertension.

Blood in the distal fistula vein flows retrograde until, at some point, the valves are able to withstand the pressure. The blood in the distal vein is carried centrally by venous collaterals, which open off the vein. With time, there is significant increase in the number of collateral vessels formed between the proximal and distal arteries and the proximal and distal veins. In the arterial system, these are stimulated by the pressure differences across the bed and, in the venous system, the hypertrophy to accommodate the large retrograde flow. Ligation of the distal fistula artery reduces the degree of development of collateral arterial vessels.

Venous collaterals develop more extensively than do arterial ones, and they accommodate the considerable retrograde venous flow that follows as incompetence of the valves occurs.

Ligation of the proximal fistula artery decreases flow through the fistula and peripheral vascular bed, an effect that is much less pronounced with a chronic fistula in which large collaterals have been stimulated to develop. These maintain blood flow through the distal vascular bed and the fistula to a much greater extent than does flow through the proximal fistula artery.

In small fistulas, there is a gradual buildup of platelets and fibrin along the fistula tract; these are replaced by smooth muscle and fibrous tissue and eventually result in fistula closure. With time, in larger fistulas, there is lengthening and dilation of the proximal and distal veins and the proximal artery, in addition to the vascular collaterals. The proximal artery develops smooth muscle hypertrophy in addition to dilation, and then it elongates. Later the muscle atrophies, and the vessel becomes tortuous and aneurysmal. In the vein, there is an increase in smooth muscle and fibrous tissue of the subintimal layer. Eventually it may develop atherosclerosis. The vein dilates for up to 8 months following construction of an AV fistula.

In addition to the foregoing changes, there is an increase in the temperature of the tissues surrounding an AV fistula because of increased flow in the adjacent collaterals. AV fistulas have been used to treat discrepancies in limb lengths in children. The increased collateral flow stimulates bone growth.

A large AV fistula may produce congestive cardiac failure. To compensate for the increased fistula flow, the pulse, stroke volume and cardiac output increase, and there is increased vasoconstriction of other parts of the vascular bed.

Blood may be 'stolen' from the vascular bed peripheral to the fistula, producing symptoms of ischemia. This happens when fistula blood flow equals about one-third of the pre-fistula cardiac output. Heart failure occurs when the fistula flow is 20%–50% of the cardiac output.

SHORT-TERM VASCULAR ACCESS

Percutaneous central venous cannulation

Although acute hemodialysis in the past was carried out primarily with external AV shunts, these have now been essentially replaced by percutaneously placed central venous catheter hemodialysis. Blood is withdrawn from the cannulated vein, passed through the dialyzer and returned to the patient via the second lumen of a double-lumen catheter.

Percutaneous subclavian vein catheterization was first reported by Aubaniac, a French military surgeon, in 1952.[6] Initially, central venous lines were used for intravenous (IV) access, central venous pressure monitoring[7] and total parenteral nutrition.[8] In addition to these three functions, this list has been expanded to include venous access for chemotherapy infusion, left heart and pulmonary artery pressure monitoring, temporary dialysis and multiple lumen vascular access channel catheters for complicated medical and surgical critical care patients.

ANATOMY

A thorough knowledge of the structures of the thoracic inlet is necessary to proceed with percutaneous central venous catheterization. The subclavian vein meets the internal jugular vein behind the sternoclavicular joint bilaterally. On the right side, this confluence forms the superior vena cava. On the left side, it forms the innominate vein, which carries the left-sided venous blood, entering the superior vena cava just cephalad to the right atrium. The cephalic vein lies uniformly in the deltopectoral groove and joins the subclavian vein in such a way that it is difficult to direct a guide wire or catheter into the proximal subclavian vein. Generally, the cephalic vein or external jugular vein is used for access by cutdown approach (Figure 54.3).

The anterior scalene muscle separates the subclavian artery and brachial plexus, which are posterior to this muscle, from the subclavian vein, which lies anterior to

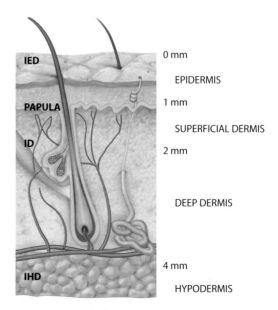

Figure 54.3 Central venous anatomy of the thoracic outlet. (From Owens ML et al., Physiology of arteriovenous fistulas, in Wilson SE and Owens ML, eds., *Vascular Access Surgery*, Year Book Medical Publishers, Chicago, IL, 1980. With permission.)

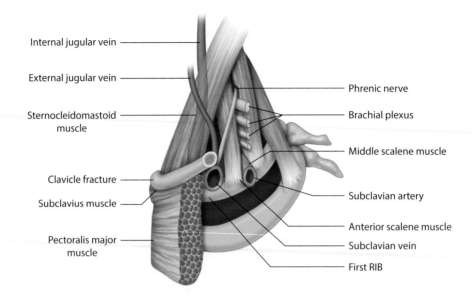

Figure 54.4 Costoclavicular scalene triangle demonstrating position of subclavian vein between clavicle and first rib.

the muscle (Figure 54.4). The scalene muscle helps protect the subclavian artery and brachial plexus from injury during needle insertion. The thoracic duct enters the left subclavian vein near its confluence with the left internal jugular vein. The lymphatic vessel on the right enters in the same position but is much smaller.

Topographically, the subclavian vein lies on a straight line between the sternal notch and the junction of the medial and middle third of the ipsilateral clavicle immediately dorsal (posterior) to the clavicle. The vein enters the thorax between the clavicle and first rib. The internal jugular vein may be found lateral to the carotid pulse and enters the thorax between the sternal and clavicular heads of the sternocleidomastoid muscle bilaterally. These surface landmarks are essential to know for safe percutaneous central venous catheter placement.

APPROACHES

There are two approaches to percutaneous central venous access. In the direct approach, the catheter enters the subclavian vein through a direct percutaneous puncture site. In the indirect approach, the catheter enters the central vein from a subcutaneous tunnel.

Direct approach

Direct central venous access is obtained by cannulating the subclavian, internal jugular or femoral vein percutaneously with a polyethylene, polyurethane or Teflon catheter and advancing the catheter into the superior or inferior vena cava. The Seldinger technique involves percutaneous vascular access by threading a catheter over a previously placed thin guide wire. The wire is advanced through a small needle that has been inserted through the skin into a vessel (artery or vein). The indication for direct vascular approach includes monitoring of central venous pressure, pulmonary artery pressure, hyperalimentation, temporary dialysis and IV access in patients with poor

peripheral veins or critical care patients in need of multiple IV portals. The available armamentarium includes single-, double- or triple-lumen catheters, each with its appropriate indication and insertion technique.

Direct subclavian vein venipuncture is usually performed in a procedure room under local anesthesia with the patient sedated and the operative site prepared and draped to maintain sterile conditions. An operating room table is useful to maintain the patient in the Trendelenburg position so as to distend the subclavian vein or internal jugular vein. If possible, IV fluid is administered to expand the venous compartment to ensure that the patient is normovolemic. A useful sign in the head-down position is that the intravascular volume is adequate if the operator can see the external jugular vein dilated with blood. A pillow may be placed in the midline of the patient's back to drop the shoulders posteriorly and to position the central veins anteriorly.

The patient's head is turned to the opposite side. Of note, the use of portable ultrasound to assist with vein cannulation should be performed in all patients and has become the standard of care at our institution.[9,10] The operator's index finger is placed in the sternal notch, and the thumb is placed under the clavicle at a point between the medial and middle third of the clavicle (Figure 54.5). A cutaneous wheal of local anesthetic is made at this area. The distance between the index finger and the thumb represents the proximal subclavian vein and its union with the internal jugular vein to form the superior vena cava behind the sternoclavicular joint.

The needle is connected to a 10 mL syringe. The needle is inserted into the skin at the wheal, directed medially toward the sternal notch, while posteriorly sliding the needle under the clavicle and aspirating on the syringe as the needle is advancing. When the subclavian vein is entered, a 'flashback' of venous blood fills the syringe. One stops for a second to be quite sure the blood is dark red and the piston of

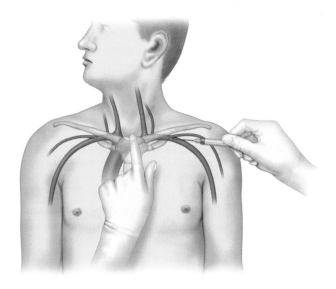

Figure 54.5 Technique for percutaneous puncture of subclavian vein. (From Owens ML et al., Physiology of arteriovenous fistulas, in Wilson SE and Owens ML, eds., *Vascular Access Surgery*, Year Book Medical Publishers, Chicago, IL, 1980. With permission.)

the syringe is not rising as it would if the subclavian artery were entered. The bevel of the needle is turned down, and the patient performs a Valsalva manoeuvre. This increases the central venous pressure and prevents air from entering the needle when the syringe is disconnected. The syringe is removed, and the guide wire is inserted into the needle and advanced. At this point, an x-ray or C arm is used to assure the correct position of the guide wire in the superior vena cava. At this point, a number 11 blade is used to enlarge the skin opening to permit the catheter to enter the skin. When the wire is in place, the needle is withdrawn from the skin, and the venotomy may be serially dilated to the correct size required for catheter placement. The catheter with its stylet is advanced into the vein using fluoroscopic guidance. Now the stylet is removed from inside the catheter, and the catheter is connected to IV fluids. Flow rates from the IV will tell the operator if the catheter is properly positioned. The plastic needle guard is sutured to the skin with 3-0 monofilament suture, and the insertion site is dressed. A post-insertion x-ray is always taken to be sure the catheter is in the superior vena cava and not turned upward into the jugular vein. In addition, one must be sure that a pneumothorax has not been created with the needle insertion.

The technique for placing the catheter in the superior vena cava from the internal jugular vein is similar. The index finger is placed in the space between the sternal and clavicular heads of the sternocleidomastoid muscle just cephalad to the clavicle. A wheal of local anesthetic is made approximately a third of the way up into the neck at the lateral border of the sternocleidomastoid muscle. The needle is inserted in the wheal at the lateral border of the muscle aimed at the index finger just deep to the clavicle. All other aspects of internal jugular cannulation

are identical to the infraclavicular subclavian approach. The internal jugular approach is easier and safer because the risk of pneumothorax is less.

Indirect approach

The indirect percutaneous catheter insertion technique to catheterize the central venous system evolved through pacemaker technology. When pacemakers were placed in subcutaneous pouches, the pacemaker lead had to be inserted under direct vision into the peripheral vein, such as the cephalic vein in the deltopectoral groove, the external jugular vein or the internal jugular vein. Occasionally, the cephalic vein was too small to accept the lead wire, or the lead wire could not be placed and advanced from the external jugular vein into the superior vena cava. At this point, a cutdown to reach the subclavian or internal jugular veins was necessary. The problem was solved with the development of the breakaway–peel-away sheath, which permitted percutaneous insertion of the pacemaker lead into the superior vena cava from the subclavian vein entry point and then allowed complete coverage of the lead in the subcutaneous pocket.

This technique is now used for routine insertion of central venous catheters through a subcutaneous tunnel for chemotherapy, hyperalimentation or vascular access. The initial procedure is similar, no matter which device is being inserted.

The J-shaped soft end of the Teflon-coated guide wire is straightened by a plastic tip deflector and inserted into the 18-gauge needle and advanced into the internal jugular or subclavian vein. At this point, an x-ray or C arm is used to assure the correct position of the guide wire in the superior vena cava. The patient should have electrocardiogram monitoring, for the guide wire may cause ventricular arrhythmias if it is advanced into the right ventricle. At this point, the insertion needle and the guide wire tip straightener are removed and the wire is left alone, care being taken not to pull it out.

A pocket or tunnel must be made for the specific device that is being inserted. For the pacemaker, self-contained reservoir or self-contained infusion pump, a subcutaneous pocket is created on the ipsilateral pectoral region. The pocket should be caudad to the incision so that the device will lie below the incision when the wound is closed and the patient is upright.

The Hickman catheter is a 90 cm silicone rubber catheter with a Dacron cuff 30 cm from the Luer lock end. The Dacron cuff is buried in a subcutaneous tunnel so that fibrous tissue will grow into the cuff for stabilization and to retard septic complications.

Two stab wounds are required to create a subcutaneous tunnel for the Hickman catheter. A stab wound is made on the precordium and at the exit site near the guide wire. Using local anesthesia, a tunnel is created between the two stab wounds. The Hickman catheter, which has been flushed with heparinized saline, 100 USP units of heparin per millilitre, is inserted into the precordial stab wound and brought out of the stab wound near the guide wire. The catheter is advanced so that the Dacron cuff is in the subcutaneous tunnel.

The Hickman catheter is now measured and cut so that the tip of the catheter following the course of the subclavian vein (plus innominate vein on the patient's left side) and superior vena cava will lie at the level of the right third rib.

With the apparatus in position (dual-lumen hemodialysis catheter, pacemaker, portacath or Hickman catheter), attention is again turned to the guide wire. Over the guide wire, insert the sheath introducer assembly. Using a twisting motion, advance the sheath introducer assembly over the guide wire under direct fluoroscopy. Leaving the sheath in place, remove the guide wire and the introducer. Venous blood will come out from inside the sheath.

From the pocket or tunnel, develop a subcutaneous path for the lead or catheter to enter the breakaway sheath. This may require a small incision where the sheath enters the skin. Introduce the catheter into the sheath and advance into position (Figure 54.6). Break the sheath by pulling it apart. Withdraw the sheath as the peeling continues. If the lead catheter withdraws from the sheath as it is being peeled and withdrawn, reinsert the catheter gently and

continue peeling. The wounds are now closed with interrupted subcuticular absorbable sutures (Figure 54.7). The central venous catheter, reservoir or pump is aspirated and flushed with heparinized saline to ensure proper function.

When using the percutaneous subclavian approach for central venous access, care must be taken when patients are obese, emphysematous or hypovolemic. The side of a patient with a healed clavicular fracture or mastectomy should be avoided for attempts at percutaneous subclavian vein access. Occasionally, a patient will be seen with occlusion of the superior vena cava. These patients are obviously poor candidates. A preoperative CT or MR venogram should be performed if the surgeon feels there is a risk of superior vena cava occlusion. It is probably best to avoid a side of the chest that has previously undergone radiation therapy.

COMPLICATIONS

Early complications of percutaneous central venous catheterization are due to technique. Pneumothorax is the most often seen. Later complications are usually related to sepsis

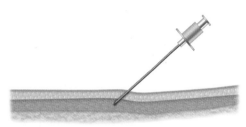

1. Introduce a thinwall percutaneous entry needle into the vessel.

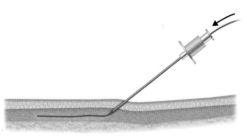

2. Pass a wire guide through the needle; advance approximately ¼ of the wire guide length into the vessel.

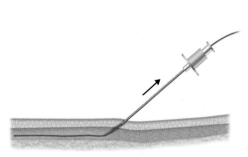

3. Leaving the wire guide in place, withdraw the needle.

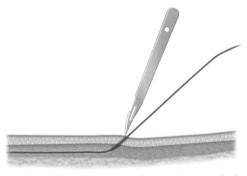

4. Enlarge the puncture site with a number 11 scalpel blade. (Optional)

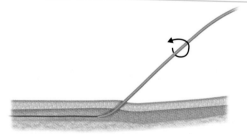

5. With a twisting motion, advance the catheter over the wire guide and into the vessel.

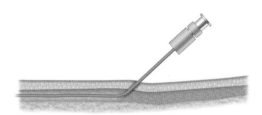

6. After the catheter is in position, remove the wire guide.

Figure 54.6 Seldinger technique for introducing catheters. (From Owens ML et al., Physiology of arteriovenous fistulas, in Wilson SE and Owens ML, eds., *Vascular Access Surgery*, Year Book Medical Publishers, Chicago, IL, 1980. With permission.)

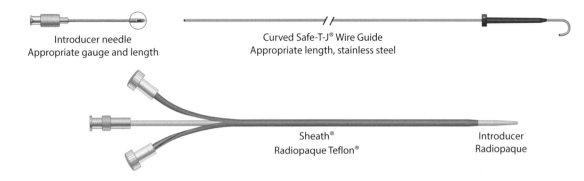

Figure 54.7 Needle, guide wire and catheter introduced. The sheath is peeled off the catheter after introduction.

or central venous thrombosis. Septic complications are more common in multiple lumen catheters and less frequent in vascular access devices that are completely buried, as compared to the Hickman or cuffed hemodialysis catheters, which exit from the patient. Catheter sepsis may be heralded only by fever, tachycardia or glucose intolerance. Treatment of catheter-related bacterial infection usually requires removal of the foreign body. Subclavian vein thrombosis is generally not symptomatic. Other complications are listed in Table 54.1.

Table 54.1 Complications of percutaneous vascular access.

Early	Late
Thoracic	Catheter obstruction
Pneumothorax	Thoracic
Tension pneumothorax	Hydrothorax
Subcutaneous emphysema	Hydromediastinum
Hemothorax	Venous
Hydrothorax	Air embolism
Hemomediastinum	Central vein thrombosis
Hydromediastinum	Superior vena cava syndrome
Arterial	Hepatic vein thrombosis
Subcutaneous hematoma	Cardiac
Arterial laceration	Arrhythmia
Pseudoaneurysm	Coronary sinus thrombosis
Venous	Lymphatic
Venous laceration	Lymphatic fistula
Air embolism	Chylothorax
Catheter embolism	Septic
Lymphatic	Catheter sepsis
Thoracic duct laceration	Septic thrombosis
Cardiac	Suppurative thrombophlebitis
Arrhythmia	
Perforation and tamponade	
Neurologic injury	
Brachial plexus	
Phrenic nerve	
Vagus nerve	
Recurrent laryngeal nerve	
Catheter misplacement	

OTHER SITES

The percutaneous access sites used for emergency hemodialysis or other procedures may include the femoral vessels. The femoral vein is cannulated in the groin using local infiltration anesthesia. Following insertion of a 16-gauge cannula into the vein, a guide wire is threaded through the cannula into the common iliac vein or the inferior vena cava. The guide wire should not be forced. If resistance is met, it is withdrawn a little and a further attempt at free passage made. The catheter is then passed over the free end of the guide wire into the iliac vein or inferior vena cava.

Percutaneous venous cannulation provides a means for the immediate dialysis of a patient. The external catheter may be removed following the course of dialysis, reducing the chance of infection. Catheter thrombosis between dialysis sessions is prevented by infusion of low-dose heparin for the duration of the catheter's use.

Blood flows of up to 200 mL/min can be achieved via these catheters, making this method of dialysis as efficient as others. The technique does not increase cardiac workload, unlike external AV shunts or internal AV fistulas.

These catheters may be changed after a period of days by reinsertion of the guide wire along the existing catheter, withdrawal of the older catheter and its replacement with a clean catheter by the Seldinger technique. With the development of Silastic catheters, which reduce the likelihood of catheter thrombosis, and because of the lower risk of infection of a catheter placed in the subclavian vein rather than in the groin, subclavian catheters can be left in situ or replaced and provide dialysis access over an interval of several weeks. This obviates the need for repeated needle punctures.

LONG-TERM VASCULAR ACCESS

The best long-term access is made by utilization of the patient's own vessels to construct an autogenous subcutaneous AV fistula. Failing this, biological conduits such as bovine carotid artery heterograft, cadaveric cryopreserved graft or synthetic materials such as polytetrafluoroethylene (PTFE) are used to bridge the distance between suitable arteries and veins.

Subcutaneous AV fistula

The autogenous AV fistula is associated with the longest useful patency and lowest rate of infection and is less likely to thrombose than prosthetic grafts. For construction, it requires an artery large enough to support a high rate of blood flow and veins that will 'arterialize' and thus dilate. The fistula is unobtrusive and does not interfere significantly with patient activities. It does, however, require 4–6 weeks following its construction for maturation of the veins into large, thick-walled vessels that can be repeatedly and reliably punctured (Figure 54.8).

It may not be feasible to construct an upper extremity autogenous fistula in a patient who has small fragile veins or a paucity of veins, possibly as the result of previous episodes of thrombophlebitis or sclerosis following IV injections. It is also difficult to construct in patients who have an obese arm. The fistula is easier to construct and more likely to remain patent in a patient who has prominent veins, such as a manual worker. The radial artery may not be large enough to maintain flow through the fistula in patients with advanced atherosclerosis. This is a pertinent consideration in the diabetic patient with renal failure. It should be determined before construction that the hand circulation can be maintained by the ulnar artery alone, using an Allen's test.

Cimino fistulas have up to a 90% useful patency rate at 12 months, which falls to about 75% at 4 years. Once failure occurs, they can, uncommonly, be surgically revised for extended longevity. Fistulas may clot during an episode of hypotension or because of restriction of the venous

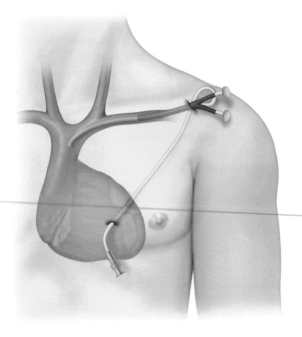

Figure 54.8 Catheter is introduced through sheath. (From Owens ML et al., Physiology of arteriovenous fistulas, in Wilson SE and Owens ML, eds., *Vascular Access Surgery*, Year Book Medical Publishers, Chicago, IL, 1980. With permission.)

outflow of the arm by clothing, a sphygmomanometer cuff or a tourniquet. In addition, flow through the fistula is reduced by advancing atherosclerosis in the feeding artery and can ultimately fall to a critically low level at which the fistula thromboses.

Following construction of an AV fistula in the arm, swelling may be seen in the hand. This is usually easily managed by elevating the hand on a pillow for a time. Rarely, severe venous hypertension follows the development of valvular incompetence in the distal fistula venous bed. Very uncommonly a forearm fistula 'steals' blood from the distal arterial circulation, leading to hand ischemia.

The fistula is constructed using local infiltration anesthesia or alternatively a brachial plexus nerve block. Patients with progressive renal failure may have their fistula formed and matured beforehand, in anticipation of the need for maintenance hemodialysis. This is done when their creatinine clearance falls to 10 mL/min.

Before constructing a Cimino fistula, the arm pulses are carefully palpated, and a tourniquet is applied around the upper arm to restrict venous outflow and aid visualization of the venous anatomy. Ultrasound vein mapping in the non-invasive vascular lab also aids with identification of available superficial veins and the calibre of the artery to be used. Extensive arterial calcification and small size may require placement of a more proximal fistula with better arterial inflow. The veins are marked out using an indelible pen. It is preferable to construct the Cimino fistula in the non-dominant arm. This aids in training the patient for regular hemodialysis, should this eventuate.

At operation, a longitudinal incision is made in the skin overlying the radial artery. The cephalic vein is dissected out from the subcutaneous fat, ligating any tributaries as necessary so that it lies alongside the radial artery without kinking or producing any stenosis. Following this, the radial artery is dissected and mobilized, taking care not to avulse any of its smaller branches since this produces a periarterial hematoma, which can interfere with the construction of an adequate fistula.

The artery and vein are anastomosed together in one of the four configurations (Figure 54.9): (1) The side-to-side anastomosis is the easiest to do well and is associated with the highest fistula flow rate. (2) The arterial end to vein side reduces turbulence and the likelihood of distal arterial steal but is associated with a lower flow rate. (3) The vein end to arterial side results in the highest proximal venous flow and minimal distal venous hypertension but is technically more difficult to construct. (4) The end-to-end anastomosis combines the least likelihood of development of distal arterial steal and venous hypertension with the lowest fistula flow rate of the four configurations.

The fistula is made utilizing about a 6–8 mm long venotomy and arteriotomy. If valves are present in the vein at the site of the venotomy, they are resected with small scissors. Fine suture material such as 6-0 Prolene is used for the anastomosis, taking care to tie the knots on the outside of the vessels. A continuous suturing technique is

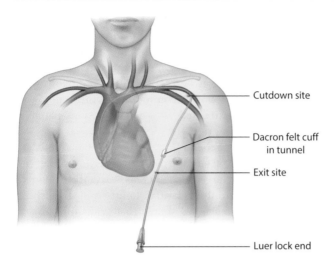

Cutdown site

Dacron felt cuff
in tunnel

Exit site

Luer lock end

Figure 54.9 Position of central venous catheter suitable for hyperalimentation placed via cephalic vein for long-term access. (From Owens ML et al., Physiology of arteriovenous fistulas, in Wilson SE and Owens ML, eds., *Vascular Access Surgery*, Year Book Medical Publishers, Chicago, IL, 1980. With permission.)

employed, starting at the midpoint of the posterior wall, with the side-to-side anastomosis.

Before completing the anastomosis, a coronary artery dilator is passed proximally in the artery and vein to ascertain that no stenosis has been produced by suturing at the vessel junctions and to relieve proximal arterial spasm. Any bleeding occurring after the vascular clamps have been released is usually controlled by the application of firm pressure for several minutes. Only if this fails is the bleeding site controlled by insertion of additional fine sutures. These can lead to further bleeding from the needle tracks and increase the likelihood of inadvertently narrowing the anastomosis.

After the operation is successfully completed, a strong thrill should be palpable. If there is vigorous arterial pulsation but no thrill, outflow obstruction is suspected, and one should confirm that there is no stenosis in the vein. Part of the anastomosis is dismantled and a small, simple rubber or Fogarty catheter is passed into the vein. If a stricture is felt, it may be dilated by bougies or by blowing up the balloon on the Fogarty catheter.

In some patients, it is not possible to construct the standard Cimino fistula at the wrist. If the patient is thin, the proximal cephalic vein is easily seen at the elbow and may be used for anastomosis to the brachial artery in the cubital fossa. A transverse incision is made a little proximal to the cubital fossa, and the brachial artery is mobilized distally to the level of the bicipital tendon. The median nerve lies medial and posterior to the artery and should be protected. The anastomosis between the artery and vein is limited to about a length of 5–7 mm to reduce the chances of developing a steal syndrome, which is more likely here.

At times, the basilic vein can be mobilized from the level of the wrist to the middle of the forearm and then tunnelled subcutaneously for anastomosis to the radial

artery. It is also possible to anastomose the basilic vein to the ulnar artery, but this should not be done if there has been a previous radiocephalic fistula in that arm because of the high chance of compromising the circulation to the hand since the radial artery is usually occluded.

Basilic vein-to-branchial artery fistulas are used when there is no available cephalic vein present. Disadvantages of the basilic vein for use as an outflow source includes its deeper anatomic location relative to the cephalic vein and its location in the medial arm. At our institution, we perform basilic vein fistulas in two separate stages. The first stage is limited to performing the AV anastomosis. Approximately 6 weeks later, if there is clinical evidence that the fistula has matured, transposition to a more superficial and lateral location is performed. Of note, transposition may assist in maturation of the fistula if large collateral branches are present in the basilic vein. Cooper and colleagues performed a recent meta-analysis which demonstrated no differences in failure and patency rates between the one- and two-stage approaches.[11]

The Cimino fistula may function for many years. Eventually it may fail due to sclerosis of the veins as a result of repeated venipuncture or following renal transplant, when changes occur in the blood that restore coagulation to normal. It is not wise to discard an AV fistula following renal transplant because dialysis may be necessary during episodes of acute rejection or if there is failure of the kidney. Reoperation to salvage a failed Cimino fistula is commonly unsuccessful. Failure is usually most expeditiously managed by construction of another access site. If another Cimino fistula cannot be constructed or the old site revised, then a prosthetic bridge fistula is constructed.

AV grafts

AV grafts (also known as bridge fistulas) constructed from alternate materials are a good alternative to the radiocephalic fistula if no autogenous vein is available. They can be formed between almost any artery and vein, are easily accessible under the skin for reliable needle puncture and can be used for dialysis earlier than the AV autogenous fistula.

These fistulas take on various configurations. If the vein and artery are close to each other, the bridge material may run in a loop or lie in a U configuration. If the artery and vein are some distance apart, the bridge graft lies in a straight or curved line. Care should be taken to avoid kinking of the fistula material, and in particular, it should not pass over joints where flexion will restrict flow and lead to graft clotting. One-year patency rates of 75%–80%, comparable to those of the Cimino fistula, have been reported with PTFE grafts.

The larger the artery used to provide flow through the fistula, the lower the rate of fistula thrombosis. For this reason, thigh fistulas, using the common or superficial femoral artery, are less likely to clot. In addition, they can be easily utilized by the patient, who has both hands free, for home dialysis, but they have the major disadvantage of a higher postoperative infection rate. Location of the fistula in the arm is almost always the first-choice site and is the mandatory position in the older patient with significant leg vessel atherosclerosis or the obese patient who has dermatitis in the groin.

A variety of biological and prosthetic materials have been used for AV graft construction. These include bovine carotid artery, human umbilical vein, homologous saphenous vein, cryopreserved cadaveric allografts, heparin-bonded ePTFE and other synthetic materials.[12–14] Of these, the PTFE graft has proved particularly successful and is currently the most commonly used material for bridge fistulas.

The bovine heterograft was developed over a decade ago, by enzyme debridement of fresh bovine carotid arteries, followed by tanning with dialdehyde.[15] A 6–10 mL internal diameter graft about 40–50 cm long results. The material is pliable and easily sutured. At one time, it was thought that bovine heterografts should be utilized primarily rather than a Cimino fistula. However, some 5 years after introduction of bovine grafts, it was evident that they were prone to infection and aneurysm formation. Progressive degeneration of the graft material occurs so that the whole graft tends to undergo aneurysmal dilation or forms nonanastomotic aneurysms. These grafts also develop stenosis at the venous anastomosis together with other prosthetic materials, which leads to graft blood flow restriction and then clotting. Recent improvements in the manufacturing and collagen cross-linking of these bioprosthetic grafts have led to recent re-evaluation of their use as hemodialysis conduits. A recent study from our institution demonstrated good functional patency compared to reported ePTFE patencies in high-risk patients who are poor candidates for placement of a native AV fistula.[16]

Expanded PTFE has become the most commonly used material for construction of AV grafts. PTFE handles well, does not require preclotting, is widely available and has a long shelf life and high patency rate. PTFE bridge fistulas are currently noted to have 12-month patency rates between 50% and 60% compared to more than 70% patency for autogenous AV fistulas over the same time frame.[17] Fortunately, should a PTFE graft thrombose, it can usually be successfully treated by either surgical and/or pharmacological thrombectomy.

The Gore Propaten® ePTFE graft (WL Gore and Associates Inc, Flagstaff, AZ) was introduced in 2006 and has a heparin-bonded inner lumen. Heparin molecules are covalently bonded to the graft surface and maintain bioactivity. Studies comparing Propaten to conventional ePTFE have been equivocal with regard to patency.[18,19] A recent randomized trial demonstrated significant lower early thrombosis rates and a trend to improved overall patency, which was not statistically significant.[13]

Infection of PTFE grafts occurs in up to 10%. Over two-thirds of these infections are found within the first 4 months of use, and the majority requires removal of the graft for resolution. To minimize chances of bacterial seeding and infecting the replacement fistula, the infected graft is removed some days before establishing another AV graft elsewhere. If the infection involves the anastomosis, it is not uncommon that the artery will need to be reconstructed with an autogenous patch or interposition vein graft.

The diameter of the graft is selected to be larger than that of the supply artery to ensure maximum fistula flow. The size, if too large, also increases the likelihood of developing high-output cardiac failure and distal limb ischemia. Experience has shown that grafts of 6 mm in diameter provide good flow and retain their patency while being uncommonly associated with the foregoing complications. In the arm, a 6 mm graft is usually selected so that the large graft–to–artery ratio provides maximal flow.

Distal limb tissue perfusion is also affected by the degree of atherosclerosis that has developed in the distal arterial tree, and this is a significant consideration in the older patient who is being prepared for a thigh AV graft. If this is a concern, then a preoperative angiogram may be helpful in planning further patient management. However, if the patient's ankle blood pressure is 80% or more of his or her brachial blood pressure and he or she has no history of claudication, then distal ischemia is unlikely to follow if an AV graft is constructed.

AV grafts have been formed between most of the suitably sized superficial arteries and veins. Puncture should be delayed for about 2 weeks until the prosthesis has been incorporated in the surrounding tissue. The puncture sites then tend to 'heal', making extravasation and perigraft hematoma formation less likely than in the unincorporated prosthesis. Puncture of a graft in the first 24 hours after implantation is possible if urgent dialysis is

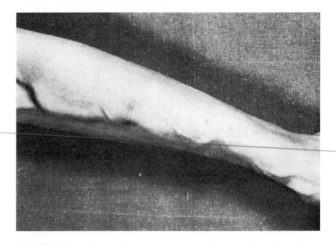

Figure 54.10 Well-developed ('arterialized') Cimino fistula. (From Owens ML et al., Physiology of arteriovenous fistulas, in Wilson SE and Owens ML, eds., *Vascular Access Surgery*, Year Book Medical Publishers, Chicago, IL, 1980. With permission.)

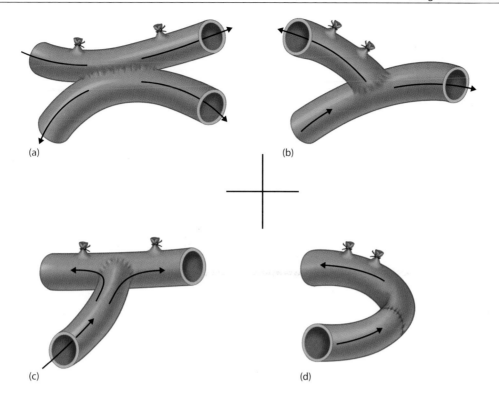

Figure 54.11 Configurations of artery and vein in Cimino fistula. (a) Side of vein to side of artery. (b) End of vein to side of artery. (c) Side of vein to end of artery. (d) End to end artery to vein. (From Owens ML et al., Physiology of arteriovenous fistulas, in Wilson SE and Owens ML, eds., *Vascular Access Surgery*, Year Book Medical Publishers, Chicago, IL, 1980. With permission.)

required; however, this is often painful for the patient and bleeding complications can develop.

In the arm, a bridge fistula can be constructed between the radial artery and cephalic or basilic vein in the cubital fossa (straight, Figure 54.10), the cephalic or basilic veins and the brachial artery (loop, Figure 54.11) and the axillary vein and brachial artery (straight, Figure 54.12). The conduit is tunnelled through the subcutaneous tissue on the radial side of the forearm to allow the arm to lie comfortably during dialysis. Bridge fistulas in the arm have a shorter useful patency than those in the thigh, since clotting is more likely because of the lower fistula flow rates. On the other hand, bridge fistulas in the arm are less likely to become infected than thigh fistulas, which are in proximity to the bacteria of the heavily colonized groin skin.

In the thigh, the initial bridge fistula is constructed between the femoral artery proximal to its exit from the adductor canal and the proximal saphenous or femoral vein (Figure 54.13). Upon failure, the arterial end of the fistula can be moved to the more proximal femoral artery.

With long-term hemodialysis, the surgeon can be called on to create multiple vascular access sites, because each will eventually fail. It is conceivable that some patients could potentially outlive their available limb access sites. Then, an AV fistula between the axillary vein and artery has been employed. Complications in this central site are serious and difficult to manage.

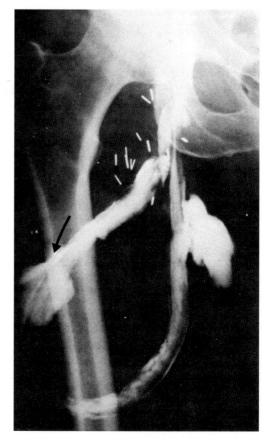

Figure 54.12 Perigraft hematoma – the result of early puncture (arrow) before the graft was tissue incorporated.

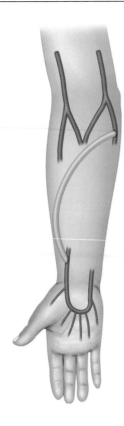

Figure 54.13 Polytetrafluoroethylene bridge fistula between radial artery and cephalic or basilic vein in cubital fossa. (From Owens ML et al., Physiology of arteriovenous fistulas, in Wilson SE and Owens ML, eds., *Vascular Access Surgery*, Year Book Medical Publishers, Chicago, IL, 1980. With permission.)

COMPLICATIONS OF AV FISTULAS

Thrombosis

The most common complication is fistula or graft thrombosis. The likelihood of this occurring depends on the type of shunt, the site of the AV anastomosis, the prosthetic material used and the diameter of patient's veins and arteries.

The autogenous Cimino fistula thromboses early following construction in about 10–15% of patients. This may be due to poor vessels (an atherosclerotic radial artery or small veins) or technical factors such as obstruction at the venous anastomosis. With time, the Cimino fistula is more likely to remain patent than a bridge fistula. However, in the initial period, the bridge fistula has a higher patency rate. Thrombosis occurring 3 months or more following construction of a Cimino fistula is commonly due to fibrosis of the veins, following the repeated trauma of needle punctures. Late thrombosis of a prosthetic graft, however, is usually due to 'intimal hyperplasia' producing stenosis of the venous outflow.

When late clotting of a Cimino fistula occurs, it may be most expedient to convert it to a bridge prosthetic fistula. Late thrombosis of a graft due to intimal hyperplasia in the vein adjacent to the prosthetic venous anastomosis occurs with PTFE and other prosthetic materials. Differences in compliance between the vein and the prosthetic material result in turbulence and hydraulic trauma to the vein.

At times, outflow obstruction is appreciated early before the graft thromboses by the dialysis nurse who observes a rise in pressure at the venous end of the conduit or notes that the blood in the venous chamber is becoming dark during dialysis. Following this observation, a 'fistulagram' may be obtained to rule out the source of the problem.

Thrombosis of an AV graft is managed by either endovascular methods (discussed later in the chapter) and/or surgical thrombectomy which can salvage between 40% and 70% of grafts. This is best performed through an incision sited near the venous end of the graft. A graft that has been in situ for a long time often has a well-formed fibrous capsule, and dissection of this can lead to tearing of the PTFE material. A 2 cm long incision is made in the graft just proximal to the venous anastomosis. The patient is heparinized, and a small Fogarty embolectomy catheter is passed into the vein to remove any thrombus. This manoeuvre has dislodged clot into the venous and pulmonary circulation.

If this fails to restore good flow in the graft, it is then necessary to explore the arterial end to remove clots. If these manoeuvres result in good flow and good pulsation with a strong thrill, then the operation may be terminated. However, if this does not occur, then an angiogram should be obtained to determine if there is any correctable stenosis at the arterial or venous ends of the fistula. Such a lesion at the venous anastomosis is managed by a patch angioplasty or constructing a more proximal venous anastomosis or grafting from the fistula to a more proximal vein.

Infection

Infection is second to cardiovascular disease as a cause of mortality and morbidity in patients on chronic dialysis. The highest rate of infection is found with tunnelled hemodialysis catheters, while the lowest is with the Cimino fistula. Needling of fistulas can produce a hematoma, which then becomes infected with skin organisms. Involvement of the anastomotic site with infection may lead to endovasculitis, septicemia and metastatic abscess formation.

Grafts may become infected at the time of implantation from skin organisms and poor aseptic technique. To lower the likelihood of this, perioperative antibiotics effective against skin organisms, particularly *Staphylococcus epidermidis* and *Staphylococcus aureus*, are routinely used. On occasion, a superficial soft tissue infection overlying a graft will resolve; however, graft infections usually require removal of the prosthetic material for complete resolution. Grafts are thought to be more resistant to infection once they have become incorporated and a pseudointimal lining has formed.

When a graft is infected and is to be removed for control of the infection, plans are made for implantation of a new graft at a different site. An interval of a few days should be allowed between removal and implantation of the new graft for resolution of the associated bacteremia and cellulitis, thus reducing the chances of 'seeding' and infecting the new graft.

In some cases of graft infection limited to a needle puncture site, a length of the graft may be excised and a replacement segment tunnelled through uninfected tissues to join the remaining proximal and distal ends.

Congestive heart failure

With a large AV communication fed by a moderately large artery, there is a considerable increase in venous return to the heart, which maintains the increased cardiac output necessary to sustain fistula flow. This can eventually lead to heart failure. When cardiac failure develops, it may be treated quite simply by 'banding' of the fistula. This is done by encircling the prosthetic graft with a 1 cm cuff of Teflon. The arterial end of the prosthesis may be narrowed by placing several interrupted sutures to achieve the same effect. The flow through the graft is reduced to a level of 300–400 mL/min. Reduction of the blood flow to lower levels is likely to lead to graft thrombosis.

Vascular insufficiency

A vascular steal syndrome occurs uncommonly. It is seen with side-to-side fistulas constructed at the wrist. Reversed flow in the distal radial artery increases as the fistula ages and the collaterals hypertrophy between the proximal and distal arteries, elevating the blood pressure in the distal artery. Thus, a significant pressure gradient develops between the distal artery and fistula itself, stealing blood from the more peripheral muscle beds.

The patient experiences ischemic pain in the hand, which is often more severe during hemodialysis. Vascular steal has also been observed in patients with fistulas formed between the femoral artery and saphenous vein in the leg. The steal may be corrected in the hand by ligation of the radial artery immediately distal to the fistula, converting it from a side-to-side to an end-to-side anastomosis.

Venous hypertension

An AV fistula is a planned means for raising pressure locally in the venous system. However, venous hypertension may occur in the tissues distal to the fistula. In the time immediately following construction of the fistula, occurrence of a significant elevation of pressure in the distal venous channels is prevented by competent venous valves. With the valvular incompetence that eventually develops, there is retrograde distal venous flow, and the higher pressure is transmitted distally up to a null point where there is no venous flow and the valves are competent. The pressure is dissipated by the opening of a large venous collateral bed. In some patients, there is marked swelling of the hand,

discoloration and pigmentation of the skin comparable to that seen in venous stasis disease in the leg. In long-standing cases, venous stasis ulceration may be seen. The treatment is ligation of the vein immediately distal to the fistula.

An end vein-to-side artery fistula, which is slightly more difficult to construct, would obviate development of this problem. However, many surgeons prefer initially to make a side venous anastomosis, reasoning that should the extremely rare problem of venous hypertension develop, the distal vein can then be easily ligated. Massive edema of the entire extremity after construction of an AV fistula signifies proximal major venous obstruction.

Vascular access neuropathy

A small number of patients with a Cimino fistula report symptoms of carpal tunnel syndrome. These symptoms are especially noticeable during the night. If this syndrome is suspected, its existence may be proved by nerve conduction velocity studies. There will be a reduction in median nerve conduction time across the carpal ligament.

Carpal tunnel syndrome possibly arises because of increased venous pressure in the hand, leading to tissue edema and compression of the median nerve. Another theory is that it is due to a vascular steal, producing ischemia of the nerve. Some evidence for this etiology comes from the observation that ligation of the radial artery distal to the AV fistula has improved the symptoms. This syndrome has been managed in a few patients by division of the carpal ligament similar to the proven treatment for the median nerve compression occurring in patients not on dialysis.

Aneurysms

Vascular prostheses may develop pseudoaneurysms secondary to needle puncture and perigraft hematoma (Figure 54.14a) formation or true aneurysmal dilation of the whole graft. The latter is thought to be the result of degeneration and 'fatigue' of the graft material itself. If the pseudoaneurysm is not infected, it can be managed by local excision and repair of the graft or excision of the graft segment with interposition of a new length of material (Figure 54.14b through d).

ENDOVASCULAR MANAGEMENT OF AV ACCESS COMPLICATIONS

A variety of endovascular techniques are available for management of threatened AV access and for restoration of flow through occluded fistulas and grafts. These minimally invasive techniques have become first-line therapy for failing or failed access, and they can be performed in the outpatient setting, under local anesthesia with minimal or no sedation.

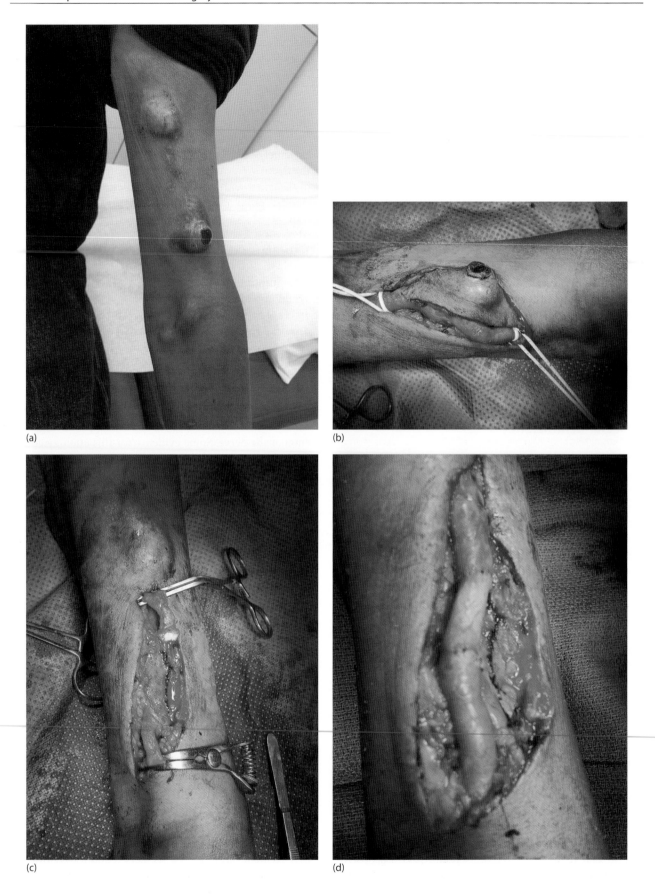

Figure 54.14 (a) Surgical management of an arteriovenous fistula aneurysm with skin erosion and impending hemorrhage (b–d). After obtaining proximal and distal control, the aneurysm with associated skin erosion is resected and an interposition bovine carotid heterograft is used to revise the fistula.

Mechanical thrombectomy

Re-establishment of flow through occluded AV fistula and grafts is the first step in salvaging occluded access sites, and this can be achieved percutaneously with minimal morbidity. Several currently available devices use a combination of pharmacologic thrombolysis with fragmentation and removal of the thrombus burden. The AngioJet thrombectomy system utilized high-speed saline jets which are injected through the catheter lumen backwards at high speed and which fragment adjacent thrombus through a Venturi effect. The fragmented thrombus is then drawn into the catheter. Thrombolytic agents can also be injected into the vessel lumen to deliver medication directly into the clot. Complications associated with AngioJet thrombectomy include embolization of the thrombus burden, intravascular hemolysis and vessel perforation. Transient hematuria resulting from hemolysis is common and should be treated with IV hydration for 48 hours.

Kakkos and colleagues demonstrated excellent results using the AngioJet device in their series of 207 declotting procedures.[20] The authors reported a 97.6% technical success rate and secondary patency rates to 62% and 47% at 2 years. No deaths were reported at 30 days. Simoni and colleagues demonstrated similar excellent results in their review of 72 patients with occluded AV access undergoing AngioJet thrombectomy.[21] Patency was restored in 88% of all grafts and native fistulas. Among autologous fistulas, 86% remained patent at 3-month follow-up. Patency for three months for prosthetic grafts was 53%. No procedural-related deaths were reported.

Balloon angioplasty and stenting

The primary cause of failure for hemodialysis fistulas and grafts is the development of intimal hyperplasia at the venous anastomosis resulting in stenosis and/or occlusion. Traditionally, open surgical thrombectomy and patch angioplasty of the venous outflow was the main method of treatment. Percutaneous balloon angioplasty and stenting are effective treatments for venous outflow stenoses and should be performed once the thrombus burden has been removed. Potential complications of these techniques include vessel perforation and migration of the stent if it is undersized. Invariably, late recurrence of intimal hyperplasia at the stent implantation site occurs and these patients frequently require repeat intervention to maintain access patency.[22]

Kakisis and colleagues reviewed outcomes following balloon angioplasty with and without nitinol stenting.[23] They demonstrated that graft thrombectomy plus angioplasty with self-expanding nitinol stent placement provided significantly higher patency rates compared with thrombectomy and angioplasty alone (24% vs. 64%, respectively).

The use of covered stents is also commonly used to treat both stenoses at the venous end of the hemodialysis fistula and central vein stenoses. According to Anaya-Ayala et al., 25 patients underwent placement of covered stents for central venous occlusive disease.[24] Technical success was achieved in 100% of patients. Primary, primary-assisted and secondary patencies were 56%, 86% and 100% at 12 months, respectively. All patients underwent prior percutaneous thrombectomy and angioplasty. Two patients developed recurrent symptoms prior to 30 days requiring repeat percutaneous transluminal angioplasty (PTA), and four patients died during the follow-up period of non-procedural-related complications.

A recent study compared the use of self-expanding bare metal stents with stent grafts for failing AV grafts.[25] Thirty-five patients underwent covered stent placement for failing AV grafts after undergoing prior angioplasty and bare metal stenting. Primary patency at 6 months was significantly improved in the stent–graft group and was 76.9% at 6 months compared with 25.7% compared with PTA and bare metal stenting alone.

The use of drug-eluting balloons for use in failed hemodialysis access is not currently the standard of care. However, some reports demonstrate early promise for this developing technology to treat outflow intimal hyperplasia in these patients. Katsanos and colleagues reported the 6-month results of a prospective randomized trial comparing paclitaxel-coated balloons vs. plain balloon angioplasty for treatment of failing AV fistulas.[26] The authors reported that primary patients for the drug-eluting balloon group were significantly higher than the plain balloon angioplasty group (70% vs. 25%, respectively). No major or minor complications were noted in either group. Larger randomized trials are needed to justify the cost difference between these two distinct modalities.

REFERENCES

1. Graham WB. Historical aspects of hemodialysis. *Transplant Proc*. 1997;9:1.
2. Quinton WE, Dillard D, Scribner BH. Cannulation of blood vessels for prolonged hemodialysis. *Trans Am Soc Artif Intern Organs*. 1960;60:104.
3. Brescia MJ, Cimino JE, Appel K, Harwich BJ. Chronic hemodialysis using venipuncture and surgically created arteriovenous fistula. *N Engl J Med*. 1966;275:1089.
4. Saran R, Li Y, Robinson B et al. US Renal Data System 2014 annual data report: Epidemiology of kidney disease in the United States. *Am J Kidney Dis*. 2015;66(1)(suppl 1):S1–S306.
5. Owens ML, Bower RW. Physiology of arteriovenous fistulas. In: Wilson SE, Owens ML, eds. *Vascular Access Surgery*. Chicago, IL: Year Book Medical Publishers; 1980.
6. Aubaniac R. L'injection Intraveineuse Sousclaviculaire: Advantages et Technique. *Presse Med*. 1952;60:1456.

7. Wilson JN, Grow JB, Demong CV et al. Central venous pressure in optimal blood volume maintenance. *Arch Surg.* 1962;85:563.

8. Dudrick SJ, Ruberg RL. Principles and practice of parenteral nutrition. *Gastroenterology.* 1971;61:901.

9. Fraqou M, Gravvanis A, Dimitrou V et al. Real-time ultrasound guided subclavian vein cannulation versus the landmark method in critical care patients: A prospective randomized study. *Crit Care Med.* 2011;39:1607–1612.

10. Karakitsos D, Labropoulos N, DeGroot E et al. Real-time ultrasound-guided catheterization of the internal jugular vein: A prospective comparison with the landmark technique in critical care patients. *Crit Care.* 2006;10:R162.

11. Cooper J, Power AH, DeRose G et al. Similar failure and patency rates when comparing one- and two-stage basilic vein transposition. *J Vasc Surg.* 2015;61:809–816.

12. May J, Tiller D, Johnson J, Ross-Sheil AG. Saphenous vein arteriovenous fistula in regular dialysis treatment. *N Engl J Med.* 1969;280:770.

13. Shemesh D, Goldin I, Hijazi J et al. A prospective randomized study of heparin-bonded graft (Propaten) versus standard graft in prosthetic arteriovenous access. *J Vasc Surg.* 2015;62:115–122.

14. Jorgensen L, Bilde T, Kristensen J et al. Human umbilical vein for vascular access in chronic hemodialysis. *Scand J Urol Nephrol.* 1985;19:49–53.

15. Sterling WA, Hazel LT, Diethelm AG. Vascular access for hemodialysis by bovine graft arteriovenous fistulas. *Surg Gynecol Obstet.* 1975;141:69.

16. Harlander-Locke M, Jimenez JC, Lawrence PF et al. Bovine carotid artery (Artegraft) as a hemodialysis access conduit in patients who are poor candidates for native arteriovenous fistulae. *Vasc Endovascular Surg.* 2014;48:497–502.

17. Culp K, Flanigan M, Taylor L, Rothstein, M. Vascular access thrombosis in new hemodialysis patients. *Am J Kidney Dis.* 1995;26:341.

18. Davidson I, Hackerman C, Kapadia A et al. Heparin bonded hemodialysis e-PTFE grafts result in 20% clot free survival benefit. *J Vasc Access.* 2009;10:153–156.

19. Charlton-Ouw KM, Nosrati N, Miller CC 3rd et al. Outcomes of arteriovenous fistulae compared with heparin-bonded and conventional grafts for hemodialysis access. *J Vasc Access.* 2012;13:163–167.

20. Kakkos SK, Haddad GK, Haddad JA et al. Secondary patency of thrombosed prosthetic vascular access grafts with aggressive surveillance, monitoring and endovascular management. *Eur J Endovasc Surg.* 2008;36:356–365.

21. Simoni E, Blitz L, Lookstein R. Outcomes of AngioJet thrombectomy in hemodialysis vascular access grafts and fistulas: PEARL I Registry. *J Vasc Access.* 2013;14:72–76.

22. Bakken AM, Protack CD, Saad WE et al. Long-term outcomes of primary angioplasty and primary stenting of central venous stenosis in hemodialysis patients. *J Vasc Surg.* 2007;45:776–783.

23. Kakisis JD, Avgerinos E, Giannakopoulos T et al. Balloon angioplasty vs nitinol stent placement in the treatment of venous anastomotic stenoses of hemodialysis grafts after surgical thrombectomy. *J Vasc Surg.* 2012;55:472–478.

24. Anaya-Ayala JE, Smolock CJ, Colvard BD et al. Efficacy of covered stent placement for central venous occlusive disease in hemodialysis patients. *J Vasc Surg.* 2011;54:754–759.

25. Karnabatidis D, Kitrou P, Spiliopoulos S et al. Stent-grafts versus angioplasty and/or bare metal stents for failing arteriovenous grafts: A cross-over longitudinal study. *J Nephrol.* 2013;26:389–395.

26. Katsanos K, Karnabatidis D, Kitrou P et al. Paclitaxel-coated balloon angioplasty vs. plain balloon dilatation for the treatment of failing dialysis access: 6-month interim results from a prospective randomized trial. *J Endovasc Ther.* 2012;19:263–272.

55

Diagnosis and management of vascular anomalies
The Yakes AVM Classification System

WAYNE F. YAKES, ALEXIS M. YAKES and ALEXANDER J. CONTINENZA

CONTENTS

Vascular anomalies constitute some of the most difficult diagnostic and therapeutic enigmas that can be encountered in the practice of medicine. The clinical presentations are extremely protean and can range from an asymptomatic birthmark to fulminant, life-threatening congestive heart failure. Attributing any of these extremely varied symptoms that a patient may present with to a vascular malformation can be challenging to the most experienced clinician. Compounding this problem is the extreme rarity of these vascular lesions. If a clinician sees one patient every few years, it is extremely difficult to gain a learning curve to diagnose and optimally treat them. Typically, these patients bounce from clinician to clinician only to experience disappointing outcomes, complications and recurrence or worsening of their presenting symptoms.

Vascular anomalies were first treated by surgeons. The early rationale of proximal arterial ligation of arteriovenous malformations (AVMs) proved totally futile as the phenomenon of neovascular recruitment reconstituted arterial inflow to the AVM nidus. Microfistulous connections became macrofistulous feeders. Complete extirpation of an AVM nidus proved very difficult and extremely hazardous, necessitating suboptimal partial resections. Partial resections could cause an initial good clinical response, but with time, the patient's presenting symptoms recurred or worsened at follow-up.[1-3] Because of the significant blood loss that frequently accompanied surgery, the skills of interventional radiologists were eventually employed to embolize these vascular lesions preoperatively. This allowed more complete resections; however, complete extirpation of an AVM was still extremely difficult and rarely possible. As catheter delivery systems and embolic agents improved, embolotherapy has since emerged as a primary mode of therapy in the management of vascular anomalies. Anatomically, vascular malformations are often in surgically difficult or inaccessible areas which have led to increased reliance on the sophisticated endosurgical skills of the interventional radiologist and interventional neuroradiologist in the management of these problematic patients.

Because the clinical and angiographic manifestations can be extremely varied, hemangiomas and vascular malformations are always difficult to classify. Moreover, numerous descriptive terms have been applied to impressive clinical examples in the hopes of distinguishing them as distinct syndromes. This has resulted in significant confusion in the categorization and treatment of these complex vascular lesions. Some of the confusing terms include congenital arteriovenous aneurysm, cirsoid aneurysm, serpentine aneurysm, capillary telangiectasia, angioma telangiectaticum, angioma arteriale racemosum, angioma simplex, angioma serpiginosum, naevus angiectoides, hemangioma simplex, lymphangioma, hemangiolymphangioma, naevus flammeus, verrucous hemangioma, capillary hemangioma, cavernous hemangioma and venous angioma. Based on the landmark research of Mulliken et al.,[4–9] a rational classification of hemangioma and vascular malformations has evolved that should be incorporated into modern clinical practice. This classification system, based on endothelial cell characteristics, has removed much of the confusion in terminology that is present in the literature today. Once all clinicians understand and utilize this important classification system, ambiguity and confusion will be removed and all clinicians can speak a common language. This classification system has been adopted by the International Society for the Study of Vascular Anomalies (ISSVA).[10]

THEORETICAL EMBRYOLOGIC ORIGINS

In the embryo, the primitive mesenchyme is nourished by an interlacing system of blood spaces without distinguishable arterial and venous channels. As the embryo matures, the interlacing system of blood spaces becomes differentiated by partial resorption of the primitive vascular spaces and the formation of mature arterial and venous vascular spaces with intervening capillary beds. The classically outlined sequence of events includes (1) the undifferentiated capillary network stage; (2) the retiform developmental stage, characterized by coalescence of the original equipotential capillaries into large, interconnecting, plexiform vascular spaces without an intervening capillary bed; and (3) the final developmental stage, characterized by the resorption of the primitive vascular elements and the formation of mature arterial, capillary, venous and lymphatic elements.[11–14]

Arrests in development or the failure of orderly resorption of embryologic primitive vascular elements results in persistence of immature vascular structures. Vascular elements retained from the undifferentiated embryonal capillary network stage reveal a strong structural similarity to venous malformations (VMs). Failure of orderly resorption of vascular elements from the retiform developmental stage results in the retention of interconnecting channels of immature arteries and veins without an intervening capillary bed. Microfistulous and macrofistulous AVMs correspond to this embryologic stage of vascular development. Other errors in embryologic morphogenesis during the retiform developmental stage could result in other types of vascular malformations. Another example would be retention of primitive capillary elements, which would explain capillary malformations found in port-wine stains. Arteriovenous fistulae (AVF) could result if there was faulty vascular morphogenesis during the later retiform stage. However, due to the constant breakdown and formation of vascular spaces in the embryo, these stages can overlap. This can lead to retained mixed vascular lesions that are complex

and contain multiple combinations of these early stages of vascular morphogenesis.

As Reid has stated:

> In view of the common development on each side of the vascular tree, and in view of the enormous constructive and destructive changes necessary before the final pattern of the vascular tree is reached, it is a marvel not that abnormal congenital communication occasionally, or rarely, occur, but that they do not occur more often.[13]

CLASSIFICATION OF HEMANGIOMAS AND VASCULAR MALFORMATIONS

Pediatric cutaneous and soft tissue vascular lesions (hemangiomas) and vascular malformations have been classified by Mulliken, Glowacki and co-workers after research into endothelial cell characteristics, numbers of mast cells present and endothelial cell in vitro characteristics.[4–9] Most pediatric hemangiomas are not present at birth, clinically manifest within the first month of life and exhibit a rapid growth phase in the first year. More than 90% of pediatric hemangiomas spontaneously regress to near complete resolution by 5–7 years of age. Hemangiomas occur with a reported incidence of 1%–2.6%.[15] Hemangiomas in the proliferative phase are characterized by rapid growth, significant endothelial cell hyperplasia forming syncytial masses, thickened endothelial basement membrane, ready incorporation of tritiated thymidine into the endothelial cells and the presence of large numbers of mast cells.[4–6] After this period of rapid expansion in the proliferative phase, hemangiomas can stabilize and grow commensurately with the child. Because of the complex nature of hemangiomas, the proliferative phase may continue as the involutive phase slowly begins to dominate. Involuting hemangiomas show diminished endothelial cellularity and replacement with fibrofatty deposits, exhibit a unilamellar basement membrane, demonstrate no uptake of tritiated thymidine into endothelial cells and have normal mast cell counts.[4–6] Other hemangioma types are congenital pediatric hemangiomas termed termed 'Rapidly Involuting Congenital Hemangioma' (RICH), 'Partially Involuting Congenital Hemangioma' (PICH), and 'Non-Involuting Congenital Hemangioma' (NICH). Kaposiform hemangioendotheliomas (KHE) of the liver can cause heart failure. KHE of soft tissue causes the Kasabach–Merritt syndrome of platelet consumption coagulopathy. These two entities have been confused with vascular malformations. Because of the landmark research of Mulliken and co-workers, studying these issues at the cellular level, not the macro-level, has allowed these diagnoses to be differentiated and defined.[4–9]

Vascular malformations are vascular lesions that are present at birth and grow commensurately with the child. Trauma, surgery, hormonal influences caused by birth control pills and the hormonal swings during puberty and pregnancy may cause a lesion to expand and grow hemodynamically. Vascular malformations demonstrate no endothelial cell proliferation, contain large vascular channels lined by flat endothelium, have a unilamellar basement membrane, do not incorporate tritiated thymidine into endothelial cells and have normal mast cell counts. They may be formed from any combination of primitive arterial, capillary, venous or lymphatic elements with or without direct arteriovenous (AV) shunts. Vascular malformations are true structural anomalies resulting from inborn errors of vascular morphogenesis and the failure of orderly resorption of these primitive vascular elements.

Vascular malformations are categorized into malformed arterial, capillary, venous, lymphatic, and combinations of these malformed primitive vascular elements. The term 'hemangioma' should be reserved for the previously described pediatric cutaneous lesions that are not present at birth, except for RICH, PICH, and NICH, manifest themselves within the first month of life, exhibit a rapid proliferative phase and then slowly involute to near complete resolution by 5–7 years of age. The old terms describing adult conditions such as 'cavernous hemangioma', 'hepatic hemangioma', 'extremity hemangioma' and 'vertebral body hemangioma' should be replaced with the term 'venous malformation'. The term `intramuscular hemangioma' should be replaced with `intramuscular capillary-venous malformation.' The typical port-wine stain, composed of dilated malformed capillary-like vessels, previously incorrectly termed 'capillary hemangioma', should instead be termed 'capillary malformation'. The old terms simple 'capillary lymphangioma', 'cavernous lymphangioma' and 'cystic hygroma' should instead be termed 'lymphatic malformations'. The old term 'hemangiolymphangioma' should be replaced with 'mixed venous lymphatic malformation'. The old terms 'arteriovenous hemangioma', 'arterial angioma', 'arteriovenous aneurysm', 'cirsoid aneurysm', 'red angioma' and 'serpentine aneurysm' should be replaced with 'arteriovenous malformation'.

Eponyms have further clouded and confused the nomenclature of hemangiomas and vascular malformations in the world's literature. Maffuci's syndrome (or Kast syndrome) has been defined as a condition whereby the patient has multiple enchondromas and coexistent hemangiomatosis.[16] In the current classification system, hemangiomatosis should be termed 'venous malformation'. The Riley–Smith syndrome has been previously characterized by macrocephaly, pseudopapilledema and multiple hemangiomas.[17] The term 'hemangioma' should be replaced with 'venous malformation'. Capillary malformations and lymphatic malformations may also be present with the Riley–Smith syndrome. The Riley–Smith syndrome, the Proteus syndrome and Bannayan's syndrome are probably a spectrum of similar congenital vascular anomalies.[17–20] Gorham syndrome, Gorham–Stout syndrome and Trinquoste syndrome are similar entities described as osteolysis (disappearing bone disease) caused by an underlying hemangiomatosis.[21] The term 'hemangiomatosis' should be replaced by 'venous malformation'. The blue rubber bleb naevus syndrome (or Bean's syndrome) is another confusing eponym, but is unusual in that it is an autosomal dominant heritable condition. It is characterized by subcutaneous (rubbery) VMs that spontaneously occur in the extremities and trunk and enlarge. More severe forms can have VMs involving the intestines and in the CNS that hemorrhage. This can cause neurological deficits or significant GI blood loss. Surgery may be required.

Another confusing group of eponyms are Klippel–Trenaunay syndrome, naevus vasculosus osteohypertrophy, naevus verrucous hypertrophycans, osteohypertrophic naevus flammeus and angioosteohypertrophy syndrome, all of which describe a congenital entity characterized by unilateral lower limb hypertrophy; cutaneous capillary malformations; lymphatic malformations; a normal, hypoplastic or atretic deep venous system; occasional extension of the vascular malformation into the trunk from the lower extremity; a retained embryonic lateral venous anomaly (Servelle's vein) of the lower extremity; and increased subcutaneous fat in the affected limb.[22–24] A similar group of eponyms (Parkes–Weber syndrome, giant limb of Robertson) represents a similar clinical entity that has the same features of the Klippel–Trenaunay syndrome with the coexistence of multiple AVF.[25] The Klippel–Trenaunay syndrome and Parkes–Weber syndrome usually occur in the lower extremity, but can also affect the upper extremity. In the upper extremity, the Parkes–Weber syndrome is more commonly seen, although the Klippel–Trenaunay syndrome is much more common overall.

These are but a few of the confusing terms used in the literature and in clinical practice. This ISSVA modern classification system can eliminate the current confusion and all clinicians can finally speak the same language. Accurate terminology will lead to precise identification of clinical entities and to enhanced patient care. The remainder of this chapter will use this modern classification system originated by Mulliken, Glowacki and co-workers, and adopted by ISSVA, as it is based on the cellular level, not the macro-level.[4–10]

CONCEPTS IN PATIENT MANAGEMENT

Vascular malformations are congenital lesions that are present at birth, whether or not evident clinically, and grow commensurately with the child. AVMs, congenital AVF, capillary malformations, VMs, lymphatic malformations and mixed malformations are grouped under the collective term vascular malformations. Post-traumatic AVF are different in that they are acquired lesions. Even without an inciting trauma, acquired AVF may occur. A common etiology in this acquired type is prior venous thrombosis and AV fistulization in the vein wall during the recanalization process.

A thorough clinical exam and history can usually establish the diagnosis of hemangioma or vascular malformation. Hemangiomas (Pediatric Hemangioma and Infantile Hemangioma are the same entity) are usually not present at birth (unless RICH, PICH, or NICH) and initially have a bright scarlet color that gradually deepens. Vascular malformations have a persistent colour, depending on the dominant arterial, capillary, venous or lymphatic component. Evaluating for skeletal abnormalities, abnormal veins, arterial abnormalities, plasticity or non-plasticity of a lesion, whether the lesion swells when dependent and flattens when elevated, disparity of limb size, warmth of the affected area, whether reflex bradycardia occurs in the Nicoladoni–Branham test of inflow arterial occlusion, along with neurologic evaluation and a good history can frequently diagnose a hemangioma or categorize a vascular malformation.

Color Doppler imaging (CDI) is an essential tool in the diagnostic workup of vascular malformations. Both high-flow lesions (AVMs, AVF) and low-flow lesions (VMs, lymphatic malformations) can be accurately diagnosed. Furthermore, CDI is also an important non-invasive method for following patients undergoing therapy. Documentation of decreased arterial flow rates in high-flow malformations and persistent venous malformation thrombosis can be accurately assessed.[26]

Computed tomography (CT), although helpful in the diagnostic workup, is less useful than magnetic resonance imaging (MRI). Unlike CT, MRI easily distinguishes between high-flow (AVMs, AVF) and low-flow (VMs, lymphatic malformations) vascular malformations utilizing STIR, T2-weighted with fat-suppression sequence and gradient echo sequence being the most useful.[27]

Furthermore, the anatomic relationship of the vascular malformation to adjacent nerves, muscles, tendons, organs, bone and subcutaneous fat allows a total assessment. MRI is also an excellent non-invasive method for following patients to determine the efficacy of therapy, often obviating repetitive arteriography and venography.[27]

MRI has proven to be a mainstay in the initial diagnostic evaluation as well as in assessing endovascular therapy at follow-up. MRI can determine and distinguish between high-flow and low-flow malformations. Further, various imaging sequences make it easy to determine relationships to adjacent anatomic structures such as organs, muscles and nerves. High-flow malformations typically demonstrate signal voids on most sequences. These flow voids are felt to be predominantly due to time-of-flight phenomenon with turbulence-related rephasing also contributing to signal loss. An additional feature to differentiate highflow lesions from low-flow lesions is the presence of enlarged feeding arteries and dilated draining veins. Gradient echo sequences show AVM as bright signal serpiginous structures. Several characteristics of low-flow malformations have been described in the literature, including a serpentine pattern with internal striations or septations associated with focal muscle atrophy or hypertrophy. Low-flow malformations, which include VMs and lymphatic malformations, demonstrate a characteristic bright signal intensity that is greater than skeletal muscle in both T1- and T2-weighted images. However, it is less than subcutaneous fat on T1-weighted images and greater than fat on T2-weighted images. STIR sequences and T2-weighted with fat-suppression sequences best image venous and lymphatic malformations.[27] Hemangiomas also are bright on T2-weighted and STIR sequences. US will show a solid mass in hemangiomas to differentiate from a venous or lymphatic lesion (Table 55.1).

ETHANOL ENDOVASCULAR THERAPY

Many endovascular occlusive agents are currently in use to treat vascular malformations. With the use of intravascular ethanol, pain control is a significant patient issue, and anesthesiologists can be of great help. Whether the anesthesiologist performs general anesthesia or intravenous sedation during the procedure, this is one less burden the interventional radiologist assumes so that he or she can concentrate on the case at hand. In pediatric patients, general anesthesia is a requirement, because children do not wish to return to that doctor that caused them to undergo a painful procedure, or repeated painful procedures. After performing thousands of procedures in all anatomic locations, general anesthesia is far better than IV sedation regarding patient safety, control and comfort. Our anesthesia team sees the same patients return for multiple procedures and no complications of multiple general anesthesia were ever documented.

Post-ethanol injection cardiopulmonary collapse has the potential for a lethal complication if not resuscitated successfully.[28] However, in our experiences and in others' experience,[29,30] if vascular injections of ethanol are limited to 0.14 mL/kg ideal body weight every 10 minutes, pulmonary hypertension and cardiopulmonary collapse can

Table 55.1 Schobinger classification of AVMs.

Stage I	*Quiescence*: Pink-bluish stain, warmth and arteriovenous shunting revealed by Doppler scanning. The AVM mimics a capillary malformation or involuting hemangioma.
Stage II	*Expansion*: Stage I plus vascular enlargement, pulsations, thrill, bruit and tortuous/tense veins (vascular engorgement).
Stage III	*Destruction*: Stage II plus dystrophic skin changes, skin ulcerations, bleeding, tissue necrosis. Bony lytic lesions may occur.
Stage IV	*Decompensation*: Stage III plus congestive cardiac failure with increased cardiac output, left ventricle hypertrophy and vascular overload due to venous hypertension and right heart decompensation.

Source: Schobinger R, In *Proceedings of the International Society for the Study of Vascular Anomalies Biennial Workshop*, Rome, Italy, June 23–26, 1996.

be totally obviated. In patients with pre-existing pulmonary hypertension for whatever cause, this caveat does not exist and Swan-Ganz monitoring of pulmonary pressures during ethanol embolizations is mandatory as this patient group has no pulmonary reserve. Ethanol embolization may even be obviated in this patient group.

Ninety-eight per cent ethyl alcohol (dehydrated alcohol injection USP, Abbott Laboratories, North Chicago, IL). Ethanol is a well-known sclerosing agent that in normal arteries induces significant thrombosis from the capillary bed backward. This results in total tissue devitalization. Ethanol induces thrombosis by denaturing blood proteins, dehydrating endothelial cells and precipitating their protoplasm, denuding the vascular wall of the endothelial cells and segmentally fracturing the vessel wall to the level of the internal elastic lamina. In the treatment of vascular malformations, ethanol has demonstrated its curative potential as opposed to the palliation seen with other embolic agents.[31-57] As with Gelfoam powder, extreme caution and superselective catheter placement are requirements when using ethanol as an endovascular occlusive agent. Ethanol can induce significant pain when injected intravascularly by stimulating the vasa nervorum. General anesthesia is required to minimize patient discomfort, especially in children. Post-embolization edema always occurs with the use of ethanol. Extreme caution must be taken with its use to minimize the possibility of nontarget embolization of normal tissues to prevent tissue necrosis and neuropathy.

YAKES AVM CLASSIFICATION SYSTEM

The world's literature certainly verifies the extreme challenges in the diagnosis and treatment of AVMs. The purpose of this chapter is to present a new Yakes AVM Classification System that has proven therapeutic implications to effectively treat complex AVMs in any anatomical area.[55-57] By employing the Yakes AVM Classification System, a physician is now able to accurately classify AVMs and determine specific endovascular treatment strategies to consistently treat AVMs, and patients can enjoy long-term excellent outcomes. Defining the angioarchitecture of the high-flow AVM determines accurately the endovascular management strategy to best permanently ablate the AVM requiring treatment. Further, employing this new Yakes AVM Classification System will lower complication rates in treating these complex congenital vascular pathologies.

The Houdart Classification of Intracranial Arteriovenous Fistulae and Malformations of high-flow lesions[58] and the Do Classification of AVMs of the peripheral arterial circulation[59] are strikingly similar despite their anatomic locational differences (CNS vs. peripheral vasculatures). Both authors also suggest similar therapeutic approaches based on their similar arteriographic classification.[58,59]

The Houdart Type a and Type b and Do Types I and II proffer retrograde approaches to occlude the vein aneurysm outflow as being a potential for curative treatment of these AVM types. Yakes illustrated retrograde vein occlusion techniques for high-flow malformations first published with 3 cases illustrated in the figures in 1990.[60] Later, Jackson et al. published the retrograde vein approach in 1996.[61] The Do Group in Seoul, Korea (also the publishers of the Do AVM Classification), published the retrograde vein approach in 2008 after Dr. Yakes demonstrated its efficacy to them in treating patients at the Samsung Medical Center in Seoul, Korea.[62]

The Yakes AVM Classification System has some similarities to both classification systems and some stark differences. The Yakes Classification System is as follows: Type I is a direct arteriovenous fistula, a direct artery to vein connection (typified by Pulmonary AVF and renal AVF, for example). This angioarchitecture type is not described in the Houdart or Do classification systems. Type II is an AVM characterized by usually multiple inflow arteries into a *nidus* pattern with direct artery–arteriolar to vein–venular structures that may, or may not, be aneurysmal. Type IIIa is characterized by multiple arteries and arterioles into an enlarged aneurysmal vein with an enlarged single outflow vein. Type IIIb is characterized by multiple arteries and arterioles into an enlarged aneurysmal vein with multiple dilated outflow veins. Type IV AVMs are microfistulous innumerable arteriolar structures shunting into innumerable venular connections that diffusely infiltrate a tissue (typified by ear AVMs that infiltrate the entire cartilage structure of the pinna). What is different in this lesion is that there are mixed among the innumerable fistulae capillary beds within the affected tissue. If the affected tissue only had AVFs, the tissue could not survive as capillary beds are required for tissue viability. No other AVM angioarchitecture has this duality. This angioarchitecture is not described in the world's literature except for these recent publications.[56,57]

Comparing Houdart's CNS Classification and the Do Peripheral Vascular Classification to the Yakes Classification has some parallels, as has been described, but has several distinct differences. Houdart Type A and Do Type I are the same and compare to the Yakes Type IIIa. Houdart Type B and Do Type II are the same and again are placed in the Yakes Type IIIa. Whether the arteriovenous (Type A/Type I) or arteriolar–venular connections (Type B/Type II) are present is not important as the same arterial physiology is present with the *nidus* being present in the vein wall itself. Regardless of the size of AVF on the vein wall, they are both treated endovascularly in the same way. Therefore, the AVF size is irrelevant. Further, even when larger AVF are present, microfistulae are also present as well and mixed with the larger connections. It never is purely one microsize only or one macrosize only.

The Houdart Type C is the same as bundling the Do Types IIIa (arteriovenous) and IIIb (arteriolar venular). This is similar to the Yakes Type II. Both authors do not explain the Yakes Type IV in their classifications. The angioarchitecture of arteriovenous shunting through arteriolar-venular innumerable fistulae, totally infiltrating a particular tissue, is another vascular phenomenon that is present that is not explained by the Houdart nor the Do

Classifications. Being that arteriographically these innumerable microfistulae are proven to infiltrate a tissue, one has to also consider that, despite the innumerable microfistulae, there is interspersed among these abnormal fistulae vascularity that is normal with capillary beds that is nutrient to the infiltrated tissue as well, or the tissue itself would be devitalized and forced to necrose. Normal capillaries must be present and admixed with the innumerable AVF in the infiltrated tissue, or it would not be viable and could not survive. Venous hypertension is usually the culprit in the injury that occurs in that infiltrated tissue. This phenomenon of arterialized veins as a vascular etiology for pathologic tissue changes was first elucidated by Jean Jacques Merland and Marie Claire Riche.[63] Thus, the *normal* vascularity of capillary beds in the infiltrated tissue to allow it to exist is not discussed in the Houdart or in the Do AVM Classifications nor are the infiltrative AVM angioarchitecture characteristics described.

The Yakes Type I AVM is a direct AV macro-connection that is characteristic of pulmonary AVF and renal AVF, but can also occur in other tissues. This direct AV connection is not described in the Houdart Classification or in the Do Classification. The Yakes Type I AV connection can also be present and interspersed in other AVM types as well (Figure 55.1).

The Yakes Type II AVM Classification possesses an angioarchitecture synonymous with the classical *nidus* pattern commonly seen in AVMs with multiple inflow arteries of varying sizes coursing towards a *nidus* (a complex tangle of vascular structures without any intervening capillaries and exiting from this *nidus* into multiple veins) (Figure 55.2). The Houdart Type C and the Do Type IIIa/Type IIIb most resemble this angioarchitecture pattern. Thus, the Yakes Type II and Yakes Type IV further define the Houdart Type C and Do Type IIIa/IIIb patterns much more specifically (Figures 55.3 and 55.4).

As an aside, the term 'nidus' is rampant in the medical literature (AVM nidus, nidus of infection, etc.). Unfortunately, the initial author was only partially familiar with the Latin language. 'Nidus' means 'nest' in Latin, and indeed, it does. However, *nidus* with the ending *us* denotes male gender. In the Latin language, the true term meaning 'nest' is, in fact, 'nidum'. The ending 'um' denotes the neuter gender which a *nest* truly is. Thus, the original author accurately describing *nest-like* conglomeration of vascular structure was woefully inaccurate penning the words as *nidus* (masculine) instead of the true word *nidum* (neuter). Being rife in the literature for decades, I do not foresee any correction of this term.

In summary, Yakes Type I is the simplest macro-direct AV connection. Yakes Type II is the common *nidum* (nest-like) AV connection. Yakes Type IIIa has multiple AV connections (arterial and arteriolar into an aneurysmal vein [*nidum* is in the vein wall]) with single outflow vein physiology. Yakes Type IIIb has multiple arterial inflow connections (arterial and arteriolar) into an aneurysmal vein (*nidum* is in the vein wall) with multiple outflow veins that is more difficult to treat by retrograde vein approaches.

Yakes Type IV angioarchitecture has innumerable micro-AV connections (with lowered vascular resistance) infiltrating an entire tissue but with concurrent normal vascular structures possessing nutrient capillary beds (with normal vascular resistance) to supply and drain the tissue that is diffusely infiltrated to allow this tissue to survive and not be devitalized. The postcapillary veins compete with AVF outflow veins that are arterialized (hypertensive) and cause the resultant non-healing pathology.[63] This infiltrative AVM entity had first been described by Yakes in the recent literature (Figure 55.5).[56,57]

Therapeutic implications of the Yakes Classification

Determining a classification system based on the AVM angioarchitecture is of little use without a practical application. For example, the Spetzler–Martin Brain AVM Classification is of importance to determine the surgical morbidity for treating Brain AVMs[64], the higher the Spetzler–Martin grade, the higher the morbidity. This allows the neurosurgeon to inform his patient accurately of the risks for treatment. The Schobinger AVM Classification for peripheral AVMs (non-neuro) is useful to quantify the degrees of symptomatology a patient possess regardless of the AVM's angioarchitecture.[65] The Yakes AVM Classification System is utilized to determine endovascular approaches and the embolic agents that will be successful to ablate these AVMs.

Embolic agents employed in the Yakes AVM Classification

Yakes Type I direct AV connections, as typically seen in pulmonary AVF and renal AVF, can be permanently ablated by occluding the AVF with mechanical devices. Coils, Amplatzer plugs, occluders, detachable balloons and the like are universally successful to cure Yakes Type I AVMs. Ethanol can also be curative in Yakes Type I AVMs if the AVF is of a small calibre.

Yakes Type II AVMs with the *nidum* nest-like angioarchitecture can be permanently ablated with absolute ethanol from a superselective transcatheter/transmicrocatheter arterial approach. Also, a direct puncture into the artery(ies) supplying the AVM immediately proximal to the AVM *nidum* and distal to any parenchymal arterial branches to then inject ethanol superselectively can be employed to circumvent catheterization obstacles when a transcatheter/transmicrocatheter positioning to achieve the same position to deliver ethanol into the *nidum* is not possible. These two transarterial approaches allow ethanol to sclerose and permanently ablate the *nidum*. Also, the *nidum* itself can be direct-punctured and ethanol (undiluted) can be injected to sclerose the *nidum* directly to effect cure in its multiple compartments as well.

Yakes AVM Classification

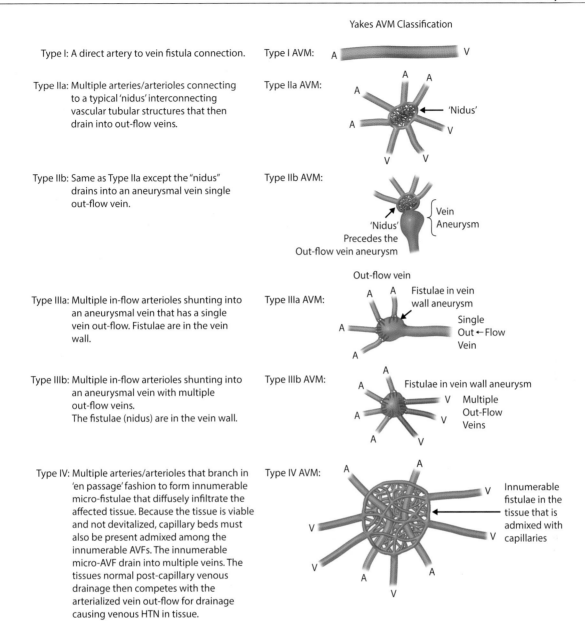

Type I: A direct artery to vein fistula connection.

Type IIa: Multiple arteries/arterioles connecting to a typical 'nidus' interconnecting vascular tubular structures that then drain into out-flow veins.

Type IIb: Same as Type IIa except the "nidus" drains into an aneurysmal vein single out-flow vein.

Type IIIa: Multiple in-flow arterioles shunting into an aneurysmal vein that has a single vein out-flow. Fistulae are in the vein wall.

Type IIIb: Multiple in-flow arterioles shunting into an aneurysmal vein with multiple out-flow veins.
The fistulae (nidus) are in the vein wall.

Type IV: Multiple arteries/arterioles that branch in 'en passage' fashion to form innumerable micro-fistulae that diffusely infiltrate the affected tissue. Because the tissue is viable and not devitalized, capillary beds must also be present admixed among the innumerable AVFs. The innumerable micro-AVF drain into multiple veins. The tissues normal post-capillary venous drainage then competes with the arterialized vein out-flow for drainage causing venous HTN in tissue.

Figure 55.1 Yakes Type I AVM. (a) Direct AV connection that can be treated with fibered coils, Amplatzer plugs and the like. Mechanical device occlusion can be curative. Ethanol injections can be curative in smaller AVFs. (b) Type I AVM: ventilator-dependent 30-year-old female with HHT and massive Lt pulmonary AVM causing O$_2$ sats of 35% despite being on 100% oxygen via the ventilator; patient sent by air ambulance emergently. Fibered coils endovascularly placed were curative and the O$_2$ saturations normalized immediately. (c) Direct artery to vein AVF connection. (d) Dilated outflow vein in the AVF. (From Yakes WF, Baumgartner I, *Gefasschirurgie*, 19, 325, 2014; Yakes WF, Yakes AM, *Egyptian J of Vasc & Endovasc Surg*, 10, 9, 2014.)

Yakes Type IIIa AVMs (multiple inflow arteries shunting into an aneurysmal vein with a single enlarged outflow vein) and Yakes Type IIIb AVMs (multiple inflow arteries into an aneurysmal vein with multiple enlarged outflow veins) can be curatively treated by several endovascular approaches. The *nidum* in this type of angioarchitecture with an aneurysmal vein is in the vein wall itself. Superselective transarterial ethanol embolization distal to all parenchymal branches via transcatheter/transmicrocatheter and direct puncture endovascular approaches to the vein wall nidus can be curative. A simpler additional curative endovascular approach for Type IIIa AVMs is to coil embolize the aneurysmal vein itself with, or without, concurrent ethanol injection into the coils within the aneurysmal vein. This is also curative when the aneurysmal vein is totally and densely packed with coils. The aneurysmal vein can be endovascularly approached by a direct 18G needle puncture and by a retrograde vein catheterization to achieve the same position within the aneurysmal vein to pack it with coils. The retrograde vein approach to curatively treat high-flow vascular lesions was first published

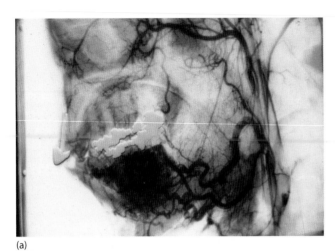

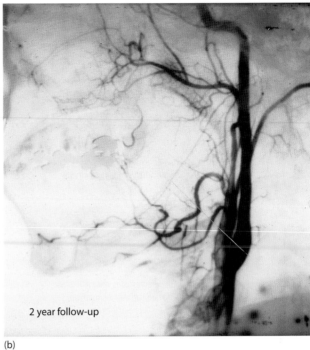

2 year follow-up

(a)

(b)

Figure 55.2 (a) Type II AVM: Typical *nidus* (Latin 'nidum' meaning 'nest') vascular angioarchitecture. Ethanol embolization super-selectively delivered by transcatheter and direct puncture techniques is curative. (b) Two year arteriographic follow-up demonstrating persistent cure of AVM.

and illustrated in 1990 by Yakes et al.[60] The second article articulating the vein approach to AVM treatment was subsequently published in 1996 by Jackson et al.[61] Cures were documented in these published patient series. Yakes et al. described cures of post-traumatic and congenital high-flow lesions.[60] Jackson et al. described cures of congenital AVMs by way of the retrograde vein approach in these publications.[61] Cho/Do et al. also published retrograde vein approach to curative AVM treatment taught to their team by Yakes.[62]

In the Yakes, Type IIIb (aneurysmal vein with enlarged multiple out-flow veins) can be cured by transarterial transcatheter ethanol embolization and can be cured by direct puncture and retrograde vein coiling techniques. However, the aneurysmal vein portion and the immediate adjacent segments of each out-flow vein must also be packed with coils completely to achieve cure. Yakes Type IIIb AVMs are more challenging to coil and cure than the Yakes Type IIIa AVMs due to the more complex multiple out-flow veins morphology.

Yakes Type IV AVMs present a unique challenge to determine curative endovascular treatment strategies. AVMs, by definition, are direct AV connections without an intervening capillary bed (Yakes Types I-IV). Thus, superselective catheter and direct puncture needle positioning distal to *all* normal branches supplying parenchyma and immediately proximal to the AVM *nidum* itself will obviate tissue necrosis, being that the capillary beds are not embolized and only the abnormal AV connections are sclerosed. However, Yakes Type IV AVMs infiltrate an entire tissue, thus, termed by

the authors as an *infiltrative* form of AVM. Being that the *infiltrated* tissue (e.g. auricular AVMs) is viable proves that capillary beds are undoubtedly interspersed along with the innumerable microfistulae throughout the involved tissue as well. Injection of ethanol by transcatheter/transmicrocatheter and direct puncture approaches will sclerose the innumerable microfistulae, but also would flood the capillary beds with ethanol devitalizing that infiltrated tissue. Necrosis of that tissue would then ensue with occlusion of the capillary beds. Thus, Yakes Type IV AVMs were a profound conundrum to treat by endovascular approaches. Polymerizing agents would also occlude AVFs, but also occlude the capillary beds as well causing massive tissue necrosis.

Thinking through this conundrum, one could rightly conclude that the only option is total surgical resection of that entire tissue as the only treatment option. After further reflection, an endovascular option for curative treatment, not palliative treatment, was considered a possibility. Capillary beds have normal peripheral resistance which has a somewhat restrictive vascular flow pattern from artery to capillary to veins. AVMs/AVF have abnormally lowered peripheral vascular resistance with rapid stunting into arterialized veins. The arterialized AVM outflow veins are hypertensive and are arterialized pressures. The postcapillary outflow normotensive veins then compete with the higher arterialized pressure AVMs outflow veins for outflow systemically. This then further restricts normal vein outflow, which in turn increases the systemic vascular resistance (SVR) of the normal arterioles immediately proximal to the capillary beds, further restricting

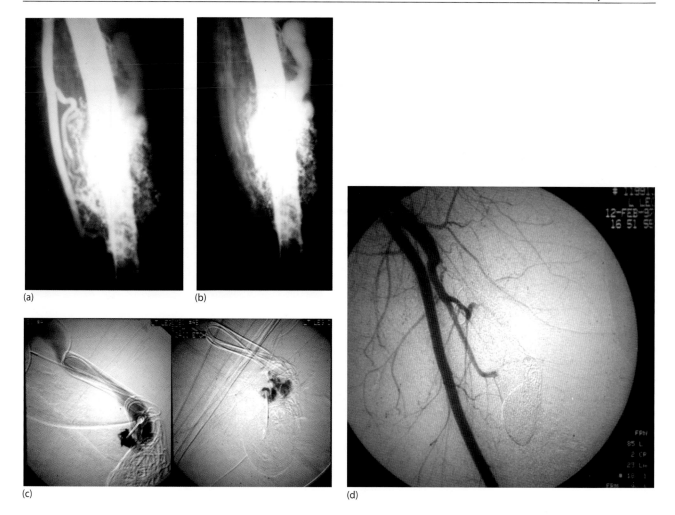

Figure 55.3 (a) Type IIIa AVM. Multiple inflow arteries into an aneurysmal vein with single vein outflow. Ethanol and/or coils directed to the outflow vein aneurysmal vein sac can be curative. YAKES Type IIIa AVM. (b) 30-year-old male with an enlarged Lt thigh, Lt thigh pain syndrome, sheets of calcifications throughout the thigh muscles and limited flexion at the Lt knee. Lt femur intraosseous AVM with single vein outflow (AVM Type IIIa). AVM *nidus* is the wall of the aneurysmal vein itself where the AVFs are present. Curative treatment can be done by total coiling of the outflow vein only. Coiling of a large vein sac followed by direct puncture of a small remnant AVF was curative at a 7-year arteriographic follow-up. (c and d) Coiling of the outflow vein and ETOH was curative at this 7-year f/up.

arteriolar inflow to the capillary beds. The increased SVR into the capillaries coupled with abnormally low resistance shunting into the admixed innumerable AVF allows for preferential vascular flow into the AVFs.

Mixing non-ionic contrast with absolute ethanol changes the viscosity and specific gravity of ethanol in this mixture. Being *thickened* and diluted allows for preferential flow to the AVFs and further restricts flow into the capillaries. Despite being 50% diluted with contrast, the ethanol can still effectively sclerose the innumerable micro-fistulae due to the small luminal diameters. This combination of preferential flow into the innumerable AVFs, the increased SVR into the capillaries restricting flow and the increased viscosity and changing of the specific gravity of the contrast with the ethanol 50% mixture all works to spare the capillaries and sclerose the innumerable AVFs. Using pure ethanol would diminish this capillary sparing effect, and the AVFs and capillaries would both be sclerosed and occluded. This does cure the AVFs but then devitalizes the tissue itself with occlusion of the capillaries. Use of various polymerizing embolic occlusive agents (nBCA, Onyx) would also cause the same devitalization of the tissues with occlusion of the capillaries. Particulate embolic agents (PVA, contour embolic, embospheres, etc.) cannot permanently occlude the AVFs and will make the capillaries ischemic with the proximal occlusion in the inflow arterioles, but will not devitalize the tissues.

Summary

Yakes Type I: Can be permanently occluded, with mechanical devices such as coils, fibered coils, Amplatzer plugs and other occluding devices. Ethanol can be curative in smaller calibre AVF.

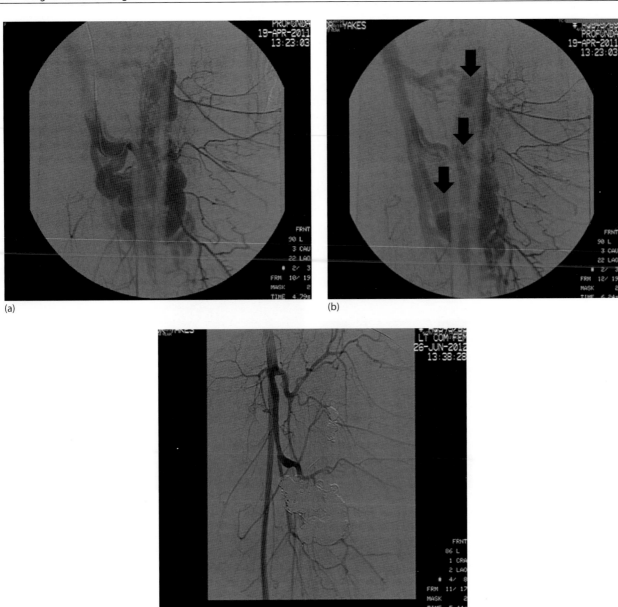

Figure 55.4 (a) Type IIIb AVM. Multiple inflow arteries–arterioles shunting into an aneurysmal vein with multiple outflow veins. The *nidus* is in the vein wall as Type IIIa AVMs. It is more challenging to treat with coils as the multiple veins must be treated. (b) Note multiple outflow veins of this femur AVM flowing into the Lt superficial femoral vein. (c) With coiling of the multiple outflow veins, complete cure is possible.

Yakes Type II: Can be permanently treated with undiluted absolute ethanol. At times, slowing the arterial inflow in the *nidum* with occlusion balloons, tourniquets and blood pressure cuffs which allows for less ethanol to be used to treat the AVM compartments. Direct puncture techniques into the inflow artery or AVM *nidum* allow ethanol to embolize and treat the AVM as well.

Yakes Type IIIa: Can be permanently occluded with transarterial embolizations with ethanol of the vein wall *nidum* the same way as in the Yakes Type II AVM. They can also be permanently occluded by dense coil packing of the vein aneurysm itself with, or without,

ethanol embolization. This can be accomplished via direct puncture of the vein aneurysm, or by retrograde vein catheterization of the vein aneurysm.

Yakes Type IIIb: Can be permanently occluded via transarterial approach as in Yakes Type II AVMs. They can be permanently occluded by treating the vein aneurysm and the multiple aneurysmal outflow veins by coil embolization.

Yakes Type IV: Can be permanently occluded via transarterial superselective 50% mixture of non-ionic contrast and ethanol that treats the micro-AVFs and spares the higher resistance capillaries. Direct puncture with

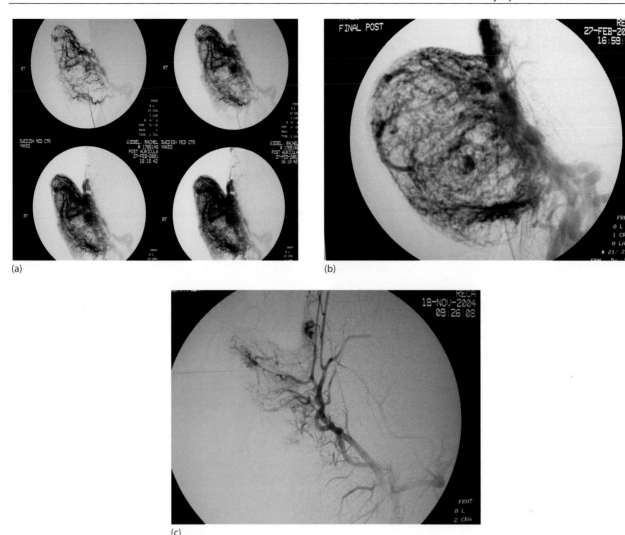

Figure 55.5 (a) Yakes Type IV AVMs. An unusual angioarchitecture for AVMs. In all AVMs, there is an artery-to-vein connection without an intervening capillary bed by definition. In this Type IV AVM, there are innumerable micro-fistulae infiltrating a tissue. But for the tissue to exist there must also be nutrient capillaries separate from the AVFs connections, arising from the same arterioles as the AVFs. Therein lies the problem of vascular occlusion of the AVFs and sparing of the needed capillaries admixed among the AVFs. (b) Note total ear tissue infiltration with innumerable AVF microfistulae admixed with capillaries or the ear would be necrotic and non-viable. (c) Note the absence of the innumerable AVFs, and the ear remains completely viable post-ethanol embolization at 3-year f/up.

23 gauge needles into the micro fistulous AV connections with 100% ethanol injections is also possible and curative.[55-57]

VENOUS AND LYMPHATIC MALFORMATIONS

VMs may be asymptomatic, cosmetically deforming, cause pain, induce neuropathy, ulcerate, hemorrhage, induce changes of abnormal bone growth, bone osteolysis and resorption, cause pathologic fractures, induce a thrombocytopenia, and have mixed venous–lymphatic components. Once it is decided that therapy is warranted, then arteriography and venography should be performed. Venography best identifies the extent of the abnormal vascular mass.[66-69] Arteriography usually shows no arterial abnormality; however, occult AVF may be present in mixed lesions and must be documented by arteriography prior to therapy. After scrutinizing all baseline studies, an appropriate treatment plan can be presented to the patient and the referring clinician (Figure 55.6).

Many authors have treated patients with VMs in all anatomic locations.[68-72] All patients were treated by direct percutaneous puncture with 18–23 gauge needles to directly access the abnormal venous vascular elements. Transarterial ablation with ethanol is never performed unless a concurrent congenital AVF is present. Ethanol will thrombose from the capillary bed backward in the arterial system, thus, sparing the venous malformation and resulting in tissue devitalization. Direct puncture techniques

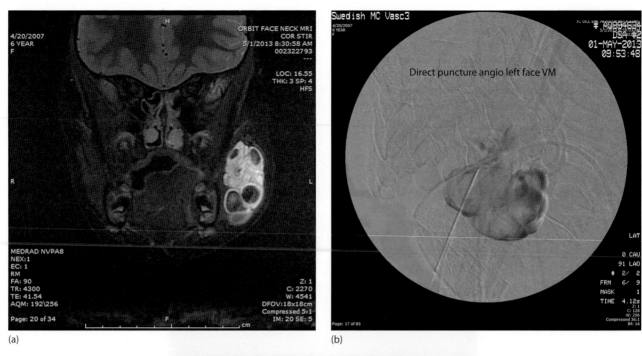

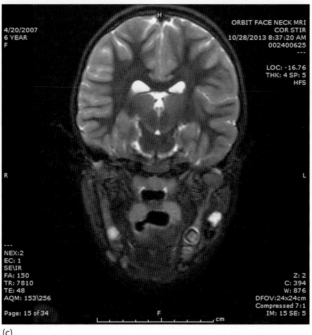

Figure 55.6 (a) Lt face venous malformation, a 6-year-old male with left facial growing compressible mass causing pain intermittently. (b and c) 5-month MRI f/up with marked reduction in size of the venous malformations with direct puncture ETOH injections.

directly attack the venous malformation itself. Thus, the inflow arterial system and capillary bed are not affected and any tissue loss will be minimized. If the venous malformation has transdermal involvement, then skin injury will always occur with eschar formation and ultimate healing by scar formation despite the type of sclerosant embolic agent injected. Several sclerosant embolic agents are used to treat VMs; bleomycin, foam sclerotherapy, polidocanol, sodium tetradecyl sulfate and doxycycline.[31–34] Ethanol is

universally successful for treatment VMs and lymphatic malformations (LMs) as other sclerosants that have shown some efficacy, if less effective than ethanol.

LMs arise from vein buds in their abnormal morphogenesis. LMs are similar histologically to VMs except that, instead of red blood cells being present within the vascular spaces, lymph fluid is present. LMs can have large saccular spaces (macrocystic) or very small luminal spaces (microcystic). LMs have the same imaging

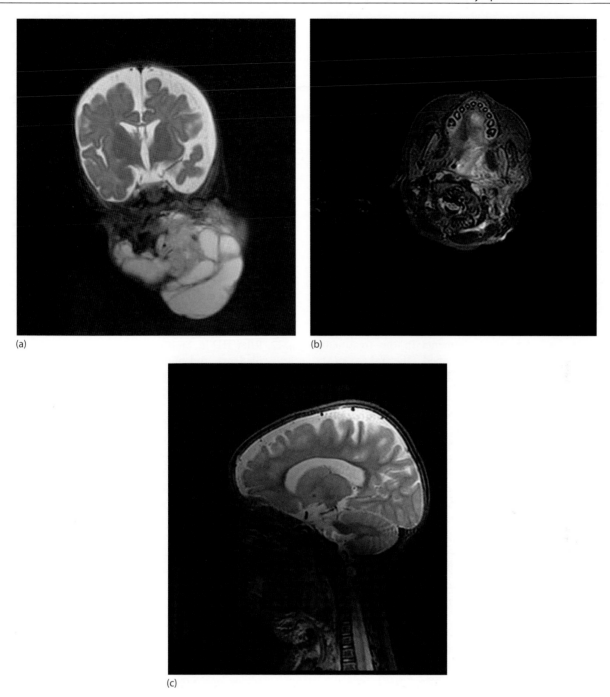

Figure 55.7 (a) A 4-year-old female, massive *cystic hygroma* (misnomer for *lymphatic malformation*, Lesion between pre-verte-bral tissues and trachea and extending laterally bilaterally, tracheostomy and G-tube since birth). (b) A 4 year old with large lymphatic malformation between cervical spine and trachea. Pt has tracheostomy and G-tube since birth. (c) Ethanol cure of the cystic lymphatic malformation at a 3-year f/up. The tracheostomy was then removed.

characteristics on MRI as do vein malformations in that they demonstrate increased signal on STIR and T2-weighted sequences. As in MRI for VMs, LMs are best imaged using STIR or T2-weighted sequences with fat suppression.[27] The old inaccurate term 'cystic hygroma' should be replaced by the more appropriate term 'lymphatic malformation'. LMs respond to percutaneous ethanol therapy in similar fashion to VMs.[45,73] Some success

in shrinkage of LMs has also been noted with bleomy-cin[75] and doxycycline (Figure 55.7).[76]

In superficial VMs, a retrospective study of a con-secutive series 167 procedures in 71 patients revealed an absence of toxic effects with ethanol if ethanol total dose notes per sessions remained below 0.14 mL/kg. Systemic complications were not related to repetitive sclerother-apy sessions.[29–30]

SUMMARY

Vascular anomalies (hemangiomas and vascular malformations) pose some of the most significant challenges in the practice of medicine today. Peripheral and neural axis vascular anomalies cause unique clinical problems with regard to their anatomic locations. Clinical manifestations of these lesions are extremely protean. Because of the rarity of these lesions, the experience of most clinicians in their diagnosis and management is limited, augmenting the enormity of the problem and leading to misdiagnoses and poor patient treatment outcomes. Vascular anomalies are best treated in medical centres where patients with these maladies are seen regularly, and the team approach is used. The occasional embolizer will never gain enough experience to adequately treat these problematic lesions, and these patients should be referred to centres that routinely deal with vascular anomalies and the dilemmas that they present. Only in this fashion can significant experience be gained, judgement in managing these lesions be improved, and definitive statements in the treatment of vascular anomalies be developed. The Yakes AVM Classification System helps clarify specific endovascular management strategies that are potentially curative specific to each AVM type.

REFERENCES

1. Decker DG, Fish CR, Juergens JL. Arteriovenous fistulas of the female pelvis: A diagnostic problem. *Obstet Gynecol.* 1968;31:799–805.
2. Szilagyi DE, Smith RF, Elliott JP, Hageman JH. Congenital arteriovenous anomalies of the limbs. *Arch Surg.* 1976;111:423–429.
3. Flye MW, Jordan BP, Schwartz MZ. Management of congenital arteriovenous malformations. *Surgery.* 1983;94:740–747.
4. Mulliken JB, Glowacki J. Hemangiomas and vascular malformations in infants and children: A classification based on endothelial characteristics. *Plast Reconstr Surg.* 1982;69:412–420.
5. Mulliken JB, Zetter BR, Folkman J. In vitro characteristics of endothelium from hemangiomas and vascular malformations. *Surgery.* 1982;92:348–353.
6. Glowacki J, Mulliken JB. Mast cells in hemangiomas and vascular malformations. *Pediatrics.* 1982;70:48–51.
7. Finn MC, Glowacki J, Mulliken JB. Congenital vascular lesions: Clinical application of a new classification. *J Pediatr Surg.* 1983;18:894–900.
8. Upton J, Mulliken JB, Murray JE. Classification and rationale for management of vascular anomalies in the upper extremity. *J Hand Surg.* 1985; 6:970–975.
9. Mulliken JB, Young AE, eds. *Vascular Birthmarks: Hemangiomas and Malformations.* Philadelphia, PA: WB Saunders; 1988.

10. Enjolras O, Wassef M, Chapot R. Introduction ISSVA classification. In: *Color Atlas of Vascular Tumors and Vascular Malformations,* 1st ed. New York: Cambridge University Press; 2007, pp. 1–12.
11. Woolard HH. The development of the principal arterial stems in the forelimb of the pig. *Contrib Embryol.* 1922;14:139–154.
12. Reinhoff WF. Congenital arteriovenous fistula: An embryological study with the report of a case. *Johns Hopkins Hosp Bull.* 1924;35:271–284.
13. Reid MR. Studies on abnormal arteriovenous communications acquired and congenital. I. Report of a series of cases. *Arch Surg.* 1925;10:601–638.
14. DeTakats G. Vascular anomalies of the extremities. *Surg Gynecol Obstet.* 1932;55:227–237.
15. Jacobs AH, Walter RC. The incidence of birthmarks in the neonate. *Pediatrics.* 1976;58:218–222.
16. Lowell SH, Mathog R. Head and neck manifestations of Maffuci's syndrome. *Arch Otolaryngol.* 1979;105:427–430.
17. Riley HD Jr., Smith WR. Macrocephaly, pseudopapilladema, and multiple hemangiomas: A previously undescribed heredofamilial syndrome. *Pediatrics.* 1960;26:293–300.
18. Wiedemann HR, Burgio GR, Aldenhoff P, Kunze J, Kaufmann HJ, Schirg E. The Proteus syndrome: Partial gigantism of the hand and/or feet, nevi, hemihypertrophy, subcutaneous tumors, macrocephaly, or other skull anomalies and possible accelerated growth and visceral affections. *Eur J Pediatr.* 1983;140:5–12.
19. Bannayan GA. Lipomatosis, angiomatosis and macrencephalia. A previously undescribed congenital syndrome. *Arch Pathol.* 1971;92:1–5.
20. Higginbottom MC, Schultz P. The Bannayan syndrome: An autosomal dominant disorder consisting of macrocephaly, lipomas, hemangiomas, and risk for intracranial tumors. *Pediatrics.* 1982;69:632–634.
21. Gorham LW, Stout AP. Massive osteolysis (acute spontaneous absorption of bone, phantom bone, disappearing bone). Its relation to hemangiomatosis. *J Bone Joint Surg.* 1955;37:985–1004.
22. Baskerville PA, Ackroyd JS, Browse NL. The etiology of the Klippel-Trenaunay syndrome. *Ann Surg.* 1985;202:624–627.
23. Gloviczki P, Hollier LH, Telander RL. Surgical implications of Klippel-Trenaunay syndrome. *Ann Surg.* 1983;197:353–362.
24. Phillips GN, Cordon DH, Martin EC, Haller JD, Casarella W. The Klippel-Trenaunay syndrome: Clinical and radiological aspects. *Radiology.* 1978;128:429–434.
25. Parkes-Weber F. Haemangiectatic hypertrophy of limbs: Congenital phlebarteriectasis and so-called congenital varicose veins. *Br J Child Dis.* 1918;15:13–17.
26. Yakes WF, Stavros AT, Parker SH et al. Color Doppler imaging of peripheral high-flow vascular malformations before and after ethanol embolotherapy.

Presented at the *76th Scientific Assembly and Annual Meeting of the Radiological Society of North America*, Chicago, IL, November 25–30, 1990.

27. Rak KM, Yakes WF, Ray RL et al. MR imaging of peripheral vascular malformations. *Am J Roentgenol.* 1992;159:107–112.

28. Jo JY, Chin JH, Park PH, Ku SW. Cardiovascular collapse due to right heart failure following ethanol sclerotherapy: A case report. *Korean J Anesthesiol.* 2014;66:388–391.

29. Ko JS, Kim JA, Do YS et al. Prediction of the effect of injected ethanol on pulmonary arterial pressure during sclerotherapy of AVMs: Relationship with dose of ethanol. *J Vasc Interv Radiol.* 2009;20:39–45.

30. Shin BS, Do YS, Cho HS et al. Effects of repeat lolus ethanol injections on cardiopulmonary hemodynamic changes during embolotherapy of AVMs of the extremities. *J Vasc Interv Radiol.* 2010;21:81–89.

31. Legiehu GM, Heran MKS. Classification, diagnosis and interventional radiologic management of vascular malformations. *Orthop Clin North Am.* 2006;37:435–474.

32. Puig S, Aref H, Chigot V, Bonin AB, Bruenelle F. Classifications of venous malformations in children and implications for sclerotherapy. *Pediatr Radiol.* 2003;33(2):99–103.

33. Lee BB, Laredo J, Lee TS, Huh S, Neville R. Terminology and classification of congenital vascular malformations. *Phlebology.* 2007;22:249–252.

34. Doppman IL, Pevsner P. Embolization of arteriovenous malformations by direct percutaneous puncture. *Am J Roentgenol.* 1983;140:773–778.

35. Yakes WF. Endovascular management of high-flow arteriovenous malformations. *Semin Intervent Radiol.* 2004;21:49–58.

36. Vogelzang RL, Yakes WF. Vascular malformations: Effective treatment with absolute ethanol. In: Pearce WH, Yao JST, eds. *Arterial Surgery: Management of Challenging Problems.* Stamford, CT: Appleton and Lange Publishers; 1997, pp. 553–560.

37. Yakes WF, Krauth L, Ecklund J et al. Ethanol endovascular management of brain arteriovenous malformations: Initial results. *Neurosurgery.* 1997;40:1145–1154.

38. Yakes WF, Luethke JM, Parker SH et al. Ethanol embolization of vascular malformations. *RadioGraphics.* 1990;10:787–796.

39. Yakes WF, Pevsner PH, Reed M, Donohue HJ, Ghaed N. Serial embolizations of an extremity arteriovenous malformation with alcohol via direct percutaneous puncture. *Am J Roentgenol.* 1986;146:1038–1040.

40. Kerber C. Balloon catheter with a calibrated leak: A new system for superselective angiography and occlusive catheter therapy. *Radiology.* 1976;120:547–550.

41. Yakes WF, Parker SH, Gibson MD et al. Alcohol embolotherapy of vascular malformations. *Semin Intervent Radiol.* 1989;6:146–161.

42. Park KB, Do YS, Kim DI et al. Predictive factors for response of peripheral arteriovenous malformations to embolization therapy: Analysis of clinical data and imaging findings. *J Vasc Interv Radiol.* 2012;23:1478–1486.

43. Yakes WF, Haas DK, Parker SH et al. Symptomatic vascular malformations: Ethanol embolotherapy. *Radiology.* 1989;170:1059–1066.

44. Yakes WF, Yakes AM. Auricular AVMs: Diagnosis and treatment. *Egypt J Vasc Endovasc Surg.* 2014;10:31–36.

45. Svendsen PA, Wikholm G, Rodriquez M et al. Orbital lymphatic malformations: Direct puncture and sclerotherapy with Sotradecol. *Intervent Neuroradiol.* 2001;7:193–199.

46. Do YS, Yakes WF, Shin SW, Lee BB, Kim DI, Liu WC, Shin ES, Kim DK, Choo SW, Choo LW. Ethanol embolization of arteriovenous malformations: Interim results. *Radiology.* 2005;235:674–682.

47. Yakes WFJ. Endovascular management of high flow arteriovenous malformations. *Chin J Stomatol.* 2008; 43:327–332.

48. Yakes WF, Yakes AM. Auricular arteriovenous malformations: Diagnosis and treatment. *Egypt J Vasc Endovasc Surg.* 2014;10:31–36.

49. Vinson AM, Rohrer DB, Wilcox CW et al. Absolute ethanol embolization for peripheral arteriovenous malformation: Report of 2 cures. *South Med J.* 1988;381:1052–1055.

50. Yakes WF. Management of high flow vascular malformations. *JVIR* 2003;14:128–133.

51. Yakes WF, Huguenot M, Yakes A, Continenza A, Kammer A, Baumgartner I. Percutaneous embolization of arteriovenous malformations of the plantar aspect of the foot. *JVS* 2015; Published On-Line Dec 2015: JVS.2015.10.092.

52. Mourao GS, Hodes JE, Gobin YP, Casasco A, Aymard A, Merland JJ. Curative treatment of scalp arteriovenous fistulas by direct puncture and embolization with absolute alcohol. *J Neurosurg.* 1991;75:634–637.

53. Rao VR, Mandalam KR, Gupta AK et al. Dissolution of isobutyl 2-cyanoacrylate on long-term follow-up. *Am J Neuroradiol.* 1989;10:135–141.

54. Yakes WF, Rossi P. Odink H. Arteriovenous malformation management: How I do it. *Cardiovasc Intervent Radiol.* 1996;19:65–71.

55. Yakes WF, Yakes AM. The Yakes classification of arteriovenous malformations. *The 40th Annual Veith Symposium Presentation*, November 19, 2013.

56. Yakes W, Baumgartner I. Interventional treatment of arterio-venous malformations. *Gefasschirurgie.* 2014;19:325–330.

57. Yakes WF, Yakes AM. Arteriovenous malformations: The Yakes Classification and its therapeutic implications. *Egypt J Vasc Endovasc Surg.* 2014;10:9–23.

58. Houdart B, Gobin YE Casasco A, Aymard A, Herbreteau D, Merland JJ. A proposed angiographic classification of intracranial arteriovenous fistulae and malformations. *Neuroradiology.* 1993;35:381–385.

59. Cho SK, Do YS, Shin SW et al. Arteriovenous malformations of the body and extremities: Analysis of therapeutic outcomes and approaches according to a modified angiographic classification. *Endovasc Ther.* 2006;13:527–538.

60. Yakes WF, Luethke JM, Merland JJ et al. Ethanol embolization of arteriovenous fistulas: A primary mode of therapy. *J Vasc Interv Radiol.* 1990;1:89–96.

61. Jackson IF, Mansfield AO, Allison DJ. Treatment of high-flow vascular malformations by venous embolization aided by flow occlusion techniques. *Cardiovasc Intervent Radiol.* 1996;19:323–328.

62. Cho SK, Do YS, Kim DI, Kim YW, Shin SW, Park KB, Ko JS, Lee AR, Choo SW, Choo IW. Peripheral arteriovenous malformations with a dominant outflow vein: Results of ethanol embolization. *Korean J Radiol.* 2008;9:258–267.

63. Merland JJ, Riche MC, Chiras J. Intraspinal extramedullary arteriovenous fistula draining into medullary veins. *J Neuroradiol.* 1980;7:271–320.

64. Spetzler RE, Martin NA. A proposed grading system for arteriovenous malformations. *J Neurosurg.* 1986;473 65:476–478.

65. Lee BB, Baumgartner I, Berlien HP et al. Consensus document of the International Union of Angiology; current concepts on the management of AVMs. *Int Angiol.* 2013;32:9–36.

66. Gieser JH, Eversmann WW. Closed-system venography in the evaluation of upper extremity hemangioma. *J Hand Surg.* 1978;3:173–178.

67. Boxt LM, Levin DC, Fellows KE. Direct puncture angiography in congenital venous malformations. *Am J Roentgenol.* 1983;140:135–136.

68. Yakes WF. Extremity venous malformations: Diagnosis and management. *Semin Intervent Radiol.* 1994;11:332–339.

69. Yakes WF. Diagnosis and management of venous malformations. In: Savader SJ, Trerotola SO, eds. *Venous Interventional Radiology with Clinical Perspectives.* New York: Thieme Medical Publishers Inc.;1996, pp. 139–150.

70. Rabe E, Panmier F. Sclerotherapy in venous malformations. *Phlebology.* 2013;1:188–191.

71. Levardi AM, Mangiri M, Vaghi M, Cazzulari A, Carrafiello G, Mattassi R. Sclerotherapy of peripheral venous malformations: A new technique to prevent serious complications. *Vasc Endovascular Surg.* 2010;44:282–288.

72. Bisdorff A, Mazighi M, Saint-Maurice JP, Chapot R, Lukaszuricz AC, Houdart E. Ethanol threshold doses for systemic complications during sclerotherapy of superficial venous malformations: A retrospective study. *Neuroradiology.* 2011;53: 891–894.

73. Impellizeri P, Romeo C, Borruto FA, Granata G, De Poute FS, Longo M. Sclerotherapy for cervical cystic lymphatic malformations in children. Our experiences with competed tomography – Guided 98% sterile ethanol insertion and review of the literature. *J Pediatr Surg.* 2010;45:2473–2478.

74. Keljo DJ, Yakes WF, Andersen JM, Timmons CF. Recognition and treatment of venous malformations of the rectum. *J Pediatr Gastroenterol Nutr.* 1996;23:442–446.

75. Malthur NN, Rana I, Bothra R, Dhawan R, Kalthuria G, Pradham T. Bleomycin sclerotherapy in congenital lymphatic and vascular malformations of the head and neck. *Int J Pediatr Otorhinolaryngol.* 2005;69:75–80.

76. Barrows PE, Mitri RK, Alomari A, Padua HM, Lord DJ, Sybria MB, Fishman SJ, Mulliken JB. Percutaneous sclerotherapy of lymphatic malformations with doxycycline. *Lymphat Res Biol.* 2008;6:109–116.

56

Vascular aspects of organ transplantation

HYNEK MERGENTAL, JEAN DE VILLE DE GOYET, JORGES MASCARO and JOHN A.C. BUCKELS

CONTENTS

INTRODUCTION

Organ transplantation is essentially a vascular surgical procedure, although with increasing complexity of procedures and subspecialization, there is a decreasing number of surgeons practising in both fields. This chapter will give an overview of the vascular aspects of organ transplantation including the procurement procedures, the current techniques of implantation and the more common vascular complications. It is intended as a general approach that should prove useful to trainees and assist vascular surgeons supporting transplantation programs; specialists in the transplant field should refer to detailed texts. Though fundamentals of thoracic organ retrieval are included, this being a frequent component of the procurement operation, details of implantation are beyond the terms of reference and will not be covered.

VASCULAR ASPECTS OF ORGAN PROCUREMENT

Organ procurement is the first step for a successful transplantation. Knowledge of the standard and aberrant vascular anatomy as well as precise surgical technique is essential to avoid graft damage. The multi-organ retrieval operation has been standardized to provide each graft with a vascular pedicle that facilities safe implantation and minimizes the risks of post-transplant thrombotic complications. With the ongoing extension of donor acceptance criteria, the organ recovery also needs to be rapid to decrease the ischemic times.

Organ donation is a multidisciplinary activity that the majority of the time involves the harvesting of the intra-thoracic and abdominal organs. A coordinated and respectful approach to the donor, theatre staff and team colleagues is paramount for a successful retrieval that will benefit the patients awaiting transplantation. The actual retrieval procedure differs according to the organs to be recovered as well as the type of donor. Depending on the way the death is declared, this is classified as donation after brain death (DBD) or circulatory death (DCD). The following sections describe multi-organ DBD procurement in a stepwise fashion in the order of standard organ removal.

The donor is placed on the operating table in the supine position and surgically prepared and draped as with any routine operation. Antibiotic prophylaxis is given based on the local protocol before the start of the procedure. In most situations, two surgical teams, thoracic and abdominal, will operate simultaneously. The chest and abdominal cavities are first entered by median sterno-laparotomy.

Heart and lung procurement

Heart and lung transplantation is an accepted therapy for the treatment of end-stage respiratory and cardiac diseases. This extends to both the adult and pediatric population who are affected by acquired or congenital heart diseases. The success of the operation is determined not only by factors that involve the recipient but also issues involving the donor. Special attention needs to be given to myocardial and lung protection, which is where most improvements have been made. This has allowed extended ischemic times and more complex operations, for example, transplantation in patients with congenital heart conditions that have or not been surgically repaired. Transplantation for acquired conditions or intra-thoracic congenital malformations and its success is subject to the appropriate management of the donor, good organ protection and a sound technique paying attention to the appropriate management of the organ and its vascular connections.

The heart or lungs can be retrieved on their own or as part of a heart–lung block for a combined heart and lung transplant.[1] If the heart needs to be split from the heart–lung block for the lungs to be sent to another centre, it is preferable to retrieve the heart first and then the lungs en bloc. Once the sterno-laparotomy incision is performed, a sternal spreader is positioned and the sternum spread apart. The upper mediastinum is exposed and dissected, the innominate vein identified and slooped. The pericardium is then opened and the edges of the pericardium are suspended to the sides of the incision with stay sutures to enhance exposure. The heart is visually inspected for major anomalies and to assess the right and left ventricle function. The coronary arteries are palpated for the presence of coronary artery disease. Both pleurae are then opened and the lungs are inspected visually for any pathology and the inflation and deflation is evaluated. Blood is aspirated from individual pulmonary veins for measuring blood gases; this gives additional information about the quality of the lungs. The heart is then prepared and left ready to clamp in case the donor deteriorates and becomes unstable. The aorta is mobilized free from the pulmonary artery and a tape is passed round it for easier manipulation and traction. The aorta should be freed to the level of the aortic pericardial reflection. This will give sufficient length of aorta for a comfortable aorta–aorta anastomosis during the implant. This is important currently, as increasing numbers of heart transplants are undertaken in patients with previous heart operations or assist devices. The main pulmonary artery is followed and freed to the level of the

pulmonary bifurcation. Attention should then be directed to the superior vena cava (SVC) and inferior vena cava (IVC), respectively. The SVC needs to be followed extra-pericardial almost to the bifurcation of the subclavian and innominate vein. The azygos vein terminating in the posterior aspect of the SVC must be tied off. Special care should be taken with the sinus node which is located at the junction of the right atrium with the SVC. The IVC needs to be mobilized free from the diaphragm and the pericardial reflection behind the IVC opened up to the right inferior pulmonary vein. To complete the dissection, the trachea is mobilized and 'slooped' behind the innominate artery in preparation for subsequent explantation of the lungs. At this stage, the cardiothoracic team may step down from the table to allow the abdominal team to proceed with the dissection of the abdominal organs before the aorta is clamped and the organs finally retrieved.

Once the abdominal team is ready to commence perfusion, 30,000 units of heparin is given IV. Purse string sutures are placed in the ascending aorta and main pulmonary artery to allow safe placement of cannulas and facilitate delivery of cardioplegia (Figure 56.1) and lung perfusion fluid, respectively. Epoprostenol is injected into the pulmonary artery, the SVC clamped and the IVC divided before the aorta is cross-clamped and the cardioplegia commenced. The right side of the heart is vented via the open IVC and the left side is best vented by amputating the tip of the left atrial appendage. The pulmonary veins are divided to include left atrial cuffs but if the lungs are also being procured, they are best taken en bloc with the back of the left atrium intact and the pulmonary artery divided (Figure 56.2). The lungs can then be separated on

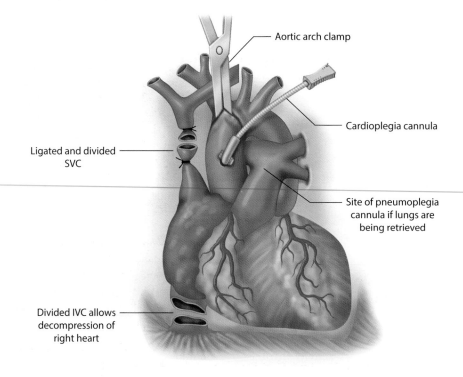

Aortic arch clamp

Cardioplegia cannula

Ligated and divided SVC

Site of pneumoplegia cannula if lungs are being retrieved

Divided IVC allows decompression of right heart

Figure 56.1 Cardiac retrieval at stage of inflow/outflow vessel division and commencement of cardioplegia perfusion.

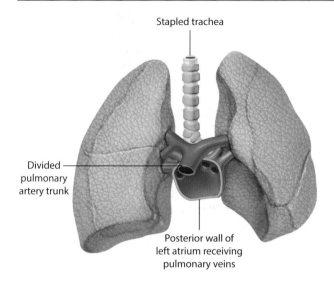

Figure 56.2 En bloc removal of lungs with back of intact left atrium intact.

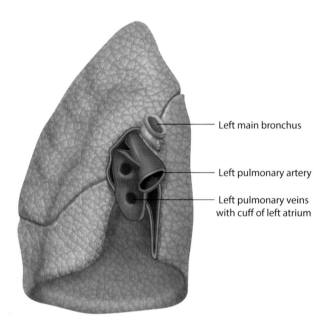

Figure 56.3 Single-lung anatomy (left) after separation from right lung.

the back table before the commencement of the recipient procedure (Figure 56.3). For combined heart–lung transplants, the organs are removed en bloc after division of the SVC, IVC, aorta and trachea.

Special consideration needs to be given to the retrieval of a heart that will be used to transplant a recipient with congenital heart disease who has or has not undergone any type of corrective surgery. In the case of hypoplastic aortic arch, the implanting team might be interested in extra donor aorta. For this, the aortic dissection of the ascending aorta needs to be extended into the aortic arch, possibly including the epiaortic vessels which will need tying off once the aortic cross-clamp has been applied. Careful attention needs to

be given to recipients with complex repairs such as Fontan operations or Glenn procedures or those with left SVC and no innominate vein where an extended length of SVC will be necessary. Sometimes, this extra dissection will require the dissection of the entire innominate vein to allow reconstruction of the latter in the recipient.

Abdominal multi-organ procurement

After entering the abdominal cavity, the umbilical ligament is tied and divided. The abdominal walls are retracted and the small bowel loops are moved upward to the left to expose the sacral promontory. The ascending colon and the root of the mesentery are mobilized to expose the right iliac vessels with the distal aorta. The aorta is dissected free and looped with two heavy ties. This initial step secures access for an immediate aortic cannulation and organ perfusion should the donor become unstable.[2]

Dissection continues with mobilization of the ascending colon, mesentery root and duodenum, which fully exposes the IVC, renal veins and abdominal aorta. The superior mesenteric artery (SMA) is identified in close proximity to the right renal vein crossing the aorta. The hepatoduodenal ligament is then dissected. After the left and right aberrant hepatic arteries are identified in the lesser omentum and on the right posterior aspect of the bile duct, respectively, the common bile duct (CBD) is dissected at the superior border of the duodenum; its distal part tied and the duct divided. The gall bladder is opened and the biliary system is well flushed. The portal vein runs medially and posteriorly to the CBD and is dissected free and encircled close to the splenic vein and superior mesenteric vein confluence for later cannulation. The gastroduodenal artery (GDA) is identified medially to the bile duct. The common hepatic artery (CHA) is dissected free towards the celiac trunk, where the splenic and left gastric arteries are visualized. The stomach and colon are retracted and the omental sac is opened allowing inspection of the pancreas and the application of topical cooling during the later organ perfusion phase. The left liver lobe is fully mobilized to expose the diaphragmatic crura. The proximal abdominal aorta is accessed and encircled here by incising the diaphragmatic muscular layer.

Provided both teams are ready for the organ perfusion, the heparin is given intravenously prior to tying and cannulating the distal aorta. The proximal abdominal aorta is cross-clamped and perfusion with pressurized preservation fluid is commenced. The most commonly used fluid for abdominal organ preservation is University of Wisconsin (UW) solution at a volume of 50 mL/kg. Immediately after starting the aortic perfusion, the IVC is opened and a suction tube is placed into the lumen for venting the blood, followed by the filling of the abdominal compartment with sterile iced saline slush for concurrent topical organ cooling. For dual liver perfusion, the portal vein is cannulated and UW perfusion under gravity commenced while the proximal end of the portal vein is completely divided to prevent pancreatic outflow congestion. The cold ischemia time commences at the moment of aortic cross-clamping.

The two crucial aspects of the warm organ procurement phase are to accurately assess the organ quality, including the identification of previously unknown donor pathology, and to visualize the key anatomical landmarks to facilitate safe and rapid organ explantation. The principal vascular structures are the CHA/GDA bifurcation, the origin of the splenic artery, the origin of the SMA and the confluence of the left renal vein with the IVC; the adrenal glands guide the dissection plane between the liver, pancreas and kidneys. The vascular techniques for the different abdominal organs will now be given in the order in which they are usually removed.

Liver retrieval

Following the removal of the heart, the supra-hepatic IVC orifice can be opened and inspected for the clarity of the preservation fluid outflow through the hepatic veins. The liver mobilization continues with the division of left and right diaphragm towards the crura and the IVC orifice, with right extension in the caudal direction towards the kidney. The ligament attaching the liver (segment 6 area) to the posterior aspect of the diaphragm is divided, and the right liver lobe mobilization is completed by division of the tissues and adrenal gland cranially to the right kidney. The infrahepatic IVC is divided at the upper level of the left renal confluence. The portal vein was divided in the initial part of the cold phase; the only remaining vascular structure is the hepatic artery. The GDA, splenic and left gastric arteries are divided, leaving at least a 5 mm long stump which could be used to create a patch for anastomosis or enabling a safe branch closure without the risk of narrowing of the main artery. The celiac trunk is followed to the aorta, where it is divided with a sufficient aortic patch.

If the right aberrant hepatic artery is present, the SMA is dissected from the aorta towards the pancreas; the hepatic artery is typically the first branch, originating within 2 cm of the distance from the aorta. In the majority of cases, it can be dissected from the pancreas without opening the gland capsule and parenchyma. In situations where this is not possible, the level of the division needs to be discussed with the accepting liver transplant surgeon. As the liver is a life-saving organ, its retrieval has priority over the pancreas, whose retrieval may be abandoned.

In situations with a left aberrant hepatic artery, the celiac trunk is dissected without division of the left gastric artery, and the lesser omentum and tissue between the stomach and liver are preserved in continuity.

After the division of the hepatic vessels, the liver dissection is completed by separation of the retrohepatic connective tissue around the IVC, and the graft is removed from the donor body and placed into a bowl with iced saline slush for inspection, bench perfusion and packing.

PARTIAL LIVER GRAFTS

Because of donor-organ shortages, new strategies to expand the donor pool have been explored. These include reducing

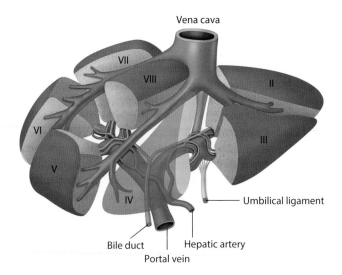

Figure 56.4 Segmental liver anatomy.

a whole organ in order to size-match it to smaller recipients, dividing a whole organ between an adult and a child, dividing a graft between two adults and living–related donation. Such procedures require a clear understanding of the segmental anatomy of the liver (Figure 56.4).

The size reduction helps the child at the expense of those adults waiting on the transplant list, therefore shifting the shortage from the pediatric population to the adult population, and is performed rarely nowadays. The technique for splitting grafts for an adult and a child and living donation of the left lateral segment to a child are similar.

Vascular structures are more easily identified, cold ischemia is minimized and the body's coagulation cascade is used most effectively in liver donation or in situ splitting, though an ex situ bench splitting is logistically easier and more common. The first vascular structure isolated is the left hepatic vein. Next, the dissection of the left hepatic artery is performed, paying special attention to the artery to segment 4. The entire left portal vein is then isolated with careful ligation of branches to the caudate lobe. The portal vein branches to segment 4 are ligated and divided to the right of the umbilical fissure. After total vascular control, the liver parenchyma is divided. The liver is split between segment 4 and segments 2 and 3 (Figure 56.5). The right graft is removed with the cava and the left graft is drained by the left hepatic vein.

Splitting of the donor organ into grafts suitable for two adults is performed with a similar technique. The parenchyma is divided along the line from the gall bladder fossa to the IVC. The left graft now comprises segments 2, 3 and 4.

LIVE DONOR LIVER DONATION

Living donation of a graft from an adult to another adult entails a formal right hepatic lobectomy or left lobectomy in the donor. The right hepatic vein with segments

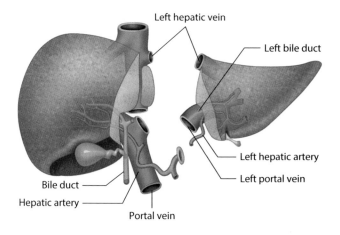

Figure 56.5 Standard liver split for sharing between adult and child recipients.

5–8 is transplanted into the recipient (Figure 56.6). Alternatively, segments 2–4 with the left hepatic vein can be used for smaller adult recipients. The technique is similar to any resection performed for other indications. Aberrant vasculature must be respected, and small arteries and veins should be reconstructed or carefully tied. The resected surface is often treated with fibrin glue before implantation.

LIVER GRAFT INJURIES

A partial cut or complete division of the aberrant right hepatic artery is the most common vascular liver injury with a possible impact on the liver graft outcome, for which back table vascular reconstruction is required. Multiple hepatic artery anastomoses are a recognized risk for hepatic artery thrombosis (HAT) and several retrospective studies advocate anticoagulant or antiplatelet prophylaxis for prevention. Damage can also be caused by division of the GDA, left gastric or splenic arteries without leaving a long enough cuff for a safe branch tie closure. Traction injury caused by inappropriate vascular handling, resulting in main hepatic artery intimal dissection, is rare, but often requires urgent retransplantation.

Parenchymal liver injuries are more common but less dangerous, and they are most often located next to the umbilical ligament (segment 3, caused by traction on the abdominal wall prior to the ligament division) and at the segment 6 area (caused by traction during the right lobe explantation). Inappropriate parenchyma handling during the liver mobilization and removal can cause large, subcapsular hematomas, which can cause major, and difficult to control, bleeding.

Pancreas retrieval

Following the liver removal, pancreas explantation commences with duodenum division. The proximal dissection line is 1–2 cm distal to the pylorus. The distal division is prepared close to the ligament of Treitz. The duodenum is divided with GIA 60–80 mm staplers. The small and large omenta are completely divided around the stomach curvatures towards the esophagus followed by division of the mesocolon from the ascending and descending colon. The ventral aspect of the gland is now fully exposed.

Vessel isolation is commenced by the division of the left renal vein on its confluence with the IVC and opening the anterior wall of the abdominal aorta to the SMA origin. Inspection of the aortic lumen allows identification of accessory renal arteries. The SMA is divided maintaining an aortic patch and the tissues on both sides of the patch are dissected through the adrenal glands. For the final pancreatic mobilization, the spleen is used as a handle and the gland is cut free from the retroperitoneum at a safe distance to prevent damage.

PANCREATIC GRAFT INJURIES

Opening the pancreatic capsule and damaging the gland are the most common injuries. This could cause late lethal post-transplant complications such as pancreatic leak and pancreatitis. Damage is often located on the pancreatic tail (injury) or the posterior aspect of the pancreatic head (isolation of aberrant right hepatic artery). A too short portal vein or injuries to the splenic artery and SMA are less common.

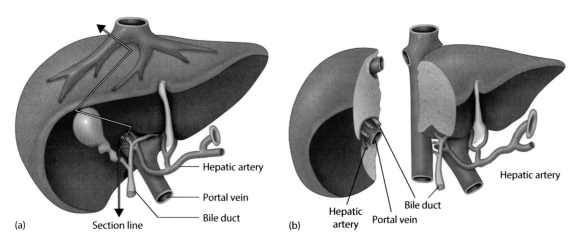

Figure 56.6 (a) Right liver graft from living donor. (b) Liver split for two adults.

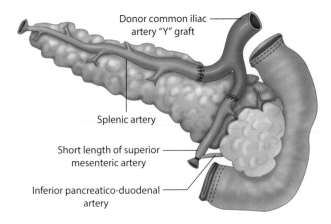

Figure 56.7 Back table preparation of pancreas graft with donor iliac graft anastomosed between splenic and superior mesenteric arteries to facilitate implantation in recipient.

BACK TABLE PROCEDURE

Preparation of the pancreatic graft requires a vascular reconstruction which is described in the surgical technique of pancreas transplantation section (Figure 56.7).

Kidney retrieval

The kidneys are mobilized from the retroperitoneum and flipped towards the midline. The posterior wall of the aorta is divided and the long aortic segment is then mobilized from the anterior aspect of the vertebral column and psoas muscles (Figure 56.8). Once the kidneys and renal vessels are mobilized individually, the ureters

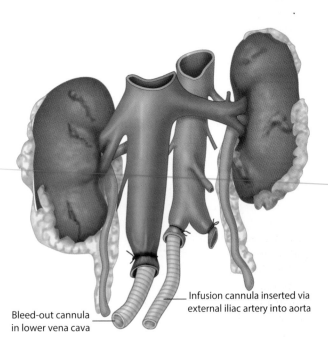

Figure 56.8 En bloc retrieval of kidneys with inflow and outflow cannulas in great vessels.

(together with periureteric tissue to avoid damaging their blood supply) are followed to the urinary bladder at which level they are divided. Once the kidneys are removed, excess perinephric fat can be excised and the kidneys double bagged and placed in a slushed ice container ready for transport.

LIVE DONOR KIDNEY DONATION

The organ shortage has been the most profound in the area of kidney transplantation. The high demand combined with the low-risk, laparoscopic surgery facilitated the development of live donor kidney techniques that represents worldwide an alternative to cadaveric transplantation. This option allows for transplantation prior to the need for renal dialysis, and this approach has been shown to have the best long-term outcomes for the recipients.

The minimally invasive donor nephrectomy can be performed laparoscopically through a retroperitoneal or intra-abdominal approach. The kidney is mobilized and separated from the adrenal gland and dissected free from the perinephric fat capsule. The renal artery and vein are skeletonized and isolated at the aorta origin and the IVC confluence, respectively. The left kidney graft provides a longer renal vein, but requires more complex dissection at the level of confluence with adrenal and lumbar vein branches. After the ureter is isolated and transected with the maximum accessible length, the renal artery and vein are divided by an endoscopic vascular stapler. The kidney is removed through a small, suprapubic (Pfannenstiel) incision and the graft is immediately flushed with ice-cold preservation solution.

KIDNEY GRAFT INJURIES

Injuries to aberrant renal arteries are the most common damage of the graft. Accidental cutting of the renal capsule on the back table is frequent but will cause less impact on the graft usability.

Small bowel retrieval

The small bowel can be procured as an isolated organ or en bloc with the liver and/or pancreas for a multi-visceral transplant.

The isolated intestinal graft vascular pedicle contains the superior mesenteric artery and vein (Figure 56.9). The proximal graft end consists of the first jejunum loop that was divided close to the ligament of Treitz. The distal end often includes the ascending colon and although the large bowel might not be transplanted, this aids graft orientation and handling during the implantation. When combined liver and small bowel grafts are indicated, the grafts are removed and transplanted en bloc with the portal vein remaining in continuity (Figure 56.10).

In situations with simultaneous procurement of isolated liver and pancreatic grafts, the retrieval also has

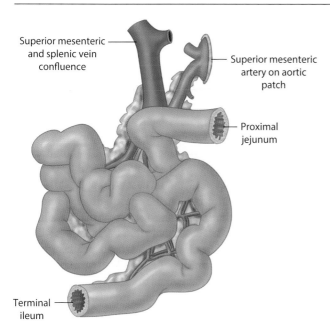

Figure 56.9 Isolated small bowel retrieval anatomy.

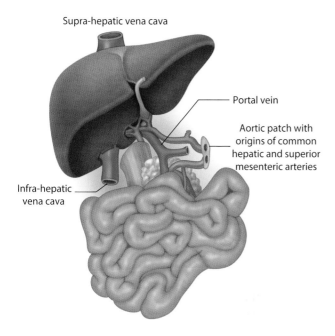

Figure 56.10 Combined liver–small bowel graft removed en bloc.

to provide adequate arteries necessary for the back table reconstruction of the blood supply for all retrieved organs. These conduits typically consist of iliac vessels, aortic arch arteries and thoracic aorta in selected circumstances. In respect to the frequently presented atypical vascular anatomy, the reconstruction has to be creative and tailored to each particular situation. The grafts for multi-visceral transplantation are often modified on case-to-case bases, and details of the implantation techniques can be found in specialized texts.

Organ retrieval after circulatory death

The persistent shortage of organs has led to the revival of the concept of organ donation from DCD donors.[3,4] There are four categories of DCD donors based on the death circumstance (Maastricht criteria classification) and controlled donors in category III (expected cardiac arrest following planned withdrawal of life support treatment) are the most commonly utilized group.

The DCD donation process starts with withdrawal of the donor's life support treatment, including vasopressor infusions and disconnection from the ventilator. Patients can receive comfort medication to prevent respiratory distress. In some countries, it is lawful to facilitate the donation by intravenous heparin administration. Following the treatment withdrawal, the donor's cardiorespiratory function gradually declines until it stops completely; this period is known as an agonal phase. A flat arterial pressure curve indicates death that can be certified following a compulsory 5 minutes 'no touch' period. The organ procurement procedure starts by rapid opening of the abdominal cavity and aortic cannulation with immediate commencement of organ perfusion. The next step is occlusion of the proximal aorta which can be secured by cross-clamping the descending aorta in the chest or by inflating the distal balloon in cases where double balloon catheter is used for the aortic cannulation. These steps are typically performed in less than 3 minutes. After commencing the organ perfusion, the operation steps are identical to the DBD donation. The procedure is performed swiftly to minimize the warm ischemia; this has been described as a super-rapid retrieval technique.[5]

The identification of the vascular anatomy without the arterial pulsations and tactile perception is often challenging, and DCD donation increases the overall risk of graft injuries. The unavoidable warm ischemia also affects the organ's quality, and the overall grafts yield per donor is less compared to DCD donors; nevertheless, DCD donors are a valuable addition to the overall donor pool. Addressing the organ quality with new technologies such as machine perfusion is an area of intensive research interest.[6,7]

The organ retrieval techniques were initially described for liver and kidney grafts and subsequently modified to enable multi-organ retrieval from each donor.[8,9] The ultimate simplification of the abdominal multi-organ retrieval technique was adopted in the 1990s following results from a trial showing no difference between the outcomes of liver transplants from grafts recovered with aortic perfusion only compared to dual liver perfusion.[10] The more recent data from a randomized controlled trial showed superior liver transplant outcomes after dual (aortic and portal) perfusion[11] (level 2 evidence).

Concerning the organ preservation, numerous studies have shown UW preservation solution to be the most efficient and to provide adequate preservation quality for all abdominal organs[12-15] (level 3 evidence).

VASCULAR ASPECTS OF ORGAN IMPLANTATION

Vascular surgical technique of kidney transplantation

The kidney is prepared on the back table under ice-cold saline with careful attention to preserve any polar vessels but to ligate venous and arterial extra-renal branches and to remove adventitia from the walls at the intended anastomotic sites.

The kidney is usually placed in an extra-peritoneal position in either iliac fossa, though many surgeons favour the right side as the iliac vessels are more superficial. The other decision is whether to utilize either the external iliac or the hypogastric (internal iliac) artery for inflow. Local lymphatics running along the vessels are traditionally ligated although there is little evidence that this reduces the risk of the subsequent development of a lymphocele. If the hypogastric artery is chosen, it initially needs to be divided at its point of distal branching. The distal end is securely ligated with the proximal end mobilized more superficially to allow an end-to-end anastomosis. An adequate length of external iliac vein is mobilized which may require ligation of small delicate side branches and can then be partially clamped with a Satinsky-type clamp. The renal vein to iliac vein end-to-side anastomosis is performed first using 5/0 monofilament non-absorbable suture such as polypropylene. Before completion, the lumens should be irrigated with a dilute solution of heparinized saline and a Blalock hook or similar instrument used to check the patency of the anastomosis. The renal artery, preferably on a small patch, can then be anastomosed end-to-side to the clamped external iliac artery, again washing the lumen with heparinized saline before completion, again with 5/0 monofilament non-absorbable suture without tension (Figure 56.11). At this stage, the clamps can be removed and any minor bleeding addressed with further sutures or diathermy.

If there are multiple renal arteries, the technique requires modification. Two larger arteries can usually be fish-mouthed together on the back table such that a single anastomosis can be performed. If there are more arteries, then the choice is to anastomose individually, preferably on Carrel patches of aorta or as a longer single patch. Isolated polar vessels can be successfully anastomosed to the inferior epigastric artery. It has been perceived that using a kidney with multiple arteries might carry a higher risk of arterial complications, particularly thrombosis. Publications give conflicting outcomes, but

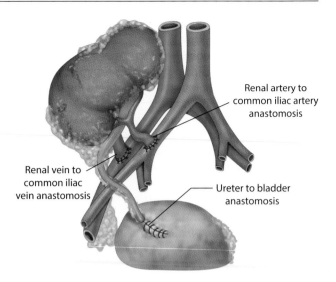

Figure 56.11 Renal transplant with vessels anastomosed to external iliac artery and vein.

some units report no difference between multiple and single vessels in both laparoscopic and non-laparoscopic retrievals[16,17] which suggests that meticulous technique may be the critical factor (level 2 evidence).

Renal vascular complications

These are uncommon but will be considered in turn.

HEMORRHAGE

Immediate hemorrhage can result from faulty anastomotic technique or more commonly from missed hilar venous or arterial branches that can easily be controlled. Late hemorrhage requires urgent exploration and if due to an infected arterial anastomosis is likely to require graft removal.

RENAL ARTERY THROMBOSIS

Early renal artery thrombosis is rare, occurring in less than 1% of transplants, and is usually suggested by a sudden decrease in urine output with a simultaneous increase in creatinine.[18] The diagnosis is confirmed by ultrasound and, if required, angiography. Early thrombosis may be the result of an intimal flap or damage incurred during procurement or implantation. Late thrombosis is usually due to rejection or progression of a stenotic segment. Occasionally, early diagnosis may allow for repair of the artery and possible salvage of the graft but in most cases graft nephrectomy will ensue.

RENAL VEIN THROMBOSIS

Renal vein thrombosis is also rare (less than 1%) but more common in patients with an underlying hypercoagulable condition. It will usually present with deteriorating kidney function, proteinuria, hematuria or pain due to sudden engorgement and stretching of the overlying peritoneum. It may result from malpositioning of the graft at the time of transplantation with twisting or kinking of the vein (too long vein length is probably a risk factor for this) or from progression of ilio-femoral vein thrombosis. There are cases of graft salvage if the thrombosis is picked up before being fully established and treated by either open thrombectomy or local thrombolytic therapy, but most grafts will be lost. There is no evidence that routine use of anticoagulation at the time of transplantation will reduce the risk except in those with hypercoagulable states.[19]

RENAL ARTERY STENOSIS

Renal artery stenosis is a late complication which manifests with hypertension, slowly rising creatinine and polycythemia. It can result from rejection, progression of atherosclerosis, clamp injury and faulty surgical technique. The diagnosis is confirmed with ultrasound and angiogram. The treatment of choice is percutaneous transluminal angioplasty.

Vascular surgical technique of liver transplantation

BENCH PREPARATION

The liver graft is inspected during the back table procedure in a bowl with ice-cold and slush saline. The redundant tissues are removed and the hepatoduodenal ligament structures are dissected free. The hepatic artery is carefully prepared to the level of the proper hepatic artery. The IVC is prepared and orifices of diaphragmatic veins and other potential bleeding points are tied or sewn. The top and bottom openings of the IVC are left open for the IVC-replacement fashion of graft implantation or may be closed for the piggyback type of transplant procedure.

Liver arterial anatomy most frequently consists of the CHA, which continues as the proper hepatic artery after division of the GDA, and its anatomical deviations do not have an impact on the whole-size liver implantation.

The right hepatic artery, originating from the SMA, is present in approximately 30% donors and requires vascular reconstruction. This is commonly done by anastomosing the artery to the splenic artery or GDA stump. The left hepatic artery from the left gastric artery is another common variation that may require the anastomosis of the celiac trunk to the donor artery. Arterial reconstruction and multiple hepatic arteries are a risk factor for the development of HAT, and transplant recipients should be given anticoagulant treatment.

IMPLANTATION PROCEDURE

The liver graft is implanted orthotopically and the implantation consists of anastomosing the hepatic artery, portal vein, bile duct and IVC. The native liver removal can be done with or without resection of the retrohepatic IVC. Implantation with replacement of the resected segment of IVC with end-to-end anastomosis of supra- and

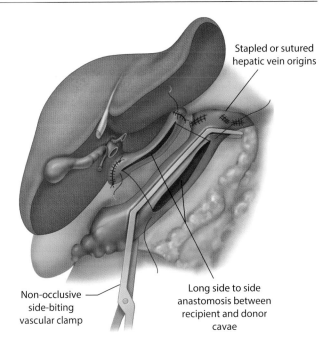

Stapled or sutured hepatic vein origins

Non-occlusive side-biting vascular clamp

Long side to side anastomosis between recipient and donor cavae

Figure 56.12 'Piggyback' liver transplant with side-to-side cavo-cavostomy.

infra-hepatic IVC is known as classical transplantation; reconstruction of the liver outflow with end-to-side or side-to-side cavo-cavostomy is called 'piggyback' implantation (Figure 56.12). The disadvantage of removing the cava with the liver is the major reduction in venous return and potential cardiovascular instability. For adults, this has usually necessitated some form of veno-venous bypass which carries its own potential problems and morbidity. The piggyback technique preserves the native cava which only requires partial clamping in order to facilitate a long side-to-side cava to caval anastomosis, and this technique has become the most widely practised.

The liver inflow is restored with end-to-end portal vein and hepatic artery anastomoses. The typical level for the arterial anastomosis is the recipient CHA/GDA patch anastomosis to the splenic/CHA patch or proper hepatic/GDA patch. Attention must be paid to prevent rotation and excessive length of both the donor artery and portal vein. The bile duct is reconstructed with end-to-end choledocho–choledocho anastomosis. In patients with primary sclerosing cholangitis or in retransplantations, the preferred bile duct reconstruction is end-to-side anastomosis to Roux-en-Y bowel loop.

AORTIC CONDUIT

An adequate arterial blood supply of the liver graft is of paramount importance for a successful transplantation. In situations with poor recipient native hepatic artery flow or compromised vessel quality which warrants a safe and long-lasting anastomosis, an aorto-hepatic conduit can provide an alternative and superior arterial supply. The conduit is created from the iliac artery which is universally provided with the graft. The common iliac artery is anastomosed end-to-side to the infrarenal aorta and directed towards the liver via the *retro-gastric, ante-pancreatic* route. The internal iliac artery is tied and the external artery end is then anastomosed to the graft artery, typically at the level of the aortic patch of the celiac trunk or splenic artery/CHA patch. There are conflicting data whether the aortic conduit represents a protective or a risk factor for a late HAT, and patients frequently receive antiplatelet treatment with aspirin[20] (level 3 evidence, recommendation level C).

Liver vascular complications

HEPATIC ARTERY THROMBOSIS

The incidence of HAT after liver transplantation ranges from 2 to 8% in adult, whole-size grafts, and it is higher in the pediatric population and partial grafts.[21] In the early post-transplant period, it can present initially with elevated liver enzymes, bile leak and bacteremia that can progress in several days to liver abscesses, fulminant hepatic necrosis and hemodynamic instability. Although several authors reported successful re-arterialization with thrombectomy, the principal treatment of HAT within the first weeks after transplantation is a super-urgent retransplantation. Late HAT presentation may be primarily biliary in nature; patients can experience cholangitis, bile duct strictures, leaks and liver abscesses, but can also be asymptomatic.[21-23] The diagnosis of HAT is made on duplex ultrasound scanning and CT angiogram. Antiplatelet therapy with aspirin may decrease the risk of HAT[20,24,25] (level 3 evidence, recommendation level C).

HEPATIC ARTERY STENOSIS

Hepatic artery stenosis is usually discovered during investigation of graft dysfunction with features of biliary complications. It may result from rejection, clamp injury or cold preservation injury. This can be treated with percutaneous transluminal angioplasty, re-arterialization or, if necessary, retransplantation.

ARCUATE LIGAMENT SYNDROME

This can be diagnosed from the pre-transplant CT angiogram or discovered during the transplantation procedure, when it causes a poor blood flow in the recipient hepatic artery (a significant reduction or disappearance of blood flow within the donor hepatic artery during the expiration phase of the respiratory cycle). Sufficient blood flow may be restored by division of the median arcuate ligament, which releases the celiac trunk origin compression. In some cases, an aorto-hepatic graft may be required.

HEPATIC ARTERY OR AORTIC CONDUIT PSEUDOANEURYSMS

This rare complication may present initially as an infection of unknown origin followed by gastrointestinal bleeding. The aneurysms usually involve local infection. The diagnosis is confirmed with CT angiogram. An endovascular intervention with a covered arterial stent together with long-term antibiotic treatment may be successful in some cases; the alternative is resection of the infected area and revascularization with an aorto-hepatic conduit. The mortality of this complication is still high, and embolization of the artery with the bleeding pseudoaneurysms followed by retransplant might be the only life-saving option in other cases.

PORTAL VEIN STENOSIS AND THROMBOSIS

This may manifest with an acute liver dysfunction with large ascites production with signs of portal hypertension such as an upper gastrointestinal bleed. The diagnosis is confirmed by venous-phase CT angiogram. The treatment is thrombectomy or percutaneous transluminal angioplasty. If unsuccessful, retransplantation is necessary.

CAVAL STENOSIS

Supra-hepatic IVC stenosis can be caused by a poor anastomotic technique or kinking. The patient may present with liver dysfunction and new-onset ascites. Infra-hepatic IVC stenosis can present with lower extremity edema and kidney dysfunction. The diagnosis is confirmed by venogram with pressure gradient measures. Treatment is with percutaneous intravascular dilatation and stenting, which can be done serially. If this fails, operative correction is necessary.

Vascular surgical technique of pancreas transplantation

BENCH PREPARATION

After unpacking and placing the pancreas in a bowel with ice-cold and slush saline, the gland is carefully inspected. Particular attention is paid to ensure the integrity of the pancreatic capsule as its injury can result in pancreatic leak, and graft pancreatitis and leaks are closely associated with intra-abdominal collections, sepsis and graft loss.

The pancreas back table is a lengthy procedure. The redundant peripancreatic tissues are dissected, tied and removed. The splenic branches at the spleen hilum are carefully tied and divided and the spleen is removed. The duodenum is trimmed by GIA staplers and the stapled ends are oversewn with PDS suture.

The pancreatic blood supply consists of SMA (pancreatic head and duodenum) and splenic artery (gland's body and tail) and the inflow vessels are routinely reconstructed on the back table to enable a single arterial anastomosis for the implantation. This is performed with a donor iliac artery bifurcation graft that should always accompany the pancreatic graft. The internal and external iliac arteries are shortened to minimize the risk of kinking, and based on the size match, these are anastomosed to the SMA and splenic artery, respectively (Figure 56.7).

IMPLANTATION PROCEDURE

The standard pancreatic graft implantation places the organ intraperitoneally, with the duodenum and gland's head pointing cranially. Such a procedure is often a part

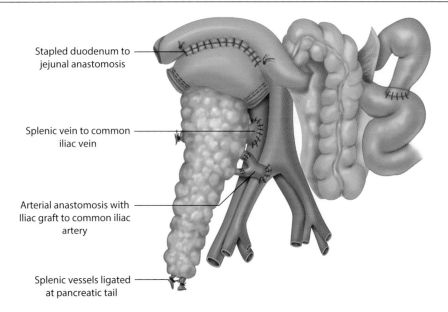

Stapled duodenum to
jejunal anastomosis

Splenic vein to common
iliac vein

Arterial anastomosis with
Iliac graft to common iliac
artery

Splenic vessels ligated
at pancreatic tail

Figure 56.13 Whole pancreas graft with vascular anastomoses to external iliac artery and vein and enteric drainage of pancreatic secretions.

of a simultaneous pancreas and kidney transplantation for diabetic patients with end-stage renal failure. During the operation, the donor common iliac artery, used for the pancreatic arterial inflow reconstruction, is anastomosed end-to-side to the recipient right common iliac artery. The venous outflow is restored via the portal vein anastomosed to the IVC, although some centres advocate a direct connection to the recipient portal system to establish a more natural pattern of glycemic control. The duodenum is attached side-to-side to the proximal jejunum with continuous PDS suture (Figure 56.13).[26]

In patients undergoing pancreas transplant alone, the gland implantation position often differs and the duodenum is anastomosed to the urinary bladder (Figure 56.14). Although this technique might cause hemorrhagic cystitis with disturbances in the recipient's acid–base balance, it might improve the graft survival by enabling the graft function and rejection monitoring by measurement of amylase levels in the urine.[26]

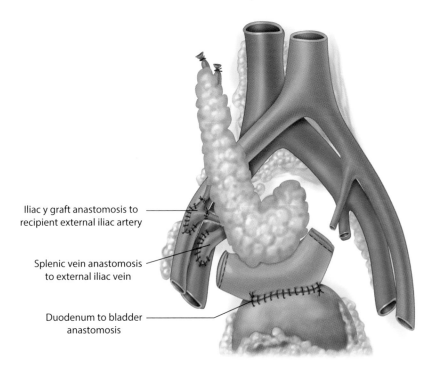

Iliac y graft anastomosis to
recipient external iliac artery

Splenic vein anastomosis
to external iliac vein

Duodenum to bladder
anastomosis

Figure 56.14 Whole pancreas graft with vascular anastomoses to external iliac artery and vein and bladder drainage of pancreatic secretions.

Pancreas vascular complications

The incidence of graft thrombosis in pancreatic transplantation ranges from 4% to 8%. It seems that grafts from DCD donors are more at risk compared to DBD organs[27] (level 3 of evidence). The clinical signs include pain and a sudden loss of the graft function (hyperglycemia). The diagnosis is confirmed by Doppler ultrasound and CT angiography. Graft pancreatitis and leak are other recognized complications in pancreatic transplantation, and all of these complications may cause life-threatening post-transplant sepsis. By its nature, pancreatic transplantation is not a life-saving operation and pancreas graft removal may often represent the safest treatment strategy in those situations.

Vascular surgical technique of small bowel transplantation

Small bowel grafts may be transplanted in isolation but often with variations including the addition of liver, pancreas or colon or as a combination of these. For a liver–bowel graft, the organs are grafted en bloc such that the arterial inflow is taken from the infer-renal aorta usually with a jump graft using donor iliac artery. The venous return is through the caval part of the liver graft, by using it either as an in situ replacement or as a piggyback graft utilizing a side-to-side cavo-cavostomy. The addition of distal stomach, pancreas and/or colon is compatible with this approach. Isolated small bowel again uses inflow from an aortic anastomosis with venous drainage ideally into the superior mesenteric vein, but if this is not technically possible, anastomosis directly onto the vena cava can be effective.

Key points

The technical challenges of transplantation have generally been met and the main obstacle now is donor shortage.

Donation after cardiac death has had a significant impact in increasing the number of available liver, kidney and lung grafts.

Living donor kidney and liver programs have been necessary in regions without deceased donation programs.

Split-liver procedures have had a dramatic impact by shortening waiting times for pediatric recipients given the lack of size-matched donors.

The increasing organ shortage leads to utilization of older donors with additional co-morbidities. Improving transplant outcomes of these organs by machine perfusion reconditioning has become an area of intensive clinical research.

REFERENCES

1. Grundy SR. Infant and paediatric cardiac transplantation. In: Franco KL, ed. *Pediatric Cardiopulmonary Transplantation*. Armonk, NY: Futura Publishing Company, Inc.; 1997, pp. 97–114.
2. Starzl TE, Miller C, Broznick B, Makowka L. An improved technique for multiple organ harvesting. *Surg Gynecol Obstet*. 1987;165(4):343–348.
3. Guidelines for the determination of death. Report of the medical consultants on the diagnosis of death to the President's Commission for the Study of Ethical Problems in Medicine and Biomedical and Behavioral Research. *J Am Med Assoc*. 1981;246(19):2184–2186.
4. Muiesan P, Girlanda R, Jassem W et al. Single-center experience with liver transplantation from controlled non-heartbeating donors: A viable source of grafts. *Ann Surg*. 2005;242(5):732–738.
5. Perera MT. The super-rapid technique in Maastricht category III donors: Has it developed enough for marginal liver grafts from donors after cardiac death? *Curr Opin Organ Transplant*. 2012;17(2):131–136.
6. Graham JA, Guarrera JV. "Resuscitation" of marginal liver allografts for transplantation with machine perfusion technology. *J Hepatol*. 2014;61(2):418–431.
7. Dutkowski P, Schlegel A, de Oliveira M, Mullhaupt B, Neff F, Clavien PA. HOPE for human liver grafts obtained from donors after cardiac death. *J Hepatol*. 2014;60(4):765–772.
8. Abu-Elmagd K, Fung J, Bueno J et al. Logistics and technique for procurement of intestinal, pancreatic, and hepatic grafts from the same donor. *Ann Surg*. 2000;232(5):680–687.
9. Ringe B, Neuhaus P, Pichlmayr R, Heigel B. Aims and practical application of a multi organ procurement protocol. *Langenbecks Arch Chir*. 1985;365(1):47–55.
10. de Ville de Goyet J, Hausleithner V, Malaise J et al. Liver procurement without in situ portal perfusion. A safe procedure for more flexible multiple organ harvesting. *Transplantation*. 1994;57(9):1328–1332.
11. D'Amico F, Vitale A, Gringeri E et al. Liver transplantation using suboptimal grafts: Impact of donor harvesting technique. *Liver Transpl*. 2007;13(10):1444–1450.
12. Stewart ZA, Cameron AM, Singer AL, Dagher NN, Montgomery RA, Segev DL. Histidine-tryptophan-ketoglutarate (HTK) is associated with reduced graft survival in pancreas transplantation. *Am J Transplant*. 2009;9(1):217–221.
13. Stewart ZA, Cameron AM, Singer AL, Montgomery RA, Segev DL. Histidine-Tryptophan-Ketoglutarate (HTK) is associated with reduced graft survival in deceased donor livers, especially those donated after cardiac death. *Am J Transplant*. 2009;9(2):286–293.

14. Stewart ZA, Lonze BE, Warren DS et al. Histidine-tryptophan-ketoglutarate (HTK) is associated with reduced graft survival of deceased donor kidney transplants. *Am J Transplant.* 2009;9(5):1048–1054.

15. O'Callaghan JM, Knight SR, Morgan RD, Morris PJ. Preservation solutions for static cold storage of kidney allografts: A systematic review and meta-analysis. *Am J Transplant.* 2012;12(4):896–906.

16. Vaccarisi S, Bonaiuto E, Spadafora N et al. Complications and graft survival in kidney transplants with vascular variants: Our experience and literature review. *Transplant Proc.* 2013;45(7):2663–2665.

17. Chedid MF, Muthu C, Nyberg SL et al. Living donor kidney transplantation using laparoscopically procured multiple renal artery kidneys and right kidneys. *J Am Coll Surg.* 2013;217(1):144–52; discussion 52.

18. Salehipour M, Salahi H, Jalaeian H et al. Vascular complications following 1500 consecutive living and cadaveric donor renal transplantations: A single center study. *Saudi J Kidney Dis Transpl.* 2009;20(4):570–572.

19. Friedman GS, Meier-Kriesche HU, Kaplan B et al. Hypercoagulable states in renal transplant candidates: Impact of anticoagulation upon incidence of renal allograft thrombosis. *Transplantation.* 2001;72(6):1073–1078.

20. Vivarelli M, La Barba G, Cucchetti A et al. Can antiplatelet prophylaxis reduce the incidence of hepatic artery thrombosis after liver transplantation? *Liver Transpl.* 2007;13(5):651–654.

21. Bekker J, Ploem S, de Jong KP. Early hepatic artery thrombosis after liver transplantation: A systematic review of the incidence, outcome and risk factors. *Am J Transplant.* 2009;9(4):746–757.

22. Silva MA, Jambulingam PS, Gunson BK et al. Hepatic artery thrombosis following orthotopic liver transplantation: A 10-year experience from a single centre in the United Kingdom. *Liver Transpl.* 2006;12(1):146–151.

23. Mourad MM, Liossis C, Gunson BK et al. Etiology and management of hepatic artery thrombosis after adult liver transplantation. *Liver Transpl.* 2014;20(6):713–723.

24. Rodriguez-Davalos MI, Arvelakis A, Umman V et al. Segmental grafts in adult and pediatric liver transplantation: Improving outcomes by minimizing vascular complications. *J Am Med Assoc Surg.* 2014;149(1):63–70.

25. Shay R, Taber D, Pilch N et al. Early aspirin therapy may reduce hepatic artery thrombosis in liver transplantation. *Transplant Proc.* 2013;45(1):330–334.

26. White SA, Shaw JA, Sutherland DE. Pancreas transplantation. *Lancet.* 2009;373(9677):1808–1817.

27. Muthusamy AS, Mumford L, Hudson A, Fuggle SV, Friend PJ. Pancreas transplantation from donors after circulatory death from the United Kingdom. *Am J Transplant.* 2012;12(8):2150–2156.

SECTION XI

Surgical Techniques

57

Vascular open surgical techniques*

FRANK J. VEITH

CONTENTS

This chapter provides illustrations and accompanying descriptions of standard techniques and operations used in vascular surgery. These include techniques for dissecting, incising and repairing injured arteries and veins; methods for vascular anastomoses and bypass grafting; and one surgeon's standard techniques for performing relatively uncomplicated, common venous and arterial operations. The methods described and illustrated represent one way of performing these operations. Other vascular surgeons may have different and even better ways of doing the same procedures, and indeed some of these are discussed and illustrated in other chapters in this volume. Moreover, the techniques that are illustrated in this chapter may not apply to every case, and certainly other special methods are required to deal with the more complex and complicated pathologic patterns of disease that seem to make up an increasing proportion of vascular surgical practice. However, the methods that are shown work well for the standard patterns of vascular pathology that require surgical treatment. The techniques shown are included to provide students and resident trainees with some of the details involved in one surgeon's way of performing these standard vascular operative procedures.

* Reprinted from Hobson/Wilson/Veith: *Vascular Surgery: Principles and Practice, Third Edition, Revised and Expanded.* DOI: 10.1081/0819-9-120024968. Copyright © 2004 by Marcel Dekker, Inc. www.dekker.com.

ARTERIAL DISSECTION

1. The periadventitial tissue is grasped with forceps and incised with scissors. This may be done in several layers.
2. The artery is then freed from its surrounding areolar tissue layers using a combination of blunt and sharp dissection. Care is taken to avoid injury to all arterial branches.
3. Small crossing veins traverse some of these periadventitial layers. These are isolated, doubly ligated and divided, as shown.

Arterial incision

4. An arterial segment is isolated between clamps in such a way that its lumen is filled with blood. A knife is then used to make the arteriotomy. Care is taken to keep the knife cut directly perpendicular to the lumen of the artery, so that the incision in the artery is straight and not skewed or tangential. The point of the knife is used to cut the artery, using light pressure and multiple strokes.
5. If the arterial wall is thickened with disease, a mosquito clamp is inserted into the artery to define the lumen, and the straight cut, which is perpendicular to the wall, is continued between the blades of the clamp as shown. If a scissors is used with a diseased, thick-walled artery, such as the one shown, then jagged, skewed openings in the artery and its various diseased layers may occur and anastomosis rendered more difficult. The ends of the arteriotomy should be fashioned at approximately 45° angles so that there is no undermining of the media or the adventitia and the intimal layer can be clearly visualized for placement of stitches.
6. If the arterial wall is relatively normal, a small Potts scissors or microscissors can be used to complete the arteriotomy.

Suture closure of arteriotomy

7. Both limbs of a double-armed atraumatic monofilament suture are placed from within outward at each end of the arteriotomy and then tied. One arm of one suture is then run to the centre of the incision. It should be noted that in performing the arteriotomy and suture closure, no excision of intima or endarterectomy is performed and all layers are cut evenly.
8. The suture originating at the other end of the arteriotomy is also run to the centre of the incision, where it is tied to the first suture.

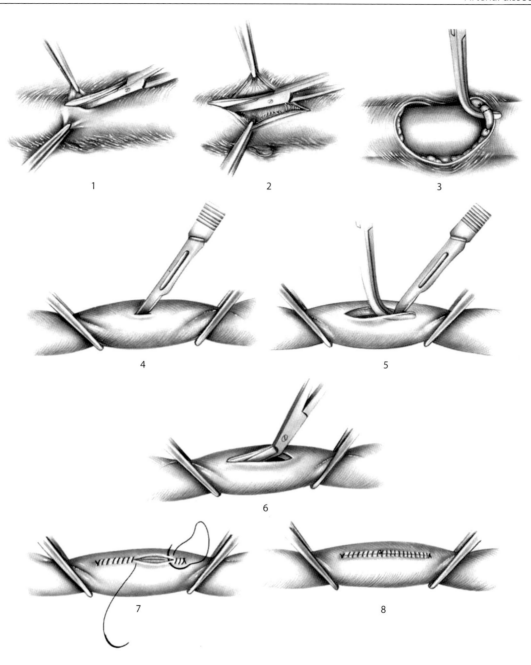

1

2

3

4

5

6

7

8

END-TO-END VASCULAR ANASTOMOSIS

1. End-to-end anastomosis of the arteries is accomplished by approximating the ends of the two arteries with occluding atraumatic clamps. A double-armed atraumatic monofilament suture is placed at either lateral side of the artery. Care is taken to include equal bites of all layers of the arterial wall in each passage of the needle. With good light and exposure, the three layers of the arterial wall can be clearly visualized.
2. The two corner stitches are tied.
3. One arm of the suture is then run along the anterior wall of the artery to the opposite corner and tied.
4. By rotating the vascular clamps and appropriately manipulating the corner sutures, the anastomosis is turned over, exposing the posterior wall. One of the sutures is then run to the opposite corner and tied to the free end of the opposite corner suture. Again, care is taken with each bite to include equal-sized portions of each layer of the arterial wall.
5. The completed anastomosis is shown.

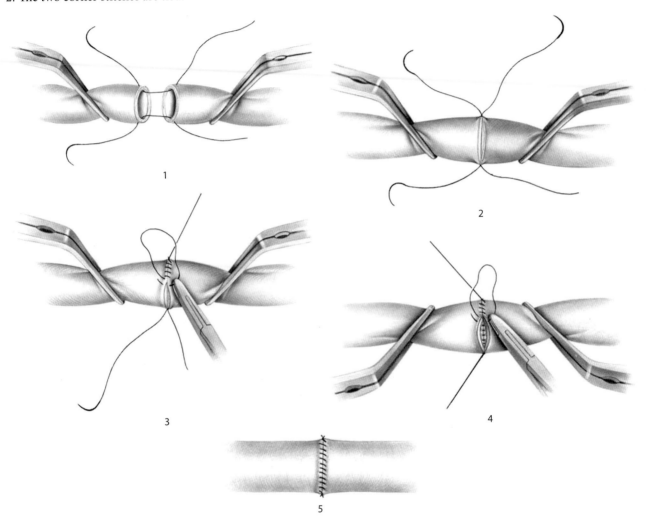

END-TO-SIDE VASCULAR ANASTOMOSIS

1. Sutures are placed at the two ends of the planned anastomosis. Care is taken to place these stitches from within outward in each structure and to catch all layers of both the vein graft and the artery. The intimal layer is particularly important in this regard. Double-armed 6-0 polypropylene atraumatic sutures are used.
2. The apex suture is tied while the opposite end suture is left untied.
3. One arm of the apex suture is run to the midportion of one side of the anastomosis. Small, even bites of all layers are taken with each stitch of the running suture.
4. The opposite limb of the suture is run along the opposite lateral margin of the anastomosis to its midportion.

5. The suture in the opposite end is tied, and both arms of this suture are run to the midportions of the anastomosis, where they are tied to the suture from the opposite end. Good visualization of the inside and the outside of the artery must be obtained when each bite is taken so that the suture will catch and fix the intimal layer. In general the arterial wall should not be grasped with forceps but should be only pushed with the closed forceps to provide visualization. It is also important that the closed or open forceps be used to stabilize the artery as the needle is being passed through it. This can be accomplished without grasping the artery, simply by using the forceps as a pusher or foil.

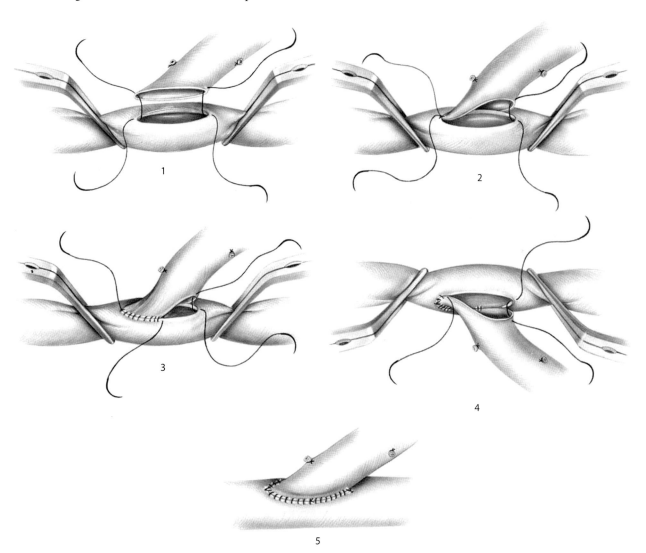

REPAIR OF LACERATED INFERIOR VENA CAVA: REPAIR OF LACERATED ARTERY OR VEIN

Repair of lacerated inferior vena cava

1. A knife wound of the inferior vena cava is shown. This is controlled by emptying the segment of cava containing the laceration by sponge stick pressure proximally and distally. Finger pressure, or pressure with a tonsil sucker, is used to control bleeding from branches entering the injured venous segment. When this is done, the vein may be dissected free proximally and distally and clamps applied, although this is often not necessary.

2. When the edges of the laceration can be clearly visualized and the adjacent wall of the vein is dissected from surrounding tissue, the edges of the laceration are grasped with a forceps and a Satinsky clamp is placed to isolate the laceration.

3. The laceration is then closed with a running 4-0 or 5-0 vascular polypropylene suture in a dry field precisely approximating the edges. If the laceration is through and through the inferior vena cava, the far wall must also be repaired. This can be accomplished after the inferior vena cava is emptied of blood by approximating the laceration in the far wall from within the vena cava through the laceration in the near wall. To accomplish this, one must get an absolutely dry field; it may be necessary to isolate the vessel proximal and distal to the injury and apply vascular clamps. It may also be necessary to isolate and ligate branches that drain into that segment. The temptation to grasp the bleeding vena cava in a pool of blood should be resisted, particularly before the vessel is cleanly dissected. Pressure control and emptying of the injured vein should be the theme of technical management.

Repair of lacerated artery or vein

TYPES OF VASCULAR INJURY AND METHODS OF REPAIR

4. A small puncture wound or minor laceration of an artery is shown. This is frequently the type of injury encountered from an arteriographic procedure. The injury is controlled by finger pressure until the artery is controlled by the application of clamps and the injury repaired.

5. Simple interrupted sutures through all layers of the arterial wall, or the adventitia and media, are adequate to control the injury and maintain patency of the artery.

6. A more extensive and somewhat jagged, although clean, laceration is shown. This can result from a knife wound or injury with a similar sharp object. Bleeding is controlled by pressure until the artery remote from the injury is isolated and controlled with clamps. All branches entering into the intervening segment also must be isolated and controlled.

7. If the laceration is clean and there is no contusion of the adjacent edges of the laceration, it may be repaired by a simple running suture. Sutures are placed from within outward at both ends of the laceration and then run to the centre, where they are tied.

8. A contused arterial wound is shown. An injury such as this can be produced by a bullet wound or other blunt trauma. In the injury depicted there is loss of arterial wall substance, and tissue adjacent to the defect is damaged. All injured artery wall must be excised by cutting the artery along the lines shown.

9. This leaves inadequate length of artery to approximate without tension.

10. Accordingly, a prosthetic graft or autologous vein graft must be used. This can be inserted as an interposition graft, as shown.

11. Alternatively, if exposure is impaired or there is excessive surrounding tissue damage or contamination, the debrided arterial ends are ligated and a remote bypass graft is carried out to restore arterial continuity.

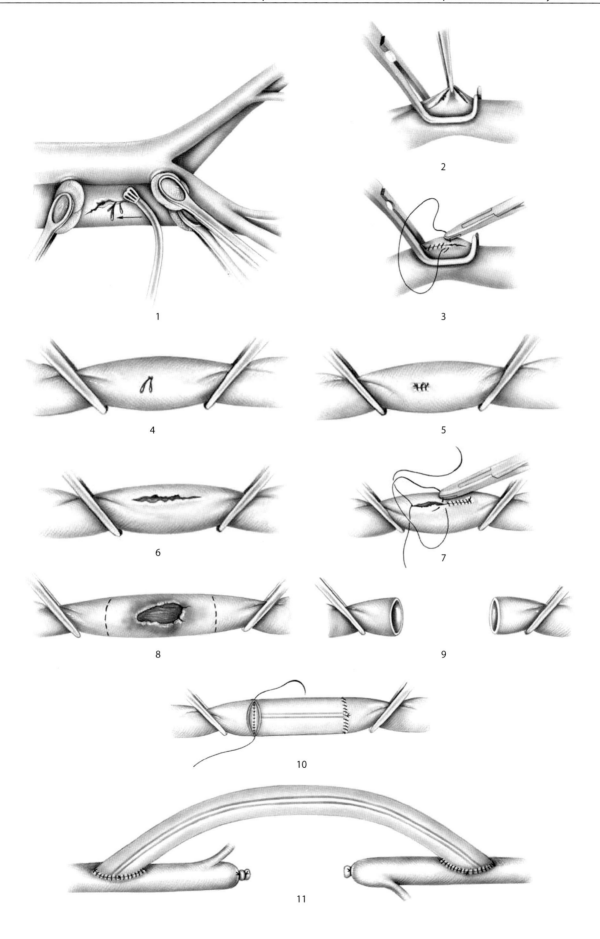

REPAIR OF LACERATED FEMORAL ARTERY

1. If the injury is thought to be complex, proximal control of the iliac artery through a suprainguinal retroperitoneal incision is advisable. While this is rapidly being accomplished, bleeding from the femoral artery laceration is controlled with finger pressure.

2. Even with occlusion of the external iliac artery, bleeding from the groin will be brisk due to the multiple branches of the deep femoral artery. However, finger pressure can control this bleeding while the superficial femoral artery is dissected and clamped.

3. It is sometimes necessary to get clamp control of the deep femoral artery as well, so that accurate approximation of the lacerated femoral artery can be accomplished. Occasionally, if only one or two sutures are required, digital or sucker pressure will control bleeding from the deep femoral artery so that the sutures can be accurately placed. More complex injuries require clamp control of all branches. In some instances of false aneurysm due to injury at the time of arteriography, the false aneurysm can simply be entered with a vertical incision in the groin and bleeding from the anterior wall of the femoral artery controlled with digital pressure. The artery can then be dissected proximally in the groin, and suture control of the bleeding point can be obtained. If the patient is obese or a complex injury is suspected, proximal control via the external iliac is advisable.

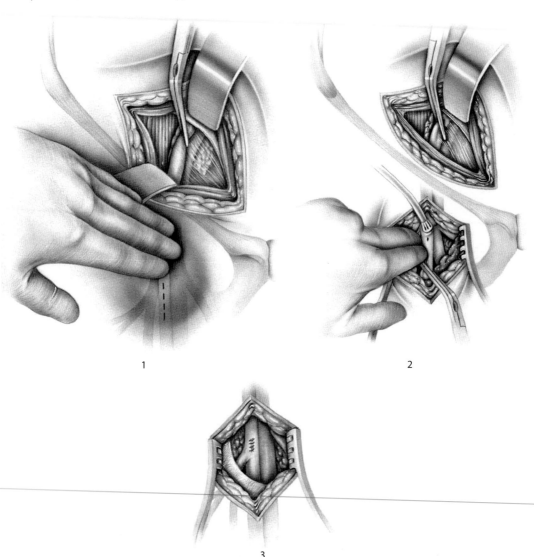

1

2

3

INFERIOR VENA CAVA PLICATION

1. A retroperitoneal incision in the right flank is made at about the level of the umbilicus, or midway between the costal margin and the iliac crest. Care is taken to extend this incision across the lateral one-half to one-third of the rectus sheaths to provide better medial exposure.
2. The three oblique abdominal muscles are cut in the direction of the skin incision, and the anterior and posterior rectus sheath is also incised. Rarely is it necessary to divide the rectus muscle.
3. After dividing the transversalis fascia, it is possible to enter the retroperitoneal plane and strip the peritoneum from the deeper layers of the abdominal wall. This is first accomplished superiorly and then inferiorly.
4. Finally, the peritoneum is swept away from the posterior parietes. In the course of this, the psoas muscle is visualized and serves as an important landmark.

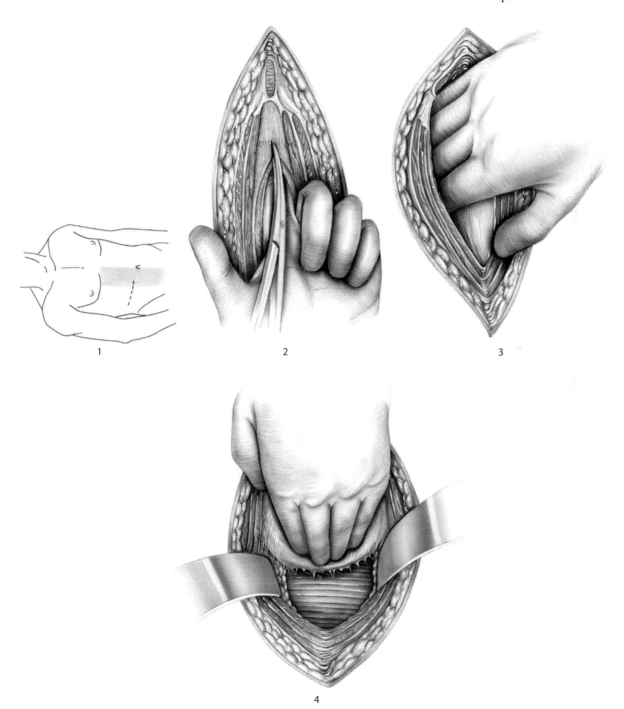

INFERIOR VENA CAVA PLICATION (CONT.)

5. By using three mechanical retractors, which are fixed to the operating table, and fitting them with appropriate 1 or 2 in. Deaver retractors, the retroperitoneal fatty tissue and edges of the incision can be retracted superiorly and inferiorly. The peritoneal cavity and its contents, along with the ureter, can be retracted strongly in a medial direction. The fatty areolar tissue overlying the inferior vena cava is then incised and dissection continued in the periadventitial plane of the inferior vena cava.

6. By pushing the inferior vena cava gently to the patient's left and putting tension on the surrounding fatty areolar tissue, the right-side lumbar veins can be visualized and protected from injury.

7. By gently holding the inferior vena cava to the patient's right, using the fingers of the surgeon's left hand, and tensioning the fatty areolar tissue to the patient's left, it is possible to visualize the left-side lumbar veins and protect them from injury.

8. Once the position of the lumbar veins is known, it is possible to compress the vena cava in the lateral plane with an atraumatic vascular forceps. A large C clamp is placed behind the vena cava to grasp a red rubber catheter, which has been cut appropriately for the purpose. Into the other end of this catheter the posterior half of the vena caval clip is inserted so that it can be drawn around the back of the cava.

9. The clip is then closed and tied, completing the operation. The retroperitoneum is allowed to collapse over the cava. The retractors are removed and the wound is closed in layers.

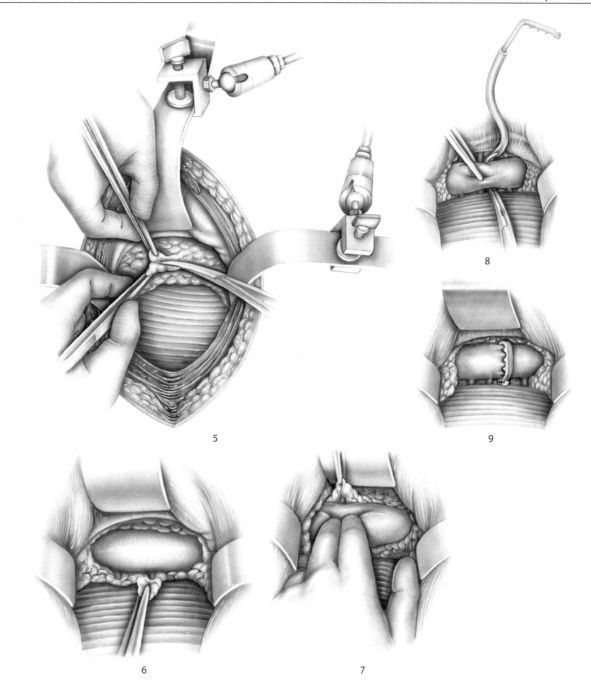

5

6

7

8

9

SAPHENOUS VEIN LIGATION AND STRIPPING

1. The anatomy of the varicose greater saphenous vein is shown, together with the three skin incisions that are typically required. The upper incision should start directly over the femoral pulse and extend medially in a diagonal fashion as shown. (All three incisions may be somewhat shorter than shown.) Additional incisions may be required if a perforator is suspected or the stripper does not pass a particular point. The position of the saphenous nerve adjacent to the vein is also shown in the ankle area. Great care must be taken to protect this from injury so as to avoid saphenous neuritis.

2. As the oblique incision in the groin is deepened in the fatty tissue, a large venous structure will be encountered. The position of the femoral artery should be carefully identified by palpating the femoral pulse; care should be taken to avoid injury to this vessel and the femoral vein. Once it has been confirmed that the first large venous structure encountered is in fact the greater saphenous vein, it can be divided between clamps as shown.

3. Both ends of the divided saphenous vein are separated and dissected free. Their branches are clamped, doubly ligated and divided. The fossa ovalis is identified by the small arterial branch that defines its lower border. The junction of the saphenous vein with the common femoral vein is clearly identified, and the saphenous vein is clamped a few millimetres away from this junction. Without pulling firmly on the saphenous vein and tenting up the adjacent walls of the common femoral vein, the vein is ligated with #00 silk.

4. A second suture is placed on the greater saphenous vein just beyond the first tie.

5. The two ligatures on the saphenous vein are shown in position, without any deformity being created in the common femoral vein.

6. A vertical incision is then made just anterior to the medial malleolus. The saphenous vein and saphenous nerve are identified, and the nerve is protected from injury. Branches in this area are ligated, and then the saphenous vein is divided between clamps. An opening is made in the proximal end of the distal saphenous vein so that the small end of the stripper can be inserted.

7. The remaining distal end of the saphenous vein is ligated and the stripper is tied in place. Traction is exerted in a cephalad direction.

8. As the stripper is being drawn toward the patient's head, a snug-fitting sterile elastic bandage is applied to the area from which the vein is being removed, thereby controlling avulsed tributaries. Positions of typical incisions in the leg are also shown.

9. Through these small incisions, previously marked clusters of varicosities can be removed. In the illustration, a twisting motion of a clamp avulses one such small cluster.

10. A slightly larger incision is made to remove a bigger cluster. Where possible, identifiable branches are ligated and the thin-walled varices are avulsed.

11. This shows the appearance of the veins as they are removed and the branches connecting with the deeper system are ligated.

12. This shows a larger incision and division and ligation of a probable communicating branch. Through these incisions, all major venous clusters are excised and avulsed.

13. A subcuticular absorbable suture is used to close all incisions. It provides the best cosmetic result.

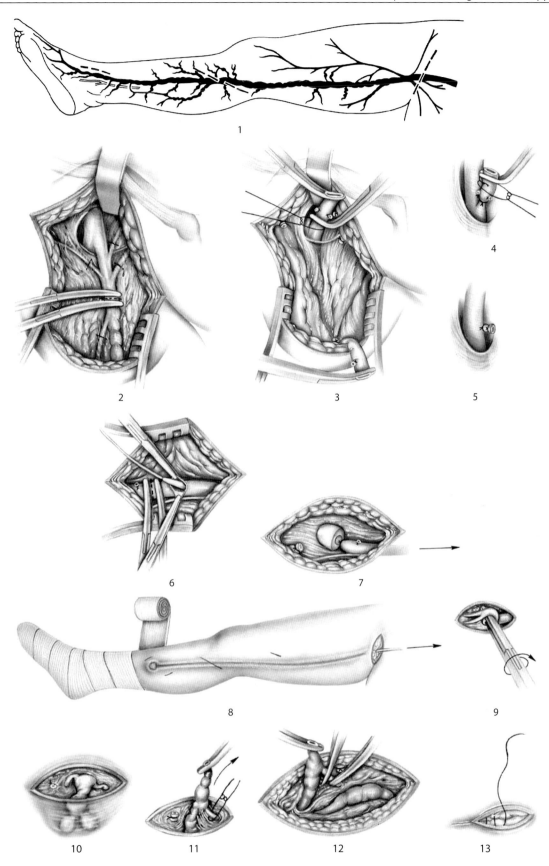

CAROTID ENDARTERECTOMY

1. The position of the patient, with the head turned away from the side of the incision, is shown. A thyroid pillow should be placed beneath the shoulders, and the head of the patient should be draped free with the anesthesiologist placed at the side of the operating table, so that the surgeon and his or her assistant can stand on either side of the table – which is rotated toward the assistant to provide equally good access to both surgeons. The incision is placed along the anterior border of the sternomastoid and curved slightly posterior in its upper portion to avoid injury to the marginal mandibular branch of the facial nerve.

2. After the incision is deepened through the subcutaneous fat and platysma, the anterior border of the sternomastoid muscle is defined and the wound edges are retracted with a self-retaining retractor. The anterior surface of the internal jugular vein is defined and the common facial branch is identified and dissected free. This vein is divided between ligatures. In the event that the vein is short, the divided ends may be oversewn.

3. Division of the common facial vein allows the internal jugular vein to be retracted laterally and posteriorly and held with the self-retaining retractor. The upper angle of the wound is then retracted with an Army Navy retractor, which can be held in a secure position with a robot arm, avoiding the need for a second assistant in this operation. The position of the common facial vein is a rough guide to the carotid bifurcation. The fascial investments of the carotid artery are then grasped with forceps, tensioned and incised to expose the underlying adventitia of the carotid artery. As this incision is extended superiorly, care is taken to identify the hypoglossal nerve and protect it from injury. Once this is identified and protected, the anterior belly of the digastric muscle is identified and retracted superiorly with the Army Navy retractor.

4. The common carotid artery, the superior thyroid artery, the external carotid artery and the internal carotid artery are then dissected free in their periadventitial plane and encircled with vessel loops. Care is taken to dissect the surrounding tissue away from the carotid artery so that it will be manipulated minimally. (This is so that the risk of embolization will be minimized.) Care should be taken to dissect the internal carotid artery as far as necessary to isolate at least 1 cm distal to the palpable disease. This upper dissection of the internal carotid artery can be facilitated by isolating, ligating and dividing small arteries and veins which hold the hypoglossal nerve posteriorly. Once these small vessels are divided, the hypoglossal nerve can be swept anteriorly and medially. This provides access to the upper reaches of the internal carotid artery. The patient is given systemic heparin [1 mg (100 IU)/kg]. Atraumatic vascular clamps are then placed gently across the common and external carotid arteries, and the superior thyroid artery is controlled with a doubled vessel loop. A needle is then inserted in the common carotid artery below palpable disease, and the stump pressure is measured. According to the surgeon's preference, the stump pressure measurement, the EKG recordings with carotid clamping and the patient's clinical and radiographic presentation, a decision is made regarding the need for shunt protection of the brain during endarterectomy.

5. A gently applied atraumatic clamp is placed across the internal carotid artery well distal to any palpable disease, and an incision is made in the common and internal carotid artery in a longitudinal direction. Entrance is gained into the lumen of the internal carotid artery distal to the disease and into the common carotid artery proximal to the disease. In between, the incision in the artery is deepened to the surface of the plaque.

6. The adventitial and a portion of the medial layers of the carotid artery are grasped with fine atraumatic forceps and the appropriate endarterectomy plane defined. Ideally, this is just deep to the circular muscle fibres within the media of the vessel. Using an endarterectomy spoon or dissector, this plane is further defined and the core of the diseased artery is dissected free proximally and distally.

7. This dissection is continued in circumferential fashion until it proceeds proximal to the obvious atheromatous plaque in the common carotid artery. The core of the artery is then transected through relatively normal intima and media. This frees the proximal end of the plaque, which can then be placed under tension to further facilitate the endarterectomy of the external carotid artery. This is accomplished by eversion with inferior traction on the clamp controlling the external carotid. Generally, the atheroma within the external carotid separates with this eversion technique. However, it is sometimes necessary to transect the atheroma sharply to end the removal of the plaque from the external carotid. Occasionally, it may be necessary to make a separate longitudinal incision in the external carotid to ensure maintenance of flow to this important vessel.

8. Following transection of the external carotid attachments of the plaque, the endarterectomy can continue up the internal carotid artery. The arteriotomy in the internal carotid artery should extend well above the upper level of the plaque, which is frequently most extensive on the posterior wall. Once the upper border of the plaque is defined, the endarterectomy may be completed by transecting the plaque through normal intima, as indicated by the dashed line in Figure 7. Sometimes, transection of the distal end of the plaque is unnecessary since it will feather out and come away from the distal intima as the plaque is freed under gentle tension. If any free intimal or medial edge is detected at the site of the upper limit of the endarterectomy, this free edge is secured with 'U' stitches placed with the knot tied on the outside of the internal carotid artery. Although some surgeons feel that placement of

these 'U' stitches is almost never necessary, we employ them frequently. If placed with care they do not distort the vessel or its lumen, and they certainly may provide protection against upward dissection of an intimal flap. After all plaque is removed and the distal end of the endarterectomy secured, care is taken to examine the endarterectomized segment of the artery to remove all loose circular muscle fragments and other debris so that no material is present which could possibly embolize. This manoeuvre is facilitated by using fine forceps and copious amounts of saline irrigation.

9. The longitudinal arteriotomy is enclosed with fine polypropylene 6-0 sutures. These are generally begun at both ends of the arteriotomy and carried to the central portion, where they are tied. If these sutures are placed carefully and encompass small bites of the endarterectomized arterial wall, the arterial closure can be accomplished without narrowing. Although some surgeons routinely use a vein or PTFE patch, we do not use it routinely in primary cases. If a patch is necessary, we favour use of an accessory saphenous vein from the thigh or PTFE. Rupture of ankle vein has been reported in a few cases, and we would not advocate use of this material. Before flow is re-established, both the internal and common carotid arteries are flushed to remove luminal debris. When the arteriotomy is closed, an effort is made to exclude all intraluminal air, and clamps are removed first from the external and common carotid artery so that debris will be carried up this vessel. Only after release of these two clamps is the internal carotid artery clamp removed.

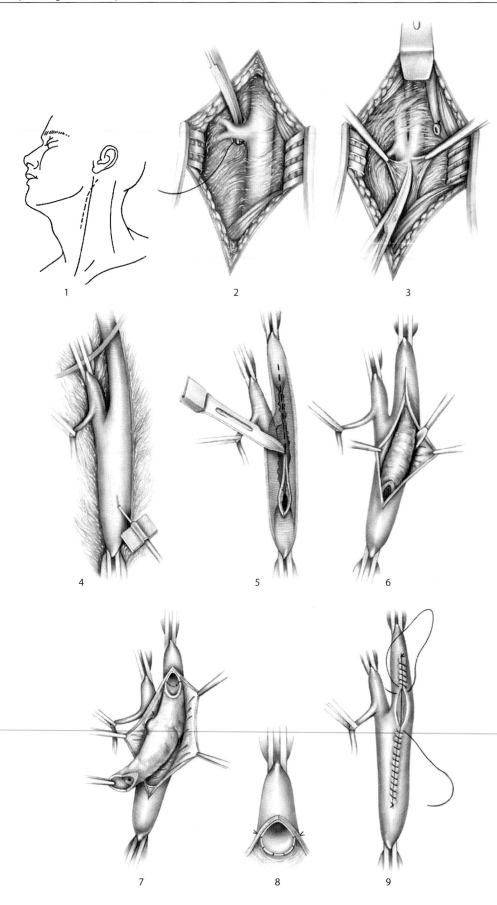

1

2

3

4

5

6

7

8

9

CAROTID ENDARTERECTOMY (CONT.)

10. In the event that a shunt is necessary, one possible technique for its insertion is shown. Small Rummel tourniquets are positioned around the internal carotid and common carotid arteries.

11. After the longitudinal incision is made in these arteries, the internal carotid artery vascular clamp is removed and the occluded shunt is gently inserted into a normal portion of this artery.

12. The Rummel tourniquet is gently tightened to secure the shunt in place, and the clamp occluding the shunt is released momentarily to assure adequate backflow from the internal carotid artery and appropriate positioning of the distal end of the shunt. The clamp on the shunt is replaced.

13. After controlling the common carotid artery with finger compression, the common carotid artery clamp is removed. The common carotid artery is then flushed by a momentary release of the finger pressure, and the proximal end of the shunt is passed down the common carotid artery between the fingers.

14. The common carotid artery Rummel tourniquet is tightened, and the clamp is removed from the shunt, restoring flow to the internal carotid artery. The endarterectomy is then performed in the standard fashion. This is somewhat more difficult with the shunt in place. However, it can be accomplished in an unhurried fashion with the same technical care as already described. If the dissection in the internal carotid artery has proceeded high enough, a very adequate end point can almost always be obtained and its adequacy assured by direct visual inspection.

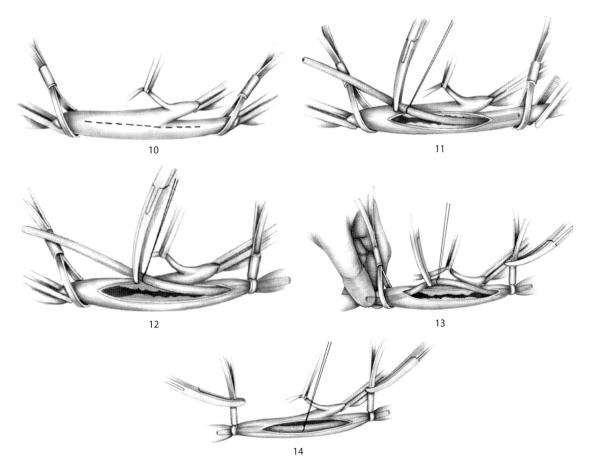

10

11

12

13

14

CAROTID ENDARTERECTOMY (CONT.)

15. To remove the shunt upon completion of the endarterectomy, the arteriotomy in the common carotid and internal carotid artery is closed for as long a distance as possible. These closures are begun at both ends of the arteriotomy and continue toward the midportion, leaving the central part of the arteriotomy open to allow removal of the shunt. The shunt is clamped in its midportion and the distal Rummel tourniquet is released. The distal end of the shunt is then carefully removed from the artery. The rush of blood aids in the removal of luminal debris. The internal carotid artery is then gently clamped.

16. With finger control of the common carotid artery again established, the proximal Rummel tourniquet on the common carotid artery is released and the shunt is removed. Clamp control of the common carotid artery is then established after flushing that vessel.

17. Traction is placed on the two suture ends defining the unclosed portion of the arteriotomy. Taking great care to avoid intraluminal air, a small partially occluding vascular clamp is placed just under the open portion of the arteriotomy. Flow is then re-established up the external carotid artery by releasing the clamps on this vessel. After a moment of this flow, the internal carotid artery clamp is released, re-establishing flow to the brain.

18. The midportion of the arteriotomy closure is then accomplished and the partially occluding clamp is removed. After securing adequate hemostasis, a few #0000 polyglycolic acid sutures are used to approximate lymphoareolar tissue over the carotid artery. The platysma and skin are then closed in layers. We generally employ a small closed suction drain for 24 hours, although this is not routinely deemed necessary.

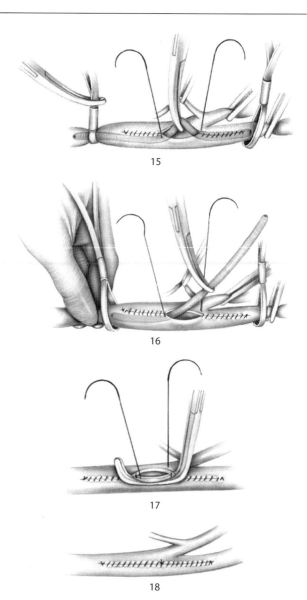

15

16

17

18

AORTIC ANEURYSM REPAIR

1. More than 95% of aortic aneurysms involve the infrarenal segment of the abdominal aorta. Aneurysms of the infrarenal aorta and iliac arteries can be approached via an anterior transperitoneal route or via a left-sided retroperitoneal route with the left side of the patient slightly elevated and the left upper extremity affixed to the ether screen. For more standard abdominal aortic and iliac aneurysms, we favour the anterior transperitoneal approach, using a long midline incision which is extended superiorly above the xiphoid in the skin and fascial layers and to the pubis inferiorly. For aortic aneurysms that involve the segment of the aorta that gives rise to the renal arteries or the superior mesenteric and celiac arteries, we favour a retroperitoneal transpleural approach with the upper lateral portion of the incision extending into the eighth or ninth intercostal space (see the section 'Aortic aneurysm repair').

2. After the abdomen is opened, the intraperitoneal and retroperitoneal viscera are explored thoroughly, the small bowel is retracted to the right and the transverse colon is retracted superiorly. This exposes the posterior peritoneum overlying the segment of the aorta below the inferior mesenteric artery. Just above this area, the ascending or fourth portion of the duodenum and the ligament of Treitz can be identified. A T-shaped incision is made in the peritoneum. This begins over the lower extent of the aortic aneurysm, which in the example shown extends inferiorly only to the aortic bifurcation. The incision is extended superiorly midway between the duodenum and the inferior mesenteric vein. In its upper portion, it is converted to a T-shaped incision which parallels the lower border of the pancreas. The inferior mesenteric vein is carefully identified, isolated and divided so that the lower border of the pancreas may be freed beneath the peritoneal incision and retracted superiorly, thereby providing access to the neck of the aneurysm, the left renal vein and the pararenal segment of the aorta if this is necessary.

3. After this incision is completed, the abdominal viscera are controlled with packs and self-retaining retraction devices. These can consist of a large ring-shaped retractor, which allows retraction of the abdominal wound laterally and the transverse colon and mesocolon superiorly, as depicted. This ring retraction device must be supplemented by two deeply placed Deaver retractors, which, with appropriate packing, allow the small bowel and duodenum to be retracted to the right and craniad and the transverse and descending colon to be retracted to the left and craniad. These two Deaver retractors may be held by surgical assistants but are best held in a fixed position by robot arm retractors, which can be affixed to the operating table. Alternatively, a special self-retaining retraction device (Omni-Tract) designed for aortic surgery can be used. This device is shaped in the form of a wishbone, which is affixed securely to the operating table. The apex of this wishbone is placed over the sternum; various retracting elements may then be secured to the wishbone. Once retraction is secured, the retroperitoneal fatty areolar tissue overlying the aneurysm is incised in the midline, using a right-angle clamp and coagulating cautery to control the small arterial and venous bleeders in this layer.

4. As dissection in this plane proceeds superiorly, the left renal vein is identified and its lower border defined. It is sometimes necessary to dissect this vein circumferentially so that it can be encircled with a loop and retracted superiorly. However, this is not always necessary. To aid in the mobilization and retraction of the left renal vein, it is sometimes necessary to divide the genital branch or branches and a posterior lumbar branch which is often present.

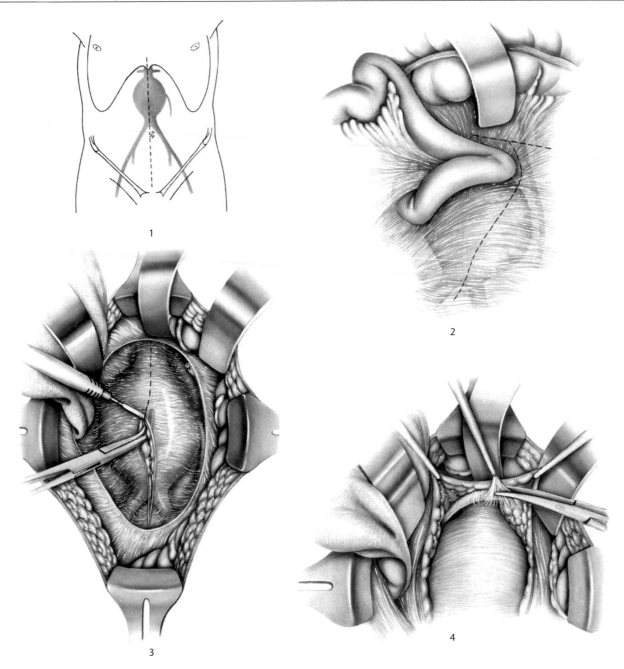

AORTIC ANEURYSM REPAIR (CONT.)

5. With the lower border of the left renal vein identified and in some cases with it appropriately retracted in a craniad direction, the fascial investing layer just outside the adventitia of the aorta is incised after elevating this layer with forceps.

6. It is then possible in most instances to dissect the lateral walls of the aorta using a combination of blunt finger dissection and occasional sharp dissection to divide resistant bands or small branches arising from this segment of the aorta. Such small branches most often represent accessory renal arteries; if these are less than 2 mm in diameter, they may be ligated and divided to facilitate aortic mobilization. It is generally not necessary to dissect the aorta completely on its posterior aspect, although some surgeons still do so. Adequate anterior and lateral mobilization of the aorta, if it is extensive enough, will usually facilitate clamp control of the aorta proximal to the aneurysm. Circumferential aortic dissection, although it may facilitate clamp control and suturing, can also lead to bleeding. For that reason, we no longer perform this dissection routinely.

7. The areolar tissue just superficial to the adventitia of the common iliac arteries is grasped with forceps, placed under tension and sharply incised. This allows periadventitial dissection of the iliac arteries anteriorly and laterally on both sides. For reasons already mentioned, we do not routinely dissect these vessels circumferentially either.

8. After administration of systemic heparin [1 mg (100 IU)/ kg], appropriate atraumatic vascular clamps are then applied to the proximal infrarenal aorta and distal common iliac arteries. A doubled vessel loop may be placed on the inferior mesenteric artery as it emerges from the aneurysm. Generally, the application of clamps is such that the aorta and iliac arteries are compressed in a lateral direction. However, if these vessels are calcified and tortuous, compression of the vessels in an anteroposterior direction may be more easily accomplished. This is particularly true if the infrarenal aorta just proximal to the aneurysm deviates to the right. An effort is made to use vascular clamps, which are shaped in such a fashion that the handles do not obscure the operative field. Some surgeons favour placement of the distal clamps first to minimize the chance of distal embolization of clot and atheromatous material. Although this is advantageous from a theoretical perspective, the placement of distal clamps before the aneurysm is decompressed by a proximal clamp is sometimes technically difficult. This is particularly true when the aneurysm is large and involves the iliac arteries. After clamp placement in a fashion that obliterates the aneurysmal pulse is completed, the aneurysm is incised along its anterior surface and this incision is extended laterally in both directions at the superior and inferior ends of the aneurysm, as indicated by the dashed lines. This incision is generally best accomplished with the coagulating cautery to minimize bleeding from small vessels in the aneurysm wall and surrounding areolar tissue. The lumen of the aneurysm is entered. It is advantageous to utilize some form of cell-saving or autotransfusion device throughout these cases to minimize the need for homologous blood transfusion.

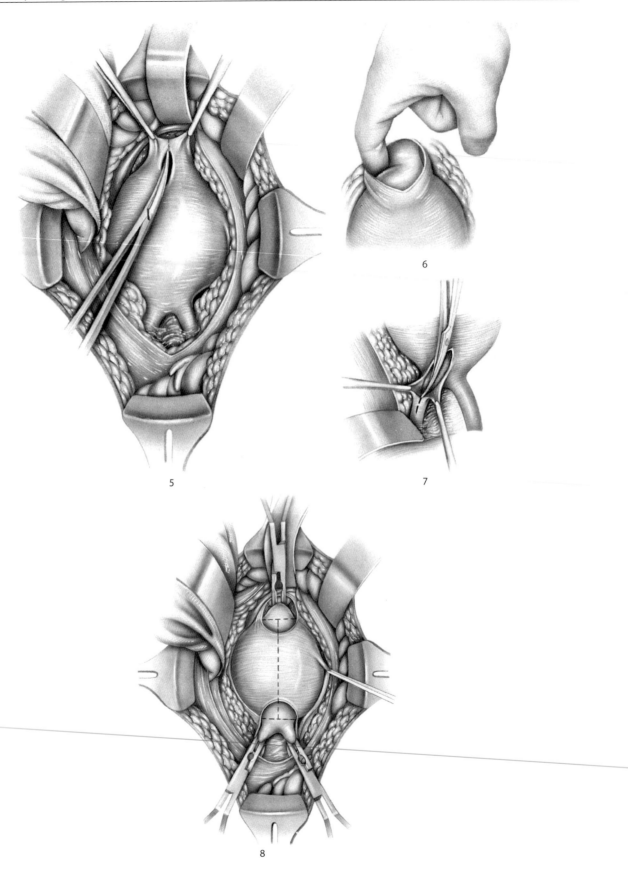

5

6

7

8

AORTIC ANEURYSM REPAIR (CONT.)

9. Clot within the lumen of the opened aneurysm is then mobilized with finger dissection and removed.

10. This exposes the orifices of lumbar arteries and other aortic branches, which can backbleed vigorously into the opened aneurysmal sac. This bleeding is controlled by oversewing the orifices of these branches with figure-of-eight #000 silk sutures. Although some large aneurysms have no patent arteries that require such control, other aneurysms have many branches. Bleeding from this source can be quite substantial. If bleeding from the inferior mesenteric artery is brisk and the inferior mesenteric artery is small, the orifice of this vessel may be oversewn as well. However, if this artery is large and there is only a trickle of backbleeding from it, consideration should be given to reimplantation of this vessel into the wall of the aortic graft. This is particularly true if there is stenotic or occlusive disease involving the celiac and superior mesenteric arteries. Often, however, the orifice of the inferior mesenteric artery is occluded; no attention need be directed to this vessel as long as flow is re-established to at least one of the internal iliac arteries.

11. An appropriate-sized aortic graft is selected for use. A variety of woven or knitted Dacron grafts or PTFE grafts may be used. If an uncoated knitted Dacron graft is employed, it must be carefully preclotted. To minimize bleeding through the graft wall, we use a collagen-coated knitted graft (Hemashield), which bleeds minimally and is easy to handle. Suturing of the graft is best accomplished with #00 polypropylene sutures with large needles. The suture is begun posteriorly as shown. This suture is tied with two or three throws, and suturing is continued laterally in both directions. The posterior wall of the aorta need not be completely divided. Some surgeons favour the loose placement of five or six of the posterior sutures in a parachute fashion followed by tensioning of these sutures to approximate the graft to the aortic wall. This technique may favour careful placement of the sutures, but care must then be taken to assure adequate tensioning of all suture loops.

12. After placement of one posterolateral quadrant of sutures, the opposite posterolateral quadrant is completed.

13. The two anterior quadrants of the suture line are then completed in similar fashion. Note the large size of the suture bites, which are placed through all layers of the aortic wall. The sutures are then tied anteriorly.

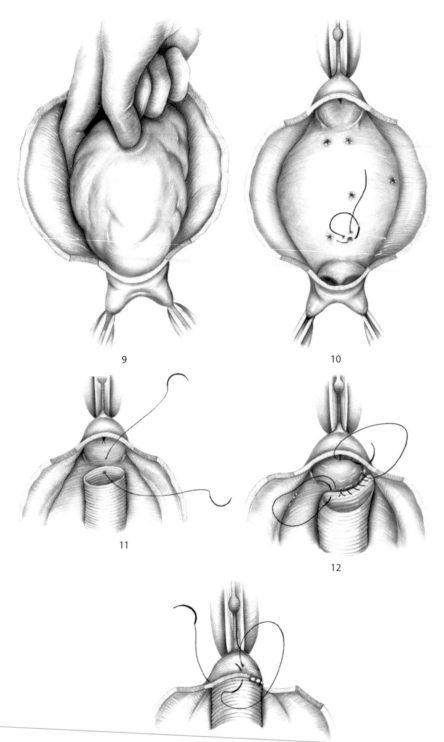

9

10

11

12

13

AORTIC ANEURYSM REPAIR (CONT.)

14. The graft is then clamped temporarily and the proximal aortic clamp released to flush debris from the lumen and to test the suture line. Any bleeding points in the suture line are reinforced and the aorta is reclamped. After appropriate tensioning of the graft, it is transected and the distal anastomosis completed in a fashion similar to the proximal anastomosis. Just before completion of this anastomosis, the iliac clamps are released to allow flushing of debris from these vessels. After suitable volume replacement, one of the iliac clamps is removed to test the anastomoses for leaks. Once both anastomoses are found to be intact, the proximal clamp is carefully released, monitoring the patient's systemic arterial pressure and replacing blood volume as needed.

15. Heparin is reversed with protamine, and the interior of the aneurysm is again checked for bleeding. Not uncommonly a well-controlled lumbar orifice will begin to bleed again with release of the aortic and iliac clamps. Once the interior of the aneurysm is free of bleeding, the aneurysm wall is closed over the graft and, where possible, the suture lines, with #000 polyglycolic acid sutures.

16. The retroperitoneum is then reapproximated so that neither the aneurysm wall nor either suture line can come into contact with the duodenum or small bowel. Closure of the retroperitoneum is often facilitated by release of the self-retaining retraction devices. It is not necessary to completely close the upper portion of the retroperitoneal incision. (In fact, this is often impossible.) In the event that a retroperitoneal layer cannot be interposed between the graft and its suture lines, it may be necessary to use a flap of retroperitoneal fat or omentum.

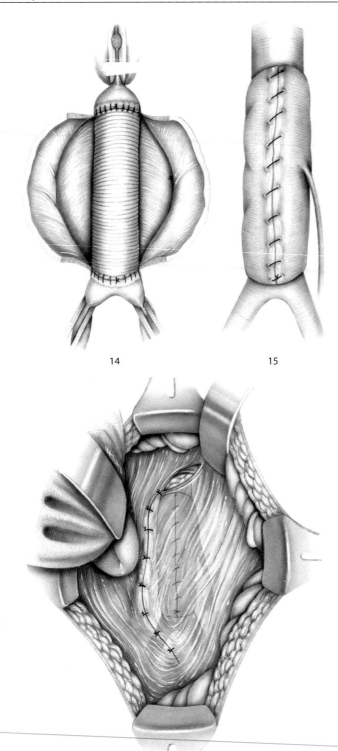

14   15

16

AORTIC ANEURYSM REPAIR (CONT.)

17. The aneurysmal incisions for managing a large right common iliac and a small left common iliac aneurysm are shown. Clamp control on the right is at the level of the internal and external iliac arteries. Often, a single Satinsky clamp can be used to accomplish the same end, particularly if the iliac aneurysm is redundant and these two branches come off posteriorly. A single atraumatic clamp is placed on the distal left common iliac artery where it is of relatively normal calibre.

18. The opened aortic and iliac aneurysms can be seen and the completed suture lines of the aortic bifurcation graft are shown. Anastomosis on the right is to the iliac bifurcation. On the left it is to the mid-common iliac artery. Similar techniques for performing these anastomoses and the aortic anastomoses are employed. Aneurysm closure and retroperitoneal closure are accomplished in the same fashion as that already outlined for a simple aortic aneurysm. Care is taken to assure adequate hemostasis before all wounds are closed.

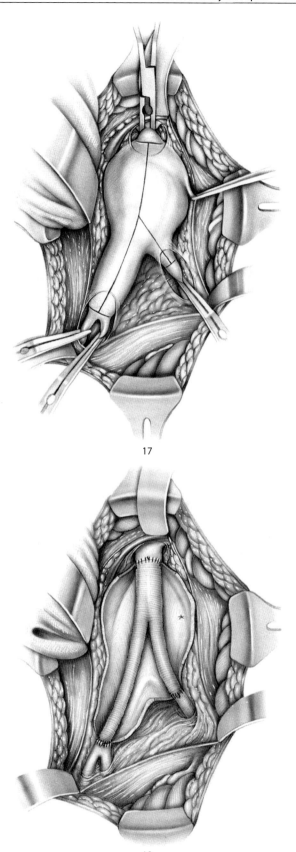

17

18

AORTIC ANEURYSM REPAIR (CONT.)

Retroperitoneal transpleural approach: The retroperitoneal transthoracic approach is particularly helpful when exposure of the pararenal or suprarenal abdominal aorta is required or when the transperitoneal approach is rendered difficult or impractical because of extreme obesity, previous operative scarring or the presence of stomas. Although infrarenal aneurysms can be approached via an incision extending into the eleventh intercostal space and not entering the pleura, we prefer a higher transpleural incision for pararenal or suprarenal aneurysms.

19. The patient is positioned to obtain 30° of elevation of the left hip and 90° of elevation of the left shoulder. A gentle S-shaped incision is made starting midway between the pubis and the umbilicus and extending across the costal margin into the left eighth or ninth intercostal space. The abdominal and thoracic muscles and fascia are cut in line with the skin incision.

20. The transversalis fascia is incised laterally to enter the retroperitoneal space.

21, 22. The peritoneum and its contents are bluntly separated from the overlying muscles and fascia, which are cut so that the peritoneal sac can be retracted medially.

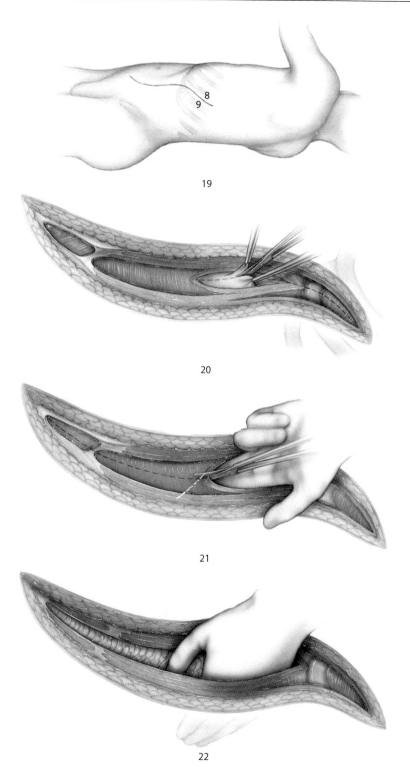

19

20

21

22

AORTIC ANEURYSM REPAIR (CONT.)

23. The intercostal muscles are divided, the pleura is entered, and the costal margin is divided.

24. The ribs are retracted with a Finochietto rib spreader. When more cranial exposure is required, it may be necessary to divide a portion of the left leaf of the diaphragm at its periphery. Below the diaphragm, further blunt dissection posteriorly, inferiorly and superiorly frees the peritoneum and its contained structures so that they can be retracted medially along with the left kidney, which is displaced anteriorly and medially. This exposes the retroperitoneal lymphoareolar tissue overlying the aorta. Self-retaining retractors are extremely helpful in maintaining this exposure. A large lumbar branch extending posteriorly from the left renal vein is often present and must be divided between ligatures (inset).

AORTIC ANEURYSM REPAIR (CONT.)

25. The fatty areolar tissue overlying the aorta contains many small vessels. This tissue is elevated with a right-angle clamp, coagulated with electrocautery and divided to expose the aorta posterolaterally. Once the periadventitial plane of the aorta below the renal arteries is entered, finger dissection permits this vessel to be cleared anteriorly and posteriorly to facilitate clamp placement if the aorta is not aneurysmal at this level (inset). Care must be exercised not to injure the inferior vena cava medially, and such injuries may be avoided by not passing a clamp circumferentially around the aorta.

To expose the anterior surface of the distal aorta, its bifurcation and the common iliac arteries, the inferior mesenteric artery has been ligated and divided to facilitate medial retraction of the ureter as well as the peritoneal sac and its contained viscera.

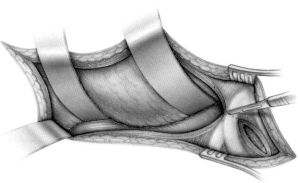

23

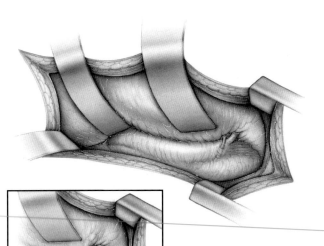

24

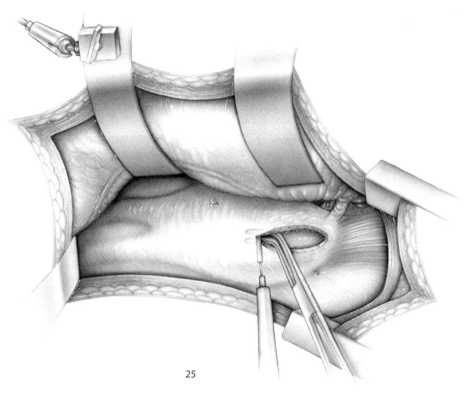

25

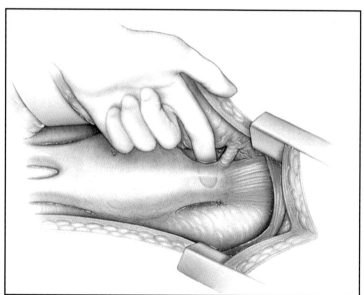

AORTIC ANEURYSM REPAIR (CONT.)

26. If further aortic exposure above the renal arteries is required, as in the case depicted, the muscle fibres from the left crus of the diaphragm are incised with electrocautery after being elevated with a right-angle clamp.

27. This gives access to the periadventitial plane of the suprarenal aorta and facilitates dissection of the superior mesenteric and celiac arteries if necessary.

28. Sufficient aortic dissection anteriorly and posteriorly can also be accomplished to allow safe clamp placement at whatever level is dictated by the nature of the patient's pathology. Inferiorly, the peritoneum, its contents and the left ureter have been mobilized and retracted medially to expose the left common iliac artery and its branches. By careful blunt finger dissection in the plane just anterior to these vessels, it is possible to free up the peritoneal sac and its contents and retract them anteriorly and to the patient's right to expose the right common iliac artery and the origins of its branches. Again, this is facilitated greatly by using appropriate self-retaining retraction techniques, which enable sufficient dissection to allow clamp placement on the right and left internal and external iliac arteries. Circumferential dissection of these vessels through this approach is dangerous and unnecessary and poses the risk of major venous injury.

After administration of heparin and application of clamps in the location dictated by the patient's pathology, the aneurysm is opened and clot is removed. Lumbar arteries are controlled by suture ligature from within, and the appropriate graft is inserted using techniques similar to those illustrated in the transperitoneal approach. In the case shown, the left renal artery would have to be reimplanted into the aortic graft or revascularized with a graft.

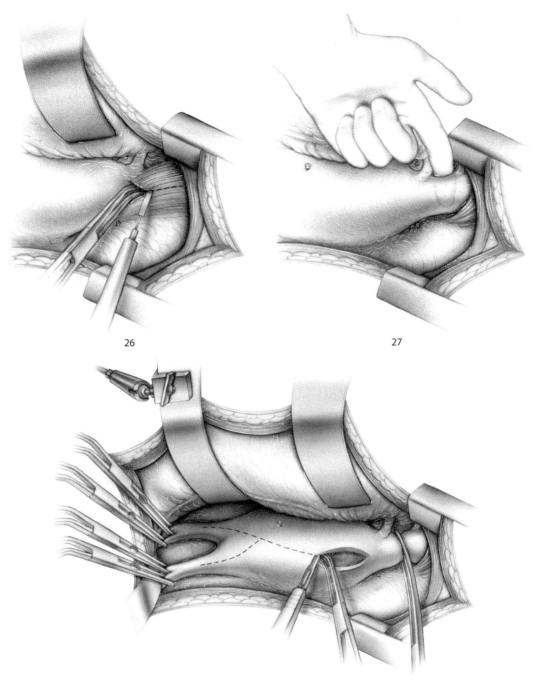

26

27

28

AORTOFEMORAL BYPASS FOR OCCLUSIVE DISEASE

1. Aortobifemoral bypass is performed on patients with aortic and extensive bilateral iliac disease, which produces severe lower extremity ischemia. A long midline incision extending upward along the xiphoid process is made.

2. The abdomen is carefully and systematically explored. The small bowel is retracted to the right, and the posterior peritoneum is incised over the aortic bifurcation. This incision is extended superiorly alongside the ascending portion of the duodenum, dividing the ligament of Treitz. This incision is placed midway between the duodenum and the inferior mesenteric vein. The retroperitoneal incision is made in the shape of a 'T' superiorly along the base of the transverse mesocolon, paralleling the lower border of the pancreas.

3. After the posterior peritoneum is incised, the small bowel and other intraperitoneal viscera are packed off within the abdominal cavity and held in place with self-retaining retractors. A ring retractor and two mechanical retractors, which are affixed to the table, are shown in the illustration. Alternatively, a Stoney retractor (Omni-Tract) can be used and is probably the best method for providing aortic exposure. These self-retaining retraction devices provide steady, safe retraction and allow optimal exposure without the requirement for multiple assistants. Once the posterior peritoneum is incised and the viscera retracted, the aorta can be seen or palpated through the retroperitoneal fatty areolar tissue.

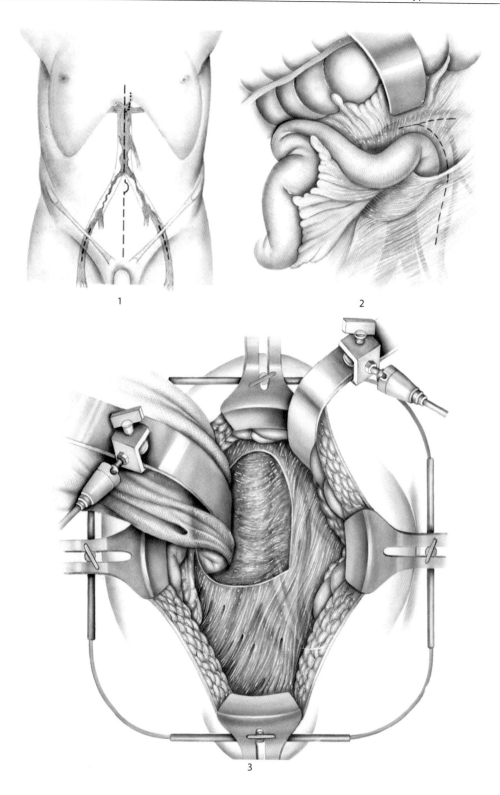

1

2

3

AORTOFEMORAL BYPASS FOR OCCLUSIVE DISEASE (CONT.)

4. This retroperitoneal fatty areolar tissue contains a number of small blood vessels and is best incised with electrocautery. The incision in this tissue is begun anterior to the aorta.

5. Once the adventitia of the aorta is visualized in the midportion of the retroperitoneal incision, the opening in the retroperitoneal fatty areolar tissue is continued cephalad and caudad by elevating this tissue with a right-angle clamp and incising it with the coagulating electrocautery.

6. The aorta is then dissected free anteriorly and laterally using a combination of blunt and sharp dissection. Superiorly, this dissection extends posteromedially and posterolaterally. However, it is not necessary to free the posterior wall of the aorta completely.

7. The common femoral artery is exposed through a vertical groin incision placed over the course of the common femoral artery. If no femoral pulse can be felt, the occluded artery can usually be palpated as a firm tubular structure. If this is not possible, the incision is made midway between the pubic tubercle and the anterior superior iliac spine. This incision is deepened through the subcutaneous tissue and fascia layers. The femoral sheath is then incised and the artery dissected free in the periadventitial plane. Care is taken to clamp and ligate all identifiable lymphatics, and lymph nodes are freed around their periphery but not transected. The skin excision extends over the groin crease. In the upper end of the wound, the inguinal ligament is identified, freed medially and laterally and retracted superiorly. Crossing venous branches may have to be clamped and ligated. The common femoral bifurcation is identified by the decreasing diameter of the femoral artery, and the superficial and deep femoral arteries are dissected free circumferentially.

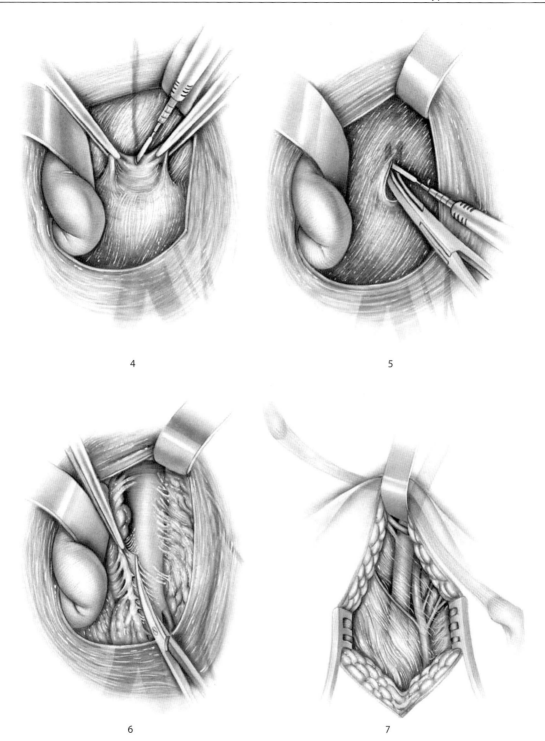

4

5

6

7

AORTOFEMORAL BYPASS FOR OCCLUSIVE DISEASE (CONT.)

8. By elevating the inguinal ligament, a tunnel between the retroperitoneal dissection within the abdomen and the groin is fashioned using primarily finger dissection. Care is taken to avoid injury to veins which may cross over the external iliac artery, as shown in Figure 7. A similar tunnel is made on the left side by passing the fingers behind the sigmoid mesentery. These tunnels should parallel the course of the subjacent arteries and should be as close to their periadventitial plane as possible. In this way, damage to the ureters and other retroperitoneal vessels is minimized.

9. Prior to occlusion of any major artery, hemostasis is assured and the patient is given 1 mg (100 IU) per kg of intravenous heparin. A large atraumatic vascular clamp is placed entirely across the aorta just below the lower border of the renal vein, which is clearly identified. A second large curved atraumatic vascular clamp is then placed (Figures 9 and 10) so as to occlude the distal aorta and all lumbar arteries entering the aortic segment posteriorly. The inferior mesenteric artery, if patent, is occluded by tensioning a doubled Silastic vessel loop and affixing it to the drapes with a clamp. The anterior wall of the aorta is then opened with a #15 scalpel blade. Once the aortic lumen is clearly identified, a small right-angle clamp is placed within the lumen to elevate all layers of the aortic wall and thereby facilitate a clean incision in this vessel. We favour side-to-end proximal aortic anastomoses so that all possible remaining pelvic circulation can be preserved. Some surgeons favour end-to-end proximal anastomosis with oversewing of the distal divided end of the aorta. There is, however, no convincing evidence that such a procedure is superior in any way to side-to-end proximal aortic anastomosis.

10. The position of the aortic clamps and their shape are clearly shown. The end sutures, which are usually of #00 or #000 polypropylene, have been placed through the aorta and the bevelled aortic bifurcation graft. In general, large atraumatic needles (MH) facilitate this procedure. These end sutures are tied, and the suture is run around from the lower and upper ends of the anastomosis and tied at the midportion on either side. Once the proximal aortic anastomosis is completed, the graft is clamped and the aortic clamps are removed. Any bleeding points at the anastomosis are controlled with interrupted sutures. Removal of the aortic clamps at this time is advisable to test the proximal anastomosis for leaks and to restore any remaining pelvic circulation. In general, smaller-sized grafts appear to perform better than larger grafts. Most patients can be treated with a 16 × 8 or 14 × 7 mm graft. We favour the use of collagen-coated knitted Dacron grafts when larger grafts are required and the use of PTFE bifurcation grafts when smaller grafts are required. In almost every instance, the proximal anastomosis is placed in the portion of the aorta between the renal arteries and the inferior mesenteric artery since the aorta below that level is so commonly involved with disease. Although one might be tempted to use a partially occluding clamp on the aorta, this is not advisable. In almost all of these patients, the aorta is thick walled, and cross-clamping is necessary to allow easy access to the lumen and adequate suture placement. When the occlusion in the aorta extends up to the renal arteries, no distal clamp is necessary. The anastomosis can still be carried out to the infrarenal aortic segment after the thrombus is removed. This is facilitated by digital control of the suprarenal aorta. More recently, we have been using suprarenal or supraceliac control to allow a more deliberate disobliteration of the infrarenal aorta in these cases. If the aorta is heavily calcified, this process usually stops below the renals and the immediate infrarenal segment can be safely cross-clamped. To occlude the distal vessels, the heavily calcified aorta often must be cracked; this can be accomplished if appropriate care is used.

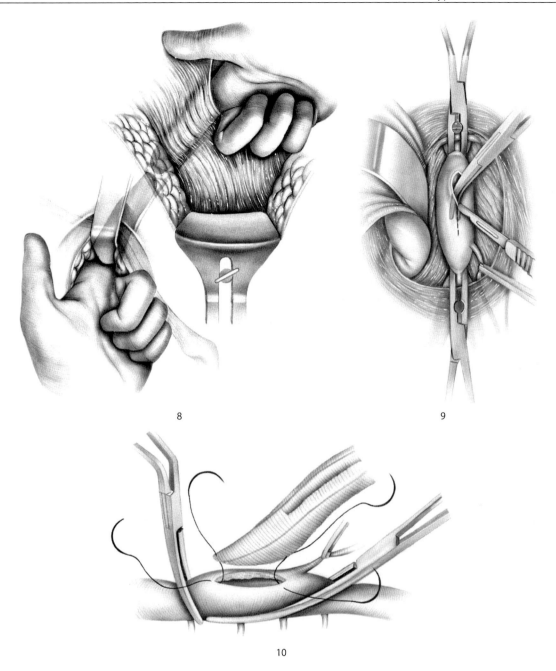

8

9

10

AORTOFEMORAL BYPASS FOR OCCLUSIVE DISEASE (CONT.)

11. Note that the single barrel of the bifurcation graft is kept short to avoid kinking of the limbs. The proximal end of the graft is cut at approximately 45° so that it will lie flush on the aorta without kinking.

12. A long, gently curved clamp is then passed, under finger control, through the previously dissected tunnels from the groin to the retroperitoneal incision where the limbs of the graft are carefully grasped within the point of the clamp so that there are no projecting stumps of the graft to catch on retroperitoneal soft tissue. The grafts are then pulled inferiorly through the tunnel and subjected to mild tension.

13. Angled atraumatic vascular clamps are then placed to occlude the common femoral, deep femoral and superficial femoral arteries. A linear arteriotomy in the common femoral artery is made to expose the origin of the deep femoral artery. If this is undiseased, a standard end-to-end anastomosis is carried out in the same fashion as shown for the proximal aortic anastomosis. However, the suture bites are much smaller and require placement with greater care, so that even bites of all layers are taken and there is no narrowing of the outflow artery lumen. Particular care is taken to be sure that all sutures catch adequate bites of intima so that no distal flaps are left. Each stitch must be placed under direct vision.

14. If there is significant disease at the origin of the deep femoral artery, as shown in the inset, the arteriotomy is extended across this disease and the graft placed over the opened lumen. We do not favour performing an endarterectomy in this circumstance, but rather prefer extending the arteriotomy across the disease and placing the graft as a patch over the stenotic segment. If a long, deep femoral artery occlusion or stenosis is present, this may be treated with a long vein patch and the graft may be placed into this. If endarterectomy is carried out, care must be taken to tack down the distal intima. After all clamps are removed, the heparin is reversed and hemostasis is assured. The wounds are then closed in layers. Care is taken to close one or more layers of fascia or fatty tissue over the graft and to obliterate dead space. The retroperitoneum is closed in such a way that a lateral peritoneal flap of connective tissue or peritoneum is interposed between the duodenum and the graft-to-aorta anastomosis. If this cannot be accomplished, omentum is interposed between the anastomosis and the duodenum.

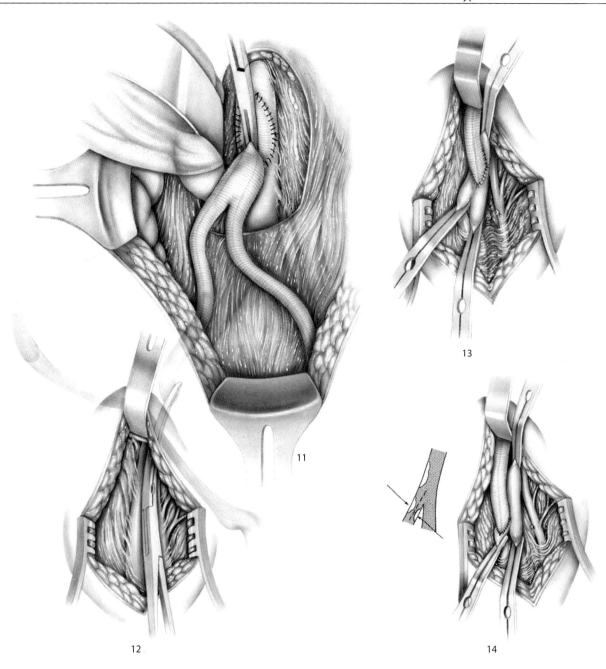

11

12

13

14

AORTOFEMORAL BYPASS FOR OCCLUSIVE DISEASE (CONT.)

Retroperitoneal approach: This approach is useful in brittle, old patients and when the standard transperitoneal approach is rendered difficult because of previous operative scarring, infection or the presence of stomas.

15. In thin patients, abdominal aortic exposure can be obtained via a curved incision beginning over the rectus muscle, halfway between the pubis and the umbilicus, and extending to the tip of the 11th rib. In fatter, more muscular patients, this incision is extended into the 10th or 11th interspace, with division of the intercostal muscles in that interspace. The pleura need not be entered. If more proximal aortic exposure is required, we favour a transpleural approach via a higher interspace (see the section 'Aortic aneurysm repair', Retroperitoneal transpleural approach, Figures 19 through 24).

16. The incision is deepened through the abdominal muscle layers until the transversalis fascia is exposed laterally and superiorly. This is incised to expose the retroperitoneal fat. The peritoneum and its contents are bluntly freed from the overlying muscles and fascia superiorly, inferiorly and medially to facilitate incision in the remaining layers of the abdominal wall (see the section 'Aortic aneurysm repair', Figures 19 through 22).

17. The peritoneum and its contained viscera are then freed from the underlying psoas muscle and retracted medially along with the accompanying left ureter. This exposes the lymphoareolar tissue overlying the aorta. This tissue contains many small vessels and is best incised using electrocautery to control troublesome bleeding.

18. Once the periadventitial plane of the aorta is entered, this vessel can be dissected anteriorly and on both sides using blunt and sharp dissection so that adequate exposure for proximal clamp placement can be obtained. Prior to administering heparin and placing these clamps, standard vertical groin incisions are made to expose the femoral arteries and usually the proximal deep femoral artery, as illustrated in the standard transperitoneal procedure.

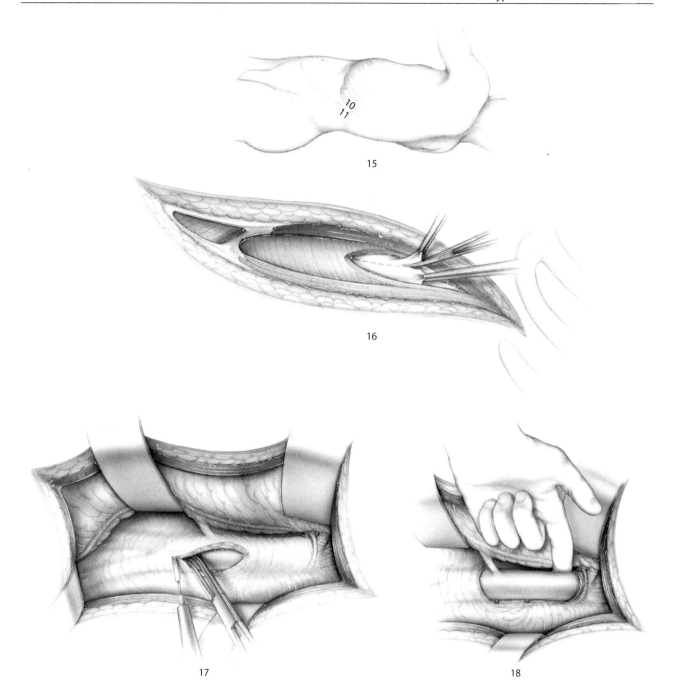

15

16

17

18

AORTOFEMORAL BYPASS FOR OCCLUSIVE DISEASE (CONT.)

19. Tunnels are created between the groin incisions and the retroperitoneal incision using blunt finger dissection and taking particular care to make the right-sided tunnel just anterior to the right common and external iliac arteries so as to avoid injury to any structures anterior to these vessels.

20. Once the dissection is completed, heparin is administered and the aorta is cross-clamped proximally. A long curved clamp is placed posteriorly to occlude retrograde bleeding from the iliac and lumbar arteries. The aorta is opened longitudinally (or transected), and the remainder of the operation is performed in a fashion similar to that illustrated and described for the transperitoneal approach.

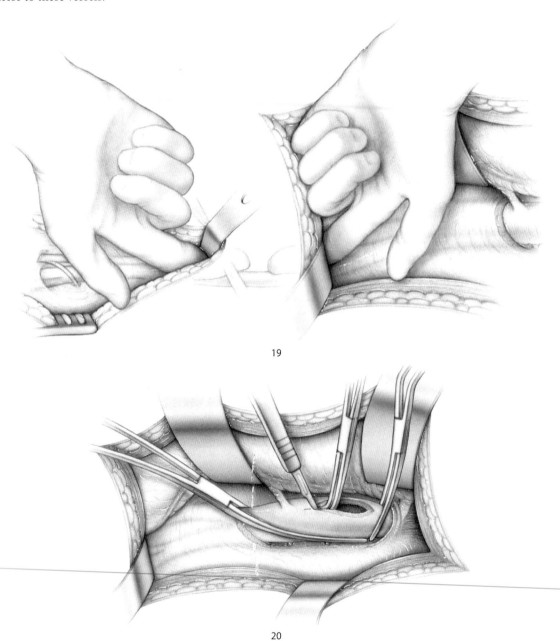

19

20

FEMOROPOPLITEAL BYPASS

1. The positioning of the extremity and location of the skin incisions are shown. If the greater saphenous vein in the thigh and upper leg is to be used as the graft, the skin incision is made directly over the course of that vein and deep subcutaneous flaps are raised to reach the appropriate arteries. Alternatively, if a prosthetic graft is to be used, skin and subcutaneous incisions placed directly over the appropriate arteries are employed. The positions for the above-knee and below-knee access routes to the popliteal artery from a medial approach are shown. The above-knee incision is placed along the anterior border of the sartorius muscle. The below-knee incision parallels the posterior border of the tibia.

2. The above-knee access route to the popliteal artery is shown after the skin and subcutaneous tissue have been incised. The fascial incision is then made along the anterior border of the sartorius muscle, just deep to which can be felt in the adductor tendon.

3. The sartorius muscle is freed from the deeper structures and retracted with a self-retaining retractor. Care is taken to avoid injury to the blood supply and nerve supply to the sartorius muscle. The deep fascia of the popliteal space is then grasped with forceps and sharply incised.

4. This exposes the popliteal fat, which is carefully separated by blunt and sharp dissection. Any crossing veins are cauterized or ligated. The popliteal neurovascular bundle can then be palpated as it emerges from the adductor muscle. By grasping the outer tissues of this bundle with forceps and elevating it, its superficial fascial investments can be incised.

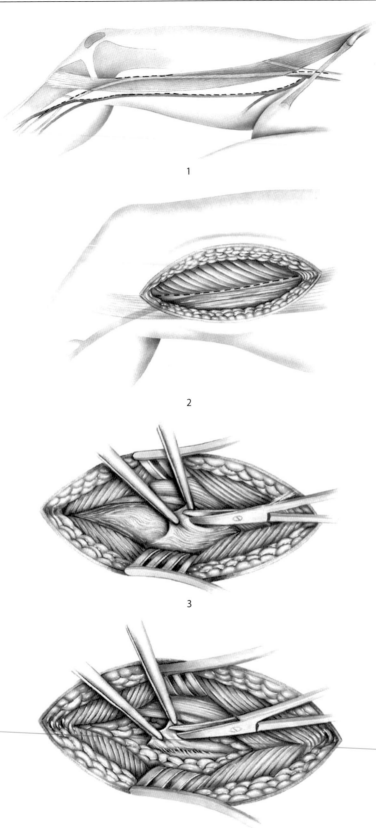

1

2

3

4

FEMOROPOPLITEAL BYPASS (CONT.)

5. Additional fascial layers overlie the periadventitial plane around the artery. In these layers course many small veins which connect the main veins that accompany the popliteal artery. By sharply dividing these fascial investments, it is possible to visualize the crossing veins. These can be carefully ligated and divided to clearly define the periadventitial plane of the popliteal artery.

6. After division of these veins, the popliteal artery can be circumferentially dissected in its periadventitial plane and elevated using Silastic loops.

7. A groin incision over the common, superficial and deep femoral arteries is made in a standard fashion. A subsartorial tunnel is then created, using blunt dissection with the fingers. If the tunnel is too long for the fingers to meet, a plastic chest tube container can be used to complete this tunnel. Once the tunnel has been created, the backs of the fingers should be in contact with the indurated surface of the diseased artery to confirm the correct location of the tunnel.

8. The greater saphenous vein is carefully harvested by a long incision placed directly over it. All branches are carefully identified and ligated so as not to constrict the vein or prevent its free enlargement as it is gently dilated. Balanced saline solution (Hank's) or chilled heparinized blood is used to irrigate the vein and gently distend it. This process is facilitated with a long plastic catheter with a well-rounded tip passed into the vein. In a sequential fashion, 2 to 3 cm segments of the vein can be isolated by gentle finger pressure and distended to identify leaks. Passage of the catheter also identifies recanalized previously thrombophlebitic segments, which cannot be found in any other way and which, if present, make a vein unsatisfactory for use. The vein is then immersed in the chilled solution until the surgeon is ready to use it.

9. After heparin is administered systemically [1 mg (100 IU)/kg], the segment of popliteal artery selected for the distal anastomosis is isolated by the careful and gentle application of atraumatic vascular clamps. Care is taken to avoid excessive closing pressure on these clamps as well as torsion, since a diseased popliteal artery can easily be injured. Small branches entering the selected segment are occluded by microclips. The area for the arteriotomy is selected by careful palpation of the vessel. An effort to use the least diseased portion of the artery is made. However, in many instances, no segment or wall of the popliteal artery is completely free of atherosclerotic involvement. The point of a new #15 scalpel blade is used to make the arteriotomy. Once the lumen of the artery has been entered, a fine mosquito clamp is inserted and opened so that the knife cut in the arterial wall will be clean and sharp and evenly placed through all layers of the diseased artery.

10. Often, the arterial incision is placed across a known stenosis in the artery to widen the stenotic area and improve outflow via the distal anastomosis. The anastomosis is then completed using 6-0 polypropylene sutures. These stitches are begun at the heel and the toe.

11. Each stitch is placed through all layers of the artery and vein, taking particular care to include even bites of the intimal layers. The suturing is continued from both ends toward the centre of the anastomosis on each side. The sutures are tied at the midportion of each wall of the anastomosis.

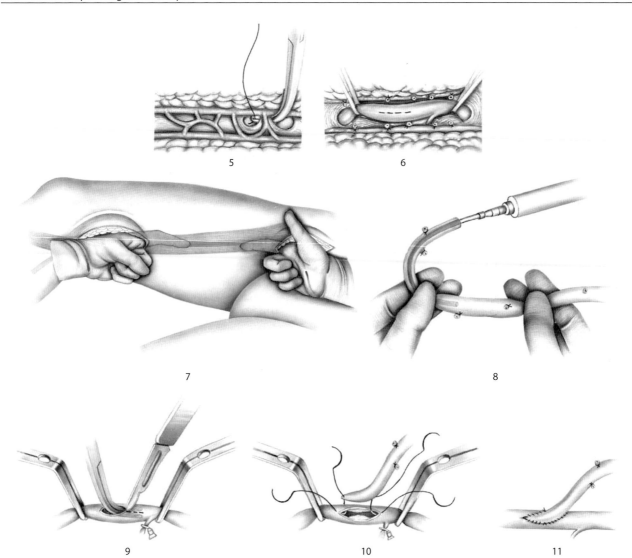

5

6

7

8

9

10

11

FEMOROPOPLITEAL BYPASS (CONT.)

12. A long, gently curved aneurysm clamp is then placed through the previously defined tunnel, and the graft is pulled retrograde from the popliteal incision through the tunnel to the groin incision, taking particular care to avoid twisting or kinking the graft. All occluding devices in the popliteal artery are removed, and the graft and outflow tract are flushed with heparinized saline solution.

13. The proximal anastomosis to the common femoral artery is completed in a fashion similar to that already described (see the section 'End-to-side vascular anastomosis', Figures 1 through 5).

14. If the proximal superficial femoral artery is free of atherosclerotic involvement, the proximal anastomosis may be constructed to the latter vessel. Use of this vessel minimizes the length of good autologous saphenous vein that is required. Grafts originating from the superficial femoral artery have acceptable long-term patency rates which are comparable to those of grafts originating from the common femoral artery.

15. Similarly, if vein length is limited, the proximal anastomosis may be constructed to the deep femoral artery as long as it is free of significant disease. If a marked stenosis is present at the origin of the deep femoral artery, the graft may be inserted across this stenosis.

16. If the common femoral artery is very thick walled and diseased, the proximal anastomosis can sometimes be facilitated by sewing a vein patch into the diseased segment and then inserting the proximal end of the vein graft into this patch. This technique is particularly useful if the proximal end of the vein (which was previously the most peripheral portion of the greater saphenous vein) is small. If suitable autologous vein is not present in the ipsilateral lower extremity or if the patient has a limited life expectancy (3–4 years), it is perfectly acceptable to use a 6 mm PTFE graft for above-knee femoropopliteal bypass. Furthermore, if the femoropopliteal bypass is inserted into an isolated or blind popliteal artery segment, the surgeon may elect to use a PTFE graft and save the vein for a simultaneous or subsequent sequential infrapopliteal bypass.

17. The position of the skin incision for access to the below-knee popliteal artery is shown. Great care must be taken to avoid injury to the greater saphenous vein, which frequently crosses the operative field. This must be carefully freed and protected from injury. The deep investing fascia of the leg is incised. As this incision extends superiorly, the tendons of the gracilis muscle and the semitendinosus muscle cross the field. These may be divided to provide better exposure.

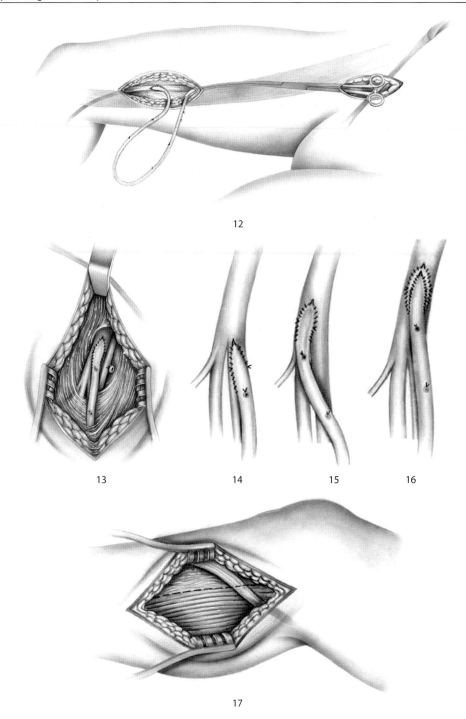

12

13   14   15   16

17

FEMOROPOPLITEAL BYPASS (CONT.)

18. The popliteal space is entered and the neurovascular bundle palpated in the upper portion of the depths of the wound. The popliteal vein is the most superficial structure. Often, dissection of the artery is facilitated by isolating the popliteal vein and retracting it with a Silastic loop. The neurovascular bundle in the inferior portion of the wound is deep to the soleus muscle. The arcing upper border of this muscle, which inserts on the posterior surface of the tibia, can clearly be seen and felt.

19. A finger or right-angle clamp can be placed deep to this muscle, and it can be incised over the finger or clamp to expose the distal popliteal artery and its trifurcation.

20. By ligating and dividing branches of the popliteal vein, this vessel can be retracted anteriorly or posteriorly to expose the underlying artery and its branches. In this view one can see the origin of the anterior tibial artery, the tibioperoneal trunk and its terminal branches and the peroneal and posterior tibial arteries. The anterior tibial artery is usually larger than shown in this drawing.

21. Any or all of these branches can be freed circumferentially and encircled with Silastic loops. The origin of the anterior tibial artery is best seen after ligation of one or more accompanying anterior tibial veins.

22. After administration of systemic heparin, suitable gentle clamp or clip application isolates the most disease-free portion of the artery. This is incised with a scalpel blade.

23. A meticulous anastomosis of the vein or PTFE graft to the artery is made. Great care is taken to visualize every suture bite and to be sure that equal portions of all layers of the artery and vein wall are caught in every stitch. PTFE grafts to the below-knee popliteal artery should be used only in poor-risk patients or in those in whom ipsilateral autologous vein is not available.

24. The completed distal anastomosis is shown after removal of all occluding instrumentation.

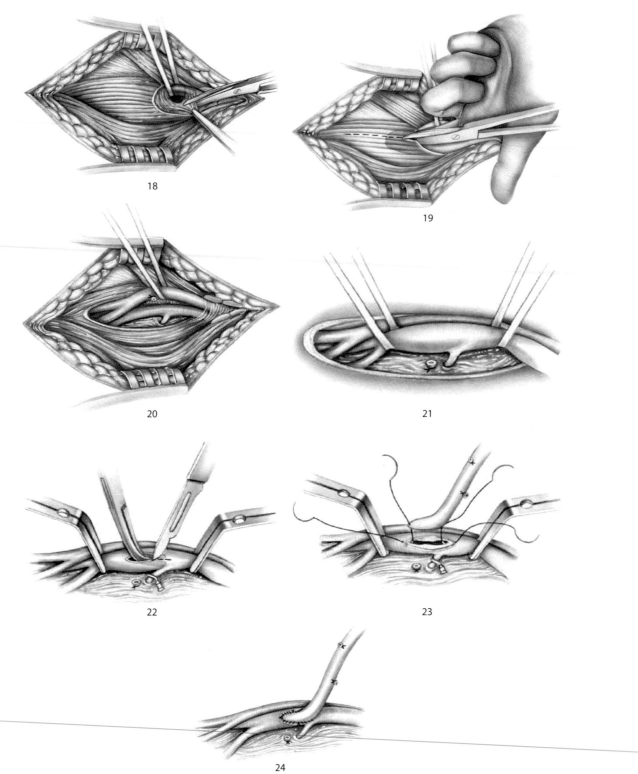

18

19

20

21

22

23

24

FEMOROPOPLITEAL BYPASS (CONT.)

25. This shows the method for constructing the portion of the tunnel behind the knee. This tunnelling should be carried out by blunt finger dissection, with the backs and tops of the fingers being placed against the popliteal vessels so that the graft will pass in the depths of the popliteal fossa. Usually, this tunnel is constructed before the patient is given heparin.

26. The graft is then passed retrograde behind the knee, using a large curved clamp, inserted under finger guidance, to draw the vein from the below-knee incision to a small above-knee incision and then to the groin.

27. This figure shows the position of the graft in its anatomic tunnel. Before performing the proximal anastomosis, the knee should be fully extended to allow appropriate tensioning of the graft and to permit the graft to be cut at precisely the right level so that it will be neither overly taut nor redundant with the knee at full extension. Heparin is reversed with protamine, and meticulous hemostasis is obtained throughout all wounds. These are then closed in layers without drainage. The in situ vein graft bypass technique has received a great deal of attention recently. There is no evidence whatsoever that this technique provides superior results in femoropopliteal bypasses. Randomized, prospective comparisons of in situ and reversed vein grafts in the femoropopliteal position have shown that the two grafting techniques produce comparable results; accordingly, we favour use of reversed vein grafts for femoropopliteal bypass. For tibial bypasses, many of which can be performed with short reversed vein grafts, we favour the latter procedure. However, it is possible that long bypasses from the upper thigh to the lower leg have better patency rates when they are performed as an in situ graft if the vein is small (<3.0 mm in distended diameter). However, this remains to be proved conclusively.

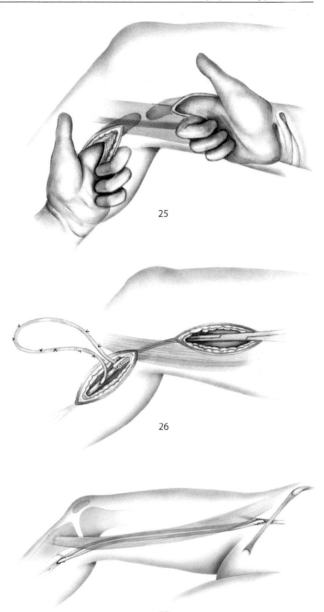

25

26

27

AXILLOFEMORAL BYPASS

1. The position of the patient and locations of the incisions are shown. The right axillary artery is less likely to be involved with significant disease and is chosen preferentially to provide inflow. However, some of our recent data have shown that approximately 25% of candidates for axillofemoral bypass have significant unsuspected axillary or subclavian artery disease, and we presently advocate preoperative arch arteriography, via a translumbar approach, to determine the presence or absence of inflow disease and to guide the surgeon in the choice of which axillary artery to use. Although many surgeons advocate the performance of routine axillobifemoral bypass even if the symptoms are restricted to one lower extremity, we have found that axillounifemoral bypasses have patency rates similar to those of axillobifemoral bypasses. We therefore perform a unilateral procedure if a patient's predominant symptoms are restricted to only one lower extremity. The pattern of disease for which an axillofemoral bypass might be employed is shown. Severe and extensive aortic and bilateral iliac disease of a sort not suitable for percutaneous transluminal angioplasty is present. The axillary incision is placed over the proximal axillary artery and is approximately parallel to the fibres of the pectoralis major muscle.

2. The skin incision is deepened through the subcutaneous tissue and the fascia of the pectoralis major muscle. The fibres of the latter muscle are separated and retracted with a self-retaining retractor. The borders of the pectoralis minor muscle are defined. A finger or right-angle clamp is then placed beneath the muscle, and this muscle is divided as close to its insertion on the coracoid process as possible. Either scissors or cautery can be used for this manoeuvre.

3. The axillary artery is identified as it courses among the components of the brachial plexus. The periadventitial plane of this artery is identified, and the artery is carefully dissected free in a circumferential manner. Silastic vessel loops are placed around the artery to elevate it and to facilitate circumferential dissection of a 5 to 7 cm segment of artery. Care is taken to avoid injury to the large thin-walled branches which arise from the proximal portion of the axillary artery. An effort is made to dissect the most proximal portion of the artery so that it can be used for the anastomosis.

4. After a groin incision is made with exposure of the inguinal ligament, as already described (see the section 'Aortofemoral bypass for occlusive disease', Figure 7), the tunnelling procedure between the two incisions is performed. This is begun by blunt finger dissection, under the pectoralis major muscle and as close to the chest wall as possible, via the axillary incision.

5. Blunt finger dissection to start the tunnel from the groin incision is also performed. This tunnel must be superficial to the inguinal ligament and aponeurosis of the external oblique muscle.

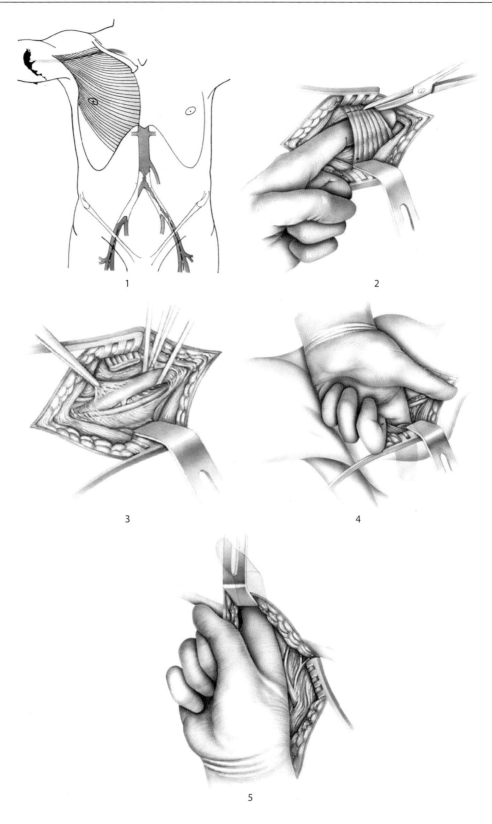

1

2

3

4

5

AXILLOFEMORAL BYPASS (CONT.)

6. Any of several varieties of tunneler may be used to join the axillary and femoral incisions. An intermediate skin incision midway along the tunnel is generally unnecessary. We have found that a plastic chest tube container serves as a very effective tunneler; this is shown in the illustration. However, a variety of other instruments can be used just as well. The tunneler is passed, under finger control, from below upward and retrieved from the axillary incision, taking care to guide the tunneler away from the axillary neurovascular structures. The closed tip of the plastic tube is then cut off with heavy scissors, as shown by the short broken line. If a bilateral femoral procedure is to be employed, the opposite groin is also opened, the femoral arteries are dissected circumferentially, and a tunnel is created in the subcutaneous plane between the two groin incisions. Care is taken to place this tunnel superficial to the inguinal ligaments and abdominal musculature and just above the pubic symphysis. The tunneler is left in place but withdrawn slightly (2–4 cm) so that it can later be retrieved for use.

7. The patient is given intravenous heparin [1 mg (100 IU)/kg]. The axillary artery is carefully elevated and occluded with gently applied atraumatic vascular clamps. The axillary artery is a very thin-walled structure that is easily damaged; these clamps should be placed with extreme care. Microclips are used to occlude the smaller branches of the axillary artery, and tensioned double-looped Silastic loops affixed to the drapes are used to occlude the larger branches.

8. The vascular clamps are rotated slightly to expose the anteroinferior portion of the axillary artery, and a longitudinal incision is made in that artery using the techniques already shown. If the artery is perfectly normal, as it often is, a scissors may be used to create the incision or extend it to its ends. If, on the other hand, the artery is diseased, the knife-and-clamp technique already illustrated (see the section 'Femoropopliteal bypass', Figure 22) should be used. Double-armed 5-0 or 6-0 polypropylene sutures are placed in the corners of the arteriotomy.

9. A 6 mm PTFE graft is anastomosed to the artery using careful suturing technique as already described for other anastomoses. The opened end of the tunneler is then pushed into the wound.

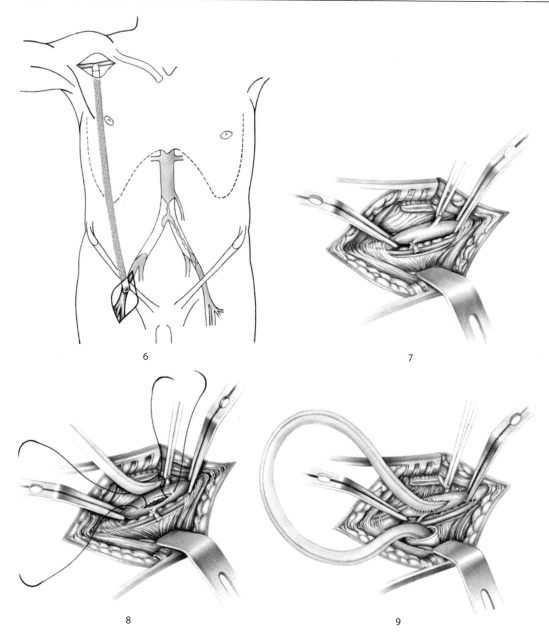

6

7

8

9

AXILLOFEMORAL BYPASS (CONT.)

10. A long bronchoscopy grasping forceps is then placed through the tunneler and the graft drawn from above downward (Figures 9 through 10).

11. The right femoral anastomosis is then completed in a standard fashion. This anastomosis either can be in the common femoral artery or extended across the origin of the deep femoral artery if there is disease at that site. Alternatively, the anastomosis can be entirely into the deep femoral artery if the proximal portion of that artery is extensively diseased. The left femoral anastomosis is completed in a similar way. Finally, the femorofemoral graft is anastomosed to the axillary limb.

12. The positions of these anastomoses are clearly shown. The nature and location of the disease in the femoral arteries determine the exact location of the graft-to-artery femoral anastomoses. If disease is present at the origin of the deep femoral artery, the arteriotomy is placed across this disease and the graft used to enlarge the orifice (see the section 'Femorofemoral bypass', Figures 3 and 5). Heparin is reversed with protamine, hemostasis is obtained, and the wounds are closed in layers, with an effort to close as much soft tissue over the anastomotic areas as is possible. This is particularly important in the groin, since the anastomosis is not deep to any muscular layers.

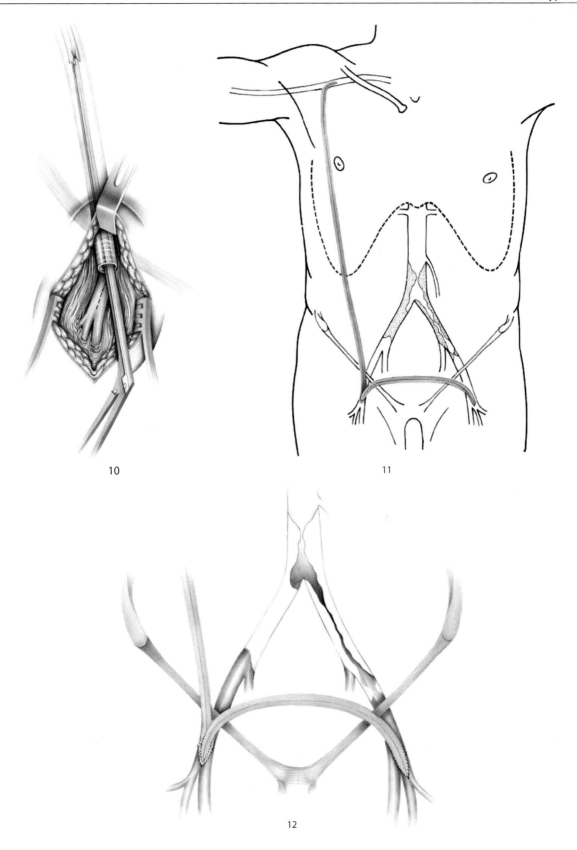

10

11

12

FEMOROFEMORAL BYPASS

1. This figure shows the typical pattern of disease for which femorofemoral bypass is an effective operative treatment. Unilateral iliac occlusive disease is present, with minimal involvement of the aorta and contralateral iliac arteries. Incisions over both femoral arteries are made and extended upward over the inguinal ligament.

2. These incisions are deepened to expose the inguinal ligaments. Once these have been identified, finger dissection is used to create a tunnel superficial to the external oblique and above the symphysis of the pubis. Care is taken to avoid dissecting deep to the inguinal ligament.

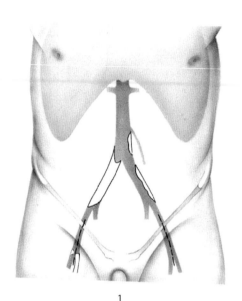

1

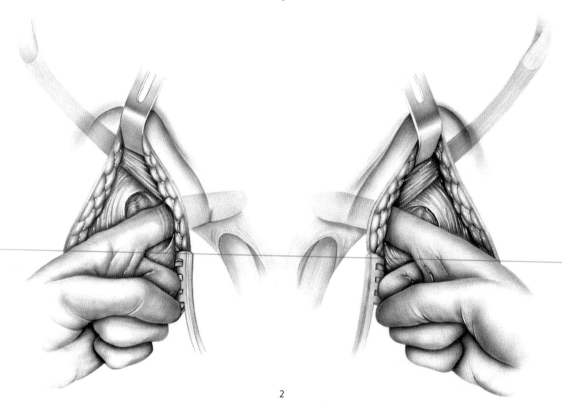

2

FEMOROFEMORAL BYPASS (CONT.)

3. Self-retaining retractors are placed to hold the edges of the wound apart and to elevate the inguinal ligament. To accomplish the latter manoeuvre, a robot arm and an Army Navy retractor can be used. After isolating the common, deep and superficial femoral arteries, control of patent arteries is obtained with atraumatic vascular clamps gently applied so as not to injure the vessels. No clamp is necessary for the occluded superficial femoral artery. Small microclips are used to occlude branch vessels without injuring them. After administration of intravenous heparin, the arteriotomy is made as already described (see the section 'Femoropopliteal bypass', Figure 22). In the instance shown, a stenosis is present at the origin of the right deep femoral artery; accordingly, the incision in the artery is made across this stenosis. No endarterectomy is carried out.

4. After the anastomosis of the 6 mm PTFE tubular graft to the right common and deep femoral artery is completed, the right-side vascular clamps are removed and the graft is clamped. It is then drawn through the tunnel, and an arteriotomy in the left common femoral artery is made along the line indicated.

5. Both anastomoses have now been completed. The position of the graft, in a gentle C-shaped arc, is shown.

   After hemostasis is assured and the heparin reversed, the wounds are carefully closed in layers, so that as many soft tissue layers as possible cover the graft and dead space is eliminated.

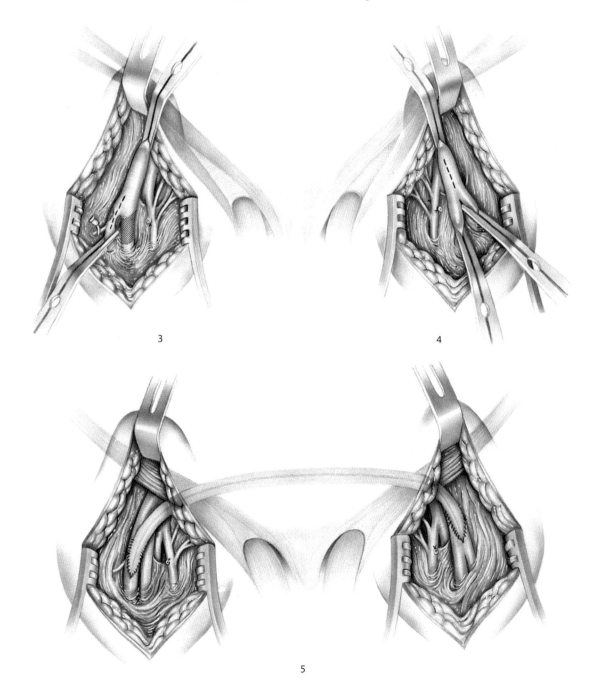

3

4

5

ACKNOWLEDGEMENT

The illustrations in this chapter were drawn by Lauren Keswick, M.S., and Charles M. Stern. Many were reproduced from the section 'Vascular Surgical Techniques', by Frank J. Veith, which appeared in an *Atlas of Surgical Techniques,* by Marvin L. Gliedman, published by McGraw-Hill in 1990.

Index

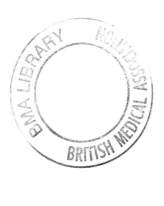